COMMUNITY/PUBLIC
HEALTH NURSING

*Promoting the Health
of Populations*

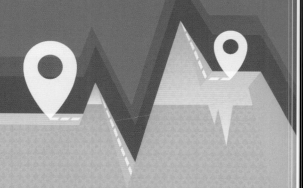

COMMUNITY/PUBLIC HEALTH NURSING

Promoting the Health of Populations

EDITION

8

Mary A. Nies, PhD, RN, FAAN, FAAHB
Special Assistant to the Dean, College of Health for Grant Writing
Tenured Professor
School of Nursing
College of Health, Joint Appointment MPH Program
Kasiska Division of Health Sciences
Idaho State University
Pocatello, Idaho

Melanie McEwen, PhD, RN, CNE, ANEF, FAAN
Distinguished Teaching Professor
University of Texas Health Science Center at Houston
Cizik School of Nursing
Houston, Texas

ELSEVIER

ELSEVIER
3251 Riverport Lane
St. Louis, Missouri 63043

COMMUNITY/PUBLIC HEALTH NURSING: PROMOTING
THE HEALTH OF POPULATIONS, EIGHTH EDITION   ISBN: 978-0-323-79531-9

Notice

Practitioners and researchers must always rely on their own experience and knowledge in evaluating and using any information, methods, compounds or experiments described herein. Because of rapid advances in the medical sciences, in particular, independent verification of diagnoses and drug dosages should be made. To the fullest extent of the law, no responsibility is assumed by Elsevier, authors, editors or contributors for any injury and/or damage to persons or property as a matter of products liability, negligence or otherwise, or from any use or operation of any methods, products, instructions, or ideas contained in the material herein.

Previous editions copyrighted 2019, 2015, 2011, 2007, 2001, 1997, and 1993.

Content Strategist: Heather Bays-Petrovic
Senior Content Development Specialist: Tina Kaemmerer
Publishing Services Manager: Deepthi Unni
Senior Project Manager: Umarani Natarajan
Design Direction: Renee Duenow

Printed in India

Last digit is the print number: 9   8   7   6   5   4   3   2

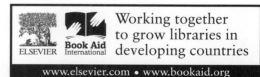

To Phil Yankovich, my husband, companion, and best friend,
whose love, caring, and true support are always there for me.
He provides me with the energy I need to pursue my dreams.

To Kara Nies Yankovich, my daughter,
for whom I wish a happy and healthy life.
Her energy, joy, and enthusiasm for life give so much to me.

To Earl Nies (who passed away October 15, 2017, at the age of 92)
and Lois Nies (who passed away January 7, 2019, at the age of 89), my parents,
for their never-ending encouragement and lifelong support.
They helped me develop a foundation for creative thinking, new ideas,
and spirited debate.

Mary A. Nies

To my husband, Scott McEwen, whose love, support, inspiration,
and encouragement have been my foundation for more than 45 years.
I can't wait to see what happens next!

Melanie McEwen

ABOUT THE AUTHORS

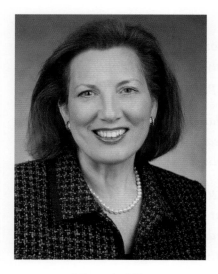

Mary A. Nies

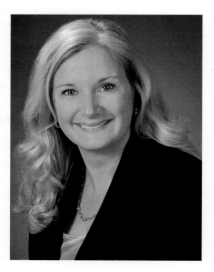

Melanie McEwen

Mary A. Nies, PhD, RN, FAAN, FAAHB, is the Special Assistant to the Dean College of Health for Grant Writing and Tenured Professor, school of nursing in the College of Health, Joint Appointment MPH Program, Kasiska Division of Health Sciences, Idaho State University. Dr. Nies received her diploma from the Bellin School of Nursing in Green Bay, Wisconsin; her BSN from the University of Wisconsin, Madison; her MSN from Loyola University, Chicago; and her PhD in Public Health Nursing, Health Services, and Health Promotion Research at the University of Illinois, Chicago. She completed a post-doctoral research fellowship in health promotion and community health at the University of Michigan, Ann Arbor. She is a fellow of the American Academy of Nursing and a fellow of the American Academy of Health Behavior. Dr. Nies co-*edited Community Health Nursing: Promoting the Health of Aggregates*, which received the 1993 Book of the Year award from the *American Journal of Nursing.* Her program of research focuses on the outcomes of health promotion interventions for minority and nonminority populations in the community. Her research is involved with physical activity and obesity prevention for vulnerable community populations. Dr. Nies received the Outstanding Researcher award at Idaho State University in 2021 and 2022. Dr. Nies was selected by the Western Institute of Nursing Board of Governors as the recipient of the 2023 Distinguished Research Lectureship Award. This prestigious annual award recognizes a senior investigator whose research career has made substantial and sustained contributions to nursing.

Melanie McEwen, PhD, RN, CNE, ANEF, FAAN, is a Distinguished Teaching Professor at the University of Texas Health Science Center at Houston's Cizik School of Nursing. Dr. McEwen received her BSN from the University of Texas School of Nursing in Austin; her Master's in Community and Public Health Nursing from Louisiana State University Medical Center in New Orleans; and her PhD in Nursing from Texas Woman's University. Dr. McEwen has been a nursing educator for 35 years and is also the co-author/editor of *Theoretical Basis for Nursing* (Wolters Kluwer, 2023).

ACKNOWLEDGMENTS

Community/Public Health Nursing: Promoting the Health of Populations could not have been written without sharing the experiences, thoughtful critique, and support of many people: individuals, families, groups, and communities. We give special thanks to everyone who made significant contributions to this book.

We are indebted to our contributing authors whose inspiration, untiring hours of work, and persistence have continued to build a new era of community health nursing practice with a focus on the population level. We thank the community health nursing faculty and students who welcomed the previous editions of the text and responded to our inquiries with comments and suggestions for the eighth edition. These people have challenged us to stretch, adapt, and continue to learn throughout our years of work. We also thank our colleagues in our respective work settings for their understanding and support during the writing and editing of this edition.

Finally, an enormous "thank you" to Elsevier editors Heather Bays-Petrovic and Tina Kaemmerer, and project manager Umarani Natarajan. Their energy, enthusiasm, encouragement, direction, and patience were essential to this project.

Mary A. Nies, PhD, RN, FAAN, FAAHB
Melanie McEwen, PhD, RN, CNE, ANEF, FAAN

I would also like to express appreciation for the chapter authors who have been with me since the very first edition of the textbook in 1993, namely:
- Patricia Burbank, Chapter 7: *Community Health Planning, Implementation, and Evaluation*
- Holly Cassells, Chapter 5: *Epidemiology;* Chapter 6: *Community Assessment*
- Jean Cozad Lyon, Chapter 9: *Case Management*

Mary A. Nies, PhD, RN, FAAN, FAAHB

CONTRIBUTORS AND REVIEWER

CONTRIBUTORS

Tonya Bragg-Underwood, DNP, PMHNP-BC, FNP-BC, CNE
Associate Professor
School of Nursing & Allied Health
Western Kentucky University
Bowling Green, Kentucky
Chapter 20: Family Health

Patricia M. Burbank, BS, MS, DNSc
Professor
College of Nursing
University of Rhode Island
Kingston, Rhode Island
Chapter 7: Community Health Planning, Implementation, and Evaluation

Holly B. Cassells, MN, MPH, PhD
Professor and Dean
Ila Faye Miller School of Nursing and Health Professions
University of the Incarnate Word
San Antonio, Texas
Chapter 5: Epidemiology
Chapter 6: Community Assessment

Christina N. DesOrmeaux, BSN, MSN, PhD
Assistant Professor
Community Nursing
The University of Texas at Houston Health Science Center
Houston, Texas
Chapter 13: Cultural Diversity and Community Health Nursing
Chapter 30: School Health

Stacy A. Drake, PhD, MPH, RN, AFN-BC, D-ABMDI, FAAN
Associate Professor
College of Nursing
Texas A&M University
Houston, Texas
Chapter 32: Forensic and Correctional Nursing

Allison P. Edwards, RN, BSN, MS, DrPH, CNE
Assistant Professor
University of Texas Health Science Center at Houston
Cizik School of Nursing
Houston, Texas
Board Member
Texas Board of Nursing
Austin, Texas
Chapter 21: Populations Affected by Disabilities

Carol G. Enderle, DNP, MBA, MSN, BSN, RN, RHCEOC
President
Administration
CommonSpirit Health / CHI St. Alexius Health—Dickinson
Dickinson, North Dakota;
VP Patient Care Services, Chief Nursing Officer/Chief Operating Officer
Administration
SCL Health / Intermountain Healthcare—Holy Rosary Healthcare
Miles City, Montana
Chapter 24: Rural and Migrant Health

Melissa Domingeaux Ethington, MSN, PhD
Assistant Dean, Admissions & Student Affairs
Assistant Professor
University of Texas Health Science Center at Houston
Cizik School of Nursing
Houston, Texas;
Chapter 16: Child and Adolescent Health

Allison Findlay, PhD, RN
Assistant Professor
Nursing
University of Colorado Colorado Springs
Colorado Springs, Colorado
Chapter 33: Faith Community Nursing

Antira Frederick, PhD, RN, CNE
Director, BSN Pacesetter Program
Assistant Professor
University of Texas Health Science Center at Houston
Cizik School of Nursing
Houston, Texas
Chapter 30: School Health

Kelli M. Galle, MSN, APRN, FNP-BC
Instructor
University of Texas Health Science Center at Houston
Cizik School of Nursing
Houston, Texas
Chapter 28: Violence

Lori A. Glenn, DNP, MS, CNM, C-EFM, RN
McAuley School of Nursing
University of Detroit Mercy;
Hurley Midwifery
Hurley Medical Center;
St. Joseph Oakland Medical Center
Huntington Woods, Michigan
Chapter 17: Women's Health

Deanna E. Grimes, DrPH, RN, FAAN
Professor Emerita
University of Texas Health Science Center at Houston
Cizik School of Nursing
Houston, Texas
Chapter 26: Communicable Disease

Karyn Leavitt Grow, MS, BSN, RN, CCM
Administrative Director of Case Management and Care Coordination
Nursing
Tahoe Forest Health System
Truckee, California;
Chief Nursing Officer
Nursing
Sierra Surgery Hospital
Carson City, Nevada;
Manager Case Management/Preadmission Screening
Nursing
Sierra Surgery Hospital
Carson City, Nevada;
Director of Care Coordination Training
Clinical
Caravan Health
Kansas City, Missouri
Chapter 9: Case Management

Barbara E. Hekel, PhD, MPH, RN
Assistant Professor
University of Texas Health Science Center at Houston
Cizik School of Nursing
Houston, Texas
Chapter 26: Communicable Disease

Lillian Felicia Jones, RN, PhD, MSN, Masters of Counseling
Lecturer, Independent Consultant
Nursing
Thomas University/Thomas Asia Pacific Institute;
Nurse
Behavioral Health
Carson Tahoe Regional Medical Center,
Carson City, Nevada
Chapter 18: Men's Health

Jean Cozad Lyon, PhD, MSN
Clinical Care Practitioner
ATOP2
HealthInsight
Reno, Nevada
Chapter 9: Case Management

Diane Cocozza Martins, PhD, RN, FAAN
Professor
College of Nursing
University of Rhode Island
Kingston, Rhode Island
Chapter 3: Thinking Upstream: Nursing Theories and Population-Focused Nursing Practice
Chapter 7: Community Health Planning, Implementation, and Evaluation

Deborah (Debbie) McCrea, EdD, APRN, FNP-BC, CNS, CNE, CEN, CFRN, EMT-P
Assistant Professor
University of Texas Health Science Center at Houston
Cizik School of Nursing
Houston, Texas
Adjunct Instructor
EMS Program
Houston Community College
Houston, Texas
Medical Case Manager
Travel Medical Assistance Department
Travelguard AID Travel Assistance
Houston, Texas
Chapter 29: Natural and Man-Made Disasters

Melanie McEwen, PhD, RN, CNE, ANEF, FAAN
Distinguished Teaching Professor
University of Texas Health Science Center at Houston
Cizik School of Nursing
Houston, Texas
Chapter 1: Health: A Community View
Chapter 2: Historical Factors: Community Health Nursing in Context
Chapter 11: The Health Care System
Chapter 12: Economics of Health Care

Cathy D. Meade, PhD, RN, FAAN, FSBM
Senior Member
Population Science, Health Outcomes & Behavior
Moffitt Cancer Center
Tampa, Florida;
Professor
Oncologic Sciences
Universiity of South Florida
Tampa, Florida
Chapter 8: Community Health Education

Mary A. Nies, PhD, RN, FAAN, FAAHB
Special Assistant to the Dean College of Health for Grant Writing;
Tenured Professor
School of Nursing
College of Health, Joint Appointment MPH Program
Kasiska Division of Health Sciences
Idaho State University
Pocatello, Idaho
Chapter 1: Health: A Community View
Chapter 4: Health Promotion and Risk Reduction
Chapter 34: Home Health and Hospice

Julie Cowan Novak, DNSc, RN, MA, CPNP, FAANP, FAAN
Adjunct Professor
Hahn School of Nursing and Health Sciences
University of San Diego
San Diego, California;
PI/Director, Pioneering a Sustainable, Innovative NP-Led Model of Care
Hillman Innovations in Care
Neighborhood House Association Head Start Health and Wellness Van
San Diego, California;
Professor Emerita
Purdue University
West Lafayette, Indiana;
Past Endowed Professorship
The University of Texas Health Houston
Houston, Texas
Chapter 15: Health in the Global Community

C. Paige Owen, MSN, RN, CEN
Instructor
University of Texas Health Science Center at Houston
Cizik School of Nursing
Houston, Texas
Chapter 28: Violence

Bridgette Crotwell Pullis, BSN, MS, PhD, CHPN
Associate Professor of Clinical Nursing
Director the Veterans' Bachelor of Science
    in Nursing Program Track
University of Texas Health Science Center
    at Houston
Cizik School of Nursing
Houston, Texas
*Chapter 4: Health Promotion and Risk
    Reduction*
Chapter 22: Veterans Health

Elda Ramirez, PhD, RN, FNP-BC, ENP-BC, FAAN, FAANP, FAEN
Dorothy T. Nicholson Distinguished
    Professor
Assistant Dean, Diversity, Equity and
    Inclusion
Track Coordinator, Emergency/Trauma
    Care
University of Texas Health Science Center
    at Houston
Cizik School of Nursing
Houston, Texas
*Chapter 29: Natural and Man-Made
    Disasters*

Tamara Rose, BSN, MSN, PhD
Associate Dean
Nursing
Oregon Health & Science University
Klamath Falls, Oregon;
Co-Director Oregon Consortium for
    Nursing Education
Nursing
Oregon Health & Science University
Klamath Falls, Oregon
Chapter 14: Environmental Health

Mary Ellen Trail Ross, DrPh, MSN, RN, GCNS-BC
Professor
University of Texas Health Science Center
    at Houston
Cizik School of Nursing
Houston, Texas
Chapter 19: Senior Health

Lisa W. Thomas, DNP, MS, CNS
Assistant Professor
University of Texas Health Science Center
    at Houston
Cizik School of Nursing
Houston, Texas
*Chapter 21: Populations Affected by
    Disabilities*

Patricia Thomas, PhD, MS, BSN, ADN
Associate Dean, Faculty Affairs
College of Nursing
Wayne State University
Detroit, Michigan
Chapter 24: Rural and Migrant Health

Meredith Troutman-Jordan, PhD, MSN
Professor
School of Nursing
University of North Carolina
Charlotte, North Carolina
*Chapter 21: Populations Affected by
    Disabilities*
Chapter 23: Homeless Populations
*Chapter 25: Populations Affected by Mental
    Illness*
Chapter 27: Substance Abuse

Tanna Woods, PhD, MSN, BSN, RN
Nursing Education Services
Nightingale College
Salt Lake City, Utah
*Chapter 10: Policy, Politics, Legislation, and
    Community Health Nursing*
Chapter 34: Home Health and Hospice

REVIEWER

Jamie Matthews, DNP, MS, RN-PHN, NE-BC
Director of Specialty Care Clinics
Veterans Administration
Minneapolis, Minnesota

More money is spent per capita for healthcare in the United States than in any other country ($10202 in 2020). The United States spent 19.7% of its gross domestic product on healthcare expenditures in 2020, reaching a record high of more than $4 trillion. It is one of the few industrialized countries in the world that lacks a program of national health services or national health insurance, so despite this spending, 9.2% of the residents lack health insurance. In addition, many countries have far better indices of health, including traditional indicators such as infant mortality rates and longevity for both men and women, than does the United States.

Over the years, the most significant improvements in the health of the population have been achieved through advances in public health using organized community efforts, such as improvements in sanitation, immunizations, and food quality and quantity. Although access to healthcare services and individual behavioral changes are important, they are only components of the larger determinants of health, such as social and physical environments. The greatest determinants of health are still equated with factors in the community, such as education, employment, housing, and nutrition. The more money put into healthcare expenditures in the United States, the less money there is to improve these community factors.

UPSTREAM FOCUS

The traditional focus of many healthcare professionals, known as a *downstream focus,* has been to deliver healthcare services to ill people and to encourage needed behavioral change at the individual level. The focus of public/community health nursing has traditionally been on health promotion and illness prevention by working with individuals and families within the community. A shift is needed to an upstream focus, which includes working with aggregates and communities in activities such as organizing and setting health policy. This focus will help aggregates and communities work to create options for healthier environments with essential components of health, including adequate education, housing, employment, and nutrition, and will provide choices that allow people to make behavioral changes, live and work in safe environments, and access equitable and comprehensive healthcare.

Grounded in the tenets of public health nursing and the practice of public health nurses such as Lillian Wald, this eighth edition of *Community/Public Health Nursing: Promoting the Health of Populations* builds on the earlier works by highlighting an aggregate focus in addition to the traditional areas of family and community health, and thus promotes upstream thinking. The primary focus is on the promotion of the health of aggregates. This approach includes the family as a population and addresses the needs of other aggregates or population subgroups. It conceptualizes the individual as a member of the family and as a member of other aggregates, including organizations and

institutions. Furthermore, individuals and families are viewed as a part of a population within an environment (i.e., within a community).

An aggregate is made up of a collective of individuals, be it a family or another group that, with others, makes up a community. This text emphasizes the aggregate as a unit of focus and how aggregates that make up communities promote their own health. The aggregate is presented within the social context of the community, and students are given the opportunity to define and analyze environmental, economic, political, and legal constraints to the health of these populations.

Community/public health nursing has been determined to be a synthesis of nursing and public health practice with goals to promote and preserve the health of populations. Diagnosis and treatment of human responses to actual or potential health problems comprise the nursing component. The ability to prevent disease, prolong life, and promote health through organized community effort is from the public health component. Community/public health nursing practice is responsible to the population as a whole. Nursing efforts to promote health and prevent disease are applied to the public, which includes all units in the community, be they individual or collective (e.g., person, family, other aggregate, community, or population).

PURPOSE OF THE TEXT

In this text, the reader is encouraged to become a student of the community, learn from families and other aggregates in the community how they define and promote their own health, and learn how to become an advocate of the community by working with it to initiate change. The student is exposed to the complexity and rich diversity of the community and is shown evidence of how the community organizes to meet change.

The use of language or terminology by clients and agencies varies in different parts of the United States, and it may vary from that used by government officials. The contributors to this text are a diverse group from various parts of the United States. Their terms vary from chapter to chapter and from those in use in local communities. For example, some authors refer to African Americans, some to blacks, some to European Americans, and some to whites. The student must be familiar with a range of terms and, most important, know what is used in his or her local community.

Outstanding features of this eighth edition include its provocative nature as it raises consciousness regarding the social inequalities that exist in the United States and how the market-driven healthcare system contributes to health disparities and prevention of the realization of health as a right for all. With a focus on social justice, this text emphasizes society's responsibility for the protection of all human life to ensure that all people have their basic needs met, such as adequate health protection and income. Attention to the merits of population-focused care, or care that covers all people residing within geographic boundaries rather than only those populations enrolled in insurance plans, highlights the need for further reform of the systems of health reimbursement. Working toward providing health promotion and population-focused care to all requires a dramatic shift in thinking from individual-focused care for the practitioners of the future. The future paradigm for healthcare is demanding that the focus of nursing moves toward population-based interventions if we are to forge toward the goals established in *Healthy People 2030.*

This text is designed to **stimulate critical thinking and challenge students to question and debate issues.** Complex problems demand complex answers; therefore, the student is expected to *synthesize prior biophysical, psychosocial, cultural, and ethical arenas of knowledge.* However, experiential knowledge is also necessary, and the student is challenged to *enter new environments within the community* and gain new sensory, cognitive, and affective experiences. The authors of this text have integrated the concept of **upstream thinking,** introduced in the first edition, throughout this eighth edition as an important conceptual basis for nursing practice of aggregates and the community. The student is introduced to the individual and aggregate roles of community health nurses as they are engaged in a collective and interdisciplinary manner, working upstream, to facilitate the community's promotion of its own health. Students using this text will be better prepared to work with aggregates and communities in health promotion and with individuals and families in illness. Students using this text will also be better prepared to see the need to take responsibility for participation in organized community action targeting inequalities in arenas such as education, jobs, and housing and to participate in targeting individual health-behavioral change. These are important shifts in thinking for future practitioners who must be prepared to function in a population-focused healthcare system.

The text is also designed to increase the **cultural awareness** and **competency** of future community health nurses as they prepare to address the needs of culturally diverse populations. Students must be prepared to work with these growing populations as participation in the nursing workforce by ethnically and racially diverse people continues to lag. Various models are introduced to help students understand the growing link between social problems and health status, experienced disproportionately by diverse populations in the United States, and understand the methods of assessment and intervention used to meet the special needs of these populations.

The goals of the text are to provide the student with the ability to assess the complex factors in the community that affect individual, family, and other aggregate responses to health states and actual or potential health problems and to help students use this ability to plan, implement, and evaluate community/public health nursing interventions to increase contributions to the promotion of the health of populations.

MAJOR THEMES RELATED TO PROMOTING THE HEALTH OF POPULATIONS

This text is built on the following major themes:
- A social justice ethic of healthcare in contrast to a market justice ethic of healthcare in keeping with the philosophy of public health as "health for all"
- Integration of the concept of *upstream thinking* throughout the text and other appropriate theoretical frameworks related to chapter topics
- The use of population-focused and other community data to develop an assessment, or profile of health, and potential and actual health needs and capabilities of aggregates
- The application of all steps in the nursing process at the individual, family, and aggregate levels
- A focus on identification of needs of the aggregate from common interactions with individuals, families, and communities in traditional environments
- An orientation toward the application of all three levels of prevention at the individual, family, and aggregate levels
- The experience of the underserved aggregate, particularly the economically disenfranchised, including cultural and ethnic groups disproportionately at risk of developing health problems.

Themes are developed and related to promoting the health of populations in the following ways:
- The commitment of community/public health nursing is to an equity model; therefore community health nurses work toward the provision of the unmet health needs of populations.
- The development of a population-focused model is necessary to close the gap between unmet healthcare needs and health resources on a geographic basis to the entire population. The contributions of intervention at the aggregate level work toward the realization of such a model.
- Contemporary theories provide frameworks for holistic community health nursing practice that help students conceptualize the reciprocal influence of various components within the community on the health of aggregates and the population.
- The ability to gather population-focused and other community data in developing an assessment of health is a crucial initial step that precedes the identification of nursing diagnoses and plans to meet aggregate responses to potential and actual health problems.
- The nursing process includes, in each step, a focus on the aggregate, assessment of the aggregate, nursing diagnosis of the aggregate, planning for the aggregate, and intervention and evaluation at the aggregate level.
- The text discusses development of the ability to gather clues about the needs of aggregates from complex environments, such as during a home visit, with parents in a waiting room of a well-baby clinic, or with elders receiving hypertension screening, and to promote individual, collective, and political action that addresses the health of aggregates.

- Primary, secondary, and tertiary prevention strategies include a major focus at the population level.
- In addition to offering a chapter on cultural influences in the community, the text includes data on and the experience of underserved aggregates at high risk of developing health problems and who are most often in need of community health nursing services (i.e., low and marginal income, cultural, and ethnic groups) throughout.

ORGANIZATION

The text is divided into seven units. *Unit 1, Introduction to Community Health Nursing*, presents an overview of the concept of health, a perspective of health as evolving and as defined by the community, and the concept of community health nursing as the nursing of aggregates from both historical and contemporary mandates. Health is viewed as an individual and collective right, brought about through individual and collective/political action. The definitions of public health and community health nursing and their foci are presented. Current crises in public health and the healthcare system and consequences for the health of the public frame implications for community health nursing. The historical evolution of public health, the healthcare system, and community health nursing is presented, as well as the evolution of humans from wanderers and food gatherers to those who live in larger groups. The text also discusses the influence of the group on health, which contrasts with the evolution of a healthcare system built around the individual person, increasingly fractured into many parts. Community health nurses bring to their practice awareness of the social context; economic, political, and legal constraints from the larger community; and knowledge of the current healthcare system and its structural constraints and limitations on the care of populations. The theoretical foundations for the text, with a focus on the concept of upstream thinking, and the rationale for a population approach to community health nursing are presented. Recognizing the importance of health promotion and risk reduction when striving to improve the health of individuals, families, groups, and communities, this unit concludes with a chapter elaborating on those concepts. Strategies for assessment and analysis of risk factors and interventions to improve health are described.

Unit 2, The Art and Science of Community Health Nursing, describes application of the nursing process—assessment, planning, intervention, and evaluation—to aggregates in the community using selected theory bases. The unit addresses the need for a population focus that includes the public health sciences of biostatistics and epidemiology as key in community assessment and the application of the nursing process to aggregates to promote the health of populations. Application of the art and science of community health nursing to meeting the needs of aggregates is evident in chapters that focus on community health planning and evaluation, community health education, and case management.

Unit 3, Factors That Influence the Health of the Community, examines factors and issues that can both positively and negatively affect health. Beginning with an overview of health policy and legislation, the opening chapter in this unit focuses on how policy is developed and the effect of past and future legislative changes on how healthcare is delivered in the United States. This unit examines the healthcare delivery system and the importance of economics and healthcare financing on the health of individuals, families, and populations. Cultural diversity and associated issues are described in detail, showing the importance of consideration of culture when developing health interventions in the community. The influence of the environment on the health of populations is considered, and the reader is led to recognize the multitude of external factors that influence health. This unit concludes with an examination of various aspects of global health and describes features of the healthcare systems and patterns of health and illness in developing and developed countries.

Unit 4, Aggregates in the Community, presents the application of the nursing process to address potential health problems identified in large groups, including children and adolescents, women, men, families, and seniors. The focus is on the major indicators of health (e.g., longevity, mortality, and morbidity), types of common health problems, use of health services, pertinent legislation, health services and resources, selected applications of the community health nursing process to a case study, application of the levels of prevention, selected roles of the community health nurse, and relevant research.

Unit 5, Vulnerable Populations, focuses on those aggregates in the community considered vulnerable: persons with disabilities, veterans of the armed forces, the homeless, those living in rural areas including migrant workers, and persons with mental illness. Chapters address the application of the community health nursing process to the special service needs in each of these areas. Basic community health nursing strategies are applied to promoting the health of these vulnerable high-risk aggregates and to reducing the numerous health disparities.

Unit 6, Population Health Problems, focuses on health problems that affect large aggregates and their service needs as applied in community health nursing. These problems include communicable disease, violence and associated issues, substance abuse, and a chapter describing nursing care during disasters.

Unit 7, Community Health Settings, focuses on selected sites or specialties for community health: school health, occupational health, faith community health, home health and hospice, and forensic and correctional nursing.

SPECIAL FEATURES

The following features are presented to enhance student learning:

- **Learning objectives.** Learning objectives set the framework for the content of each chapter.
- **Key terms.** A list of key terms for each chapter is provided at the beginning of the chapter. The terms are highlighted in

blue within the chapter. The definitions of these terms are found in the glossary located on the book's Evolve website.

- **Chapter outline.** The major headings of each chapter are provided at the beginning of each chapter to help locate important content.
- **Theoretical frameworks.** The use of theoretical frameworks common to nursing and public health will aid the student in applying familiar and new theory bases to problems and challenges in the community.
- *Healthy People 2030.* Goals and objectives of *Healthy People 2030* are presented in a special box throughout the text (The updated *Healthy People 2030* information is new to this edition and based on the proposed objectives.).
- **Upstream thinking.** This theoretical construct is integrated into chapters throughout the text.
- **Case studies and application of the nursing process at individual, family, and aggregate levels.** The use of case studies and **clinical examples** throughout the text is designed to ground the theory, concepts, and application of the nursing process in practical and manageable examples for the student.
- **Research highlights.** The introduction of students to the growing bodies of community health nursing and public health research literature is enhanced by special boxes devoted to specific research studies.
- **Active learning exercises.** Selected learning activities are interspersed throughout the chapter to test students' knowledge of the content they've just read, helping provide clinical application and knowledge retention.
- **Photo novellas.** Numerous stories in photograph form depicting public healthcare in a variety of settings and with different population groups.

- **Ethical insights boxes.** These boxes present situations of ethical dilemmas or considerations pertinent to particular chapters.

NEW CONTENT IN THIS EDITION

- Discussion of the effect of COVID-19 on the health and wellbeing of the population is presented in many chapters, within the topical context (e.g., the epidemiology of COVID-19 in Chapter 5; how COVID-19 affects elders in Chapter 19; and COVID-19 immunization in Chapter 26).
- Most chapters contain new or updated **Research Highlights boxes** highlighting timely, relevant examples of the topics from recent nursing literature and **Ethical Insights boxes** that emphasize specific ethical issues.

TEACHING AND LEARNING PACKAGE

Evolve website: The website at http://evolve.elsevier.com/Nies/ community is devoted exclusively to this text. It provides materials for both instructors and students.

- **For Instructors:** PowerPoint lecture slides, image collection, Case Studies, more than 900 test bank questions with alternative item questions, new Next-Generation NCLEX® (NGN)—Style Case Studies, and TEACH for Nurses, which contains detailed chapter Lesson Plans, including references to curriculum standards.
- **For Students:** NCLEX-style multiple-choice review questions with correct answer rationales

CONTENTS

1

Health: A Community View

Melanie McEwen and Mary A. Nies

OBJECTIVES

Upon completion of this chapter, the reader will be able to do the following:

1. Compare and contrast definitions of health from a public health nursing perspective.
2. Define and discuss the focus of public health.
3. Discuss determinates of health and indicators of health and illness from a population perspective.
4. List the three levels of prevention and give examples of each.
5. Explain the difference between public/community health nursing practice and community-based nursing practice.

6. Describe the purpose of *Healthy People 2030* and give examples of the leading health indicators, social determinants of health and topic areas for the national health objectives.
7. Discuss public/community health nursing practice in terms of public health's core functions and essential services.
8. Discuss public/community health nursing interventions as explained by the Intervention Wheel.

OUTLINE

KEY TERMS

aggregates
community
community health
community health nursing
disease prevention
health

health promotion
health-related quality-of-life (HRQOL)
Healthy People 2030
population
population-focused nursing

primary prevention
public health
public health nursing
secondary prevention
tertiary prevention

1

As a result of recent and anticipated changes related to healthcare reform and the long-term consequences of the COVID-19 pandemic, community/public health nurses are in a position to assist the US healthcare system in the transition from a disease-oriented system to a health-oriented system. Costs of caring for the sick account for the majority of escalating healthcare dollars, which increased from 5.7% of the gross domestic product in 1965 to almost 18% in 2018 (National Center for Health Statistics [NCHS], 2019). Alarmingly, national annual healthcare expenditures reached nearly $3 trillion in 2017, or an astonishing $10,700 per person.

♥ **HEALTHY PEOPLE 2030**

Major Topic Areas and Selected Subtopics
Health Conditions
Arthritis
Cancer
Dementias
Diabetes
Heart Disease
Sexually Transmitted Infections

Health Behaviors
Child and Adolescent Development
Drug and Alcohol Use
Emergency Preparedness
Family Planning
Nutrition and Healthy Eating
Tobacco Use
Vaccination

Populations
Adolescents
Children
LGBT
Older Adults
People with Disabilities

Settings and Systems
Environmental Health
Healthcare
Health Insurance
Health Policy
Hospital and Emergency Services
Schools

From US Department of Health and Human Services: *Healthy People 2030: browse objectives.* Available from: https://health.gov/healthypeople/objectives-and-data/browse-objectives.

Health expenditures in the United States reflect a focus on the care of the sick. In 2017, $0.39 of each healthcare dollar supported hospital care, $0.23 supported physician/professional services, and $0.11 was spent on prescription drugs (more than double the proportion since 1980). The vast majority of these funds were spent providing care for the sick, and less than $0.03 of every healthcare dollar was directed toward preventive public health activities (NCHS, 2018). Despite high hospital and physician expenditures, US health indicators such as life expectancy and infant mortality rate remain considerably below

the health indicators of many other countries. This situation reflects a relatively severe disproportion of funding for preventive services and social and economic opportunities. Furthermore, the health status of the population within the United States varies markedly across areas of the country and among different cohorts. For example, it is widely recognized that the economically disadvantaged and many cultural and ethnic groups have poorer overall health status compared with middle-class Caucasians.

Nurses constitute the largest segment of healthcare workers; therefore, they are instrumental in creating a healthcare delivery system that will meet the health-oriented needs of the people. According to a survey of registered nurses (RNs) conducted by the National Council of State Boards of Nursing (NCSBN, 2018), about 55.7% of approximately 2.8 million RNs employed full-time in the United States worked in hospitals during 2017 (down from about 66.5% in 1992). This survey also found that about 11%, of all RNs worked in home, hospice, school, public/community health, or correctional facilities; 9.4% worked in ambulatory care settings; and 5.3% worked in nursing homes or other extended care or assisted living facilities (NCSBN, 2018).

Between 1980 and 2018, the number of nurses employed in community, health, and ambulatory care settings more than doubled (NCSBN, 2018; US Department of Health and Human Services [USDHHS], Health Resources and Services Administration [HRSA], 2010). The decline in the percentage of nurses employed in hospitals and the subsequent increase in nurses employed in community settings suggests a shift in focus from illness and institution-based care to health promotion and preventive care. This shift will likely continue into the future as alternative delivery systems, such as ambulatory, home care, and hospice employ more nurses (American Nurses Association (ANA), 2016; Institute of Medicine (IOM), 2011; Rosenfeld & Russell, 2012).

Community/public health nursing is the synthesis of nursing practice and public health practice. The major goal of community/public health nursing is to preserve the health of the community and surrounding populations by focusing on health promotion and health maintenance of individuals, families, and groups within the community. Thus, community/public health nursing is associated with health and the identification of populations at risk rather than with an episodic response to patient demand.

Public health is often described as the art and science of preventing disease, prolonging life and promoting health through organized community efforts to benefit each citizen (Winslow, 1920). **The mission of public health is social justice, which entitles all people to basic necessities such as adequate income and health protection and accepts collective burdens to make it possible.** Public health, with its egalitarian tradition and vision, often conflicts with the predominant US model of market justice that largely entitles people to what they have gained through individual efforts. Although market justice respects individual rights, collective action and obligations are minimal. An emphasis on technology and curative medical services within the market justice system has limited the evolution of a health system designed to protect and preserve the health of the population. Public health assumes that it is society's responsibility to meet the basic needs of the people. Thus, there is a greater need for public funding of prevention efforts to enhance the health of our population.

Current US health policies advocate changes in personal behaviors that might predispose individuals to chronic disease or accidents. These policies promote exercise, healthy eating, tobacco use cessation, and moderate consumption of alcohol. However, simply encouraging the individual to overcome the effects of unhealthy activities lessens focus on collective behaviors necessary to change the determinants of health stemming from such factors as poor air and water quality, workplace hazards, unsafe neighborhoods, and unequal access to healthcare. Because living arrangements, work/school environment, and other sociocultural constraints affect health and well-being, public policy must address societal and environmental changes, in addition to lifestyle changes, which will positively influence the health of the entire population.

With ongoing and very significant changes in the healthcare system and increased employment in community settings, there will be greater demands on community and public health nurses to broaden their population health perspective. The Code of Ethics of the ANA (2015) promotes social reform by focusing on health policy and legislation to positively affect accessibility, quality, and cost of healthcare. Community and public health nurses therefore must align themselves with public health programs that promote and preserve the health of populations by influencing sociocultural issues such as human rights, homelessness, violence, disability, and stigma of illness. This principle allows nurses to be positioned to promote the health, welfare, and safety of all individuals.

This chapter examines health from a population-focused, community-based perspective. Therefore, it requires understanding of how people identify, define, and describe related concepts. The following section explores six major ideas:
1. Definitions of "health" and "community"
2. Determinants of health and disease
3. Indicators of health and disease
4. Definition and focus of public and community health
5. Description of a preventive approach to health
6. Definition and focus of "public health nursing," "community health nursing," and "community-based nursing"

DEFINITIONS OF HEALTH AND COMMUNITY
Health
The definition of **health** is evolving. The early, classic definition of health by the World Health Organization (WHO) set a trend toward describing health in social terms rather than in medical terms. Indeed, the WHO (1958, p. 1) defined health as "a state of complete physical, mental, and social well-being and not merely the absence of disease or infirmity."

Social means "of or relating to living together in organized groups or similar close aggregates" (American Heritage College Dictionary, 1997, p. 1291) and refers to units of people in communities who interact with one another. "Social health" connotes community vitality and is a result of positive interaction among groups within the community, with an emphasis on health promotion and illness prevention. For example, community groups may sponsor food banks in churches and civic organizations to help alleviate problems of hunger and nutrition. Other community groups may form to address problems of violence and lack of opportunity, which can negatively affect social health.

In the mid-1980s, the WHO expanded the definition of health to emphasize recognition of the social implications of health. Thus, health is

> the extent to which an individual or group is able, on the one hand, to realize aspirations and satisfy needs; and, on the other hand, to change or cope with the environment. Health is, therefore, seen as a resource for everyday life, not the objective of living; it is a positive concept emphasizing social and personal resources, and physical capacities.
> **WHO (1986, p. 73)**

The WHO definition considers several dimensions of health. These include physical (structure/function), social, role, mental (emotional and intellectual), and general perceptions of health status. It also conceptualizes health from a macroperspective, as a resource to be used rather than a goal in and of itself (Saylor, 2004).

The nursing literature contains many varied definitions of health. For example, health has been defined as "a state of well-being in which the person is able to use purposeful, adaptive responses and processes physically, mentally, emotionally, spiritually, and socially" (Murray et al., 2009, p. 53); "the individual's total well-being, the regular patterns of people and their environments that result in maintaining wholeness and human integrity" (Roy, 2009, p. 3); "realization of human potential through goal-directed behavior, competent self-care, and satisfying relationships with others, while adapting to meet the demands of everyday life within one's social and physical environment" (Murdaugh et al., 2019, p. 14); and a "state of physical, mental, spiritual and social functioning that realizes a person's potential and is experienced within a developmental context" (Ross & Kleman, 2018, p. 5).

The variety of characterizations of the word illustrates the difficulty in standardizing the conceptualization of health. Commonalities involve description of "goal-directed" or "purposeful" actions, processes, responses, functioning, or behaviors and the possession of "integrity," "wholeness," and/or "well-being." Problems can arise when the definition involves a unit of analysis. For example, some writers use the individual or "person" as the unit of analysis and exclude the community. Others may include additional concepts, such as adaptation and environment, in health definitions, and then present the environment as static and requiring human adaptation rather than as changing and enabling human modification.

For many years, community and public health nurses have favored Dunn's (1961) classic concept of wellness, in which family, community, society, and environment are interrelated and have an impact on health. From his viewpoint, illness, health, and peak wellness are on a continuum; health is fluid and changing. Consequently, within a social context or environment, the state of health depends on the goals, potentials, and performance of individuals, families, communities, and societies.

 ACTIVE LEARNING EXERCISE

Interview several community/public health nurses and several clients regarding their definitions of health. Share the results with your classmates. Do you agree with their definitions? Why or why not?

Community

The definitions of *community* are also numerous and variable. Baldwin and colleagues (1998) outlined the evolution of the definition of community by examining community health nursing textbooks. They determined that, before 1996, definitions of community focused on geographic boundaries combined with social attributes of people. Citing several sources from the later part of the decade, the authors observed that geographic location became a secondary characteristic in the discussion of what defines a community.

In recent nursing literature, community has been defined as "a collection of people who interact with one another and whose common interests or characteristics form the basis for a sense of unity or belonging" (Rector, 2018, p. 6); "a group of people who share something in common and interact with one another, who may exhibit a commitment with one another and may share a geographic boundary" (Lundy & Janes, 2016, p. 13); and "a locality-based entity, composed of systems of formal organizations reflecting society's institutions, informal groups and aggregates" (Shuster, 2012, p. 398).

Maurer and Smith (2013) further addressed the concept of community and identified three defining attributes: people; place; and social interaction or common characteristics, interests, or goals. Combining ideas and concepts, in this text, **community** is seen as a group or collection of individuals interacting in social units and sharing common interests, characteristics, values, and goals.

Maurer and Smith (2013) noted that there are two main types of communities: geopolitical communities and phenomenological communities. Geopolitical communities are those most traditionally recognized or imagined when the term *community* is considered. *Geopolitical communities* are defined or formed by natural and/or human-made boundaries and include cities, counties, states, and nations. Other commonly recognized geopolitical communities are school districts, census tracts, zip codes, and neighborhoods. *Phenomenological communities*, on the other hand, refer to relational, interactive groups. In phenomenological communities, the place or setting is more abstract, and people share a group perspective or identity based on culture, values, history, interests, and goals. Examples of phenomenological communities are schools,

colleges, and universities; churches, synagogues, and mosques; and various groups and organizations, such as social networks.

A community of solution is a type of phenomenological community. A *community of solution* is a collection of people who form a group specifically to address a common need or concern. The Sierra Club, whose members lobby for the preservation of natural resource lands, and a group of disabled people who challenge the owners of an office building to obtain equal access to public buildings, education, jobs, and transportation are examples. These groups or social units work together to promote optimal "health" and to address identified actual and potential health threats and health needs.

Population and *aggregate* are related terms that are often used in public health and community health nursing. **Population** is typically used to denote a group of people with common personal or environmental characteristics. It can also refer to all of the people in a defined community (Williams, 2020). **Aggregates** are subgroups or subpopulations that have some common characteristics or concerns (Gibson & Thatcher, 2020). Depending on the situation, needs, and practice parameters, community health nursing interventions may be directed toward a community (e.g., residents of a small town), a population (e.g., all elders in a rural region), or an aggregate (e.g., pregnant teens within a school district).

DETERMINANTS OF HEALTH AND DISEASE

The health status of a community is associated with a number of factors, such as healthcare access, economic conditions, social and environmental issues, and cultural practices, and it is essential for the community health nurse to understand the determinants of health and recognize the interaction of the factors that lead to disease, death, and disability. It has been estimated that individual behaviors are responsible for about 50% of all premature deaths in the United States (Elbel et al., 2019). Indeed, individual biology and behaviors influence health through their interaction with each other and with the individual's social and physical environments. Thus, policies and interventions can improve health by targeting detrimental or harmful factors related to individuals and their environment. Fig. 1.1 shows the model developed for *Healthy People 2020*. This model depicts the interaction of these determinants and shows how they influence health.

In a seminal work, McGinnis and Foege (1993) described what they termed "actual causes of death" in the United States, explaining how lifestyle choices contribute markedly to early deaths. Their work was updated a decade later (Mokdad et al., 2004). Leading the list of "actual causes of death" was tobacco, which was implicated in almost 20% of the annual deaths in the United States—approximately 435,000 individuals. Poor diet and physical inactivity were deemed to account for about 16.6% of deaths (about 400,000 per year), and alcohol consumption was implicated in about 85,000 deaths because of its association with accidents, suicides, homicides, and cirrhosis and chronic liver disease. Other leading causes of death were microbial agents (75,000), toxic agents (55,000), motor vehicle

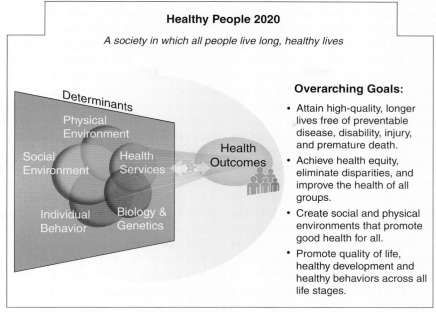

Fig. 1.1 Model: Healthy People 2020. (From US Department of Health and Human Services: *Healthy People 2030: browse objectives.* Available from: https://www.healthypeople.gov/sites/default/files/HP2020Framework.pdf.)

crashes (43,000), firearms (29,000), sexual behaviors (20,000), and illicit use of drugs (17,000).

Although all of these causes of mortality are related to individual lifestyle choices, they can also be strongly influenced by population-focused policy efforts and education. For example, the prevalence of smoking has fallen dramatically during the past two decades, largely because of legal efforts (e.g., laws prohibiting sale of tobacco to minors and much higher taxes), organizational policy (e.g., smoke-free workplaces), and education. Likewise, concerns about the widespread increase in incidence of overweight and obesity have led to population-based measures to address the issue (e.g., removal of soft drink and candy machines from schools, regulations prohibiting the use of certain types of fats in processed foods).

Public health experts have observed that health has improved over the past 100 years largely because people become ill less often (McKeown, 2003; Russo & Gourevitch, 2019). Indeed, at the population level, better health can be attributed to higher standards of living, good nutrition, a healthier environment, and having fewer children. Furthermore, public health efforts, such as immunization and clean air and water, and medical care, including management of acute episodic illnesses (e.g., pneumonia, tuberculosis) and chronic disease (e.g., cancer, heart disease), have also contributed significantly to the increase in life expectancy.

Community and public health nurses should understand these concepts and appreciate that health and illness are influenced by a web of factors, some that can be changed (e.g., individual behaviors such as tobacco use, diet, physical activity) and some that cannot (e.g., genetics, age, gender). Other factors (e.g., physical and social environment) may require changes that will need to be accomplished from a policy perspective. Public health nurses must work with policy-makers and community leaders to identify patterns of disease and death and to advocate for activities and policies that promote health at the individual, family, aggregate, and population levels.

INDICATORS OF HEALTH AND ILLNESS

A variety of health indicators are used by health providers, policy-makers, and community health nurses to measure the health of the community. Local or state health departments, the Centers for Disease Control and Prevention (CDC), and the National Center for Health Statistics (NCHS) provide morbidity, mortality, and other health status–related data. State and local health departments are responsible for collecting morbidity and mortality data and forwarding the information to the appropriate federal-level agency, which is often the CDC. Some of the more commonly reported indicators are life expectancy, infant mortality, age-adjusted death rates, and cancer incidence rates.

Indicators of mortality in particular illustrate the health status of a community and/or population because changes in mortality reflect a number of social, economic, health service, and related trends (Shi & Singh, 2019). These data may be useful in analyzing health patterns over time, comparing communities from different geographic regions, or comparing different aggregates within a community.

When the national health objectives for *Healthy People 2030* were being revised, a total of 23 "leading health indicators" (LHIs) were identified that reflected the major public health concerns in the United States (see *Healthy People 2030* box).

The LHIs are noted to be a subset of "high-priority" HP 2030 objectives that were selected to direct provider and population responses to improve health and well-being. Among the LHIs are individual behaviors (e.g., cigarette smoking, consumption of calories from added sugars, annual vaccination against influenza), physical and social environmental factors (e.g., household food insecurity and hunger, exposure to unhealthy air, homicides), and health systems issues (e.g., persons with medical insurance). In addition, there are population or group specific indicators (e.g., infant mortality, children and adolescents with obesity, maternal mortality, new cases of diagnosed diabetes). Each of these indicators can affect the health of individuals and communities and can be correlated with leading causes of morbidity and mortality. For example, tobacco use is linked to heart disease, stroke, and cancer; substance abuse is linked to accidents, injuries, and violence; irresponsible sexual behaviors can lead to unwanted pregnancy as well as sexually transmitted diseases, including human immunodeficiency virus/acquired immunodeficiency syndrome (HIV/AIDS); and lack of health insurance can contribute to poor pregnancy outcomes, untreated illness, and disability.

❤ HEALTHY PEOPLE 2030

Selected Leading Health Indicator Topics

All Ages
- Children, adolescents, and adults who use the oral healthcare system
- Drug overdose deaths
- Exposure to unhealthy air
- Homicides
- Household food insecurity and hunger

Infants
- Infant deaths

Children and adolescents
- Adolescents with major depressive episodes who receive treatment
- Children and adolescent with obesity

Adults and older adults
- Adults engaging in binge drinking of alcoholic beverages during the past 30 days
- Adults who receive a colorectal cancer screening based on the most recent guidelines
- Adults with hypertension whose blood pressure is under control
- Cigarette smoking in adults
- Maternal deaths

From US Department of Health and Human Services: *Healthy People 2030 leading health indicators.* Available from: https://health.gov/healthypeople/objectives-and-data/leading-health-indicators.

Public health nurses should be aware of health patterns and health indicators within their practice. Each nurse should ask relevant questions, including the following: What are the leading causes of death and disease among various groups served? Which groups have been most affected by COVID-19? How do infant mortality rates and teenage pregnancy rates in my community compare with regional, state, and national rates? What are the most serious health threats in my neighborhood? What are the most serious environmental risks in my city? The public health nurse may identify areas for further investigation and intervention through an understanding of health, disease, and mortality patterns. For example, if a school nurse learns that the teenage pregnancy rate in their community is higher than regional and state averages, the nurse should address the problem with school officials, parents, and students. Likewise, if an occupational health nurse discovers an apparent high rate of chronic lung disease in an industrial facility, the nurse should work with company management, employees, and state and federal officials to identify potential harmful sources. Finally, if a public health nurse works in a state-sponsored AIDS clinic and recognizes an increase in the number of women testing positive for HIV, the nurse should report all findings to the designated agencies. The nurse should then participate in investigative efforts to determine what is precipitating the increase and work to remedy the identified threats or risks.

DEFINITION AND FOCUS OF PUBLIC HEALTH AND COMMUNITY HEALTH

C. E. A. Winslow is known for the following classic definition of public health:

> *Public health is the Science and Art of (1) preventing disease, (2) prolonging life, and (3) promoting health and efficiency through organized community effort for:*
> *(a) sanitation of the environment,*
> *(b) control of communicable infections,*
> *(c) education of the individual in personal hygiene,*
> *(d) organization of medical and nursing services for the early diagnosis and preventive treatment of disease, and*
> *(e) development of the social machinery to ensure everyone a standard of living adequate for the maintenance of health, so organizing these benefits as to enable every citizen to realize his birthright of health and longevity.*
>
> *Hanlon (1960, p. 23)*

A key phrase in this definition of public health is "through organized community effort." The term *public health* connotes organized, legislated, and tax-supported efforts that serve all people through health departments or related governmental agencies.

The public health nursing tradition, begun in the late 1800s by Lillian Wald and her associates, clearly illustrates this phenomenon (Wald, 1971; see Chapter 2). After moving into the immigrant community in New York City to provide care for individuals and families, these early public health nurses saw that neither administering bedside clinical nursing nor teaching family members to deliver care in the home adequately addressed the true determinants of health and disease. They resolved that collective political activity should focus on advancing the health of aggregates and improving social and environmental conditions by addressing the social and environmental determinants of health, such as child labor,

From Institute of Medicine: *The future of public health,* Washington, DC, 1988, National Academy Press.

BOX 1.1 Core Public Health Functions

Assessment: Regular collection, analysis, and information sharing about health conditions, risks, and resources in a community.

Policy development: Use of information gathered during assessment to develop local and state health policies and to direct resources toward those policies.

Assurance: Focuses on the availability of necessary health services throughout the community. It includes maintaining the ability of both public health agencies and private providers to manage day-to-day operations and the capacity to respond to critical situations and emergencies.

pollution, and poverty. Wald and her colleagues affected the health of the community by organizing the community, establishing school nursing, and taking impoverished mothers to testify in Washington, DC (Wald, 1971).

In a key action, the National Academy of Medicine (NAM), formerly called the IOM (1988), identified the following three primary functions of public health: *assessment, assurance,* and *policy development.* Box 1.1 lists each of the three primary functions and describes them briefly. All nurses working in community settings should develop knowledge and skills related to each of these primary functions.

The term **community health** extends the realm of public health to include organized health efforts at the community level through both government *and* private efforts. Participants include privately funded agencies such as the American Heart Association and the American Red Cross. A variety of private and public structures serves community health efforts.

Public health efforts focus on prevention and promotion of population health at the federal, state, and local levels. These efforts at the federal and state levels concentrate on providing support and advisory services to public health structures at the local level. The local-level structures provide direct services to communities through two avenues:

- Community health services, which protect the public from hazards such as polluted water and air, tainted food, and unsafe housing
- Personal healthcare services, such as immunization and family planning services, well-infant care, and sexually transmitted disease (STD) treatment

Personal health services may be part of the public health effort and often target the populations most at risk and in need of services. Public health efforts are multidisciplinary because they require people with many different skills. Community health nurses work with a diverse team of public health professionals, including epidemiologists, local health officers, and health educators. Public health science methods that assess biostatistics, epidemiology, and population needs provide a method of measuring characteristics and health indicators and disease patterns within a community. In 1994, the American Public Health Association drafted a list of 10 essential public health services, which the US Department of Health and Human Services later adopted. The updated list of essential services (CDC, 2020) appears in Box 1.2.

PREVENTIVE APPROACH TO HEALTH

Health Promotion and Levels of Prevention

Contrasting with "medical care," which focuses on disease management and "cure," public health efforts focus on health promotion and disease prevention. **Health promotion** activities enhance resources directed at improving well-being, whereas **disease prevention** activities protect people from disease and the effects of disease. Leavell and Clark (1958) identified three levels of prevention commonly described in nursing practice: primary prevention, secondary prevention, and tertiary prevention (Fig. 1.2 and Table 1.1).

Primary prevention relates to activities directed at preventing a problem before it occurs by altering susceptibility or reducing exposure for susceptible individuals. Primary prevention consists of two elements: general health promotion and specific protection. Health promotion efforts enhance resiliency and protective factors and target essentially well populations. Examples include promotion of good nutrition, provision of adequate shelter, and encouraging regular exercise. Specific protection efforts reduce or eliminate risk factors and include

BOX 1.2 Essential Public Health Services

Assessment
- Assess and monitor population health status, factors that influence health, and community needs and assets.
- Investigate, diagnose, and address health problems and hazards affecting the population.

Policy Development
- Communicate effectively to inform and educate people about health, factors that influence it, and how to improve it.
- Strengthen, support, and mobilize communities and partnerships to improve health.
- Create, champion, and implement policies, plans, and laws that impact health.
- Utilize legal and regulatory actions designed to improve and protect the public's health.

Assurance
- Assure an effective system that enables equitable access to the individual services and care needed to be healthy.
- Build and support a diverse and skilled public health workforce.
- Improve and innovate public health functions through ongoing evaluation, research, and continuous quality improvement.
- Build and maintain a strong organizational infrastructure for public health.

From Centers for Disease Control and Prevention, Public Health Professionals Gateway: Available from: https://www.cdc.gov/publichealthgateway/publichealthservices/essentialhealthservices.html.

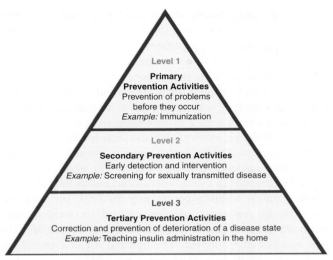

Fig. 1.2 The three levels of prevention.

such measures as immunization, seat belt use, and water purification.

Secondary prevention refers to early detection and prompt intervention during the period of early disease pathogenesis. Secondary prevention is implemented after a problem has begun, but before signs and symptoms appear, and targets those populations that have risk factors. Mammography, blood pressure screening, COVID-19 testing, and prostate-specific antigen (PSA) tests are examples of secondary prevention.

Tertiary prevention targets populations that have experienced disease or injury and focuses on limitation of disability and rehabilitation. Aims of tertiary prevention are to keep health problems from getting worse, to reduce the effects of disease and injury, and to restore individuals to their optimal level of functioning. Examples include teaching how to perform insulin injections and disease management to a patient with diabetes, referral of a patient with spinal cord injury for occupational and physical therapy, and leading a support group for grieving parents.

Much of public health nursing practice is directed toward preventing the progression of disease at the earliest period or phase feasible using the appropriate level(s) of prevention. For example, when applying "levels of prevention" to a client with HIV/AIDS, a nurse might perform the following interventions:

- Educate students on the practice of sexual abstinence or "safer sex" by using barrier methods (primary prevention).
- Encourage testing and counseling for clients with known exposure or who are in high-risk groups; provide referrals

TABLE 1.1 Examples of Levels of Prevention and Clients Served in the Community

	LEVEL OF PREVENTION		
Definition of Client Served[a]	**Primary (Health Promotion and Specific Prevention)**	**Secondary (Early Diagnosis and Treatment)**	**Tertiary (Limitation of Disability and Rehabilitation)**
Individual	Dietary teaching during pregnancy Immunizations	HIV testing Screening for cervical cancer	Teaching new clients with diabetes how to administer insulin Exercise therapy after stroke Skin care for incontinent patients
Family (two or more individuals bound by kinship, law, or living arrangement and with common emotional ties and obligations [see Chapter 20])	Education or counseling regarding smoking, dental care, or nutrition Adequate housing	Dental examinations COVID-19 testing for family potentially exposed	Mental health counseling or referral for family in crisis (e.g., grieving or experiencing a divorce) Dietary instructions and monitoring for family with overweight members
Group or aggregate (interacting people with a common purpose or purposes)	Birthing classes for pregnant teenage mothers AIDS and other STI education for high school students	Vision screening of a first-grade class Mammography van for screening of women in a low-income neighborhood Hearing tests at a senior center	Group counseling for grade-school children with asthma Swim therapy for physically disabled elders at a senior center Alcoholics anonymous and other self-help groups Mental health services for military veterans
Community and populations (aggregate of people sharing space over time within a social system [see Chapter 6]; population groups or aggregates with power relations and common needs or purposes)	Fluoride water supplementation Environmental sanitation Removal of environmental hazards	Organized screening programs for communities (e.g., health fairs) Lead screening for children by school district	Shelter and relocation centers for fire or earthquake victims Emergency medical services Community mental health services for chronically mentally ill Home care services for chronically ill

[a]Note that terms are used differently in literature of various disciplines. There are not any clear-cut definitions; for example, families may be referred to as an aggregate, and a population and subpopulations may exist within a community.
AIDS, Acquired immunodeficiency syndrome; *HIV*, human immunodeficiency virus; *STI*, sexually transmitted infection.

for follow-up for clients who test positive for HIV (secondary prevention).

- Provide education on management of HIV infection, advocacy, case management, and other interventions for those who are HIV positive (tertiary prevention).

Thinking Upstream

The concepts of prevention and population-focused care figure prominently in a conceptual orientation to nursing practice referred to as *thinking upstream*. This orientation is derived from an analogy of patients falling into a river upstream and being rescued downstream by health providers overwhelmed with the struggle of responding to disease and illness. The river as an analogy for the natural history of illness was first coined by McKinlay (1979), with a charge to health providers to refocus their efforts toward preventive and "upstream" activities. In a description of the daily challenges of providers to address health from a preventive versus curative focus, McKinlay differentiates the consequences of illness (*downstream* endeavors) from its precursors (*upstream* endeavors). The author then charges health providers to critically examine the relative weights of their activities toward illness response versus the prevention of illness.

A population-based perspective on health and health determinants is critical to understanding and formulating nursing actions to prevent disease. By examining the origins of disease, nurses identify social, political, environmental, and economic factors that often lead to poor health options for both individuals and populations. The call to refocus the efforts of nurses "upstream, where the real problems lie" (McKinlay, 1979) has been welcomed by community health nurses in a variety of practice settings. For these nurses, this theme provides affirmation of their daily efforts to prevent disease in populations at risk in schools, work sites, and clinics throughout their local communities and in the larger world.

ETHICAL INSIGHTS

Inequities: Distribution of Resources

In the United States, it has been established that inequities in the distribution of resources pose a threat to the common good and a challenge for community and public health nurses. Factors that contribute to wide variations in health disparities include education, income, and occupation. Lack of health insurance is a key factor in this issue and a major rationale for healthcare reform efforts. Lack of health insurance is damaging to population health, as low-income, uninsured individuals are much less likely than insured individuals to receive timely primary healthcare and preventive dental care.

Public health nurses are regularly confronted with the consequences of the fragmented healthcare delivery system. They diligently work to improve the circumstances for populations who have not had adequate access to resources largely because of who they are and where they live.

Ethical questions commonly encountered in community and public health nursing practice include the following: Should resources (e.g., free or low-cost immunizations) be offered to all, even those who have insurance that will pay for the care? Should public health nurses serve anyone who meets financial need guidelines, regardless of medical need? Should the health department provide flu shots to persons of all ages or just those most likely to be affected by the disease? Should nonresidents in the United States illegally or persons working on "green cards" receive the same level of healthcare services that are available to citizens? Who should have free or reduced-cost access to extremely expensive drugs such as those that treat hepatitis C, multiple sclerosis, or many forms of cancer, and who should bear the financial burden?

Access to healthcare is a goal for all. To this end, community and public health nurses must face the challenges and dilemmas related to these and other questions, as they assist individuals, families, and communities dealing with the uneven distribution of health resources and the associated costs of healthcare.

Prevention Versus Cure

Spending additional dollars for cure in the form of healthcare services does little to improve the health of a population, whereas spending money on prevention does a great deal to improve health. Getzen (2013) and others (Russo & Gourevitch, 2019; Shi & Singh, 2019) note that there is an absence of convincing evidence that the amount of money expended for healthcare improves the health of a population. The real determinants of health, as mentioned, are prevention efforts that provide education, housing, food, a decent minimal income, and safe social and physical environments, as well as encouraging positive lifestyle choices. The United States spends more than one-sixth of its wealth on healthcare or "cure" for individuals, likely diverting money away from the needed resources and services that would make a greater impact on health (NCHS, 2019; Shi & Singh, 2019).

US policy-makers must become committed to achieving improved health outcomes for the poor and vulnerable populations. With a limited health workforce and monetary resources, the United States cannot continue to spend vast amounts on healthcare services when the investment fails to improve health outcomes. In industrialized countries, life expectancy at birth is not related to the level of healthcare expenditures; in developing countries, longevity is closely related to the level of economic development and the education of the population (Russo & Gourevitch, 2019; Shi & Singh, 2019).

The current healthcare system is currently in a flux following implementation of the Affordable Care Act (ACA) and subsequent efforts to "repeal and replace" it. Some of these endeavors have actually been detrimental to the health of the population, as the focus on obtaining health insurance for more people has deferred a large investment of the country's wealth from education and other developmental efforts that would positively affect the health of the population as a whole. Managed care organizations (MCOs) focus on prevention and have determined that the rate of healthcare cost increases has slowed among employees of large firms (Kongstvedt, 2020). Prevention programs may help reduce costs for those enrolled in MCOs, but it remains unclear who will provide services for those who are required to purchase insurance, those who are currently uninsured and may remain so, the poor, and other vulnerable populations. In addition, still to be determined is who will provide adequate schooling, housing, meals, wages, and a safe environment for the disadvantaged. Increasing healthcare spending may negatively affect efforts to address economic disparities by reducing investments in sufficient housing, employment, education, nutrition, and safe environments.

Healthy People 2030

In 1979, the US Department of Health and Human Services (USDHHS) published a national prevention initiative titled *Healthy People: The Surgeon General's Report on Health Promotion and Disease Prevention*. The 1979 version established goals that would reduce mortality among infants, children, adolescents and young adults, and adults and increase independence among older adults. In 1990, the mortality of infants, children, and adults declined sufficiently to meet the goal. Adolescent mortality did not reach the 1990 target, and data systems were unable to adequately track the target for older adults (USDHHS, 2000).

Published in 1989, *Healthy People 2000* built on the first surgeon general's report. *Healthy People 2000* contained the following broad goals (USDHHS, 1989):

1. Increase the span of healthy life for Americans.
2. Reduce health disparities among Americans.
3. Achieve access to preventive services for all Americans.

The purpose of *Healthy People 2000* was to provide direction for individuals wanting to change personal behaviors and to improve health in communities through health promotion policies. The report assimilated the broad approaches of health promotion, health protection, and preventive services and contained more than 300 objectives organized into 22 priority areas. Although many of the objectives fell short, the initiative was extremely successful in raising providers' awareness of health behaviors and health promotional activities. States, local health departments, and private sector health workers used the objectives to determine the relative health of their communities and to set goals for the future.

Healthy People 2010 emerged in January 2000. It expanded on the objectives from *Healthy People 2000* through a broadened prevention science base, an improved surveillance and data system, and a heightened awareness of and demand for preventive health services. This reflects changes in demographics, science, technology, and disease. *Healthy People 2010* listed two broad goals:

Goal 1: Increase quality and years of healthy life.
Goal 2: Eliminate health disparities.

The first goal moved beyond the idea of increasing life expectancy to incorporate the concept of **health-related quality-of-life (HRQOL)**. This concept of health includes aspects of physical and mental health and their determinants and measures functional status, participation, and well-being. HRQOL expands the definition of health—beyond simply opposing the negative concepts of disease and death—by integrating mental and physical health concepts (USDHHS, 2000).

The final review and analysis of the *Healthy People 2010* objectives showed decidedly mixed progress for the nation. Some 23% of the objectives were met or exceeded, and another 48% "moved toward target." Conversely, 24% of the objectives "moved away from target" (i.e., the indicators were worse than in the previous decade), and another 5% showed no change. Particularly concerning were the poor responses in two of the focus areas:

arthritis, osteoporosis and chronic back conditions (focus area 2) and nutrition and overweight (focus area 19) "moved toward" or "achieved" less than 25% of their targets (USDHHS, 2012).

The fourth version of the nation's health objectives, *Healthy People 2020,* was published in 2010. *Healthy People 2020* was divided into 42 topic areas and contained numerous new objectives and updates for hundreds of objectives from the previous editions (USDHHS, 2017). Per the 2020 midcourse review (CDC/NCHS, 2017), more than 20% of the objectives set in 2010 had met or exceeded their 2020 targets. Furthermore, almost 20% were "improving," 27.3% showed "little or no detectable change," 11% were "worse," and 18% had baseline data only. Among the target areas meeting or exceeding the most goals were genomics, heart disease and stroke, medical product safety, occupational health and safety, and oral health. Among the target area in which progress for objectives was "worse" were early and middle childhood, mental health and mental disorders, older adults, and sleep health.

The latest iteration of the national health objectives—*Healthy People 2030*—was launched in August of 2020. *Healthy People 2030* consists five "overarching goals." These are as follows:

- Attain healthy, thriving lives, and well-being free of preventable disease, disability, injury, and premature death.
- Eliminate health disparities, achieve health equity, and attain health literacy to improve the health and well-being of all.
- Create social, physical, and economic environments that promote attaining the full potential for health and well-being for all.
- Promote healthy development, healthy behaviors, and well-being across all life stages.
- Engage leadership, key constituents, and the public across multiple sectors to take action and design policies that improve the health and well-being of all.

To help achieve these goals, there are 355 "data-driven" objectives, which are intended "to improve health and well-being over the next decade" (USDHHS, 2020). Furthermore, the initiative provides a wealth of resources and information designed to help health professionals address health priorities and monitor progress. All healthcare practitioners, particularly those working in the community, should review the *Healthy People 2030* objectives and focus on the relevant areas in their practice. Practitioners should incorporate these objectives into programs, events, and publications whenever possible and should use them as a framework to promote healthy cities and communities. Selected relevant objectives are presented throughout this book to acquaint future community health nurses with the scope of the *Healthy People 2030* initiative and to enhance awareness of current health indicators and national goals (see www.healthypeople.gov for more information).

? ACTIVE LEARNING EXERCISE

Become familiar with *Healthy People 2030* (www.healthypeople.gov). Review objectives from several of the topics covered. How does your community compare with the groups, aggregates, and populations described? What objectives should be targeted for your community?

DEFINITION AND FOCUS OF PUBLIC HEALTH NURSING, COMMUNITY HEALTH NURSING, AND COMMUNITY-BASED NURSING

The terms *community health nursing* and *public health nursing* are often used synonymously or interchangeably. Like the practice of community/public health nursing, the terms are evolving. In past debates and discussions, definitions of "community health nursing" and "public health nursing" have indicated similar yet distinctive ideologies, visions, or philosophies of nursing. These concepts and a third related term—*community-based nursing*—are discussed in this section.

Public and Community Health Nursing

Public health nursing has frequently been described as the synthesis of public health and nursing practice. Freeman (1963) provided a classic definition of public health nursing:

> *Public health nursing may be defined as a field of professional practice in nursing and in public health in which technical nursing, interpersonal, analytical, and organizational skills are applied to problems of health as they affect the community. These skills are applied in concert with those of other persons engaged in health care, through comprehensive nursing care of families and other groups and through measures for evaluation or control of threats to health, for health education of the public, and for mobilization of the public for health action (p. 34).*

Through the 1980s and 1990s, most nurses were taught that there was a distinction between "community health nursing" and "public health nursing." Indeed, "public health nursing" was seen as a subspecialty nursing practice generally delivered within "official" or governmental agencies. In contrast, "community health nursing" was considered to be a broader and more general specialty area that encompassed many additional subspecialties (e.g., school nursing, occupational health nursing, forensic nursing, home health). In 1980, the ANA defined **community health nursing** as "the synthesis of nursing practice and public health practice applied to promoting and preserving the health of populations" (ANA, 1980, p. 2). This viewpoint noted that a community health nurse directs care to individuals, families, or groups; this care, in turn, contributes to the health of the total population.

The ANA has revised the standards of practice for this specialty area (ANA, 2013). In the updated standards, the designation was again "public health nursing," and the ANA used the definition presented by the American Public Health Association (APHA) Committee on Public Health Nursing (1996). Thus, public health nursing is defined as "the practice of promoting and protecting the health of populations using knowledge from nursing, social, and public health sciences" (APHA, 1996, p. 5). The ANA (2013) elaborated by explaining that public health nursing practice "is population-focused, with the goals of promoting health and preventing disease and disability for all people through the creation of conditions in which people can be healthy" (p. 5).

Some nursing writers will continue to use *community health nursing* as a global or umbrella term and *public health nursing* as a component or subset. Others, as stated, use the terms interchangeably. This book uses the terms interchangeably.

ACTIVE LEARNING EXERCISE

Ask several neighbors or consumers of healthcare about their views of the role of public health and community health nursing. Share your results with your classmates.

RESEARCH HIGHLIGHTS

Public Health Nursing Research Agenda

A national conference was held to set a research agenda that would advance the science of public health nursing (PHN). The conference employed a multistage, multimethod, and participatory developmental approach, involving many influential PHN leaders. Following numerous meetings and discussions, an agenda was proposed. The agenda was structured around four "High Priority Themes": (1) public health nursing interventions models, (2) quality of population-focused practice, (3) metrics of/for public health nursing, and (4) comparative effectiveness and public health nursing outcomes. The aim of the agenda is to help PHN scholars contribute to an understanding of how to improve health and reduce population health disparities by advancing the evidence base regarding the outcomes of practice and by influencing related health policy. The group encouraged the agenda's use to guide and inform programs of research, to influence funding priorities, and to be incorporated into doctoral PHN education through course and curriculum development. Ultimately, it is anticipated that PHN research will proactively contribute to the effectiveness of the public health system and create healthier communities.

Data from Issel LM, Bekemeier B, Kneipp S: A public health nursing research agenda, *Public Health Nurs* 29:330–342, 2012.

Community-Based Nursing

The term *community-based nursing* has been identified and defined in recent years to differentiate it from what has traditionally been seen as community and public health nursing practice. Community-based nursing practice refers to "application of the nursing process in caring for individuals, families and groups where they live, work or go to school or as they move through the healthcare system" (McEwen & Pullis, 2009, p. 6). Community-based nursing is setting specific, and the emphasis is on acute and chronic care and includes such practice areas as home health nursing and nursing in outpatient or ambulatory settings.

Zotti, Brown, and Stotts (1996) compared community-based nursing and community health nursing and explained that the goals of the two are different. Community health nursing emphasizes preservation and protection of health, and community-based nursing emphasizes managing acute or chronic conditions. In community health nursing, the primary client is the community; in community-based nursing, the primary clients are the individual and the family. Finally, services in community-based nursing are largely direct, but in community health nursing, services are both direct and indirect (Williams, 2020).

Community and Public Health Nursing Practice

Community and public health nurses practice disease prevention and health promotion. It is important to note that public health nursing practice is collaborative and is based in research and theory. It applies the nursing process to the care of individuals, families, aggregates, and the community. Box 1.3 provides an overview of the Standards for Public Health Nursing (ANA, 2013).

As discussed, the core functions of public health are assessment, policy development, and assurance. In 2003, the Quad Council of Public Health Nursing Organizations (Quad Council) closely examined the core functions and used them to develop a set of public health nursing competencies. These competencies were updated in 2018 and are summarized in Table 1.2 (Quad Council Coalition Competency Review Task Force, 2018). Current and future community health nurses should study these competencies to understand the practice parameters and skills required for public health nursing practice.

 ACTIVE LEARNING EXERCISE

Interview several community/public health nurses regarding their opinions on the focus of community/public health nursing. Do you agree?

BOX 1.3   The Scope and Standards of Practice for Public Health Nursing

The Scope and Standards of Practice for Public Health Nursing is the result of the collaborative effort between the American Nurses Association and the Quad Council of Public Health Nursing Organizations. The standards were originally developed in 1999 and were updated in 2013. The Scope and Standards of Practice, which are divided into Standards of Practice and Standards of Professional Performance, describe specific competencies relevant to the public health nurse and the public health nurse in advanced practice.

The Standards of Practice include six standards that are based on the critical thinking model of the nursing process, with competencies addressing each nursing process step. The implementation step is further broken down into specific public health areas, including coordination of services, health education and health promotion, consultation, and regulatory activities. The Standards of Professional Performance include the leadership competencies necessary in the professional practice of all registered nurses, but with additional standards specific to the public health nurse and advanced public health nurse roles. These standards include evidence-based practice and research, collaboration, resource utilization, and advocacy, with competencies specific to public health, such as building coalitions and achieving consensus in public health issues, assessing available health resources within a population, and advocating for equitable access to care and services.

Data from American Nurses Association: *Public health nursing: scope and standards of practice*, ed 2, Silver Spring, MD, 2013, Author. The standards can be purchased at: http://www.nursesbooks.org/Homepage/Hot-off-the-Press/Public-Health-Nursing-2nd.aspx.

POPULATION-FOCUSED PRACTICE AND COMMUNITY/PUBLIC HEALTH NURSING INTERVENTIONS

Community/public health nurses must use a population-focused approach to move beyond providing direct care to individuals and families. **Population-focused nursing** concentrates on specific groups of people and focuses on health promotion and disease prevention, regardless of geographic location (Baldwin et al., 1998). The goal of population-focused nursing is "to provide evidence-based care to targeted groups of people with similar needs in order to improve outcomes" (Curley, 2020, p. 6). In short, population-focused practice (Minnesota Department of Health, 2003):

- Focuses on the entire population
- Is based on assessment of the population's health status
- Considers the broad determinants of health
- Emphasizes all levels of prevention
- Intervenes with communities, systems, individuals, and families

Whereas community and public health nurses may be responsible for a specific subpopulation in the community (e.g., a school nurse may be responsible for the school's pregnant teenagers), population-focused practice is concerned with many distinct and overlapping community subpopulations. The goal of population-focused nursing is to promote healthy communities.

Population-focused public health nurses would not have exclusive interest in one or two subpopulations, but instead would focus on the many subpopulations that make up the entire community. A population focus involves concern for those who do, and for those who do not, receive health services. A population focus also involves a scientific approach to community health nursing. Thus, a thorough, systematic assessment of the community or population is necessary and basic to planning, intervention, and evaluation for the individual, family, aggregate, and population levels.

Public health nursing practice requires the following types of data for scientific approach and population focus: (1) the epidemiology, or body of knowledge, of a particular problem and its solution and (2) information about the community. Each type of knowledge and its source appear in Table 1.3. To determine the overall patterns of health in a population, data collection for assessment and management decisions within a community should be ongoing, not episodic.

Public Health Interventions

Public health nurses focus on the care of individuals, groups, aggregates, and populations in many settings, including homes, clinics, worksites, and schools. In addition to interviewing clients and assessing individual and family health, public health nurses must be able to assess a population's health needs and resources and identify its values. Public health nurses must also work with the community to identify and implement programs that meet health needs and to evaluate the effectiveness of programs after implementation. For example, school nurses

TABLE 1.2 Selected Tier 1 Public Health Nursing (PHN) Competencies (Generalist Public Health Nurses)

Domain	Community and Public Health Nursing Competencies
1. Assessment and analytic skills	Assess the health status and health literacy of individuals and families, including determinants of health, using multiple sources of data. Use an ecological perspective and epidemiological data to identify health risks for a population. Select variables that measure health and public health conditions. Interpret valid and reliable data that impacts the health of individuals, families and communities to make comparisons that are understandable to all who were involved in the assessment process. Applies ethical, legal, and policy guidelines and principles in the collection, maintenance, use, and dissemination of data and information. Use evidence-based strategies of promising practices from across disciplines to promote health in communities and populations.
2. Policy development/program planning skills	Identify local, state, national, and international policy issues relevant to the health of individuals, families, and groups. Describe the implications and potential impacts of public health programs and policies on individuals, families, and groups within a population. Identify outcomes of health policy relevant to public health nursing practice for individuals, families, and groups. Provide information that will inform policy decisions. Function as a team member in developing organizational plans while assuring compliance with established policies and program implementation guidelines. Participate in quality improvement teams by using quality indicators and core measures to identify and address opportunities for improvement in services for individuals, families, and groups.
3. Communication skills	Determine the health, literacy, and the health literacy of the population served to guide health promotion and disease prevention activities. Apply critical thinking and cultural awareness to all communication modes (i.e., verbal, nonverbal, written, and electronic) with individuals, the community, and stakeholders. Use input from individuals, families, and groups when planning and delivering healthcare programs and services. Use a variety of methods to disseminate public health information to individuals, families, and groups within a population. Create a presentation of targeted health information.
4. Cultural competency skills	Use determinants of health effectively when working with divers individuals, families, and groups. Use data, evidence, and information technology to understand the impact of determinants of health on individuals, families, and groups. Deliver culturally responsive public health nursing services for individuals, families, and groups practice. Explain the benefits of a diverse public health workforce that supports a just and civil culture.
5. Community dimensions of practice skills	Use assessments, develop plans, and implement and evaluate interventions for public health services for individuals, families, and groups. Use formal and informal relational networks among community organizations and systems conducive to improving the health of individuals, families, and groups within communities. Select stakeholders needed to address public health issues impacting the health of individuals, families, and groups within the community. Use community assets and resources including the government, private, and nonprofit sectors to promote health and to deliver services to individuals, families, and groups. Identify evidence of the effectiveness of community engagement strategies on individuals, families, and groups.
6. Public health sciences skills	Use the determinants of health and evidence-based practices from public health and nursing science when planning health promotion and disease prevention interventions for individuals, families, and groups. Determine the relationship between access to clean, sustainable water, sanitation, food, air, and energy quality on individual, family, and population health. Use evidence-based practice in population-level programs to contribute to meeting core public health functions and the 10 essential public health services. Participate in research activities impacting the health of populations. Use a wide variety of sources and methods to access public health information (i.e., GIS, mapping, community health assessment, local/state/ national sources). Demonstrate compliance with the requirements of patient confidentially and human subject protection.

Continued

TABLE 1.2   Selected Tier 1 Public Health Nursing (PHN) Competencies (Generalist Public Health Nurses)—cont'd

Domain	Community and Public Health Nursing Competencies
7. Financial planning, evaluation, and management skills	Explain the interrelationships among local, state, tribal, and federal public health and healthcare systems.
	Explain the public health nurse's role in emergency preparedness and disaster response during public health events (i.e., infectious disease outbreak, natural or human-made disasters).
	Implement operational procedures for public health programs and services.
	Interpret the impact of budget constraints on the delivery of public health nursing services to individuals, families, and groups.
	Explain implications of organizational budget priorities on individuals, groups. and communities.
	Deliver public health nursing services to individuals, families, and groups based on reported evaluation results. Use public health informatics skills pertaining to public health nursing services of individuals, families, and groups.
8. Leadership and systems thinking skills	Identify internal and external factors affecting public health nursing practice and opportunities for interprofessional collaboration.
	Use individual, team, and organizational learning opportunities for personal and professional development as a public health nurse.
	Identify organizational quality improvement initiatives that provide opportunities for improvement in public health nursing practice.
	Interpret organization dynamics of collaborating agencies.
	Select advocacy strategies to address the needs of diverse and underserved populations.
	Identify organizational policies and procedures that meet practice and public health accreditation requirements.

Modified from Quad Council Coalition Competency Review Task Force: *Community/public health nursing competencies, 2018.* Available at: https://www.cphno.org/wp-content/uploads/2020/08/QCC-C-PHN-COMPETENCIES-Approved_2018.05.04_Final-002.pdf.

TABLE 1.3   Information Useful for Population Focus

Type of Information	Examples	Sources
Demographic data	Age, gender, race/ethnicity, socioeconomic status, education level	Vital statistic data (national, state, county, local); census
Groups at high risk	Health status and health indicators of various subpopulations in the community (e.g., children, elders, those with disabilities)	Health statistics (morbidity, mortality, natality); disease statistics (incidence and prevalence)
Services/providers available	Official (public) health departments; healthcare providers for low-income individuals and families; community service agencies and organizations (e.g., Red Cross, Meals on wheels)	City directories; phone books; local or regional social workers; low-income providers' lists; local community health nurses (e.g., school nurses)

were once responsible only for running first aid stations and monitoring immunization compliance. Now they are actively involved in assessing the needs of their population and defining programs to meet those needs through activities such as health screening and group health education and promotion. The activities of school nurses may be as varied as designing health curricula with a school and community advisory group, leading support groups for elementary school children with chronic illness, advocating for emergency equipment (e.g., automatic external defibrillators) in gyms and athletic fields, and monitoring the health status of teenage mothers.

Similarly, occupational health nurses are no longer required to simply maintain an office or dispensary. They are involved in many different types of activities. These activities might include maintaining records of workers exposed to physical or chemical risks, monitoring compliance with Occupational Safety and Health Administration standards, teaching classes on health issues, acting as case managers for workers with chronic health

conditions, and leading support group discussions for workers with health-related problems.

Private associations, such as the American Diabetes Association or the Red Cross, employ public health nurses for their organizational ability and health-related skills. Other public health nurses work with multidisciplinary groups of professionals, serve on boards of voluntary health associations such as the American Heart Association, work as case managers for insurance companies, and are members of health planning agencies and councils.

GENETICS IN PUBLIC HEALTH

Community-Based Research for the Prevention of Cardiovascular Disease

Cardiovascular disease (CVD) is the leading cause of death among Americans, and prevention of CVD should be a priority for all nurses. It has been established that CVD results from a complex interaction among modifiable factors including lifestyle choices and environmental influences, and nonmodifiable factors such as age and race/ethnicity or genetics. A group of nurse researchers led by Fletcher (2011) presented a "call to action for nursing" to promote community-based research that focuses on the genetic factors that contribute to CVD. The team described the need to build capacity for participation in genetics research within communities through community engagement, particularly among vulnerable ethnic minority groups. The importance of identifying the genetic–environmental interactions that may lead to clinical manifestation of CVD was stressed, and a number of community-based interventions to prevent CVD were described.

Fletcher BJ, Himmelfarb CD, Lira MT, Meininger JC, Pradhan SR, Sikkema J: Global cardiovascular disease prevention: a call to action for nursing, *J Cardiovasc Nurs* 26(45): 535–545, 2011.

The Public Health Intervention Wheel

The Public Health Intervention Model was initially proposed in the late 1990s by nurses from the Minnesota Department of Health to describe the breadth and scope of public health nursing practice (Keller et al., 1998). This model was later revised and termed the *Intervention Wheel* (Fig. 1.3) (Keller et al., 2004a; Keller et al., 2004b), and it has become increasingly recognized as a framework for community and public health nursing practice.

The Intervention Wheel contains three important elements: (1) it is population based; (2) it contains three levels of practice (community, systems, and individual/family); and (3) it identifies and defines 17 public health interventions. The levels of practice and interventions are directed at improving population health (Keller et al., 2004a). Within the Intervention Wheel, the 17 health interventions are grouped into five "wedges." These interventions are actions taken on behalf of communities, systems, individuals, and families to improve or protect health status. Table 1.4 provides definitions.

The Intervention Wheel is further dissected into levels of practice, in which the interventions may be directed at an entire population within a community, a system that would affect the health of a population, and/or the individuals and families within the population. Thus, each intervention can and should be applied at each level. For example, a systems-level intervention within "disease investigation" might be the community health nurse working with the state health department and federal

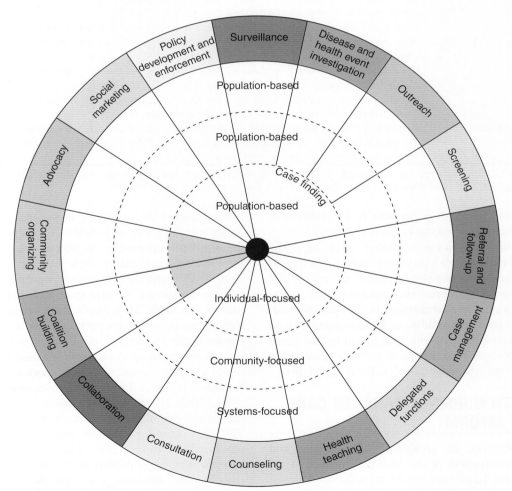

Fig. 1.3 Public health intervention wheel. (Modified from Minnesota Department of Health: *Public health interventions* 2019. Available from: https://www.health.state.mn.us/communities/practice/research/phncouncil/docs/PHInterventionsHandout.pdf.)

TABLE 1.4   Public Health Interventions and Definitions

Public Health Intervention	Definition
Surveillance	Describes and monitors health events through ongoing and systematic collection, analysis, and interpretation of health data for the purpose of planning, implementing, and evaluating public health interventions
Disease and other health event investigation	Systematically gathers and analyzes data regarding threats to the health of populations, ascertains the source of the threat, identifies cases and others at risk, and determines control measures
Outreach	Locates populations of interest or populations at risk and provides information about the nature of the concern, what can be done about it, and how services can be obtained
Screening	Identifies individuals with unrecognized health risk factors or asymptomatic disease conditions
Case finding	Locates individuals and families with identified risk factors and connects them with resources
Referral and follow-up	Assists individuals, families, groups, organizations, and/or communities to identify and access necessary resources to prevent or resolve problems or concerns
Case management	Optimizes self-care capabilities of individuals and families and the capacity of systems and communities to coordinate and provide services
Delegated functions	Carries out direct care tasks under the authority of a healthcare practitioner as allowed by law
Health teaching	Communicates facts, ideas, and skills that change knowledge, attitudes, values, beliefs, behaviors, and practices of individuals, families, systems, and/or communities
Counseling	Establishes an interpersonal relationship with a community, a system, and a family or individual, with the intention of increasing or enhancing their capacity for self-care and coping
Consultation	Seeks information and generates optional solutions to perceived problems or issues through interactive problem solving with a community system and family or individual
Collaboration	Commits two or more persons or organizations to achieve a common goal by enhancing the capacity of one or more of the members to promote and protect health
Coalition building	Promotes and develops alliances among organizations or constituencies for a common purpose
Community organizing	Helps community groups to identify common problems or goals, mobilize resources, and develop and implement strategies for realizing the goals they collectively have set
Advocacy	Pleads someone's cause or acts on someone's behalf, with a focus on developing the community, system, and individual or family's capacity to plead their own cause or act on their own behalf
Social marketing	Utilizes commercial marketing principles and technologies for programs designed to influence the knowledge, attitudes, values, beliefs, behaviors, and practices of the population of interest
Policy development and enforcement	Places health issues on decision-makers' agendas, acquires a plan of resolution, and determines needed resources, resulting in laws, rules, regulations, ordinances, and policies. Policy enforcement compels others to comply with laws, rules, regulations, ordinances, and policies

Modified from Keller LO, Strohschein S, Lia-Hoagberg B, Schaffer MA: *Population-based public health interventions: practice-based and evidence-supported. Part I*, St. Paul, MN, 2004, Minnesota Department of Health, Center for Public Health Nursing.

vaccine program to coordinate a response to an outbreak of measles in a migrant population. An example of a population- or community-level intervention for "screening" would be public health nurses working with area high schools to give each student a profile of his or her health to promote nutritional and physical activity lifestyle changes to improve the student's health.

Finally, an individual-level implementation of the intervention "referral and follow-up" would occur when a nurse receives a referral to care for an individual with a diagnosed mental illness who would require regular monitoring of his or her medication compliance to prevent rehospitalization (Keller et al., 2004b).

PUBLIC HEALTH NURSING, MANAGED CARE, AND HEALTH REFORM

Shifts in reimbursement, the growth of managed care, and implementation and revision of the ACA have revitalized the notion of population-based care. Health insurance companies, governmental financing entities (e.g., Medicare, Medicaid), and MCOs use financial incentives and organizational structures in an attempt to increase efficiency and decrease healthcare costs.

The foundation for managed care is management of healthcare for an enrolled group of individuals. This group of enrollees is the population covered by the plan who receive health services from managed care plan providers (Kongstvedt, 2020).

An understanding of enrolled populations and healthcare patterns is essential for managing healthcare services and resources effectively. Most MCOs have become sophisticated in identifying key subgroups within the population of enrollees at risk for health problems. Typically, managed care systems target subgroups according to characteristics associated with risk or use of expensive services, such as selected clinical conditions, functional status, and past service use patterns.

In March 2010, President Obama signed the Patient Protection and Affordable Care Act (ACA) (PL 111-148) into law. The ACA served to expand insurance coverage for those uninsured and to help control healthcare costs. Expansion of coverage was accomplished by requiring individuals to purchase health insurance for themselves and their families, implementation of "exchanges" to increase options for individuals to purchase health insurance, and requiring more employers to offer health insurance to employees. Public programs (e.g., Medicaid and State Children's Health Insurance Program) were expanded to cover healthcare for those who could not afford to buy their own insurance. With the change of administration in 2021, significant revisions of the ACA are likely to be implemented with new federal- and state-sponsored initiatives. Public health nurses must stay informed of these changes and work with groups and organizations to support legislation that will promote population health, reduce disparities, and better manage the costs of care.

The purpose of public health is to improve the health of the public by promoting healthy lifestyles, preventing disease and injury, and protecting the health of communities. In the past, shrinking public health resources have supported personal health services over community health promotion. In public health practice, the community is the population of interest. With the proposed changes to healthcare financing, the personal healthcare system will be under increasing pressure to provide the services that health departments previously provided. Traditionally served by public health, the most vulnerable populations will pose tremendous challenges for private healthcare providers. Public health agencies and providers will be responsible for partnering with private providers to care for these populations.

Providing population-based care requires a dramatic shift in thinking from individual-based care. Some of the practical demands of population-based care are the following:

1. It must be recognized that populations are not homogeneous; therefore, it is necessary to address the needs of special subpopulations within populations.
2. High-risk and vulnerable subpopulations must be identified early in the care delivery cycle.
3. Nonusers of services often become high-cost users; therefore, it is essential to develop outreach strategies.
4. Quality and cost of all healthcare services are linked together across the healthcare continuum (Kaiser Family Foundation, 2013a,b).

Nurses in community and public health have an opportunity to share their expertise regarding population-based approaches to healthcare for groups of individuals across healthcare settings. Today, healthcare practitioners require additional skills in assessment, policy development, and assurance to provide community public health practice and population-based service. Healthcare professionals should focus attention on promoting healthy lifestyles, providing preventive and primary care, expanding and ensuring access to cost-effective and technologically appropriate care, participating in coordinated and interdisciplinary care, and involving patients and families in the decision-making process. Public health nurses must work in partnership with colleagues in managed care settings to improve community health. Partnerships may address information management, cultural values, healthcare system improvement, and the physical environment roles in health and may require complex negotiations to share data. The partners may need to develop new community assessment strategies to augment epidemiological methods that often mask the context or meaning of the human experience of vulnerable populations.

SUMMARY

The healthcare system has been evolving from focusing on individuals in acute care settings to being more community based and population health directed. Nursing practice has changed in response, and today, a growing proportion of nurses is working outside of hospitals. Public and community health nursing practice includes population-focused interventions that seek to improve the health and well-being of groups, aggregates, and communities.

This chapter has presented information on key concepts, including "health" and "community," and described the vital importance of addressing societal needs to improve population health. With widely recognized changes in population demographics, it is necessary that nurses be attuned to the determinants and indicators of health, health-promoting activities, and changes in the healthcare system. This includes efforts to promote access to more individuals and to understand the need to contain costs. With this knowledge and skills, public and community health nurses can influence health practices and policies that will positively affect the future health of individuals, families, groups, and communities.

EVOLVE WEBSITE

http://evolve.elsevier.com/Nies/community.
- NCLEX Review Questions
- Case Studies

BIBLIOGRAPHY

American Heritage College Dictionary, ed 3, New York, 1997, Houghton Mifflin.

American Nurses Association: *A conceptual model of community health nursing*, Kansas City, MO, 1980, ANA.

American Nurses Association: *Public health nursing: scope and standards of practice*, Silver Spring, MD, 2013, American Nurses Publishing.

American Nurses Association: *Code of ethics for nurses, with interpretive statements*, Silver Spring, MD, 2015, American Nurses Publishing.

American Nurses Association: *ANA's nurses by the numbers*, 2016. Available from: http://assets.1440n.net/16-238/10/.

American Public Health Association: *Ad Hoc Committee on Public Health Nursing: the definition and role of public health nursing practice in the delivery of health care*, Washington, DC, 1996, American Public Health Association.

Baldwin JH, Conger CO, Abegglen JC, et al: Population-focused and community-based nursing: moving toward clarification of concepts, *Public Health Nurs* 15:12−18, 1998.

Centers for Disease Control and Prevention/National Center for Health Statistics: *Healthy People 2020 midcourse review*, 2017.

Available from: https://www.cdc.gov/nchs/healthy_people/hp2020/hp2020_midcourse_review.htm.

Centers for Disease Control and Prevention (CDC): *10 essential public health services*, 2020. Available from: https://www.cdc.gov/publichealthgateway/publichealthservices/essentialhealthservices.html.

Curley ALC: Introduction to population-pased nursing. In Curley ALC, editor: *Population-based nursing: concepts and competencies for advanced practice*, ed 3, New York, 2020, Springer Publishing Co.

Dunn HL: *High level wellness*, Arlington, VA, 1961, RW Beatty.

Elbel B, Cassidy EF, Trujillo MD, Orleans CT: Health and behavior. In Knickman JR, Elbel B, editors: *Health care delivery in the United States*, ed 12, New York, 2019, Springer Publishing.

Freeman RB: *Public health nursing practice*, ed 3, Philadelphia, 1963, WB Saunders.

Getzen T: *Health economics and financing*, ed 5, Hoboken, NJ, 2013, John Wiley & Sons.

Gibson ME, Thatcher EJ: Community as client: assessment and analysis. In Stanhope M, Lancaster J, editors: *Public health nursing: population-centered health care in the community*, ed 10, St. Louis, 2020, Elsevier.

Hanlon JJ: *Principles of public health administration*, ed 3, St. Louis, 1960, Mosby.

Institute of Medicine: *The future of public health*, Washington, DC, 1988, National Academy Press.

Institute of Medicine: *The future of nursing*, Washington, DC, 2011, National Academy Press.

Kaiser Family Foundation: *Health reform source*, 2013a. Available from: http://kff.org.

Kaiser Family Foundation: *Summary of the new health reform law*, Pub No. 8061, 2013b. Available from: http://kff.org/health-reform/factsheet/summary-of-the-affordable-care-act/.

Keller LO, Strohschein S, Lia-Hoagberg B, et al: Population-based public health interventions: a model for practice, *Public Health Nurs* 15:207–215, 1998.

Keller LO, Strohschein S, Lia-Hoagberg B, et al: Population-based public health interventions: practice-based and evidence-supported. Part I, *Public Health Nurs* 21:453–468, 2004a.

Keller LO, Strohschein S, Schaffer MA, et al: Population-based public health interventions: innovations in practice, teaching and management. Part II, *Public Health Nurs* 21:469–487, 2004b.

Kongstvedt PR: *Health insurance and managed care: what they are and how they work*, ed 5, Burlington, MA, 2020, Jones and Bartlett.

Leavell HR, Clark EG: *Preventive medicine for the doctor in his community*, New York, 1958, McGraw-Hill.

Lundy KS, Janes S: *Community health nursing: caring for the public's health*, ed 3, Boston, 2016, Jones & Bartlett.

Maurer FA, Smith CM: *Community/public health nursing practice: health for families and populations*, ed 5, St. Louis, 2013, Elsevier.

McEwen M, Pullis B: *Community-based nursing: an introduction*, ed 3, St. Louis, 2009, WB Saunders.

McGinnis MJ, Foege W: Actual causes of death in the United States, *JAMA* 270:2207–2212, 1993.

McKeown T: Determinants of Health. In Lee PR, Estes CL, editors: *The nation's health*, ed 7, Boston, 2003, Jones & Bartlett.

McKinlay JB: A case for refocusing upstream: the political economy of illness. In Jaco EG, editor: *Patients, physicians, and illness*, ed 3, New York, 1979, The Free Press.

Minnesota Department of Health: *Definitions of population based practice*, 2003. Available from: http://www.health.state.mn.us/divs/opi/cd/phn/docs/0303phn_popbasedpractice.pdf.

Mokdad AH, Marks JS, Stroup DF, et al: Actual causes of death in the United States, *JAMA* 291:1238–1245, 2004.

Murdaugh CL, Parsons MA, Pender NJ: *Health promotion in nursing practice*, ed 8, New York, NY, 2019, Pearson Education.

Murray RB, Zentner JP, Yakimo R: *Health promotion strategies through the life span*, ed 8, Upper Saddle River, NJ, 2009, Prentice Hall.

National Center for Health Statistics: *Health, United States, 2018*, 2019. Available from: https://www.cdc.gov/nchs/data/hus/hus18.pdf# Highlights.

National Council for State Boards of Nursing (NCSBN): The 2017 national nursing workforce survey, *Jnl of Nsg Reg* 9(3), 2018.

Quad Council Coalition Competency Review Task Force: *Community/Public health nursing [C/PHN] competencies*, 2018. Available from: https://www.cphno.org/wp-content/uploads/2020/08/QCC-C-PHN-COMPETENCIES-Approved_2018.05.04_Final-002.pdf.

Rector C: *Community and public health nursing: promoting and protecting the public's health*, ed 9, Philadelphia, PA, 2018, Wolters Kluwer.

Rosenfeld P, Russell D: A review of factors influencing utilization of home and community-based long-term care: trends and implications to the nursing workforce, *Policy Polit Nurs Pract* 13:72–80, 2012.

Ross R, Kleman CC: Health defined: health promotion, protection and prevention. In Edelman CL, Kudzma EC, editors: *Health Promotion throughout the Life Span*, ed 9, St. Louis, 2018, Elsevier.

Roy C: *The Roy adaption model*, ed 3, Upper Saddle River, NJ, 2009, Pearson.

Russo P, Gourevitch MN: Population health. In Kovner AR, Knickman JR, editors: *Health care delivery in the United States*, ed 12, New York, 2019, Springer Publishing.

Saylor C: The circle of health: a health definition model, *J Holist Nurs* 22:98–115, 2004.

Shi L, Singh DA: *Delivering health care in America: a systems approach*, ed 7, Boston, 2019, Jones & Bartlett.

Shuster GR: Community as client: assessment and analysis. In Stanhope M, Lancaster J, editors: *Public health nursing: population-centered health care in the community*, ed 8, St. Louis, 2012, Elsevier.

US Department of Health and Human Services, Health Resources and Services Administration: *The registered nurse population: initial findings 2008 national sample survey of registered nurses*, 2010. Available from: https://bhw.hrsa.gov/healthworkforce/rnsurvey/initialfindings2008.pdf.

US Department of Health and Human Services: *Healthy People 2000 objectives*, Washington, DC, 1989, Author.

US Department of Health and Human Services: *Healthy People 2010 objectives*, Washington, DC, 2000, Author.

US Department of Health and Human Services: *Healthy People 2010: final review*, Washington, DC, 2012, Author. Available from: http://www.cdc.gov/nchs/data/hpdata2010/hp2010_final_review.pdf.

US Department of Health and Human Services: *Healthy People 2020 objectives*, 2017. Available from: http://www.healthypeople.gov/2020/about/default.aspx.

US Department of Health and Human Services: *Healthy People 2030 objectives*, 2021. Available from: https://health.gov/healthypeople/objectives-and-data.

Wald LD: *The house on Henry street*, New York, 1971, Dover Publications.

Williams CA: Public health foundations and population health. In Stanhope M, Lancaster J, editors: *Public health nursing: population-centered health care in the community*, ed 10, St. Louis, 2020, Elsevier.

Winslow CEA: The untilled field of public health, *Mod Med* 2:183, March 1920.

World Health Organization: The first 10 years of the World Health Organization, *Chron WHO* 1:1–2, 1958.

World Health Organization: A discussion document on the concept and principles of health promotion, *Health Promot* 1:73–78, 1986.

Zotti ME, Brown P, Stotts RC: Community-based nursing versus community health nursing: what does it all mean? *Nurs Outlook* 44:211–217, 1996.

Historical Factors: Public Health Nursing in Context

Melanie McEwen

OBJECTIVES

Upon completion of this chapter, the reader will be able to do the following:

1. Describe the impact of aggregate living on population health.
2. Identify approaches to population health promotion from prerecorded historic to present times.
3. Understand historical events that have influenced population health.
4. Compare the application of public health principles to the nation's major health problems at the turn of the 20th century (i.e., acute disease) with that at the beginning of the 21st century (i.e., chronic disease).
5. Describe two leaders in nursing who had a profound impact on addressing population health.
6. Discuss major contemporary issues facing community/public health nursing, and trace the historical roots to the present.

OUTLINE

KEY TERMS

district nursing
Edward Jenner
Edwin Chadwick
Elizabethan Poor Law
endemic
epidemic
Flexner Report

Florence Nightingale
health visiting
House on Henry Street
John Snow
Joseph Lister
Lemuel Shattuck
Lillian Wald

Louis Pasteur
pandemic
Robert Koch
Sanitary Revolution
stages in disease history

An understanding of the historical factors that have influenced the evolution of population health may help explain current health challenges. This chapter examines the health of Western populations from early historic times to recent times and describes the evolution of modern health care. The role of public health nurses and concurrent challenges for improving the health of groups, aggregates, and communities are also discussed.

EVOLUTION OF HEALTH IN WESTERN POPULATIONS

Medical anthropologists use paleontological records and disease descriptions of primitive societies to speculate on the interrelationship of early humans, probable diseases, and their environment. Historians have also documented the existence of public health activity (i.e., an organized community effort to prevent disease, prolong life, and promote health) since before recorded historical times. This section describes how aggregate living patterns and early public health efforts have affected the health of Western populations.

Aggregate Impact on Health

Polgar (1964) defined the following **stages in disease history**: hunting and gathering stage, settled villages stage, preindustrial cities stage, industrial cities stage, and present stage (Fig. 2.1). In these stages, growing populations, increased population density, and imbalanced human ecology resulted in changes in

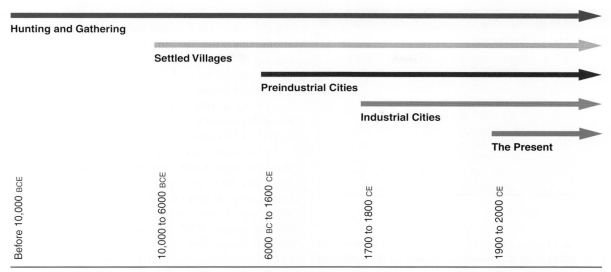

Fig. 2.1 Stages in the disease history of humankind. Stages overlap, and time periods are widely debated in the field of anthropology. Some form of each stage remains evident in the world today.

cultural adaptation. In each stage, humans created an ecological imbalance by altering their environment to accommodate group living. This imbalance subsequently had a significant effect on aggregate health.

Although these stages are associated with the evolution of civilization, it is important to note that the information is limited by cultural bias. The stages depict the evolution of civilization from the perspective of the Western world. They consist of overlapping historical time periods, which anthropologists widely debate. However, the stages of human disease can provide a frame of reference to aid in determining the relationship among humans, disease, and environment from early historical times to the present. Furthermore, although the stages chronicle the general evolution in the Western world, it is important to realize that each stage still exists in civilization today. For example, Australian aborigines continue to hunt and gather food, and "settled villages" can readily be found in developing countries.

Public health nurses should be aware that populations from each stage consist of a variety of people with distinct cultural traditions and a broad range of health care practices and beliefs. For example, a nurse currently practicing in an American community may need to plan care for immigrants or refugees from a settled village or a preindustrial city. Public and community health nurses must recognize that the environment, the population's health risks, and the host culture's strengths and challenges affect the health status of each particular group.

Hunting and Gathering Stage

During the Paleolithic period, or Old Stone Age, nomadic and seminomadic people engaged in hunting and gathering, with generations of small aggregate groups wandering in search of food. Armelagos and Dewey (1978) reviewed how the size, density, and relationship to the environment of such people

probably affected their health. These groups may have avoided many contagious diseases because the scattered groups were small, nomadic, and separated from other groups. Under these conditions, diseases would not spread among the groups. Evidently the disposal of human feces and waste was not a great problem; the nomadic people most likely abandoned the caves they used for shelter once waste accumulated.

Settled Village Stage

Small settlements were characteristic of the Mesolithic period, or Middle Stone Age, and the Neolithic period, or New Stone Age. Wandering people became more sedentary and formed small encampments and villages. The concentration of people in these small areas caused new health problems. For example, people began to domesticate animals and live close to their herds, a practice that probably transmitted diseases such as salmonella, anthrax, Q fever, and tuberculosis (TB) (Polgar, 1964). These stationary people also domesticated plants, a change that may have reduced the range of consumable nutrients and may have led to deficiency diseases. They had to secure water and remove wastes, often leading to the cross-contamination of the water supply and the spread of waterborne diseases such as dysentery, cholera, typhoid, and hepatitis A.

Preindustrial Cities Stage

In preindustrial times, large urban centers formed to support the expanding population. Populations inhabited smaller areas; therefore exposure to preexisting problems expanded. For example, the urban population had to resource increased amounts of food and water and remove increased amounts of waste products. Some cultures developed elaborate water systems. However, waste removal via the water supply led to

TABLE 2.1   Disease Definitions

Types of Disease	Definition
Endemic	Diseases that are always present in a population (e.g., colds and pneumonia)
Epidemic	Diseases that are not always present in a population but flare up on occasion (e.g., diphtheria and measles)
Pandemic	The existence of disease in a large proportion of the population: a global epidemic (e.g., human immunodeficiency virus, acquired immunodeficiency syndrome, and annual outbreaks of influenza type A)

diseases such as cholera. Further, with the development of towns, rodent infestation increased and facilitated the spread of plague. People had more frequent close contact with one another; therefore the transmission of diseases spread by direct contact increased, and diseases such as mumps, measles, influenza, and smallpox became endemic (Polgar, 1964). Of significance, a population must reach a certain size to maintain a disease in endemic proportions (Table 2.1); for example, approximately 1 million people are needed to sustain measles at an endemic level (Cockburn, 1967).

Industrial Cities Stage

Industrialization caused urban areas to become denser and even more heavily populated. Increased industrial wastes, air and water pollution, and harsh working conditions took a toll on health. During the 18th and 19th centuries, there was an increase in respiratory diseases such as TB, pneumonia, and bronchitis and in epidemics of infectious diseases such as diphtheria, smallpox, typhoid fever, typhus, measles, malaria, and yellow fever (Armelagos and Dewey, 1978). Furthermore, exploration and imperialism spread epidemics of many diseases to susceptible populations throughout the world because settlers, traders, and soldiers moved from one location to another, introducing communicable diseases into native population groups.

Present Stage

Although infectious diseases no longer account for a majority of deaths in the Western world, they continue to cause many deaths in the non-Western world. This trend persists despite the very significant impact of COVID 19 through 2020 and into 2021. For the most part, infectious diseases remain prevalent among low-income populations and some ethnic minority groups in the West. Western diseases such as cancer, heart disease, obesity, hypertension, and diabetes are less common among populations from nonindustrial communities. These diseases typically appear when cultures adopt Western customs and transition into urban environments. Epidemiological studies suggest that common risk factors that contribute to

chronic health conditions are changes in diet (e.g., increases in refined sugar and fats and lack of fiber), environmental alterations (e.g., use of motorized transportation and climate-controlled living and work sites), and occupational hazards. A rise in population and greater population density also increase mental and behavioral disorders. Importantly, some of the risk factors for chronic diseases (e.g., diabetes, obesity) and other social disparities were also implicated in poorer outcomes from COVID 19—obviously an infectious disease.

In summary, disease patterns and environmental demands changed when wandering, hunting, and gathering aggregates grew into large populations and became sedentary. Humans had to adapt to more densely populated, largely urban existence with marked consequences for health. As a result, over time, the leading causes of death changed from infectious disease to chronic illness. Due to the effect of globalization, however, as COVID 19 has demonstrated, infectious disease remain a threat.

Evolution of Early Public Health Efforts

Traditionally, historians believed that organized public health efforts were 18th- and 19th-century activities associated with the Sanitary Revolution. However, modern historians have shown that organized community health efforts to prevent disease, prolong life, and promote health have existed since early human history.

Public health efforts developed slowly over time. The following sections briefly trace the evolution of organized public health and highlight the periods of prerecorded historical times (i.e., before 5000 BCE), classical times (i.e., 3000 to 200 BCE), the Middle Ages (i.e., 500 to 1500 CE), the Renaissance (i.e., 15th, 16th, and 17th centuries), the 18th century, the 19th century, and into the present day. It is important to note that, like the disease history of humankind, public health efforts exist in various stages of development throughout the world, and this brief history suggests a Western viewpoint.

Prerecorded Historic Times

From the early remains of human habitation, anthropologists recognize that early nomadic humans became domesticated and tended to live in increasingly larger groups. Aggregates ranging from extended families to larger communities inevitably shared episodes of life, health, sickness, and death. Whether based on superstition or sanitation, health practices evolved to ensure the survival of many aggregates. For example, primitive societies used elements of medicine (e.g., voodoo), isolation (e.g., banishment), and fumigation (i.e., use of smoke) to manage disease and thus protect the community for thousands of years (Hanlon and Pickett, 1990).

Classical Times

In the early years of the period 3000 to 1400 BCE, the Minoans devised ways to flush water and construct drainage systems. Circa 1000 BCE, the Egyptians constructed elaborate drainage systems, developed pharmaceutical preparations, and embalmed the dead. Pollution is an ancient problem. The biblical book of Exodus reported that "all the waters that were in the river stank," and in the book of Leviticus (believed to be written around 500 BCE), the Hebrews formulated the first written hygiene code. This hygiene code protected water and food by creating laws that governed personal and community hygiene such as contagion, disinfection, and sanitation.

Greece. Greek literature contains accounts of communicable diseases such as diphtheria, mumps, and malaria. The Hippocratic book *On Airs, Waters and Places,* a treatise on the balance between humans and their environment, may have been the only volume on this topic until the development of bacteriology in the late 19th century (Rosen, 2015). Diseases that were always present in a population, such as colds and pneumonia, were called **endemic**. When diseases such as diphtheria and measles presented fairly widespread outbreaks, the diseases were termed **epidemic**.

In practice, the Greeks emphasized the preservation of health, or good living, which the goddess Hygeia represented, and curative medicine, which the goddess Panacea personified. Human life had to be in balance with environmental demands; therefore the Greeks weighed the importance of exercise, rest, and nutrition according to age, sex, constitution, and climate (Rosen, 2015).

Rome. Although the Romans readily adopted Greek culture, they far surpassed Greek engineering by constructing massive aqueducts, bathhouses, and sewer systems. For example, at the height of the Roman Empire, Rome provided its 1 million inhabitants with 40 gallons of water per person per day, which is comparable to modern consumption rates (Rosen, 2015). Inhabitants of the overcrowded Roman slums, however, did not share in public health amenities such as sewer systems and latrines, and their health suffered accordingly.

The Romans also observed and addressed occupational health threats. In particular, they noted the pallor of the miners, the danger of suffocation, and the smell of caustic fumes (Rosen, 2015) (Box 2.1). For protection, miners devised safeguards by using masks made of bags, sacks, membranes, and bladder skins.

In the early years of the Roman Republic, priests were believed to mediate diseases and often dispensed medicine. Public physicians worked in designated towns and earned money to care for the poor. In addition, they were able to charge wealthier patients a service fee. Much as in a modern health maintenance organization or group practice, several families paid a set fee for yearly services. Hospitals, surgeries, infirmaries, and nursing homes appeared throughout Rome. In the 4th century, a Christian woman named Fabiola established a hospital for the sick poor. Others repeated this model throughout medieval times (Donahue, 2011).

Middle Ages

The decline of Rome, which occurred circa 500 CE, led to the Middle Ages. Monasteries promoted collective activity to protect public health, and the population adopted protective measures such as building wells and fountains, cleaning streets, and disposing of refuse. The commonly occurring communicable diseases were measles, smallpox, diphtheria, leprosy, and bubonic plague. Physicians had little to offer in the management of diseases such as leprosy. The church took over by enforcing the hygienic codes from Leviticus and establishing isolation and leper houses, or leprosaria (Rosen, 2015).

A **pandemic** is the existence of disease in a large proportion of the population. One such pandemic, the bubonic plague, ravaged much of the world in the 14th century. This plague, or Black Death, claimed close to half the world's population at that time (Hanlon and Pickett, 1990). For centuries, medicine and science did not recognize that fleas, which were attracted to the large number of rodents inhabiting urban areas, were the transmitters of plague. Modern public health practices such as isolation, disinfection, and ship quarantines emerged in response to the bubonic plague (Box 2.2).

BOX 2.2 Human Plague Cases in the United States

Between 1900 and 2012, more than 1000 cases of human plague occurred in the United States (CDC, 2015). A recent analysis of the historical epidemiology of the disease described how it evolved over the 113 years, changing from an illness that was largely located in port cities of California and the Gulf Coast between 1900 and 1925, to being primarily found in the "four corners" regions of the American Southwest, with periodic outbreaks in the mid-1980s and mid-1990s. Although many of the very early (pre-1925) cases affected Asian immigrants and sailors and were believed to have been transmitted person to person, the later outbreaks (post-1965) affected a high percentage of American Indians and were most commonly associated with working with animals and known flea bites.

Recently, two cases of plague were reported to have occurred after visits to Yosemite National Park in 2015 (CDC, 2016). A comprehensive investigation indicated that the two individuals likely contracted the disease from rodent droppings, but from different locations within the park. Significant changes and interventions were undertaken by park staff and education initiatives for the public were proposed to reduce the risk for further plague transmission.

Data from Centers for Disease Control and Prevention: Plague in the United States, 2019. Available from: https://www.cdc.gov/plague/maps/, https://wwwnc.cdc.gov/eid/article/21/1/pdfs/14-0564.pdf. Centers for Disease Control and Prevention: investigation of and response to 2 plagues cases, Yosemite National Park, California, USA, 2015, *Emerg Infect Diseases* 22(12):2045–2053, 2016. Available from: https://wwwnc.cdc.gov/eid/article/22/12/pdfs/16-0560.pdf.

BOX 2.1 Romans Provided Public Health Services

The ancient Romans provided public health services that included the following:
- A water board to maintain the aqueducts
- A supervisor of the public baths
- Street cleaners
- Supervision of the sale of food

Data from Rosen G: *A history of public health,* expanded ed, Baltimore, MD, 2015, Johns Hopkins Press.

During the Middle Ages, clergymen often acted as physicians and treated kings and noblemen. Monks and nuns provided nursing care in small houses designated as structures similar to today's small hospitals. Medieval writings contained information on hygiene and addressed such topics as housing, diet, personal cleanliness, and sleep (Rosen, 2015). Box 2.3 presents an account of living conditions in the 16th century.

The Renaissance

Although the cause of infectious disease remained undiscovered, two events important to public health occurred during the Renaissance. In 1546, Girolamo Fracastoro presented a theory that infection was a cause and epidemic a consequence of the "seeds of disease." Then, in 1676, Anton van Leeuwenhoek described microscopic organisms, although he did not associate them with disease (Rosen, 2015).

The **Elizabethan Poor Law**, enacted in England in 1601, held the church parishes responsible for providing relief for the poor. This law governed health care for the poor for more than two centuries and became a prototype for later US laws.

Eighteenth Century

Great Britain. The 18th century was marked by imperialism and industrialization. Unsanitary conditions remained a huge problem. During the Industrial Revolution, a gradual change in industrial productivity occurred. The industrial boom sacrificed many lives for profit. In particular, it forced poor children into labor. Under the Elizabethan Poor Law, parishes established workhouses to employ the poor. Orphaned and poor children were wards of the parish; therefore the parish forced these young children to labor in parish workhouses for long hours (George, 1925). At 12 to 14 years of age, a child became a master's apprentice. Those apprenticed to chimney sweeps reportedly suffered the worst fate because their masters forced them into chimneys at the risk of being burned and suffocated.

Vaccination was a major discovery of the times. In 1796, **Edward Jenner** observed that people who worked around cattle were less likely to contract smallpox. He concluded that immunity to smallpox resulted from an inoculation with the cowpox virus. Jenner's contribution was significant because approximately 95% of the population suffered from smallpox

BOX 2.3 Life in an English Household in the Sixteenth Century

In the following account, Erasmus described how life in the sixteenth century must have affected health. Such accounts appeared in literature throughout the sixteenth century.

As to floors, they are usually made with clay, covered with rushes that grow in the fens and which are so seldom removed that the lower parts remain sometimes for 20 years and has in it a collection of spittle, vomit, urine of dogs and humans, beer, scraps of fish, and other filthiness not to be named.

Quotation from Hanlon JJ, Pickett GE: *Public health administration and practice*, ed 9, Mosby, St. Louis, MO, 1990, p. 25.

and approximately 10% of the population died of smallpox during the 18th century. Frequently, the faces of those who survived the disease were scarred with pockmarks.

The **Sanitary Revolution's** public health reforms were beginning to take place throughout Europe and England. In the 18th century, scholars used survey methods to study public health problems (Rosen, 2015). These surveys mapped "medical topographies," which were geographic factors related to regional health and disease. A health education movement provided books and pamphlets on health to the middle and upper classes, but it neglected "economic factors" and was not concerned with the working classes.

Nineteenth Century

Europe. During the 19th century, communicable diseases ravaged the population that lived in unsanitary conditions, and many lives were lost. For example, in the mid-1800s, typhus and typhoid fever claimed twice as many lives each year as the Battle of Waterloo (Hanlon and Pickett, 1990).

Edwin Chadwick called attention to the consequences of unsanitary conditions that resulted in health disparities that shortened life spans of the laboring class in particular. Chadwick contended that death rates were high in large industrial cities such as Liverpool, where more than half of all children born of working-class parents died by age 5. Laborers lived an average of 16 years. In contrast, tradesmen lived 22 years, and the upper classes lived 36 years (Richardson, 1887). In 1842, Chadwick published his famous *Report on an Inquiry Into the Sanitary Conditions of the Labouring Population of Great Britain*. The report furthered the establishment of the General Board of Health for England in 1848. Legislation for social reform followed, addressing prevailing concerns such as child welfare; factory management; education; and care for the elderly, sick, and mentally ill. Clean water, sewers, fireplugs, and sidewalks emerged as a result.

In 1849, a German pathologist named Rudolf Virchow argued for social action—bettering the lives of the people by improving economic, social, and environmental conditions—to attack the root social causes of disease. He proposed "a theory of epidemic disease as a manifestation of social and cultural maladjustment" (Rosen, 2015, p. 62). He further argued that the public was responsible for the health of the people; that social and economic conditions heavily affected health and disease; that efforts to promote health and fight disease must be social, economic, and medical; and that the study of social and economic determinants of health and disease would yield knowledge to guide appropriate action.

These principles were embodied in a public health law submitted to the Berlin Society of Physicians and Surgeons in 1849 (Rosen, 2015). According to this document, public health has as its objectives (1) the healthy mental and physical development of the citizen, (2) the prevention of all dangers to health, and (3) the control of disease.

A very critical event in the development of modern public health occurred in 1854, when an English physician, anesthetist, and epidemiologist named **John Snow** demonstrated that cholera was transmissible through contaminated water. In a large population afflicted with cholera, he shut down the community's water resource by removing the pump handle from a well on Broad Street and carefully documented changes as the number of cholera cases fell dramatically (Rosen, 2015).

United States. In the United States during the 19th century, waves of epidemics continued to spread. As in Europe, diseases such as yellow fever, smallpox, cholera, typhoid fever, and typhus particularly affected the poor. These illnesses spread because cities grew and the poor crowded into inadequate housing with unsanitary conditions.

Lemuel Shattuck, a Boston bookseller and publisher with an interest in public health, organized the American Statistical Society in 1839 and issued a *Census of Boston* in 1845. The census showed high overall mortality and very high infant and maternal mortality rates. Living conditions for the poor were inadequate, and communicable diseases were widely prevalent (Rosen, 2015). Shattuck's 1850 *Report of the Sanitary Commission of Massachusetts* outlined the findings and recommended modern public health reforms that included keeping vital statistics and providing environmental, food, drug, and communicable disease control information. Shattuck called for well-infant, well-child, and school-aged—child health care; mental health care; vaccination; and health education. Unfortunately, the report fell on deaf ears, and little was done to improve population health for many years. For example, a state board of health was not formed until 19 years after the report was issued.

ADVENT OF MODERN HEALTH CARE

Early public health efforts evolved slowly throughout the mid-19th century. Administrative efforts, initial legislation, and debate regarding the determinants of health and approaches to health management began to appear on a social, economic, and medical level. The advent of "modern" health care occurred around this time, and nursing made a large contribution to the progress of health care. The following sections discuss the evolution of modern nursing, the evolution of modern medical care and public health practice, the evolution of the community caregiver, and the establishment of public health nursing.

Evolution of Modern Nursing

Florence Nightingale, the woman credited with establishing "modern nursing," began her work during the mid-19th century. Historians remember Florence Nightingale for contributing to the health of British soldiers during the Crimean War and establishing nursing education. However, many historians failed to recognize her remarkable use of public health principles and distinguished scientific contributions to health care reform (Cohen, 1984; Grier and Grier, 1978).

Nightingale was from a wealthy English family, was well educated, and traveled extensively. She studied with Adolphe Quetelet, a Belgian statistician who taught her the discipline of social inquiry (Goodnow, 1933). Nightingale also had a passion for hygiene and health, and in 1851, at the age of 31 years, she

trained in nursing at Kaiserswerth Hospital in Germany. She later studied the organization and discipline of the Sisters of Charity in Paris. Nightingale wrote extensively and published analyses of the nursing systems she studied in France, Austria, Italy, and Germany (Dock and Stewart, 1925).

In 1854, Nightingale responded to distressing accounts of a lack of care for wounded soldiers during the Crimean War. She and 40 other nurses traveled to Scutari, which was then a part of the Ottoman Empire. Nightingale was accompanied by lay nurses, Roman Catholic sisters, and Anglican sisters. Upon their arrival, the nurses learned that the British army's methods for treating the sick and wounded had created conditions that resulted in extraordinarily high death rates among soldiers. Indeed, one of Nightingale's greatest achievements was improving the management of these ill and wounded soldiers (Dossey, 2010).

During the Crimean War, cholera and "contagious fever" were rampant. Equal numbers of men died of disease and battlefield injury (Cohen, 1984). Nightingale found that allocated supplies were bound in bureaucratic red tape; for example, supplies were "sent to the wrong ports or were buried under munitions and could not be got" (Goodnow, 1933, p. 86).

Nightingale encountered problems reforming the army's methods for care of the sick because she had to work through eight military affairs departments related to her assignment. She sent reports of the appalling conditions of the hospitals to London. In response to her actions, governmental and private funds were donated to set up kitchens and a laundry and provided food, clothing, dressings, and laboratory equipment (Dock and Stewart, 1925).

Major reforms occurred during the first 2 months of her assignment. Aware that an interest in keeping social statistics was emerging, Nightingale realized that her most forceful argument would be statistical in nature. She reorganized the methods of keeping statistics and was the first to use shaded and colored coxcomb graphs of wedges, circles, and squares to illustrate the preventable deaths of soldiers. Nightingale compared the deaths of soldiers in hospitals during the Crimean War with the average annual mortality in Manchester and with the deaths of soldiers in military hospitals in and near London at the time (Fig. 2.2). Through her statistics she also showed that, by the end of the war, the death rate among ill soldiers during the Crimean War was no higher than that among well soldiers in Britain (Cohen, 1984). Indeed, Nightingale's careful statistics revealed that the death rate for treated soldiers decreased from 42% to 2%. Furthermore, she established community services and activities to improve the quality of life for recovering soldiers. These included rest and recreation facilities, study opportunities, a savings fund, and a post office. She also organized care for the families of the soldiers (Dock and Stewart, 1925).

After returning to London at the close of the war in 1856, Nightingale devoted her efforts to sanitary reform. At home, she surmised that if the sanitary neglect of the soldiers existed in the battle area, it probably existed at home in London. She prepared statistical tables to support her suspicions (Table 2.2).

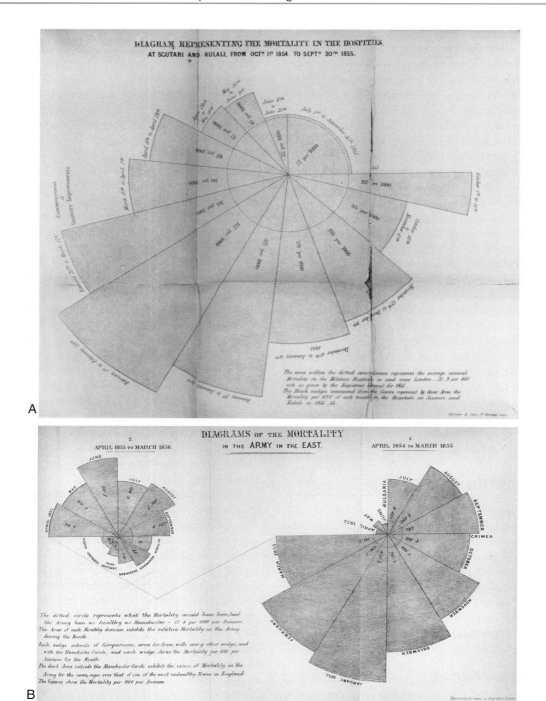

Fig. 2.2 (A) Coxcomb charts by Florence Nightingale. (B) Photographs of large, foldout charts from an original preserved at the University of Chicago Library. (A, From Nightingale F: *Notes on matters affecting the health, efficiency and hospitalization of the British army,* London, 1858, Harrison and Sons. B, Public domain; courtesy University of Chicago Library.)

In one study comparing the mortality of men aged 25 to 35 years in the army barracks of England with that of men the same age in civilian life, Nightingale found that the mortality of the soldiers was nearly twice that of the civilians. In one of her reports, she stated that "our soldiers enlist to death in the barracks" (Kopf, 1978, p. 95). Nightingale was very political and distributed her reports to members of Parliament and to the medical and commanding officers of the army (Kopf, 1978). Prominent leaders of the time challenged her reports. Undaunted, she rewrote them in greater depth and redistributed them.

In her efforts to compare the hospital systems in European countries, Nightingale discovered that each hospital kept

TABLE 2.2 Nightingale's Crimean War Mortality Statistics: Nursing Research That Made a Difference[a]

Year	Deaths That Would Have Occurred in Healthy Districts Among Males of the Soldiers' Ages[b]	Actual Deaths of Noncommissioned Officers and Men	Excess of Deaths Among Noncommissioned Officers and Men
1839	763	2,914	2,151
1840	829	3,300	2,471
1841	857	4,167	3,310
1842	888	5,052	4,164
1843	914	5,270	4,356
1844	920	3,867	2,947
1845	911	4,587	3,676
1846	930	5,125	4,195
1847	981	4,232	3,251
1848	987	3,213	2,226
1849	954	4,052	3,098
1850	919	3,119	2,200
1851	901	2,729	1,828
1852	915	3,120	2,205
1853	920	3,392	2,472
Total	13,589	58,139	44,550

[a]Number of deaths of noncommissioned officers and men also shows the number of deaths that would have occurred if the mortality were 7.7 per 1000—such as it was among Englishmen of the soldiers' age in healthy districts, in the years 1849 to 1853—which fairly represent the average mortality.
[b]The exact mortality in the healthy districts is 0.0077122, with use of the logarithm of 3.8871801.
From Grier B, Grier M: Contributions of the passionate statistician, *Res Nurs Health* 1:103–109, 1978. Copyright ©1978 by John Wiley & Sons, Inc. Reprinted by permission of John Wiley & Sons, Inc.

incomparable data and that many hospitals used various names and classifications for diseases. She noted that these differences prevented the collection of similar statistics from larger geographic areas. These statistics would create a regional health–illness profile and allow for comparison with other regions. She printed common statistical forms that some hospitals in London adopted on an experimental basis. A study of the tabulated results revealed the promise of this strategy (Kopf, 1978) (Box 2.4).

Nightingale also stressed the need to use statistics at the administrative and political levels to direct health policy. Noting the ignorance of politicians and those who set policy regarding the interpretation and use of statistics, she emphasized the need to teach national leaders to use statistical facts. Nightingale continued the development and application of statistical procedures, and she won recognition for her efforts. The Royal Statistical Society made her a fellow in 1858, and the American Statistical Association made her an honorary member in 1874 (Kopf, 1978).

It is interesting to note that the paradigm for nursing practice and nursing education that evolved through Nightingale's work did not incorporate her emphasis on statistics and a sound research base. It is also curious that nursing education did not consult her writings and did not stress the importance of determining health's social and environmental determinants until much later.

BOX 2.4 Nightingale's Use of Statistical Methods in Community Assessment

London's Southeastern Railway planned to remove St. Thomas' Hospital to enlarge the railway's right of way between London Bridge and Charing Cross. Nightingale applied her statistical method to the health needs of the community by conducting a community assessment. She plotted the cases served by the hospital, analyzed the proportion by distance, and calculated the probable impact on the community if the hospital were relocated to the proposed site. In her view, hospitals were a part of the wider community that served the needs of humanity. Kopf (1978) noted that this method of health planning and matching resources to the needs of the population was visionary and was not reapplied until the twentieth century.

? ACTIVE LEARNING EXERCISE

Find two recent articles about Florence Nightingale. After reading the articles, list Nightingale's contributions to public health, public health nursing, and community health nursing.

Establishment of Modern Health Care and Public Health Practice

To place Nightingale's work in perspective, it is necessary to consider the development of health care in light of common education and practice during the late 19th and early 20th centuries. Goodnow (1933) called this time a "dark age." Health sciences were underdeveloped, and bacteriology was unknown. Few medical schools existed at the time, thus apprenticeship was the path to medical education. The majority of physicians believed in the "spontaneous generation" theory of disease causation, which stated that disease organisms grew from nothing (Najman, 1990). Typical medical treatment included bloodletting, starving, using leeches, and prescribing large doses of metals such as mercury and antimony (Goodnow, 1933).

Nightingale's uniform classification of hospital statistics focused on the importance of tabulating the classification of diseases in hospital patients and the need to identify the diseases that patients contracted in the hospital. These diseases, such as gangrene and septicemia, were later called *iatrogenic* diseases (Kopf, 1978). Considering the lack of surgical sanitation in hospitals at the time, it is not surprising that iatrogenic infection was rampant. For example, Goodnow (1933) illustrates the following unsanitary operating procedures:

Before an operation the surgeon turned up the sleeves of his coat to save the coat and would often not trouble to wash his hands, knowing how soiled they soon would be! The area of the operation would sometimes be washed with soap and water, but not always, for the inevitability of corruption made it seem useless. The silk or thread used for stitches or ligatures was hung over a button of the surgeon's coat, and during the operation, a convenient place for the knife to rest was between his lips. Instruments .. used for .. lancing abscesses were kept in the vest pocket and often only wiped with a piece of rag as the surgeon went from one patient to another. (pp. 471–472)

During the 19th century, the following important scientists were born: **Louis Pasteur** in 1822, **Joseph Lister** in 1827, and **Robert Koch** in 1843. Their research had a profound impact on health care, medicine, and nursing. Pasteur was a chemist, not a physician. While experimenting with wine production in 1854, he proposed the theory of the existence of "germs." Although his colleagues ridiculed him at first, Koch applied his theories and developed his methods for handling and studying bacteria. Subsequently, Pasteur's colleagues gave him acknowledgment for his work (Kalisch and Kalisch, 2004).

Lister, whose father perfected the microscope, observed the healing processes of fractures. He noted that when the bone was broken but the skin was not, recovery was uneventful. However, when both the bone and the skin were broken, fever, infection, and even death were frequent. He postulated the answer to his observation from Pasteur's work and suggested that something outside the body entered the wound through the broken skin, causing the infection (Goodnow, 1933). Lister's surgical successes eventually improved when he soaked the dressings and instruments in mixtures of carbolic acid (i.e., phenol) and oil.

In 1882, Koch discovered the causative agent for cholera and the tubercle bacillus. Pasteur discovered immunization in 1881 and the rabies vaccine in 1885. These discoveries were significant to the development of public health and medicine. However, physicians accepted these discoveries slowly (Rosen, 2015). For example, TB was a major cause of death in late 19th-century America and often afflicted its victims with chronic illness and disability. It was a highly stigmatized disease, and most physicians thought it was a hereditary, constitutional disease associated with poor environmental conditions. Hospitalization for TB was rare because the stigma caused families to hide their infected relatives. Without treatment, the communicability of the disease increased. The most common treatment was a change of climate (Rosen, 2015). Although Koch had announced the discovery of the tubercle bacillus in 1882, it was 10 years before the emergence of the first organized community campaign to stop the spread of the disease.

The case of puerperal (i.e., childbirth) fever illustrates another example of slow innovation stemming from scientific discoveries. Although Pasteur showed that *Streptococcus* caused puerperal fever, it was years before physicians accepted his discovery. However, medical practice eventually changed, and physicians no longer delivered infants after performing autopsies of puerperal fever cases without washing their hands (Goodnow, 1933).

Debates over the causes of disease occurred throughout the 19th century. Scientists discovered organisms during the latter part of the century, supporting the theory that specific contagious entities caused disease. This discovery challenged the earlier miasmic theory that environment and atmospheric conditions caused disease (Greifinger and Sidel, 1981). The new scientific discoveries had a major impact on the development of public health and medical practice. The emergence of the germ theory of disease focused diagnosis and treatment on the individual organism and the individual disease.

State and local governments felt increasingly responsible for controlling the spread of microorganisms. A community outcry for social reform forced state and local governments to take notice of the deplorable living conditions in the cities. In the New York City riots of 1863, the populace expressed their disgust for overcrowding; filthy streets; lack of provisions for the poor; and lack of adequate food, water, and housing. Local boards of health formed, taking responsibility for safeguarding food and water stores and managing the sewage and quarantine operation for victims of contagious diseases (Greifinger and Sidel, 1981).

The New York Metropolitan Board of Health formed in 1866, and state health departments formed shortly thereafter. States built large public hospitals that treated TB and mental disease with rest, diet, and quarantine. In 1889, the New York City Health Department recommended the surveillance of TB and TB health education, but physicians did not welcome either recommendation (Rosen, 2015). Despite their objections, in 1894 the New York City Health Department required institutions to report cases of TB and required physicians to do the same by 1897.

In 1883, The Johns Hopkins University Medical School in Baltimore, Maryland, formed under the German model that promoted medical education on the principles of scientific discovery. In the United States, the Carnegie Commission appointed Abraham Flexner to evaluate medical schools throughout the country on the basis of the German model. In 1910, the **Flexner Report** outlined the shortcomings of US medical schools that did not use this model. Within a few years, the report caused philanthropic organizations such as the Rockefeller and Carnegie foundations to withdraw funding of poor-performing and scientifically "inadequate" medical schools, ensuring their closure. A "new breed" of physicians emerged who had been taught about "germ theory" and the "single agent theory" of disease causation (Greifinger and Sidel, 1981, p. 132) (Box 2.5).

Philanthropic foundations continued to influence health care efforts. For example, the Rockefeller Sanitary Commission for the Eradication of Hookworm formed in 1909. Hookworm was an occupational hazard among Southern workers. Implementation of preventive efforts to eradicate hookworm kept the workers healthy and thus proved to be a great industrial benefit. The model was so successful that the Rockefeller Foundation established the first school of public health, The Johns Hopkins School of Hygiene and Public Health, in 1916. The focus of this institution was the preservation and improvement of individual and community health and the prevention of disease through multidisciplinary activities.

Community Caregiver

The traditional role of the community caregiver or the traditional healer has nearly vanished in the West. However, medical and nurse anthropologists who have studied primitive and Western cultures are familiar with the community healer and caregiver role (McFarland and Wehbe-Alamah, 2018). The traditional healer (e.g., shaman, midwife, herbalist, or priest) is common in non-Western, ancient, and underdeveloped societies. Although traditional healers have always existed, professionals and many people throughout industrialized societies may overlook or minimize their role. The role of the healer is often integrated into other institutions of society, including religion, medicine, and morality. The notion that one person acts alone in healing may be foreign to many cultures; healers can be individuals, kin, or entire societies (Hughes, 1978).

BOX 2.5 Scientific Theory/Single-Agent Theory

The emphasis on the use of scientific theory, or single-agent theory, in medical care developed into a focus on disease and symptoms rather than a focus on the prevention of disability and care for the "whole person." The old-fashioned family doctor viewed patients in relation to their families and communities and apparently helped people cope with problems in personal life, family, and society. American medicine adopted science with such vigor that these qualities faded away. Science allowed the physician to deal with tissues and organs, which were much easier to comprehend than the dynamics of human relationships or the complexities of disease prevention. Many physicians made efforts to integrate the various roles, but society was pushing toward academic science.

Societies retain folk practices because they provide some repeated successes. Most cultures have a pharmacopeia and maintain therapeutic and preventive practices, and it is estimated that one-fourth to one-half of folk medicines are empirically effective. Indeed, many modern drugs are based on the medicines of primitive cultures (e.g., eucalyptus, coca, and opium) (Hughes, 1978).

Since ancient times, folk healers and cultural practices have both positively and negatively affected health. The late 19th- and early 20th-century practice of midwifery illustrates modern medicine's arguably sometimes negative impact on traditional healing in many Western cultures (Smith, 1979). For example, traditional midwifery practices made women rise out of bed within 24 h of delivery to help "clear" the lochia. Throughout the mid-1900s, in contrast, "modern medicine" recommended keeping women in bed after delivery, often for fairly extended periods (Smith, 1979).

RESEARCH HIGHLIGHTS

Historical Methodology for Nursing Research
Historiography is the methodology of historical research. It involves specialized techniques, principles, and theories that pertain to historical matters. *Historical research* involves interpreting history and contributing to understanding through data synthesis. It relies on existing sources or data and requires the researcher to gain access to sources such as libraries, librarians, and databases.

Historical research should be descriptive. It should answer the questions of who, what, when, where, how, and the interpretive why. Historians reconstruct an era using primary sources and interpret the story from that perspective. Historical research in nursing will enhance the understanding of current nursing practice and will help prepare for the future.

Adapted from Lusk B: Historical methodology for nursing research, *Image J Nurs Sch* 29:3555–3560, 1997.

Establishment of Public Health Nursing

Public health nursing as a holistic approach to health care developed in the late 19th and early 20th centuries. Public and community health nursing in its current form evolved from home nursing practice, community organizations, and political interventions on behalf of families, groups, and populations as explained in this section.

England

Public health nursing developed from providing nursing care to the sick poor and furnishing information and through channels of community organization that enabled the poor to improve their own health status.

District Nursing. **District nursing** was first established in England. Between 1854 and 1856, the Epidemiological Society of London developed a plan that trained selected poor women to provide nursing care to the disadvantaged families within a community. The society theorized that nurses belonging to their patients' social class would be more effective caregivers and that more nurses would be available to improve the health of community residents (Rosen, 2015).

A similar plan was implemented by William Rathbone in Liverpool in 1859. After experiencing the excellent care a nurse gave his sick wife in his home, Rathbone strongly believed that nurses could offer the same care throughout the community. He developed a plan that divided the community into 18 districts and assigned a nurse and a social worker to each district. This team met the needs of their communities with respect to nursing, social work, and health education. The community widely accepted the plan. To further strengthen it, Rathbone consulted Nightingale about educating the district nurses. She assisted him by providing training for the district nurses, referring to them as "health nurses." The model was successful, and eventually voluntary agencies adopted the plan on the national level (Rosen, 2015).

Health Visiting. **Health visiting** to provide information to improve health is a parallel service based on the district nursing tradition. The Ladies Section of the Manchester and Salford Sanitary Association originated health visiting in Manchester in 1862. Prior to that time, it had been observed that providing health pamphlets alone had little effect on improving health; therefore this service enlisted home visitors to distribute health information to the poor.

In 1893, Nightingale pointed out that the district nurse should be a health teacher and a nurse for the sick in the home. She believed that teachers should educate "health missioners" for this purpose. The model charged the district nurse with providing care for the sick in the home and the health visitor with providing health information in the home. Eventually, government agencies sponsored health visitors, medical health officers supervised them, and the municipality paid them. Thus a collaborative model developed between government and voluntary agencies.

United States

In the United States, public health nursing developed from the British traditions of district nursing, health visiting, and home nursing. In 1877, the Women's Board of the New York City Mission sent a graduate nurse named Frances Root into homes to provide care for the sick. The innovation spread, and nursing associations, later called *visiting nurse associations,* were implemented in Buffalo in 1885 and in Boston and Philadelphia in 1886.

In 1893, nurses **Lillian Wald** and Mary Brewster established a district nursing service on the Lower East Side of New York City called the **House on Henry Street**. This was a crowded area teeming with unemployed and homeless immigrants who needed health care. The organization, later called the Visiting Nurse Association of New York City, played an important role in establishing public health nursing in the United States. Box 2.6 contains Wald's compelling account of her early exposure to the community where she identified public health nursing needs.

Wald (1971) described a range of services that evolved from the House on Henry Street. Nurses provided home visits, and patients paid carfare or a cursory fee. Physicians were consultants

to Henry Street, and families could arrange a visit by calling the nurse directly, or a physician could call the nurse on the family's behalf. The nursing service adopted the philosophy of meeting the health needs of the population, which included the many evident social, economic, and environmental determinants of health. By necessity, this effort involved an aggregate approach that empowered people of the community.

Helen Hall, who later directed the House on Henry Street, wrote that the settlement's role was "one of helping people to help themselves" (Wald, 1971) through the development of centers of social action aimed at meeting the needs of the community and the individual. Community organization led to the formation of a great variety of programs, including youth clubs, a juvenile program, sex education for local schoolteachers, and support programs for immigrants.

Additional programs such as school nursing were based on individual observations and interventions. Wald reported the following incident that preceded her successful trial of school nursing (1971):

I had been downtown only a short time when I met Louis. An open door in a rear tenement revealed a woman standing over a washtub, a fretting baby on her left arm, while with her right she rubbed at the butcher's aprons which she washed for a living.

"Louis," she explained, "was bad." He did not "cure his head of lice and what would become of him, for they would not take him into the school because of it?" Louis said he had been to the dispensary many times. He knew it was awful for a twelve-year-old boy not to know how to read the names of the streets on the lamp-posts, but "every time I go to school Teacher tells me to go home."

It needed only intelligent application of the dispensary ointments to cure the affected area, and in September, I had the joy of securing the boy's admittance to school for the first time in his life. The next day, at the noon recess, he fairly rushed up our five flights of stairs in the Jefferson Street tenement to spell the elementary words he had acquired that morning. (pp. 46—47)

Overcrowded schools, an uninformed and uninterested public, and an unaware Department of Health all contributed to social health neglect. Wald and the nursing staff at the settlement kept anecdotal notes on the sick children teachers excluded from school. One nurse found a boy in school whose skin was desquamating from scarlet fever and took him to the president of the Department of Health in an attempt to place physicians in schools. A later program had physicians screen children in school for 1 h each day.

Twentieth Century. In 1902, Wald persuaded Dr. Ernest J. Lederle, Commissioner of Health in New York City, to try a school nursing experiment. Henry Street lent a public health nurse named Linda Rogers to the New York City Health Department to work in a school (Dock and Stewart, 1925). The experiment was successful, and schools adopted nursing on a

BOX 2.6 Lillian Wald: The House On Henry Street

The following highlights from *The House on Henry Street*, published in 1915, bring Lillian Wald's experience to life:

A sick woman in a squalid rear tenement, so wretched and so pitiful that, in all the years since, I have not seen anything more appalling, determined me, within half an hour, to live on the East Side.

I had spent 2 years in a New York training-school for nurses ... After graduation, I supplemented the theoretical instruction, which was casual and inconsequential in the hospital classes 25 years ago, by a period of study at a medical college. It was while at the college that a great opportunity came to me.

While there, the long hours "on duty" and the exhausting demands of the ward work scarcely admitted freedom for keeping informed as to what was happening in the world outside. The nurses had no time for general reading; visits to and from friends were brief; we were out of the current and saw little of life saved as it flowed into the hospital wards. It is not strange, therefore, that I should have been ignorant of the various movements which reflected the awakening of the social conscience at the time.

Remembering the families who came to visit patients in the wards, I outlined a course of instruction in home nursing adapted to their needs, and gave it in an old building in Henry Street, then used as a technical school and now part of the settlement. Henry Street then as now was the center of a dense industrial population.

From the schoolroom where I had been giving a lesson in bedmaking, a little girl led me one drizzling March morning. She had told me of her sick mother, and gathering from her incoherent account that a child had been born, I caught up the paraphernalia of the bedmaking lesson and carried it with me.

The child led me over broken roadways—there was no asphalt, although its use was well established in other parts of the city—over dirty mattresses and heaps of refuse—it was before Colonel Waring had shown the possibility of clean streets even in that quarter—between tall, reeking houses whose laden fire-escapes, useless for their appointed purpose, bulged with household goods of every description. The rain added to the dismal appearance of the streets and to the discomfort of the crowds which thronged them, intensifying the odors which assailed me from every side. Through Hester and Division Street[s] we went to the end of Ludlow; past odorous fishstands, for the streets were a market-place, unregulated, unsupervised, unclean; past evil-smelling, uncovered garbage-cans; and—perhaps worst of all, where so many little children played—past the trucks brought down from more fastidious quarters and stalled on these already overcrowded streets, lending themselves inevitably to many forms of indecency.

The child led me on through a tenement hallway, across a court where open and unscreened closets were promiscuously used by men and women, up into a rear tenement, by slimy steps whose accumulated dirt was augmented that day by the mud of the streets, and finally into the sickroom.

All the maladjustments of our social and economic relations seemed epitomized in this brief journey and what was found at the end of it. The family to which the child led me was neither criminal nor vicious. Although the husband was a cripple, one of those who stand on street corners exhibiting deformities to enlist compassion, and masking the begging of alms by a pretense at selling; although the family of seven shared their two rooms with boarders—who were literally boarders, since a piece of timber was placed over the floor for them to sleep on—and although the sick woman lay on a wretched, unclean bed, soiled with a hemorrhage 2 days old, they were not degraded human beings, judged by any measure of moral values.

In fact, it was very plain that they were sensitive to their condition, and when, at the end of my ministrations, they kissed my hands (those who have undergone similar experiences will, I am sure, understand), it would have been some solace if by any conviction of the moral unworthiness of family I could have defended myself as a part of a society which permitted such conditions to exist. Indeed, my subsequent acquaintance with them revealed the fact that, miserable as their state was, they were not without ideals for the family life, and for society, of which they were so unloved and unlovely a part.

That morning's experience was a baptism of fire. Deserted were the laboratory and the academic work of the college. I never returned to them. On my way from the sickroom to my comfortable student quarters my mind was intent on my own responsibility. To my inexperience, it seemed certain that conditions such as these were allowed because people did not know, and for me there was a challenge to know and to tell. When early morning found me still awake, my naive conviction remained that, if people knew things—and "things" meant everything implied in the condition of this family—such horrors would cease to exist, and I rejoiced that I had had a training in the care of the sick that in itself would give me an organic relationship to the neighborhood in which this awakening had come.

To the first sympathetic friend to whom I poured forth my story, I found myself presenting a plan which had been developing almost without conscious mental direction on my part.

Within a day or two a comrade from the training-school, Mary Brewster, agreed to share in the venture. We were to live in the neighborhood as nurses, identify ourselves with it socially, and, in brief, contribute to it our citizenship.

I should like to make it clear that from the beginning we were most profoundly moved by the wretched industrial conditions which were constantly forced upon us ... I hope to tell of the constructive programmes that the people themselves have evolved out of their own hard lives, of the ameliorative measures, ripened out of sympathetic comprehension, and finally, of the social legislation that expresses the new compunction of the community.

From Wald L: *The House on Henry Street*, New York, 1971, Dover Publications (original work published 1915, Henry Holt), pp. 1–9.

widespread basis. School nurses performed physical assessments, treated minor infections, and taught health to pupils and parents.

In 1909, Wald mentioned the efficacy of home nursing to one of the officials of the Metropolitan Life Insurance Company. The company decided to provide home nursing to its industrial policyholders, and soon the United States and Canada used the program successfully (Wald, 1971).

The growing demand for public health nursing was hard to satisfy. In 1910, the Department of Nursing and Health formed at the Teachers College of Columbia University in New York City. A course in visiting nursing placed nurses at the Henry Street settlement for fieldwork. In 1912, the newly formed National Organization for Public Health Nursing elected Lillian Wald its first president. This organization was open to public health nurses and to those interested in public health nursing. In 1913, the Los Angeles Department of Health formed the first Bureau of Public Health Nursing (Rosen, 2015). That same year, the Public Health Service appointed its first public health nurse.

At first, many public health nursing programs used nurses in specialized areas such as school nursing, TB nursing, maternal-child health nursing, and communicable disease nursing. In later years, more generalized programs have become acceptable. Efforts to contain healthcare costs include reducing the number of hospital days. With the advent of shortened hospital stays, private home health agencies provide home-based illness care across the United States.

The second half of the century saw a shift in emphasis to cost containment and the provision of healthcare services through managed care. Traditional models of public health nursing and visiting nursing from home health agencies became increasingly common over the next several decades, but

RESEARCH HIGHLIGHTS

Example of Historical Nursing Research

Thompson and Keeling (2012) presented an historical examination describing how public health nurses contributed to a significant decline in infant mortality in New England between 1884 and 1925. Analyzing archived data and documents from Providence, Rhode Island, they estimated that in the late 19th century, the mortality rate of children younger than 2 was between 15% and 20%. Furthermore, they reported that the health officials believed that of those infants and small children who died during those years, 40%–50% died from digestive-related diseases (e.g., diarrhea).

The germ theory was not widely accepted until the early 1900s. Thus, in the late 19th century, nurses were trained to understand "elements of modern hygiene" (e.g., good nutrition, light, cleanliness). But following acceptance of the germ theory and epidemiological techniques for data analysis in the early 1900s, public health efforts shifted to consideration of factors, including biological, environmental, and economic, that contributed to the high infant mortality rate.

To address the problem of infant/child mortality, public health nurses focused on teaching low-income mothers how to care for and feed their children. The nurses worked in homes, "milk stations," and other creative settings to meet the identified needs. They set up and participated in "milk dispensaries," which provided pasteurized milk (rather than the widely available unrefrigerated milk—which was frequently days old). They also promoted breast-feeding and provided information on "infant hygiene" along with the milk. These and other efforts, including developing the role of a "children's special nurse," were effective, and the infant mortality rate dropped from 142/1000 to 102/1000 between 1907 and 1917.

From Thompson ME, Keeling AA: Nurses' role in the prevention of infant mortality in 1884–1925: health disparities then and now, *J Pediatr Nurs* 27:471–478, 2012.

waned toward the end of the century due to changes in healthcare financing.

ACTIVE LEARNING EXERCISE

1. Research the history of the health department or visiting nurse association in a particular city or county.
2. Discuss with peers how Lillian Wald's approach to individual and community health care provides an understanding of how to facilitate the empowerment of aggregates in the community.

CONSEQUENCES FOR THE HEALTH OF POPULATIONS

An understanding of the consequences of the healthcare delivery system for population health is necessary to form conclusions about public health nursing from a historical perspective. Implications for the health of aggregates relate to new causes of mortality (i.e., *Hygeia,* or health promotion/care, vs. *Panacea,* or cure) and additional theories of disease causation.

Twenty-First Century
New Causes of Mortality

Since the middle of the 20th century, the focus of disease in Western societies has changed from mostly infectious diseases to chronic diseases. Increased food production and better nutrition during the 19th and early 20th centuries contributed to the decline in infectious disease—related deaths. Other factors were better sanitation through water purification, sewage disposal, improved food handling, and milk pasteurization. According to McKeown (2001) and Schneider (2021), the components of "modern" medicine, such as antibiotics and immunizations, had little effect on health until well into the 20th century. Indeed, widespread vaccination programs began in the late 1950s, and antibiotics came into use after 1945.

The advent of chronic disease in Western populations puts selected groups at risk, and those groups need health education, screening, and programs to ensure occupational and environmental safety. Too often modern medicine still focuses on the single cause of disease (i.e., germ theory) and treating the acutely ill. As a result, many health providers treat the chronically ill with an acute care approach even though preventive care, health promotion, and restorative care are necessary and would likely be more effective in combating chronic disease. This expanded approach may develop under new systems of cost containment.

Hygeia Versus Panacea

The Grecian Hygeia (i.e., healthful living) versus Panacea (i.e., cure) dichotomy still exists today. Although the change in the nature of health "problems" is certain, the roles of individual and collective activities in the prevention of illness and premature death are slow to evolve.

In 2010, about two-thirds of the active physicians in the United States were specialists (U.S. Department of Health and Human Services, Agency for Healthcare Research and Quality [USDHHS/AHRQ], 2011). In recent years, medical education has increasingly focused on enhancing the education of primary care physicians (e.g., those specializing in internal medicine, obstetrics-gynecology, family medicine, and pediatrics) to meet the growing need for primary care. In addition to primary care, Hygeia (health promotion) requires a coordinated system that addresses health problems holistically with the use of multiple approaches and planning of outcomes for aggregates and populations. A redistribution of interest and resources to address the major determinants of health, such as food, housing, education, and a healthy social and physical environment, is critical (Shi and Singh, 2019).

Additional Theories of Disease Causation

As mentioned, the germ theory of disease causation is a unicausal model that evolved in the late 19th century. Najman (1990) reviewed the following theories of disease causation: the multicausal view, which considers the environment multidimensionally, and the general susceptibility view, which considers stress and lifestyle factors. Najman contended that each theory accounts for some disease under some conditions, but no single theory accounts for all disease. Other factors, such as literacy and nutrition, may reduce disease morbidity and mortality to a greater extent than medical interventions alone.

SOCIAL CHALLENGES AND PUBLIC HEALTH NURSING

Several social and political changes have occurred in the United States that have affected the development of public health nursing practice. Throughout the 20th century, the health of the client, nursing, health, and the environment were influenced by the development of health insurance and an emphasis on population-based focus.

The advent of and changes in health insurance dramatically altered health care delivery. The greatest health concerns at the beginning of the 20th century were lost wages associated with sickness. The cost of health care was so low that there was little understanding of the need for health insurance. Between 1900 and 1920, there were minimal technological advances. Treatments available at the time, including surgery, were often performed in private homes.

During the 1920s and 1930s, the costs of health care rose. As the population moved from rural to urban settings, the delivery points for much of health care changed, moving from private homes to hospitals. Improved therapeutic options, more medications, the acceptance of medicine as a science, and the closure of underperforming medical schools during the 1920s increased the demand for health care and raised the associated cost (Rosenberg, 1987).

As hospitals began to expand and organize, they formed the American Hospital Association, whose leaders encouraged the development of health insurance plans. In 1929, the Committee of the Costs of Medical Care, a national group, produced a report that promoted voluntary insurance in the United States. That same year, Baylor Hospital in Dallas, Texas, joined with a local teachers' association to provide health care for those agreeing to pay a small monthly premium. In a short time, this relationship grew to include more employers and evolved into Blue Cross (Getzen, 2013; Sparer and Thompson, 2015). Improvements in medical technology and the growing practice of employers' offering health insurance in place of employee compensation during and after World War II further supported the expansion of private health insurance.

During the 1960s, politicians supported the development of federal and state health insurance for the poor and the elderly populations, subsequently enacting Medicare and Medicaid. As a result, since the 1970s most health care has been paid for with either public or private insurance plans. As a result of "third-party" reimbursement, costs grew steadily as much of the public paid little attention to charges because they were not directly responsible for payment. Consequently, the growth in available treatments because of improving technological advances, chronic disease associated with an aging population, and negative lifestyle choices and other factors led to a dramatic number of individuals and families who were not able to afford health care because they could not afford health insurance.

The Patient Protection and Affordable Care Act (ACA) was passed in 2010 to help reduce some of the problems associated with access to health care. After implementation, the number of uninsured dropped dramatically, but costs continued to increase and access was still problematic for some.

With the new administration in 2020, updates to the ACA are anticipated, but problems with costs and access will likely persist. Indeed, considerable attention on current public health initiatives, such as the *Healthy People 2030* campaign and further health care reform, focus on ensuring elimination of health disparities and working toward equity in health care. Box 2.7 provides a summary of some of the dramatic effects of public health activities on the health of Americans during the last 100 years. The photo novella in this chapter illustrates community health nursing in the early and mid-20th century.

RESEARCH HIGHLIGHTS

Example of Historical Nursing Research

Fairman's (1996) review of 150 fictional novels from 1850 to 1995 revealed how the image of nursing has changed over the past 140 years. The results showed that the image of nursing improved dramatically from the negative perception of the 1850s. Trained nurses became more common in the early 1900s, and novels began to depict strong, independent, female nurses. The positive image continued until the 1960s and 1970s, when novels presented the negative image of "bed hopping honeys." Popular literature showed the most negative image of nurses, and classics and children's literature showed a more positive image.

Adapted from Fairman PL: *Analysis of the image of nursing and nurses as portrayed in fictional literature from 1850 to 1995*, San Francisco, CA, 1996, University of San Francisco Dissertation Abstracts.

ACTIVE LEARNING EXERCISE

Obtain copies of early articles from nursing journals (e.g., *American Journal of Nursing* dates from 1900). Discuss the health problems, medical care, and nursing practice these articles illustrated.

Collect copies of early nursing textbooks. Discuss the evolution of thoughts on pathology, illness management, and health promotion.

CHALLENGES FOR PUBLIC HEALTH NURSING

Public health nurses face the challenge of promoting the health of populations. They must accomplish this goal with a broadened understanding of the multiple causes of morbidity and mortality. The specialization of medicine and nursing has affected the delivery of nursing and health care. Well-prepared nurses must be aware of the increased technological advances that specialization has contributed to. These advances have resulted in an increase in the number of advanced practice nurses in the past several decades. It is anticipated that this growth will persist and likely expand (IOM, 2011).

The community need for a focus on prevention, health promotion, and home care may become more widespread with

BOX 2.7 Ten Great Public Health Achievements—United States, 1900–2010

During the 20th century, the health and life expectancy of persons living in the United States improved dramatically. It is important for nurses to realize that of the 30 years of life expectancy gained during the century, 25 years were attributable to public health efforts. During 1999, the Centers for Disease Control and Prevention published a series of articles outlining 10 of the great public health achievements of the twentieth century. In 2011, the agency published an update of highlights from the ensuing decade. Summarized here are the "Public Health Achievements" presented:

Vaccination/vaccine-preventable diseases—Widespread vaccination programs resulted in eradication of smallpox; elimination of polio in the Americas; and control of measles, rubella, tetanus, diphtheria, and a number of other infectious diseases in the United States. In the first decade of the 21st century, new vaccines (e.g., rotavirus, herpes zoster, hepatitis A, and human papilloma virus) were introduced and are having a significant, positive impact on population health.

Motor vehicle safety—Improvements in motor vehicle safety contributed to large reductions in traffic deaths. Improvements included efforts to make both vehicles and highways safer and to change personal behaviors (e.g., increase use of seat belts and child safety seats, reduce driving under the influence [DUI] offenses). Between 2000 and 2009, the death rate from motor vehicle accidents continued to decline, largely as a result of safer vehicles, safer roads, safer road use, and related policies (e.g., graduated driver's licenses).

Safer workplaces—Work-related health problems (e.g., coal worker's pneumoconiosis [black lung] and silicosis) were very significantly reduced during the twentieth century, as were severe injuries and deaths related to mining, manufacturing, construction, and transportation. Following legislation in 1980, safer workplaces resulted in further reduction of 40% in the rate of fatal occupational injuries by the end of the century.

Control of infectious diseases—Since the early 1900s, control of infectious diseases has resulted from clean water and better sanitation. Cholera and typhoid were major causes of illness and death in the early twentieth century and have been virtually eliminated today. Additionally, the discovery of antimicrobial therapy has been very successful in helping efforts to control infections such as TB, sexually transmitted infections, and influenza. Much of the efforts in the last decade of the twentieth century and the first of the 21st century focused on prevention and treatment of human immunodeficiency virus/acquired immunodeficiency syndrome (HIV/AIDS). Prevention/education efforts, along with enhanced screening for HIV, early diagnosis, and effective treatment,

have resulted in reduction in transmission of the virus, along with enabling access to lifesaving treatment and care for those who are HIV positive and their partners.

Decline in deaths from coronary heart disease (CHD) and stroke—Since 1972, the death rate for CHD has decreased 51%. This improvement is largely the result of risk factor modification (e.g., smoking cessation, blood pressure control) coupled with early detection and better treatment. In the last decade, CHD deaths continued to decline, going from 195/100,000 to 126/100,000. Contributing to the ongoing reduction are better control of hypertension, reduction in elevated cholesterol and smoking, and improvement in treatment and available medications.

Safer and healthier foods—Since 1900, reduction in microbial contamination and increases in nutritional content have led to safer and healthier foods. Food fortification programs and enhanced availability of nutritional options have almost eliminated major nutritional deficiency diseases in the United States.

Healthier mothers and babies—Since 1900, infant mortality in the United States has decreased 90% and maternal mortality has decreased 99%. These improvements are the result of better hygiene and nutrition, availability of antibiotics, access to better health care, and advances in maternal and neonatal medicine. During the early 21st century, there has been a significant reduction in the number of infants born with neural tube defects, a change attributable to mandatory folic acid fortification of cereal grain products.

Family planning—Access to family planning and contraceptives has provided women with better social and economic opportunities and health benefits, including smaller families and longer intervals between children.

Fluoridation of drinking water—Fluoridation of drinking water began in 1945, and by 1999 about half of all Americans had fluoridated water. This achievement positively and inexpensively benefited both children and adults by preventing tooth decay. Indeed, fluoridation has been credited for reducing tooth decay by 40%–70% in children and tooth loss by 40%–60% in adults.

Tobacco control—Recognition in 1964 that tobacco use is a health hazard resulted in behavior and policy changes that eventually led to a dramatic decline in the prevalence of smoking among adults. The rate of smoking peaked in the 1960s, and by 2009 only about 20% of adults and youths were current smokers. Health policy efforts (e.g., prohibition of smoking in worksites, restaurants, and bars), dramatic increases in cigarette taxes, and prohibition of selling to youths have contributed to much of the recent decline.

Data from Centers for Disease Control and Prevention: 10 great public health achievements—United States, 1900–1999, *MMWR Morb Mortal Wkly Rep* 48(12):241–243, 1999 and Centers for Disease Control and Prevention: 10 great public health achievements—United States, 2001–2010, *MMWR Morb Mortal Wkly Rep* 60(19):619–623, 2001.

the changing patterns of healthcare cost reimbursement. Holistic care requires multiple dimensions and must have more attention in the future. Further, as evidenced by the COVID 19 pandemic, more attention needs to be given to identification of communicable disease threats and development of rapid community interventions to mitigate them.

The need for education in public health nursing calls for a curriculum that prepares students to meet the needs of aggregates through population-based strategies that include an understanding of statistical data and epidemiology. Such a curriculum would move the focus from the individual to a broader population approach. Strategies would promote literacy, nutrition programs, prevention of overweight school-aged

children, decent housing and income, education, and safe social and physical environments.

Healthcare services to individuals alone cannot solve today's health problems. All healthcare workers must learn to work with and on behalf of aggregates and help them build a constituency for the consumer issues they face.

A population focus for nursing addresses the health of all in the population through the careful gathering of information and statistics. A population focus will better enable community health nurses to contribute to the ethic of social justice by emphasizing society's responsibility for health (Beauchamp, 1986). Helping aggregates help themselves will empower people and create avenues for addressing their concerns.

IMAGES OF COMMUNITY HEALTH NURSING IN THE EARLY AND MID-TWENTIETH CENTURY

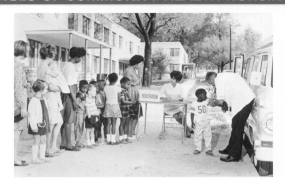

Group Immunization. Multiracial group of women and children in a housing project mobile clinic waiting for and receiving vaccinations. Scene contains a doctor and a nurse. (1972). (Courtesy of the Centers for Disease Control and Prevention Public Health Image Library [PHIL] Image #1661. Source: CDC/ Reuel Waldrop.)

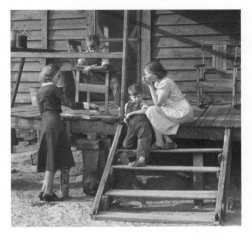

A visiting nurse outside a shack with a mother and two children. (Courtesy of the US National Library of Medicine, History of Medicine Division. Order No. A017986.)

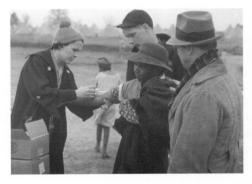

A public health nurse immunizes farm and migrant workers in the 1940s. (Courtesy of the Library of Congress, Washington, DC.)

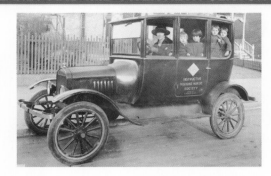

A public health nurse transports children to a clinic. (Courtesy of MedStar Visiting Nurse Association.)

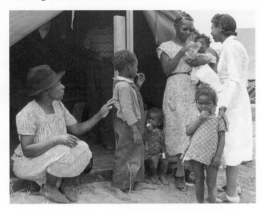

A public health nurse performs health teaching. (Courtesy of the Library of Congress, Washington, DC.)

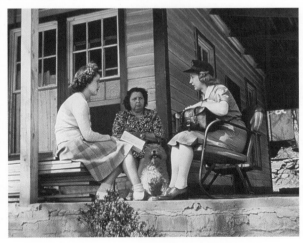

A public health nurse talks to a young woman and her mother about childbirth. (Courtesy of the US National Library of Medicine, History of Medicine Division. Order No. A029980.)

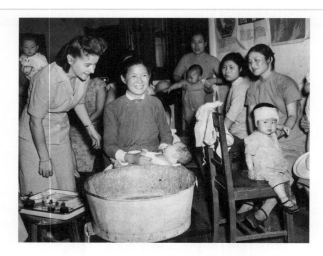

The Shanghai Mother's Club of the Child Welfare and Maternal Health Clinic. United Nations Relief and Rehabilitation Administration (UNRRA) Public Health Nurse Irene Muir instructs Nurse S. U. Zee on child bathing techniques. (Courtesy of the US National Library of Medicine, History of Medicine Division. Order No. A016681.)

RESEARCH HIGHLIGHTS

Example of Historical Nursing Research

An in-depth examination of all of the issues from 115 years of the *American Journal of Nursing* was undertaken to "explore the nurse's historical and contemporary role in promoting patient safety" (Kowalski and Anthony, 2017, p. 34). A detailed content analysis of almost 1100 articles outlined the evolution of nursing's emphasis and interventions related to safety.

The authors described how the "safety" focus moved from asepsis and the "newly understood germ theory" in the early decades of the 20th century to preventing medication errors in the 1930s. During and after World War II, improving patient survival rates was emphasized, and in the 1950s, attention moved to progressive patient care and various levels of care (intensive,

intermediate, long term, or home care). During the 1960s and 1970s, focus turned to the increasing complexity of care related to technology and enhanced medication regimens and the associated safety problems. Hospital-acquired infections and medication and nursing procedure safety were emphasized in the 1980s and 1990s. Since 2000, safety attention has moved to systematic factors such as communication, patient–nurse ratios, provider skill mix, and shift work.

The authors identified three major themes related to patient safety throughout the 115 years: infection prevention, medication safety, and technology response. They described the concurrent processes and procedures that were implemented to improve patient safety, but concluded that much more work is needed.

Kowalski SL, Anthony M: Nursing's evolving role in patient safety, *Am J Nurs* 117(2):34–50, 2017.

SUMMARY

Western civilization evolved from the Paleolithic period to the present, and people began to live in increasingly closer proximity to one another; therefore they experienced a change in the nature of their health problems.

In the mid-19th and early 20th centuries, public health efforts and the precursors of modern and public health nursing began to improve societal health. Nursing pioneers such as Nightingale in England and Wald in the United States focused on the collection and analysis of statistical data, health care reforms, home health nursing, community empowerment, and nursing education. They established the groundwork for today's public health nurses.

Modern public health nurses must recognize and try to understand the philosophical controversies that influence society and ultimately their practice. These controversies include different opinions about what "intervention" means—specifically in regard to "cure" versus "care."

Controversy also surrounds the significance of maintaining a focus on individuals, families, groups, or populations. Finally, public health nurses need to understand social determinants of health and to be part of the solution with regard to coming up with ways to address persistent health problems while addressing the critical problem of escalating health care costs.

EVOLVE WEBSITE

http://evolve.elsevier.com/Nies/community

- NCLEX Review Questions
- Case Studies

BIBLIOGRAPHY

Armelagos GK, Dewey JR: Evolutionary response to human infectious diseases. In Logan MH, Hunt EE, editors: *Health and the human condition*, North Scituate, MA, 1978, Duxbury Press.

Beauchamp DE: Public health as social justice. In Mappes T, Zembaty J, editors: *Biomedical ethics*, ed 2, New York, 1986, McGraw-Hill.

Centers for Disease Control and Prevention: Plague in the United States, 2019. Available from: https://www.cdc.gov/plague/maps/.

Centers for Disease Control and Prevention: Investigation of and response to 2 plagues cases, Yosemite National Park, California, USA, 2015, *Emerg Infect Dis* 22(12):2045–2053, 2016. Available from: https://wwwnc.cdc.gov/eid/article/22/12/pdfs/16-0560.pdf.

Cockburn TA: The evolution of human infectious diseases. In Cockburn T, editor: *Infectious diseases: their evolution and eradication*, Springfield, IL, 1967, Charles C Thomas.

Cohen IB: Florence nightingale, *Sci Am* 250:128–137, 1984.

Dock LL, Stewart IM: *A short history of nursing: from the earliest times to the present day*, New York, 1925, Putnam.

Donahue MP: *Nursing: the finest art*, ed 3, St. Louis, MO, 2011, Mosby/Elsevier.

Dossey BM: *Florence nightingale: mystic, visionary, healer*, Philadelphia, 2010, F.A. Davis Co.

Duffus RL: *Lillian wald: neighbor and crusader*, New York, 1938, Macmillan.

Fairman PL: *Analysis of the image of nursing and nurses as portrayed in fictional literature from 1850 to 1995*, Dissertation Abstracts, 1996, University of San Francisco.

Garn SM: Culture and the direction of human evolution, *Hum Biol* 35:221–236, 1963.

George MD: *London life in the XVIIIth century*, New York, 1925, Knopf.

Getzen T: *Health economics and financing*, ed 5, Hoboken, NJ, 2013, John Wiley & Sons.

Goodnow M: *Outlines of nursing history*, Philadelphia, 1933, WB Saunders.

Greifinger RB, Sidel VW: American medicine: charity begins at home. In Lee P, Brown N, Red I, editors: *The nation's health*, San Francisco, 1981, Boyd and Fraser.

Grier B, Grier M: Contributions of the passionate statistician, *Res Nurs Health* 1:103–109, 1978.

Hanlon JJ, Pickett GE: *Public health administration and practice*, ed 9, St. Louis, 1990, Mosby.

Hughes CC: Medical care: ethnomedicine. In Logan MH, Hunt EE, editors: *Health and the human condition*, North Scituate, MA, 1978, Duxbury Press.

Institute of Medicine (IOM): *The future of nursing*, Washington, DC, 2011, National Academies Press.

Kalisch PA, Kalisch BJ: *American nursing: a history*, ed 4, Philadelphia, 2004, Lippincott, Williams & Wilkins.

Kopf EW: Florence nightingale as statistician, *Res Nurs Health* 1:93–102, 1978.

Kowalski SL, Anthony M: Nursing's evolving role in patient safety, *Am J Nurs* 117(2):34–50, 2017.

McFarland MR, Wehbe-Alamah HB: *Leininger's transcultural nursing: concepts theories, research & practice*, ed 4, United States, 2018, McGraw-Hill.

McKeown T: Determinants of Health. In Lee P, Estes CL, editors: *The nation's health*, ed 6, Boston, MA, 2001, Jones & Bartlett.

Najman JM: Theories of disease causation and the concept of a general susceptibility: a review, *Soc Sci Med* 14A:231–237, 1990.

Nightingale F: *Notes on matters affecting the health, efficiency and hospitalization of the British Army*, London, 1858, Harrison and Sons.

Polgar S: Evolution and the ills of mankind. In Tax S, editor: *Horizons of anthropology*, Chicago, 1964, Aldine.

Richardson BW: *The health of nations: a review of the works of Edwin Chadwickl* (vol 2), London, 1887, Longmans.

Rosen G: *A History of public health, revised expanded edition*, Baltimore, MD, 2015, Johns Hopkins University Press.

Rosenberg CE: *The care of strangers*, New York, 1987, Basic Books.

Schneider MJ: *Introduction to public health*, ed 6, Burlington, MA, 2021, Jones & Bartlett.

Shi L, Singh DA: *Delivering health care in America: a systems approach*, ed 7, Boston, MA, 2019, Jones & Bartlett.

Smith FB: *The people's health 1830–1910*, London, 1979, Croom Helm.

Sparer MS, Thompson FJ: Government and health insurance. In Knickman JR, Kovner AR, editors: *Health care delivery in the United States*, ed 11, New York, 2015, Springer Publishing Co.

Thompson ME, Keeling AA: Nurse's role in the prevention of infant mortality in 1884e1925: health disparities then and now, *J Pediatr Nurs* 27:471e478, 2012.

U.S. Department of Health and Human Services, Agency for Healthcare Research and Quality: *The number of practicing primary care physicians in the United States*, 2015. Available from: http://www.ahrq.gov/research/findings/factsheets/pcwork1.html.

Wald L: *The house on Henry Street*, New York, 1971, Dover Publications (original work published 1915, Henry Holt).

3

Thinking Upstream: Nursing Theories and Population-Focused Nursing Practice

Diane Cocozza Martins

It may seem as if many community/public health challenges are so complex, so multifaceted, and so deep that it is impossible for a nurse to make substantial improvements in health. Although nurses see persons in whom cancer, cardiovascular disease, or pulmonary disease has just been diagnosed, we know that their diseases began years or even decades ago. In many cases, genetic risks for diseases are interwoven with social, economic, and environmental risks in ways that are difficult to understand and more difficult to change. In the face of all these challenges, how can nurses hope to affect the health of the public in a significant way? How can the actions nurses take today to reduce the current burden of illness and prevent illness in the next generation of citizens?

When nurses work on complex community/public health issues, they need to think strategically. They need to know where to focus their time, energy, and programmatic resources. Most likely

they will be up against health problems that have existed for years, with other layers of foundational problems that may have existed for generations. If nurses use organizational resources in an unfocused manner, they will not solve the problem at hand and may create new problems along the way. If nurses do not build strong relationships with community partners (e.g., parent groups, ministers, local activists), it will be difficult to succeed. If nurses are unable to advocate for their constituencies in a scientifically responsible, logical, and persuasive manner, they may fail. In the face of these challenges and many more, how can nurses succeed in their goal to improve public health?

Fortunately, there are road maps for success. Some of those road maps can be found by reading a nursing history book or an archival work that tells the story of a nurse who succeeded in improving health by leveraging diplomacy skills or neighborhood power, such as Lillian Wald. Other road maps may be found in "success stories" that provide an overview of how a nurse approached a problem, mobilized resources, and moved strategically to promote change. This chapter addresses another road map for success: the ability to think conceptually, almost like a chess player, to formulate a plan to solve complex problems. Thinking conceptually is a subtle skill that requires you to understand the world at an abstract level, seeing the manifestations of power, oppression, justice, and access as they exist within our communities. Most of all, thinking conceptually means that you develop a "critical eye" for the community or the population and understand how change happens at the micro and macro levels.

This chapter begins with a brief overview of nursing theory, which is followed by a discussion of the scope of community health nursing in addressing population health concerns. Several theoretical approaches are compared to demonstrate how different conceptualizations can lead to different conclusions about the range of interventions available to the nurse.

THINKING UPSTREAM: EXAMINING THE ROOT CAUSES OF POOR HEALTH

I am standing by the shore of a swiftly flowing river and hear the cry of a drowning man. I jump into the cold waters. I fight against the strong current and force my way to the struggling man. I hold on hard and gradually pull him to shore. I lay him out on the bank and revive him with artificial respiration. Just when he begins to breathe, I hear another cry for help. I jump into the cold waters. I fight against the strong current and swim forcefully to the struggling woman. I grab hold and gradually pull her to shore. I lift her out onto the bank beside the man and work to revive her with artificial respiration. Just when she begins to breathe, I hear another cry for help. I jump into the cold waters. Fighting again against the strong current, I force my way to the struggling man. I am getting tired, so with great effort I eventually pull him to shore. I lay him out on the bank and try to revive him with artificial respiration. Just when he begins to breathe, I hear another cry for help. Near exhaustion, it occurs to me that I'm so busy jumping in, pulling them to shore, and applying artificial respiration that I have no time to see who is upstream pushing them all in.

Adapted from McKinlay (2012)

In his description of the frustrations in medical practice, McKinlay (1979) used the image of a swiftly flowing river to represent illness. In this analogy, doctors are so busy rescuing victims from the river that they fail to look upstream to see who is pushing patients into the perilous waters. Many things could cause a patient to fall (or be pushed) into the waters of illness. Refocusing upstream requires nurses to look beyond individual behavior or characteristics to what McKinlay terms the "manufacturers of illness." McKinlay discusses factors such as tobacco products companies, companies that profit from selling products high in saturated fats, the alcoholic beverage industry, the beauty industry, exposure to environmental toxins, and

occupationally induced illnesses. "Manufacturers of illness" are what push clients into the river. Cigarette companies are a good example of manufacturers of illness—their product causes a change for the worse in the health status of their consumers, and they take little to no responsibility for it. McKinlay used this analogy to illustrate the ultimate futility of "downstream endeavors," which are characterized by short-term, individual-based interventions, and challenged healthcare providers to focus more of their energies "upstream, where the real problems lie" (McKinlay, 1979, p. 9). Downstream healthcare takes place in our emergency departments, critical care units, and many other healthcare settings focused on illness care. Upstream thinking actions focus on modifying economic, political, and environmental factors that are the precursors of poor health throughout the world. Although the story cites medical practice, it is equally fitting to the dilemmas of nursing practice. Nursing has a rich history of providing preventive and population-based care, but the current U.S. health system emphasizes episodic and individual-based care. According to the Centers of Disease Control and Prevention (CDC) *six in 10 Americans live with at least one chronic disease, like heart disease and stroke, cancer, or diabetes. These and other chronic diseases are the leading causes of death and disability in America, and they are also a leading driver of health care costs* (CDC, 2021).

HISTORICAL PERSPECTIVES ON NURSING THEORY

Many scholars agree that Florence Nightingale was the first nurse to formulate a conceptual foundation for nursing practice. Nightingale believed that clean water, clean linens, access to adequate sanitation, and quiet would improve health outcomes (Ali Parani, 2016). However, in the years after her leadership, the nursing practice became less theoretical and was based primarily on reacting to the immediacy of patient situations and the demands of medical staff. Thus hospital and medical personnel defined the boundaries of nursing practice. Once nursing leaders saw that others were defining their profession, they became proactive in advancing the theoretical and scientific foundations of nursing practice. Some of the early nursing theories were extremely narrow and depicted healthcare situations that involved only one nurse and one patient. Family members and other health professionals were noticeably absent from the context of care. Historically, this characterization may have been an appropriate response to the constraints of nursing practice and the need to emphasize the medically dependent activities of the nursing profession.

Although somewhat valuable, theories that address health from a microscopic, or individual, rather than a macroscopic, or global/social, perspective have limited applicability to community/public health nursing. Such perspectives are inadequate because they do not address social, political, and environmental factors that are central to an understanding of communities. More recent advances in nursing theory development address the dynamic nature of health-sustaining and/or health-damaging environments and address the nature of a collective (e.g., school, worksite) versus an individual client.

HOW THEORY PROVIDES DIRECTION TO NURSING

Nursing theory-guided practice helps improve the quality of nursing care because it allows nurses to articulate what they do for patients and why they do it (Younas and Quennell, 2019).

Theory-based practice guides data collection and interpretation in a clear and organized manner; therefore, it is easier for the nurse to diagnose and address health problems. Through the process of integrating theory and practice, the student can focus on factors that are critical to understanding the situation. The student also has an opportunity to analyze the realities of nursing practice in relation to a specific theoretical perspective, in a process of ruling in and ruling out the fit of particular concepts (Schwartz-Barcott et al., 2002). Barnum (1998) stated, "A theory is like a map of a territory as opposed to an aerial photograph. The map does not give the full terrain (i.e., the full picture); instead, it picks out those parts that are important for its given purpose" (p. 1).

As with other abstract concepts, different nursing writers have defined and interpreted theory in different ways. The lack of uniformity among these definitions reflects the evolution of thought and the individual differences in the understanding of relationships among theory, practice, and research. The definitions also reflect the difficult job of describing complex and diverse theories within the constraints of a single definition. Reading several definitions can foster an appreciation for the richness of theory and help the reader identify one or two particularly meaningful definitions. Within the profession, definitions of theory typically refer to a set of concepts and relational statements and the purpose of the theory. This chapter presents theoretical perspectives that are congruent with a broad interpretation of theory and correspond with the definitions proposed by Chinn and Kramer (2019).

MICROSCOPIC VERSUS MACROSCOPIC APPROACHES TO THE CONCEPTUALIZATION OF COMMUNITY HEALTH PROBLEMS

Each nurse must find her or his own way of interpreting the complex forces that shape societies to understand population health. The nurse can best achieve this transformation by integrating population-based practice and theoretical perspectives to conceptualize health from a macroscopic rather than microscopic perspective. Table 3.1 differentiates these two approaches to conceptualizing health problems.

The individual patient is the **microscopic focus**, whereas society or social economic factors influencing health status are the **macroscopic focus**. When the individual is the focus, the microfocus contains the health problem of interest (e.g., pediatric exposure to lead compounds). In this context, a microscopic approach to assessment would focus exclusively on individual children with lead poisoning. Nursing interventions would focus on the identification and treatment of the child and family. However, the nurse can broaden his or her view of this problem by addressing the removal of lead sources in the home and by examining interpersonal and intercommunity factors that perpetuate lead poisoning on a national scale. A macroscopic approach to lead exposure may incorporate the following activities: examining trends in the prevalence of lead poisoning over time, estimating the percentage of older homes in a neighborhood that may contain lead pipes or lead-based paint surfaces, and locating industrial sources of lead emissions. These efforts usually involve the collaborative efforts of nurses from school, occupational, government, and community settings. Burbank and Martins (2019) discussed macro-level perspectives that provide nurses with the conceptual tools that empower clients to make health decisions on the basis of the interests of the community at large.

One common dilemma in community health practice is the tension between working on behalf of individuals and working on behalf of a population. For many nurses, this tension is exemplified by the need to reconcile and prioritize multiple daily tasks. Population-directed actions are often more global than the immediate demands of ill people; therefore, they may

TABLE 3.1 Microscopic Versus Macroscopic Approaches to the Delineation of Community Health Nursing Problems

Microscopic Approach	Macroscopic Approach
Examines individual, and sometimes family, responses to health and illness	Examines interfamily and intercommunity themes in health and illness
	Delineates factors in the population that perpetuate the development of illness or foster the development of health
Often emphasizes behavioral responses to an individual's illness or lifestyle patterns	Emphasizes social, economic, and environmental precursors of illness
Nursing interventions are often aimed at modifying an individual's behavior by changing his or her perceptions or belief system	Nursing interventions may include modifying social or environmental variables (i.e., working to remove care barriers and improving sanitation or living conditions)
	May involve social or political action

sink to the bottom of the priority list. A community health nurse or nursing administrator may plan to spend the day on a community project directed at preventive efforts, such as screening programs, updating the surveillance program, or meeting with key community members about a specific preventive program. However, the nurse may actually end up spending the time responding to the emergency of the day. This type of reactive rather than proactive nursing practice prevents progress toward "big picture" initiatives and population-based programs. When faced with multiple demands, nurses must be vigilant in devoting a sustained effort toward population-focused projects. Daily pressures can easily distract the nurse from population-based nursing practice. Several nursing organizations focus on this population, and one organization, the Council of Public Health Nurse Organizations (CPHNO), represents seven member organizations:

- Alliance of Nurses for Healthy Environments (ANHE)
- Association of Community Health Nursing Educators (ACHNE)
- Association of Public Health Nurses (APHN)
- American Public Health Association (APHA), Public Health Nursing Section
- American Nurses Association (ANA)
- National Association of School Nurses (NASN)
- Rural Nurse Organization (RNO)

See https://www.cphno.org/ for more information on each of the public health nursing organizations.

A theoretical focus on the individual level of care can preclude the understanding of a larger perspective. Dreher (1982) used the term conservative scope of practice in describing frameworks that focus energy exclusively on intrapatient and nurse-patient factors. She stated that such frameworks often adopt psychological explanations of patient behavior. This mode of thinking attributes low compliance, missed appointments, and reluctant participation to problems in patient motivation or attitude. Nurses are responsible for altering patient attitudes toward health rather than altering the system itself, "even though such negative attitudes may well be a realistic appraisal of healthcare" (Dreher, 1982, p. 505). This perspective does not entertain the possibility of altering the system or empowering patients to make changes.

ASSESSING A THEORY'S SCOPE IN RELATION TO COMMUNITY HEALTH NURSING

The theoretical scope is especially important to community health nursing because there are many levels of practice within this specialty area. For example, a home health nurse who is caring for ill people after hospitalization has a very different scope of practice from that of a nurse epidemiologist or health planner. Unless a given theory is broad enough in scope to address health and the determinants of health from a population perspective, the theory will not be very useful to community health nurses. *Healthy People 2030* integrated social determinants of health into the nation's health objectives (U.S. Department of Health and Human Services, 2021). (Kaiser

Family Foundation 2018) addressed the need to understand social determinants in promoting health and health equity (Aritga and Hinton, 2018). Social determinants include factors like socioeconomic status, education, neighborhood and physical environment, employment, and social support networks, as well as access to healthcare (Artiga and Hinton, 2018, p. 2) (Box 3.1). Applying the terms *microscopic* and *macroscopic* to health situations may help nurses guide and stimulate theory development in community health nursing.

Although the concept of macroscopic is similar to the upstream analogy, the term *macroscopic* refers to a broad scope that incorporates many variables to aid in understanding a health problem. Upstream thinking would fall within this domain. Viewing a problem from this perspective emphasizes the variables that precede or play a role in the development of health problems. Macroscopic is the broad concept, and upstream is a more specific concept. These related concepts and their meanings can help nurses develop a critical eye in evaluating a theory's relevance to population health.

⑦ ACTIVE LEARNING EXERCISE

Review the ANA's definition of public health nursing practice and the APHA's Public Health Nursing Section's definition of public health nursing practice. What do these definitions indicate about the theoretical basis of community health nursing? How does the theoretical basis of community health nursing practice differ from that of other nursing specialty areas?

REVIEW OF THEORETICAL APPROACHES

The differences among theoretical approaches demonstrate how a nurse may draw very diverse conclusions about the reasons for client's decisions and the range of available interventions. The following section uses two theories to exemplify individual microscopic approaches to community/public health nursing practice; one originates within nursing and one is based on social psychology. Two other theories demonstrate the examination of nursing practice from a macroscopic perspective; one originates from nursing and another has roots in critical social theory.

The format for this review is as follows:
1. The individual is the focus of change (i.e., microscopic).
   a. Orem's self-care deficit theory of nursing
   b. The health belief model (HBM)
2. Thinking upstream: Society is the focus of change (i.e., macroscopic).
   a. Milio's framework for prevention
   b. Critical social theory perspective

The Individual Is the Focus of Change
Orem's Self-Care Deficit Theory of Nursing

In 1958, Dorothea Orem, a staff and private duty nurse who later became a faculty member at the Catholic University of America, began to formalize her insights about the purpose of

BOX 3.1 Social Determinants of Health

Economic Stability	Neighborhood and Physical Environment	Education	Food	Community and Social Context	Healthcare System
Employment	Housing	Literacy	Hunger	Social integration	Health coverage
Income	Transportation	Language	Access to healthy	Support systems	Provider availability
Expenses	Safety	Early childhood	options	Community engagement	Provider linguistic and cultural
Debt	Parks	education		Discrimination	competency
Medical bills	Playgrounds	Vocational training		Stress	Quality of care
Support	Walkability	Higher education			
	Zip code/Geography				

From kff.org.

nursing activities and why individuals required nursing care (Berbiglia and Banfield, 2014). Her theory is based on the assumption that self-care needs and activities are the primary focus of nursing practice. Orem outlined her self-care deficit theory of nursing and stated that this general theory is actually a composite of the following related constructs: the theory of self-care deficits, which provides criteria for identifying those who need nursing; the theory of self-care, which explains self-care and why it is necessary; and the theory of nursing systems, which specifies nursing's role in the delivery of care and how nursing helps people (Orem, 2001).

Application of Self-Care Deficit Theory. During a discussion about theory-based initiatives, a British occupational health nurse lamented over her nursing supervisor's intention to adopt Orem's self-care deficit theory. She was frustrated and argued that much of the model's assumptions seemed incongruous with the realities of her daily practice. Kennedy (1989) maintained that the self-care deficit theory assumes that people are able to exert purposeful control over their environments in the pursuit of health; however, people may have little control over the physical or social aspects of their work environment. On the basis of this thesis, she concluded that the self-care model is incompatible with the practice domain of occupational health nursing.

The Health Belief Model

The second theory that focuses on the individual as the locus of change is the health belief model (HBM). The model evolved from the premise that the world of the perceiver determines action. The model had its inception during the late 1950s when America was breathing a collective sigh of relief after the development of the polio vaccine. When some people chose not to bring themselves or their children into clinics for immunization, social psychologists and other public health workers recognized the need to develop a more complete understanding of factors that influence preventive health behaviors. Their efforts resulted in the HBM.

Kurt Lewin's work lent itself to the model's core dimensions. He proposed that behavior is based on current dynamics confronting an individual rather than prior experience (Maiman and Becker, 1974). Fig. 3.1 outlines the variables and relationships in the HBM. The HBM is based on the assumption that the major determinant of preventive health behavior is disease avoidance. The concept of disease avoidance includes perceived susceptibility to disease "X," perceived seriousness of disease "X," modifying factors, cues to action, perceived benefits minus perceived barriers to preventive health action, perceived threat of disease "X," and the likelihood of taking a recommended health action. Disease "X" represents a particular disorder that a health action may prevent. It is important to note that actions that relate to breast cancer will be different from those relating to measles. For example, in breast cancer, a cue to action may involve a public service advertisement encouraging women to make an appointment for a mammogram. However, for measles, a cue to action may be news of a measles outbreak in a neighboring town.

Application of the Health Belief Model. Over the years, a number of writers have proposed broadening the scope of the HBM to address health promotion and illness behaviors (Kirscht, 1974; Pender et al., 2019) and to merge its concepts with other theories that describe health behavior (Cummings et al., 1980). The following section contains a brief personal account of the author's perceptions addressing the strengths and limitations of the model.

During my nursing education classes at the undergraduate level, I was exposed to a large number of nursing theories. The HBM was probably my least favorite. Most of the content was interesting, but I found it difficult to apply the concepts to patients in the community and home settings. The model's focus on compliance was something that nurses with a critical theoretical perspective would have difficulty applying in their own clinical practice. My perception of the model changed a few years ago when my younger brother had pancreatic cancer diagnosed. This experience allowed me to see how the HBM could offer some insight into an individual's health behaviors. It helped me organize ideas about why people choose to accept or reject the instructions of well-intended nurses and doctors. Concepts such as perceived seriousness, perceived susceptibility, and cue to action afforded new insights into the dynamics of health decision making. I began to apply the model's concepts to guide my work with my family. My brother who became ill had smoked much of his life. Another brother also

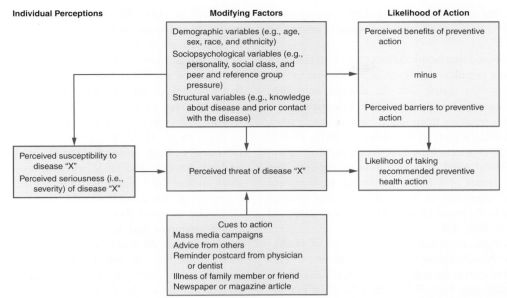

Fig. 3.1 Variables and relationships in the health belief model (HBM). (Redrawn from Rosenstock IM: Historical origins of the health belief model. In Becker MH, editor: *The health belief model and personal health behavior,* Thorofare, NJ, 1974, Charles B. Slack.)

smoked. My family members believed that you are destined to follow a path of life and death, but this experience clearly modified their health beliefs. Until this point, my family members did not quit smoking because they did not perceive the susceptibility and seriousness of smoking; they belonged to a reference group that disdained most traditional medical practices and favored inaction over action. During the next several weeks, my siblings requested information on strategies that would help them quit smoking and hopefully decrease their chances for the development of cancer.

Over the years, I have become more skilled in assessing and identifying patient needs and issues and have gained a better appreciation for the strengths and limitations that any theoretical framework imposes on a situation.

Studies Using the Health Belief Model. Studies have used use the predictive abilities of HBM concepts (Shmueli, 2021). In this study, the author explored the intentions, motivators, and barriers of the general public to vaccinate against COVID-19, using both the Health Belief Model (HBM) and the Theory of Planned Behavior (TPB) model. The researcher found that providing data on the public perspective and predicting intention for COVID-19 vaccination using HBM and TPB is important for health policymakers and healthcare providers and can help better guide compliance with the COVID-19 vaccine. In another study, the HBM constructs of perceived threat, perceived barriers, perceived benefits, perceived self-efficacy, and cues to action were used to reinforce COVID-19 behaviors such as social distancing and remaining home whenever possible. community pharmacists were shown to have a direct role in combating misinformation and helping patients select healthy behaviors (Carico et al., 2021).

The HBM may effectively promote behavioral change by altering patients' perspectives, but it does not acknowledge the health professional's responsibility to reduce or ameliorate healthcare barriers. The model reflects the type of theoretical perspective that dominates behavioral health. The narrow scope of the model is its strength and its limitation: nurses are not challenged to examine the root causes of health opportunities and behaviors in the communities and with the populations we serve.

The Upstream View: Society Is the Focus of Change

Milio's Framework for Prevention

Nancy Milio (1985) conducted extensive research on tobacco policy. Milio's (1981) approach to advancing people's health is seen in her seminal book, *Promoting Health Through Public Policy,* and through her detailed studies of tobacco policy and Norwegian farm food policy (Draper, 1986). **Milio's framework for prevention** (Milio, 1976) provides a complement to the HBM and a mechanism for directing attention upstream and examining opportunities for nursing intervention at the population level. Nancy Milio outlined six propositions that relate an individual's ability to improve healthful behavior to a society's ability to provide accessible and socially affirming options for healthy choices. Milio used these propositions to move the focus of attention upstream by challenging the notion that the main determinant for unhealthful behavioral choices is lack of knowledge. She said that government and institutional policies set the range of health options, so community health nursing needs to examine a community's level of health and attempt to influence it through public policy. She noted that the range of available health choices is critical in shaping a society's overall health status. Milio believed that national-level policy-making was the best way to favorably affect the health of most Americans rather than concentrating efforts on imparting information in an effort to change individual patterns of behavior.

Milio (1976) proposed that health deficits often result from an imbalance between a population's health needs and its health-sustaining resources. She stated that the diseases associated with excess (e.g., obesity and alcoholism) afflict affluent societies and that the diseases resulting from inadequate or unsafe food, shelter, and water afflict the poor. Within this context, the poor in affluent societies may experience the least desirable combination of factors. Milio (1976) cited the socioeconomic realities that deprive many Americans of a health-sustaining environment despite the fact that "cigarettes, sucrose, pollutants, and tensions are readily available to the poor" (p. 436). Propositions proposed by Milio are listed in Table 3.2.

Personal and societal resources affect the range of health-promoting or health-damaging choices available to individuals. Personal resources include the individual's awareness, knowledge, and beliefs and the beliefs of the individual's family and friends. Money, time, and the urgency of other priorities are also personal resources. Community and national locale strongly influence societal resources. These resources include the availability and cost of health services, environmental protection, safe shelter, and the penalties or rewards for failure to select the given options.

Milio (1976) challenged health education's assumption that knowledge of health-generating behaviors implies an act in accordance with that knowledge. She proposed that "most human beings, professional or nonprofessional, provider or consumer, make the easiest choices available to them most of

the time" (p. 435). Health-promoting choices must be more readily available and less costly than health-damaging options for individuals to gain health and for society to improve its health status. Milio's framework can enable a nurse to reframe this view by understanding the historical play of social forces that have limited the choices available to the parties involved.

Comparison of the HBM and Milio's Conceptualizations of Health. Milio's health resources bear some resemblance to the concepts in the HBM. The purpose of the HBM is to provide the nurse with an understanding of the dynamics of personal health behaviors. The HBM specifies broader contextual variables, such as the constraints of the healthcare system, and their influence on the individual's decision-making processes. The HBM also assumes that each person has unlimited access to health resources and free will. In contrast, Milio based her framework on an assessment of community resources and their availability to individuals. By assessing such factors upfront, the nurse is able to gain a more thorough understanding of the resources people actually have. Milio offered a different set of insights into the health behavior arena by proposing that many low-income individuals are acting within the constraints of their limited resources. furthermore, she investigated beyond downstream focus and population health by examining the choices of significant numbers of people within a population.

Compared with the HBM, Milio's framework provides for the inclusion of economic, political, and environmental health determinants; therefore, the nurse is given a broader range in the diagnosis and interpretation of health problems. Whereas the HBM allows only two possible outcomes (i.e., "acts" or

TABLE 3.2   Application of Milio's Framework in Public Health Nursing

Milio's Proposition Summary	Population Health Examples
Population health results from deprivation and/or excess of critical health resources.	Individuals and families living in poverty have poorer health status compared with middle- and upper-class individuals and families.
Behaviors of populations result from selection from limited choices; these arise from actual and perceived options available, as well as beliefs and expectations resulting from socialization, education, and experience.	Positive and negative lifestyle choices (e.g., smoking, alcohol use, safe sex practices, regular exercise, diet/nutrition, seatbelt use) are strongly dependent on culture, socioeconomic status, and educational level.
Organizational decisions and policies (both governmental and nongovernmental) dictate many of the options available to individuals and populations and influence choices.	Health insurance coverage and availability are largely determined and financed by federal and state governments (e.g., Medicare and Medicaid) and employers (e.g., private insurance); the source and funding of insurance very strongly influence health provider choices and services.
Individual choices related to health-promoting or health-damaging behaviors are influenced by efforts to maximize valued resources.	Choices and behaviors of individuals are strongly influenced by desires, values, and beliefs. For example, the use of barrier protection during sex by adolescents is often dependent on peer pressure and the need for acceptance, love, and belonging.
Alteration in patterns of behavior resulting from decision making of a significant number of people in a population can result in social change.	Some behaviors, such as tobacco use, have become difficult to maintain in many settings or situations in response to organizational and public policy mandates. As a result, tobacco use in the United States has dropped dramatically.
Without concurrent availability of alternative health-promoting options for investment of personal resources, health education will be largely ineffective in changing behavior patterns.	Addressing persistent health problems (e.g., overweight/obesity) is hindered because most people are very aware of what causes the problem, but are reluctant to make lifestyle changes to prevent or reverse the condition. Often, "new" information (e.g., a new diet) or resources (e.g., a new medication) can assist in attracting attention and directing positive behavior changes.

Adapted from Milio N: A framework for prevention: changing health-damaging to health-generating life patterns, *Am J Pub Heath* 66:435–439, 1976.

"fails to act" according to the recommended health action), Milio's framework encourages the nurse to understand health behaviors in the context of their societal milieu.

Implications of Milio's Framework for Current Health Delivery Systems. Through its broader scope, Milio's model provides direction for nursing interventions at many levels. Nurses may use this model to assess the personal and societal resources of individual patients and to analyze social and economic factors that may inhibit healthy choices in populations. Population-based interventions may include such diverse activities as working to improve the nutritional content of school lunches and encouraging political activity to improve health outcomes.

Overall, current healthcare delivery systems perform best when responding to people with diagnostic-intensive and acute illnesses. Those people who experience chronic debilitation or have less intriguing diagnoses generally fare worse in the healthcare system despite efforts by the community- and home-based care to "fill the gaps." Nurses in both hospital and community-based systems often feel constrained by profound financial and service restrictions imposed by third-party payers. These third parties often terminate nursing care after the resolution of the latest immediate health crisis and fail to cover care aimed toward long-term health improvements. Many health systems use nursing standards and reimbursement mechanisms that originate from a narrow, compartmentalized view of health.

Personal behavior patterns are not simply "free" choices about "lifestyle" that are isolated from their personal and economic context. Lifestyles are patterns of choices made from available alternatives according to people's socioeconomic circumstances and how easily they are able to choose some over others (Milio, 1981). It is therefore imperative to practice nursing from a broader understanding of health, illness, and suffering. Public health nurses must often work at both the individual and societal levels. As Milio suggested, it is not only individual behaviors but the economic context as well. This can be seen in Table 3.3, which shows that the focus of change can be at the individual or societal level.

Critical Theoretical Perspective

Similar to Milio's framework for prevention, a critical theoretical perspective uses societal awareness to expose social inequalities that keep people from reaching their full potential. This perspective is devised from the belief that social meanings structure life through social domination. "A critical perspective can be used to understand the linkages between the healthcare system and the broader political, economic, and social systems of society" (Waitzkin, 1983, p. 5). According to Navarro (1976), in *Medicine Under Capitalism*, the healthcare system mirrors the class structure of the broader society. According to Conrad and Leiter (2019), a critical theoretical perspective is one that does not regard the present structure of healthcare as sacred. A critical theoretical perspective accepts no truth or fact merely because it has been accepted as such in the past. The social aspects of health and illness are too complex to use only one

TABLE 3.3 **Comparison of Individual and Societal Levels of Change**	
Individual Level	**Societal Level**
The individual is the focus of change	Society/community is the focus of change
Microscopic	Macroscopic
Downstream activities emphasized	Upstream activities emphasized
Theories:	Theories:
1. Orem's self-care deficit theory of nursing	a. Milio's framework for prevention
2. The health belief model (HBM)	b. Critical social theory perspective

perspective. The critical theoretical perspective assumes that health and illness entail societal and personal values and that these values have to be made explicit if illness and healthcare problems are to be satisfactorily dealt with. This perspective is informed by the following values and assumptions:

- The problems and inequalities of health and healthcare are connected to the particular historically located social arrangements and the cultural values of society.
- Healthcare should be oriented toward the prevention of disease and illness.
- The priorities of any healthcare system should be based on the needs of the clients/population and not the healthcare providers.
- Ultimately, society itself must be changed for health and medical care to improve (Conrad and Leiter, 2019).

Stevens and Hall (1992) used a critical theoretical perspective in nursing to address unsafe neighborhoods as well as the economic, political, and social disadvantages of the communities we serve. They advocate for emancipator nursing actions for our communities. Proponents of this theoretical approach maintain that social exchanges that are not distorted by power imbalances will stimulate the evolution of a more just society (Allen et al., 1986). The critical theoretical perspective assumes that truth standards are socially determined and that no form of scientific inquiry is value free. Allen et al. (1986) stated, "One cannot separate theory and value, as the empiricist claims. Every theory is penetrated by value interests" (p. 34).

Application of Critical Theoretical Perspective. Critical theory has been applied to nursing in communities. Application of a critical theoretical perspective can be seen when healthcare is used as a form of social control. The social control function in healthcare is used to get patients to adhere to norms of appropriate behavior. This is accomplished through the medicalization of a wide range of psychological and socioeconomic issues. *Medicalization* is the identification or categorization of (a condition or behavior) as being a disorder requiring medical treatment or intervention. Examples include medicalization related to sexuality, family life, aging, learning disabilities, and dying (Conrad, 1975, 1992; Zola, 1972). Medicalization can incorporate many facets of health and illness care, from childbirth and allergies to hyperactivity and hospitals that have become dominated by the medical profession and its explanation of health and illness. When social problems are medicalized, there is often profit to be made. This can be seen when a patient readily receives a prescription for medication before the root social cause of the illness is addressed by the healthcare provider. Using medical treatments for "undesirable behavior" has been implemented throughout history, including lobectomies for mental illness and synthetic stimulants for classroom behavior problems.

In this context, the nurse may examine how the concepts of power and empowerment influence access to quality childcare (Kuokkanen and Leino-Kilpi, 2000). The nurse may contrast an organization's policies with interviews with workers who believe the organization is an impediment to achieving quality childcare. Data analysis may also include an examination of the interests of workers and administration in promoting social change versus maintaining the status quo.

Wild (1993) used critical social theory to analyze the social, political, and economic conditions associated with the cost of prescription analgesics and the corresponding financial burden on clients who require these medications. Wild compared the trends in pharmaceutical pricing with the inflation rates of other commodities. The study stated that pharmaceutical sales techniques, which market directly to physicians, the distance the needs of ill clients from the pharmaceutical industry. Wild's analysis specified nursing actions that a downstream analysis would not consider, such as challenging pricing policies on behalf of client groups.

Challenging Assumptions About Preventive Health Through Critical Theoretical Perspective.
The HBM and Milio's prevention model focuses on personal health behaviors from a disease avoidance or preventive health perspective; nurses may also analyze this phenomenon using critical social theory. Again, McKinlay's upstream analogy refers to health workers who were so busy fishing sick people out of the river that they did not look upstream to see how they were ending up in the water. Later in the same article, McKinlay (1979) used his upstream analogy to ask the rhetorical question, "How preventive is prevention?" (p. 22). He used this tactic to critically examine different intervention strategies aimed at enhancing preventive behavior. Fig. 3.2 illustrates McKinlay's model, which contrasts the different modes of prevention. He linked health professionals' curative and lifestyle modification interventions to a downstream conceptualization of health; the majority of alleged preventive actions fail to alter the process of illness at its origin. Political-economic interventions remain the

most effective way to address population determinants of health and to ameliorate illness at its source.

McKinlay (1979) delineated the activities of the "manufacturers of illness—those individuals, interest groups, and organizations which, in addition to producing material goods and services, also produce, as an inevitable by-product, widespread morbidity and mortality" (pp. 9, 10). The manufacturers of illness embed desired behaviors in the dominant cultural norm and thus foster the habituation of high-risk behavior in the population. Unhealthy consumption patterns are integrated into everyday lives; for example, the American holiday dinner table offers concrete examples of "the binding of at-riskness to culture" (p. 12). The existing U.S. healthcare system, in a misguided attempt to help, devotes its efforts to change the products of the illness manufacturers and neglects the processes that create the products. Manufacturers of illness include the tobacco industry, the alcohol industry, and multiple corporations that produce environmental carcinogens.

Waitzkin (1983) continued this theme by asserting that the healthcare system's emphasis on lifestyle diverts attention from important sources of illness in the capitalist industrial environment and "it also puts the burden of health squarely on the individual rather than seeking collective solutions to health problems" (p. 664). Salmon (1987) supported this position by noting that the basic tenets of Western medicine promote an understanding of individual health and illness factors and obscure the exploration of their social and economic roots. He stated that critical social theory "can aid in uncovering larger dimensions impacting health that are usually unseen or misrepresented by ideological biases. Thus the social reality of health conditions can be both understood and changed" (p. 75).

In the past decade, a critical theoretical perspective has been used with *symbolic interactionism,* a theory that focuses predominantly on the individual and the meaning of situations. **Critical interactionism** brings the two theories together to address some issues at both upstream and downstream levels to make healthcare system changes Burbank and Martins (2019). Nurses can use both upstream and downstream approaches to address health issues through critical interactionism (Table 3.4).

Nurses in all practice settings face the challenge of understanding and responding to collective health within the context of a health system that allocates resources at the individual

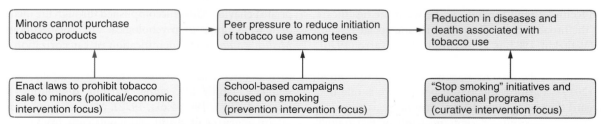

Fig. 3.2 McKinlay's model of continuum of health behaviors and corresponding interventions foci applied to tobacco use. (Data from McKinlay J: A case for refocusing upstream: the political economy of illness. In Gartley J, editor: *Patients, physicians and illness: a sourcebook in behavioral science and health,* New York, 1979, Free Press, pp. 9–25.)

TABLE 3.4   Critical Interactionism: Comparison of Upstream and Downstream Focuses

Issue	Downstream Focus	Upstream Focus	Critical Interactionism: An Upstream/Downstream Approach
Clients: Obesity rates	Individual behavior strategies to reduce weight Lifestyle changes Bariatric surgery nursing care	Health policy changes Vending machines in schools with healthier choices School lunch program modifications Target corporations that profit from obesity	Individual strategies with weight loss in conjunction with system changes Social marketing at both levels
Client or nurse: Workplace violence	Behavior change at individual level Workplace programs to reduce violence	Address organizational factors that promote workplace violence What organizational structures perpetuate workplace violence?	Change needed in knowledge and skills to address issue of workplace violence at both the downstream and upstream levels
Nurse: Workplace errors	Focus on individual: Root-cause analysis that has the individual as the focus Change the behavior of the individual nurse Reeducation of nurse with workplace error	System changes needed What system-level factors lead to workplace errors? What organizational structures perpetuate workplace errors?	A dual approach: Providers need changes in knowledge and skills to address root causes of workplace errors that move from individual to system level

Data from Martins DC, Burbank P: Critical interactionism: an upstream-downstream approach to healthcare reform, *Adv Nur Sci* 34(4):315–329, 2011.

level. The Tavistock Group (1999) released a set of ethical principles that summarizes this juxtaposition by noting that "the care of individuals is at the center of healthcare delivery but must be viewed and practiced within the overall context of continuing work to generate the greatest possible health gains for groups and populations" (pp. 2, 3). This perspective is an accurate reflection of Western-oriented thought, which generally gives individual health precedence over collective health. Although nurses can appreciate the concept of individual care at the center of health delivery, they should also consider transposing this principle. Doing so allows the nurse to consider a healthcare system that places the community in the center of healthcare and holds the goal of generating health gains for individuals. Fortunately, these worldviews of health delivery systems are not mutually exclusive, and nurses can understand the duality of healthcare needs in individuals and populations.

activities. Although social justice activities are alive and well in nursing practice, many leaders think that the continuing struggle for resources is taking its toll on the scope of social action within community health systems. In addition, the policies of the current federal administration often emphasize market justice values over social justice values. *Market justice* refers to the principle that people are entitled to valued ends (e.g., status, income) when they acquire them through fair rules of entitlement. In contrast, *social justice* refers to the principle that all citizens bear equitably the benefits and burdens of society (Drevdahl et al., 2001). These are complex concepts that cannot be easily distilled into a clear set of rules or nursing policies. However, in the context of community health nursing, health (and consequently healthcare) is considered a right rather than a privilege. To the extent that certain citizens, by virtue of their income, race, health needs, or any other attribute, are unable to access healthcare, our society as a whole suffers. Nurses are well positioned to "stand on the shoulders" of yesterday's nursing leaders and act on behalf of justice in healthcare access for all citizens.

ACTIVE LEARNING EXERCISE

- Select a theory or conceptual model. Evaluate its potential for understanding health in individuals, families, a population of 400 children in an elementary school, a community of 50,000 residents, and 2000 workers within a corporate setting.
- Identify one health problem (e.g., opioid overdoses, intimate partner violence, or cardiovascular disease) that is prevalent in the community or city. Analyze the problem using two different theories or conceptual models. One should emphasize individual determinants of health, and another should emphasize population determinants of health. What are some differences in the way these different perspectives inform nursing practice?

ETHICAL INSIGHTS

Social Injustice in Community-Based Practice

Chafey (1996) refers to "putting justice to work in community-based practice" and notes that nursing has a rich historical legacy in social justice

Healthy People 2030

Healthy People 2030 continued to integrate the population level with social determinants of health and emphasized the need to eliminate health disparities, achieve health equity, and attain health literacy to improve the health and well-being of all. To ensure that all Americans have that opportunity to have improved health outcomes, advances are needed not only in healthcare but also in the areas of housing and neighborhoods, income, education, healthy food, and discrimination. Making these advances would involve working together to explore how programs, practices, and policies in these areas affect the health of individuals, families, and populations (U.S. Department of Health and Human Services, 2021).

The pictures in this chapter's photo novella present environmental health issues and efforts being taken by nurses to address them.

NURSES WORK IN ENVIRONMENTAL HEALTH IN A VARIETY OF WAYS

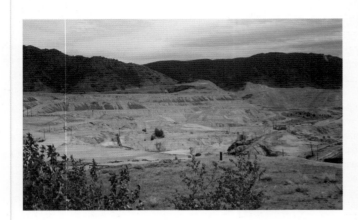

Open mine waste in the rural West can pose a continuing threat to local citizens. Nurses have been involved in advocacy efforts to ensure that citizens receive periodic screening for exposure to lead. Nurses can be active in policy efforts to prevent environmental disasters in the future.

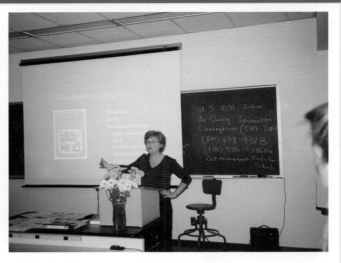

A public health nurse teaches a class on environmental health for local nurses. Environmental health is an important part of community health nursing's expanding practice.

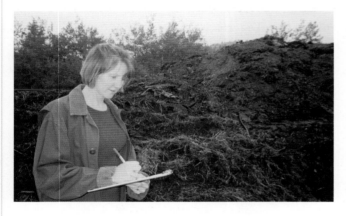

A public health nurse inspects the site of an asphalt spill off a rural railway car. Hazardous materials spills often occur in remote areas away from healthcare services. Broad conceptual frameworks allow nurses to think upstream and incorporate environmental risks into the consideration of community health issues.

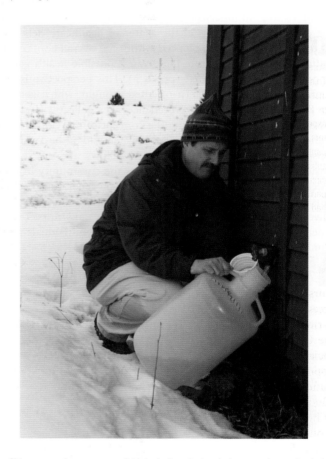

Citizens can be unaware of biological and chemical contaminants in their drinking water. Nurses are playing more active roles in water testing and in communicating the results of such tests to community members. When health is conceptualized broadly, nurses understand and view risk in new ways.

Continued

NURSES WORK IN ENVIRONMENTAL HEALTH IN A VARIETY OF WAYS—cont'd

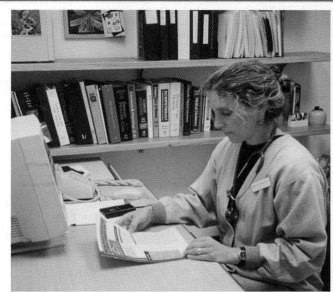

A nurse practitioner reviews educational materials addressing occupational and environmental health risks. By providing guidance, the nurse is working to reduce risks and empower her clients to reduce their personal and community-based risks.

RESEARCH HIGHLIGHTS

Assessment of Hunger With the Homeless Populations

This study examined the relationship between nutritional status, food insecurity, and health risk among the population experiencing homelessness in Rhode Island (RI). A correlational study used a sample of 319 adults experiencing homelessness surveyed for access to emergency foods, shelters, and the Supplemental Nutrition Assistance Program (SNAP). Participants completed a U.S. Department of Agriculture Food Security Module subset. Anthropometric measures included height, weight, and waist circumference. A 24-h food diary was also collected. Findings indicated that participants had insufficient vegetables, fruit, dairy, and meat/beans but they had excessive amounts of fats. Almost 70% were overweight or obese.

Ninety-four percent were food insecure, with 64% of this subset experiencing hunger. Only 55% were currently receiving SNAP benefits. Participants expressed concern about having no kitchen or ability to store or prepare food with their SNAP benefit.

The study results led to policy change in RI. The SNAP was expanded to include a *Restaurant Meals Program* so that the homeless, elderly, and disabled could use their SNAP benefits for prepared foods. This is now utilized across the state.

Adapted from Martins DC, et al.: Assessment of food intake, obesity and health risk among the homeless in Rhode Island, *Publ Health Nurs* 32(5):453–461, 2015.

SUMMARY

Nursing and health service literature often focuses on healthcare access issues. This topic is interesting because tremendous disparities in access exist between insured and uninsured people in the United States. Access to care is associated with economic, social, and political factors, and, depending on individual and population needs, it can be a primary determinant of health status and survival. Structural variables, such as race-ethnicity, educational status, gender, and income, maybe highly predictive of health status. These types of factors, which are also strongly grounded in the sociopolitical and economic milieu, identify risk factors for poor health and opportunities for community-based interventions.

Community/public health nurses have been instrumental in making many of the lifesaving advances in sanitation, communicable diseases, and environmental conditions that today's society takes for granted. Community/public health practice helps develop a broad context of nursing practice because community environments are inherently less restrictive than hospital settings.

In a discussion addressing the future of community/public health nursing, Bellack (1998) differentiates between "nursing in the community" and "nursing with the community." This subtle reframing of the nursing role reinforces the notion that the health agenda originates from natural leaders, church members, local officials, parents, children, teens, and other community members. Forming and advancing a shared vision of health can be a formidable challenge for the nurse; as with any other complex issue, multiple viewpoints are the norm. Even "naming" health problems can be difficult because different constituents are likely to see issues differently and pursue different lines of reasoning. However, allowing the genesis of change to occur from within the community is the essential challenge of nursing with the community. "Nursing with the community" efforts allow the nurse to create agendas that arise from community members rather than those imposed on community members. Listening, being patient, providing accurate and scientifically sound information, and respecting the experiences of community members are essential to the success of these efforts.

The nursing profession has advanced and with it so has the need to develop nursing theories that formalize the scientific base of community health nursing. The richness of community health nursing comes from the challenge of conceptualizing and implementing strategies that will enhance the health of many people. Likewise, nurses in this practice area must have access to theoretical perspectives that address the social, political, and environmental determinants of population health. The integration of population-based theory with practice gives nurses the means to favorably affect the health of the global community.

EVOLVE WEBSITE

http://evolve.elsevier.com/Nies/community
- NCLEX Review Questions
- Case Studies

BIBLIOGRAPHY

Ali Pirani SS: Application of Nightingale's theory in nursing practice, *Ann Nurs Pract* 3(1):1040, 2016.

Allen DG, Diekelmann N, Benner P: Three paradigms for nursing research: methodologic implications. In Chinn P, editor: *Nursing research methodology: issues and implementation*, Rockville, MD, 1986, Aspen Publishers.

Artiga S, Hinton E: *Beyond health care: the role of social determinants in promoting health and health equity*, In Kaiser Family Foundation's Racial Equity & Health Policy, 2018. Available from: www.kff.org/racial-equity-and-health-policy/issue-brief/beyond-health-care-the-role-of-social-determinants-in-promoting-health-and-health-equity/2021.

Barnum BS. In *Nursing theory: analysis, application, evaluation*, ed 5, Philadelphia, 1998, Lippincott.

Bellack JP: Community-based nursing practice: necessary but not sufficient, *J Nurs Educ* 37(3):99–100, 1998.

Berbiglia V, Banfield B: Self-care deficit theory of nursing. In Alligood M, editor: *Nursing theorists and their work*, ed 8, St. Louis, MO, 2014, Elsevier Mosby.

Berwick D, Davidoff F, Hiatt H, et al.: Refining and implementing the Tavistock principles for everybody in health care, *Br J Med* 323:616–620, 2000.

Burbank P, Martins DC: Critical interactionism: a theoretical bridge for understanding complex human conditions. In Jacobsen MH, editor: *Critical and cultural interactionism: insights from sociology and criminology*, London, 2019, Routledge, Ch. 5.

Carico R, Sheppard J, Thomas B: Community pharmacists and communication in the time of COVID-19: applying the health belief model, *Res Soc Adm Pharm* 17(1):1984–1987, 2021.

Centers for Disease Control and Prevention: *National Center for Chronic Disease Prevention and Health Promotion: chronic disease prevention*, 2021. Available from: https://www.cdc.gov/chronicdisease/index.htm.

Chafey K: Caring is not enough: ethical paradigms for community-based care, *N HC Perspect Communit* 17(1):10–15, 1996.

Chinn P, Kramer M. In *Knowledge development in nursing: theory and process*, ed 10, St Louis, MO, 2019, Elsevier.

Conrad P: The discovery of hyperkinesis: notes on the medicalization of deviant behavior, *Soc Probl* 23:12–21, 1975.

Conrad P: Medicalization and social control, *Annu Rev Sociol* 18:209–232, 1992.

Conrad P, Leiter V. In *The sociology of heath and illness: critical perspectives*, ed 10, Thousand Oaks, California, 2019, Sage.

Cummings KM, Becker MH, Malie MC: Bringing the models together: an empirical approach to combining variables to explain health actions, *J Behav Med* 3:123–145, 1980.

Draper P: Nancy Milio's work and its importance for the development of health promotion, *Health Promot Int* 1(1):101–106, 1986.

Dreher M: The conflict of conservatism in public health nursing education, *Nurs Outlook* 30(9):504–509, 1982.

Drevdahl D, Kneipp S, Canales M, et al.: Reinvesting in social justice: a capital idea for public health nursing? *ANS Adv Nurs Sci* 24(2):19–31, 2001.

Kaiser Family Foundation: *Beyond Health Care: The Role of SDOH in Promoting Health and Health Equity*, 2018. Retrieved 26 May 2022, https://files.kff.org/attachment/issue-brief-beyond-health-care.

Kennedy A: How relevant are nursing models? *Occup Health* 41(12):352–354, 1989.

Kirscht JP: The health belief model and illness behavior. In Becker MH, editor: *The health belief model and personal health behavior*, Thorofare, NJ, 1974, Charles B. Slack.

Kuokkanen L, Leino-Kilpi H: Power and empowerment in nursing: three theoretical approaches, *J Adv Nurs* 31(1):235–241, 2000.

Maiman LA, Becker MH: The health belief model: origins and correlates in psychological theory. In Becker MH, editor: *The health belief model and personal health behavior*, Thorofare, NJ, 1974, Charles B. Slack.

Martins DC, Gorman K, Miller R, et al.: Assessment of food intake, obesity and health risk among the homeless in Rhode Island, *Publ Health Nurs* 32(5):453–461, 2015.

McKinlay J: A case for refocusing upstream: the political economy of illness. In Gartley J, editor: *Patients, physicians and illness: a sourcebook in behavioral science and health*, New York, 1979, Free Press.

McKinlay JB: A case for refocusing upstream: the political economy of illness. In Conrad P, Leiter V, editors: *The sociology of health and illness: critical perspectives*, ed 9, New York, 2012, Worth Publishing.

Milio N: A framework for prevention: changing health-damaging to health-generating life patterns, *Am J Publ Health* 66:435–439, 1976.

Milio N: *Promoting health through public policy*, Philadelphia, 1981, FA Davis.

Milio N: Health policy and the emerging tobacco reality, *Soc Sci Med* 21(6):603–613, 1985.

Navarro V: *Medicine under capitalism*, New York, 1976, Prodist.

Orem DE. In *Nursing: concepts of practice*, ed 6, New York, 2001, Mosby.

Pender N, Parsons M, Murdaugh C. In *Health promotion in nursing practice*, ed 8, New York, 2019, Pearson.

Salmon JW: Dilemmas in studying social change versus individual change: considerations from political economy. In Duffy M, Pender NJ, editors: *Conceptual issues in health promotion: a report of proceedings of a wingspread conference*, Indianapolis, IN, 1987, Sigma Theta Tau.

Shmueli L: Predicting intention to receive COVID-19 vaccine among the general population using the health belief model and the theory of planned behavior model, *BMC Publ Health* 21:804, 2021. https://doi.org/10.1186/s12889-021-10816-7.

Schwartz-Barcott D, Patterson BJ, Lusardi P, et al.: From practice to theory: tightening the link via three fieldwork strategies, *J Adv Nurs* 39(3):281—289, 2002.

Stevens PE, Hall JM: Applying critical theories to nursing in communities, *Publ Health Nurs* 9(1):2—9, 1992.

Tavistock Group: A shared statement of ethical principles for those who shape and give health care: a working draft from the Tavistock group, *Image—J Nurs Scholarsh* 31(2—3), 1999.

U.S. Department of Health and Human Services: *Healthy People 2030: social determinants of health*, 2021. Available from: https://health.gov/healthypeople.

Waitzkin H: A Marxist view of health and health care. In Mechanic D, editor: *Handbook of health, health care, and the health professions*, New York, 1983, Free Press.

Wild LR: Caveat emptor: a critical analysis of the costs of drugs used for pain management, *Adv Nurs Sci* 16:52—61, 1993.

Younas A, Quennell S: Usefulness of nursing Theory-guided practice: an integrative review, *Scand J Caring Sci* 33(3):540—555, 2019. https://doi.org/10.1111/scs.12670. Epub 2019 Mar 13. PMID: 30866078.

Zola I: Medicine as an institution of social control, *Sociol Rev* 20(4):487—504, 1972.

4

Health Promotion and Risk Reduction

Bridgette Crotwell Pullis and Mary A. Nies

OBJECTIVES

Upon completion of this chapter, the reader will be able to do the following:

1. Discuss various theories of health promotion, including Pender's Health Promotion Model, the Health Belief Model, the Transtheoretical Theory, and the Theory of Reasoned Action.
2. Discuss definitions of health.
3. Demonstrate an understanding of the difference between health promotion and health protection.
4. Define risk.
5. Discuss the relationship of risk to health and health promotion activities.
6. Demonstrate an understanding of the stratification of risk factors by age, race, and gender.
7. Discuss the influence of various factors on health.
8. List health behaviors for health promotion and disease prevention.
9. Relate the clinical implications of health promotion activities.

OUTLINE

KEY TERMS

determinants of health
health
health promotion

health protection
portion distortion
risk

risk communication
risk reduction

HEALTH PROMOTION AND COMMUNITY HEALTH NURSING

Since its inception, nursing has focused on helping individuals, groups, and communities maintain and protect their health. Florence Nightingale and other nursing pioneers recognized the importance of nutrition, rest, and hygiene in maximizing and protecting one's state of health. Though people are responsible for their health and medical care, they often seek advice from nurses in the community regarding health promotion and to help them make sense of the many, often competing recommendations that appear daily on TV, online, and in newspapers and magazines.

Green and Kreuter (1991) define health promotion as "any combination of health education and related organizational, economic, and environmental supports for behavior of individuals, groups, or communities conducive to health" (p. 2). Parse (1990) states that health promotion is that which is motivated by the desire to increase well-being and to reach the best possible health potential. This chapter's photo novella provides some examples of nurses engaging in health promotion.

Consider the clinical example of Jamie R. in Clinical Example 4.1. Jamie exemplifies this motivation to stay in her best health, at least at first glance. Let's look further into Jamie's health history.

HEALTH PROMOTION IN THE COMMUNITY

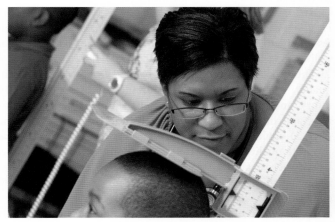

Elementary school screening: A nursing student takes height and weight measurements, which serve as a baseline to measure the growth rate of students.

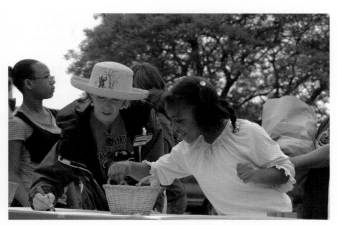

A Veggie Fair in the community teaches children and their parents about the benefits of eating vegetables.

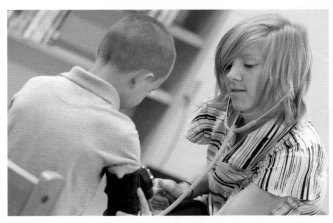

Elementary school screening: A nursing student securely holds the cuff as she takes this little boy's blood pressure.

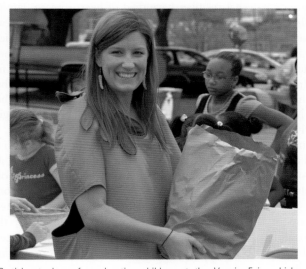

Participants have fun educating children at the Veggie Fair, which will hopefully lead children and their parents to enjoy vegetables as a nutritious part of their daily diet.

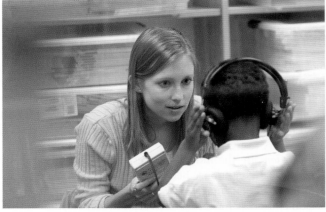

Elementary school screening: A nursing student watches and listens as she gives a hearing test.

Clinical Example 4.1

Jamie R. is a lifelong athlete. Married with three grown children, she rises at 4:20 each morning to go to the gym to swim for an hour before going to her job as an executive with a large company. A nonsmoker, Jamie rarely drinks alcohol and eats a diet consisting mostly of vegetables, grains, and fruit. Jamie's body mass index is in the normal range, and though her cholesterol and triglyceride levels are elevated, she does not require medication for this issue. After work, Jamie and her husband relax by walking their two dogs and reading. An early riser, Jamie is in bed by 9:30 almost every night. At 50 years of age, Jamie is youthful and energetic.

We all have friends like Jamie—people who seem to have an endless amount of energy and self-discipline. The rest of us, however, are typically less successful in achieving our health promotion goals.

When it comes to health practices, Jamie is a study in contradictions. Jamie's father had a myocardial infarction (MI) at the age of 48 years and died of an MI at the age of 50 years. Many of Jamie's paternal relatives have died of heart disease. Jamie's mother and one maternal aunt were each diagnosed with breast cancer in their early 50s. Though she has an annual physical examination by her family doctor and monitors her blood cholesterol and triglycerides, Jamie has never been screened for cardiac disease. Jamie receives the flu vaccine every year but has not had a tetanus-diphtheria vaccine booster in 14 years and has not had the shingles vaccine; though she sees her gynecologist yearly, she has had only one mammogram, 3 years ago.

In skipping annual mammograms and in not pursuing cardiac screening despite her high risk, Jamie is neglecting an important step in maintaining her health—health protection. Health protection consists of those behaviors in which one engages with the specific intent to prevent disease, detect disease in the early stages, or maximize health within the constraints of disease (Parse, 1990). Immunizations and cervical cancer screening are examples of health protection activities.

In discussing health promotion, it is helpful to define what is meant by health. One definition states that health is "being sound in body, mind, and spirit: freedom from physical disease or pain" (Merriam-Webster, 2009). As health promotion has become an important strategy to improve health, the way health is defined has shifted from a focus on the curative model to a focus on multidimensional aspects such as the social, cultural, and environmental facets of life and health (Benson, 1996). The well-known definition by the World Health Organization (WHO) states that health is "a state of complete physical, mental and social well-being, and not merely the absence of disease" (WHO, 2009). WHO also states that health is the extent to which an individual or group is able to realize aspirations, satisfy needs, and change or cope with the environment. In this aspect, health is viewed not only as an important goal but also as a resource for a living (WHO, 1986).

 Healthy People 2030

Healthy People is a health promotion initiative for the nation. Developed through a consortium and managed by the U.S. Department of Health and Human Services (USDHHS), *Healthy People* "challenges individuals, communities, and professionals, to take specific steps to ensure that good health, as well as long life, are enjoyed by all" (USDHHS, 2012).

The broad goals of *Healthy People 2030* are to attain high-quality, longer lives free of preventable disease, disability, injury, and premature death; achieve equity, eliminate disparities, and improve the health of all groups; create social and physical environments that promote good health for all; and promote quality of life, healthy development, and healthy behaviors across all life stages. There are 355 objectives toward achieving these goals organized into the topic areas of health conditions, health behaviors, populations, settings and systems, and social determinants of health. Leading Health Indicators (LHIs) are a small subset of high-priority *Healthy People 2030* objectives selected to motivate progress toward improving health and well-being. Most LHIs address factors that impact major causes of death and disease in the United States. The LHIs guide organizations, communities, and states to focus their resources and efforts where they will improve the health and well-being of most people. Healthy People 2030 includes 23 LHIs. The homepage for *Healthy People 2030* can be accessed at https://health.gov/healthypeople.

❓ ACTIVE LEARNING

1. How have *Healthy People* changed? Get to know the *Healthy People 2030* proposed objectives at https://health.gov/healthypeopleRead over the new objectives and compare them with the *Healthy People 2020* objectives at https://www.cdc.gov/nchs/healthy_people/hp2020.htm.
2. How did Americans do in meeting the *Healthy People 2020* objectives? Choose a focus area from *Healthy People 2020*, and access the periodic reviews for *Healthy People 2020*. What are the challenges to meeting the objectives? What are the strategies for meeting the objectives? Did the objective change for *Healthy People 2030*?

DETERMINANTS OF HEALTH

Biology is an individual's genetic makeup, family history, and any physical and mental health problems developed in the course of life. Aging, diet, physical activity, smoking, stress, alcohol or drug abuse, injury, violence, or a toxic or infectious agent may produce illness or disability, changing an individual's biology.

Behaviors are the individual's responses to internal stimuli and external conditions. Behaviors interact with biology in a common relationship, as one may influence the other. If a person chooses behaviors such as alcohol abuse or smoking, his or her biology may be changed as a result (e.g., liver cirrhosis, chronic obstructive pulmonary disease [COPD]). On the other hand, if an individual has a history of colon cancer in his or her family, the individual may choose to have regular screenings, thereby preventing advanced cancer and possibly death and changing his or her biology for the better. One's biology may affect behavior; if a person has hypertension or diabetes, he or she may choose to begin an exercise regimen and eat more healthfully.

The *social environment* includes interactions and relationships with family, friends, coworkers, and others in the community. Social institutions, such as law enforcement, faith communities, schools, and government agencies, are also part of the social environment, as well as housing, safety, public transportation, and availability of resources. The social environment has a great impact on the health of individuals, groups, and communities, yet it is complex in nature because of different cultures and practices.

The *Physical environment* is what is experienced with the senses—what is smelled, seen, touched, heard, and tasted. The physical environment can affect health negatively or positively. If there are toxic or infectious substances in the environment, this is certainly a negative influence on health. If the environment is clean with areas to recreate and play, this is a good influence on health.

Policies and interventions can have a profound effect on the health of individuals, groups, and communities. Positive effects such as policies against smoking in public places, seatbelt and child restraint laws, litter ordinances, and enhanced healthcare promote health. Policies are implemented at local, state, and national levels by many agencies, such as Transportation, Health and Human Services, Veterans' Affairs, Housing, and Justice Departments.

Expansion of access to quality healthcare is essential to decrease health disparities and to improve the quality of life and the number of years of healthy life (USDHHS, 2013).

THEORIES IN HEALTH PROMOTION

Health promotion activities are broad in scope and in the setting. Community health nurses and their clients engage in health promotion activities in workplace settings, schools, clinics, and communities. The theories that are used most in health promotion are very diverse to accommodate the variety of settings, clients, and activities in community health. Working knowledge of theory is important in understanding why people act as they do and why they may or may not follow the advice given to them by medical professionals and in helping clients progress from knowledge to behavior change. Some of the most frequently used health promotion theories and models are discussed here.

Pender's Health Promotion Model

Developed in the 1980s and revised in 1996, Pender's Health Promotion Model (HPM) explores the myriad biopsychosocial factors that influence individuals to pursue health promotion activities. The HPM depicts the complex multidimensional

factors with which people interact as they work to achieve optimum health. This model contains seven variables related to health behaviors, as well as individual characteristics that may influence a behavioral outcome.

Pender's model does not include threat as a motivator, as a threat may not be a motivating factor for clients in all age groups (Pender et al., 2011). The HPM is depicted in Fig. 4.1.

Let's relate the HPM to Jamie R. in Clinical Example 4.1. The experience of having relatives who died of heart disease and cancer has probably increased her desire to engage in healthful behavior. Similarly, her busy schedule and lack of communication with her doctor may be reflected in her failure to obtain screenings or immunizations. Jamie has a habit of engaging in exercise and a high self-efficacy related to her success with exercise in the past. Jamie feels better after exercise, and she receives positive comments from significant others regarding her appearance, also increasing her motivation to exercise. Jamie works out in a lovely gym and is very committed to her workout routine. Jamie has found that working out first thing in the morning minimizes the competing demands that may keep her from exercising.

The Health Belief Model

Initially proposed in 1958, the Health Belief Model (HBM) provides the basis for much of the practice of health education and health promotion today. The HBM was developed by a group of social psychologists to attempt to explain why the public failed to participate in screening for tuberculosis (Hochbaum, 1958). Hochbaum and his associates had the same questions that perplex many health professionals today: *Why do people who may have a disease reject health screening? Why do individuals participate in screening if it may lead to the diagnosis of disease?* This research documented that information alone is rarely enough to motivate one to act. Individuals must know what to do and how to do it before they can take action. Also, the information must be related in some way to the individual's needs. One of the most widely used conceptual frameworks in health behavior, the HBM has been used to explain behavior change and maintenance of behavior change and to guide health promotion interventions (Champion and Skinner, 2008).

The HBM has several constructs: perceived seriousness, perceived susceptibility, perceived benefits of treatment, perceived barriers to treatment, cues to action, and self-efficacy. These components can be found in Table 4.1. All of these constructs relate to the client's perception. How does the client perceive the seriousness of the condition? His or her susceptibility to the condition? The benefits of prevention or treatment? The barriers to prevention or treatment? The HBM is depicted in Fig. 4.2 (McEwen and Pullis, 2009).

Let's apply the HBM to Jamie. She may not perceive that she is susceptible to heart disease or breast cancer, or she may not perceive that there is a benefit of screening, or treatment for heart disease or cancer—thus her failure to take up screening for these diseases.

Individual Characteristics and Experiences   Behavior-Specific Cognitions and Affect   Behavioral Outcome

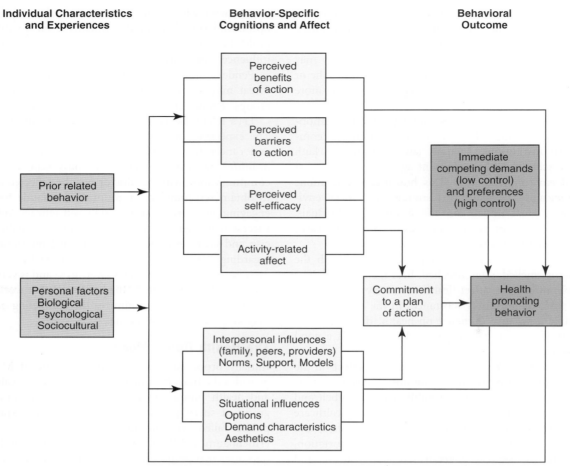

Fig. 4.1 The health promotion model. (From Pender N: *The health promotion model*, 2009, The University of Michigan School of Nursing. Available from: www.nursing.umich.edu/faculty/pender/chart.gif.)

TABLE 4.1   Key Concepts and Definitions of the Health Belief Model

Concept	Definition
Perceived susceptibility	One's belief regarding the chance of getting a given condition
Perceived severity	One's belief regarding the seriousness of a given condition
Perceived benefits	One's belief in the ability of an advised action to reduce the health risk or seriousness of a given condition
Perceived barriers	One's belief regarding the tangible and psychological costs of an advised action
Cues to action	Strategies or conditions in one's environment that activate readiness to take action
Self-efficacy	One's confidence in one's ability to take action to reduce health risks

From Janz JK, Champion VL, Stretcher VJ: The health belief model. In Glanz K, Rimer BK, Lewis FM, editors: *Health behavior and health education: theory, research, and practice*, San Francisco, CA, 2002, Jossey-Bass.

The Transtheoretical Model

The Transtheoretical Model (TTM) combines several theories of intervention, giving its name. Table 4.2 lists the core constructs of the model, which also include the constructs of self-efficacy and the processes of change. The TTM is depicted in Fig. 4.3.

The TTM is based on the assumption that behavior change takes place over time, progressing through a sequence of stages. It also assumes that each of the stages is both stable and open to change. In other words, one may stop in one stage, progress to the next stage, or return to the previous stage.

The Transtheoretical Model and Change

Change is difficult, even for the most motivated of individuals. People resist change for many reasons. Change may:
- Be unpleasant (exercising)
- Require giving up pleasure (eating desserts or watching TV)
- Be painful (insulin injections)
- Be stressful (eating new foods)
- Jeopardize social relationships (gatherings with friends and family that involve food)

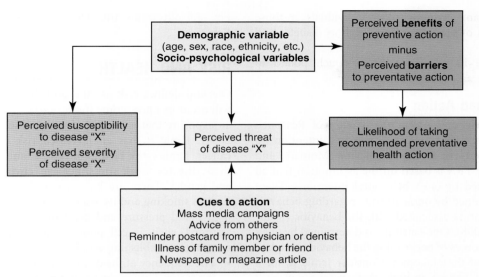

Fig. 4.2 The health belief model. (From Becker MH, Maiman LA: Sociobehavioral determinants of compliance with health and medical care recommendations, *Med Care* 13:10, 1975.)

TABLE 4.2	**The Transtheoretical Model**
Constructs	**Description**
Stages of Change	
Precontemplation	The individual has no intention to take action toward behavior change in the next 6 months. May be in this phase because of a lack of information about the consequences of the behavior or failure on previous attempts at change.
Contemplation	The individual has some intention to take action toward behavior change in the next 6 months. Weighing pros and cons to change.
Preparation	The individual intends to take action within the next month and has taken steps toward behavior change. Has a plan of action.
Action	The individual has changed overt behavior for less than 6 months. Has changed behavior sufficiently to reduce risk of disease.
Maintenance	The individual has changed overt behavior for more than 6 months. Strives to prevent relapse. This phase may last months to years.
Decisional Balance	
Pros	The benefits of behavior change
Cons	The costs of behavior change

Modified from Prochaska JO, Redding CA, Evers KE: The transtheoretical model and stages of change. In Glanz K, Rimer B, Viswanath K, editors: *Health behavior and health education: theory, research, and practice,* San Francisco, CA, 2008, Jossey-Bass, pp 97–121.

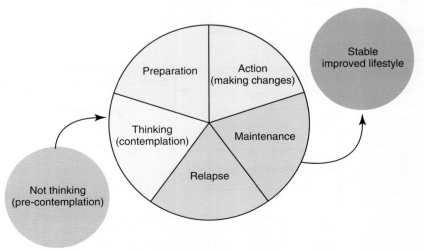

Fig. 4.3 The transtheoretical model. (From Prochaska J, DiClemente C: Transtheoretical therapy: toward a more integrative model of change, *Psychother: Theor Res & Pract* 19:276–288, 1982.)

- Not seem important anymore (older individuals or those with the ill effects of lifestyle choices, such as diabetes and hypertension)
- Require a change in self-image (from couch potato to athlete) (Westberg and Jason, 1996).

Theory of Reasoned Action

Developed by Fishbein and Ajzen, the Theory of Reasoned Action (TRA) attempts to predict a person's intention to perform or not to perform a certain behavior (Montano and Kasprzyk, 2008). The TRA is based on the assumption that all behavior is determined by one's behavioral intentions. These intentions are determined by one's attitude regarding behavior and the subjective norms associated with the behavior (Montano and Kasprzyk, 2008). One's attitude is determined by one's beliefs about the outcomes of performing the behavior, weighed by one's assessment of the outcomes. Consider Jamie R. for a moment. Jamie must believe strongly that exercise will have positive results, as she rises early and takes time from her busy schedule to work out daily. Conversely, Jamie may believe strongly that routine immunizations or health screenings will have negative results.

One's subjective norm is determined by one's normative beliefs, or whether or not important people in one's life approve or disapprove of the behavior under consideration, weighed by one's motivation to comply with those important persons (Montano and Kasprzyk, 2008). If Jamie believes that her husband or children think that she should get a mammogram, and if she is motivated to comply with their wishes, Jamie will have a positive subject norm regarding getting a mammogram.

Recently, the variable of perceived control has been added to the TRA to account for the amount of control an individual may have over whether or not he or she performs the behavior. With the addition of perceived control, the Theory of Planned Behavior was developed (Montano and Kasprzyk, 2008).

Fig. 4.4 illustrates the TRA and the Theory of Planned Behavior.

RISK AND HEALTH

Oleckno defines risk as "the probability that a specific event will occur in a given time frame" (2002, p. 352). A risk factor is an exposure that is associated with a disease (Friis and Sellers, 2004). Jamie R. has an increased risk of heart disease and cancer. Jamie's risk factors include a family history of both of these diseases, work stress, her age, environmental exposures, and gender. There are known risk factors for some diseases, such as smoking and its association with lung cancer, as well as high blood pressure and heart disease. Some risk factors are assumed, such as cell phones and brain tumors. The three criteria for establishing a risk factor are as follows:

- The frequency of the disease varies by category or amount of the factor. Lung cancer is more likely to develop in cigarette smokers than in nonsmokers and in those who smoke heavily than in those who smoke little.
- The risk factor must precede the onset of the disease. Cigarette smokers have lung cancer after they have been smoking for a while. If smokers had lung cancer before starting to smoke, this fact would cast doubt on smoking as a risk factor for lung cancer.
- The association of concern must not be due to any source of error. In any research study (especially one involving human behavior), there are many sources of error, such as study design, data collection methods, and data analysis. Other criteria that have been noted in the literature include the strength of the association, consistency with repetition, specificity, and plausibility (Friis and Sellers, 2004).

In order to determine the health risks to individuals, groups, and populations, a risk assessment may be conducted. A *risk assessment* is a systematic way of distinguishing the risks posed by potentially harmful exposures. The four main steps of a risk

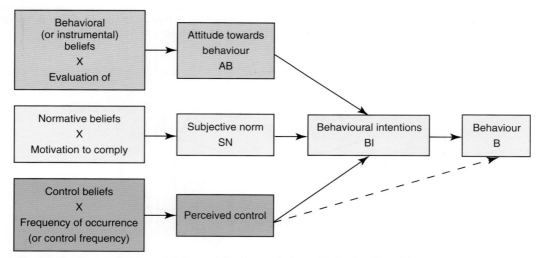

Fig. 4.4 The theory of reasoned action and the theory of planned behavior. (From Montano DE, Kaspryzk D: Theory of reasoned action, theory of planned behavior, and the integrated behavioral model. In Glanz K, Rimer BK, Viswanath K, editors: *Health behavior and health education*, San Francisco, CA, 2008, Jossey-Bass, pp 67—96.)

assessment are hazard identification, risk description, exposure assessment, and risk estimation (Savitz, 1998).

THE RELATIONSHIP OF RISK TO HEALTH AND HEALTH PROMOTION ACTIVITIES

Health is directly related to the activities in which we participate, the food we eat, and the substances to which we are exposed daily. Where we live and work and our gender, age, and genetic makeup also affect health. In the assessment of risk regarding health and health promotion activities, there are two types of risks: modifiable risks and nonmodifiable risks. *Modifiable risk factors* are those aspects of a person's health risk over which he or she has control. Examples include smoking, leading a sedentary or active lifestyle, the type and amount of food eaten, and the type of activities in which he or she engages (skydiving is riskier than bowling). *Nonmodifiable risk factors* are those aspects of one's health risk over which one has no or little control. Examples include genetic makeup, gender, age, and environmental exposure. A useful tool to help clients assess their family history for possible health risks is available at the U.S. Surgeon General's website at http://www.hhs.gov/familyhistory/. This assessment is easy to use and can create a dialogue between family members to discuss family health history. As the nurse assesses the various aspects of a client's health, it is important to evaluate behaviors that have a positive effect on the client's health, not only those behaviors that are detrimental to health. Healthful behaviors, such as maintaining an exercise regimen and following an eating plan, build self-efficacy and self-esteem. Positive health behaviors also provide a foundation on which a nurse can build to address unhealthful behaviors. If a client has been successful at smoking cessation, the confidence and self-efficacy learned from this change can be drawn upon to help him or her stick to a low-sodium, low-fat diet to address hypertension.

Risk reduction is a proactive process in which individuals participate in behaviors that enable them to react to actual or potential threats to their health (Pender, 1996). Risk communication is the process through which the public receives information regarding possible or actual threats to health. Risk communication is affected by the way individuals and communities perceive, process, and act on their understanding of risk (Finnigan and Vinswanath, 2008). Individuals, groups, and communities receive information on health risks from many sources besides healthcare professionals today. The Internet is a newer source of risk communication for many community members, with 60% of Internet users accessing it for health information (Atkinson et al., 2009). Internet use vastly increased during the COVID pandemic with users accessing health information and news, and interacting with family and friends (Schumacher and Kent, 2020). Newspapers, periodicals, radio, TV, and billboards are long-standing sources of health information in public health. Though there are many sources of information on health risks available to the public, the quality varies widely in terms of the accuracy of the information presented. The use of social media to communicate with audiences has also increased among public and private entities. Chat rooms, forums, Facebook, Twitter, and many specialized websites such as *Five Wishes*, which offers information on advance care planning, and nutrition websites such as *Eating Well* provide a wide range of information. Healthcare professionals are endeavoring to make risk communication as personalized and specific as possible for individuals, groups, and communities in an effort to improve uptake of screening and behavior change. Research has not shown personalized risk communication to be any more effective than traditional methods of risk communication (Edwards et al., 2013).

Approximately 50% of annual U.S. deaths occur as a result of modifiable or lifestyle factors (McGinnis and Foege, 1993; Mokdab et al., 2004). Fig. 4.5 depicts the leading causes of death and the numbers of deaths related to each. Those causes of death with the highest mortality (heart disease, cancer, stroke, and chronic respiratory disease) are all related to lifestyle factors (McGinnis and Foege, 2004; NRC and IOM, 2015). The relationship of lifestyle factors to mortality is so strong that medical care has been found to play a minor role in preventing premature deaths (Schroeder et al., 2007). Table 4.3 details the relationship between the leading causes of death and common risk factors. A 2012 study found that people adopting healthful behaviors such as exercising, eating a healthful diet, not using tobacco, and maintaining a normal weight had a 66% lower risk of death than did those who did not adopt these behaviors (Loef and Walach, 2012).

Unfortunately, many people experience a clustering of unhealthy lifestyle behaviors such as poor diet, physical inactivity, obesity, and smoking. The American Heart Association has developed a useful self-assessment of cardiovascular health. Life's Simple Seven (LS7) (http://www.heart.org/HEARTORG/Conditions/My-Life-Check—Lifes-Simple-7_UCM_471453_Article.jsp#.WOKWg2ckq70) is based on physical activity, diet, tobacco use, body weight, cholesterol, blood pressure, and blood sugar. This tool uses data entered by the user to derive a score and to offer feedback on areas needing improvement.

Tobacco and Health Risk

Smoking cessation is an important step in achieving optimum health. In the United States, smoking is the leading cause of preventable death, accounting for approximately one out of every five deaths, or 438,000 deaths, per year. Smoking is a causal factor in cancers of the esophagus, bladder, stomach, oral cavity, pharynx, larynx, cervix, and lungs, with more than 90% of lung cancers in men and 80% of lung cancers among women attributable to smoking. Over 16 million Americans are currently living with a disease caused by smoking. Smoking harms nearly every organ in the body Smoking also has an economic impact, costing $170 billion annually in healthcare and lost productivity.

Most smokers are between the ages of 18 and 44 years, and more men than women smoke. In 2019, 15.3% of adult men and 12.7% of adult women were smokers. The prevalence of smoking is highest among American Indians/Alaskan Natives and Caucasians. Smoking is most common among adults who

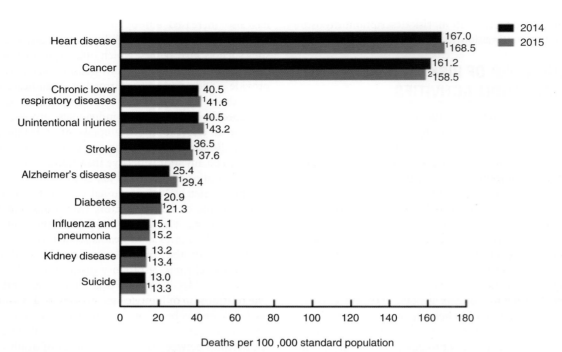

Fig. 4.5 Leading causes of death, United States, 2014–2015. (From Centers for Disease Control and Prevention, National Center for Chronic Disease: *Age-adjusted death rates for the 10 leading causes of death in 2015: United States, 2014 and 2015.* NCHS, National vital statistics system, Mortality. Available from: https://www.cdc.gov/nchs/products/databriefs/db267.htm.)

TABLE 4.3 **Relationship Between Risk Factors and 10 Leading Causes of Death**

Cause of Death	Percentage of Total Deaths	Smoking	High-Fat, Low-Fiber Diet	Sedentary Lifestyle	High Blood Pressure	Elevated Cholesterol	Obesity	Diabetes	Alcohol Abuse
Heart disease	25	X	X	X	X	X	X	X	X
Cancer	23	X	X	X			X		X
Stroke	6	X	X		X	X	X		
Chronic obstructive pulmonary disease (COPD)	5	X							
Unintentional injury	5	X							X
Diabetes	3		X	X			X	X	
Alzheimer disease	3		X	X					
All other causes	29	X							

From Centers for Disease Control and Prevention. *Health United States 2010.* Available from: http://www.cdc.gov/heartdisease/statistical_reports.htm.

are less educated and adults who live below the poverty level. Smoking rates are higher in the Midwest and lowest in the western US. Persons with a disability smoke at a higher rate than do persons without a disability. Gay, lesbian, and bisexual adults are more likely to smoke than straight Americans (CDC, 2020).

More than 70% of current smokers report that they would like to quit smoking (CDC, n.d.a,b). Nicotine addiction is the most common form of chemical dependence in the United States. Smokers who are trying to quit experience withdrawal symptoms such as anxiety, increased appetite, irritability, and difficulty concentrating. These symptoms make quitting diffi-cult, and most people relapse several times before being able to quit successfully. Nicotine replacement, pharmaceutical alter-natives, hypnosis, and acupuncture may be helpful in the attempt to quit smoking. The American Cancer Society rec-ommends the following steps to quit smoking:

- Make the decision to quit. Any change is scary, and smoking cessation is a big change, requiring a long-term commitment.
- Set a date to quit and choose a plan.
- Mark the date on your calendar.
- Tell your family and friends about the date, and ask for their support.
- Get rid of all tobacco products, ashtrays, and lighters in your environment.
- Stock up on oral substitutes such as sugarless gum, hard candy, fruit, and carrot sticks.
- Decide on a plan and prepare to implement it; register for the stop-smoking class, or see your doctor about nicotine replacement therapy or pharmaceutical alternatives.
- Practice saying "No thank you, I don't smoke."
- Think back to your previous attempts to quit and see what worked and what did not work.
- If you are taking bupropion or varenicline, take your medi-cation each day of the week leading up to your quit day. Deal with withdrawal by:
- Avoiding temptation.
- Changing your habits. Walk when you are stressed or dur-ing breaks. Use hard candy, carrot sticks, or gum to satisfy the need to put something in your mouth. If you feel the urge to light up, tell yourself that you are going to wait 10 min before giving in. Usually, the urge will pass within that time.
- Staying off of tobacco is a lifelong process. Many former smokers state that they experienced strong desires to smoke after weeks, months, or even years of smoking cessation. These unexpected cravings can be difficult to deal with.
- Remind yourself of the reasons why you quit.
- Wait out the craving. There is no such thing as just one ciga-rette or just one puff.
- Avoid alcohol.
- Begin an exercise program and work on eating a healthy diet to avoid gaining weight (American Cancer Society, 2016).

Information on quitting can be accessed at the CDC website at http://www.cdc.gov/tobacco/quit_smoking/how_to_quit/index.htm. The American Lung Association also has information on smoking cessation at http://www.lung.org/stop-smoking/. The American Cancer Society offers a quit-smoking guide at https://www.cancer.org/healthy/stay-away-from-tobacco/guide-quitting-smoking/deciding-to-quit-smoking-and-making-a-plan.html.

It is important to remember that smokers who are trying to quit smoking need support, and most families and loved ones want to help. The American Cancer Society has suggestions for supporting someone who is quitting smoking at https://www.cancer.org/healthy/stay-away-from-tobacco/helping-a-smoker-quit.html.

Teens are a population of concern regarding smoking. Though the rate of smoking has declined among Americans since the 1990s, more high school juniors and seniors smoke than do adults. Half of high school-aged smokers have tried to quit at least once. Those who start using tobacco in their teens have a harder time giving up smoking later in life. Most smokers pick up the habit at age 18, with very few initiating smoking after the age of 25 (American Cancer Society, 2012). A resource for teens who are trying to quit smoking is available at https://www.lung.org/quit-smoking/helping-teens-quit/kids-and-smoking.

Only 4% to 7% of smokers are able to quit smoking in any attempt without pharmaceutical or other interventions to help them, so nurses must provide information and referrals to help clients access resources that help them to get off and to stay off tobacco.

Smokeless tobacco also poses a health threat. Commonly called *spit tobacco,* smokeless tobacco is a significant health threat and is not a safe substitute for smoking tobacco. Smokeless tobacco is known to be a cause of cancer and oral health problems. Smokeless tobacco causes nicotine addiction and dependence, and adolescents who use smokeless tobacco are more likely to take up smoking (CDC, 2020). In the United States, about 2% of adults use smokeless tobacco, with 4.7% of men being smokeless tobacco users. Non-Hispanic whites accounted for most smokeless tobacco users. Wyoming had the highest rate of smokeless tobacco use with New Jersey having the lowest. It is estimated that 4.8% of high school students use smokeless tobacco. Smokeless tobacco use is more common among young white males, with its heaviest use among blue-collar workers, service workers, and laborers as well as the unemployed. School nurses are in an important position to intervene early in the use of smokeless tobacco. Most smokeless tobacco use begins in middle school, and interventions to prevent or stop this habit are essential in the school setting.

The clinical implications of tobacco use are clear. First, community health nurses must ask about tobacco use at every clinic visit or home visit and look for teachable moments, when the client may be interested in discussing his or her tobacco habit (a respiratory illness or a scare with an oral lesion may prompt the client to reconsider the habit). Assess the client's tobacco use: "Do you use tobacco?" "What kind of tobacco (cigarettes, cigars, chewing tobacco, pipe) do you use?" "How much do you smoke (dip, chew)?" "Have you thought about quitting?" Explore with the client why he or she may or may not have considered giving up the tobacco habit and what options are available to help should he or she desire to quit. Refer the client to smoking cessation websites or other healthcare professionals for assistance in quitting. Chances are great that the client is very well acquainted with the health risks posed by tobacco but not with the options for helping him or her to quit. Encourage the client to attempt to give up tobacco, and encourage him or her in any attempts to decrease or stop the use of tobacco.

Alcohol Consumption and Health

Alcohol use is very common in our society. In 2018, more than half of Americans reported being current drinkers, with 7% reporting being heavy drinkers and 17% engaging in binge drinking. Though only 6% of the U.S. population is addicted to alcohol, about 25% of the population drinks excessively. One in five adults reported drinking five or more drinks per day. Men are more likely (63%) than women (55%) to be current drinkers and to binge drink. Men are also more than twice as likely to suffer death or injury related to drinking. Nationally, women are nearly twice as likely as men to be lifetime abstainers, yet one in two women of childbearing age drinks alcohol. An emerging trend in alcohol abuse is high-intensity drinking. High-intensity drinking is the consumption of two or more times the gender-specific binge drinking threshold. This practice is dangerous. Compared with people who did not binge drink, people who engaged in high-intensity drinking were 70 times more likely to have an alcohol-related emergency department (ED) visit. Those who consumed three times the gender-specific binge thresholds for alcohol were 93 times more likely to have an alcohol-related ED visit.

Binge drinking is an unrecognized problem among women and girls. One in five high school-aged girls and one in eight adult women reported binge drinking. The intensity and frequency of binge drinking are similar among pregnant and nonpregnant women: about three times per month and six drinks per occasion. It takes less alcohol for females to become impaired than males because of body size and differences in the way alcohol is processed by females. About 7.6% of women use alcohol while pregnant, with about one in 20 women using alcohol heavily before discovering that they are pregnant. For both men and women, those aged 25 to 44 years had the highest prevalence of drinking. The drinking prevalence declines at age 44 years and declines steadily with age thereafter. Non-Hispanic white people have the highest drinking prevalence, with non-Hispanic white men being the heaviest drinkers.

Alcohol use, particularly heavy alcohol use, is responsible for many health problems such as liver disease and for unintentional injuries. *Excessive alcohol use* is drinking more than two drinks per day on average for men or more than one drink per day for women; *binge drinking* is drinking five or more drinks on a single occasion for men or four or more drinks in a single occasion for women. Binge drinking is the most common form of excessive alcohol use in America. Most people who binge drink are not alcohol dependent. A *drink* is any drink containing 0.6 ounces or 1.2 tablespoons of pure alcohol. A drink is:

- 12 ounces of beer or wine cooler
- 8 ounces of malt liquor
- 5 ounces of wine
- 1.5 ounces of 80-proof distilled spirits or liquor (gin, rum, vodka, whiskey)

The *Dietary Guidelines for Americans* state that alcohol should be consumed in moderation—no more than one drink per day for women and no more than two drinks per day for men (USDHHS, 2015). People who should not drink are those who:

- Are less than 21 years of age
- Are taking medications that can cause harmful reactions when mixed with alcohol
- Are pregnant or trying to become pregnant
- Are recovering from alcoholism or are unable to control the amount that they drink
- Have a medical condition that may be worsened by alcohol
- Are driving or planning to drive or to perform activities requiring coordination and concentration (USDHHS, 2015)

Responsible for 95,000 deaths annually, alcohol use is the third leading lifestyle-related cause of death in the nation. In 2010, excessive alcohol use cost the US economy $249 billion, or $2.05 per drink. The short-term risks of alcohol consumption are usually due to binge drinking or excess drinking and include risky sexual behavior, violence, unintentional injuries from motor vehicle accidents, falls, firearms, and drowning. Miscarriage or stillbirth and alcohol poisoning are also possible immediate effects of excessive alcohol use. The long-term risks of alcohol use are neurological conditions such as dementia and stroke; cardiovascular problems such as MI, hypertension, and cardiomyopathy; psychiatric problems such as depression and anxiety; social problems such as unemployment and family dysfunction; cancer of the mouth, throat, liver, and breast; and liver disease, including cirrhosis and hepatitis. Pancreatitis and gastritis are other gastrointestinal consequences of long-term alcohol consumption (CDC, 2020).

The prevalence of underage drinking declined significantly when states established the minimum legal drinking age as 21 years, and those states with more stringent drinking laws have a lower prevalence of adult and underage binge drinking. Despite age limits for legal consumption of alcohol, alcohol is the number-one used and abused drug among U.S. youth. Underage drinking is a significant public health problem in the U.S. and is responsible for more than 3500 deaths and 210,000 years of potential life lost among people under age 21 each year. Underage drinking cost the U.S. $24 billion in 2010 and accounted for approximately 119,000 emergency room visits by persons aged 12 to 21, and approximately 19% of youth aged 12 to 20 reported drinking alcohol in 2019. Initiation to alcohol begins early: a national report found that 33% of eighth-graders had tried alcohol and 13% had drunk alcohol in the previous month. Youth who start drinking prior to age 15 are six times more likely to experience alcohol dependence or abuse than those who begin drinking at or after 21 years of age. The prevalence of adult binge drinking behavior is strongly predictive of binge drinking behavior by college students living in the same state (CDC, 2020).

Clinical implications for health promotion related to alcohol consumption emphasize the prevention of underage drinking and identifying and assisting groups and individuals at risk for alcohol abuse and dependence. A helpful resource for locating and contacting local agencies for alcohol treatment is the

National Drug and Alcohol Treatment Referral Routing Service, available at 1-800-662-HELP. Alcohol Screening and Brief Intervention (SBI) consists of screening those who are at risk for excessive alcohol consumption and providing brief counseling. In trauma centers and EDs where SBI has been implemented, medical costs and readmissions related to alcohol have been reduced (CDC, 2015).

Preventing underage drinking is a public health priority. Enforcement of the legal drinking age, as well as enforcement of bans on sales of alcohol to minors, is an important aspect of prevention. Increased excise tax on alcoholic beverages has also been found to decrease underage drinking. Education of both adults and youth regarding alcohol and the myriad of risks posed by underage alcohol consumption must accompany enforcement efforts. The CDC (2020) has an alcohol program aimed at preventing excessive alcohol use. With interventions at the individual, local, and national levels, the program emphasizes evidence-based recommendations to prevent alcohol misuse. The program can be found at https://www.cdc.gov/alcohol/fact-sheets/prevention.htm.

Preventing excessive alcohol consumption must consider several prominent environmental factors:
- Alcohol is cheap.
- Alcohol is readily available.
- Americans are exposed to $4 billion of alcohol advertising per year.
- New alcohol products cater to youthful tastes and may promote underage drinking (U.S. Department of Justice, 2002).

Decreasing the morbidity and mortality related to overconsumption of alcohol requires a community-wide effort to address the problem on several fronts. Youth tend to model their drinking behavior after adults, and adults are often the source of alcohol for many youths, meaning that interventions must be aimed at the population across the lifespan. Interventions supported by research include:
- Increase taxes on alcohol—a 10% increase in price results in a 7% decrease in alcohol consumption.
- Decrease alcohol outlet density—higher outlet density is associated with greater alcohol consumption and negative impacts of alcohol.
- Hold alcohol retailers responsible for harm caused by inebriated or underage drinkers.

Diet and Health

Diet is one of the most modifiable of risk factors. A healthy diet contributes to the prevention of such chronic diseases as type 2 diabetes, hypertension, heart disease, and some cancers. With 21% of U.S. children 2 to 19 years and 42.5% of U.S. adults being obese (CDC, 2021), diet is an important topic in health promotion. Americans are bombarded with nutrition information, and many are confused and have no idea how to apply the information regarding the diet that they have received. As portion sizes get larger, Americans of all ages are spending more time engaged in inactive pursuits such as watching TV and using a computer. Commonly, the terms "portion" and "serving" are misused. A *portion* is the "amount of a single

food item served in a single eating occasion." A meal or a snack is a single eating occasion, with the number of green beans or roast beef on your plate being the portion. A *serving* is a "standardized unit of measuring foods" used in dietary guidelines. A cup or an ounce is an example of serving size (CDC, 2006).

What does it mean to be overweight or obese? Both of these terms are used to indicate a condition of excess weight for height. Both terms also identify ranges of weight that have been found to be associated with an increased risk of certain diseases or conditions. The body mass index (BMI) is used to determine weight status in adults and children. The BMI takes both height and weight into account and has been found to correlate well with the amount of body fat present. An adult with a BMI of 25 to 29.9 is considered overweight, and an adult with a BMI of 30 or higher is considered obese. Though there are many contributing factors to overweight and obesity, controlling one's weight is a matter of balancing caloric intake with physical activity. Too many calories in and too few calories out eventually result in being overweight. Fig. 4.6 illustrates this energy balance.

The rate of obesity in the United States increased from 30.5% to 42.4% from 2017 to 2018. The Midwest (33.9%) and South (33.3%) had the highest prevalence of obesity, followed by the Northeast (29.0%), and the West (27.4%) All states and territories had more than 20% of adults with obesity (CDC, 2021). To access a map to see how your state rates in obesity go to https://www.cdc.gov/obesity/data/prevalence-maps.html.

Non-Hispanic black adults (49.6%) had the highest prevalence of obesity, followed by Hispanic adults (44.8%), non-Hispanic white adults (42.2%), and non-Hispanic Asian adults (17.4%). The rate of obesity varies with age. The prevalence of obesity was 40.0% among adults aged 20 to 39 years, 44.8% among adults aged 40 to 59 years, and 42.8% among adults aged 60 and older (CDC, 2021).

The burden of obesity is greater among people with lower education and low-income levels.

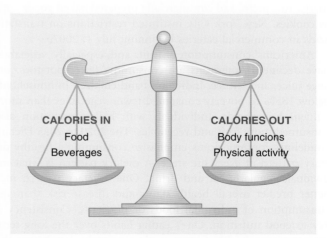

Fig. 4.6 Caloric balance equation. (From Centers for Disease Control and Prevention: *Overweight and obesity: an overview*, 2009. Available from: www.cdc.gov/nccdphp/dnpa/obesity/contributing_factors.htm.)

Overall, men and women with college degrees had lower obesity prevalence compared with those with less education. Among men, obesity prevalence was lower in the lowest and highest income groups compared with the middle-income group. Among women, obesity prevalence was lower in the highest income group than in the middle and lowest income groups (CDC, 2021).

Obesity is also a concern for children. The prevalence of obesity among children was 19.3% and affected about 14.4 million children and adolescents. Obesity prevalence was 13.4% among 2- to 5-year-olds, 20.3% among 6- to 11-year-olds, and 21.2% among 12- to 19-year-olds. Childhood obesity is also more common among certain populations with Hispanic and non-Hispanic black children having the highest rates of obesity. The prevalence of obesity decreased as the head of household's level of education increased (CDC, 2021).

As rates of obesity have risen, so has the cost associated with the health comorbidities of obesity. It is well known that obesity is related to the most common causes of death—heart disease, stroke, some cancers, and type 2 diabetes. In 2008, medical costs associated with obesity were estimated to be approximately $147 billion, with obese persons each costing $1429 more in medical expenditures than individuals of normal weight. It is estimated that about 27% of the increase in healthcare spending between 1987 and 2001 was related to obesity, and about half of this cost was paid for by Medicare and Medicaid. An obese beneficiary costs Medicare more than $600 more annually than a beneficiary of normal weight.

Fats are an essential nutrient for energy and serve many purposes in the body, but too much fat in the diet, especially transfats, saturated fats, and cholesterol, may increase the risk of heart disease (U.S. Department of Agriculture [USDA]/USDHHS, 2010). Transfatty acids are deleterious to health, leading to an increased risk for heart disease and stroke. The Food and Drug Administration revoked the "generally recognized as safe" status for transfatty acids on June 16, 2015, and gave food manufacturers until June 2018 to remove transfats from their products. Most transfats are found in fried foods, margarine, pizza, and commercially prepared baked goods such as cookies. New York City instituted restrictions on transfatty acids in commercial eateries beginning July 1, 2007.

Americans' consumption of fruits and, especially, vegetables have declined. Americans are consuming fewer potatoes, orange juice, and lettuce. Individuals and children in households below 185% of poverty consumed fewer vegetables than more affluent households. Individuals with higher education also consumed more fruit and vegetables. The 2020 to 2025 Dietary Guidelines for Americans emphasize consuming a healthy dietary pattern at every life stage. A dietary pattern is what individuals regularly eat and drink. One's dietary pattern may better predict overall health status and disease risk than the consumption of individual foods or nutrients. Consistency is key to good nutrition. One's eating habits over the long term impact many health factors such as weight, cardiovascular disease risk, diabetes, cancer risk, and bone health and muscle strength. The new guidelines recommend that adults consume two cups of fruits and two to three cups of vegetables per day. Most Americans do not follow a healthy eating pattern with 10% to 20% meeting the recommended allowance of fruit and vegetables. Rather than focusing on the intake of individual food groups or nutrients, the new guidelines emphasize the importance of eating a healthful diet regularly. Fig. 4.7 lists the key concepts and recommendations in the new guidelines (USDA, 2020).

The CDC has information on incorporating fruits and vegetables into a daily diet at https://www.cdc.gov/healthyweight/healthy_eating/index.html.

The USDA recommends that all Americans go to http://www.choosemyplate.gov/to develop a personalized eating plan based on individual needs and preferences. *My Plate* (Fig. 4.8) was released in 2011, replacing the Food Guide Pyramid. This tool helps users easily translate the USDA guidelines into the kinds and amounts of food to eat each day. *My Plate* is applicable to children as well as adults and is simple and fun enough that children can use it themselves. *My Plate* illustrates a healthful eating plan in a simple and familiar format—a place setting. The key messages of *My Plate* are that half of the plate should be fruits and vegetables; a quarter of the plate should be grains, and half of the grains consumed daily should be whole grain; one-quarter of the plate should be protein; and a serving of a low-fat or nonfat dairy product should be included in each meal. Oils, a source of essential nutrients, are also included in *My Plate,* with the emphasis on oils low in transfats. The Choose My Plate homepage at http://www.choosemyplate.gov/ contains information on eating on a budget, weight management, and a food and activity tracker to help users balance food intake with activity. Many popular foods, such as pizza and spaghetti, are mixed dishes in that they do not fit into only one food group.

Americans eat and drink about one-third of their calories from foods prepared away from home. Usually, these foods contain more calories, saturated fat, and sodium than meals prepared at home. To help individuals make informed and healthy decisions, many restaurants list calories in foods or beverages on menus and offer additional nutrition information upon request. More information is available at fda.gov/CaloriesOnTheMenu. You can find out how many calories you need daily by looking at the table at https://www.fda.gov/media/112972/download. Studies confirm that eating away from home is associated with an increased likelihood of being overweight (Bauer et al., 2012; Rafferty). Busy families have more opportunities to eat away from home as the number of eateries has increased in recent years. The latest findings indicate that from 1987 to 2017, American families spent 45% of their food budget on foods eaten away from home eating away from home 4 to 5 times per week. American families spend more on food eaten away from home than on food eaten at home. Consumers choose food based on affordability, time constraints, and their tastes and preferences. Though parental employment is a benefit to families, the stresses of balancing family and work demands affect nutrition and the kinds of foods consumed. Families with parents who work full time

Key recommendations

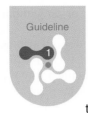

Follow a healthy dietary pattern at every life stage.
At every life stage—infancy, toddlerhood, childhood, adolescence, adulthood, pregnancy, lactation, and older adulthood—it is never too early or too late to eat healthfully.

- **For about the first 6 months of life**, exclusively feed infants human milk. Continue to feed infants human milk through at least the first year of life, and longer if desired. Feed infants iron-fortified infant formula during the first year of life when human milk is unavailable. Provide infants with supplemental vitamin D beginning soon after birth.

- **At about 6 months**, introduce infants to nutrient-dense complementary foods. Introduce infants to potentially allergenic foods along with other complementary foods. Encourage infants and toddlers to consume a variety of foods from all food groups. Include foods rich in iron and zinc, particularly for infants fed human milk.

- **From 12 months through older adulthood**, follow a healthy dietary pattern across the lifespan to meet nutrient needs, help achieve a healthy body weight, and reduce the risk of chronic disease.

Customize and enjoy nutrient-dense food and beverage choices to reflect personal preferences, cultural traditions, and budgetary considerations.
A healthy dietary pattern can benefit all individuals regardless of age, race, or ethnicity, or current health status. The *Dietary Guidelines* provides a framework intended to be customized to individual needs and preferences, as well as the foodways of the diverse cultures in the United States.

Focus on meeting food group needs with nutrient-dense foods and beverages, and stay within calorie limits.
An underlying premise of the *Dietary Guidelines* is that nutritional needs should be met primarily from foods and beverages—specifically, nutrient-dense foods and beverages. Nutrient-dense foods provide vitamins, minerals, and other health-promoting components and have no or little added sugars, saturated fat, and sodium. A healthy dietary pattern consists of nutrient-dense

forms of foods and beverages across all food groups, in recommended amounts, and within calorie limits.

The core elements that make up a healthy dietary pattern include:

- Vegetables of all types—dark green; red and orange; beans, peas, and lentils; starchy; and other vegetables

- Fruits, especially whole fruit

- Grains, at least half of which are whole grain

- Dairy, including fat-free or low-fat milk, yogurt, and cheese, and/or lactose-free versions and fortified soy beverages and yogurt as alternatives

- Protein foods, including lean meats, poultry, and eggs; seafood; beans, peas, and lentils; and nuts, seeds, and soy products

- Oils, including vegetable oils and oils in food, such as seafood and nuts

Limit foods and beverages higher in added sugars, saturated fat, and sodium, and limit alcoholic beverages.
At every life stage, meeting food group recommendations—even with nutrient-dense choices—requires most of a person's daily calorie needs and sodium limits. A healthy dietary pattern doesn't have much room for extra added sugars, saturated fat, or sodium—or for alcoholic beverages. A small amount of added sugars, saturated fat, or sodium can be added to nutrient-dense foods and beverages to help meet food group recommendations, but foods and beverages high in these components should be limited. **Limits are:**

- **Added sugars**—Less than 10 percent of calories per day starting at age 2. Avoid foods and beverages with added sugars for those younger than age 2.

- **Saturated fat**—Less than 10 percent of calories per day starting at age 2.

- **Sodium**—Less than 2300 milligrams per day—and even less for children younger than age 14.

- **Alcoholic beverages**—Adults of legal drinking age can choose not to drink or to drink in moderation by limiting intake to 2 drinks or less in a day for men and 1 drink or less in a day for women, when alcohol is consumed. Drinking less is better for health than drinking more. There are some adults who should not drink alcohol, such as women who are pregnant.

Fig. 4.7 Key recommendations in the dietary guidelines for Americans, 2020 to 2025. (From https://www. dietaryguidelines.gov/sites/default/files/2021-03/Dietary_Guidelines_for_Americans-2020-2025.pdf.)

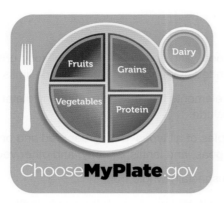

Fig. 4.8 *My Plate* logo. (From the United States Department of Agriculture: *My Plate* 2013, (n.d.). Available from: http://www.choosemyplate.gov/print-materials-ordering/graphic-resources.html.)

spend less time on food preparation, eat fewer family meals, eat more fast food, and spend less time encouraging healthful eating behaviors. Men between the ages of 40 and 59 years consume the most food prepared away from home (Van der Horst et al., 2011). (This author can attest to the fact that when her 57-year-old husband is left to fend for himself at mealtime, he will most likely eat out.) Adolescents also consume a large amount of fast food, with 30% of adolescent males and 27% of adolescent females reporting eating fast food at least three times per week (Bauer et al., 2009). Among adults, the percentage of calories consumed from fast food rises as weight status increases, with obese adults consuming the highest percentage of their calories from fast food (Fryar and Ervin, 2013). Economics can also determine the quality of a family's diet, with families with lower incomes having a poorer-quality diet than do families with higher incomes. Research has found that families with less money to spend on food eating diets lower in fruits and vegetables than do families who have more money to spend on food (USDA, 2018).

Portions served in restaurants are larger than portions served at home, in some cases up to 40% larger. Convenience foods and prepackaged foods contain larger portion sizes than in the 1970s. When presented with large portion size, individuals often unknowingly eat larger amounts than they would usually eat or than they intend to eat. This phenomenon, called **portion distortion,** occurs frequently when people are dining out (NHLBI, 2013). Portion control is an important aspect of weight management, and distortion of portion sizes makes this difficult task harder. There are several reasons why we tend to overeat when we eat away from home: foods presented in restaurants are high in energy density (high number of calories for a particular weight of food); restaurant foods are very palatable and there is a wide variety of this great-tasting food to choose from, and we want to get more food for our money, so we order the larger entrées (The Keystone Center, 2006).

For many people, eating at home all the time is impossible or impractical, and food is central to many social interactions. In order to consume fewer calories when eating out, one may:
- Patronize establishments that offer a variety of food choices and are willing to make substitutions or changes

- Order lower-fat steamed, broiled, baked, roasted, or poached items, or ask that an item be prepared in a lower-calorie way, such as grilled rather than fried
- Choose lower-calorie sauces or condiments, or do without them altogether
- Substitute colorful vegetables for other side dishes (such as French fries)
- Ask for half of the meal to be boxed to take home before the meal is brought to the table
- Share an entrée with someone
- Order a vegetarian meal
- Select fruit for dessert

To decrease reliance on away-from-home foods, plan ahead and:
- Pack healthy snacks to avoid the use of vending machines
- Cook a healthful dinner at home, and make extra to pack for lunch the next day
- Purchase healthful foods when grocery shopping to pack for lunch, such as prepackaged salads, fresh fruits, vegetables, and low-calorie soups
- For travel or longer excursions, bring along nutritious foods that will not spoil, such as fresh fruits and vegetables, or pack a cooler with healthy foods

Various online communities and other support groups are available to help individuals manage their weight. Social media is harnessing the power of the Internet to help the public meet fitness goals. Sites such as Sparkpeople and Livestrong offer interactive and social networking opportunities. Group support is helpful for those who want them, whereas others prefer to have programs that they can implement on their own. The cost to join a weight management community ranges from free to moderate in price. Another popular option for weight control is the large selection of applications for mobile devices. With these applications, it is possible to easily track foods eaten and calories expended throughout the day. Many are free and available for mobile devices.

Physical Activity and Health

There are many reasons why people engage in physical activity and exercise: for weight management, increased energy, or better appearance; to fit into those favorite jeans; to prevent the development or worsening of a chronic health condition; to manage stress; to improve mood and self-esteem; or any combination of these reasons.

Several factors acting individually and in concert can affect the likelihood that one is physically active. Men are a little more likely to engage in leisure physical activity and are more likely to engage in strength training than women. The percentage of adults who engage in leisure-time physical activity decreases with age, from its highest among adults aged 18 to 24 years. White adults and Asian adults are more likely to engage in leisure-time physical activity than are black and Hispanic adults. The percentage of adults participating in leisure-time physical activity increases with the level of education; adults with advanced degrees are twice as likely to engage in some physical activity than are high school graduates. The percentage of adults who engage in regular leisure-time physical activity also increases with income level. Adults whose income is four times the federal poverty level are nearly twice more likely to engage in some form of regular leisure-time physical activity than adults whose income is below the poverty level. Adults living in the southern region of the United States get the least amount of leisure-time physical activity (CDC, 2021).

As has been previously mentioned, one's surroundings also affect whether one will choose to exercise. The Walk Score has ranked cities across the United States for suitability for walking. So what makes a city walkable?

- A center: It may be a shopping center, park, or main street.
- Mixed-use, mixed-income: Businesses are located next to homes at all price points.
- Pedestrian-centric design: Businesses are close to the street to encourage foot traffic with parking in the back.
- Density: The city is compact enough to allow businesses to flourish and for public transportation to run frequently.
- Parks and public spaces: There are plenty of public areas in which to gather.
- Nearby schools and workplaces: Schools and workplaces are close enough that most people can walk from home (Walk Score, 2013).

Research has found that one's environment is a significant factor in health promotion. Adults and adolescents living in neighborhoods with high walkability engage in significantly more walking and cycling than those living in neighborhoods with low walkability. As a result, the rates of obesity are lower in communities that are walkable than in communities that do not encourage physical activity (Brown et al., 2013; CDC, 2015; Slater et al., 2013).

How much exercise do I need? What counts as exercise? Nurses in the community hear these questions commonly as they educate the public on the need to increase physical activity. The answers to these questions depend on the age, physical condition, and gender of the client. The CDC website at https:// www.cdc.gov/physicalactivity/basics/index.htm presents the amount of exercise recommended for adults and children. Videos on the website further explain and illustrate the use of these guidelines. People may feel overwhelmed by the idea that they must add one more demand to an already busy schedule, and some think, "I'm in such bad shape, I'll never be able to exercise." The most important idea is that one must take the first step to try exercise. Walking, biking, taking the stairs, swimming—there is something for everyone, and any exercise is better than none. Exercise may also be broken up into smaller blocks of time during the day if it is not possible or convenient to do it all at once. Physical activity can also be a family affair, with the entire family using the time to reconnect and have fun together. Walking has been found to be one of the most beneficial exercises. It does not require special skills or expensive equipment, and many people with disabilities are able to participate in a walking program using assistive devices. Walking is an easy form of physical activity to perform and maintain. Walking is a safe activity with a lower likelihood of

injury than more vigorous forms of exercise. And it is a good activity for those who are physically inactive, as it can be adapted to one's abilities, time, and circumstances.

? ACTIVE LEARNING

1. How is your community doing in comparison with other communities? Prevalence and incidence rates for diseases or health conditions allow us to make comparisons between communities. Rates of activities such as smoking and physical activity allow us to make comparisons between communities regarding other areas of health promotion. Consider a community of which you are a member (e.g., your state, your county, your age group, or your school). Choose a health promotion topic that is of particular importance to your community of interest, such as sexual health, obesity, communicable disease, or physical activity. How does your community compare with a similar community in a different area of the state or the country? How does your community compare with a similar community in another part of the world?

2. View the Institute of Medicine series *Weight of the Nation* at https://www.imdb.com/title/tt2220150/#: ~ :text=The%20Weight%20of%20the%20Nation%20examines%20the%20long-term,heart%20disease%2C%20the%20negative%20impact%20of%20high%20weight. As you watch the series consider the following: What is the largest contributing factor to obesity among children? What interventions can you think of that would be effective in preventing or reducing obesity prevalence in your community? What are common barriers to preventing or reducing obesity among people across the lifespan? What negative effects will the United States as a whole face due to obesity?

Sleep

Sleep is an essential component of chronic disease prevention and health promotion, yet 74% of adults report having a sleeping problem one or more nights per week. One-quarter of the U.S. population reports that they occasionally do not get enough sleep, 39% report getting less than 7 h of sleep per night, and 37% report being so sleepy during the day that it interferes with daily activities. Insufficient sleep is associated with diabetes, heart disease, obesity, and depression. Insufficient sleep contributes to 100,000 motor vehicle crashes each year and 15,000 deaths. Sleep requirements change as people age (Table 4.4), and depending on life circumstances, one may require more than the minimum hours listed. If a person is so tired or sleepy that it interferes with his or her daily activities, that person probably needs more sleep (National Sleep Foundation, n.d.).

As we age, sleep is often interrupted by pain, trips to the bathroom, medications, medical conditions, and sleep disorders. In order to get enough sleep, we must plan to set aside enough time for sleep. Preferably, this means that we can awaken naturally, without an alarm clock, ensuring adequate rest. The need for sleep is regulated by two processes. One is the number of hours we are awake. The longer we are awake, the stronger the desire is to sleep. The other process is the circadian biological clock in the brain, the suprachiasmatic nucleus, which responds to light. This clock makes us tend to be sleepy

TABLE 4.4 How Much Sleep Do We Really Need?

Age	Sleep Needs
Newborns (1—2 months)	10.5—18 h
Infants (3—11 months)	9—12 h during night and 30-min to 2-h naps, 1—4 h a day
Toddlers (1—3 years)	12—14 h
Preschoolers (3—5 years)	11—13 h
School-aged children (5—12 years)	10—11 h
Teens (11—17 years)	8.5—9.25 h
Adults	7—9 h
Older adults	7—9 h

Used with permission of the National Sleep Foundation. For further information, please visit www.sleepfoundation.org/how-much-sleep-do-we-really-need.

at night when it is dark and to be active during the day when it is light. The circadian rhythm is why we are sleepiest between 2:00 and 4:00 a.m. and 1:00 and 3:00 p.m. The circadian rhythm also regulates the 24-h cycle of the body. While we sleep, important hormones are released, memory is consolidated, blood pressure is decreased, and kidney function changes (National Sleep Foundation, n.d.).

One of the results of lack of sleep is drowsy driving. More than one-third of U.S. drivers admit to having fallen asleep while driving, and 4% have had an accident due to driving while drowsy. An estimated 1550 deaths result from driver fatigue annually. Sleep-related motor vehicle accidents are most common among young people, shift workers, men, and adults with children. Adults between 18 and 29 years of age are the most likely to drive when sleepy. The lesser the people sleep, the greater their risk of being involved in a vehicular crash. People who sleep 6 to 7 h per night are twice as likely to be involved in a crash as those sleeping 8 h per night or more. People sleeping 4 to 5 h have a four to five times higher risk of being involved in a sleep-related accident. Being awake for 18 h produces the same degree of impairment as being legally intoxicated.

Practicing sleep hygiene will help achieve optimum sleep, as follows:

- Avoid caffeine and nicotine close to bedtime.
- Avoid alcohol, as it can cause sleep disruptions.
- Go to bed and get up at the same time every day.
- Exercise regularly, but finish all exercise and vigorous activity at least 3 h before bedtime.
- Establish a regular, relaxing bedtime routine (a warm bath, reading a book).
- Create a dark, quiet, cool sleep environment.
- Have a comfortable mattress and bedding.
- Use the bed for sleep only; do not read, listen to music, or watch TV in bed.

- Avoid large meals before bedtime (National Sleep Foundation, n.d.).

Sleep assessment is an important nursing function. If a client reports snoring, apnea, restlessness, or insomnia, he or she may have a sleep disorder. Recommend keeping a sleep log that details how many hours are spent in sleep each night and any problems with sleep. If insufficient sleep is causing trouble concentrating or completing daily activities, recommend consulting a doctor, as a sleep disorder may be to blame. A sleep assessment tool and a list of sleep disorders and descriptions of each may be found on the National Sleep Foundation's website, at http://www.sleepfoundation.org/.

Because of the 24-hour-per-day nature of nursing, nurses are among many workers who must work night shifts. Negative physical effects of working nights include an increased risk for stroke and heart disease, increased development of metabolic syndrome, and irregular menstrual cycles. Sleep deprivation related to shift work can cause practice errors related to a lack of attention to detail, impaired psychomotor skills, and reduced coordination, among others.

Those who work night shifts often experience *shift work disorder*. Shift work disorder is caused by night shifts, rotating shifts, and sometimes morning shifts. It causes chronic sleep deprivation in which a person never catches up on needed sleep. This sleep deprivation affects one's health, safety, productivity, and quality of life. Many shift workers struggle with excess sleepiness during work or leisure hours that interfere with their ability to work, study, or engage in social activities.

The National Sleep Foundation has helpful ways to cope with shift work disorder at https://sleepfoundation.org/shift-work/content/living-coping-shift-work-disorder.

An important benefit of sleep is an improved immune system to prevent or limit infection in. Healthy sleep can support boosting the body's immune defense and may prevent one from getting sick as often.

Sleep not only increases your immune system function but it also has been shown to play a role in improving antibody responses to vaccinations. Getting enough sleep before and after receiving vaccinations can boost the body's response to the vaccine (National Sleep Foundation, 2021).

? ACTIVE LEARNING

How do people, groups, and populations meet health promotion goals? Interview someone who is successful at meeting his or her health promotion goals. For example: How did the person manage to keep his or her weight at a healthy level? How did the person stop smoking? How does he or she make time to exercise daily? Does the individual have a philosophy of health that helps him or her stay on track with health promotion goals? How does the individual incorporate health promotion into daily life? What advice does he or she have for others striving to achieve better health?

SUMMARY

Health promotion is an essential component to ongoing good health and well-being, yet many Americans have difficulty with one or more of the components of health promotion. Exercise, diet, sleep, and tobacco and alcohol use all affect our health. Nurses, particularly community health nurses, are in a position to assess and counsel clients on their health habits. Community health nurses also possess the unique combination of community familiarity and the knowledge and training to affect health at the policy level. As the environment is made safer and more walkable, or with a lower density of available alcohol or fast food, the community as a whole will benefit.

EVOLVE WEBSITE

http://evolve.elsevier.com/Nies/community
- NCLEX Review Questions
- Case Studies

BIBLIOGRAPHY

American Cancer Society: *Child and teen tobacco use*, November 8, 2012. Available from: http://www.cancer.org/cancer/cancercauses/tobaccocancer/childandteentobaccouse/child-and-teen-tobacco-use-child-and-teen-tobacco-use. Accessed February 27, 2013.

American Cancer Society: *Guide to quitting smoking*, April 19, 2016. Available from: https://www.cancer.org/healthy/stay-away-from-tobacco/guide-quitting-smoking/deciding-to-quit-smoking-and-making-a-plan.html. (Accessed April 7 2017).

American Cancer Society: *Helping a smoker quit. October 2016*, April 7, 2017. Available from: https://www.cancer.org/healthy/stay-away-from-tobacco/helping-a-smoker-quit.html.

American Lung Association: *Quit smoking*, n.d. Available from: http://www.lung.org/stop-smoking/. (Accessed 9 January 2014).

Atkinson LN, Saperstein LS, Pleis J: Using the internet for health-related activities: findings from a national probability sample, *J Med Internet Res* 11(1):e4, 2009.

Bauer KW, Hearst MO, Escoto K: Parental environments and work-family stress: associations with family food environments, *Soc Sci Med* 75:496−504, 2012.

Bauer KW, Larson NI, Nelson MC: Fast food intake among adolescents: secular and longitudinal trends from 1999−2004, *Prev Med* 48:284−287, 2009.

Benson H: *Timeless healing: the power and biology of belief*, New York, 1996, Scribner.

Brown BB, Smith KR, Hanson H: Neighborhood design for walking and biking: physical activity and body mass index, *Am J Prev Med* 44:23−238, 2013.

Burger KS, Kern M, Coleman KJ: Characteristics of self-selected portion sizes in young adults [electronic version], *J Am Diet Assoc* 107:611−1608, 2007.

https://www.cdc.gov/alcohol/fact-sheets/prevention.htm.

https://www.cdc.gov/nchs/fastats/obesity-overweight.htm.

https://www.cdc.gov/chronicdisease/resources/publications/factsheets/alcohol.htm.

https://www.cdc.gov/obesity/data/childhood.html.

https://www.cdc.gov/tobacco/data_statistics/fact_sheets/smokeless/use_us/index.htm#adult-national.

https://www.cdc.gov/obesity/data/adult.html.

https://www.cdc.gov/obesity/data/prevalence-maps.html.

https://www.cdc.gov/physicalactivity/data/inactivity-prevalence-maps/index.html.

https://www.cdc.gov/tobacco/data_statistics/fact_sheets/smokeless/health_effects/index.htm.

https://www.cdc.gov/alcohol/fact-sheets/underage-drinking.htm.

Centers for Disease Control and Prevention. Available: https://www.ncbi.nlm.nih.gov/pubmed/?term=Ogden+CL%2C+Carroll+MD%2C+Lawman+HG%2C+Fryar+CD%2C+Kruszon-Moran+D%2C+Kit+BK%2C+et+al.+Trends+in+Obesity+Prevalence+Among+Children+and+Adolescents+in+the+United+States%2C+1988-1994+Through+2013-2014.+Jama+2016%3B315(21)%3A2292

Centers for Disease Control and Prevention: *Alcohol screening*, April 21, 2015. Available from: https://www.cdc.gov/features/alcoholscreening/index.html (Accessed 13 April 2017).

Centers for Disease Control and Prevention: *Alcohol use and health*, July 25, 2016a. Available from: https://www.cdc.gov/alcohol/fact-sheets/alcohol-use.htm (Accessed 13 April 2017).

Centers for Disease Control and Prevention: *Binge drinking*, October 16, 2016. Available from: https://www.cdc.gov/alcohol/fact-sheets/binge-drinking.htm (Accessed 13 April 2017).

Centers for Disease Control and Prevention: *Current cigarette smoking among adults in 2015*, December 1, 2016. Available from: https://www.cdc.gov/tobacco/data_statistics/fact_sheets/adult_data/cig_smoking/index.htm (Accessed 3 April 2017).

Centers for Disease Control and Prevention: *Do increased portion sizes affect how much we eat? Nutrition resources for health professionals*, May 2006. Available from: www.cdc.gov/nccdphp/dnpa/nutrition/pdf/portion_size_research.pdf (Accessed 20 April 2009).

Centers for Disease Control and Prevention: *Excessive alcohol use and risks to women's health*, October 1, 2012. Available from: http://www.cdc.gov/alcohol/fact-sheets/womens-health.htm (Accessed 28 February 2012).

Centers for Disease Control and Prevention: *Facts about physical activity*, 2014. Available from: https://www.cdc.gov/physicalactivity/data/facts.htm (Accessed 17 April 2017).

Centers for Disease Control and Prevention: *Incorporating eaten-away-from-home food into a healthy eating plan: nutrition resources for health professionals*, December 22, 2008. Available from: www.cdc.gov/nccdphp/dnpa/nutrition/pdf/r2p_away_from_home_food.pdf (Accessed 13 April 2009).

Centers for Disease Control and Prevention: *National center for chronic disease prevention and health promotion: state indicator report on fruits and vegetables 2013*, November 6, 2008. Available from: https://www.cdc.gov/nutrition/downloads/state-indicator-report-fruits-vegetables-2013.pdf   apps.nccd.cdc.gov/5ADaySurveillance/displayV.asp (Accessed 13 April 2009).

Centers for Disease Control and Prevention: *Prevalence of childhood obesity in the United States*, April 10, 2017. Available from: https://www.cdc.gov/obesity/data/childhood.html (Accessed 14 April 2017).

Centers for Disease Control and Prevention: *Prevalence of obesity among adults and youth: United States 2011−2014*. Available from: https://www.cdc.gov/nchs/data/databriefs/db219.pdf. (Accessed 13 April 2017).

Centers for Disease Control and Prevention: *Preventing excessive alcohol use*, October 17, 2016. Available from: https://www.cdc.gov/alcohol/fact-sheets/prevention.htm (Accessed 13 April 2017).

Centers for Disease Control and Prevention: *Quick stats: age 21 legal minimum drinking age. alcohol and public health*, September 3, 2008. Available from: www.cdc.gov/alcohol/quickstats/mlda.htm (Accessed 4 May 2009).

Centers for Disease Control and Prevention: *Smoking cessation (n.d.)*, January 2, 2013a. Available from: http://www.cdc.gov/tobacco/data_statistics/fact_sheets/cessation/quitting/index.htm (Accessed 22 August 2013).

Centers for Disease Control and Prevention: *Smokeless tobacco use in the United States*, 2014a. Available from: https://www.cdc.gov/tobacco/data_statistics/fact_sheets/smokeless/use_us/index.htm (Accessed 7 April 2017).

Centers for Disease Control and Prevention: *Trends in the prevalence of extreme obesity among US preschool-aged children living in low-income families, 1998–2010*. Available from: http://www.cdc.gov/obesity/data/childhood.html/. (Accessed March 2013).

Centers for Disease Control and Prevention: *Underage drinking*, October 20, 2016. Available from: https://www.cdc.gov/alcohol/fact-sheets/underage-drinking.htm (Accessed 10 April 2017).

Centers for Disease Control and Prevention: *US obesity trends 1985–2007: overweight and obesity*, July 24, 2008a. Available from: www.cdc.gov/nccdphp/dnpa/obesity/trend/maps/index.htm (Accessed 19 April 2009).

Centers for Disease Control and Prevention: *Ways to reduce cancer risk*, January 2, 2013. Available from: http://www.cdc.gov/cancer/dcpc/prevention/other.htm (Accessed 25 February 2013).

Champion VL, Skinner CS: The health belief model. In Glanz K, Rimer BK, Viswanath K, editors: *Health behavior and health education: theory, research, and practice*, San Francisco, 2008, Jossey-Bass.

De Castro JM, King GA, Duarte-Gardea M: Overweight and obese humans overeat away from home, *Appetite* 59:204–211, 2012.

https://www.dietaryguidelines.gov/.

https://www.ers.usda.gov/webdocs/publications/90228/eib-196_ch3.pdf?v=8116.5.

Edwards A, Naik G, Ahmed H: Personalised risk communication for informed decision making about screening tests (Review) [update], *The Cochr Lib* 2:CD001865, 2013.

https://www.fda.gov/media/112972/download.

Finklestein EA, Trogdon JG, Cohen JW: Annual medical spending attributable to obesity: payer- and service-specific estimates, *Health Aff* 289(5):w822–w831, 2009.

Finnigan JR, Vinswanath K: Communication theory and health behavior change. In Glanz KR, Rimer BK, Vinswanath K, editors: *Health behavior and health education*, ed 4, San Francisco, 2008, Jossey-Bass, pp 363–384.

Flegal K, Carroll O: Johnson prevalence and trends among US adults, 1999–2000, *JAMA* 288:1723–1727, 2002.

Frank LS: Linking objectively measured physical activity with objectively measured urban form: findings from SMARTRAQ, *Am J Prev Med* 28:117–125, 2005.

Friis R, Sellers: *Epidemiology for public health practice*, London, 2004, Jones & Bartlett.

Fryar CD, Ervin RB: *Caloric intake from fast food among adults: United States, 2007–2010. NCHS data brief no. 114*, 2013. Available from: www.cdc.gov/nchs/data/databriefs/db114.htm (Accessed March 2013).

Fulkerson JA, Farbakhsh K, Lytle L: Away-from-home family dinner sources and associations with weight status, body composition and related biomarkers of chronic disease among adolescents and their parents, *J Am Diet Assoc* 111(112):1892–1897, 2011.

Green L, Kreuter M: *Health promotion and planning: an educational and environmental approach*, Mountain View, CA, 1991, Mayfield.

Hendrick PA, Ahmed OH, Bankier SS: Acute low back pain information online: an evaluation of quality, content, accuracy and readability of related websites, *Man Ther* 17:318–324, 2012.

Hochbaum G: *Public participation in medical screening programs: a socio-psychological study*, Washington, DC, 1958, U.S. Public Health Service.

Kupferberg N, Protus B: Accuracy and completeness of drug information in Wikipedia: an assessment, *J Med Libr Assoc* 99:310–313, 2011.

Lin B-H, Jean C, Buzby, Tobenna D, Anekwe, Bentley J, editors: *U.S. food commodity consumption broken down by demographics, 1994–2008*, March 2016, USDA, Economic Research Service.

Loef M, Walach H: The combined effects of healthy lifestyle behaviors on all cause mortality: a systematic review and meta-analysis, *Prev Med* 55:163–170, 2012.

Marchetta CM, Denny CH, Floyd L: Alcohol use and binge drinking among women of childbearing age—United States, 2006–2010, *Morb Mortal Wkly Rep* 61:534–538, 2012.

McCrory MA, Fuss PJ, Hays NP, et al.: Overeating in America: association between restaurant food consumption and body fatness in healthy adult men and women, *Obes Res* 92:564–571, 1999.

McEwen M, Pullis B: *Community-based nursing: an introduction*, St. Louis, 2009, Saunders.

McGinnis JM, Foege WH: Actual causes of death in the United States, *JAMA* 270:2207–2212, 1993.

McGinnis JM, Foege WH: The immediate and the important, *JAMA* 291:1263–1264, 2004.

Medscape: *Help me make it through the night (shift)*. Available from: http://www.medscape.com/viewarticle/757050. (Accessed March 2013).

Merriam-Webster Online Dictionary: *Health*, March 2009. Available from: www.merriam-webster.com/dictionary/health (Accessed 23 March 2009).

Mokdab AH, Marks JS, Stroup DF, et al.: Actual causes of death in the United States 2000, *JAMA* 291:1238–1245, 2004.

Montano D, Kasprzyk D: Theory of reasoned action, theory of planned behavior, and the integrated behavioral model. In Glanz KR, editor: *Health behavior and health education: theory, research, and practice*, ed 4, San Francisco, 2008, Jossey-Bass, pp 67–96.

National Heart, Lung, and Blood Institute (NHLBI): *Portion distortion*. February 2013. http://www.nhlbi.nih.gov/health/public/heart/obesity/wecan/portion/index.htm Accessed January 2014, January 2014.

National Institutes of Health: *Alcohol facts and statistics*, February 2017. Available from: https://pubs.niaaa.nih.gov/publications/AlcoholFacts&Stats/AlcoholFacts&Stats.htm (Accessed 10 April 2017).

National Research Council (NRC) and Institute of Medicine (IOM): Measuring the risks and causes of premature death: summary of workshops. In Rhodes HG, editor: *Rapporteur, committee on population, division of behavioral and social sciences and education and board on health care services*, Washington, DC, 2015, Institute of Medicine, The National Academies Press.

National Sleep Foundation: *Drowsy driving: facts and stats*. Available from: http://drowsydriving.org/about/facts-and-stats/. (Accessed March 2013).

National Sleep Foundation: *How much sleep do we really need?*, 2013. Available from: http://www.sleepfoundation.org/article/how-sleep-works/how-much-sleep-do-we-really-need (Accessed 28 January 2010).

IA https://www.nia.nih.gov/health/online-health-information-it-reliable. https://www.niaaa.nih.gov/publications/brochures-and-fact-sheets/alcohol-facts-and-statistics. https://www.niaaa.nih.gov/alcohols-effects-health/special-populations. https://www.niaaa.nih.gov/alcohols-effects-health.

Office of Applied Studies: *The NSDUH report: alcohol dependence or abuse and age at first use*, Rockville, MD, Substance Abuse and Mental Health Services Administration.

Ogden C, Carroll C, Curtin LR, et al.: Prevalence of overweight and obesity in the United States, 1999–2004, *JAMA* 295:1545–1599, 2006.

Ogden C, Carroll MD, Flegal KM: *Prevalence of obesity in the United States: 2009–2010. NCHS Data Brief #82.* Available from: http://www.cdc.gov/obesity/data/adult.html. (Accessed March 2013).

Ogden CL, Carroll MD, Lawman HG, et al.: Trends in obesity prevalence among children and adolescents in the United States, 1988-1994 through 2013-2014, *JAMA* 315(21):2292–2299, 2016.

Ogden CL, Lamb MM, Carroll MD: *Obesity and socioeconomic status in adults: United States, 2005–2008, NCHS data brief no. 50,* 2010. Available from: http://www.cdc.gov/nchs/data/databriefs/db50.pdf.

Oleckno W: Essential epidemiology. Prospects Heights, IL: Waveland Press.

https://www.pewresearch.org/fact-tank/2020/04/30/from-virtual-parties-to-ordering-food-how-americans-are-using-the-internet-during-covid-19/.

Parse R: Health promotion and prevention: two distinct cosmologies, *Nurs Sci Q* 3:101, 1990.

Pender N. In *Health promotion and disease prevention*, ed 3, Stamford, CT, 1996, Appleton & Lange.

Pender N, Murdaugh CL, Parsons MA. In *Health promotion in nursing practice*, ed 6, Upper Saddle River, NJ, 2011, Pearson.

Rehm CD, Monsivais P, Drewnowski A: Relation between diet cost and Healthy Eating Index 2010 scores among adults in the United States 2007–2010, *Prev Med* 73:70–75, 2015.

Saelens B, Salis JF, Black JB, et al.: Neighborhood-based differences in physical activity: an environment scale evaluation, *Resear & Pract* 93:43–54, 2003.

Savitz DR: Methods in chronic epidemiology. In Brownson RC, Remington PL, Davis JR, editors: *Chronic disease epidemiology and control*, Washington, DC, 1998, American Public Health Association, pp 27–54.

Schroder H, Fito M, Cavas M: Association of fast food consumption with energy intake, diet quality, body mass index, and the risk of obesity in a representative Mediterranean population, *Br J Nutr* 98:1274–1280, 2007.

Schroeder SA: We can do better—improving the health of the American people, *N Engl J Med* 357:1221–1228, 2007. https://doi.org/10.1056/NEJMsa073350.

Schumacher S, Kent N: *8 Charts on internet use as countries grapple with COVID 19*, 2020. Accessed at, https://www.pewresearch.org/fact-tank/2020/04/02/8-charts-on-internet-use-around-the-world-as-countries-grapple-with-covid-19/.

Schwartz J, Byrd-Bredbrenner C: Portion distortion: typical portion sizes selected by young adults, *J Am Diet Assoc* 106:1412–1418, 2006.

Slater DJ, Nicholson L, Chriqui J: Walkable communities and adolescent weight, *Am J Prev Med* 44:164–168, 2013.

The Keystone Center: *The Keystone forum on away-from-home foods: opportunities for preventing weight gain and obesity*, 2006. Washington, DC.

U.S. Department of Agriculture: *Choose my plate.gov*, 2020. Available from: http://www.choosemyplate.gov/ (Accessed March, 2013).

U.S. Department of Agriculture. In *Center for nutrition policy and promotion: 2010 dietary guidelines for Americans*, ed 8, 2015, Author. Available from: https://health.gov/dietaryguidelines/2015/guidelines/.

U.S. Department of Agriculture and U.S. Department of Health and Human Services: Chapter 3. Foods and food components to reduce. In *Dietary guidelines for Americans, Washington, DC*, 2010, US Government Printing Office, pp 30–32.

U.S. Department of Health and Human Services: *About healthy people*, December 17, 2012. Available from: http://www.healthypeople.gov/2020/about/default.aspx (Accessed March 2013).

U.S. Department of Health and Human Services: *Healthy People 2020: topics and objectives*, March 8, 2013. Available from: http://www.healthypeople.gov/2020/topicsobjectives2020/default.aspx (Accessed March 2013).

U.S. Department of Health and Human Services: *Step it up! the surgeon general's call to action to promote walking and walkable communities*, 2015. Available from: www.surgeongeneral.gov (Accessed April 2017).

U.S. Department of Justice: *Drinking in America: myths, realities and prevention policies*, 2002. Available from: http://www.udetc.org/documents/Drinking_in_America.pdf (Accessed 28 February 2013).

Van der Horst K, Brunner TA, Siegrist M: Fast food and take-away food consumption are associated with different lifestyle characteristics, *J Hum Nutr Diet* 24:596–602, 2011.

Walk Score: *What makes a city walkable? Walkscore: find a walkable place to live*, 2013. Available from: www.walkscore.com/rankings/what-makes-a-city-walkable.shtml (Accessed 9 January 2014).

Westberg J, Jason H: Fostering healthy behavior: the process. In Woolf SH, Jonas S, Lawrence RS, editors: *Health promotion and disease prevention in clinical practice*, Baltimore, 1996, Williams & Wilkins.

World Health Organization: Health promotion: a discussion document on the concept and principles, *Public Health Rev* 14:245–254, 1986.

World Health Organization: *Mental health*, 2009. Available from: www.who.int/topics/mental_health/en/ (Accessed 23 March 2009).

5

Epidemiology

Holly B. Cassells

OBJECTIVES

Upon completion of this chapter, the reader will be able to do the following:

1. Identify epidemiological models used to explain disease and health patterns in populations.
2. Use epidemiological methods to describe the state of health in a community or aggregate.
3. Calculate epidemiological rates in order to characterize population health.
4. Understand the use of epidemiological methods in primary, secondary, and tertiary prevention.
5. Evaluate epidemiological study designs for researching health problems.

OUTLINE

KEY TERMS

age adjustment of rates
age-specific rates
analytic epidemiology
attack rates
cause-and-effect relationship
crude rates
descriptive epidemiology
ecosocial epidemiology
epidemiological triangle

epidemiology
incidence rates
infant mortality rate
morbidity rates
mortality rates
natural history of disease
person—place—time model
prevalence rate
proportionate mortality ratio

rates
risk
risk factors
screening
screening programs
standardization of rates
surveillance
web of causation

Epidemiology is the study of the distribution and determinants of health and disease in human populations and is the principal science of public health. It entails a body of knowledge derived from epidemiological research and specialized epidemiological methods and approaches to scientific research. Community health nurses use epidemiological concepts to improve the health of population groups by identifying risk factors and optimal approaches that reduce disease risk and promote health. Epidemiological methods are important for accurate community assessment and diagnosis, and in planning and evaluating effective community interventions. This chapter discusses the uses of epidemiology and its specialized methodologies.

USE OF EPIDEMIOLOGY IN DISEASE CONTROL AND PREVENTION

Although epidemiological principles and ideas originated in ancient times, formal epidemiological techniques developed in the 19th century. Early applications focused on identifying factors associated with infectious diseases and the spread of disease in the community. Public health practitioners hoped to improve preventive strategies by identifying critical factors in disease development.

Specifically, investigators attempted to identify characteristics of people who had a disease such as cholera or plague and compared them with characteristics of those who remained healthy. These differences might include a broad range of personal factors, such as age, gender, socioeconomic status, and health status. Investigators also questioned whether there were differences in the location or living environment of ill people compared with healthy individuals and whether these factors influenced disease development. Finally, researchers examined whether common time factors existed (i.e., when people acquired disease). Use of this **person-place-time model** organized epidemiologists' investigations of the disease pattern in the community (Box 5.1). This study of the amount and distribution of disease constitutes **descriptive epidemiology**. Identified patterns frequently indicate possible causes of disease that public health professionals can examine with more advanced epidemiological methods.

In addition to investigating the person, place, and time factors related to disease, epidemiologists examine complex relationships among the many determinants of disease. This investigation of the causes of disease, or etiology, is called *analytic epidemiology.*

Even before the identification of bacterial agents, public health practitioners recognized that single factors were insufficient to cause disease. For example, while exploring the cholera epidemics in London in 1855, Dr. John Snow collected data about social and physical environmental conditions that might favor disease development. He specifically examined the contamination of local water systems. Snow also gathered information about people who became ill—their living patterns, water sources, socioeconomic characteristics, and health status. A comprehensive database helped him develop a theory about the possible cause of the epidemic. Snow suspected that a single biological agent was responsible for the cholera infection, although the organism, *Vibrio cholerae,* had yet to be discovered. He compared the death rates among individuals using one water well with those among people using a different water source. His findings suggested an association between cholera and water quality (Box 5.2).

The epidemiologist examines the interrelationships between host and environmental characteristics and uses an organized method of inquiry to derive an explanation of disease. This model of investigation is called the **epidemiological triangle** because the epidemiologist must analyze the following three elements: agent, host, and environment (Fig. 5.1). The development of disease depends on the extent of the host's exposure to an agent, the strength or virulence of the agent, and the host's genetic or immunological susceptibility. Disease also depends on the environmental conditions existing at the time of exposure, which include the biological, social, political, and physical environments (Table 5.1). The model implies that the rate of disease will change when the balance among these three factors is altered. By examining each of the three elements, a community health nurse can methodically assess a health problem, determine protective factors, and evaluate the factors that make the host vulnerable to disease.

Conditions linked to clearly identifiable agents, such as bacteria, chemicals, toxins, and other exposure factors, are readily explained by the epidemiological triangle. However, other models that stress the multiplicity of host and environmental interactions have developed and understanding of disease has progressed. The "wheel model" is an example of such a model (Fig. 5.2). The wheel consists of a hub that represents the host and its human characteristics, such as genetic makeup, personality, and immunity. The surrounding wheel represents the environment and comprises biological, social, and physical dimensions. The relative size of each component in the wheel depends on the health problem. A relatively large genetic core represents health conditions associated with heredity. Origins of other health conditions may be more dependent on environmental factors (Mausner & Kramer, 1985). This model subscribes to multiple-causation rather than single-causation disease theory; therefore it is more useful for analyzing complex chronic conditions and identifying factors that are amenable to intervention.

After the discovery of the causative agents of many infectious diseases, public health interventions eventually resulted in a decline in widespread epidemic mortality, particularly in developed countries. The focus of public health then shifted to chronic diseases such as cancer, coronary heart disease, and diabetes during the past few decades. The development of these chronic diseases tends to be associated with multiple interrelated factors rather than single causative agents.

In studying chronic diseases, epidemiologists use methods that are similar to those used in infectious disease investigation, thereby developing theories about chronic disease control. Risk factor identification is of particular importance to chronic disease reduction. **Risk factors** are variables that increase the rate of disease in people who have them (e.g., a genetic predisposition) or in people exposed to them (e.g., an infectious agent or a diet high in saturated fat). Therefore, their identification is critical to identifying specific prevention and

---

BOX 5.1   Person–Place–Time Model

Person: "Who" factors, such as demographic characteristics, health, and disease status

Place: "Where" factors, such as geographic location, climate and environmental conditions, and political and social environment

Time: "When" factors, such as time of day, week, or month and secular trends over months and years

BOX 5.2   Example of the Epidemiological Approach

An early example of the epidemiological approach is John Snow's investigation of a cholera epidemic in the 1850s. He analyzed the distribution of person, place, and time factors by comparing the death rates among people living in different geographic sectors of London. His geographic map of cases, shown here, is an early example of the use of geographic information to formulate a hypothesis about the causes of an epidemic. Snow noted that people using a particular water pump had significantly higher mortality rates from cholera than people using other water sources in the city. Although the cholera organism was yet unidentified, the clustering of disease cases around one neighborhood pump suggested new prevention strategies to public health officials (i.e., that cholera might be reduced in a community by controlling contaminated drinking water sources). As an immediate response, in September 1854, Snow persuaded local leaders to remove the handle of the pump, which to this day can be seen on Broadwick Street in London (Snow, 1855).

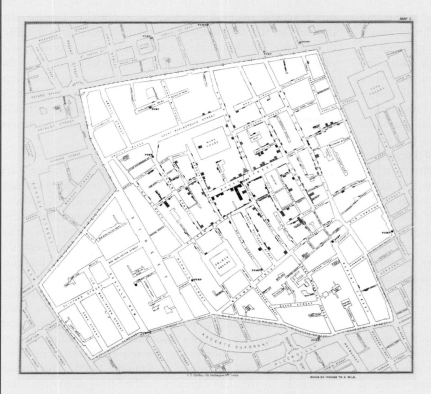

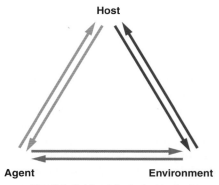

(Replica of the famous Broad Street pump, Broadwick Street, London. Photo courtesy of http://commons. wikimedia.org/wiki/File:John_Snow_memorial_and_ pub.jpg, Creative Commons Attribution-Share Alike 2.0 Generic [CC BY-SA 2.0].)

John Snow's map of London neighborhood showing location of cholera case cluster surrounding the Broad Street water pump. (Published by Cheffins CF: Lith, Southampton Buildings, London, England, 1854. In Snow J, editor: *On the mode of communication of cholera*, ed 2, London, 1855, John Churchill. Available from: www.ph.ucla.edu/epi/snow/ snowmap1_1854_lge.htm.)

Host

Agent   **Environment**

Fig. 5.1 Epidemiological triangle.

intervention approaches that effectively and efficiently reduce chronic disease morbidity and mortality. For example, the identification of cardiovascular disease risk factors has suggested lifestyle modifications that could reduce the morbidity risk before disease onset. Primary prevention strategies, such as dietary saturated fat reduction, smoking cessation, and hypertension control, were developed in response to epidemiological studies that identified these risk factors (Box 5.3). The **web of causation** model illustrates the complexity of relationships among causal variables for heart disease (Fig. 5.3).

A newer paradigm, **ecosocial epidemiology**, challenges the more individually focused risk factor approach to

TABLE 5.1   A Classification of Agent, Host, and Environmental Factors That Determine the Occurrence of Diseases in Human Populations

Factors	Examples
Agents of Disease—Etiological Factors	
A. Nutritive elements:	
Excesses	Cholesterol, saturated fat
Deficiencies	Vitamins, proteins
B. Chemical agents:	
Poisons	Carbon monoxide, carbon tetrachloride, drugs
Allergens	Ragweed, poison ivy, medications
C. Physical agents:	
Ionizing radiation	Sun exposure, medical imaging
Mechanical	Repetitive motion injury
D. Infectious agents:	
Metazoa	Hookworm, schistosomiasis, onchocerciasis
Protozoa	Amebae, malaria
Bacteria	Rheumatic fever, lobar pneumonia, typhoid, tuberculosis, syphilis
Fungi	Histoplasmosis, athlete's foot
Rickettsia	Rocky Mountain spotted fever, typhus, Lyme disease
Viruses	Measles, mumps, chickenpox, smallpox, poliomyelitis, rabies, yellow fever, human immunodeficiency virus, SARS-Coronavirus
Host Factors (i.e., Intrinsic Factors)—Susceptibility or Response Influence Exposure to Agent	
A. Genetic	Cystic fibrosis, Huntington disease
B. Age	Alzheimer disease
C. Sex	Rheumatoid arthritis
D. Ethnic group	Tay-Sachs disease, sickle cell disease
E. Physiological state	Fatigue, pregnancy, puberty, stress, nutritional state
F. Prior immunological experience:	Hypersensitivity, protection
Active	Prior infection, immunization
Passive	Maternal antibodies, gamma globulin prophylaxis
G. Intercurrent or preexisting disease	Diabetes, liver dysfunction, hypertension
H. Human behavior	Personal hygiene, food handling, diet, interpersonal contact, mask-wearing, occupation, recreation, use of health resources, tobacco use
Environmental Factors (i.e., Extrinsic Factors)—Influence Existence of the Agent, Exposure, or Susceptibility to Agent	
A. Physical environment	Geology, climate
B. Biological environment	
Human populations	Density
Flora	Sources of food, influence on vertebrates and arthropods, as a source of agents
Fauna	Food sources, vertebrate hosts, arthropod vectors
C. Socioeconomic environment	
Occupation	Exposure to chemical agents
Urbanization and economic development	Urban crowding, tension and pressures, use of public transportation, cooperative efforts in health and education
Disruption	Wars, floods, famine

Modified from Lilienfeld DE, Stoley PD: *Foundations of epidemiology*, New York, NY, 1994, Oxford University Press.

understanding disease origins. This ecosocial approach emphasizes the role of evolving macro-level socioenvironmental factors, including complex political and economic forces, along with microbiological processes, in understanding health and illness. Investigating the context of health necessitates alternative research approaches, such as qualitative and ecological studies and studies of social institutions and processes. In turn, the examination of social and contextual origins expands the range of public health interventions and supports an emphasis on the social determinants of health.

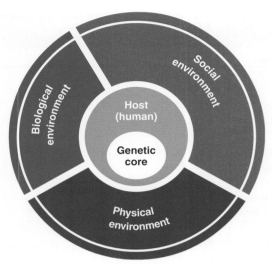

Fig. 5.2 Wheel model of human—environment interaction. (Redrawn from Mausner JS, Kramer S: *Mausner and Bahn Epidemiology: An Introductory Text*, ed 2, Philadelphia, 1985, Saunders.)

For example, Mehra et al. (2020) applied an ecosocial and intersectional perspective, along with the biopsychosocial model of health, to gain insight into the "gendered racism" experiences of Black pregnant women. Specifically, they sought to glean new information to explain the disparities leading to poor maternal and infant outcomes among Blacks in the U.S. Following detailed interviews of 24 pregnant Black women, they uncovered what was termed "racialized pregnancy stigma."

BOX 5.3   Cardiovascular Disease Risk Factors Supported by Epidemiologic Studies

Traditional Risk Factors
- Age
- Gender (male; postmenopausal women)
- Current cigarette smoking
- Hypertension
- High level of low-density lipoprotein (LDL) cholesterol
- Low level of high-density lipoprotein (HDL) cholesterol
- Diabetes
- Family history of premature coronary heart disease

Newer Risk Factors
- High-risk race/ethnicity
- Chronic kidney disease
- Increased inflammation (C-reactive protein [CRP])
- Elevated lipoprotein a (Lp(a))
- Elevated apoB (apoB) (as an alternative to LDL cholesterol)

Arnett DK, Blumenthal RS, Albert MA, et al.: 2019 ACC/AHA guideline on the primary prevention of cardiovascular disease: a report of the American College of Cardiology/American Heart Association Task Force on Clinical Practice Guidelines, *Circulation* 140:e596—e646, 2019. https://dx.doi.org/10.1161/CIR.0000000000000678.

They reported that Black pregnant women felt they were not valued by society and felt judged based on negative assumptions. This stigmatization affected access to health care, social services, and housing and was seen as a source of stress that ultimately could contribute to poor outcomes. The authors concluded that health care and social service providers should receive antibias training to address gendered racism. In addition, Black pregnant women should be screened for the presence of stressors that could lead to poor outcomes and offered assistance and information on assistive resources and coping strategies. Finally increased social discourse to address the systematic problems of health disparities was strongly advocated.

In another study, Phillips (2011) applied an ecosocial perspective when examining the effects of social/contextual factors on adherence to antiretroviral therapy (ART) among Black men who tested positive for human immunodeficiency virus (HIV). He examined both individual factors (e.g., psychological state of mind, psychological distress, illicit drug use) and interpersonal/social contextual factors (e.g., partner status, housing status, patient—provider relationship, social capital [groups/networks]). He concluded that adherence to the medication regimen was strongly associated with homelessness and how well the individual tolerated the ART. Other factors included the individual's state of mind and illicit drug use. Practice implications included the observation that providers should assess social and behavioral factors and intervene accordingly. This would include identification of psychological distress or presence of substance abuse. He also suggested assessment of housing status and facilitation of effective patient—provider relationships to mitigate tolerability issues with ART.

CALCULATION OF RATES

The community health nurse must analyze data about the health of the community to determine disease patterns. The nurse may collect data by conducting surveys or compiling data from existing records (e.g., data from clinic facilities or vital statistics records). Assessment data often are in the form of counts or simple frequencies of events (e.g., the number of people with a specific health condition). Community health practitioners interpret these raw counts by transforming them into rates.

Rates are arithmetic expressions that help practitioners consider a count of an event relative to the size of the population from which it is extracted (e.g., the population at risk). Rates are population proportions or fractions in which the numerator is the number of events occurring in a specified period. The denominator consists of those in the population at the specified time period (e.g., per day, per week, or per year), frequently drawing on demographic data from the U.S. census. This proportion is multiplied by a constant *(k)* that is a multiple of 10, such as 1000, 10,000, or 100,000. The constant usually converts the resultant number to a whole

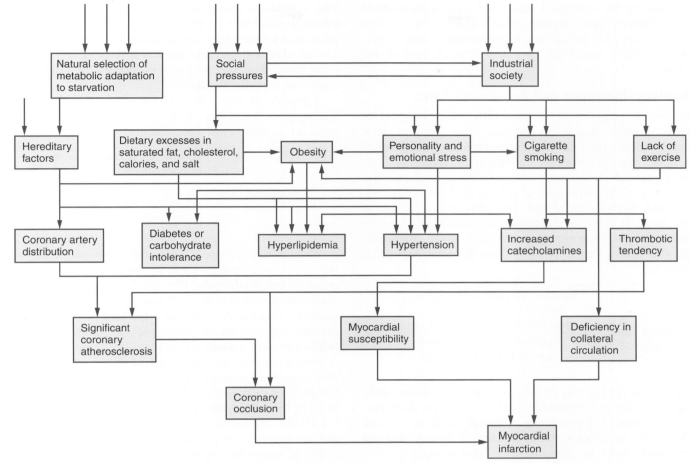

Fig. 5.3 The web of causation for myocardial infarction. (From Friedman GD: *Primer of epidemiology*, ed 5, New York, 2004, McGraw-Hill.)

number, which is larger and easier to interpret. Thus, a rate can be the number of cases of a disease occurring for every 1000, 10,000, or 100,000 people in the population, as follows:

$$\text{Rate} = \frac{\text{Numerator}}{\text{Denominator}}$$
$$= \frac{\text{Number of health events in a specified period}}{\text{Population in same area in same specified period}}$$

When raw counts or numbers are converted to rates, the community health nurse can make meaningful comparisons with rates from other cities, counties, districts, or states; from the nation; and from previous periods. These analyses help the nurse determine the magnitude of a public health problem in a given area and allow more meaningful and reliable tracking of trends in the community over time (Box 5.4).

Sometimes a ratio is used to express a relationship between two variables. A *ratio* is obtained by dividing one quantity by another, and the numerator is not necessarily part of the

---

BOX 5.4 Using Rates in Everyday Community Health Nursing Practice

The following school situation exemplifies the value of rates:

A community health nurse screened 500 students for tuberculosis (TB) in Southside School and identified 15 students with newly positive tuberculin test results. The proportion of Southside School students affected was 15/500, or 0.03 (3%), or a rate of 30/1000 students at risk for TB. Concurrently, the nurse conducted screening in Northside School and again identified 15 students with positive tuberculin test results. However, this school was much larger than the Southside School and had 900 potentially at-risk students. To place the number of affected students in perspective relative to the size of the Northside School, the nurse calculated a proportion of 15/900, or 0.017 (1.7%), or a rate of 17/1000 students at risk in Northside School.

On the basis of this comparison, the nurse concluded that although both schools had the same number of tuberculin conversions, Southside School had the greater rate of tuberculin test conversions. To determine whether rates are excessively high, the nurse should compare rates with the city, county, and state rates and then explore reasons for the difference in these rates.

denominator. For example, a ratio could contrast the number of male births to that of female births. *Proportions* can describe characteristics of a population. A proportion is often a percentage, and it represents the numerator as part of the denominator.

Morbidity: Incidence and Prevalence Rates

The two principal types of **morbidity rates**, or rates of illness, in public health are incidence rates and prevalence rates. **Incidence rates** describe the occurrence of new cases of a disease (e.g., tuberculosis, influenza) or condition (e.g., teen pregnancy) in a community over a given period relative to the size of the population at risk for that disease or condition during that same period. The denominator consists of only those at risk for the disease or condition; therefore known cases or those not susceptible (e.g., those immunized against a disease) are subtracted from the total population (Table 5.2):

$$\text{Incidence rate} = \frac{\text{Number of new cases or events occurring in the population in a specified period}}{\text{Population at risk during same specified period}} \times k$$

The incidence rate may be the most sensitive indicator of the changing health of a community because it captures the fluctuations of disease in a population. Although incidence rates are valuable for monitoring trends in chronic disease, they are particularly useful for detecting short-term changes in acute disease—such as those that occur with influenza or measles—in which the duration of the disease is typically short.

If a population is exposed to an infectious disease at a given time and place, the nurse may calculate the attack rate, a specialized form of the incidence rate. **Attack rates** document the number of new cases of a disease in those exposed to the disease. A common example of the application of the attack rate is food poisoning; the denominator is the number of people exposed to a suspect food, and the numerator is the number of people who were exposed and became ill. The nurse can calculate and compare the attack rates of illness among those exposed to specific foods to identify the critical food sources or exposure variables.

A **prevalence rate** is the number of all cases of a specific disease or condition (e.g., deafness) in a population at a given point in time relative to the population at the same point in time:

$$\text{Prevalence rate} = \frac{\text{Number of existing cases in population at specified point in time}}{\text{Population at same specified point in time}} \times k$$

When prevalence rates describe the number of people with the disease at a specific point in time, they are sometimes called *point prevalences*. For this reason, cross-sectional studies frequently use them. *Period prevalences* represent the number of existing cases during a specified period or interval of time and include old cases and new cases that appear within the same period.

Prevalence rates are influenced by the number of people who experience a particular condition (i.e., incidence) and the duration of condition. A nurse can derive the prevalence rate *(P)* by multiplying incidence *(I)* by duration *(D)*: (P = I × D). An increase in the incidence rate or the duration of a disease increases the prevalence rate of a disease. With the advent of life-prolonging therapies (e.g., insulin for treatment of type 1 diabetes and antiretroviral drugs for treatment of HIV), the prevalence of a disease may increase without a change in the incidence rate. Those who survive a chronic disease without cure remain in the "prevalence pot" (Fig. 5.4). For conditions such as cataracts, surgical removal of the cataracts permits many people to recover and thereby move out of the prevalence pot. Although the incidence has not

TABLE 5.2 **Examples of Rate Calculations**		
Morbidity Rates	**Crude Rates**	**Specific Rates**
Incidence Rate	**Crude Death Rate**	**Infant Mortality Rate**
$\frac{\text{Number of new cases in a given time period}}{\text{Population atrisk in the same time period}} \times 10,000$	$\frac{\text{Number of deaths in a year}}{\text{Total population size}} \times 100,000$	$\frac{\text{Number of infant deaths} < 1 \text{ year of age}}{\text{Number of births in same year}} \times 1000$
$\frac{75}{(4000-250 \text{ old cases})} = 0.02$	$\frac{1720}{200,000} = 0.0086$	$\frac{300}{45,000} = .00666 \times 1000 = 6.66 \text{ per 1000 live births}$
$0.02 \times 1000 = 20 \text{ per 1000 per time period}$	$0.0086 \times 100,000 = 860 \text{ per } 100,000 \text{ per year}$	
Prevalence Rate	**Crude Birth Rate**	**Fertility Rate**
$\frac{\text{Number of existing cases}}{\text{Total population}} \times 1000$	$\frac{\text{Number of births in a year}}{\text{Total population size}} \times 100,000$	$\frac{\text{Number of live births}}{\text{Number of women aged 15-44 years}} \times 1000$
$\frac{250}{4000} = .0625$	$\frac{2900}{200,000} = 0.0145$	$\frac{35,000}{500,000} = .07 \text{ per women aged 15-44 years}$
$.0625 \times 1000 = 62.5 \text{ per 1000}$	$0.0145 \times 100,000 = 1450 \text{ per } 100,000 \text{ per year}$	$.07 \times 1000 = 70 \text{ per 1000 women aged 15-44 years}$

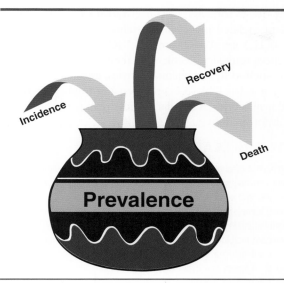

Fig. 5.4 Prevalence pot: The relationship between incidence and prevalence. (Redrawn from Morton RF, Hebel JR, McCarter RJ: *A study guide to epidemiology and biostatistics*, ed 3, Gaithersburg, MD, 1990, Aspen Publishers.)

necessarily changed, the reduced duration of the disease (because of surgery) lowers the prevalence rate of cataracts in the population.

Morbidity rates are not available for many conditions because surveillance of many chronic diseases is not widely conducted. Furthermore, morbidity rates may be subject to underreporting when they are available. Routinely collected birth and death rates, or **mortality rates**, are more widely available. Table 5.2 provides examples of calculating selected rates.

Other Rates

Numerous other rates are useful in characterizing the health of a population. For example, **crude rates** summarize the occurrence of births (i.e., crude birth rate), mortality (i.e., crude death rates), or diseases (i.e., crude disease rates) in the general population. The numerator is the number of events, and the denominator is the average population size or the population size at midyear (i.e., usually July 1) multiplied by a constant.

The denominators of crude rates represent the total population and not the population at risk for a given event; therefore these rates are subject to certain biases in interpretation. Crude death rates are sensitive to the number of people at the highest risk for dying. A relatively older population will probably produce a higher crude death rate than a population with a more evenly distributed age range. Conversely, a young population will have a somewhat lower crude death rate. Similar biases can occur for crude birth rates (e.g., higher birth rates in young populations).

This distortion occurs because the denominator reflects the entire population and not exclusively the population at risk for

giving birth. Age is one of the most common confounding factors that can mask the true distribution of variables. However, many variables, such as race and socioeconomic status, can also bias the interpretation of biostatistical data. Therefore, the nurse may use several approaches to remove the confounding effect of these variables on rates.

Age-specific rates characterize a particular age group in the population and usually consider deaths and births. Determining the rate for specific subgroups of a population and using a denominator that reflects only that subgroup remove age bias:

$$\text{Age specific rate} = \frac{\begin{array}{c}\text{Number of cases in specific}\\\text{age category in population}\\\text{at specified time}\end{array}}{\begin{array}{c}\text{Population in the same}\\\text{age category at the}\\\text{same specified time}\end{array}} \times k$$

To characterize a total population using age-specific rates, one must compute the rate for each category separately. The reason is that a single summary rate, such as a mean, cannot adequately characterize a total population. Specific rates for other variables can be determined in a similar fashion (e.g., race-specific or gender-specific rates) (Table 5.3).

Age adjustment or **standardization of rates** is another method of reducing bias when there is a difference between the age distributions of two populations. The nurse uses either the direct method or the indirect standardization method. The direct method selects a standard population, which is often the population distribution of the United States. This method essentially converts age-specific rates for age categories of the two populations to those of the standard population, and it

TABLE 5.3 Comparison of US Mortality Rates—2019

Death Rate	Rate Per 100,000
Crude death rate	869.7
Age-adjusted death rate	715.2
Age-specific death rates (years):	
<1 (infant)	558.0
1–4	23.3
5–14	13.4
15–24	69.7
25–34	128.8
35–44	199.2
45–54	392.4
55–64	883.3
65–74	1764.6
75–84	4308.3
≥85	13,228.6

Modified from National Center for Health Statistics: Mortality in the United States, 2019, Data Brief No 395, 2020. Available from https// www.cdc.gov/nchs/products/databriefs/db395.htm.

calculates a summary age-adjusted rate for each of the two populations of interest. This conversion enables the nurse to compare the two rates as if both had the standard population's age structure (i.e., without the prior problem of age distortion).

The **proportionate mortality ratio** (PMR) method also describes mortality. It represents the percentage of deaths resulting from a specific cause relative to deaths from all causes. It is often helpful in identifying areas in which public health programs might make significant contributions to reducing deaths. In some situations, a high PMR may reflect a low overall mortality or reduced number of deaths resulting from other causes. Therefore, the PMR requires consideration in the context of the mortality experience of the population.

$$PMR = \frac{\text{Number of deaths resulting from specific cause in a specified period}}{\text{Total number of deaths in same time period}} \times k$$

Table 5.4 summarizes the advantages and disadvantages of crude, specific, and adjusted rates. Numerous other rates assess particular segments of the population. One that is followed closely by public health professionals is the **infant mortality rate**, calculated by dividing the number of deaths in infants less than 1 year old by the number of live births for that period. This rate is considered a particularly sensitive indicator of the health of a community or nation and reflective of the care provided to women and children. Disparities in infant mortality rates can be seen within subgroups of the U.S. population, and the rate ranks 34 among 38 developed countries (Organisation for Economic Cooperation and Development [OECD], 2021). Although the United States achieved its *Healthy People 2020* goal of 6.0 per 1000, the 2018 rate, 5.7 per 1000, masks disparities within the population. Black infants experienced an infant mortality rate 2.35 times higher than White infants (10.8 vs. 4.6 per 1000 in 2018) (Centers for Disease Control and Prevention [CDC], 2020). Socioeconomic status and racial disparities, which are frequently associated with inadequate prenatal care, prematurity, adolescent pregnancy, and smoking,

are key risk factors. Recent concern focuses on the steep rise in pregnancy-related maternal mortality from 10 per 100,000 in 1990 to 17.3 per 100,000 in 2017 (CDC, 2021). Again, racial differences were significant, with the presence of chronic conditions such as hypertension, diabetes, and heart disease likely playing a role. Table 5.5 provides a summary of the major public health rates. A standard epidemiology textbook contains more information.

❓ ACTIVE LEARNING EXERCISE

1. Compile a database of relevant demographic and epidemiological data for your community by examining census reports, vital statistics reports, city records, and other sources in libraries and agencies.
2. Using numerators from vital statistics and denominators from census data, compute crude death and birth rates for your community.
3. Compare morbidity and mortality rates for your community with those of the state and the nation. Determine whether your community rates are higher or lower, and hypothesize about reasons for any disparities.

CONCEPT OF RISK

The concepts of risk and risk factor are familiar to community health nurses whose practices focus on disease prevention. **Risk** refers to the probability of an adverse event (i.e., the likelihood that healthy people exposed to a specific factor will acquire a specific disease). *Risk factor* refers to the specific exposure factor, such as cigarette smoke, hypertension, high cholesterol, excessive stress, high noise levels, or an environmental chemical. Frequently, the exposure factor is external to the individual. Risk factors may include fixed characteristics of people, such as age, sex, and genetic makeup. Although these intrinsic risk factors are not alterable, certain lifestyle changes may reduce their effect. For example, weight-bearing exercise and taking calcium and hormonal supplements may reduce the risk of osteoporosis for susceptible women.

Epidemiologists describe disease patterns in aggregates and quantify the effects of exposure to particular factors on the disease rates. To identify specific risk factors, epidemiologists

TABLE 5.4   Advantages and Disadvantages of Crude, Specific, and Adjusted Rates

Rate	Advantages	Disadvantages
Crude	Actual summary rates Readily calculable for international comparisons (widely used despite limitations)	Populations vary in composition (e.g., age); therefore differences in crude rates are difficult to interpret
Specific	Homogeneous subgroup Detailed rates useful for epidemiological and public health purposes	Cumbersome to compare many subgroups of two or more populations
Adjusted	Summary statements Differences in composition of group "removed," permitting unbiased comparison	Fictional rates Absolute magnitude dependent on chosen standard population Opposing trends in subgroups masked

Modified from Mausner JS, Kramer S: *Mausner and Bahn epidemiology: an introductory text*, ed 2, Philadelphia, 1985, W. B. Saunders.

TABLE 5.5 Major Public Health Rates

Rate Denominator	Rates		Usual	Factor Rate for United States, 2017[a]
Total population	Crude birth rate $=$	$\dfrac{\text{Number of live births during the year}}{\text{Average (midyear) population}}$	Per 1000 population	11.8
	Crude death rate $=$	$\dfrac{\text{Number of deaths during the year}}{\text{Average (midyear) population}}$	Per 100,000 population	823.7[b]
	Age $-$ specific death rate $=$	$\dfrac{\text{Number of deaths among people of a given age group during the year}}{\text{Average (midyear) population of the same age group}}$	Per 100,000 population	74 (15—24 yr)[c] 401.5 (45—54 yr)[c] 1790.9 (65—75 yr)[c]
	Cause $-$ specific death rate $=$	$\dfrac{\text{Number of deaths from a stated cause during the year}}{\text{Average (midyear) population of the same age group}}$	Per 100,000 population	165.0 (heart diseases) 152.5(malignant neoplasms)
Women aged 15—44 yr	Fertility rate $=$	$\dfrac{\text{Number of live births during the year}}{\text{Number of women 15—44 years of age in the same year}}$	Per 1000 women aged 15—44 yr	60.3
Live births	Infant mortality rate $=$	$\dfrac{\text{Number of deaths during the year of children younger than 1 year of age}}{\text{Number of live births in the same year}}$	Per 1000 live births	5.8
	Neonatal mortality rate $=$	$\dfrac{\text{Number of deaths during the year of children younger than 28 days}}{\text{Number of live births in the same year}}$	Per 1000 live births	3.9
	Maternal mortality rate (puerperal) $=$	$\dfrac{\text{Number of deaths from puerperal causes during the year}}{\text{Number of live births in the same year}}$	Per 100,000 live births	17.3[c]
Live births and fetal deaths	Fetal death rate $=$	$\dfrac{\text{Number of fetal deaths during the year}}{\text{Number of live births in the same year}}$	Per 1000 live births and fetal deaths	5.9
	Perinatal mortality rate $=$	$\dfrac{\text{Number of fetal deaths(28 \textit{weeks plus infant} < 7\textit{days}) during the year}}{\text{Number of live births} > 28 \textit{ weeks} \text{ in the same year}}$	Per 1000 live births and fetal deaths	6.2

[a]2017 rates from National Center for Health Statistics: *Health, United States, 2018.* Available from http://www.cdc.gov/nchs/data/hus/hus18.pdf.
[b]2019 rate from Centers for Disease Control and Prevention: *FastStats: Deaths and Mortality*, National Center for Health Statistics. Available from https//www.cdc.gov/nchs/fastats/deaths.htm.
[c]Rate from Centers for Disease Control and Prevention: *Mortality in the United States, 2018*, National Center for Health Statistics Data Brief 355, 2020. Available from www.cdc.gov/nchs/data/databrief/db355-h.pdf.
Modified from Mausner JS, Kramer S: *Mausner and Bahn epidemiology: an introductory text*, ed 2, Philadelphia, 1985, Saunders. Rates from U.S. Department of Health and Human Services/National Center for Health Statistics: *Health, United States, 2018.* Available from: http://www.cdc.gov/nchs/data/hus/hus18.pdf

compare rates of disease for those exposed with those not exposed. One method for comparing two rates is subtracting the rate of nonexposed individuals from the exposed. This measure of risk is called the *attributable risk*; it is the estimate of the disease burden in a population. For example, if the rate of non—insulin-dependent diabetes were 5000 per 100,000 people in the obese population (i.e., those weighing more than 120% of ideal body weight) and 1000 per 100,000 people in the

nonobese population, the attributable risk of non—insulin-dependent diabetes resulting from obesity would be:

$$4000 \text{ per } 100,000 \text{ people } \left(\text{i.e., } \frac{5000}{100,000} - \frac{1000}{100,000} \right)$$

This means that 4000 cases per 100,000 people may be attributed to obesity. Thus, a prevention program designed to reduce obesity could theoretically eliminate 4000 cases per 100,000 people in the population. Attributable risks are particularly important in describing the potential impact of a public health intervention in a community.

A second measure of the excess risk caused by a factor is the *relative risk ratio*. The relative risk is calculated by dividing the incidence rate of disease in the exposed population by the incidence rate of disease in the nonexposed population. In the previous example, a relative risk of five was obtained by dividing 5000/100,000 by 1000/100,000. This risk ratio suggests that an obese individual has a fivefold greater risk of diabetes than a nonobese individual. In general, a relative risk of 1 indicates no excessive risk from exposure to a factor; a relative risk of 1.5 indicates a 50% increase in risk; a relative risk of 2 indicates twice the risk; and a relative risk of less than 1 suggests that a factor may have a protective effect associated with a reduced disease rate.

The relative risk ratio forms the statistical basis for the risk factor concept. Relative risks are valuable indicators of the excess risk incurred by exposure to certain factors. They have been used extensively in identifying the major causal factors of many common diseases, and direct public health practitioners' efforts to reduce health risks.

Community health nurses may apply the concept of relative risk to suspected exposure variables to isolate risk factors associated with community health problems. For example, a community health nurse might investigate an outbreak of probable foodborne illness. The nurse may compare the incidence rate among those exposed to potato salad in a school cafeteria with the incidence rate among those not exposed. The relative risk calculated from the ratio of these two incidence rates indicates the amount of excess risk for disease incurred by eating the potato salad. A community health nurse might also determine the relative risks for other suspected foods and compare them with the relative risk for potato salad. Attack rates are the calculated incidence rates for foods involved in foodborne illnesses. A food with a markedly higher relative risk than other foods might be the causal agent in a foodborne epidemic. The identification of the causal agent, or specific food, is critical to the implementation of an effective prevention program such as teaching proper food-handling techniques.

USE OF EPIDEMIOLOGY IN DISEASE PREVENTION

Primary Prevention

The central goals of epidemiology are describing the disease patterns, identifying the etiological factors in disease development, and taking the most effective preventive measures. These preventive measures are specific to the stage of disease progression, or the **natural history of disease**, from prepathogenesis through resolution of the disease process. When interventions occur before disease development, they are called *primary prevention*. Primary prevention relies on epidemiological information to indicate those behaviors that are protective, or those that will not contribute to an increase in disease, and those that are associated with increased risk.

Two types of activities constitute primary prevention. Those actions that are general in nature and designed to foster healthful lifestyles and a safe environment are called *health promotion*. Actions aimed at reducing the risk of specific diseases are called *specific protection*. Public health practitioners use epidemiological research to understand practices that are likely to reduce or increase disease rates. For example, numerous research studies have confirmed that regular exercise is an important health promotion activity that has positive effects on general physical and mental health. Immunizations exemplify specific protection measures that reduce the incidence of particular diseases.

Secondary and Tertiary Prevention

Secondary prevention occurs after pathogenesis. Those measures designed to detect disease at its earliest stage, namely screening and physical examinations that are aimed at early diagnosis, are *secondary prevention*. Interventions that provide for early treatment and cure of disease are also in this category. Again, epidemiological data and clinical trials determining effective treatments are crucial in disease identification. Mammography, guaiac testing of feces, and the treatment of infections and dental caries are all examples of secondary prevention.

Tertiary prevention focuses on limitation of disability and the rehabilitation of those with irreversible diseases such as diabetes and spinal cord injury. Epidemiological studies examine risk factors affecting function and suggest optimal strategies in the care of patients with chronic advanced disease.

Establishing Causality

As discussed earlier, a principal goal of epidemiology is to identify etiological factors of diseases to encourage the most effective prevention activities and develop treatment modalities. During the last few decades, researchers recognized that many diseases have not one but multiple causes. Epidemiologists who examine disease rates and conduct population-focused research often find multiple factors associated with health problems. For example, cardiovascular disease rates may vary by location, ethnicity, and smoking status. Even infectious diseases often require not only an organism but also certain behaviors or conditions to cause exposure. Determining the extent that these correlates represent associative or causal relationships is important for public health practitioners who seek to prevent, diagnose, and treat disease.

Definitively establishing causality—particularly in chronic disease—is a challenge. The following six criteria establish the existence of a **cause-and-effect relationship:**

1. **Strength of association:** Rates of morbidity or mortality must be higher in the exposed group than in the nonexposed group. Relative risk ratios, or odds ratios, and correlation coefficients indicate whether the relationship between the exposure variable and the outcome is causal. For example, epidemiological studies demonstrated a higher relative risk for heart disease among smokers than among nonsmokers.

2. **Dose–response relationship:** An increased exposure to the risk factor causes a concomitant increase in disease rate. Indeed, the risk of heart disease mortality is higher for heavy smokers than for light smokers.

3. **Temporally correct relationship:** Exposure to the causal factor must occur before the effect, or disease. For heart disease, smoking history must precede disease development.

4. **Biological plausibility:** The data must make biological sense and represent a coherent explanation for the relationship. Nicotine and other tobacco-derived chemicals are toxic to the vascular endothelium. In addition to raising low-density lipoprotein and decreasing high-density lipoprotein cholesterol levels, cigarette smoking causes arterial vasoconstriction and platelet reactivity, which contribute to platelet thrombus formation.

5. **Consistency with other studies:** Varying types of studies in other populations must observe similar associations. Numerous studies using different designs have repeatedly supported the relationship between smoking and heart disease.

6. **Specificity:** The exposure variable must be necessary and sufficient to cause disease; there is only one causal factor. Although specificity may be strong causal evidence in the case of infectious disease, this criterion is less important today. Diseases do not have single causes; they have multifactorial origins.

The exposure variable of smoking is one of several risk factors for heart disease. Few factors are linked to a single condition. Furthermore, smoking is not specific to heart disease alone. It is a causal factor for other diseases such as lung and oral cancers. Additionally, smoking is not "necessary and sufficient" to the development of heart disease, because there are nonsmokers who also have coronary heart disease. Therefore, the causal criterion of specificity more frequently pertains to infectious diseases.

Although these criteria are useful in evaluating epidemiological evidence, it is important to note that causality is largely a matter of judgment. In reality, absolute causality is only rarely established. Rather, epidemiologists more commonly refer to suggested causal and associated factors. The effect of confounding variables makes it difficult to ascertain true relationships between the exposure and outcome variables. Confounding variables must be independently related to both the dependent variable and the independent variable. Therefore these third variables can distort the true relationship between the dependent and independent variables. For example, researchers frequently control for the confounding effect of exercise and age when they examine the relationship between diet and coronary heart disease. This is because persons with heart disease may exercise less and be older than those without heart disease; that is, there is both an independent relationship between exercise and heart disease and also between age and heart disease. Without controlling for these factors, it is not possible to know if the association between dietary fat and heart disease is real or if it can be attributed to differences in physical activity and age.

By measuring the confounding variable, the researcher can statistically account for its effect in the analysis (e.g., by using multiple logistical regression analysis or stratification). A biostatistics text contains a discussion of these methods. Alternatively, matching subjects in treatment and control groups with respect to the confounding variable minimizes the effects of the confounder. Again, standardization for variables such as age is another method for managing spurious associations, which makes true relationships more apparent. An understanding of such relationships facilitates the practitioner's interpretation and application of findings.

Screening

As explained previously, a central aim of epidemiology is to describe the course of disease according to person, place, and time. Observations of the disease process may suggest factors that aggravate or ameliorate its progress. This information also assists in determining effective treatment and rehabilitation options (i.e., secondary or tertiary prevention approaches).

The purpose of **screening** is to identify risk factors and diseases in their earliest stages. Screening is usually a secondary prevention activity because indications of disease appear *after* a pathological change has occurred. In all forms of secondary and tertiary prevention, the identification of illness prompts the nurse to consider which forms of upstream prevention could have interrupted disease development.

Community health nurses commonly conduct **screening programs**. Community health nurses may devote a large portion of their work activities to performing physical examinations; promoting client self-examination; or conducting screening programs in schools, clinics, or community settings. Although secondary prevention activities are important and provide vital information on community health status, they focus on detecting existing disease. In contrast, primary prevention and anticipatory guidance, which are hallmarks of community health nursing practice, attempt to prevent the development of disease.

Community health nurses should consider several guidelines for screening programs. First, nurses must plan and execute adequate and appropriate follow-up treatment for patients who test positive for the disease. It is critical that nurses identify how to contact patients with positive findings and where to refer them and then follow up with patients to determine whether they accessed care. Health fairs have been criticized for the lack of consistent follow-up of screening activities. Second, in the planning phase, the nurse should determine whether early disease diagnosis constitutes a real benefit to clients in terms of improved life expectancy or quality of life. Third, a critical prerequisite to screening is the existence of acceptable and medically sound treatment and follow-up. In the past, public health providers debated the ethical and practical arguments for implementing widespread HIV screening. Concern exists regarding the potential for stigmatic consequences for and discrimination against those who screen positively for a test; therefore people implementing screening programs should establish procedures for ensuring confidentiality. These procedures, in conjunction with the development of effective antiviral treatments, have encouraged earlier and more widespread identification of HIV-positive individuals.

A screening program's procedures must also be cost effective and acceptable to clients. Although colonoscopy is a routine and effective screening procedure for colon cancer, it is neither simple nor inexpensive. Although it is recommended periodically for all Americans with no known risk factors beginning at age 50 years, about a third of the population was not up-to-date with colorectal screening in 2018 (CDC, 2021). Annual screening using home fecal immunochemical tests (FIT) are not only cheaper but do not require bowel preparation, anesthesia, or transportation. Therefore, non-DNA FITs are suggested by the U.S. Preventive Services Task Force as a more acceptable alternative to colonoscopy (Lin et al., 2016). In short, a nurse should consider whether or not to screen a population on the basis of the significant costs of screening programs and procedures, follow-up for clients who test positive, and subsequent medical care (Box 5.5).

When developing a screening program, the community health nurse also must evaluate issues related to the validity of the screening test. Detecting clients with disease is the purpose of screening, and *sensitivity* is the test's ability to do so correctly. Conversely, *specificity* is the extent to which a test can correctly identify those who do not have disease. To obtain estimates of these two dimensions, the nurse must compare screening results with the best available diagnostic procedure. For a given test, the sensitivity and specificity tend to be inversely related to each other. When a test is highly sensitive, individuals without disease may be incorrectly labeled as testing positive. These false-positive results may cause stress and worry for clients and require further expense in the form of testing to confirm a diagnosis. With a highly sensitive test, specificity may be lower, and the test may identify people as having the disease who are in fact disease free (i.e., more false-positive results). If the sensitivity is low (and the specificity high), more patients who have the disease will have negative test results. These patients will not be diagnosed and thus presumably will receive care later in the disease process.

Optimally, a screening test should be maximally sensitive and specific. To a large extent, this depends on the precision of the test and the stringency of the cutoff point established for determining a positive result. In the past, for example, the tuberculosis skin testing criterion was based exclusively on a skin reaction of 10 mm of induration. As a result, some persons with the disease were missed because their skin reactions were less than 10 mm (false-negative results), and some with 10 mm of reaction were identified as having the disease but further testing showed they did not have it (false-positive results). More recently, risk factors have been considered in addition to induration, creating a more sensitive and specific TB screening algorithm. Currently, high-risk individuals, such as those with HIV disease, are considered to have a positive skin test result with 5 mm of induration, which is more sensitive than the criteria of 15 mm set for those of low risk. Use of the more stringent 5-mm criterion among those with HIV will lead to fewer false-negative results, and use of the 15-mm cut point among low-risk individuals will lead to fewer false-positive results (CDC, 2021). Box 5.6 shows the formula for calculating sensitivity and specificity.

Sensitivity and specificity reflect the *yield* of a screening test, which is the amount of detected disease. One measure of yield is the *positive predictive value* of a test, which is the proportion of true-positive results relative to all positive test results. On the basis of Box 5.6, the formula is $\frac{a}{a+b}$. The positive predictive value depends on the prevalence of undetected disease in a population. Screening for a rare disease such as phenylketonuria will yield a lower predictive value and more false-positive results. In phenylketonuria, a low predictive value is acceptable, because the false-negative result has very serious consequences. The predictive value is also affected by the nature of the screened population. Screening only the individuals at high risk for a disease will produce a higher predictive value and can be a more efficient way to identify those with health problems. For example, diabetes screening in an American Indian, Mexican

---

BOX 5.5   Guidelines for Screening Programs

- Screen for conditions in which early detection and treatment can improve disease outcome and quality of life.
- Screen populations that have risk factors or are more susceptible to the disease.
- Select a screening method that is simple, safe, inexpensive to administer, acceptable to clients, and has acceptable sensitivity and specificity.
- Plan for the timely referral and follow-up of clients with positive results.
- Identify referral sources that are appropriate, cost-effective, and convenient for clients.
- Refer to evidenced-based screening recommendations published by the U.S. Preventive Services Taskforce (http://www.uspreventiveservicestaskforce.org/Page/Name/recommendations) and other organizations.

BOX 5.6 Sensitivity and Specificity of a Screening Test

Screening Test Result	Those With Disease	Those Without Disease
Positive	True-positives (a)	False-positives (b)
Negative	False-negatives (c)	True-negatives (d)

$$\text{Sensitivity (in percent)} = \frac{\text{True positives}}{\text{All with disease}} - \frac{(a)}{(a+c)} \times 100$$

$$\text{Sensitivity (in percent)} = \frac{\text{True negative}}{\text{All without disease}} - \frac{(d)}{(b+d)} \times 100$$

American, or African American adult population should produce a higher predictive value than screening the general adult population.

Surveillance

In addition to screening, **surveillance** is a mechanism for the ongoing collection of community health information. Monitoring for changes in disease frequency is essential to effective and responsive public health programs. Identifying trends in disease incidence or identifying risk factor status by location and population subgroup over time allows the community health nurse to evaluate the effectiveness of existing programs and to implement interventions targeted to high-risk groups. Again, identifying new cases for calculating incidence rates is particularly useful in evaluating morbidity trends. However, this form of surveillance data is more difficult to collect, and public health practitioners can access the data only for selected diseases. Prevalence rates, mortality data, risk factor data, and hospital and health service data can help indicate a program's successes or deficiencies.

The Centers for Disease Control and Prevention (CDC) coordinates a system of data collection among federal, state, and local agencies. These groups compile numerous sets of data and base some of these data sets on the entire population (e.g., vital statistics data) and other collections on subsamples of the population (e.g., the National Health Interview Survey). The completeness of data reporting is variable because not all diseases are reportable. For example, practitioners are required to report only four sexually transmitted infections (i.e., HIV/AIDS, syphilis, gonorrhea, and chlamydia) to local and state health departments. Furthermore, not all practitioners report cases on a regular basis, and not all people with sexually transmitted infections actually seek care. Studies have indicated that practitioners also underreport childhood communicable diseases, such as chickenpox and mumps. The CDC conducts studies that estimate the magnitude of this underreporting problem.

Practitioners have a continuing need for comprehensive and systematically collected surveillance data that describe the health status of national and local subgroups. They use this information to evaluate the impact of programs on specific groups in a community.

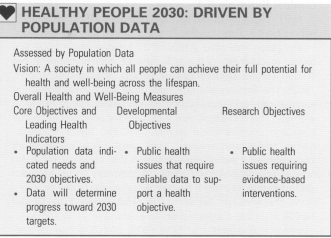

HEALTHY PEOPLE 2030: DRIVEN BY POPULATION DATA

Assessed by Population Data
Vision: A society in which all people can achieve their full potential for health and well-being across the lifespan.
Overall Health and Well-Being Measures

Core Objectives and Leading Health Indicators	Developmental Objectives	Research Objectives
• Population data indicated needs and 2030 objectives. • Data will determine progress toward 2030 targets.	• Public health issues that require reliable data to support a health objective.	• Public health issues requiring evidence-based interventions.

Adapted from U.S. Department of Health and Human *Services: Healthy people, 2030.* https://health.gov/healthypeople/objectives-and-data/about-objectives/healthy-people-2030-objectives-and-measures.

The effectiveness of *Healthy People (2030)* depends on the availability of reliable baseline and continuing data to characterize health problems and evaluate objective achievement as listed in the *Healthy People 2030* box (U.S. Department of Health and Human Services, n.d.). For example, simply documenting children's mortality rates resulting from injury is insufficient for the development of specific methods of injury prevention. Data on the number of injured children and the nature of injury (e.g., motor vehicle accidents, drowning, abuse) across the nation increase the usefulness of surveillance information. The Health Indicators Warehouse and HealthData.gov compile indicator data for initiatives like *Healthy People 2030*, the Center for Medicare and Medicaid Services, and for current health issues such as COVID-19 so that health status and service quality can be monitored. Databases such as Health, United States, and *Healthy People 2030* Objectives and Data, available at the CDC webpage, will be the primary source of evaluative information.

Nurses need to describe trends in health and illness according to a community's locale, demographics, and risk factor status to intervene effectively on behalf of the people. They must compare the data for their locale with those of a relevant neighboring area (e.g., a census tract, city, county, state, or nation) to gain perspective on the magnitude of a local problem (see Clinical Example 5.1). Ideally, the nurse should have access to surveillance data at several different levels over a given period. In some instances, community health nurses find it necessary to construct their own surveillance systems that are tailored to specific health conditions or available programs in their community. These smaller data collection systems help nurses evaluate programs when the data are readily accessible and are compatible with data from large city or statewide surveillance systems.

Clinical Example 5.1

In 1991, a cluster of neural tube defects (NTDs) occurred in babies born in Brownsville, Texas, within a span of 6 weeks. Investigation indicated a rate of 27.1 cases per 10,000 live births, in contrast to the U.S. rate of approximately 8 per 10,000 (Texas Department of Health, unpublished report, 1992). The Brownsville rate was more than three times the national rate and represented an increased risk in Hispanic women. This increased risk was partially attributable to cultural and environmental factors, including lower socioeconomic status and migrant farm work. The investigators implemented a surveillance program that obtained more accurate population-based data. Additionally, the program implemented folic acid supplementation in Texas counties along the Mexican border. NTD rates dropped to 13 per 10,000 after the supplementation effort.

Research suggests that 50%–70% of NTDs may be preventable with folic acid supplementation. This finding supports the fortification of bread and cereal products; in January 1998, the U.S. Food and Drug Administration (FDA) mandated the addition of 140 µg of vitamin B per 100 g of most grain products. It is estimated that there has been a 24% reduction in the number of NTDs since grain fortification with folic acid began.

Dietary intake alone may be insufficient; also, the greatest risk to the fetus occurs within the first 3–8 weeks of pregnancy, a time when many women do not yet recognize their pregnancies. Therefore, the CDC and U.S. Preventive Services Task Force recommend that all women of reproductive age consume 400 µg (0.4 mg) to 800 µg (0.8 mg) daily of synthetic folic acid in addition to dietary sources such as cereal or grain products, leafy green vegetables, and vitamin supplements.

From U.S. Preventive Services Task Force: Folic acid for the prevention of neural tube defects: preventive medication, 2017. Available from: Final Recommendation Statement: Folic Acid for the Prevention of NTDs: Preventive Medication, United States Preventive Services Taskforce (uspreventiveservicestaskforce.org).

RESEARCH HIGHLIGHTS

Reducing Infant Mortality Rates Using the Perinatal Periods of Risk Model

The infant mortality rate is an accepted indicator for measuring a nation's health. The rate is representative of the health status and social well-being of any nation. Despite decreases in the past 50 years, infant mortality rates in the United States remain higher than in other industrialized countries. Using overall infant mortality rates to determine the effectiveness of interventions does not help communities focus on particular underlying factors contributing to the rates. Targeting interventions to the factors most responsible for the infant mortality rate should help reduce the rate more rapidly and effectively.

The Perinatal Periods of Risk (PPOR) model was developed to provide direction, focus, and suggestions for effective interventions. The model helps users identify and rank four factors as they contribute to the overall infant mortality rate: (1) mother's health before and between pregnancies, (2) maternal health care systems, (3) neonatal health care systems, and (4) infant health during the first year of life. The PPOR model is based on two major theoretical constructs: age of fetus-infant at death and birth weight. The PPOR model maps each death in a geographic region on the basis of birth weight and age at death, including fetal, neonatal, and postneonatal periods. The lowest birth weight infant deaths are combined into one cell named the maternal health cell. The three remaining groups are put into cells suggesting the primary preventive focus for that group: maternal health, newborn health, and infant health. Multiple interventions are important in reducing infant mortality, and the PPOR model guides prioritizing interventions based on the cell contributing the most to infant mortality rates (Peck et al., 2010).

The PPOR model has been used in several programs and research studies to improve mother and infant health. In one intervention study (Chao et al., 2010) the PPOR model was successfully used to improve birth outcomes in very-high-risk populations in the Antelope Valley area of Los Angeles County. On the basis of assessment findings per PPOR directives, efforts were made to infuse resources into the community and expand case management initiatives for high-risk mothers. Long-term findings indicated that the PPOR model was useful for identifying risk and social factors and that it helped mobilize community partnerships that resulted in widely improved birth outcomes. In another example, a study conducted in Kalamazoo, Michigan used the PPOR model to assess factors associated with excess mortality in Black infants (Kothari et al., 2017). They determined that while high socioeconomic status did not entirely mitigate maternal risks, persistent inequities, and lack of preconception and prenatal care impacted prematurity and complications of birth. The PPOR infant health category identified poverty as a key factor in that most postneonatal deaths in Black infants were due to unsafe sleep conditions. Thus, community interventions focused on underlying social causes of racial disparities such as access to information and resources, social stress, and poverty, were targeted to Black women of all income levels, poor women, and those with prior negative birth outcomes. The PPOR assists in identifying population-specific risks and the interpretation of community epidemiologic data.

Data from Chao SM, Donatoni G, Bemis C, et al. Integrated approaches to improve birth outcomes: perinatal periods of risk, infant mortality review and the Los Angeles mommy and baby project, *Mater & Child Health J* 14:827–837, 2010; Kothari CL, Romph C, Bautista T, Lenz D: Perinatal periods of risk analysis: disentangling race and socioeconomic status to inform a black infant mortality community initiative, *Mater & Child Health J* 21:49–58, 2017; Peck MG, Sappenfield WM, Skala J: Perinatal periods of risk: a community approach for using data to improve women and infants' health, *Mater & Child Health J* 14:864–874, 2010.

As stated, epidemiologists describe the course of disease over time. These secular trends are changes that occur over years or decades, such as the fairly recent, significant decline in lung cancer deaths in men and the gradual increase in lung cancer deaths in women. Frequently, epidemiologists document the associated patterns of treatment and intervention. In many instances, studies conducted by clinical epidemiologists provide this information. Cancer registries are a form of surveillance that document the prevalence and incidence of cancer in a community and document its course, treatment, and associated survival rates. The Surveillance, Epidemiology, and End Results program of the National Cancer Institute compiles national cancer data from existing cancer registries covering approximately 28% of the U.S. population (National Cancer Institute, 2021).

Public health practitioners need to conduct community surveys of population segments to plan for the segments' health. For example, a survey of the disabled population that assesses prevalence may also evaluate the adequacy of current services and project future needs.

USE OF EPIDEMIOLOGY IN HEALTH SERVICES

Epidemiological approaches, such as the ones presented here, can be used to describe the distribution of disease and its determinants in populations. However, epidemiological principles are also useful in studying population health care delivery and in describing and evaluating the use of community health services. For example, analyzing the ratio of healthcare providers to population size helps determine the system's ability to provide care. The clients' reasons for seeking care, the clients' payment methods, and the clients' satisfaction with care are also informative. Regardless of whether community health nurses or other health services professionals collect these data, the information is essential for those who strive to improve clients' access to quality health care.

Health services epidemiology focuses on the population's healthcare patterns. In particular, public health practitioners are concerned with the accessibility and affordability of services and the barriers that may contribute to excess morbidity in at-risk groups. Traditionally, children are a vulnerable group, and they are a particular focus of health services research. Studies examining poverty rates and care access have underscored the need to expand insurance coverage to those who do not have private medical insurance and do not qualify for Medicaid programs or the State Children's Health Insurance Program.

Ultimately, nurses must apply epidemiological findings in practice. It is essential that they incorporate study results into prevention programs for communities and at-risk populations. Furthermore, the philosophy of public health and epidemiology dictates that nurses extend their application into major health policy decisions, because the aim of health policy planning is to achieve positive health goals and outcomes for improved population health.

A goal of policy development is to bring about desirable social changes. Epidemiological factors, history, politics, economics, culture, and technology influence policy development. The complex interaction of these factors may explain the challenges with application of epidemiological knowledge. Lung disease in the United States exemplifies the incomplete progress in implementing effective health policy. In the early 1950s, studies identified and conclusively linked cigarette smoking to lung cancer and heart disease (Doll & Hill, 1952). Beginning in the 1950s, public policies to address this health threat have included cigarette taxes, cigarette package warning labels, smoking restrictions in public areas, the institution of smoke-free workplaces, and restrictions on selling tobacco to minors. Despite the successes of the past 70 years, approximately 20% of Americans continue to smoke, with rates particularly high among young adults, suggesting a continued

need for focused and effective public health policy. Community health nurses should exercise "social responsibility" in applying epidemiological findings, but doing so will require the active involvement of the consumer. Community health nurses collaborating with community members can combine epidemiological knowledge and aggregate-level strategies to effect change on the broadest scale.

❓ ACTIVE LEARNING EXERCISE

Consult *Healthy People 2030* to find the national goals for selected causes of morbidity and mortality. Identify groups at an increased risk for these selected diseases. What are the approaches suggested by these documents for reducing the rates of disease? How can this information be useful in planning for your community?

EPIDEMIOLOGICAL METHODS

Two epidemiological methods—descriptive epidemiology and analytic epidemiology—are used by community health nurses. This section describes both and gives examples of how they are used in population health.

Descriptive Epidemiology

Descriptive epidemiology focuses on the amount and distribution of health and health problems within a population. Its purpose is to describe the characteristics of both people who are protected from disease and those who have a disease. Factors of particular interest are age, sex, ethnicity or race, socioeconomic status, occupation, and family status. Epidemiologists use morbidity and mortality rates to describe the extent of disease and to determine the risk factors that make certain groups more prone to acquiring disease.

In addition to "person" characteristics, the place of occurrence describes disease frequency. For example, certain parasitic diseases, such as malaria and schistosomiasis, occur in tropical areas. Other diseases may occur in certain geopolitical entities. For example, gastroenteritis outbreaks often occur in communities with lax water quality standards. Time is the third parameter that helps define disease patterns. Epidemiologists may track incidence rates over a period of days or weeks (e.g., epidemics of infectious disease such as COVID-19 which were tracked daily, weekly, and monthly) or over an extended period of years (e.g., secular trends in the cancer death rate).

These person, place, and time factors can form a framework for disease analysis and may suggest variables associated with high versus low disease rates. Descriptive epidemiology can then generate hypotheses about the cause of disease, and *analytic epidemiology* approaches can test these hypotheses (Box 5.7).

Analytic Epidemiology

Analytic epidemiology investigates the causes of disease by determining why a disease rate is lower in one population group than in another. This method tests the hypotheses

BOX 5.7 An Example of Descriptive Epidemiology

The **p**erson-**p**lace-**t**ime model is illustrated by one of the first outbreaks of coronavirus 2019 (COVID-19) outside of Wuhan, China. This occurred on a cruise ship sailing among ports in Southeast Asia.

- *Person:* Initially two passengers developed symptoms of COVID-19 on January 22 and 23, 2020. One disembarked in Singapore and tested positive on February 1, after which the ship was notified and testing arranged for symptomatic passengers arriving in Yokohama, Japan. Ultimately, of the 3711 passengers and crew, 710 or 19.2% tested positive. Of these, 46.5% were asymptomatic, 37 required hospitalization, and 9 died.
- *Place:* Diamond Princess cruise ship that made stops in six South Asian ports and was quarantined in Yokohama, Japan, on February 3. Passengers with negative COVID-19 tests were confined to cabins for 14 days, while those who tested positive were either hospitalized, transferred from the ship for land-based or home-country quarantines. Asymptomatic crew continued to perform on-board duties and live in the quarters assigned to staff.
- *Time:* The index case is likely one of the two passengers who developed symptoms on January 22 and 23, 2020.

From Centers for Disease Control and Prevention: public health responses to COVID-19 outbreaks on cruise ships—Worldwide, February-March 2020, *Morb and Mort Rep* 69(12):347–352, 2020. https://doi.org/10.15585/mmwr.mm6912e33xternal_icon.
Centers for Disease Control and Prevention: investigation of transmission of COVID-19 among crew members during quarantine of a cruise ship — Yokohama, Japan, 69(11):312–313, 2020. https://doi.org/10.15585/mmwr.mm6911e2external_icon.

generated from descriptive data and either accepts or rejects them on the basis of analytic research. The epidemiologist seeks to establish a cause-and-effect relationship between a preexisting condition or event and the disease (see previous section on causality). To determine this relationship, the epidemiologist may undertake two major types of research studies: *observational* and *experimental.*

Observational Studies

Epidemiologists frequently use *observational studies* for descriptive purposes, but they also use them to discover the etiology of disease. The investigator can begin to understand the factors that contribute to disease by observing disease rates in groups of people differentiated by experience or exposure. For example, differences in disease rates may occur in the obese compared with the nonobese, in smokers compared with nonsmokers, and in those with high stress levels compared with those with low stress levels. These characteristics (i.e., obesity, smoking, and stress) are called *exposure* variables.

Unlike experimental studies, observational studies do not allow the investigator to manipulate the specific exposure or experience or to control or limit the effects of other extraneous factors that may influence disease development. For example, life stress is related to depression. People with low socioeconomic status also have high depression rates. People with low socioeconomic status frequently experience greater life stresses; therefore, the confounding factor of socioeconomic status makes it more difficult to demonstrate the effect of stress on depression. The three major study designs used in observational research are cross-sectional, retrospective, and prospective studies.

Cross-Sectional Studies. Cross-sectional studies, sometimes called *prevalence* or *correlational studies,* examine relationships between potential causal factors and disease at a specific time (Fig. 5.5). Surveys that simultaneously collect information about risk factors and disease exemplify this design. For example, the National Health and Nutrition Examination

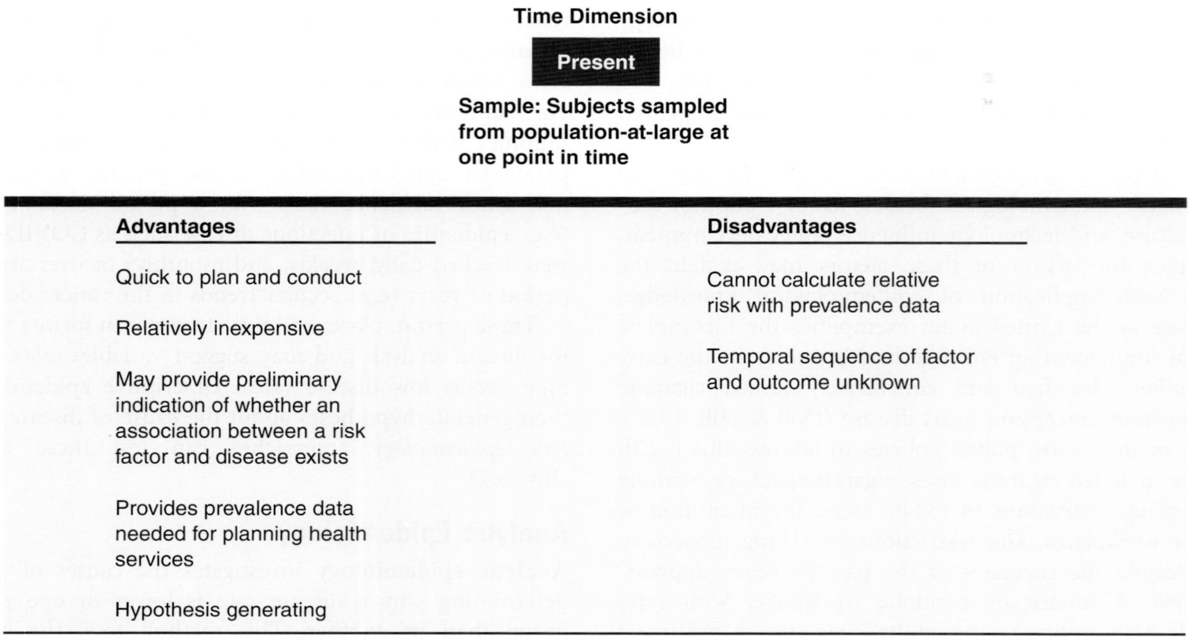

Time Dimension

Present

Sample: Subjects sampled from population-at-large at one point in time

Advantages	Disadvantages
Quick to plan and conduct	Cannot calculate relative risk with prevalence data
Relatively inexpensive	Temporal sequence of factor and outcome unknown
May provide preliminary indication of whether an association between a risk factor and disease exists	
Provides prevalence data needed for planning health services	
Hypothesis generating	

Fig. 5.5 Cross-sectional, or prevalence, study.

Survey (NHANES) has collected cross-sectional data regarding current dietary practices, physical status, and health in adults and children in the United States since the early 1960s (CDC, 2021). Data from the NHANES studies have been analyzed and compared over the years by a number of researchers and have provided important health information.

For example, NHANES studies have tracked contemporary behavior issues such as unsweetened beverage consumption in U.S. youth (Marriott et al., 2019) and fast food in adults, showing recent declines in the total daily calories consumed from these sources that lead to increased intake of carbohydrates, fat, and sodium. Although overall fast-food consumption has declined, 36.6% of adults consumed fast food on a given day during the period 2013–16. Non-Hispanic Black adults (42.4%) were the most frequent consumers, followed by non-Hispanic White and then Hispanic adults. On the whole those of higher income consumed more fast food, with men eating it for lunch and women as snacks (Fryar et al., 2018). NHANES has conducted interviews and physical examinations on youth, nutrient studies on children, and dietary surveys of older Americans, contributing important data that suggest risk factors that can be examined through more rigorous study designs.

Although a cross-sectional study can identify associations among disease and specific factors, it is impossible to make causal inferences because the study cannot establish the temporal sequence of events (i.e., the cause preceded the effect). For example, the NHANES was unable to determine whether high salt intake precedes hypertension—thus making it a causal factor—or whether they are unrelated. Therefore, cross-sectional studies have limitations in discovering etiological factors of disease. These studies can help identify preliminary relationships that other analytic designs may explore further; therefore, they are hypothesis-generating studies.

Retrospective Studies. *Retrospective studies* compare individuals with a particular condition or disease and those who do not have the disease. These studies determine whether cases, or a diseased group, differ in their exposure to a specific factor or characteristic relative to controls, or a nondiseased group. To make unambiguous comparisons, investigators select the cases according to explicitly defined criteria regarding the type of case and the stage of disease. Investigators also select a control group from the general population that is characteristically similar to the cases (Fig. 5.6).

Frequently, people hospitalized for diseases that are not under study become controls if they do not share the

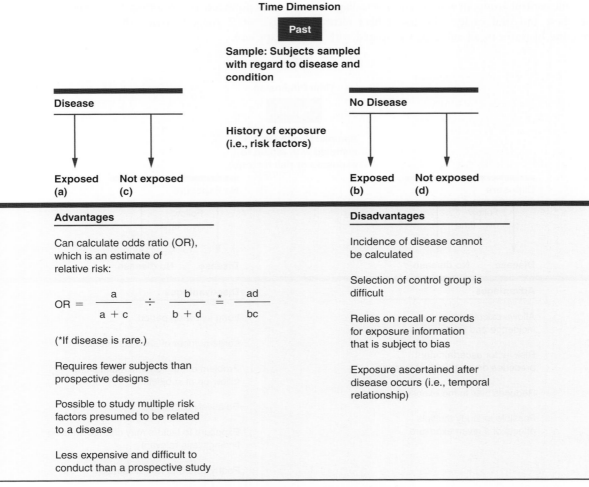

Time Dimension

Past

Sample: Subjects sampled with regard to disease and condition

Disease   **No Disease**

History of exposure (i.e., risk factors)

Exposed **Not exposed**   **Exposed** **Not exposed**
(a)   **(c)**   **(b)**   **(d)**

Advantages	Disadvantages
Can calculate odds ratio (OR), which is an estimate of relative risk:	Incidence of disease cannot be calculated
$$OR = \frac{a}{a+c} \div \frac{b}{b+d} \stackrel{*}{=} \frac{ad}{bc}$$	Selection of control group is difficult
(*If disease is rare.)	Relies on recall or records for exposure information that is subject to bias
Requires fewer subjects than prospective designs	Exposure ascertained after disease occurs (i.e., temporal relationship)
Possible to study multiple risk factors presumed to be related to a disease	
Less expensive and difficult to conduct than a prospective study	

Fig. 5.6 Retrospective, or case–control, study.

exposure or risk factor under study. For example, a researcher may select patients with heart disease to be controls in a study of patients with lung cancer. However, this choice may introduce serious bias because the two groups often share the risk factor of smoking. The methods of data collection must be the same for both groups to prevent further introduction of bias into the study. Therefore, it is desirable for interviewers to remain unaware of which subjects are cases and which are controls.

In retrospective studies, data collection extends back in time to determine previous exposure or risk factors. Investigators analyze study data by comparing the proportion of subjects with disease, or cases, who possess the exposure or risk factors with the corresponding proportion in the control group. A greater proportion of exposed cases than of exposed controls suggests a relationship between the disease and the risk factor.

Investigators often use retrospective study designs because these designs address the question of causality better than cross-sectional studies. Retrospective studies also require fewer resources and less data collection time than prospective studies. Many examples of *retrospective,* or *case–control,* studies exist in the literature. One classic example is Doll and Hill's (1952) investigation of risk factors for lung cancer. They compared exposure rates for cases in which lung cancer was diagnosed with those in the control group, in whom cancer was diagnosed outside the chest and oral cavity. The researchers recorded detailed smoking histories in all subjects. Compared with the controls, a significantly higher proportion of patients with lung cancer smoked. This study yielded the hypothesis that smoking may be etiologically related to lung cancer.

Prospective Studies. *Prospective studies* monitor a group of disease-free individuals to determine whether and when disease occurs (Fig. 5.7). These individuals, or the *cohort,* have a common experience within a defined period. For example, a birth cohort consists of all people born within a given period. The study assesses the cohort with respect to an exposure factor associated with the disease and thus classifies it at the beginning of the study. The study then monitors the cohort for disease development. The investigator compares the disease rates for those with a known exposure and the disease rates for those who remain unexposed. The study observes subjects prospectively; therefore, it summarizes data collected over time by the incidence rates of new cases (Box 5.8). Again, comparing two incidence rates produces a measure of relative risk:

$$\text{Realtive risk} = \frac{\text{Incidence rate among exposed}}{\text{Incidence rate among unexposed}}$$

The relative risk indicates the extent of excess risk incurred by exposure relative to nonexposure. A relative risk of 1 suggests no excess risk resulting from exposure, whereas a relative risk of 2 suggests twice the risk of having disease from exposure.

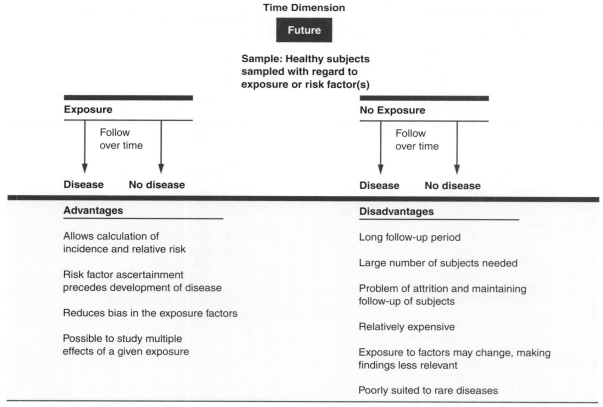

Fig. 5.7 Prospective, or cohort, study.

BOX 5.8 Comparison of Time Factors in Retrospective and Prospective Study Designs

Cohort Study
Girls with bacteriuria → Women with renal disease
Girls with sterile urine → Women without renal disease

Case–Control Study
Girls with bacteriuria ← Women with renal disease
Girls with sterile urine ← Women without renal disease
PAST————————PRESENT (BEGINNING)————————FUTURE
Comparison of time factors in prospective design (i.e., cohort) and retrospective design (i.e., case–control) approaches to studying the possible effect of childhood bacteriuria on renal disease in adult women.

Prospective studies, or *longitudinal*, *cohort*, or *incidence* studies, are advantageous because they obtain more reliable information about the cause of disease than do other study methodologies. These studies establish a stronger temporal relationship between the presumed causal factors and the effect than do retrospective and cross-sectional studies. Calculations of incidence rates and relative risks provide a valuable indicator of the level of risk that exposure creates.

ETHICAL INSIGHTS

The Tuskegee Syphilis Study
In 1932 the U.S. Public Health Service (PHS) began a longitudinal-experimental study of 600 African American sharecroppers, 399 of whom had syphilis and 201 who did not. The study was conducted in one of the poorest counties of Alabama, and the subjects were unaware that they had syphilis; they were told they were being treated for "bad blood." Enticed by the promise of free medical care and meals, the subjects joined the study without knowledge of their disease, its treatment, or the study procedures. The experimental group was initially treated with ineffective doses of the treatments of the time—bismuth or mercury—and later with aspirin. Even when penicillin became available in the late 1940s, these subjects were actively denied treatment. For 40 years, these men were followed up by PHS investigators affiliated with the Tuskegee Institute and Hospital, who claimed to be observing the differences in the progression of the disease in Blacks in comparison with the control group. During the course of the study, many subjects died of syphilis or other causes, numerous wives became infected, and children were born with congenital syphilis.

In 1972, a former venereal disease interviewer, Peter Buxtun, "blew the whistle" on the study, and reports were published in newspapers. Only after the public became outraged about the unethical nature of the study did the CDC and the PHS move to end it. In 1973, the National Association for the Advancement of Colored People won a $10 million class action suit on behalf of the subjects. In 1997, President Bill Clinton formally apologized to the few survivors and their families for the harm inflicted on these men and their families in the name of public health research.

The Tuskegee Study raises questions about how a study could proceed without informing and seeking consent of participants, how available treatment could be withheld, and how government researchers could pursue an unethical research plan without periodic review and questioning. Furthermore, the racial and discriminatory issues suggest disturbing questions for researchers and practicing nurses to contemplate, one being that the Tuskegee Study contributes to a legacy of distrust that minorities may harbor toward both the health care delivery system and research programs.

Data from Centers for Disease Control and Prevention: *The Tuskegee timeline*, 2021. Available from: http://www.cdc.gov/tuskegee/timeline.htm; Infoplease: *The Tuskegee syphilis experiment*, 2021, Pearson Education. Available from: https://www.infoplease.com/history/black-history/the-tuskegee-syphillis-experiment.

However, certain disadvantages are inherent in the prospective design. It is costly in terms of resources and staff to monitor a cohort over time, and lengthy studies result in subject attrition. Problems arising from the nature of chronic diseases may compound these logistical dilemmas. Frequently, chronic diseases have long latency periods between exposure and symptom manifestation. Furthermore, the onset of chronic conditions may be insidious, making it extremely difficult to document the incidence of disease. In addition, many diseases do not have a unifactorial cause (i.e., single variable) because many interacting factors influence disease. These problems do not negate the benefits of prospectively designed epidemiological studies; rather, they suggest a need to carefully plan and tailor a study specifically to the disease and the study's purpose.

The literature contains numerous prospective studies. In many cases, these studies have been instrumental in substantiating causal links between specific risk factors and disease. A classic example is a Doll and Hill cohort study of subjects who eventually developed lung cancer during the follow-up period (1956). Doll and Hill originally completed questionnaires on a cohort of physicians in Great Britain. Next, they classified the subjects according to several variables, emphasizing the number of cigarettes smoked. In 4½ years, they accessed death certificate data. These data revealed a higher mortality rate resulting from lung cancer and coronary thrombosis among smoking physicians compared with nonsmokers. The death rate for heavy smokers was 166 per 100,000 versus 7 per 100,000 for nonsmokers. Combining these two incidence rates in a measure of excess risk indicated that heavy smokers were 23.7 times more likely to develop lung cancer than nonsmokers:

$$\text{Relative risk} = \frac{\frac{166}{100,000} \div 7}{100,000} = 23.7$$

These findings in a prospective study provided strong epidemiological support for smoking as a risk factor for lung cancer.

Another well-known prospective study is the Framingham Heart Study, which has followed an essentially healthy cohort of Framingham, Massachusetts residents for more than 50 years. Findings from the study suggested that serum cholesterol level and other risk factors are associated with the future development of cardiovascular disease (Kramarow et al., 2013). The Framingham Study and subsequent "offspring studies" helped form the basis for later experimental studies aimed at reducing serum cholesterol through diet modification or drug therapy to ultimately lower the incidence rate of coronary heart disease.

The Nurses' Health Study was initiated in 1976 with 121,700 registered nurses, with the intent of examining the long-term consequences of oral contraceptives. The initial cohort still returns questionnaires every 2 years, and data have been collected on diet and nutrition, smoking, hormone use, and menopause as well as various chronic illnesses. In 1989, the Nurses' Health Study II was initiated to study lifestyle issues, contraception, and illness patterns in younger women, and in 2008 a third study was begun looking at similar issues in another cohort.

These studies continue to monitor nurses' changing health status and risk factors and to examine factors associated with the development of numerous health conditions in women, such as breast cancer, heart disease, and other conditions (Nurses' Health Study, 2021). For example, research using Nurses' Health Study data has identified associations between air pollutants and breast cancer (Hart et al., 2018), and outdoor light at night and breast cancer (James et al., 2017) that will stimulate further investigations. The Nurses' Health Study also identifies negative associations with disease as exemplified by determining that regular use of powder in the genital area was not associated with increased ovarian cancer (O'Brien et al., 2020). Important findings from the Nurses' Health Study suggested the deleterious effects of exposure to foods containing transfats. Groundbreaking research found a 50% increase in cardiovascular disease risk for women who consumed the highest transfat intakes (Willet et al., 1993). This initial finding set the stage for sweeping policy changes in FDA labeling of these fats on Nutrition Facts boxes on food packages, on restaurant menus in many cities, and an ultimate 2015 FDA determination that partially hydrogenated oils are not "Generally Recognized as Safe" (Curtis et al., 2016). These changes have led to a reduction in population levels of serum cholesterol.

Experimental Studies

Another type of analytic study is the experimental design, called the *randomized clinical trial* (Fig. 5.8). Epidemiological investigations apply experimental methods to test treatment and prevention strategies. The investigator randomly assigns subjects at risk for a particular disease to an experimental or a control group. The investigator observes both groups for the occurrence of disease over time, but only the experimental group receives intervention, although often the control group receives a placebo. The primary statistical analysis is based on "intention to treat," that is, all subjects remain assigned to the original treatment group, regardless of whether subjects may have decided on their own to discontinue or change their therapy. For example, if a subject in a drug trial who is assigned to the active medication experiences side effects possibly from this medication and therefore discontinues the medication, this subject still is considered to be within the active drug group for the purpose of statistical testing. The change in category from treatment to no treatment, or vice versa, is called a *crossover* and may decrease the likelihood of finding a significant effect for the active treatment.

Theoretically, it is possible to introduce a harmful exposure or risk factor as the experimental factor; however, ethical considerations usually prohibit the use of human subjects for these purposes. For example, it is unacceptable to require an experimental group to smoke cigarettes in an experiment; therefore the investigator uses case-control or cohort epidemiological designs. This limitation usually restricts experimental epidemiological

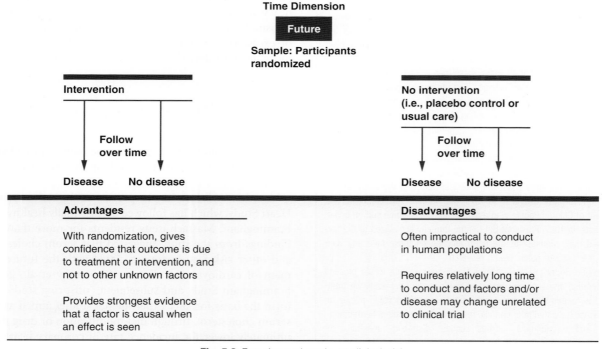

Fig. 5.8 Experimental study, or clinical trial.

studies to prophylactic and therapeutic clinical trials. Experimental studies testing vaccines and medications for safety and efficacy are examples.

The experimental design is also useful for investigating chronic disease prevention. Thus experimental studies may help evaluate community health nursing interventions. For example, they may help determine the effectiveness of a sex education program in preventing high rates of teenage pregnancy or the feasibility of an AIDS prevention program among intravenous drug users. Randomized trials were used to evaluate the Nurse-Family Partnership program, which established the long-term positive effects nurse home visits had on high-risk pregnant women and their children in comparison with those who did not receive home visits (Olds et al., 2014).

CASE STUDY Application of the Nursing Process

Using an Epidemiological and Public Health Approach to Managing a Foodborne Outbreak

Nurses working in schools, daycare centers, camps, and other facilities where food is served must be cognizant of safe food-handling principles. Furthermore, they must be aware of the potential for transmitting disease if proper procedures are not followed. Outbreaks of foodborne illness must be assessed and managed, and often it is the community health nurse who initiates and participates in this process. The following is a scenario in which the nurse utilized the nursing process to analyze and intervene in such an epidemic.

Assessment

On Wednesday, October 4, the school nurse at Greenly Elementary School saw eight students who complained of abdominal cramping, diarrhea, and fever. Parents of the sick students were called, and the students were sent home. On Thursday, the nurse was alerted to a large number of absent students and teachers. Specifically, 62 students and 10 teachers were absent. Most reported diarrhea symptoms. Because the absentee rate of 10% exceeded the average daily rate of 4% for the 620-student school and because the nurse determined that the large number of diarrhea cases suggested an epidemic, the local public health department was notified.

Public health officials arrived at the school and began to assess students still at school and those who were recovering at home. Stool culture specimens were collected and sent to the state laboratory. Results indicated that the organism causing illness was in most cases *Shigella sonnei*, the most commonly found form of the bacteria. Persons with severe symptoms were referred to their physicians for possible antibiotic therapy. Food histories of meals eaten both at school and outside of school were taken.

Friday saw a continuing increase in absenteeism of students and staff reporting gastrointestinal illness. Public health specialists defined the criteria for identifying cases on the basis primarily of positive laboratory results, symptoms of diarrhea or vomiting, fever with nausea or abdominal pain, or all of these. Cafeteria staff were interviewed, and it was determined that one staff member had had diarrhea over the previous weekend but had returned to work on Monday. Public health staff continued to take dietary histories of affected and unaffected persons and constructed rates of illness for all foods served in the cafeteria beginning on Friday of the previous week. These data are displayed in the following table.

From the data, it can be seen that students who ate lunch at school on Tuesday and ate fajitas and salad had higher rates of illness than those who did not. Therefore it was concluded that the outbreak of *Shigella* could be attributed to a food source.

Diagnosis

Determining the likely cause of the outbreak was important in specifying a diagnosis and directing the planning of an intervention. The following diagnosis was formulated:

Increased risk for infectious diarrhea among elementary school children related to inadequate hygiene and food-handling practices as evidenced by a 19% increase in reported cases within a 4-day period.

Planning

The school nurse, in conjunction with public health specialists, determined that several groups should be targeted in order to eliminate the further spread of disease. They identified a need to assist families in understanding the nature of the disease, how to care for their children who were ill, and how to prevent the spread at home. Within the school, there was a need to review food-handling practices and the training that cafeteria workers received. Staff, including teachers, also required information about *Shigella* and how it should be prevented in the everyday lives of students. Needs of special ages and developmental levels of children were also important. A formal plan of what needed to be done, by whom, and when was drawn up. Research into the nature and prevention of *Shigella* was gathered from the CDC and the local health department, among other sources. Health department staff developed a plan to release information to the public about the prevention of gastrointestinal illnesses, as many of these diseases are easily spread and so many students were already ill.

Long-Term Goal
- An absence of cases of infectious diarrhea

Short-Term Goals
- Treatment and recovery of all identified cases of diarrhea
- Implementation of an effective program of hygienic practices among students and staff
- Implementation of a food-handling program for all cafeteria workers
- Adequate informing of the larger community in order to prevent spread of the epidemic

Intervention

The school nurse took a central leadership role, directing action within the school aimed at staff, students, and student families. Teaching of appropriate hand washing was stressed. Hand-washing facilities were inspected for soap, paper towels, and running water. Food preparation guidelines were reviewed with staff, and policies regarding remaining at home when ill were reiterated. The health department staff provided technical assistance and made recommendations. They informed community physicians about surveillance and reporting requirements and provided information regarding case identification and treatment regimens. Daycare centers and preschools were advised to watch for diarrhea outbreaks and to adhere to strict hand-washing and diaper-handling practices, as these facilities tend to be high-risk areas for the transmission of organisms such as *Shigella*. The media were contacted to elicit their help in disseminating correct and useful information to the community.

Evaluation

Immediate evaluation involved monitoring the decline in *Shigella* cases both within the school and in the larger community. The school nurse noted that rates of absenteeism returned to normal on the following Monday. She determined that all classes had received hygiene instruction within the following 2 weeks and that all teachers had received a flyer with specific information about

CASE STUDY   Application of the Nursing Process

Using an Epidemiological and Public Health Approach to Managing a Foodborne Outbreak—cont'd

Shigella, its care, and its prevention. She observed that bathrooms had filled soap dispensers, that friendly signs reminding students to wash hands were posted near sinks, and that students were given the opportunity to wash hands before lunch and snacks. The public health department likewise continued surveillance activities after encouraging physicians to collect and submit stool culture specimens for suspected cases and to report cases to the health department. Rates of diarrhea declined rapidly in the week after the school outbreak. The infection did not spread to other schools or community groups. This outcome can be attributed to successful epidemic management, yet surveillance remains critical if the public's health is to be protected.

Levels of Prevention
Primary
- Teach students and staff about hand washing and hygienic practices.

- Maintain a system that promotes safe food-handling practices.
- Exclude those with symptoms from school or food handling.

Secondary
- Collect stool culture specimens from all symptomatic individuals.
- Treat those with advanced diarrhea symptoms with antibiotics.
- Exclude those with positive culture results from food handling, and exclude those with symptoms from school.
- Advise families and individuals in the care of those with diarrhea.

Tertiary
- Treat and counsel those determined to be carriers of *Shigella.*

Information on *Shigella* infections is available at https://www.cdc.gov/shigella/index.html.

Number Exposed by Meal and Food Item (*N* = 143).

Exposure Variable (Food Eaten)	NUMBER WHO ATE		NUMBER WHO DID NOT EAT		Odds Ratio[a]
	III (A)	Not III (B)	III (C)	Not III (D)	
Ate on Monday	47	60	18	18	0.78
Ate on Tuesday:	63	57	3	20	7.37
Fajitas	57	52	8	26	4.56
Salad	44	21	24	54	4.7
Salsa	26	29	40	48	1.07
Tortillas	48	53	16	26	1.47
Beans	29	32	34	48	1.28
Milk	53	56	11	23	1.98
Ate on Wednesday	21	64	43	15	0.11

[a]Odds ratios were calculated with the formula: ad/bd.

Modified from Texas Department of Health: *Shigella* outbreak in an elementary school, *Dis Prev News* 55(6):1–3, 1995.

⚕ GENETICS IN PUBLIC HEALTH

Community-Based Research for the Prevention of Anencephaly

A nurse-led investigation in Washington State exposed a cluster of infants born with anencephaly in a three county region between 2010 and 2017. Subsequent investigation revealed almost five times greater incidence of anencephaly in the counties in question when compared with rates of the U.S. (9.5 per 10,000 in select Washington counties vs. 2.1 per 10,000 nationwide). Preliminarily review showed that cases were much more commonly identified among Hispanic infants, suggesting that cultural and genetic factors were contributory. Among the risk factors identified was increased dietary consumption of nonfortified corn-based foods, rather than wheat-based products. Also noted were defects in folic acid metabolism among mothers of Hispanic ancestry.

Strategies to address and ultimately reduce the number of babies born with anencephaly were to enhance surveillance activities including both active and passive case finding, counseling to reduce risk factors including stressing the importance of folic acid intake, participating in research, and advocating policy change to protect patients from preventable birth defects.

Barron S: Anencephaly: An ongoing investigation in Washington state. *AJN* 116(3):60—66; Washington State Department of Health: Anencephaly investigation, n.d. Available from: https://www.doh.wa.gov/YouandYourFamily/IllnessandDisease/BirthDefects/Anencephaly Investigation.

SUMMARY

Epidemiology offers the community health nurse methods to quantify the extent of health problems in the community and provides a body of knowledge about risk factors and their association with disease. At each step of the nursing process, epidemiological applications support the practice of the community health nurse. Compiling descriptive data from surveys or studies contributes to the nurse's understanding of the community's health level. In assessing community problems, epidemiological rates describe the magnitude of disease and provide support for community diagnoses. Epidemiological studies suggest interventions and their potential efficacy—information that is useful in planning prevention and intervention approaches. Evaluation studies using epidemiological methods, either reported in the literature or conducted by community health nurses, are essential for providing optimal research-based care.

EVOLVE WEBSITE

http://evolve.elsevier.com/Nies/community

- NCLEX Review Questions
- Case Studies.

BIBLIOGRAPHY AND REFERENCES

Centers for Disease Control and Prevention: Deaths: preliminary report for 2014, *Natl Vital Stat Rep* 65(4):1—122, 2016. Available from: http://www.cdc.gov/nchs/data/nvsr/nvsr65/nvsr65_04.pdf.

Centers for Disease Control and Prevention: Infant mortality in the United States, 2018: data from the period linked birth/infant death file, *Natl Vital Stat Rep* 69(7):1—17, 2020. Available from: www.cdc.gov/nchs/data/nvsr/nvsr69/NVSR-69-7-508.pdf.

Centers for Disease Control and Prevention: *About the national health and nutrition examination survey*, 2021. Available from: www.cdc.gov/nchs/nhanes/about_nhanes.htm.

Centers for Disease Control and Prevention: *Pregnancy mortality surveillance system*, 2021. Available from: www.cdc.gov/reproductivehealth/maternal-mortality/index.html.

Centers for Disease Control and Prevention: *The Tuskegee timeline*, 2021. Available from: http://www.cdc.gov/tuskegee/timeline.htm.

Centers for Disease Control and Prevention: *Tuberculosis skin testing*, 2021. Available from: http://www.cdc.gov/tb/publications/factsheets/testing/skintesting.htm.

Centers for Disease Control and Prevention: *Use of colorectal cancer screening tests*, 2021. Available from: www.cdc.gov/cancer/colorectal/statistics/use-screening-tests-BRFSS.htm.

Curtis CJ, Clapp J, Goldstein G, et al.: How the nurses' health study helped Americans take the trans fat out, *Am J Public Health* 106:1537—1539, 2016.

Doll R, Hill AB: Study of the aetiology of carcinoma of the lung, *BMJ* 2:1271—1285, 1952.

Doll R, Hill AB: Lung cancer and other causes of death in relation to smoking, *BMJ* 2:1071—1081, 1956.

Friedman GD: *Primer of epidemiology*, ed 4, New York, McGraw-Hill.

Fryar CD, Hughes JP, Herrick KA, et al.: *Fast food consumption among adults in the United States, 2013—2016*. National Center for Health Statistics Data Brief, 322, 2018. Available from: http://stacks.cdc.gov/view/cdc/59582.

Hart JE, Bertrand KA, DuPre N, et al.: Exposure to hazardous air pollutants and risk of incident breast cancer in the Nurses' Health Study ll, *Environ Health* 17(28):28, 2018. https://doi.org/10.1186/s12940-018-0372-3.

James P, Bertrand KA, Hart JA, et al.: Outdoor light at night and breast cancer incidence in the Nurses' Health Study ll, *Environ Health Perspect* 125, 2017. https://doi.org/10.1289/EHP935.

Kramarow E, Lubitz J, Francis R: Trends in the coronary heart disease risk profile of middle-aged adults, *Ann Epidemiol* 23:31—34, 2013.

Lin JS, Piper MA, Perdue LA, et al. Screening for colorectal cancer: updated evidence report and systematic review for the US preventive services task force, *JAMA* 315(23):2576—2594, 2016. https://doi.org/10.1001/jama.2016.3332.

Marriott BP, Hunt KJ, Lalek A, Newman N: Trends in intake of energy and total sugar from sugar-sweetened beverages in the United States among children and adults, NHANES 2003—2016, *Nutrients* 11, 2019. https://doi.org/10.3390/nu11092004.

Mausner JS, Kramer S: *Mausner and Bahn epidemiology: an introductory text*, ed 2, Philadelphia, 1985, Saunders.

Mehra R, Boyd LM, Magriples U, Kershaw TS, Ickovics JR, Keene DE: Black pregnant women "get the most judgment": a qualitative study of the experiences of black women at the intersection of race, gender and pregnancy, *Wom Health Issues* 30(6):484—492, 2020.

Morton RF, Hebel JR, McCarter RJ: *A study guide to epidemiology and biostatistics*, ed 3, Gaithersburg, MD, 1990, Aspen Publishers.

National Cancer Institute: *Surveillance, epidemiology and end results program*, 2021. Available from: http://seer.cancer.gov/.

Nurses' Health Study: *History*, 2021. Available from: http://www.nurseshealthstudy.org/about-nhs/history.

O'Brien KM, Tworoger SS, Harris HR, et al.: Association of powder use in the genital area with risk of ovarian cancer, *JAMA* 323(1):49—59, 2020. Available from: https://doi.org/10.1001/jama.2019.20079.

Olds DL, Kitzman HJ, Knudtson MD, et al.: Effect of home visiting by nurses on maternal and child mortality: results of a 2-decade follow-up of a randomized clinical trial, *JAMA Pediatr* 168(9):800—806, 2014. https://doi.org/10.1001/jamapediatrics.2014.472.

Organisation for Economic Cooperation and Development (OECD): *Health status: infant mortality rates*, 2021. Available from: https://data.oecd.org/healthstat/infant-mortality-rates.htm.

Peck MG, Sappenfield WM, Skala J: Perinatal periods of risk: a community approach for using data to improve women and infants' health, *Mater & Child Health J* 14:864e874, 2010.

Phillips JC: Antiretroviral therapy adherence: testing a social context model among black men who use illicit drugs, *J Assoc Nurs AIDS Care* 22:100—127, 2011.

Snow J: *On the mode of communication of cholera*, ed 2, London, 1855, Churchill, p 18.

Texas Department of Health: Shigella outbreak in an elementary school, *Dis Prev News* 55(6):1—3, 1995.

U.S. Department of Health and Human Services: *Healthy people 2030*, 2021. Available from: https://health.gov/healthypeople/objectives-and-data/about-objectives.

Willet WC, Stampfer MJ, Manson JE, et al.: Intake of trans fatty acids and risk of coronary heart disease among women, *Lancet* 341:581—585, 1993.

6

Community Assessment

Holly B. Cassells

OBJECTIVES

Upon completion of this chapter, the reader will be able to do the following:

1. Discuss the major dimensions of a community.
2. Identify sources of information about a community's health.
3. Describe the process of conducting a community assessment.
4. Formulate community and aggregate diagnoses.
5. Identify uses for epidemiological data at each step of the nursing process.

OUTLINE

KEY TERMS

aggregate
census tracts
community diagnosis
community of solution

geographic community
metropolitan statistical areas
needs assessment
social system

vital statistics
windshield survey

The primary concern of community health nurses is to improve the health of the community. To address this concern, community health nurses employ the principles and skills of both nursing and public health practice. This process involves using demographic and epidemiological methods to assess the community's health and diagnose its health needs.

Before beginning this process, the community health nurse must define the community of interest. The nurse may wonder how he or she can provide services to such a large and nontraditional "client," but there are smaller and more circumscribed entities than towns and cities that constitute "communities." A principal aspect of public health practice is the application of approaches and solutions to health problems that ensure the majority of people receive the maximum benefit. To this end, the nurse works to use time and resources efficiently for the good of community or population.

Despite the desire to provide services to each individual in a community, the community health nurse recognizes the impracticality of this task. An alternative approach considers the community itself to be the unit of service and works collaboratively with the community using the steps of the nursing process. Therefore, the community is not only the context or place where community health nursing occurs; it is

the focus of community health nursing care. The nurse partners with community members to identify community problems and develop solutions to ultimately improve the community's health.

Another central goal of public health practitioners is primary prevention, which protects the public's health and prevents disease development. Chapter 3 discusses how these "upstream efforts" are intended to reduce the pain, suffering, and huge expenditures that occur when significant segments of the population essentially "fall into the river" and require downstream resources to resolve their health problems. In a society greatly concerned about increasingly high healthcare costs, the need to prevent health problems becomes dire. In addition to reducing the occurrence of disease in individuals, community health nurses must examine the larger aggregate—its structures, environments, and shared health risks—to develop improved upstream prevention programs.

This chapter addresses the first steps in adopting a community- or population-oriented practice. A community health nurse must define a community and describe its parameters before applying the nursing process. Then, the nurse can launch the assessment and diagnosis phase of the nursing process at the aggregate level and incorporate epidemiological approaches. Comprehensive assessment data are essential to directing effective primary prevention interventions within a community.

Gathering these data is one of the core public health functions identified in the Institute of Medicine's (2002) report on the future of public health, and a key dimension of the 10 Essential Public Health Services (Centers for Disease Control and Prevention, 2020) (Fig. 6.1). The community health nurse participates in assessing the community's health and its ability to deal with health needs. With sound data, the nurse makes a valuable contribution to health policy development and population-based interventions.

THE NATURE OF COMMUNITY

There are numerous ways to define and/or describe a community. These include an aggregate of people, a location in space and time, and a social system (Box 6.1).

Aggregate of People

An aggregate is a community composed of people who have common characteristics. For example, members of a community may share residence in the same city, membership in the same religious organization, or similar demographic characteristics such as age and ethnic background. The aggregate of

senior citizens, for example, comprises primarily retirees who frequently share ages, economic pressures, life experiences, interests, and concerns. This group lived through the many societal changes of the past 50 years; therefore, they may possess similar perspectives on current issues and trends. Many elderly people share concern for the maintenance of good health, the pursuit of an active lifestyle, and the security of needed services to support a quality life. These shared interests translate into common goals and activities, which also are defining attributes of a common interest community. Communities also may consist of overlapping aggregates, in which case some community members belong to multiple aggregates.

Many human factors help delineate a community. Health-related traits, or risk factors, are one aspect of "people factors" to be considered. People who have impaired health or a shared predisposition to disease may join together in a group or community to learn from and support each other. Parents of disabled infants, people with acquired immunodeficiency syndrome (AIDS), or those at risk for a second myocardial infarction may consider themselves a community. Even when these individuals are not organized, the nurse may recognize that their unique needs constitute a form of community, or aggregate.

A community of solution may form when a common problem unites individuals. Although people may have little

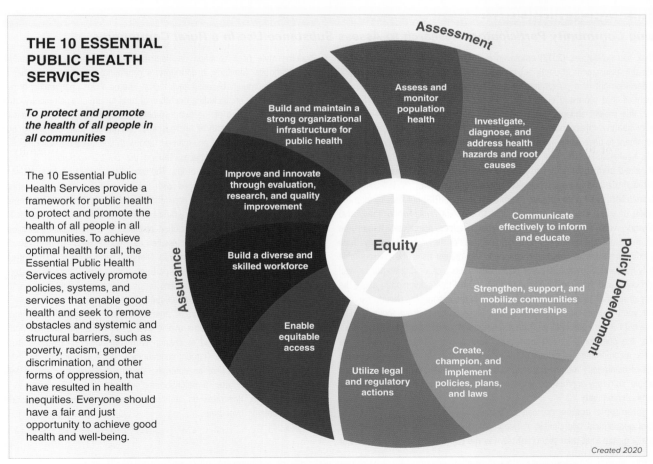

Fig. 6.1 10 Essential Public Health Services. (From the Centers for Disease Control and Prevention, 2021. Available from: https://www.cdc.gov/publichealthgateway/publichealthservices/essentialhealthservices.html.)

BOX 6.1 Major Features of a Community

- Aggregate of people
  The "who": personal characteristics and risks
- Location in space and time
  The "where" and "when": physical location frequently delineated by boundaries and influenced by the passage of time
- Social system
  The "why" and "how": interrelationships of aggregates fulfilling community functions

---

else in common with each other, their desire to redress problems brings them together. Such problems may include a shared hazard from environmental contamination, a shared health problem arising from a soaring rate of teenage suicide, or a shared political concern about an upcoming city council election. The community of solution often disbands after problem resolution, but it may subsequently identify other common issues.

Each of these shared features may exist among people who are geographically dispersed or in close proximity to one another. However, in many situations, proximity facilitates the recognition of commonality and the development of cohesion among members. This active sharing of features fosters a sense of community among individuals.

Location in Space and Time

Regardless of shared features, geographic, or physical location may define communities of people. Traditionally, a community is an entity delineated by geopolitical boundaries; this view best exemplifies the dimension of location. These boundaries demarcate the periphery of cities, counties, states, and nations. Voting precincts, school districts, water districts, and fire and police protection precincts set less visible boundary lines.

Census tracts subdivide larger communities. The U.S. Census Bureau uses them for data collection and population assessment. Census tracts facilitate the organization of resident information in specific community geographic locales. In densely populated urban areas, the size of tracts tends to be small; therefore data for one or more census tracts frequently describe neighborhood residents. Although residents may not be aware of their census tract's boundaries, census tract data help define and describe neighborhood communities.

Social System

A third major feature of a community is the relationships that community members form with one another. Community

---

RESEARCH HIGHLIGHTS

Using Community Participatory Research to Assess Substance Use in a Rural Community

Kulbok and colleagues (2012) employed a Community Participatory Model to guide the assessment of youth substance abuse in a rural Virginia county and the development of a prevention model. They integrated multiple assessment modalities that represent current public health nursing competencies. Specifically, this project engaged local community members and leaders with community health professionals in every step of the project, from planning the assessment to developing and evaluating the intervention. This process allowed public health nurses to integrate their knowledge of the local community with that gained from community partners and to develop a deeper understanding of substance use and its local ecological and cultural context.

Researchers used a geographic information system (GIS) not only to map the location of youth substance use but also to pinpoint areas where preventive behaviors were more common. These maps helped specifically target the location for preventive interventions. Perspectives of the youth about key "teen places" were also geographically mapped. The project used the photographic charity Photovoice to capture participants' descriptions of local strengths as well as concerns and then employed the images to facilitate conversation about the nature of alcohol, tobacco, and substance use in the community. Qualitative data about youth beliefs about substance use were gathered from focus groups. These data were combined with descriptive information about the local population, the community environment, and local social systems and beliefs to develop a comprehensive picture of the local community. Involvement of a broad range of community members throughout the project planning enabled a more effective, culturally appropriate, and sustainable intervention to be developed for this rural community.

A **geographic community** can encompass less formalized areas that lack official geopolitical boundaries. A geographic landmark may define neighborhoods (e.g., the East Lake section of town or the North Shore area). A particular building style or a common development era also may identify community neighborhoods. Similarly, a dormitory, a communal home, or a summer camp may be a community because each facility shares a close geographic proximity. Geographic location, including the urban or rural nature of a community, strongly influences the nature of the health problems a community health nurse might find there. Public health is increasingly recognizing that the interaction of humans with the natural environment and with constructed environments consisting of buildings and spaces, termed the *built environment*, is critical to healthy behavior and quality of life. The spatial location of health problems in a geographic area can be mapped with the use of GIS software, assisting the nurse to identify vulnerable populations and public health departments to develop programs specific to geographic communities. For example, public health practitioners can map the distribution of smoking, the prevalence of hypertension, or the presence of areas classified as "food deserts" to help specifically target areas for intervention (Fig. 6.2). Mapping tools such as those offered by the Community Commons and their partners allow one to select parameters and build maps for local geographic areas (https://communitycommons.org/entities/60847319-e438-44be-a5c3-5b8d298845e1, 2021).

Location and the dimension of time define communities. The community's character and health problems evolve over time. Although some communities are very stable, most tend to change with the members' health status and demographics and the larger community's development or decline. For example, the presence of an emerging young workforce may attract new industry, which can alter a neighborhood's health and environment. A community's history illustrates its ability to change and how well it addresses health problems over time.

Data from Kulbok PA, Thatcher E, Park E, et al.: Evolving public health nursing roles: focus on community participatory health promotion and prevention, *Online J Issues Nurs* 17(2):1, 2012. Available from: https://pubmed.ncbi.nlm.nih.gov/22686109/.

Current Smokers, Percent of Adults by tract, BRFSS 500 Cities Project 2014

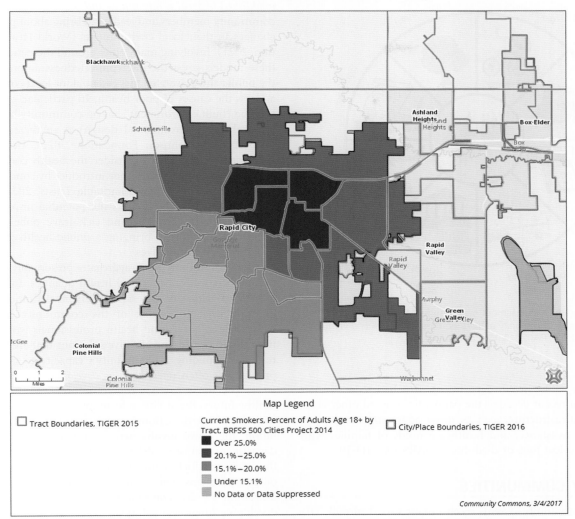

Fig. 6.2 Current smokers, percent of adults by tract, BRFSS 500 Cities Project, 2014. Location, Rapid City, South Dakota. Community Commons. Available from: www.communitycommons.org.

members fulfill the essential functions of community by interacting in groups. These functions provide socialization, role fulfillment, goal achievement, and member support. Therefore a community is a complex social system, and its interacting members constitute various subsystems within the community. These subsystems are interrelated and interdependent (i.e., the subsystems affect one another and affect various internal and external stimuli). These stimuli consist of a broad range of events, values, conditions, and needs.

A healthcare system is an example of a complex system that consists of smaller, interrelated subsystems. A healthcare system can also be a subsystem because it interacts with and depends on larger systems such as the city government. Changes in the larger system can cause repercussions in many subsystems. For example, when local economic pressures cause a health department to scale back its operations, many subsystems are affected. The health department may eliminate or cut back programs, limit service to other healthcare providers, reduce access to groups that normally use the system, and deny needed care to families who constitute subsystems in society. Almost every subsystem in the community must react and readjust to such a financial constraint.

Prevalent health problems also can have a severe impact on multiple systems. For example, the coronavirus (COVID 19) pandemic required significant national, state and local funds for screening, contact investigation, vaccination, and public health education. However, in addition to placing intense

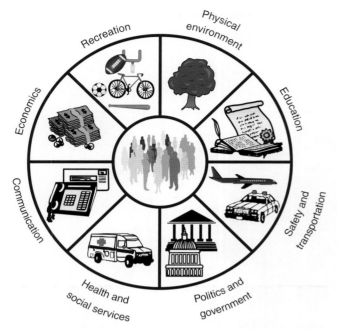

Fig. 6.3 Diagram of assessment parameters. (Modified from Anderson ET, McFarlane J: *Community as partner: theory and practice in nursing,* ed 8, Philadelphia, PA, 2019, Wolters Kluwer.)

pressure on public health departments that had reduced their personnel in recent decades, the pandemic strained other areas of public infrastructure such as those addressing unemployment, food assistance, and healthcare needs of families with workers who lost jobs or died due to SARS-COVID-19.

HEALTHY COMMUNITIES

Complex community systems receive many varied stimuli. The community's ability to respond effectively to changing dynamics and meet the needs of its members indicates productive functioning. Examining the community's functions and subsystems provides clues to existing and potential health problems. Examples of a community's functions include the provision of accessible and acceptable health services; educational opportunities; and safe, crime-free environments.

The model in Fig. 6.3 suggests assessment parameters that can help a nurse develop a more complete list of critical community functions. The community health nurse can then prioritize these functions from a particular community's perspective. Americans' views on health and healthy communities frequently reflect concern for quality-of-life issues over the absence of disease, and in particular safety and low levels of crime are of high priority. These findings are echoed in city-sponsored health surveys across the nation: ensuring safe and healthy environments that allow for healthy lifestyles, which include activity and nutritious food, is as important to residents as accessing quality healthcare.

Movements such as *Healthy Cities and Healthy Communities established by local communities and philanthropic partners* urge community members and leaders to bring about positive health changes in their local environments (World Health Organization, 2021). Involving many cities around the nation and world, these models stress the interconnectedness among people and the public and private sectors essential for local communities to address the causes of poor health. In particular, examining the role the "built environment" has on community health (e.g., its physical and environmental design) is an increasing priority (Robert Wood Johnson Foundation, 2021). Urban communities are encouraged to consider the health consequences of new policies and programs they introduce by conducting health impact assessments (Pew Charitable Trusts, 2021). These assessments of projects, such as the potential impact of zoning decisions, transit systems, and sick leave policies, serve the important function of bringing a public health perspective to urban and civic initiatives.

Each community and aggregate presumably will have a unique perspective on critical health qualities. Indeed, a community or aggregate may have divergent definitions of health, differing even from that of the community health nurse. Nevertheless, nurses and health professionals work with communities in developing effective solutions that are acceptable to residents. Building a community's capacity to address future problems is often referred to as *developing community competence*. The nurse assesses the community's commitment to a healthy future, the ability to foster open communication and to elicit broad participation in problem identification and resolution, the active involvement of structures such as a health department that can assist a community with health issues, and the extent to which members have successfully worked together on past problems. This information provides the nurse with an indication of the community's strengths and potential for developing long-term solutions to identified problems.

ASSESSING THE COMMUNITY: SOURCES OF DATA

The community health nurse becomes familiar with the community and begins to understand its nature by traveling through the area. The nurse begins to establish certain hunches or hypotheses about the community's health, strengths, and potential health problems through this down-to-earth approach, called *shoe leather epidemiology*. The community health nurse must substantiate these initial assessments and impressions with more concrete or defined data before he or she can formulate a community diagnosis and plan.

Community health nurses often perform a community windshield survey by driving or walking through an area and making organized observations. See illustrations depicting an actual "windshield survey" in this chapter's photo novella. The nurse can gain an understanding of the environmental layout,

WINDSHIELD SURVEY

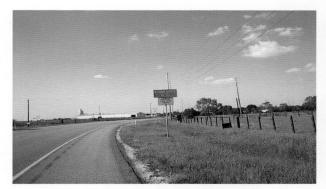

Brookshire is a town of about 3500 in Southeast Texas.

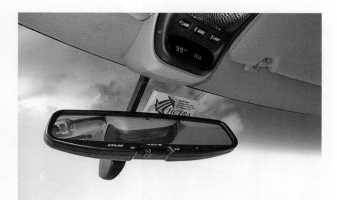

The car's thermometer shows 99°, evidence of a pervasive health threat in the summertime.

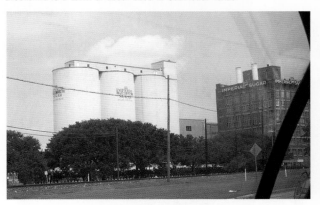

Sugar mills and farms are the source of most jobs.

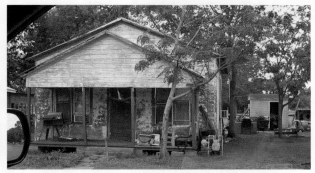

Much of the housing is substandard and suggests low-income families.

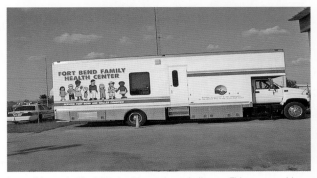

Accessible and affordable healthcare is a challenge. This van provides services to unskilled workers and area elders.

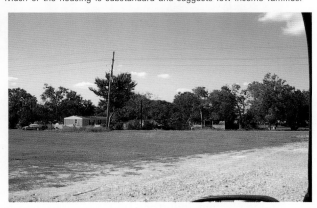

Many people live in small homes on multiple-acre lots.

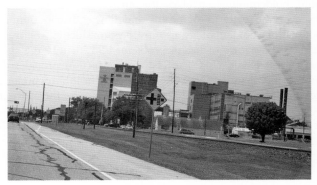

The economy of the town is predominantly agriculture and processing.

Continued

WINDSHIELD SURVEY—cont'd

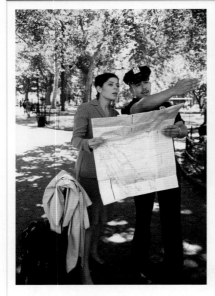
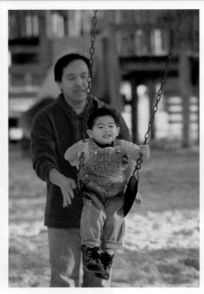
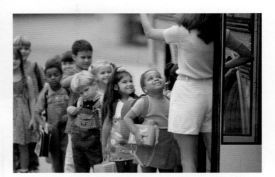
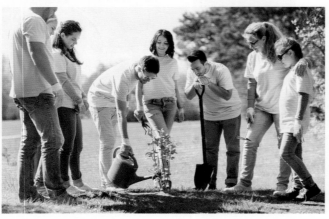
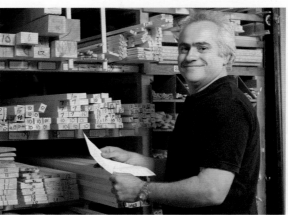

The important determinants of a health community include a low crime rate, a good place to bring up children, good schools, a strong family life, good environmental quality, and a healthy economy (iStock 540095516, 683792276, 504534788, 470237304, 638480042). Photos courtesy of University of Texas Health Science Center at Houston, School of Nursing, Community Health Division.

including geographic features and the location of agencies, services, businesses, and industries, and can locate possible areas of environmental concern through "sight, sense, and sound." The windshield survey offers the nurse an opportunity to observe people and their role in the community. Box 6.2 provides examples of questions to guide a windshield survey assessment.

In addition to direct observational methods, certain public health tools become essential to an aggregate-focused nursing practice. The analysis of demographic information and statistical data provides descriptive information about the population. Epidemiology involves the analysis of health data to discover the patterns of health and illness distribution in a population. Epidemiology also involves conducting research to explain the nature of health problems and identify the aggregates at increased risk. The rest of this section provides data sources and describes how the community health nurse can use demographic and epidemiological data to assess the aggregate.

BOX 6.2 Questions to Guide Community Observations During a Windshield Survey

1. Community vitality:
   - Are people visible in the community? What are they doing?
   - Who are the people living in the neighborhood? What is their age range? What is the predominant age (e.g., elderly, preschoolers, young mothers, or school-aged children)?
   - What ethnicity or race is most common?
   - What is the general appearance of those you observed? Do they appear healthy? Do you notice any people with obvious disabilities, such as those using walkers or wheelchairs, or those with mental or emotional disabilities? Where do they live?
   - Do you notice residents who are well nourished or malnourished, thin or obese, vigorous or frail, unkempt or scantily dressed, or well dressed and clean?
   - Do you notice tourists or visitors to the community?
   - Do you observe any people who appear to be under the influence of drugs or alcohol?
   - Do you see any pregnant women? Do you see women with strollers and young children?

2. Indicators of social and economic conditions:
   - What is the general condition of the homes you observe? Are these single-family homes or multifamily structures? Is there any evidence of dilapidated housing or of areas undergoing urban renewal? Is there public housing? What is its condition?
   - What forms of transportation do people seem to be using? Is there public transit? Are there adequate bus stops with benches and shade? Is transportation to healthcare resources available?
   - Are there any indicators of the kinds of work available to residents? Are there job opportunities nearby, such as factories, small businesses, or military installations? Are there unemployed people visible, such as homeless people?
   - Do you see men congregating in groups on the street? What do they look like, and what are they doing?
   - Is this a rural area? Are there farms or agricultural businesses?
   - Do you note any seasonal workers, such as migrant or day laborers?
   - Do you see any women hanging out along the streets? What are they doing?
   - Do you observe any children or adolescents out of school during the daytime?
   - Do you observe any interest in political campaigns or issues, such as campaign signs?
   - Do you see any evidence of health education on billboards, advertisements, signs, radio stations, or television stations? Do these methods seem appropriate for the people you observed?
   - What kinds of schools and day care centers are available?

3. Health resources:
   - Do you notice any hospitals? What kind are they? Where are they located?
   - Are there any clinics? Whom do they serve? Are there any family planning services?
   - Are there doctors' and dentists' offices? Are they specialists or generalists?
   - Do you notice any nursing homes, rehabilitation centers, mental health clinics, alcohol or drug treatment centers, homeless or abused shelters, wellness clinics, health department facilities, urgent care centers, mobile health vehicles, blood donation centers, or pharmacies?
   - Are these resources appropriate and sufficient to address the kinds of problems that exist in this community?

4. Environmental conditions related to health:
   - Do you see evidence of anything that might make you suspicious of ground, water, or air pollutants?
   - What is the sanitary condition of the housing? Is housing overcrowded, dirty, or in need of repair? Are windows screened?
   - What is the condition of the roads? Are potholes present? Are drainage systems in place? Are there low water crossings, and do they have warning signals? Are there adequate traffic lights, signs, sidewalks, and curbs? Are railroad crossings fitted with warnings and barriers? Are streets and parking lots well lit? Is this a heavily trafficked area, or are roads rural? Are there curves or features that make the roads hazardous?
   - Is there handicapped access to buildings, sidewalks, and streets?
   - Do you observe recreational facilities and playgrounds? Are they being used? Is there a YMCA/YWCA or community center? Are there any daycare facilities or preschools?
   - Are children playing in the streets, alleys, yards, or parks?
   - Do you see any restaurants?
   - Is food sold on the streets? Are people eating in public areas? Are there trash receptacles and places for people to sit? Are public restrooms available?
   - What evidence of any nuisances such as ants, flies, mosquitoes, or rodents do you observe? Are there stray animals wandering in the neighborhood?

5. Social functioning:
   - Do you observe any families in the neighborhoods? Can you observe their structure or functioning? Who is caring for the children? What kind of supervision do they have? Is more than one generation present?
   - Are there any identifiable subgroups related to one another either socially or geographically?
   - What evidence of a sense of neighborliness can you observe?
   - What evidence of community cohesiveness can you observe? Are there any group efforts in the neighborhood to improve the living conditions or the neighborhood? Is there a neighborhood watch? Do community groups postsigns for neighborhood meetings?
   - How many and what type of churches, synagogues, and other places of worship are there?
   - Can you observe anything that would make you suspicious of social problems, such as gang activity, juvenile delinquency, drug or alcohol abuse, and adolescent pregnancy?

6. Attitude toward health and healthcare:
   - Do you observe any evidence of folk medicine practice, such as a botánica or herbal medicine shop? Are there any alternative medicine practitioners, such as healers or curanderos?
   - Do you observe that health resources are well utilized or underutilized?
   - Is there evidence of preventive or wellness care?
   - Do you observe any efforts to improve the neighborhood's health? Planned health fairs? Do you see advertisements for health-related events, clinics, or lectures?

Census Data

Every 10 years, the U.S. Census Bureau undertakes a massive survey of all American families. In addition to this decennial census, intermediate surveys collect specific types of information. These collections of statistical data describe the population characteristics of the nation within progressively smaller geopolitical entities (e.g., states, counties, and census tracts). The census also describes metropolitan areas that extend beyond formal city boundaries, called **metropolitan and micropolitan statistical areas**. A metropolitan statistical area consists of a central city with more than 50,000 people and includes the associated suburban or adjacent counties to form a large metropolitan area. A micropolitan statistical area clusters around one or more smaller urban areas of 10,000 people but is not larger than 50,000 persons. A census tract is one of the smallest reporting units. It usually consists of 3000 to 6000 people who share characteristics such as ethnicity, socioeconomic status, and housing class.

The census is extremely helpful to community health nurses familiarizing themselves with a new community. The census tabulates many demographic variables, including population size and the distribution of age, sex, race, and ethnicity. The American Community Survey, conducted annually, and the decennial census report social data such as income, poverty, and occupational factors. Both data sets can be accessed through use of the U.S. Census Bureau's website at https://data.census.gov/cedsci/. Here the nurse can view variables which have a bearing on health (e.g., age and ethnicity), and construct a community profile and compare trends with those in other communities. Note that variables that describe the community's health are not part of census data. However, census numbers are frequently used as denominators for morbidity and mortality rates (see Chapter 5).

The nurse analyzes and interprets data by comparing current and local census data with previous data and information from various locations to pinpoint key local differences and changes over time. The nurse can identify the attributes that make each community unique by comparing data for one census unit, such as a zip code or a city, with those of another community or the entire nation. These attributes provide clues to the community's potential vulnerabilities or health risks. For example, a community health nurse may review census reports and discover that a community has many elderly people. This knowledge directs the nurse toward further assessment of the social resources (i.e., housing, transportation, and community centers), health resources (i.e., hospitals, nursing homes, and geriatric clinics), and health problems common to aging people. By identifying the trends in the population over time, the community health nurse can modify public health programs to meet the changing needs of the community.

Vital Statistics

The official registration records of births, deaths, marriages, divorces, and adoptions form the basis of data in **vital statistics**. Every year, city, county, and state health departments aggregate and report these events for the preceding year. When compared with those from previous years, vital statistics provide indicators of population growth or reduction. In addition to supplying information about the number of births and deaths, registration certificates record the causes of death, which is useful in determining morbidity and mortality trends. Similarly, birth certificates document birth information (e.g., cesarean delivery, prenatal care, and teen mothers) and the occurrence of any congenital malformations. This information also is important in assessments of the community's health status.

Other Sources of Health Data

The U.S. Census Bureau conducts numerous surveys on subjects of government interest, such as crime, housing, and labor. Results of these surveys, the census reports, and vital statistics reports are usually available through public libraries and on the Internet. The National Center for Health Statistics (NCHS) compiles annual National Health Interview Survey data, which describe health trends in a national sample. The NCHS publishes reports on the prevalence of disability, illness, and other health-related variables. Specifically, the Behavioral Risk Factor Surveillance System is the world's largest telephone survey of U.S. citizens' health behaviors and risk factors. It tracks trends by nation, state, and year, with the goal of identifying emerging health problems. Data also are used to evaluate achievement of health objectives and develop prevention strategies. The Behavior Risk Factor Surveillance System's website allows one to compile graphs and maps to describe specific risk behaviors by state (http://www.cdc.gov/brfss/).

In addition to these important sources of information, community health nurses can access a broad range of local, regional, and state government reports that contribute to the comprehensive assessment of a population. Local agencies, chambers of commerce, and health and hospital districts collect invaluable information on their community's health. Local health planning agencies also compile and analyze statistical

data during the planning process. The community health nurse can use these formal and informal resources in learning about a community or aggregate (Table 6.1). Box 6.3 lists additional information about sources of population health data.

Formal data collection does not exist for all community aspects; therefore, many community health nurses must perform additional data collection, compilation, and analysis. For example, school nurses regularly use aggregate data from student records to learn about the demographic composition of

TABLE 6.1 Community Assessment Parameters

Parameter	Importance to CHN	Source of Information
Geography Topography Climate (e.g., extreme heat or cold)	Influences nature of health problems and access to healthcare	Almanac Chamber of commerce
Population Size Demographic character (e.g., aged or young) Trends Migration Density	Describes population served; suggests their health risks and needs Suggests growth or decline Increases stress; may increase exposure to communicable disease	Census documents Chamber of commerce
Environment Water (e.g., source, fluoridated) Sewage and waste disposal Air quality (e.g., ozone, pollutants) Food quality and access Housing (e.g., single-family or multifamily dwellings) Animal control (e.g., exposure to rabies and other zoonotic diseases)	Affects quality of life and nature of environmental health problems Reflects community resources Suggests socioeconomic issues	Local and state health departments Newspapers Local environmental action group Census documents
Industry Employment levels Manufacturing White collar versus blue collar Income levels	Affects social class, access to healthcare, and resources Influences nature of health problems	Chamber of commerce Almanac Employment commission Census documents
Education Schools (e.g., physical plant, playground safety) Types of education Literacy rates Special education Health services Sex education School lunch programs (e.g., nutritious diets) After-school programs Daycare Access to higher education	Influences socioeconomic status, access to healthcare, and ability to read and understand health information	Census documents School districts and nurses
Recreation Parks and playgrounds Libraries Public and private recreation Special facilities	Reflects quality of life, resources available to community, and concern for the young and disadvantaged	Parks and recreation departments Newspapers
Religion Churches and synagogues Denominations Community programs Health-related programs and parish health programs Community organizations	Influences values in community by organizing common interests and concerns Reflects involvement of members, community skills, and resources for community needs	Chamber of commerce Newspapers Community center newsletters

Continued

Community Assessment Parameters—cont'd

Parameter	Importance to CHN	Source of Information
Communication Newspapers Neighborhood news Radio and television Telephone Internet Hotlines Medical media Public service announcements	Reflects concerns and needs of the community Contains networks and resources available for health-related use	Local libraries Newspapers Internet resources Local health department Medical and nursing societies
Transportation Intercity and intracity Handicapped Emergency transport	Affects access to services, food, and other resources Reflects resources available to community	Local bus and train services Local hospital emergency service
Public Services Fire protection Police protection Emergency medical services Rape treatment centers Utilities	Affects community security Reflects available resources	Local police department
Political Organization Structure Method for filing positions Responsibilities of positions Sources of revenue Voter registration	Reflects level of citizen activism, involvement, values, and concerns Mechanism for nurse activism and lobbying	Newspapers Local political party organization Local board of elections Local representatives
Community Development or Planning Activities Major issues	Reflects community needs and concerns Affects level of professionals' involvement in issues	Newspapers Local and state planning board Local community organizations
Disaster Programs American Red Cross Disaster plans Potential sources of disaster	Offers a level of preparedness, coordination, and available resources Influences resources and plans	Local American Red Cross office Local emergency coordinating council Local fire department
Health Statistics Mortality Morbidity Leading causes of death Births	Reflects health problems, trends, and state of community health Affects resources needed and CHN services provided	Local and state health department Health facilities and programs National vital statistics reports National Center for Health Statistics reports Morbidity and Mortality weekly report
Social Problems Mental health issues Alcoholism and drug abuse Suicide Crime School dropout Unemployment Gangs	Affects health problems and amounts of required services Influences CHN program priorities	Local and state department of social services Local mental health centers Local hotlines Libraries
Health Professionals Number of physicians, dentists, and nurses per population	Influences available health resources and nature of CHN practice	Local and state health planning agencies Health professional organizations Telephone directory Community service director
Health Professional Organizations	Provides support for CHN practice	Public health association
Community Services (e.g., cost and eligibility, accessibility, and acceptability) Institutional care (e.g., hospitals and nursing homes) Mental healthcare Ambulatory care Preventive health services Nursing services Welfare services	Reflect available resources	Local United Way organization Local voluntary service directory County hospital Local health department Telephone directory/Internet resources

CHN, Community health nursing.

BOX 6.3 Descriptive Statistics: Percent, Mean, Median, Mode, and Percent Change

To interpret sets of data, descriptive statistics may be used by the community health nurse to interpret the general trends, particularly those among demographic factors. For example, this set of patient data might be analyzed to identify the central tendencies in the sample.

Patient/Resident/ Subject	Sex (Male, Female, Other)	Age in Years
1	M	21
2	F	45
3	F	52
4	F	72
5	M	44
6	M	55
7	F	67
8	O	59
9	M	59
10	M	68
11	M	38
12	M	48
13	F	52
14	F	70
15	M	33
16	F	75
17	M	61
18	M	59
19	F	70
20	F	36

Percent is useful to calculate when subjects can be separated into categories. Example: Calculate the percent of patients of female gender:
Percent = Total number of females ÷ Total number in sample.
  Percent of females = 9 ÷ 20 = 45%
Mean is the average value of a variable or characteristic in the sample. Example: Calculate the average age in the patient sample:
Mean = Sum of all ages ÷ Total size of the sample.
  Mean age = 1084 ÷ 20 = 54.2 years.
Median is the middle value in the distribution of values. Arrange the values in order from lowest to highest and then identify the mid-value in the group. Example: Determine the median age in the patient sample:
Median = Midpoint in the range of values.
  Median of all 20 ages arranged from 21–75 is 55 years, or the 10th age in the range.
Mode is the most frequently occurring value in a sample. Example: Determine the mode for age in the patient sample:
Mode = The age that occurs most often in the sample.
  Mode is 59 since three persons have this same age.
Percent Change is useful when data for two time periods are available. Then the amount of growth, shrinkage, or other alteration can be determined. Example: determine the percent change in a population size from Time 1 to Time 2.
Percent change = (Value at Time 2 − Value at Time 1) ÷ Value at Time 1
  Percent change in population = (1200 in year 2020 − 1000 in year 2010) ÷ 1000 in 2010.
    200 ÷ 1000 = 0.2 or 20% increase.

their population. They conduct ongoing surveys of classroom attendance and causes of illness, which are essential to an effective school health program. Sometimes the nurse must screen the entire school population to discover the extent of a disease. Thus the school nurse is both a consumer of existent data and a researcher who collects new data for the assessment of the school community. See Box 6.4 for descriptive statistics that a nurse can use to discover the central trends in self-collected data or in data compiled from other data bases.

NEEDS ASSESSMENT

The nurse must understand the community's perspective on health status, the services it uses or requires, and its concerns. Most official data do not capture this type of information. Data collected directly from an aggregate may be more insightful and accurate; therefore community health nurses sometimes conduct community needs assessments. There are several approaches to gathering subjective data; however, a nurse's careful planning of the process will contribute to its reliability and utility regardless of the method. Box 6.5 presents the required steps in conducting a needs assessment.

The strategy chosen for collecting needs assessment data depends on the size and nature of the aggregate, the purpose for collecting information, and the resources available to the nurse. In some cases, the nurse may survey a small sample of clients to measure their satisfaction with a program. In other situations, a large-scale community needs assessment may help the nurse determine gaps in service. Although the process of needs assessment can indicate a program's strengths and weaknesses, it can also raise expectations for new services on the part of community members. Involving community members in the planning of the assessment builds trust and ownership in the process, and subsequently in the improvements that result. With the implementation of the U.S. Patient Protection and Affordable Care Act, nonprofit hospitals must conduct comprehensive community health needs assessments, often called *CHNAs*, which create an important opportunity to coordinate with public health agencies to more effectively make decisions and strategically plan to address local health needs (Centers for Disease Control and Prevention, 2021a. Available from: https://cdc.gov/publichealthgateway/cha/plan.html; National Association of County and City Health Officials [NACCHO], 2021).

A first approach to gathering data is to interview *key informants* in the community. These may be knowledgeable residents, elected officials, or healthcare providers. It is essential that the community health nurse recognize that the views of these people may not reflect the views of all residents. A second approach is to hold a *community forum* to discuss selected questions. It is important for the nurse to carefully plan the meeting in advance to gain the most useful information. The community health nurse can also mail surveys to community

BOX 6.4   Retrieval of Data

Current data on U.S. population health are stored in many places. Finding the latest statistics at the local, state, or national level can be a challenging experience for a student, community health nurse, graduate student, or nurse researcher. However, statistics provide a necessary comparison in identifying the health status of an aggregate or population in a community. The following guidelines suggest places to begin a search.

Reference Librarian

The best place to start is in a school or community library or in a large university's health sciences library. Cultivate a relationship with the reference librarian and learn how to access the literature of interest (e.g., government documents) or how to perform computer-guided literature searches.

Government Documents

Local libraries have a listing of government depository libraries, which house government documents for the public. If the government document is not available at a local library, ask the reference librarian to contact a regional or state library for an interlibrary loan. The Library of Congress in Washington, D.C., has a *Directory of U.S. Government Depository Libraries.*

Health, United States

An annual publication of the National Center for Health Statistics (2019), *Health, United States* reports the latest health statistics for the country. It presents statistics in areas such as maternal–child health indicators (e.g., prenatal care, low birth weight, and infant mortality), life expectancy, mortality, morbidity (e.g., cancer incidence and survival, AIDS, and diabetes), environmental health indicators (e.g., air pollution and noise exposure), and health system use (e.g., national health expenditures, health insurance coverage, physician contacts, and diagnostic and surgical procedures). Graphs and tables are easy to read and interpret with accompanying texts. Many statistics include a selected number of years to illustrate trends. Some statistics are compared with those from other countries and U.S. minority populations (For more information, visit http://www.cdc.gov/nchs/hus/index.htm).

Morbidity and Mortality Weekly Report (MMWR)

The CDC in Atlanta, Georgia, prepares this publication. State health departments compile weekly reports for the publication that outline the numbers of cases of notifiable diseases such as AIDS, gonorrhea, hepatitis, measles (rubeola), pertussis, rubella, syphilis, tuberculosis, and rabies and reports the deaths in 122 U S. cities by age. It also reports accounts of interesting cases, environmental hazards, disease outbreaks, or other public health problems. Local and state health departments and many local and health sciences libraries house this weekly publication. A subscription is available at http://www.cdc.gov/mmwr/.

Centers for Disease Control and Prevention

The CDC compiles information on a range of topics, including health behavior, educational and community-based programs, unintentional injuries, occupational safety and health, environmental health, oral health, diabetes and chronic disabling conditions, communicable disease, immunizations, clinical preventive services, and surveillance and data systems. Data are reported in several publications and on the website: http://www.cdc.gov/.

BOX 6.5   Steps in the Needs Assessment Process

1. Identify aggregate for assessment.
2. Engage community in planning the assessment.
3. Identify required information.
4. Select method of data gathering.
5. Develop questionnaire or interview questions.
6. Develop procedures for data collection.
7. Train data collectors.
8. Arrange for a sample representative of the aggregate.
9. Conduct needs assessment.
10. Tabulate and analyze data.
11. Identify needs suggested by data.
12. Develop an action plan.

members to elicit information from a more diverse group of people who may be unwilling or unable to attend a community forum. *Focus groups* are a third approach; these can be very effective in gathering community views, particularly for remote and vulnerable segments of a community and for those with underdeveloped opinions. Nurses who conduct focus groups must carefully select participants, formulate questions, and analyze recorded sessions (University of Kansas, 2021). These sessions can produce greater interaction and expression of ideas than surveys and may provide more insight into an aggregate's opinions. In addition to encouraging community participation in the identification of assets and needs, focus groups may lay the groundwork for community involvement in planning the solutions to identified problems.

DIAGNOSING HEALTH PROBLEMS

The next step of the nursing process is synthesizing assessment data, in which the nurse examines data and creates a list of all actual and potential problems. Then the nurse develops diagnostic statements about the community's health. These statements, or diagnoses, specify the nature and cause of an actual or potential community health problem and direct the community health nurses' plans to resolve the problem. Muecke (1984) developed a format that assists in writing a community diagnosis. The diagnosis consists of four components: the identification of the health problem or risk, the affected aggregate or community, the etiological or causal statement, and the evidence or support for the diagnosis (Fig. 6.4). Each of these components has an important role to play in the nursing process. The problem represents a synthesis of all assessment data. The "among" phrase specifies the aggregate that will be the beneficiary of the nurse's action plan and whose health is at risk. The "related to" phrase describes the cause of the health problem and directs the focus of the intervention. All plans and interventions will be aimed at

Increased risk of _____
(disability, disease, etc.)

among _____ related to
(community or population)

_____ as demonstrated
(etiological statement)

in _____ .
(health indicators)

Fig. 6.4 Format for community health diagnosis. (Redrawn from Muecke MA: Community health diagnosis in nursing, *Public Health Nurs* 1:23—35, 1984. Used with permission of Blackwell Scientific Publications.)

addressing this underlying cause. Last, the health indicators are the supporting data or evidence drawn from the completed assessment. These data can suggest the magnitude of the problem and have a bearing on prioritizing diagnoses. Other factors that assist the nurse in ranking the importance of diagnoses include the nature of the diagnosis, its potential impact on a broad range of community residents, and the community's perceptions of the health issue.

NURSING CARE GUIDELINES

Wellness Diagnosis

Sometimes nurses develop *wellness diagnoses*. These often focus on the individual, but can make a positive statement about the community's strengths. They are a variant on the North American Nursing Diagnosis Association's health promotion diagnoses. Wellness diagnoses address the potential of a segment of the population of the community to move toward a higher level of wellness and presume a certain level of readiness to change. For example, a wellness diagnosis might be written to describe a strength that should be reinforced and supported, as follows: ***Increased potential*** for positive infant outcomes ***among*** teenage mothers ***related to*** effective parenting ***as evidenced by*** increased participation in mother—baby practice sessions and positive newborn-care behaviors.

As in a community diagnosis, four components lead to a cohesive statement about health status.

With a clear statement of the problem in the form of a diagnosis, the community health nurse is ready to begin the planning phase of the nursing process. Inherent in this phase is a plan for the intervention and its evaluation. Once again, epidemiological data can be useful as a basis for determining success. By comparing baseline data, national and local data, and other relevant indicators, the nurse can construct benchmarks to gauge achievement of program objectives. This step may entail the calculation of incidence rates if the goal is to reduce the development of disease, or primary prevention. Comparing data with national rates or with prevalence rates found in a local community may be other indicators of success. Reducing the presence of risk

factors and documenting patterns of healthy behavior are other objective indices of successful programs.

It is evident that epidemiological data and methods are essential to each phase of the nursing process. The community health nurse compiles a range of assessment data that support the nursing diagnosis. Epidemiological studies support program planning by establishing the effectiveness of certain interventions and their specificity for different aggregates. Finally, epidemiological data are important for the community health nurse's documentation of a program's long-term effectiveness. Box 6.6 provides an evaluation example.

❓ ACTIVE LEARNING EXERCISE

1. Walk through a neighborhood and compile a list of variables that are important to describe with demographic and epidemiological data. Write down hunches or preconceived notions about the nature of the community's population. Compare ideas with the collected statistical data.
2. Compile a range of relevant demographic and epidemiological data for the community by examining census reports, vital statistics reports, city records, and other library and agency sources.
3. Using the collected data, identify three community health problems and formulate three community health diagnoses.

BOX 6.6 Example of Outcomes Evaluation: A Community-Based Intervention to Promote Smoking Cessation

Matthews and colleagues (2013) reported the results of a community-based and culturally tailored smoking cessation program designed for lesbian, gay, bisexual, transgender (LGBT) people, a population with more than double the rate of smoking as heterosexuals and an increased risk for respiratory and cardiac disease. A series of smoking cessation classes designed for and marketed to the LGBT community were conducted for 198 individuals. Adapted from the American Lung Association's Freedom from Smoking curriculum, the intervention incorporated LGBT concerns related to the role of smoking in LGBT culture, stress due to homophobia as a smoking trigger, relationship between bar culture and smoking and alcohol, and the targeting of LGBT persons by the tobacco industry. Thirty separate small treatment groups were conducted in eight weekly sessions. Three of these included a peer-buddy program in the Call it Quits groups, and free nicotine replacement was available to all. Although only 42% completed treatment, 32.3% selfreported smoking cessation upon completion, with the 24% who used nicotine replacement having the highest cessation rates. These rates were consistent with general community programs; however, the authors cited the benefits of a tailored, culturally specific program and stressed the need to continue to address the formidable barriers to abstention faced by LGBT smokers in preventing relapses.

Data from Matthews AK, Chien-Ching L, Kuhns LM, et al.: Results from a community-based smoking cessation program for LGBT smokers, *J Environ Public Health*, 2013. Available from: https://www.ncbi.nlm.nih.gov/pmc/articles/PMC3694499/. https://doi.org/10.1155/2013/984508.

CASE STUDY   Application of the Nursing Process

Assessment and Diagnosis

The following example demonstrates the process of collecting and analyzing data and deriving community diagnoses. It also exemplifies the multiple care levels within which community health nurses function: the individual client, the family, and the aggregate or community levels. In this scenario, the nurse identified an individual client health problem during a home visit, which provided the initial impetus for an aggregate health education program. Data collection expanded from the assessment of the individual to a broad range of literature and data about the nature of the problem in populations. The nurse then formulated a community-level diagnosis to direct the ensuing plan. This was subsequently implemented at the aggregate level and then evaluated.

School nurses frequently address a broad range of student health problems. In the West San Antonio School District, school nurses generally reserve several hours a week for home visits. In a recent case, a teacher expressed concern for a high school junior named "John" whose brother was dying of cancer. In a health class, John shared his personal fears about cancer, which caused his classmates to question their own cancer risks and how they might reduce them.

Assessment

The school nurse visited John's family and learned that the 25-year-old son had testicular cancer. Since his diagnosis 1 year earlier, he had undergone a range of therapies that were palliative but not curative; the cancer was advanced at the time of diagnosis. The nurse spent time with the family discussing care, answering questions, and exploring available support for the entire family.

At a school nurse staff meeting, the nurse inquired about her colleagues' experiences with other young clients with this type of cancer. Only one nurse remembered a young man with testicular cancer. The nurses were not familiar with its prevalence, incidence, risk factors, prevention strategies, or early detection approaches. The nurse recognized the high probability that high school students would have similar questions and could benefit from reliable information.

The school nurse embarked on a community assessment to answer these questions. The nurse first collected information about testicular cancer. Second, the nurse reviewed the nursing and medical literature for key articles discussing client care, diagnosis, and treatment. Epidemiological studies provided additional data regarding testicular cancer's distribution pattern in the population and associated risk factors.

The nurse learned that young men aged 20–35 years were at the greatest risk. Other major risk factors were not identified. It was learned that healthy young men do not seek testicular cancer screening and regular healthcare; they may be apprehensive about conditions affecting sexual function. These factors contribute to delays in detection and treatment. Although only an estimated 9470 new cases of testicular cancer will have been diagnosed in the United States in 2021, it is one of the most common tumors in young men. Furthermore, this cancer is amenable to treatment with early diagnosis (American Cancer Society (ACS), 2021).

On the basis of these facts, the nurse reasoned that a prevention program would benefit high school students. However, to perform a comprehensive assessment, it was important that the nurse clarified what students did know, how comfortable they were discussing sexual health, and how much the subject interested them. Therefore, the nurse approached the junior and senior high school students and administered a questionnaire to elicit this information. The nurse also queried the health teacher about the amount of pertinent cancer and sexual development information the students received in the classroom. The nurse considered the latter an important prerequisite to dealing with the sensitive subject of sexual health. According to the health teacher, the students did receive instruction about physical development and psychosexual issues. Students expressed a strong desire for more classroom instruction on these subjects and more information on cancer prevention. However, they did not have sufficient knowledge of the beneficial health practices related to cancer prevention and early detection.

Key Assessment Data

- Health status of John's brother
- Knowledge, coping, and support resources of family
- Testicular cancer, its natural history, treatment and prevention, incidence, prevalence, mortality, and risk factors
- High school students' knowledge about cancer and its prevention
- Students' comfort level with discussing sexual health issues

Community Diagnosis

There is an increased risk of undetected testicular cancer among young men related to insufficient knowledge about the disease and the methods for preventing and detecting it at an early stage, as demonstrated by high rates of late initiation of treatment.

Planning

Clarifying the problem and its cause helped the nurse direct the planning phase of the nursing process and determine both long-term and short-term goals.

The long-term goal was:

- Students will identify testicular lesions at an early stage and seek care promptly.

The short-term goals were:

- Students will understand testicular cancer and self-detection techniques.
- Students will exhibit comfort with sexual health issues by asking questions.
- Male students will report regular testicular self-examination.

Planning encompassed several activities, including the discovery of recommended healthcare practices regarding testicular cancer. The nurse also sought to determine the most effective and appropriate educational approaches for male and female high school students. Identifying helpful community agencies was also an essential part of the process. The local chapter of the American Cancer Society provided valuable information, materials, and consulting services. A nearby nursing school's media center and faculty were also very supportive of the program.

After formalizing her objectives and plan, the nurse presented the project to the high school's teaching coordinator and principal. Their approval was necessary before the nurse could implement the project. After eliciting their enthusiastic support, the nurse proceeded with more detailed plans. She selected and developed classroom instruction methods and activities that would maximize high school students' involvement. The nurse also ordered a film and physical models for demonstrating and practicing testicular selfexamination. She prepared group exercises designed to relax students and help them be comfortable with the sensitive subject matter. The nurse scheduled two 40-min sessions dealing with testicular cancer for the junior-level health class. In a final step of the planning phase, she designed evaluation tools that assessed knowledge levels after each class session and measured the extent to which students integrated these health practices into their lifestyles at the end of their junior and senior years.

The nurse was now ready to proceed with the implementation of a testicular cancer prevention and screening program. She initiated the assessment phase by identifying an individual client and family with a health need, and she extended the assessment to the high school aggregate. Her data collection at the aggregate level, for both the general and local high school populations, assisted in her community diagnosis. The diagnosis directed the development of a community-specific health intervention program and its subsequent implementation and evaluation.

Intervention

The nurse conducted the two sessions in a health education class. At the beginning of the class period, students participated in a group exercise, and the nurse asked them about their knowledge of testicular cancer. The nurse showed a film and led a discussion about cancer screening. In the second session, she demonstrated the selfexamination procedure using testicular models and supervised the students while they practiced the procedure on the models. The

CASE STUDY Application of the Nursing Process Assessment and Diagnosis—cont'd

nurse advised the male students about the frequency of selfexamination. With the females, she discussed the need for young men to be aware of their increased risk, drawing a parallel to breast selfexamination.

Evaluation

After completing the class sessions, the nurse administered the questionnaires she had developed for evaluation purposes. Analysis of the questionnaires indicated that knowledge levels were very high immediately after the classes. Students were pleased with the frank discussion, the opportunity to ask questions, and the clear responses to a sensitive subject. Teachers also offered positive feedback. Consequently, the nurse became a knowledgeable health resource in the high school.

Intermediate-term evaluation occurred at the end of the students' junior and senior years. The nurse arranged a 15-min evaluation during other classes, which assessed the integration of positive health practices and testicular self-examinations into the students' lifestyles. At the end of the school year, the prevalence of regular selfassessment was significantly lower than knowledge levels. However, 30% of male students reported regularly practicing self-examinations at the end of 1 year, and 70% reported they had performed self-examination at least once during the past year.

The compilation of incidence data is ideal for long-term evaluation, and it documents the reduction of a community health problem. Testicular cancer is

very rare; therefore, incidence data are not reliable and may not be feasible to collect. However, for more prevalent conditions, objective statistics help reveal increases and decreases in disease rates, and these may be related to the strengths and deficiencies of health programs.

Levels of Prevention

The following are examples of the three levels of prevention as applied to this case study.

Primary
- Promotion of healthy lifestyles and attitudes toward sexuality
- Education about sexual health and the care of one's body

Secondary
- Selfexamination to detect testicular cancer in its earliest stage
- Referral for medical care as soon as a lump or symptom is discovered
- Medical and surgical care to treat and cure testicular cancer

Tertiary
- Advanced care, including hospice services for those with incurable disease
- Support services and grief counseling to help families cope with loss of a loved one

SUMMARY

Communities form for a variety of reasons and can be homogeneous or heterogeneous in composition. To help assess the nature of a given community, community health nurses study and interpret data from sources such as local government agencies, census reports, morbidity and mortality reports, and vital statistics. Nurses can gather valuable information about the causes and prevalence of health and disease in a community through epidemiological studies. On the basis of this information, the community health nurse can apply the nursing process, expanding assessment, diagnosis, planning, intervention, and evaluation from the individual client level to a targeted aggregate in the community.

EVOLVE WEBSITE

http://evolve.elsevier.com/Nies/community
- NCLEX Review Questions
- Case Studies

BIBLIOGRAPHY

ACS 2021 -American Cancer Society. Facts about testicular cancer. Available from: Facts About Testicular Cancer | Testicular Cancer Statistics.

Boutain DM: Social justice in nursing: a review of the literature. In de Chesnay M, editor: *Caring for the vulnerable: perspectives in nursing*, Boston, 2020, Jones and Bartlett.

Centers for Disease Control and Prevention: *Community health assessments and health improvement plans*, 2021a. Available from: https://www.cdc.gov/publichealthgateway/cha/plan.html.

Centers for Disease Control and Prevention: *10 Essential public health services*, 2021b. Available from: https://www.cdc.gov/publichealthgateway/publichealthservices/essentialhealthservices.html.

Community Commons: *Vulnerable population footprint*, 2021. Available from: https://communitycommons.org/entities/60847319-e438-44be-a5c3-5b8d298845e1.

Institute of Medicine: *The future of the public's health in the 21st century*, Washington, DC, 2002, National Academies Press.

Kulbok PA, Thatcher E, Park E, et al.: Evolving public health nursing roles: focus on community participatory health promotion and prevention, *Online J Issues Nurs* 17(2):1, 2012. Available from: https://pubmed.ncbi.nlm.nih.gov/22686109/.

Matthews AK, Chien-Ching L, Kuhns LM, et al.: Results from a community-based smoking cessation program for LGBT smokers, *J Environ Public Health*, 2013. Available from: https://www.ncbi.nlm.nih.gov/pmc/articles/PMC3694499/ https://doi.org/10.1155/2013/984508.

Muecke MA: Community health diagnosis in nursing, *Publ Health Nurs* 1:23—35, 1984.

National Association of County and City Health Officials: *Community health assessment and improvement planning*, 2021. Available from: http://www.naccho.org/programs/public-health-infrastructure/performance-improvement/community-health-assessment.

National Center for Health Statistics. Health, United States, 2019. Available from: Health, United States 2019 (www.cdc.gov).

Pew Charitable Trusts: *Health impact project*, 2021. Available from: http://www.pewtrusts.org/en/projects/health-impact-project/health-impact-assessment.

Robert Wood Johnson Foundation: *Built environment and health*, 2021. Available from: http://www.rwjf.org/en/our-focus-areas/topics/built-environment-and-health.html.

University of Kansas: *The community toolbox: assessing community needs and resources*, 2021. Available from: http://ctb.ku.edu/en/table-of-contents/assessment/assessing-community-needs-and-resources/conduct-focus-groups/main.

World Health Organization: *Healthy cities*, 2021. Available from: https://who.int/healthpromotion/healthy-cities/en/.

7

Community Health Planning, Implementation, and Evaluation

Diane Cocozza Martins and Patricia M. Burbank

OBJECTIVES

Upon completion of this chapter, the reader will be able to do the following:

1. Describe the concept "community as client."
2. Apply the nursing process to the larger aggregate within a system's framework.
3. Describe the steps in the Health Planning Model.
4. Identify the appropriate prevention level and system level for nursing interventions in families, groups, aggregates, and communities.
5. Recognize major health planning legislation.
6. Analyze factors that have contributed to the failure of health planning legislation to control healthcare costs.
7. Describe the community health nurse's role in health planning, implementation, and evaluation.

OUTLINE

KEY TERMS

certificate of need
community as client
health planning
Health Planning Model

Hill-Burton Act
key informant
National Health Planning and Resources Development Act

Partnership for Health Program
Regional Medical Programs

Health planning for and with the community is an essential component of community health nursing practice. The term health planning seems simple, but the underlying concept is quite complex. Like many of the other components of community health nursing, health planning tends to vary at the different aggregate levels. Health planning with an individual or a family may focus on direct care needs or selfcare responsibilities. At the group level, the primary goal may be health education, and at the community level, health planning may involve population disease prevention or environmental hazard control. Clinical Example 7.1 illustrates the interaction of community health nursing roles with health planning at a variety of aggregate levels.

Clinical Example 7.1

Maria Guitierrez is a registered nurse in a suburban middle school. During the course of the school year, she noted an increased incidence of sexually transmitted infections (STIs) among the middle school students. After reviewing information in nursing journals, other professional journals, and Internet sources, Maria understood that there was a national increase in STIs among young adolescents. She found that significant numbers of adolescents are initiating sexual activity at age 13 and younger. The school nurse reviewed the Centers for Disease Control and Prevention

(CDC) site on "Adolescent and School Health—Sexual Risk Behavior" (CDC, 2021). The CDC reported:

Many young people engage in sexual risk behaviors that can result in unintended health outcomes. For example, among U.S. high school students surveyed in 2019

- 38% had ever had sexual intercourse.
- 27% had sexual intercourse during the previous 3 months, and, of these
  - 46% did not use a condom the last time they had sex.
  - 12% did not use any method to prevent pregnancy.
  - 21% had drunk alcohol or used drugs before last sexual intercourse.
- Less than 10% of sexually experienced students have ever been tested for human immunodeficiency virus (HIV).

Sexual risk behaviors place teens at risk for HIV infection, other STIs, and unintended pregnancy:

- Young people (aged 13–24) accounted for an estimated 21% of all new HIV diagnoses in the United States in 2018.
- Among young people (aged 13–24) diagnosed with HIV in 2018, 81% were gay and bisexual males.
- Half of the nearly 20 million new STIs reported each year were among young people, between the ages of 15–24.
- Nearly 180,000 babies were born to teen girls aged 15–19 years in 2018 (CDC, 2021).
- Among students who had any sexual contact with people of the same sex (LGB), the percentage who were threatened or injured with a weapon (17.4%) or who seriously considered suicide (54.2%) significantly increased from 2015 to 2019 (CDC, 2019).

Maria reviewed the reasons for the increased STIs. Her assessment of the problem had several findings. LGBT sexual health issues were not being addressed. Sexually active teenagers do not use contraception regularly. Also, a variety of sexual misconceptions lead teens to believe they are invulnerable to STIs. Adolescents also find it difficult or embarrassing to obtain contraceptives that protect from not only pregnancy but also STIs. The suburb does not have a local family planning clinic, and area primary care providers are reluctant to counsel teenagers or prescribe contraceptives without parental permission. The nurse also discovered that several years earlier a group of parents had stopped an attempt by the local school board to establish sex education in the school system. The parents believed this responsibility belonged in the home.

Maria considered all of these factors in developing her plan of action. She met with teachers, officials, and parents. Teachers and school officials were willing to deal with this sensitive issue if parents could recognize its validity. In meetings, many parents revealed they were uncomfortable discussing sexuality with their adolescent children and welcomed assistance. However, they were concerned that teachers might introduce the mechanics of reproduction without giving proper attention to the moral decisions and obligations involved in relationships. The parents expressed their desire to participate in curriculum planning and to meet with the teachers instead of following a previous plan that required parents to sign a consent form for each student. In support of the parents, Maria asked a nearby urban family planning agency to consider opening a part-time clinic in the suburb.

Implementing such a comprehensive plan is time-consuming and requires community involvement and resources. The nurse enlisted the aid of school officials and other community professionals. Time will reveal the plan's long-term effectiveness in reducing teen pregnancy.

This example shows how nurses can and should become involved in health planning. Teen pregnancy is a significant health problem and often results in lower education and lower socioeconomic status, which can lead to further health problems. The nurse's assessment and planned interventions involved individual teenagers, parents and families, the school system, and community resources.

This chapter provides an overview of health planning and evaluation from a nursing perspective. It also describes a model for student involvement in health planning projects and a review of significant health planning legislation.

OVERVIEW OF HEALTH PLANNING

One of the major criticisms of community health nursing practice involves the shift in focus from the community and larger aggregate to family caseload management or agency responsibilities. When focusing on the individual or family, nurses must remember that these clients are members of a larger population group or community and that environmental factors influence them. Nurses can identify these factors and plan health interventions by implementing an assessment of the entire aggregate or community. Fig. 7.1 illustrates this process.

The concept of "community as client" is not new. Lillian Wald's work at New York City's Henry Street settlement in the late 1800s exemplifies this concept. At the Henry Street settlement, Miss Wald, Mary Brewster, and other public health nurses worked with extremely poor immigrants.

The increased focus on community-based nursing practice yields a greater emphasis on the aggregate as the client or care unit. However, the community health nurse should not neglect nursing care at the individual and family levels by focusing on healthcare only at the aggregate level. Rather, the nurse can use this community information to help him or her understand individual and family health problems and improve their health status. Table 7.1 illustrates the differences in community health nursing practice at the individual, family, and community levels. However, before nurses can participate in healthcare planning, they must be knowledgeable about the process and comfortable with the concept of community as client or care focus.

HEALTH PLANNING MODEL

A model based on Hogue's (1985) group intervention model was developed in response to this need for population focus. The Health Planning Model aims to improve aggregate health and applies the nursing process to the larger aggregate within a systems framework. Fig. 7.2 depicts this model. Incorporated

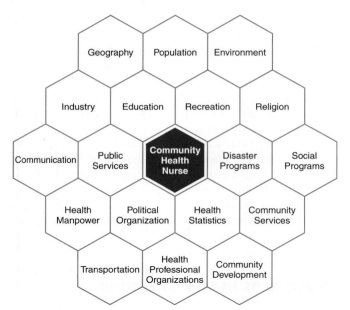

Fig. 7.1 The community as client. Chapter 6, Table 6.1, provides assessment parameters that help identify the client's assets and needs.

health intervention. For example, an urban area might have a variety of industrial and business settings that need assistance, whereas a suburban community may offer a choice of family-oriented organizations, such as boys' and girls' "clubs" and parent-teacher associations that would benefit from intervention.

A nurse should also consider personal interests and strengths in selecting an aggregate for intervention. For example, the nurse should consider whether he or she has an interest in teaching health promotion and preventive health or in planning for organizational change, whether his or her communication skills are better suited to large or small groups, and whether he or she has a preference for working with older adults or with children. Thoughtful consideration of these and other variables will facilitate assessment and planning.

Assessment

As discussed in Chapter 6 on assessment, it is essential to establish a professional relationship with the selected aggregate, which requires that a community health nurse first gain entry into the group. Good communication skills are essential to making a positive first impression. The nurse should make an appointment with the group leaders to set up the first meeting.

The nurse must initially clarify his or her position, organizational affiliation, knowledge, and skills. The nurse should also clarify mutual expectations and available times. Once entry into the aggregate is established, the nurse continues negotiation to maintain a mutually beneficial relationship.

Meeting with the aggregate on a regular basis will allow the nurse to make an in-depth assessment. Determining socio-demographic characteristics (e.g., distribution of age, sex, and race) may help the nurse ascertain health needs and develop appropriate intervention methods. For example, adolescents

into a health planning project, the model can help students view larger client aggregates and gain knowledge and experience in the health planning process. Nurses must carefully consider each step in the process, using this model. Box 7.1 outlines these steps. In addition, Box 7.2 provides the systems framework premises that nurses should incorporate.

Several considerations affect how nurses choose a specific aggregate for study. The community may have extensive or limited opportunities appropriate for nursing involvement. Additionally, each community offers different possibilities for

TABLE 7.1 Levels of Community Health Nursing Practice

Client	Example	Characteristics	Health Assessment	Nursing Involvement
Individual	Lisa McDonald	An individual with various needs	Individual strengths, problems, and needs	Client—nurse interaction
Family	Moniz family	A family system with individual and group needs	Individual and family strengths, problems, and needs	Interactions with individuals and the family group
Group	Boy Scout troop Alzheimer support group	Common interests, problems, and needs Interdependency	Group dynamics Fulfillment of goals	Group member and leader
Population group	Patients with acquired immunodeficiency syndrome (AIDS) in a given state Pregnant adolescents in a school district	Large, unorganized group with common interests, problems, and needs	Assessment of common problems, needs, and vital statistics	Application of nursing process to identified needs
Organization	A workplace A school	Organized group in a common location with shared governance and goals	Relationship of goals, structure, communication, patterns of organization to its strengths, problems, and needs	Consultant and/or employee application of nursing process to identified needs
Community	Immigrant neighborhood Anytown, USA	An aggregate of people in a common location with organized social systems	Analysis of systems, strengths, characteristics, problems, and needs	Community leader, participant, and healthcare provider

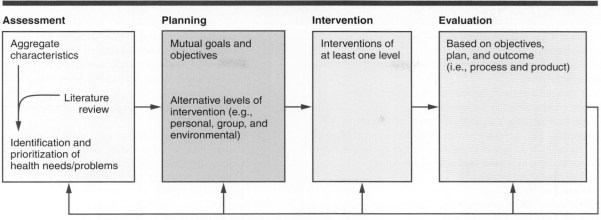

Fig. 7.2 Health planning model.

need information regarding nutrition, abuse of drugs and alcohol, and relationships with the opposite sex. They usually do not enjoy lectures in a classroom environment, but the nurse must possess skills to initiate small-group involvement and participation. An adult group's average educational level will affect the group's knowledge base and its comfort with formal versus informal learning settings. The nurse may find it more difficult to coordinate time and energy commitments if an organization is the focus group, because the aggregate members may be more diverse.

The nurse may gather information about sociodemographic characteristics from a variety of sources. These sources include observing the aggregate, consulting with other aggregate workers (e.g., the factory or school nurse, a Head Start teacher, or the resident manager of a high-rise senior citizen apartment building), reviewing available records or charts, interviewing members of the aggregate (i.e., verbally or via a short questionnaire), and interviewing a key informant. A **key informant** is a formal or informal leader in the community who provides data that are informed by his or her personal knowledge and experience with the community.

In assessing the aggregate's health status, the nurse must consider both the positive and negative factors. Unemployment or the presence of disease may suggest specific health problems,

---

BOX 7.1   Health Planning Project Objectives

I. Assessment
   A. Specify the aggregate level for study (e.g., group, population group, or organization). Identify and provide a general orientation to the aggregate (e.g., characteristics of the aggregate system, suprasystem, and subsystems). Include the reasons for selecting this aggregate and the method for gaining entry.
   A. Describe specific characteristics of the aggregate.
      1. *Sociodemographic characteristics:* Including age, sex, race or ethnic group, religion, educational background and level, occupation, income, and marital status.
      2. *Health status:* Work or school attendance, disease categories, mortality, healthcare use, and population growth and population pressure measurements (e.g., rates of birth and death, divorce, unemployment, and drug and alcohol abuse). Select indicators appropriate for the chosen aggregate.
      3. *Suprasystem influences:* Existing health services to improve aggregate health and the existing or potential positive and negative impact of other community-level social system variables on the aggregate. Identify the data collection methods.
   B. Provide relevant information from the literature review, especially in terms of the characteristics, problems, or needs within this type of aggregate. Compare the health status of the aggregate with that of similar aggregates, the community, the state, and the nation.
   C. Identify the specific aggregate's health problems and needs on the basis of comparative data collection analysis and interpretation and literature

review. Include input from clients regarding their need perceptions. Give priorities to health problems and needs, and indicate how to determine these priorities.

II. Planning
   A. Select one health problem or need, and identify the ultimate goal of intervention. Identify specific, measurable objectives as mutually agreed on by the student and aggregate.
   B. Describe the alternative interventions that are necessary to accomplish the objectives. Consider interventions at each system level where appropriate (e.g., aggregate/target system, suprasystem, and subsystems). Select and validate the intervention(s) with the highest probability of success. Interventions may use existing resources, or they may require the development of new resources.

III. Intervention
   A. Implement at least one level of planned intervention when possible.
   B. If intervention was not implemented, provide reasons.

IV. Evaluation
   A. Evaluate the plan, objectives, and outcomes of the intervention(s). Include the aggregate's evaluation of the project. Evaluation should consider the process, product, appropriateness, and effectiveness.
   B. Make recommendations for further action based on the evaluation, and communicate them to the appropriate individuals or system levels. Discuss implications for community health nursing.

BOX 7.2   Systems Framework Premises

I. Each system is a goal-directed collection of interacting or interdependent parts, or subsystems.

II. The whole system is continually interacting with and adapting to the environment, or suprasystem.

III. There is a hierarchical structure (suprasystem, system, subsystems).

IV. Each system is characterized by the following:

  A. *Structure:* Arrangement and organization of parts, or subsystems.

    1. Organization and configuration (e.g., traditional vs. nontraditional; greater variability [no right or wrong and no proper vs. improper form]).

    2. Boundaries (open vs. closed; regulate input and output).

    3. Territory (spatial and behavioral).

    4. Role allocation.

  B. *Functions:* Goals and purpose of system and activities necessary to ensure survival, continuity, and growth of system.

    1. General.

      a. *Physical:* Food, clothing, shelter, protection from danger, and provision for health and illness care.

      b. *Affectional:* Meeting the emotional needs of affection and security.

      c. *Social:* Identity, affiliation, socialization, and controls.

    2. Specific: Each family, group, or aggregate has its own individual agenda regarding values, aspirations, and cultural obligations.

  C. Process and dynamics.

    1. *Adaptation:* Attempt to establish and maintain equilibrium; balance between stability, differentiation, and growth; selfregulation and adaptation (equilibrium and homeostasis).

      a. *Internal:* Families, groups, or aggregates.

      b. *External:* Interaction with suprasystem.

    2. Integration: Unity and ability to communicate.

    3. Decision making: Power distribution, consensus, accommodation, and authority.

---

but low rates of absenteeism at work or school may suggest a need to focus more on preventive interventions. The specific aggregate determines the appropriate health status measures. Immunization levels are an important index for children, but nurses rarely collect this information for adults. However, the nurse should consider the need for influenza and/or pneumonia vaccines with older adults. Similarly, the nurse would expect a lower incidence of chronic disease among children, whereas older adults have higher rates of long-term morbidity and mortality.

Public health nursing (PHN) competencies include applying systems theory to PHN practice with communities and populations. This includes integrating systems thinking into public health practice and evaluating new approaches to public health practice that integrate organizational and systems theories (Council of Public Health Nursing Organizations [CPHNO]).

A systems analysis is needed when one is assessing the aggregate. The three levels of the system are the subsystem, the system, and the suprasystem. For example, a community health nurse working with incarcerated women in a prison needs to work at the three levels of the system to assist women planning to reunite with their children at release. The system is the group of women, the subsystem consists of the individual women, and the suprasystem would be the department of corrections and/or the state's department of social services.

The aggregate's suprasystem may facilitate or impede health status. Different organizations and communities provide various resources and services to their members. Some are obviously health related, such as the presence or absence of hospitals, clinics, private practitioners, emergency facilities, health centers, home health agencies, and health departments. Support services and facilities such as group meal sites or Meals on Wheels (MOW) for older adults and recreational facilities and programs for children, adolescents, and adults are also important. Transportation availability, reimbursement mechanisms or sliding-scale fees, and community-based volunteer groups may determine the use of services. An assessment of

these factors requires researching public records (e.g., town halls, telephone directories, and community services directories) and interviewing health professionals, volunteers, and key informants in the community. The nurse should augment existing resources or create a new service rather than duplicating what is already available to the aggregate.

A literature review is an important means of comparing the aggregate with the norm. For example, children in a Head Start setting, day care center, or elementary school may exhibit a high rate of upper respiratory tract infections during the winter. The nurse should review the pediatric literature and determine the normal incidence for this age range in group environments. Furthermore, the nurse should research potential problems in an especially healthy aggregate (e.g., developmental stresses for adolescents or work or family stresses for adults) or determine whether a factory's experience with work-related injury is within an average range. Comparing the foregoing assessment with research reports, statistics, and health information will help determine and prioritize the aggregate's health problems and needs.

The last phase of the initial assessment is identifying and prioritizing the specific aggregate's health problems and needs. This phase should relate directly to the assessment and the literature review and should include a comparative analysis of the two. Most important, this step should reflect the aggregate's perceptions of need. Depending on the aggregate, the nurse may consult the aggregate members directly or may interview others who work with the aggregate (e.g., a Head Start teacher). Interventions are seldom successful if the nurse omits or ignores the clients' input.

During the needs assessment, four types of needs should be assessed. The first is the expressed need or the need expressed by the behavior. This is seen as the demand for services and the market behavior of the targeted population. The second need is normative, which is the lack, deficit, or inadequacy as determined by expert health professionals. The third type of need is the perceived need expressed by the audience. Perceived needs include the population's wants and preferences. The final need is the relative need, which is the gap showing health disparities between the advantaged and disadvantaged populations (Issel et al., 2021).

Finally, the nurse must prioritize the identified problems and needs to create an effective plan. The nurse should consider the following factors when determining priorities:

- The aggregate's preferences
- Number of individuals in the aggregate affected by the health problem
- Severity of the health need or problem
- Availability of potential solutions to the problem
- Practical considerations such as individual skills, time limitations, and available resources

In addition, the nurse may further refine the priorities by applying a framework such as Maslow's (1968) hierarchy of needs (i.e., lower-level needs have priority over higher-level needs) or Leavell and Clark's (1965) levels of prevention (primary, secondary, and tertiary prevention). Primary prevention consists of health promotion and activities that protect the client from illness or dysfunction. Secondary prevention includes early diagnosis and treatment to reduce the duration and severity of disease or dysfunction. Tertiary prevention applies to irreversible disability or damage and aims to rehabilitate and restore an optimal level of functioning. Plans should include goals and activities that reflect the identified problem's prevention level.

Assessment and data collection are ongoing throughout the nurse's relationship with the aggregate. However, the nurse should proceed to the planning step once the initial assessment is complete. It is particularly important to link the assessment stage with other stages at this point in the process. Planning should stem directly and logically from the assessment, and implementation should be realistic.

An essential component of health planning is to have a strong level of community involvement. The nurse is responsible for advocating for client empowerment throughout the assessment, planning, implementation, and evaluation steps of this process. Community organization reinforces one of the field's underlying premises, as outlined by Nyswander (1956): "Start where the people are." Moreover, Labonte (1994) stated that the community is the engine of health promotion and a vehicle of empowerment. He describes five spheres of an empowerment model that focus on the following levels of social organization: interpersonal (personal empowerment), intragroup (small-group development), intergroup (community collaboration), interorganizational (coalition building), and political action. Paying attention to collective efforts and support of community involvement and empowerment, rather than focusing on individual efforts, will help ensure that the outcomes reflect the needs of the community and truly make a difference in people's lives.

Labonte's (1994) multilevel empowerment model allows us to consider both macrolevel and microlevel forces that combine to create both health and disease. Therefore it seems that both micro- and macroviewpoints on health education provide

nurses with multiple opportunities for intervention across a broad continuum. In summary, health education activities that have an "upstream" focus examine the underlying causes of health inequalities through multilevel education and research. This allows nurses to be informed by a critical social perspective from education, anthropology, and public health and through community-based participatory research (Israel et al., 2012).

Successful health programs rely on empowering citizens to make decisions about individual and community health. Empowering citizens causes power to shift from health providers to community members in addressing health priorities. Collaboration and cooperation among community members, academicians, clinicians, health agencies, and businesses help ensure that scientific advances, community needs, sociopolitical needs, and environmental needs converge in a humanistic manner.

❓ ACTIVE LEARNING EXERCISE

You are working with U.S. veterans who have served in Iraq and Afghanistan. Refer to the U.S. Department of Veterans Affairs website (http://www.va.gov/health/) to review some health issues you should consider in your assessment.

Planning

As already stated, the nurse should determine which problems or needs require intervention in conjunction with the aggregate's perception of its health problems and needs and on the basis of the outcomes of prioritization. Then the nurse must identify the desired outcome or ultimate goal of the intervention. For example, the nurse should determine whether to increase the aggregate's knowledge level and whether an intervention will cause a change in health behavior. It is important to have specific and measurable goals and desired outcomes. Doing so will facilitate planning the nursing interventions and determining the evaluation process.

Planning interventions is a multistep process. First, the nurse must determine the intervention levels (e.g., subsystem, aggregate system, and/or suprasystem). A system is a set of interacting and interdependent parts (subsystems) organized as a whole with a specific purpose. Just as the human body can be viewed as a set of interacting subsystems (e.g., circulatory, neurological, integumentary), a family, a worksite, or a senior high rise can also be viewed as a system. Each system then interacts with, and is further influenced by, its physical and social environment, or suprasystem (e.g., the larger community).

Second, the nurse should plan interventions for each system level, which may center on the primary, secondary, or tertiary level of prevention. These levels apply to aggregates, communities, and individuals.

Third, the nurse should validate the practicality of the planned interventions according to available personal as well as aggregate and suprasystem resources. Although teaching is often a major component of community health nursing, the nurse should consider other potential forms of intervention (e.g., personal counseling, policy change, or community service development). Input from other disciplines or community agencies may also be helpful. Finally, the nurse should coordinate the planned interventions with the aggregate's input to maximize participation.

Goals and Objectives

Development of goals and objectives is essential. The goal is generally where the nurse wants to be, and the objectives are the steps needed to get there. *Measurable objectives* are the specific measures used to determine whether the nurse is successful in achieving the goal. The objectives are instructions about what the nurse wants the population to be able to do. In writing the objectives, the nurse should use verbs and include specific conditions (how well or how many) that describe to what degree the population will be able to demonstrate mastery of the task.

Because the objectives are specific and can be quantified, they may be used to measure outcomes. Objectives may also be referred to as *behavioral objectives* or *outcomes* because they describe observable behavior rather than knowledge. An example of the goals and measurable objectives for a city with a high rate of childhood obesity is shown in Box 7.3.

Intervention

The intervention stage may be the most enjoyable stage for the nurse and the clients. The nurse's careful preliminary assessment and planning should help ensure the aggregate's positive response to the intervention. Although implementation should follow the initial plan, the nurse should prepare for unexpected problems (e.g., bad weather, transportation problems, poor attendance, or competing events). If the nurse is unable to complete the intervention, the reasons for its failure should be analyzed. Interventions should be included from a range of strategies, including mass media (public service announcements, radio, television, billboards), general information dissemination (e.g., pamphlets, DVDs, CDs, posters), electronic information dissemination (e.g., websites, blogs, tweets, video stream), and public forums (e.g., town meetings, focus groups, discussion groups).

Evaluation

Evaluation is an important component for determining the success or failure of a project and understanding the factors that contributed to its success or failure. The evaluation should include the participant's verbal or written feedback and the nurse's detailed analysis. Evaluation includes reflecting on each previous stage to determine the plan's strengths and weaknesses (*process evaluation*). Process evaluation is also referred to as *formative evaluation*. It allows one to evaluate both positive and negative aspects of each experience honestly and comprehensively and whether the desired outcomes were achieved (*product evaluation*). Product evaluation is summative and can consist of end-of-intervention surveys and other tools that measure whether objectives have been met. *Summative evaluation* is another term for product evaluation and looks at outcomes. Evaluation should include adequacy, efficiency, appropriateness, and cost-benefit analysis. During both process and product evaluations, the nurse may ask the following questions:

- Was the assessment adequate?
- Were plans based on an incomplete assessment?
- Did the plan allow adequate client involvement?
- Were the interventions realistic or unrealistic in terms of available resources?
- Did the plan consider all levels of prevention?
- Were the stated goals and objectives accomplished?
- Were the participants satisfied with the interventions?
- Did the plan advance the knowledge levels of the aggregate and the nurse?

The intervention may have limited impact if the nurse fails to communicate follow-up recommendations to the aggregate upon completion of the project. Although follow-up activity is not necessary for all plans, most require additional interventions within the aggregate using community agencies and resources. A comprehensive health planning project involves a close working relationship with the aggregate and careful consideration of each step. Long-term evaluation may need to be done by those professionals working continuously with the aggregate to determine behavior changes and/or changes in health status.

BOX 7.3   Program Goals and Objectives for Reduction of Childhood Obesity

Goal
Reduce the rate of childhood obesity in the city of New Bedford.

Objectives
The percentage of children whose body weight exceeds the 98th percentile for age and height will be reduced to 5%.
All the children will be invited to join a 5, 2, 1 program:
- Five fruits and vegetables per day
- Two-hour limit on screen time (TV, video games, and computer) per day
- One hour of physical activity per day
The food pyramid will be taught to all school nurses and health educators by the end of the school year.
The food pyramid will be presented and distributed to parents at all the summer health fairs.

🔲 RESEARCH HIGHLIGHTS

What About the Children Playing Sports? Pesticide Use on Athletic Fields.

Children come in contact with athletic fields on a daily basis. How these fields are maintained may have an impact on children's potential exposure to pesticides and associated health effects.

This is a cross-sectional, descriptive study that utilized a survey to assess playing field maintenance practices regarding the use of pesticides. Athletic fields ($N = 101$) in Maryland were stratified by population density and randomly selected.

A survey was administered to field managers ($n = 33$) to assess maintenance practices, including the use of pesticides. Analysis included descriptive statistics and generalized estimating equations.

Managers of 66 fields (65.3%) reported applying pesticides, mainly herbicides (57.4%). Managers of urban and suburban fields were less likely to apply pesticides than were managers of rural fields. Combined cultivation practice was also a significant predictor of increased pesticide use.

The use of pesticides on athletic fields presents many possible health hazards. Results indicate that there is a significant risk of exposure to pesticides for children engaged in sports activities. Given that children are also often concurrently exposed to pesticides as food residues and from home pest management, we need to examine opportunities to reduce their exposures. Both policy and practice questions are raised.

Data from Gilden R, Friedmann E, Sattler B, et al.: Potential health effects related to pesticide use on athletic fields, *Publ Health Nurs* 29(3):198–207, 2012.

HEALTH PLANNING PROJECTS

Successful Projects

Student projects have used this health planning model with group, organization, population group, and community aggregates. Table 7.2 describes interventions with these aggregates at the subsystem, aggregate system, and suprasystem levels. Clinical Example 7.2 describes a successful project at a textile plant. Clinical Example 7.3 describes a crime watch program, and Clinical Example 7.4 involves clients in a rehabilitation group.

Clinical Example 7.2
Textile Industry

A nursing student studied a textile plant that had approximately 470 employees but did not have an occupational health nurse. The student nurse collected data and identified three major problems or needs by collaborating with management and union representatives. First, the student nurse observed that the most common, costly, and chronic work-related injury in plant workers was lower back injury. Second, some employees had concerns about possible undetected hypertension. Third, the first-aid facilities were disorganized and without an accurate inventory system. The student nurse planned and implemented interventions for all three areas.

Continued

On the suprasystem level, the student nurse formulated plans with the company's physicians and lobbied management to enact an employee training program on proper lifting techniques. The student nurse proposed creating specific and concise job descriptions and requirements to facilitate potential employees' medical assessments. In addition, the student nurse organized and clearly labeled the first-aid supplies and developed an inventory system. On the aggregate system level, the student nurse planned and conducted a hypertension screening program. Approximately 85% of the employees underwent screening, and 10 people had elevated blood pressure readings. These 10 people were referred for follow-up care, and hypertension was subsequently diagnosed in several of them.

In evaluating the project, management representatives recognized that a variety of nursing interventions could improve or maintain workers' health. Consequently, management hired the student nurse upon graduation to be the occupational health nurse.

Clinical Example 7.3
Crime Watch

Another nursing student was concerned with the rising incidence of crime in a community and organized a crime watch program. The student nurse met periodically with the police and local residents, or aggregate system. Interventions included posting crime watch signs in the neighborhood and establishing more frequent police patrols at the suprasystem level. Evaluation of the program revealed that the residents had greater awareness of and concern for neighborhood safety.

Clinical Example 7.4
Rehabilitation Group

After working at a senior citizens center for a few weeks, a student nurse began a careful assessment of the center's clients. The student nurse interviewed the center's clients and visited its homebound clients served by social workers and the MOW program. Several of the homebound clients identified a need for socialization and rehabilitation. The center had recently purchased a van equipped to transport handicapped people in wheelchairs, which was a necessary factor in fulfilling this need.

After the student nurse assessed the clients' health and functional status and determined mutual goals, four of these homebound clients expressed a desire to attend a rehabilitation program at the center. The student nurse and the center's management initiated a weekly program based on the clients' needs, which included van transportation, a coffee hour, a noontime meal, an exercise class, and a craft class. Although some members were initially reluctant to participate and one man withdrew from the group, the group ultimately functioned very well. Evaluating this new program showed clearly that the student nurse made progress in meeting the goals of increased socialization and rehabilitation among elders at the center.

TABLE 7.2 Interventions by Type of Aggregate and System Level

Project	Type of Aggregate	System Level for Intervention
Rehabilitation group	Group, organization	Subsystem and aggregate system
Textile industry	Population group	Aggregate system and suprasystem
Crime watch	Group, organization, and population group	Aggregate system and suprasystem
Bilingual students (case study)	Community	Aggregate system and suprasystem

Unsuccessful Projects

Project failure is usually caused by problems with one or more steps of the nursing process. Usually the student does not discover problems until the evaluation phase. The following unsuccessful projects illustrate failures at different steps in the nursing process. Table 7.3 summarizes the identified problem areas for Clinical Examples 7.5 to 7.7.

Clinical Example 7.5
Group Home for Developmentally Delayed Adults

A nursing student worked with an aggregate of six women living in a group home for developmentally delayed citizens. The nursing student observed that the clients were all overweight, and she decided to establish a weight reduction program. She proceeded to meet with the women, chart their weight, and discuss their food choices on a weekly basis. After 8 weeks, her evaluation revealed that none of the women had lost weight and a few had actually gained weight. During the assessment phase the student failed to consider the women's perceptions of need. The women did not consider their weight a priority health problem, and their boyfriends provided positive reinforcement regarding their appearance.

Clinical Example 7.6
Safe Rides Program

One student nurse assessed a university student community through a questionnaire and identified a drinking and driving problem. Of those she surveyed, 77% admitted to driving under the influence of alcohol, and 16.5% stated they had been involved in an alcohol-related car accident. After identifying the problem and determining student interest, the student nurse worked with the campus alcohol and drug resource center to plan and implement a program called Safe Rides. In this program, student volunteers would work a hotline and dispatch "on-call" drivers to pick up students who were unsafe to drive.

The student nurse resolved many potential complications before implementation (e.g., liability coverage for all participating individuals and expense funds for gasoline). The student nurse formulated a 12-h training program that lasted 3 weeks to prepare student volunteers for the Safe Rides program. By the end of the semester, Safe Rides was ready to begin. However, the student nurse graduated at the semester's end, and her commitment had been the program's prime motivating force. Although others were committed and involved, the student nurse did not arrange for a replacement to coordinate and continue the program upon her departure. The Safe Rides program required ongoing coordination efforts, and no one fully implemented the program in the student nurse's absence.

Clinical Example 7.7
Manufacturing Plant

Even careful planning cannot always eliminate potential obstacles. For example, one student nurse chose to work in an

Clinical Example 7.7—cont'd

occupational setting involving heavy industry. The occupational health nurse and the nurse's personnel supervisor both approved the student nurse's entry into the organization. After reviewing the literature, working with the nurse for several weeks, and assessing the organization and its employees, the student nurse concluded that back injury risk was a primary problem. She planned to reduce the risk factors involved in back injuries by distributing information about proper body mechanics in a teaching session.

The personnel manager resisted this plan. Although he recognized the need for education, he was initially unwilling to allow employees to attend the session on company time. The student nurse and manager reached a compromise by allowing attendance during extended coffee breaks. The personnel manager, however, canceled the program before the student nurse could implement the class; negotiations for a new union contract were forming, and there was high probability of a strike. This situation led management to deny any changes in the usual routine.

The student nurse proceeded appropriately and received clearance from the proper officials, but she could not anticipate or circumvent union problems. The student nurse could only share her information and concern with the nurse and the personnel manager and encourage them to implement her plan when contract negotiations were complete.

Discussion

Each of these projects attempted to address a particular level of prevention. Most of these examples focused on primary prevention and health promotion because they were conducted by students and limited by time available due to the length of the academic semester. Table 7.4 lists these projects and their prevention levels. However, the full-time community health nurse working with an aggregate (e.g., in the occupational health setting) would target interventions for all three levels of prevention at a variety of system levels. It is useful to view nursing interventions with aggregates within a matrix structure to address all intervention opportunities. The matrix in Table 7.5 gives examples of how the occupational health nurse may intervene at all system levels and all prevention levels.

In practice, most interventions occur at the individual level and include all prevention levels. Interventions at the aggregate

TABLE 7.3 Unsuccessful Projects	
Project	**Problematic Step of Nursing Process**
Group home for developmentally delayed	Assessment (i.e., mutual identification of health problems and needs)
Safe rides program	Planning (i.e., mutual identification of goals and objectives)
Manufacturing plant	Evaluation (i.e., recommendations for follow-up)
	Implementation

TABLE 7.4	Level of Prevention for Each Project	
Primary Prevention	**Secondary Prevention**	**Tertiary Prevention**
Textile industry	Textile industry	Rehabilitation group
Crime watch	Group home for developmentally delayed	
Manufacturing plant		
Safe rides program		

level are usually less common. For many community health nurses, time does not allow intervention at the suprasystem level. However, schools and schoolchildren are integral parts of the community system. Factors that affect the community's health also affect schoolchildren's health. For school nurses in these school districts, interventions at the suprasystem level may become a reality and improve the health of the community and the students. The suprasystem intervention can be used to reduce hunger and food insufficiency for all schoolchildren in a district. A school nurse working with students in the school office may note that the students are presenting with dizziness, headaches, or abdominal pain in the morning and may keep intervention at the individual level by treating the symptoms presented (e.g., with acetaminophen or food). However, the school nurse may investigate why the students are presenting with the symptoms especially on Monday mornings and may realize that lack of food in the homes is an issue. The nurse then would work to develop a breakfast program for the school district. This strategy is a good example of refocusing upstream by addressing the real source of problems.

These projects illustrate the variety of available opportunities for aggregate health planning. In addition, they exemplify the application of the nursing process within various aggregate types, at different systems levels, and at each prevention level. These examples demonstrate the vital importance of each step of the nursing process:

1. Aggregate assessments must be thorough. The textile industry project exemplifies this point. Assessments should elicit answers to key questions about the aggregate's health and demographic profile and should compare this information with information for similar aggregates presented in the literature.
2. The nurse must complete careful planning and set goals that the nurse and the aggregate accept. The rehabilitation group project illustrates the importance of mutual planning.
3. Interventions must include aggregate participation and must meet the mutual goals. The crime watch project exemplifies this point.
4. Evaluation must include process and product evaluation and aggregate input.

HEALTH PLANNING MODELS IN PUBLIC HEALTH

According to Issel et al. (2021), many planning programs to address public health problems began as environmental planning of water and sewer systems. Additional population-based planning became necessary with the advent of immunizations. Blum (1974) was the first to suggest how public health planning should be done. Perspectives on health planning range from systematic problem solving and an epidemiological approach to a social awareness approach.

Beginning in the mid-1980s the CDC began to develop and promote systematic methods for health planning in public health. These models were important for a structured approach to public health planning.

The PRECEDE-PROCEED model (Fig. 7.3) provides a structure for assessing health and quality-of-life needs. It also assists in designing, implementing, and evaluating health promotion and public health programs to meet those needs. PRECEDE (*Predisposing, Reinforcing, and Enabling Constructs in Educational Diagnosis and Evaluation*) assesses the diagnostic and planning process to assist in the development of

TABLE 7.5	Occupational Health: Levels of Prevention for System Levels		
System Level	**Primary Prevention**	**Secondary Prevention**	**Tertiary Prevention**
Subsystem	Yearly physical examination for each employee	Regular blood pressure monitoring and diet counseling for each employee with elevated blood pressure	Referral for job retraining for employee with a back injury
Aggregate and group system	Incentive program to encourage departments to use safety devices	Weight reduction group for overweight employees	Support group for employees who are recovering from problems with alcohol or drug use
Suprasystem	Health fair open to the community and employees	Counseling and referral of community members with elevated blood pressure or cholesterol on the basis of health fair findings	Media advertising to encourage people with substance abuse problems to seek help and use community resources that provide assistance

NURSES INVOLVEMENT IN RALLIES/PROTESTS

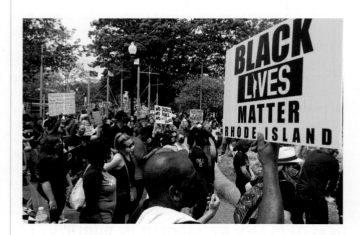

Nurses can support the health planning to improve population healthcare with awareness of, and involvement in, the political process. This involvement can consist of being an informed voter, contacting legislators on issues of concern, and participating in rallies and protests.

Food donation sites have increased need during the Covid-19 pandemic. Food insufficiency and hunger during the pandemic create the need for expanded SNAP benefits as well as food donation sites.

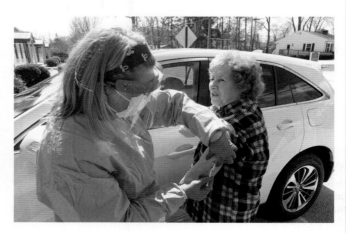

Nurses participate in Covid vaccine efforts.

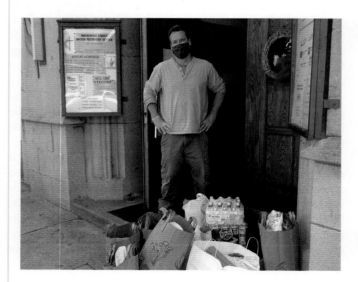

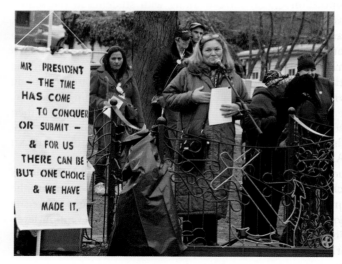

Nurses speak out for healthcare as a right. (Photo courtesy Anthony Ricci, MD.)

focused public health programs. PROCEED (*Policy, Regulatory, and Organizational Constructs in Educational and Environmental Development*) guides the implementation and evaluation of the programs (Green and Kreuter, 2005).

The PRECEDE-PROCEED framework is an approach to planning that examines factors contributing to behavior change. They are:

Predisposing factors: The knowledge, attitudes, behavior, beliefs, and values before intervention that affect willingness to change.

Enabling factors: The environment or community of an individual that facilitates or presents obstacles to change.

Reinforcing factors: The positive or negative effects of adopting new behavior (including social support).

These factors require that individuals be considered in the context of their community and social structures, and not in isolation, in the planning of communication or health education strategies (Green and Kreuter, 2005).

Patch

The Planning Approach to Community Health (PATCH) model was based on Green's PRECEDE (Green et al., 1980; Green and Kreuter, 2005; Porter, 2016). This model encouraged the idea that health promotion is a process that enables the

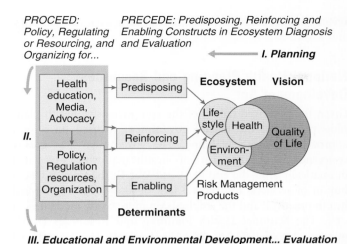

PROCEED: *PRECEDE: Predisposing, Reinforcing and*
Policy, Regulating *Enabling Constructs in Ecosystem Diagnosis*
or Resourcing, and *and Evaluation*
Organizing for...   *I. Planning*

III. Educational and Environmental Development... Evaluation

Fig. 7.3 Green's PRECEDE-PROCEED Model. Green's website provides assistance in guiding use and applications of this model at http://www.lgreen.net/precede.htm. (From Green LW, Kreuter MW: *Health program planning: An educational and ecological approach*, ed 4, 2004, McGraw-Hill.)

population to have more control over its own health. An essential element of the PATCH model is community participation. Another element is the use of data to develop comprehensive health strategies. The PATCH model achieved this through mobilizing the community, collecting health data, selecting health priorities, developing a comprehensive intervention plan, and evaluating the process (Issel et al., 2021).

APEX-PH Program

The Assessment Protocol for Excellence in Public Health (APEX-PH) program began in 1987 as a cooperative project of the American Public Health Association, the Association of Schools of Public Health, the Association of State and Territorial Health Officials, the CDC, the National Association of County and City Health Officials (NACCHO, 2022), and the United States Conference of Local Health Officers. The APEX-PH is a voluntary process for organizational and community selfassessment, planned improvements, and continuing evaluation and reassessment. It is a true self-assessment and is intended to be more of a public endeavor involving the community as well as the public organizations (NACCHO, 2007).

MAPP Model

More recently, the CDC and NACCHO have released the MAPP (Mobilizing for Action through Planning and Partnerships) model. The MAPP model is a health planning model that helps public health leaders facilitate community priorities about health issues and identify sources to address them. The first phase of MAPP is to mobilize the community; the second is to guide the community toward a shared vision for long-range planning; and the third is to conduct four assessments: identifying community strengths, local health systems, health status, and forces of change within the population (NACCHO, 2021).

⚡ ACTIVE LEARNING EXERCISE

Select one of the following community diagnoses from your community: increased rates of violence, asthma, lead poisoning, SDIs, pediculosis, infected tattoos/piercings, childhood obesity, food insufficiency, or homelessness. Write a plan on how to address that diagnosis, including goals and objectives. What resources will be needed?

HEALTH PLANNING FEDERAL LEGISLATION

Health planning at the national, state, and local levels is another example of aggregate planning. Planning at any of these levels can be a broader extension of the suprasystem level and affects the individual, family, group, population, and organization levels. Again, upstream change can occur on these levels; for example, individual consumers and consumer groups have protested some managed-care practices at the suprasystem level because health policy can directly affect patient care.

Historically, nurses have influenced health planning only minimally at the community level, but health planning has a tremendous effect on nurses and nursing practice. It is necessary to understand planning on a suprasystem level; therefore, the following section contains a review of past health planning efforts with projections for the future.

Hill-Burton Act

In 1946, Congress passed the Hospital Survey and Construction Act (Hill-Burton Act, PL 79-725) to address the need for better hospital access. This act provided federal aid to states for hospital facilities. A state had to submit a plan documenting available resources and need estimates to qualify for hospital construction and modernization funds under the **Hill-Burton Act** (Young and Kroth, 2017). In addition, each state had to designate a single agency for the development and implementation of the hospital construction plan. The Hill-Burton Act caused the expenditure of vast sums of money and resulted in an increase in the number of beds, especially in general hospitals. The act and its amendments focused only on construction.

Regional Medical Programs

The Hill-Burton Act provided construction-related planning, but it did not address coordination and care delivery directly. In response to recommendations from Dr. Michael DeBakey's national commission, the Heart Disease, Cancer, and Stroke Amendments of 1965 (PL 89-239) were enacted. This legislation was more comprehensive and established regional medical programs (RMPs).

The **RMPs** intended to make the latest technology for the diagnosis and treatment of heart disease, cancer, stroke, and related diseases available to community healthcare providers through the establishment of regional cooperative arrangements among medical schools, research institutions, and hospitals. The goals of these cooperative arrangements were to improve the health manpower and facilities available to the communities. The intent was to avoid interfering with methods of financing, hospital administration, patient care, or professional practice.

Although RMPs have been credited with the regionalization of certain services and the introduction of innovative approaches to organization and care delivery, some observers believed the reforms were not comprehensive enough. The RMPs did not partner with the existing federal and state programs; therefore, there were gaps and duplication in service delivery, personnel training, and research (National Institute of Health, 2021).

Comprehensive Health Planning

Congress signed the Comprehensive Health Planning and Public Health Services Amendments of 1966 (PL 89-749) into law to broaden the previous legislation's categorical approach to health planning. Combined with the Partnership for Health Amendments of 1967 (PL 90-174), these amendments created the Partnership for Health Program (PHP). The PHP provided federal grants to states to establish and administer a local agency program to enact local comprehensive healthcare planning. The PHP's objectives were promoting and ensuring the highest level of health for every person and not interfering with the existing private practice patterns (Shonick, 1995).

To meet these objectives, the PHP formulated a two-level planning system. Under this system, each state had to designate a single health planning agency, or "A" agency. To play a statewide coordinating role, the "A" agency had to partner with an advisory council, which consisted largely of healthcare consumers. Meanwhile, the local "B" agencies formulated plans to meet designated local community needs, which could be any public or nonprofit private agency or organization. "A" agencies were to encourage the formation of local, comprehensive health planning "B" agencies, and federal grants were made available for that purpose (Shonick, 1995).

Although the comprehensive health plans were the first of these programs to mandate consumer involvement, they may have failed in their basic intent. The possible failure may have resulted from funding shortage, conflict avoidance in policy formulation and goal establishment, political absence, and provider opposition (e.g., American Medical Association, American Hospital Association, and major medical centers) (Shonick, 1995).

Certificate of Need

In response to increased capital investments and budgetary pressures, state governments developed the idea of obtaining prior governmental approval for certain projects through the use of a certificate of need (CON). New York State passed the first CON law in 1964, which required government approval of hospitals' and nursing homes' major capital investments. Eventually all states supported this CON requirement, and it ultimately became a component of health legislation (PL 93-641). In practice, state CON programs differ in structure and goals. These differences include program focus, decision-making levels,

review standard scope, and appeals process exemption (Young and Kroth, 2017).

National Health Planning and Resources Development Act

Given the perceived failure of the comprehensive health planning programs, the federal government focused on a new approach to health planning. The government was greatly concerned with the cost of healthcare, which escalated dramatically after the end of World War II; the uneven distribution of services; the general lack of knowledge of personal health practices; and the emphasis on more costly modalities of care. The National Health Planning and Resources Development Act of 1974 (PL 93-641) (Endicott, 1975) combined the strengths of the Hill-Burton Act, RMPs, and the comprehensive health planning program to forge a new system of single-state and area-wide health planning agencies (Harlow, 2006).

The goals and purposes of the new law were to increase accessibility to as well as acceptability, continuity, and quality of health services; control over the rising costs of healthcare services; and prevention of unnecessary duplication of health resources. The new law addressed the needs of the underserved and provided quality healthcare. The provider and consumer were to be involved in planning and improving health services, and the law placed the system of private practice under scrutiny.

At the center of the program was a network of local health planning agencies, which developed health systems plans for their geographic service areas. The local agencies then submitted these plans to a state health planning and development agency, which integrated the plans into a preliminary state plan. The state agency presented this preliminary plan to a statewide health coordinating council for approval. The law required that the council consist of at least 16 governor-appointed members and that 50% of these members represent health system agencies and 50% represent consumers. One major function of this council was to prepare a state health plan that reflected the goals and purposes of the act. Once the council formulated a tentative plan, they presented it at public hearings throughout the state for discussion and possible revisions (Thorpe, 2002).

Despite careful deliberations by health planners with input from consumers, not all states accepted the health system plan at the grassroots level. A number of problems were encountered, and in time, the legislation failed to effect major change in the healthcare system. A significant problem was that the legislation had grandfathered in the entire healthcare system (i.e., healthcare delivery methods did not change). Although legislation mandated consumer involvement in the health system agency, it was often difficult to implement this aspect. Additionally, despite the mandated efforts by CON and required reviews, costs continued to rise and the healthcare system remained essentially unchanged (Thorpe, 2002).

Changing Focus of Health Planning

Health planning legislation is heavily influenced by the politics of the administration in power at any given time. The Reagan administration encouraged competition within the healthcare system. During the 1980s, the administration emphasized cost shifting and cost reduction with greater state power, less centralization of functions, and less national control. This approach represented the government's philosophical shift and combined it with a funding cutback from the Omnibus Budget Reconciliation Act in 1981. The result was a curtailment on federal health planning efforts at that time (Mueller, 1993). The cutbacks caused health system agencies to redefine their roles, and the federal government recommended eliminating these agencies.

A reduction in federal funding and the influence of medical lobbies caused the closure of some health system agencies. Those that remained open experienced a decrease in staff, a resulting drop in overall board functioning, and a reordering of priorities. In an effort to compensate for the decrease in federal funding, some health system agencies sought nonfederal funding or built coalitions to provide the necessary power base for change. Although the administration did not renew federal health planning legislation in the 1980s, it used other regulatory approaches to control costs. These included basing payments to Medicare on diagnosis-related groups, and, in the 1990s, the requirement by many individual states that their Medicaid recipients enroll in health maintenance organizations.

The Clinton administration's plan for healthcare reform included mechanisms to revitalize planning at the national level. The failure of Congress to pass the plan in 1994 gave planning efforts back to state and local agencies. As a result, most states became very involved in various aspects of health planning. Indeed, there is considerable variation as many have statewide health plans, local health plans, and some other type of local health planning.

The National Conference of State Legislators (NCSL, 2021) provides a state by state map on CON. It is anticipated that state CON programs will continue to assume a stronger role because states must increasingly monitor and report the quality of, cost of, and access to healthcare that managed care promised.

? ACTIVE LEARNING EXERCISE

1. Attend remotely or in person, a state or local health planning meeting. Observe the number of healthcare providers and consumers in attendance. Compare the meeting's issues with the goals of improving care quality and reducing healthcare costs.
2. Review current journal articles on the CPHNO website https://www.cphno.org/. Discuss which action may improve public health in your community.

Affordable Care Act (ACA) of 2010

The ACA law, also referred to as Obamacare, has three primary goals:

1. Make affordable health insurance available to more people. The law provides consumers with subsidies ("premium tax credits") that lower costs for households with incomes between 100% and 400% of the federal poverty level (FPL). Note: If your income is above 400% FPL, you may still qualify for the premium tax credit in 2021.
2. Expand the Medicaid program to cover all adults with income below 138% of the FPL. (Not all states have expanded their Medicaid programs.)
3. *Support innovative medical care delivery methods designed to lower the costs of healthcare generally* Healthcare.gov (2021). This act placed individuals, families, and small business owners in control of their healthcare. It reduced premium costs for millions of working families and small businesses by providing hundreds of billions of dollars in tax relief—the largest middle-class tax cut for healthcare in history. It also reduced what families paid for healthcare by capping out-of-pocket expenses and requiring preventive care to be fully covered without any out-of-pocket expense. It attempted to keep insurance companies honest by setting clear rules that rein in the worst insurance industry abuses. And it prohibited insurance companies from denying insurance coverage because of a person's preexisting medical conditions while giving consumers new power to appeal insurance company decisions that deny doctor-ordered treatments covered by insurance (Rambur, 2022).

According to the Center on Budget and Policy Priorities (2021), the COVID-19 pandemic brought economic devastation with millions of people losing their jobs or reductions in income. The economic loss increased the uninsured rate due to the large numbers of people lost job-based health coverage since the start of the pandemic. Although the ACA has had multiple legal challenges, it has survived a third challenge on a seven to two ruling, in 2021, where the Supreme Court found that the states and individuals challenging the law lacked standing (Zinberg, 2021). Current President Biden had proposed to strengthen the ACA, for example, by shifting the health insurance exchange benchmark and adding a public option. Biden's plan to expand U.S. health programs as part of a broad domestic spending bill has receded by pandemic related concerns associated with the infrastructure bill passed in November of 2021 (Lovelace, 2021).

To help achieve improved health status for all, health planning needs a coordinated approach that combines public and private cooperation with an emphasis on supplies and services. Advances in planning models and the sophistication level of planners will affect future health planning efforts. These efforts are supported by the *Healthy People 2030* in section "Explore the impact of community health assessment and improvement planning efforts objectives" (Healthy People, 2030).

? ACTIVE LEARNING EXERCISE

Review the ACA and your state's plans for action if repealed.

Case Study Application of the Nursing Process

School Bilingual Program

José Mendez, a bilingual community health nursing student, worked with the school system in a community that had a large Portuguese subsystem. His primary responsibility was for students enrolled in the town's bilingual program. His contacts included the school nurse and the program teachers.

Assessment

José included the specific group of students, the members of the school system's organizational level, and the population group of the town's Portuguese-speaking residents in his assessment of the aggregate's health needs. José identified the subsystem's lack of primary disease prevention, specifically related to hygiene, dental care, nutrition, and lifestyle choices, by observing the children, interviewing teachers and community residents, and reviewing the literature. José's continued assessment and prioritization revealed that the problem was related to a lack of knowledge and not a lack of concern.

Diagnosis
Individual
- Inadequate preparation at home regarding basic hygiene, dental care, nutrition, and healthy lifestyles

Family
- Developing strengths toward selfcare regarding basic hygiene, dental care, nutrition, and healthy lifestyles

Community
- Inadequate resources for communicating basics of hygiene, dental care, nutrition, and healthy lifestyles to the Portuguese community

Planning
The teachers and staff of the bilingual program helped contract and set goals, which reinforced the need for mutuality at this step in the process. A variety of alternative interventions were necessary to accomplish the following goals.

Individual
Long-Term Goal
- Students will regularly practice good hygiene, preventive dental care, good nutrition, exercise, and adequate sleep habits.

Short-Term Goal
- Students will learn the basics of good hygiene, preventive dental care, good nutrition, exercise, and adequate sleep habits.

Family
Long-Term Goal
- Families will regularly practice and teach their children good hygiene, preventive dental care, good nutrition, exercise, and adequate sleep habits.

Short-Term Goal
- Families will learn the basics of good hygiene, preventive dental care, good nutrition, exercise, and adequate sleep habits.

Community
Long-Term Goal
- Systematic programs will provide families and their children with education and information regarding the basics of good hygiene, preventive dental care, good nutrition, exercise, and adequate sleep habits.

Short-Term Goal
- Bilingual personnel will translate information into Portuguese, and program teachers will distribute it to families. This information will cover the basics of good hygiene, preventive dental care, good nutrition, exercise, and adequate sleep habits.

Intervention
- Sometimes nursing students' projects are more limited than the planning stage's ideal; in this case, interventions assessed only one grade level.

Individual
- The student nurse taught children many healthy lifestyle basics, including nutrition, hygiene, and dental care. Classes presented information in Portuguese and English.

Family
- All parents received a summary of the class content in both languages and in pictures.

Community
- The local teachers communicated the student nurse's activities to their state-level coordinators, and the coordinators incorporated the student nurse's materials into the bilingual program throughout the state.

Evaluation
Individual, Family, Community
This community health planning project had an impact on the individuals in the specific aggregate and had broader implications for the family system and the community suprasystem. The outcomes, or product, were hugely successful. Mutually identified goals and objectives influenced the development of the process and incorporated input from a variety of sources. The student nurse believed the resources and support for the bilingual program were adequate. Although the student nurse addressed only primary prevention, the continuing nature of the project will allow the teachers, the school nurse, and the families to assess problems related to the program's content. Future implementation may address secondary and tertiary prevention.

Questions
1. How would you evaluate this project?
2. How would you determine process and product evaluation?
3. What would you do differently?

NURSING IMPLICATIONS

Nurses must work collaboratively with health planners to improve aggregate health. Nurses can influence health planning at the local, state, or community level by fusing current technology with their knowledge of healthcare needs and skills gained through working with individuals, families, groups, and population groups. This is an example of "upstream interventions." Indeed, nurses may become directly involved in the planning process by participating in CON reviews or gaining membership on health planning councils. Even as students, nurses can begin to participate by engaging in aggregate-level projects, such as those outlined in this chapter, and by tracking healthcare legislation and contacting their legislators about important issues.

Increased nursing involvement is one method of strengthening local and national health planning. Nurses can use the Health Planning Model presented in this chapter to facilitate a systematic approach to improve aggregate healthcare. Nurses can assess aggregates from small groups through population groups; identify the group's health needs; and perform planning, intervention, and evaluations by applying this model. The health of individuals, families, and groups would improve if nurses reemphasized the larger aggregate.

■ SUMMARY

Community health nurses are responsible for incorporating health planning into their practice. Nurses' unique talents and skills, augmented by the comprehensive application of the nursing process, can facilitate population health improvement at various aggregate levels. Health planning policy and process constitute part of the knowledge base of the baccalaureate-prepared nurse. Systems theory provides one framework for nursing process application in the community. Interventions are possible at subsystem, system, and suprasystem levels using all three levels of prevention.

EVOLVE WEBSITE

http://evolve.elsevier.com/Nies/community
- NCLEX Review Questions
- Case Studies

BIBLIOGRAPHY

American Health Planning Association. In *National directory of health planning, policy, and regulatory agencies*, ed 22, VA, 2016, Falls Church. AHPA.

American Planning Association: *Planning and community health research center*, 2021. Available from: http://www.planning.org/nationalcenters/health/.

Blum HL: *Planning for health*, New York, 1974, Human Sciences Press.

Center on Budget and Policy Priorities: *Health care lifeline: the affordable care act and the COVID-19 pandemic*, 2021. Available from: https://www.cbpp.org/research/health/health-care-lifeline-the-affordable-care-act-and-the-covid-19-pandemic.

Center of Disease Control (CDC): *Suicidal Ideation and Behaviors Among High School Students — Youth Risk Behavior Survey, United States*, 2019. Morbidity and Mortality Weekly Report, https://www.cdc.gov/mmwr/volumes/69/su/su6901a6.htm. Retrieved 26 May 2022.

Centers for Disease Control and Prevention: *Adolescent and school health: sexual risk behavior*, 2021. Available from: https://www.cdc.gov/healthyyouth/sexualbehaviors.

Congressional Budget Office: *American Health Care Act of 2017*, 2021. Available at: www.cbo.gov/publication/52752, https://www.cbo.gov/.

Endicott KL: National Health Planning and Resources Development Act of 1974: PL 93-641, *Publ Health Rep* 90(3):i2, 1975. Available from: http://www.ncbi.nlm.nih.gov/pmc/articles/PMC1435675/.

Gilden R, Friedmann E, Sattler B, et al.: Potential health effects related to pesticide use on athletic fields, *Publ Health Nurs* 29(3):198—207, 2012.

Green LW, Kreuter MW. In *Health promotion planning: an educational and ecological approach*, ed 4, New York, 2005, McGraw-Hill.

Green LW, Kreuter MW, Deeds SG, et al.: *Health education planning: a diagnostic approach*, Palo Alto, CA, 1980, Mayfield Publishing.

Harlow JM: Government and other types of oversight. In Garber KM, editor: *The U.S. Health Care Delivery System: fundamental facts, definitions, and statistics*, Chicago, 2006, American Hospital Association.

Healthcare.gov: *Affordable Care Act*, 2021. Available from: https://www.healthcare.gov/.

Heart disease: cancer, and stroke amendments of 1965: PL, 1965, pp 89—239.

Healthy People 2030, *Explore the impact of community health assessment and improvement planning efforts*, Available from: https://health.gov/healthypeople/objectives-and-data/browse-objectives/public-health-infrastructure/explore-impact-community-health-assessment-and-improvement-planning-efforts-phi-r09.

Hogue C: An epidemiologic approach to distributive nursing practice. In Hall JE, Weaver BR, editors: *Distributive nursing practice: a systems approach to community health*, ed 2, Philadelphia, 1985, Lippincott Williams & Wilkins.

Hospital Survey and Construction Act of 1946 (Hill-Burton Act): PL 79-725.

Israel BA, Eng E, Schulz AJ, Parker EA: *Methods in community-based participatory research for health*, ed 2, San Francisco, 2012, Jossey-Bass.

Issel LM, Wells R, Williams M: *Health program planning and evaluation*, ed 5, Burlington, MA, 2021, Jones and Bartlett.

Kaiser Family Foundation: *Health reform source, 2017*, 2017. Available from: http://www.kff.org/health-reform/video/health-reform-hits-main-street/.

Labonte R: Health promotion and empowerment: reflections on professional practice, *Health Educ Q* 21:253—268, 1994.

Leavell HR, Clark EG: *Preventive medicine for the doctor in his community*, New York, 1965, McGraw-Hill.

Lovelace B: *Biden outlines plans to expand U.S. health programs as part of broad domestic spending plan. Health and Science*, 2021. CNBC. Available from: https://www.cnbc.com/2021/10/28/biden-outlines-plan-to-expand-us-health-programs-as-part-of-broad-domestic-spending-bill.html.

Maslow AH: *Toward a psychology of being*, New York, 1968, Van Nostrand Reinhold.

Mueller K: *Health care policy in the United States*, Lincoln, NE, 1993, University of Nebraska Press.

National Association of County and City Health Officials (NACCHO): *MAPP*, 2017. Available from: http://archived.naccho.org/topics/infrastructure/mapp/.

National Association of County and City Health Officials (NACCHO): *MAPP*, 2017. Available from: http://archived.naccho.org/topics/infrastructure/mapp/.

National Association of County and City Health Officials (NAC-CHO) (2021) Mobilizing for Action through Planning and Partnerships (MAPP). https://www.naccho.org/programs/public-health-infrastructure/performance-improvement/community-health-assessment/mapp Retrieved 26 May 2022

National Association of County and City Health Officials (NACCHO) 2022 Mission Statement. https://www.naccho.org/about/our-mission. Retrieved May 26, 2022.

National Conference of State Legislatures (NCSL), 2021. Available from: https://www.ncsl.org/research/health/con-certificate-of-need-state-laws.aspx.

National Institute of Health: *Regional medical programs*, Washington, DC, 2021, US National Library of Medicine. Available from: https://profiles.nlm.nih.gov/spotlight/rm/feature/briefhistory.

Nyswander DB: Education for health: some principles and their application, *Health Educ Monogr* 14:65—70, 1956.

Partnership for Health: *Amendments of 1967*, 1967, PL, pp 90—174.

Porter C: Revisiting Precede—Proceed: a leading model for ecological and ethical health promotion, *Health Educ J* 75(6):753—764, 2016.

Rambur B: *Health care finance, economics and policy for nurses: a foundational guide*, ed 2, New York, 2022, Springer Publishing Co.

Shonick W: *Government and health services: government's role in the development of U.S. health services*, New York, 1995, Oxford University Press, 1930—1980.

Silverstein NG: Lillian Wald at Henry Street: 1893—1895, *ANS Adv Nurs Sci* 7(1—12), 1985.

Thorpe K: Cost containment. In Kovner A, Jonas S, editors: *Health care delivery in the United States*, ed 7, New York, 2002, Springer.

U.S. Department of Health and Human Services: *About the affordable care act*, 2017. Available from: https://www.hhs.gov/healthcare/about-the-aca/index.html. Accessed November 9, 2021.

U.S. Department of Veterans Affairs: Veterans Health Administration. Available at: https://www.va.gov/health/.

U.S. Social Security Administration: compilation of the social security laws: comprehensive health planning and public health services amendments of 1966: PL 89—749. Available from: https://www.ssa.gov/OP_Home/ssact/ssact-toc.htm.

Young K, Kroth P: *Sultz & Young's healthcare USA: understanding its organization and delivery*, ed 9 Burlington, MA, 2017, Jones and Bartlett.

Zinberg J: *Obamacare survives a third (and likely final) challenge*, 2021, Health Care Politics and Law. Available: https://www.city-journal.org/obamacare-survives-a-third-and-likely-final-challenge.

Community Health Education and Engagement

Cathy D. Meade, PhD, RN, FAAN FSBM FAACE

OBJECTIVES

Upon completion of this chapter, the reader will be able to do the following:

1. Describe the goals of health education within the community setting.
2. Examine the nurse's role in community education within a sociopolitical, environmental, and cultural context.
3. Select a learning theory, and describe its application to the individual, family, or aggregate.
4. Examine innovative and effective teaching and learning strategies that exemplify community-centered health education for the individual, family, or aggregate/group.
5. Compare and contrast Freire's approach to health education with an individualistic health education model.
6. Examine the importance of community engagement for impacting health disparities toward health equity.
7. Highlight the role of health literacy in community health education and engagement.
8. Outline a systematic process for developing culturally and literacy relevant health education materials, messages, media, and programs.
9. Relate and apply factors that enhance the suitability of health education materials, messages, digital media, and programs for an intended audience.
10. Prepare a meaningful teaching plan and evaluation criteria for the individual, family, and/or group.

OUTLINE

KEY TERMS

autonomy
cognitive theory
community engagement
community empowerment
community-based participatory research (CBPR) methods
culturally effective and responsive care

health disparities
health education
health equity
health literacy
humanistic theories
learner verification
learning
literacy

materials, media, digital technologies, and messages
participatory action research (PAR)
Paulo Freire
problem-solving education
social justice
social learning theory

CONNECTING WITH EVERYDAY REALITIES

The nurse may be tempted to ask the following questions:

- Why does Ms. Lee keep smoking? She is pregnant.
- Why doesn't Mr. Bonne (a 63-year-old) get his follow-up colonoscopy? His fecal immunochemical test (FIT) was abnormal.
- Why doesn't Carlos (15 years old and newly diagnosed with diabetes) take his insulin shots each day?
- Why aren't the parents thinking about the human papilloma virus (HPV) series for their kids? The twins are about to turn 11 years old.
- Why don't more women attend the clinic's cervical cancer screening? It's free!
- Why does the community have such an alarming rate of obesity?

Although these questions show the nurse's desire and good intentions to understand the link between health behavior and health education, they do not yield actionable answers or empower individuals, families, or groups. In fact, such questions negate critical root health issues and, rather, create a "blaming the victim" approach as recounted by Israel and colleagues (1994, 2013). Instead, the nurse should try to reframe the questions to get at reasons that help explain the behavior and that lend themselves to nursing actions. Consider the questions the nurse might ask instead:

- What life stressors might be going on with Ms. Lee? What social support could I offer to help her quit?
- What structural, communication or cultural factors might be preventing Mr. Bonne from getting a colonoscopy? For example, is transportation a problem? Are the instructions clear? Might he view the colonoscopy procedure as scary? What beliefs might he have about the test, for example, "that it has to do with my manhood?" Does he have money for the preparation? What can I do better to verify that he understands the importance of the test?
- How does Carlos like to learn? What makes it difficult for him to remember to take his insulin? Are the needles a concern? Does he have worries about how his diabetes might affect his soccer game? Could text reminders or an app be helpful? What can I do to better connect my instructions to what is important to him in his everyday school and sports activities?
- What might be hindering the parents from planning to get HPV immunizations for their kids? What have they heard about HPV? Could their religious beliefs play a role? Do they think their children will be sexually active sooner? Might they be worried about side effects of the immunizations that they heard about from their relatives? How could I do a better job of explaining the importance of the HPV series in consideration of these concerns?
- What outreach methods might better attract the women to the free cervical cancer screening? Could a promotora help engage women and help them navigate the process? Are the educational materials and promotional flyers language specific and easy to understand?
- What social, physical, cultural, language, linguistic, or structural factors should be considered when developing nutrition messages? What role can I play to develop links with schools, grocery stores, churches, and community centers to better reach and teach families about nutritional interventions? How can community capacity be strengthened to advocate for greater access to healthier food in the neighborhood grocery stores?

HEALTH EDUCATION IN THE COMMUNITY

Historically, teaching has been a significant nursing responsibility since Florence Nightingale's (1859) early work. Gardner (1936) emphasized that health teaching is one of the most fundamental nursing principles and that "a nurse, in even the most obscure position must be a teacher of no mean order." There is much support for the nurse's involvement in health education and health communications, including nurse practice acts, professional statements from the American Nurses Association (2021); Association of Community Health Nursing Educators Association of Public Health Nurses; American Public Health Association—Public Health Section; the Alliance of Nursing for Healthy Environments (https://www.nursingworld.org/practice-policy/workforce/public-health-nursing/); and the National Association of School Nursing to name a few. Healthy People 2030 also endorses a strong vision for health promotion, disease prevention, and wellness in our communities—(See Healthy People, 2030 objectives—U.S. Department of Health and Human Services [USDHHS], n.d., https://health.gov/healthypeople). Further, in the National Academies of Sciences, Engineering and Medicine report (2021) titled: The Future of Nursing 2020–30: Charting a Path to Achieve Health Equity, the critical role of nurses over the next decade is underscored since "nurses live and work at the intersection of **health, education, and communities.**"

Health education is an integral part of the nurse's role in the community for promoting health, preventing disease, and maintaining optimal wellness (Box 8.1). Moreover, the community is a vital link for the delivery of effective healthcare and offers the nurse multiple opportunities to provide appropriate health education and transformational community engagement within the context of a setting that is familiar to people (Jones et al., 2020; Meade et al., 2011). The role of the nurse as health educator is especially important considering the increasing diversity and demographically changing population in the United States and globally. Additionally, the increased pace of technological advancements and digital communications enable wider and quicker dissemination of new knowledge. The COVID-19 pandemic is an example of the need for a "rapid response" to new information requirements. As such, nurses are pivotal in their education roles to improve the connection between scientific discovery and the delivery of responsive and credible interventions in the community to advance **health equity** and **social justice** (Alcaraz et al., 2016; Freeman, 2004; Marmot and Wilkinson 2005; Quinn et al., 2015; Thurman Pfitzinger-Lippe, 2017).

BOX 8.1 Health Education Roles and Activities of the Nurse in the Community

- Advocate
- Administrator
- Caregiver
- Case manager
- Catalyst
- Change agent
- Coach
- Collaborator
- Consultant
- Counselor
- Culture broker
- Educator
- Facilitator
- Implementer
- Information agent and knowledge broker
- Innovator
- Liaison
- Mediator
- Navigator
- Negotiator
- Policy analyst, policy maker
- Promoter of collaborative partnerships
- Promoter of self-care and self-efficacy
- Referral resource
- Resource Steward
- Researcher
- Sensitizer
- Social activist

Note: Can you think of any other roles of the nurse in the community setting?

American Nurses Association: *Nursing: scope and standards of practice*, ed 4. Silver Spring, MD, 2021, American Nurses Association. Available from: chrome-extension://oemmndcbldboiebfnladdacbdfmadadm/https://www.nursingworld.org/~49d755/globalassets/practiceandpolicy/scope-of-practice/3sc-booklet-2021-june.pdf; Quad Council Coalition Competency Review Task Force (2018); Redman BK: *The practice of patient education: a case study approach*, ed 10, St. Louis, Missouri, 2007, Elsevier.

More than ever before, health education and community engagement activities are taking place outside the walls of hospitals in such settings as missions, community centers, beauty salons and barbershops, grocery stores, truck stops, youth centers, homeless shelters, food banks, Veterans of Foreign Wars halls, churches, community-based clinics, health maintenance organizations, schools, worksites, shopping malls, senior centers, adult education/literacy centers, mobile health units, homes, libraries, etc. Health education activities also are increasingly occurring in home settings via social media, and/or other digital communication channels (e-health, telehealth, etc.) (Glanz et al., 2015; Koskan et al., 2014; Kuwabara et al., 2020). At the core of community health education is the development of trustworthy relationships based on nurturing and healing interactions that heavily rely on **community-based participatory methods**. Such methods highlight community strengths and sustainable collaborations and trustworthy partnerships that aim for a co-learning (patient-community centric) relationship (Braun et al., 2015; Gwede et al., 2010; Simmons et al., 2015; Tucker et al., 2017; Ward et al., 2018).

Health education is any combination of learning experiences designed to predispose, enable, and reinforce voluntary behavior conducive to health in individuals, groups, or communities and society. Its goal is to understand health behavior and to translate knowledge into relevant interventions and strategies for health enhancement, disease prevention, and chronic illness management. Health education aims to enhance wellness and decrease disability; attempts to actualize the health potential of individuals, families, communities, and society;

and includes a broad and varied set of strategies aimed at influencing individuals within their social environment for improved health and well-being (Green and Kreuter, 2005).

Kleinman (1978) described a social and cultural community healthcare system as one that bridges external factors (e.g., economic, political, and epidemiological) to internal factors (e.g., behavioral and communicative). This view of a sociocultural healthcare system firmly grounds health education activities within sociopolitical structures especially within local environmental settings, and views the *community* as client (Emerson et al., 2019; Holt et al., 2017; Kuehnert et al., 2021; Meade et al., 2011; Quinn et al., 2020). As such, because the community level is often the location of health prevention and health promotion programs, it is a significant and enriching venue for obtaining positive health outcomes. Nurses are uniquely qualified to influence the health and well-being of community members' health behaviors through original and inventive activities that incorporate culturally, linguistically, and literacy relevant health education and messaging. Due to nurses' knowledge, competencies, and skills, they can take on leadership and advocacy roles to expertly assess community assets, identify information gaps and system-level obstacles, and put forward effective solutions to complex, multicausal community concerns for advancing social justice and health equity (Thurman and Pfitzinger-Lippe, 2017; Vamos et al., 2021).

It is paramount that community nurse educators address the myriad sociopolitical conditions that affect community health by placing value on the contributions of community members' strengths. Sustained cognitive and behavioral changes often rely heavily on engaging learners in becoming partners in their own health behavior and practice. For example, look at the following community interventions directed toward the use of empowering and participatory approaches:

- Aranda and colleagues (2018) reported that the use of participatory methods (15 focus groups among young people, ages 11 to 19) was helpful to generate discussions about sexual health. By making the topic more visible, they addressed the complex tensions in designing and delivering acceptable sexual healthcare services. As a result, the school nurse was instrumental in promoting a positive sexual health culture within the school setting.
- Holliday and colleagues (2018), in a pilot project, based on a strong reciprocal relationship between community and university partners, clarified the learning needs of tribal community members by determining strengths, assets and resources available to the community to address youth suicide and substance abuse on a reservation. Using a variety of CBPR-driven processes (e.g., photovoice, digital storytelling and community capacity surveys), the team refined a strength-based intervention based on the "Gathering of Native American's (GONA) curriculum (As background, the GONA curriculum was first developed and published in 1990s as a culture-based intervention through a special initiative of the US Center for Substance Abuse Prevention, in collaboration with a team of Native American trainers and

curriculum developers from across the US: https://www.ojp.gov/ncjrs/virtual-library/abstracts/gathering-native-americans-gona-substance-abuse-prevention).

- Kelly and colleagues (2017) carried out in-depth interviews with incarcerated women to examine their experiences with Pap tests and how they followed up on abnormal results. Several contextual factors elucidated in this work included Pap test abnormality as an all-inclusive phrase for women's health problems, the nature of women's changing and often unstable lives, and the structural challenges of money, and competing demands—all of which played a role in whether they followed up on abnormal Pap test results or with other health problems.

- Gwede and colleagues. (2019) illustrated how a community—academic partnership led to the development of improved colorectal cancer screening rates among Spanish-preferring Latinos receiving care in community clinics. This randomized pilot intervention was conceptualized, designed, and implemented based on CBPR principles within the context of the Tampa Bay Community Cancer Network (TBCCN), an established community-academic network aimed at tackling health disparities. It was found that the provision of low-literacy, linguistically salient educational materials (i.e., fotonovella) plus a FIT kit improved CRC screening uptake (87%) and exceeded national screening targets.

- Jiao and colleagues (2021) reported findings from a thematic analysis of 35 interviews with indoor sex workers, clients, and third parties to understand the role of information and communication technologies (ICTs) in sex workers' occupational health and safety. Three key themes related to the intersection of sex work, technology use, and occupational health and safety were: (1) screening; (2) confidentiality, privacy, and disclosure; and (3) malice. Findings suggested that ICTs strongly shaped occupational health and safety and that prevailing socio-political contexts must be considered in the development of interventions that build capacities of sex workers' health and safety.

- Singh and Nichols (2020) highlighted the value of a Nurse-led Led Education and Engagement Study for Diabetes Care (called NEEDS) involving a mixed-methods protocol to develop a sustainable program for diabetes prevention and management for patients with type 2 diabetes mellitus in sub-Saharan Africa. Methods used included surveys, key informant interviews, focus group discussions, and ethnography to derive a practical collaborative and empowering protocol for managing diabetes among Ghanaian patients. Findings informed a multisystems effort to address the severe shortage of health workers through a task-shifting strategy and leveraging of mobile technology and set the foundation for an m-health intervention.

- Overall, these studies reinforce that nurses have significant roles in providing contextually appropriate health education, which involves practical, useful, and scientifically sound methods that can fit the lives and learning needs of groups across the lifespan in the US and globally.

LEARNING THEORIES, PRINCIPLES, AND HEALTH EDUCATION MODELS

Learning Theories

Learning theories are helpful to understand how individuals, families, and groups learn. The field of psychology provides the basis for most of these theories and illustrates how environmental stimuli elicit specific responses. Such theories can aid nurses to recognize the mechanisms that potentially modify knowledge, attitude, and behavior. Bigge and Shermis (2004) assert that **learning** is an enduring change that involves the modification of insights, behaviors, perceptions, or motivations. Although psychology textbooks describe learning theories in greater detail, the following broad categories relate to the nursing application in a community setting: stimulus-response (S-R) conditioning (i.e., behavioristic), cognitive, humanistic, and social learning.

The nurse should remember that theories are not completely right or wrong. Different theories work well in different situations. Knowles (1989) relates that behaviorists program individuals through S-R mechanisms to behave in a certain fashion. **Humanistic theories** help individuals develop their potential in self-directing and holistic manners. Cognitive theorists recognize the brain's ability to think, feel, learn, and solve problems and train the brain to maximize these functions. Although social learning theory is largely a **cognitive theory**, it also includes elements of behaviorism (Bandura, 1977a). **Social learning theory's** premise is based on the idea that behavior

RESEARCH HIGHLIGHTS

An Examination of Intimate Partner Violence (IPV) and Sexual Relationship Power among Adolescents in South Africa.

A nurse-led team (Teitelman et al., 2016) sought to explore the associations of IPV and relationship power about sexual-risk behaviors and determine if these associations differed by gender among adolescents in South Africa. Their work required careful understanding of the landscape of gender-based sexual norms that often reflect social construction of masculinities and femininities. This perspective was important to understand possible gender inequities and associated sexual risks faced by adolescents. As background, the study built on prior work by Jemmott et al. (2010, 2015) that described a systematic approach to developing and testing an HIV/sexually transmitted infection health education intervention. This 12-h Xhosa-language educational intervention delivered to sixth graders was based on social cognitive theory, the theory of planned behavior, and extensive formative research. The intervention ($n = 1057$) was carried out in 18 schools in Cape Province, South Africa. Results showed that students retained risk-reduction knowledge, self-efficacy, and outcome expectancies and kept engaging in safer sexual behavior during follow-up at multiple time points.

The current large scale community randomized study (Teitelman et al., 2016) reported data from the 54-month follow-up among 786 adolescents who reported sexual debut (mean age = 16.9). The rationale for exploring this aspect of sexual health (IPV and sexual relationship power) is based on literature showing that low relationship power and victimization by IPV is linked to increased HIV risks among adult females and adolescent girls. The study assessed self-reported adolescents' sexual risk behaviors (e.g., multiple partners in 3 months, condom use at last sex, IPV, and relationship power).

IPV victimization was operationalized as "things that happened to you with a sexual partner while you were having an argument, for example, physical, sexual and psychological threatening." Results showed that adolescent boys were less likely to report condom use at last sex ($P = .001$) and more likely to report multiple partners ($P < .001$). Also, as IPV increased, reported condom use decreased at last sex for girls, but for boys, it increased. Overall, boys reported lower total relationship power than girls, which may suggest a shift toward more progressive gender norms and gender parity in sexual decision-making power. Findings suggest that sexual risk-reduction interventions for adolescents in South Africa should consider social context to reduce adolescent partner violence and sexual relationship power imbalances, integrate individual attitudes about IPV and interpersonal gender power dynamics, as well as draw on community-level intervention approaches to change harmful social gender norms that perpetuate inequalities. Also, HIV risk-reduction policies and programs should address IPV to promote gender equity and respectful and safe relationships among adolescents. Collectively, these studies point to the value of nurse-delivered health education and reinforce the need for future studies (both globally and here in the US) that test the utility of theoretically driven health education interventions that discern key features that contribute to healthy behaviors.

Data from Teitelman AM, Jemmott AM, Bellamy SL, et al.: Partner violence, power and gender differences in South African adolescents' HIV/STI behaviors, *Health Psychol* 35(7):751–760, 2016. https://doi.org/10.1037/hea0000351; Jemmott JB, Jemmott LS, O'Leary A, et al.: School-based randomized controlled trial of an HIV/STD risk-reduction intervention for South African adolescents, *Arch Pediatr Adolesc Med* 164(10):923–929, 2010. https://doi.org/10.1001/archpediatrics.2010.176; Jemmott JB, Jemmott LS, O'Leary A, et al.: HIV/STI risk-reduction-intervention efficacy with South African adolescents over 54 months, *Health Psychol* 34(6):610–621, 2015. https://doi.org/10.1037/hea0000140

explains and enhances learning through the concepts of efficacy, outcome expectation, and incentives. Clinical Example 8.1 applies various theories to a community intervention.

Clinical Example 8.1

Application of Characteristics of Adult Learners to the Development of a Community Support Group.

This example illustrates the long-standing value of incorporating theoretical underpinnings in the development of community-engaged activities designed to meet specific learning needs. It provides a description of how nurses played an active role in bolstering the community capacity and health of their community. Although this account dates to the 1980s, it is an important reminder of the value of applying learning theories to one's work and how such application leads to sustainability of efforts (a key goal of nursing actions!). It is common for nurses based in community settings to be educational resources for patients, families, and community members as they cope with health, wellness, and disease. Later in the chapter, another example is discussed, LUNA (Latinas Unidas por un Nuevo Amanecer, Inc.), a nonprofit organization whose mission is to provide support and offer culturally and linguistically relevant education to Hispanic breast cancer survivors and their families, and it is based on similar tenets.

As background, the author, and another nursing colleague initiated a community education support group for individuals with amyotrophic lateral sclerosis (ALS), more commonly known as *Lou Gehrig's disease*, on the basis of an identified

community need. ALS is an incurable degenerative neuromuscular disease that affects nerve and muscle function and the brain's ability to control muscle movement (see http://alsawi.org/ for more information about ALS). The support group was open to family members and friends. At that time, Southeast Wisconsin did not have a support group. Community members provided feedback and identified the need for specific education topics and support for people with ALS. This foundational dialogue provided the organizing framework for the inception of the first support group, and based on observations and interactions at the monthly meetings, an illustration of Knowles' assumptions follows:

Need to know: At the first support group meetings, the facilitators, both nurses, introduced possible topics by describing the reason for the discussion and the rationale for the selected subjects (e.g., common concerns of patients and family members and informal assessments based on conversations and the literature). To prepare for discussion, group members introduced themselves, and the nurses asked what they hoped to learn from the sessions. In some cases, members were unsure why they might want more information on given topics but indicated that they wanted to listen. Progression of the disease is variable; therefore the *need to know* was often facilitated by the nurses and other patients who already noted the importance of specific learning needs (e.g., need for supportive care, assistive walking devices, financial planning, or information on assistive breathing devices).

Self-concept: A comfortable, informal, and trusting environment allowed patients to express feelings, emotions, and frustrations about the disease. Patients, family members, caregivers, and support persons were encouraged to express themselves. Over time, participants cultivated mutual respect and trust for one another due to shared commonalities and experiences. Hugs were common as members began to understand that others had similar situations and concerns. Group members had an opportunity to share and speak about ways that they managed and coped with their disease (e.g., decisions about life support and feeding tubes). Even if their choices were not the same, participants recognized and acknowledged these decisions without imposing their own value judgments. Facilitators and group members soon became equal partners in the learning process (colearners). At the core of the meetings was the formation of therapeutic healing and respectful relationships.

Experiences: Some patients and family members had gone through other difficult life experiences and stressors (e.g., other illnesses or deaths in the family) and helped others cope with the management of ALS. Patients shared their strengths gained from such experiences with other support group members. Additionally, individuals and family members who were going through varying stages of the disease process shared their experiences (e.g., obtaining home care, selecting a computer, and managing swallowing and eating). They shared tips and time-saving strategies with one another and with newly diagnosed families and all learned from those collective experiences.

Readiness to learn: Family members often take on many roles when someone becomes ill, especially with a chronic illness such as ALS. This redefinition of roles creates new

Continued

Clinical Example 8.1—cont'd

learning opportunities; however, it can hinder learning if it is too overwhelming. For example, the well partner may assume the roles of caregiver, parent, and financial supporter. It is helpful for nurses to identify resources to help the family cope with new roles (e.g., respite care).

Orientation to learning: Learning a variety of psychomotor skills is necessary to care for the patient with ALS (e.g., communication, suctioning, positioning, using a feeding tube, and toileting). The time frame for learning such skills varies depending on the course of illness. Presenting information about such skills too early in the course of the disease may cause fear and anxiety. Families may be resistant to learning such tasks until the need is apparent. In some cases, the need may be evident at a crisis point (e.g., a fall, a choking incident, or severe respiratory distress). However, nurse facilitators of support groups can introduce these topics slowly by providing information via educational sessions, newsletters, e-mail, telephone calls, the Internet, printed brochures, blogs, FaceTime, discussion boards, one-on-one discussions, or other digital health technologies

Motivation: Individuals and families often experience a shift in life goals when faced with ALS. Such shifts create new learning opportunities aimed at enhancing quality of life, promoting survivorship, and maintaining self-esteem. For example, a college professor with ALS kept his link to the university. He was highly motivated to continue his research work and supervise his graduate students. To continue his academic work, he learned to manage his breathing by using a ventilator, arranged transportation to the university, obtained nursing care, and created communication methods by using a computer to ensure that his students' work continued.

As a result of this initial local support group, the ALS Association Wisconsin Chapter evolved and became an official ALS Association chapter in 1987. The chapter's mission is to "lead the fight to cure and treat ALS through global, cutting-edge research, and to empower people with ALS and their families to live fuller lives by providing them with compassionate care and support." Today, there are seven ALS Association Wisconsin Chapter–sponsored patient/caregiver support groups in Wisconsin as well as five additional support groups and meetings in Wisconsin. This is the result from just one meeting held by two nurses on a Saturday several decades ago in response to an unmet need in the community. Over the years, many community and family activities, health education programs, and fundraising events have brought significant awareness and visibility, scientific advancements, and patient services to individuals with ALS and their loved ones.

For more information on services, go to ALS national and state websites.

❓ ACTIVE LEARNING

In groups of three to four students, discuss how theoretical frameworks help explain health behavior. Identify the strengths and limitations of models that focus on individual health determinants versus models that encompass sociopolitical, environmental, and structural factors.

Knowles' Assumptions About Adult Learners

Knowles (1988, 1989) outlines several assumptions about adult learners. He contends that adults, like children, learn better in a facilitative, nonrestrictive, and nonstructured environment. Nurses who are familiar with these assumptions can develop teaching strategies that motivate and interest individuals, families, and groups and encourage active and full participation in the learning process. Nurses can help create a self-directing, self-empowering learning environment. The following characteristics affect learning: the client's need to know, concept of self, readiness to learn, orientation to learning, experience, and motivation. Table 8.1 expands on these characteristics.

Health Education Models

In addition to learning theories, the application of education theories and principles to situations involving individuals, families, and groups illustrates how ideas fit together, offers explanations for health behaviors or actions, and helps direct community nursing interventions. Such theoretical elements form the basis of understanding health behavior. Theoretical frameworks offer nurses an intervention blueprint that promotes learning and provides them with an organized approach to explaining concept relationships (Padilla and Bulcavage, 1991). This roadmap gives nurses the ability to assess an intervention's strength and impact. Importantly, theory and practice need to coexist, and the best theory is one often rooted from practice (Glanz et al., 2015).

Models of Individual Behavior

Two models that explain preventive behavior determinants are the health belief model (HBM), which is presented in Table 8.2 (Becker et al., 1977; Hochbaum, 1958; Kegeles et al., 1965; Rosenstock, 1966), and the health promotion model (HPM) (Murdaugh et al., 2019; Pender et al., 2015). Both models are multifactorial; are based on value expectancy; and address individual perceptions, modifying factors, and likelihood of action. The HBM is based on social psychology and has undergone much empirical testing to predict compliance on singular preventive measures. The initial purpose of the HBM was to explain why people did not participate in health education programs to prevent or detect disease, in particular tuberculosis screening programs (Hochbaum, 1958). Subsequent studies addressed other preventive actions and factors related to adherence to medical regimens (Becker, 1974). Primarily, the HBM is a value expectancy theory that addresses factors that promote health-enhancing behavior. It is disease specific and focuses on avoidance orientation. The HBM considers perceived susceptibility, perceived severity, perceived benefits, perceived barriers, and cues to action and other sociopsychological and structural variables (modifying factors). Self-efficacy, defined as the notion that an individual can act successfully on a given behavior to produce the desired outcome (Bandura, 1977a,b), was later added to the HBM (Rosenstock et al., 1988; Strecher et al., 1986). In a meta-analysis (data combined from 18 studies with 2702

TABLE 8.1 Characteristics of Adult Learners

Characteristics	Application to Health Education
Need to Know Adults must know why they need to learn.	The nurse explores reasons that individuals, families, and groups want to learn and identifies learning needs.
Concept of Self Adults have a self-concept that develops from dependence to independence. It moves from others' direction to self-direction. Adults want to be capable of self-direction.	The nurse acknowledges that individuals, families, and groups can make choices and decisions. The nurse creates an environment in which patients can express themselves. The nurse recognizes that individuals, families, and groups can learn from their selected actions and can take self-direction and responsibility for their behaviors.
Learning From Experience Adults can draw on many life experiences. Such experiences are enriching and are powerful learning resources.	The nurse assesses individuals, families, and groups for life and worldview experiences related to health issues. The nurse helps facilitate connections between previous and present experiences. The nurse allows individuals, families, and groups to share experiences with others in a supportive and trustworthy manner. The nurse leverages experiential-learning methods, problem solving, and case-studies to uncover learners' experiences. The nurse clarifies previous and present experiences; this is especially helpful with negative and/or positive past experiences that may impact learning outcomes.
Readiness to Learn Developmental tasks and social roles affect readiness to learn. The timing of learning experiences with developmental tasks is important.	The nurse assesses and identifies individual, family, and group roles (e.g., caregivers, or single parents) and key developmental tasks. The nurse finds out what matters. The nurse seeks to understand the impact of roles and tasks on learning. The nurse supports individuals, families, and groups to learn according to their social, work or family roles and developmental age the nurse creates role-modeling experiences.
Orientation to Learning Learning is often present oriented and "now" based. Learning is directed to the immediate need and is problem centered to immediate application to everyday life.	The nurse assesses the learning needs of individuals, families, and groups based on learning priority. The nurse recognizes everyday stresses and hassles and addresses them within the learning context. The nurse provides health information, gives responses to their immediate needs, offers/provides health information, and offers problem-solving skills.
Motivation Internal drivers and factors are powerful motivators (e.g., self-esteem, life goals, quality of life, and responsibility).	The nurse determines individual, family, and group internal motivators. The nurse assesses for impediments that block motivation (e.g., poor self-esteem or lack of resources) and provides appropriate education, counseling, support, and referrals to optimize motivation

Modified from Knowles MS: *The making of an adult educator: an autobiographical journey*, San Francisco, 1989, Jossey-Bass; Knowles MS: *The modern practice of adult education: from pedagogy to andragogy*, Chicago, 1988, Cambridge Press.

TABLE 8.2 Health Belief Model (HBM)[a]

Components	Example and Explanation
Perceived susceptibility[a]	Belief that disease state or a health problem is present or likely to occur
Perceived severity[a]	Perception that disease state or health problem/condition is harmful and has serious consequences
Perceived benefits[a]	Belief that health action is of value and has efficacy, for example, walking contributes to fitness
Perceived barriers[a]	Belief that health action is associated with hindrances (e.g., cost, fear of cancer)
Self-efficacy	Belief that actions can be performed to achieve the desired outcome (one's confidence in carrying out a behavior).
Modifying factors (demographic, psychosocial, structural)	Such as age, gender, race/ethnicity, educational attainment, socio-economic status, experience, motivation, discrimination/racism, where one lives ("place") etc.
Cues to action	Influencing factors to get ready for action (e.g., educational materials, text messaging, billboards, newspapers, computer apps, blogs, reminders, etc.)

[a]For a more detailed description of the HBM and the original components, see Becker MH, editor: *The health belief model and personal health behavior*, Thorofare, NJ, 1974, Charles B. Slack.

subjects), it was found that benefits and barriers were the strongest predictors of behaviors over time (Carpenter, 2010).

Champion and Skinner (2008) point out that one of the limitations of the HBM is the variability in measurement of the central HBM constructs, which include the inconsistent measurement of HBM concepts and the failure to establish the validity and reliability of the measures before testing. For example, applying similar construct measures across different behaviors, such as barriers for mammography and colonoscopy, may be quite different. The past decades have produced some good examples of HBM scale development (Champion et al., 2008a,b, 2016; Rawl et al., 2012, 2015), yet caution in the application of the HBM to multicultural settings is warranted. It would be important to determine whether the overall assumptions of the HBM—assumptions related to the value of health and illness—are like those of the racial/ethnic group under study. Although the HBM identifies an array of variables important in explaining individual health, nurses should view these variables within a larger societal perspective. Checking for cultural distinctions is especially critical to the model's usefulness among diverse racial/ethnic groups (Brenner et al., 2015) and is even more important today considering our demographically changing landscape.

Pender's HPM is a competence- or approach-oriented model first appearing in the nursing literature in 1982. The HPM brings together numerous constructs from expectancy-value theory and social cognitive theory within a holistic nursing framework. Unlike the HBM, it does not rely on personal threat as a motivating factor. Rather, it aims to explain why individuals engage in health actions. The central focus of the model is based on individual characteristics and experience, behavior-specific cognitions and affect, and behavioral outcomes that can be assessed by the nurse and that serve as key points for nursing intervention (Pender et al., 2015; Murdaugh et al., 2019). The model is contextually driven with wide applicability across the lifespan and has been used to examine the multidimensional nature of persons interacting with their physical and interpersonal environments. For example, it was used in studies to identify factors that enhance health-promoting behaviors of military spouses (Padden et al., 2013); to investigate the effect of a 17-week *Girls on the Move* (GOTM) intervention on increasing moderate-to-vigorous physical activity (MVPA) among fifth- to eighth-grade girls ($n = 1519$) in racially/ethnically diverse public schools in urban, underserved areas of the Midwestern US (Robbins et al., 2019). Or see how the HPM was applied to predict and detect factors among older adults' participation in community-based health promotion activities. Data collected among 139 older adults who attended a community care center in Taoyuan City, Taiwan (mean age 72.7 years) indicated that age, perceived benefits, and self-efficacy were significant predictors of participation in health promotion activities with "perceived benefits" having the strongest association (Chen et al., 2021).

Table 8.3 lists the main components of the HPM and supplies their definitions. The HBM and HPM can facilitate community health nurses in examining an individual's health choices and decisions for influencing health-related behaviors. The models offer nurses a cluster of variables and helpful cues that provide insights into explaining health behavior. The nurse can consider them in planning programs, but should not try to fit an individual into all the categories. Simply put, models are frameworks that guide nurses in assessing patients and groups for the development, selection, and implementation of relevant educational nursing interventions.

Try applying the model to your own life and health behaviors. Consider the following questions:

- Do you continually strive for improved health?
- Are you or your family susceptible to heart disease, diabetes, or obesity?
- Does a family history of cardiovascular disease motivate you or your family to exercise?
- What are your cholesterol and triglyceride numbers? What is your BP?
- Does looking fit and toned and having energy motivate you to exercise?
- Do work, school, or family responsibilities get in the way of your exercise plans?
- Has a family member, friend, or health provider recently reminded you of the benefits of exercise and encouraged you to start exercising?
- Do you believe you can initiate and incorporate a walking or running into your lifestyle, or do you need external reinforcement and cues?
- Do money, safety, or school commitments pose any impediments to exercise?
- What would make exercise more appealing, such as a "running app or having a running partner?"
- What do you see as the benefits to exercise, for example, looking and feeling better and having more energy?
- In modifying your health behaviors, how important is exercise compared with other behaviors (e.g., getting relief from work and school stresses, cutting down on snacks, spending quality and fun time with your family and friends)?

Think about these questions and consider your answers. Talk about this behavior with a peer and develop an exercise *action* plan that is personalized to your own priorities, needs, abilities, available time, and interests. Be specific in creating a plan and goals. Importantly, make it enjoyable and sustainable!

Model of Health Education Empowerment

The HBM and HPM focus on individual strategies for achieving optimal health and well-being. The models are similar in that they are multifactorial; are based on the idea of value expectancy; and address individual perceptions, modifying factors, and likelihood of action. Although such approaches may be quite appropriate in changing individual behaviors, they do not necessarily address the complex relationships among social, structural, and physical factors in the environment, such as inadequate social support systems, racism, discrimination, and inaccessibility of health services (Devia et al., 2017; Israel et al., 2013; Minkler, 2012). Van Wyk (1999) suggests that nurses cannot assign power and control to the individual within the community, but, rather, that the "power" must be taken on by the individual and community with the nurse *guiding* this dynamic process. This process includes examination of such factors as education, health literacy, gender, racism, discrimination, social justice, and class and recognition of the structural and foundational changes, etc., that are needed to elicit change for socially and politically disenfranchised groups. Thus knowledge is produced in a social context, and it is inextricably bound to relations of power. Therefore an appropriate and more relevant health education

TABLE 8.3 Health Promotion Model (HPM) Components and Definitions[a]

Component	Definition and Example
Individual Characteristics and Experiences	
Prior behaviors	Amount and frequency of same/similar past behaviors
Personal factors (biological, psychological, and sociocultural)	Age, gender, sex, race/ethnicity, income, personality, socioeconomic status
Behavior—Specific Cognitions and Affect	
Activity-related affect (positive/negative)	Subjective feeling of emotions before, during, or after the health behavior
Interpersonal influences	Interactions with family, peers, and nurses: Influence on and perceptions about the behaviors
Situational factors	Perceptions of compatibility of life context or environmental determinants that make health-promoting options available and engaging
Perceived self-efficacy	Perceived ability to perform the necessary behaviors to achieve an outcome—judgment of personal capability
Perceived benefits of health-promoting behaviors	Perception of positive outcomes that can occur from health-promoting behavior (e.g., feel fit and toned)
Perceived barriers to health-promoting behaviors	Perception of things that obstruct health-promoting behaviors (e.g., money and transportation)
Commitment to plan of action	Intention to carry out a specific health behavior and identification of successful strategies to achieve it
Immediate competing demands and preferences	Competing demands and preferences are alternative behaviors that influence a course of action just before intended occurrence of planned behavior
	Competing demands are alternative behaviors over which people have low control versus competing preferences are alternative behaviors over which people have high control
Behavioral outcome	
Health-promoting behavior	Desired behavioral outcome, such as weight loss, improved decision making, screening, improved physical activity, etc.

[a]For a more comprehensive description and explanation of the HPM, see Pender NJ, Murdaugh CL, Parsons MA, Pender NJ: *Health promotion in nursing practice*, ed 8, Englewood Cliffs, NJ, 2019, Prentice Hall; Pender NJ, Murdaugh C, Parsons MA., et al.: *Health promotion in nursing practice*, ed 7, 2015, Pearson.

model may be one that embraces a broader definition of *health* and addresses social, political, and economic aspects of health. Such a theoretical perspective is highly congruent with current community health education practices because it supports learner participation, highlights community engagement, and emphasizes empowerment. In a consensus paper from the Academy of Nursing authored by Kuehnert and colleagues (2021), a conceptual framework is described that advances planetary health equity and planetary health equity quality of life and the importance of linking environmental concepts with social determinants of health as key influencers on health.

This framework, drawing from nursology, provides direction for nursing roles and actions at the individual, family, and population levels with an eye on supporting upstream, midstream and downstream nursing education actions for health policy change and with an emphasis on addressing systemic and structural racism.

Freire: A Focus on Problem-Solving Education

Empowerment and literacy are two concepts that have a common history. The concept of empowerment can be traced back to **Paulo Freire**, a Brazilian educator in the 1950s who sought to promote literacy among the poorest of the poor and most oppressed members of the population. He based his work on a problem-solving approach to education, which contrasts with what he called the "banking education approach," which often places the learner in a passive role. **Problem-solving education** allows active participation and ongoing dialogue and encourages learners to be critical of and reflective about health issues. Freire suggested that when individuals assume the role of objects, they often become powerless and allow the environment to control them. However, when individuals become *subjects*, they influence environmental factors that affect their lives and community. Thus community members, or subjects, are the best resources to elicit change (Freire, 2005).

Freire's methodology, often referred to as *critical consciousness*, involves not only education but also activism on the part of the educator. The basic tenet of Freire's work centers on empowerment; the contextualization of peoples' daily experiences; and collaborative, collegial dialog in adult education. Freire's work speaks to a variety of action research applications, including those that relate to improving community health of marginalized populations. Freire's approach to health education increases health knowledge through a participatory group process and emphasizes establishing sustainable lateral relationships. This process explores the problem's nature and addresses the problem's deeper issues. The nurse serves as a central resource person and becomes an equal partner with other group members. Listening is a first essential step to understanding the issues. This exchange of ideas and concerns then creates a problem-posing dialogue to identify core problems or generative themes. As this process moves along, the group further delves into the root causes. Finally, the group cocreates relevant action plans that are suitably aligned with their lives (Freire, 2000).

Nurses can use health education as an empowering strategy to help people develop skills in problem solving, critical thinking, networking, negotiating, lobbying, advocacy, policy-making, and information seeking to enhance health. Freire's approach may seem like health education's emphasis on helping people take responsibility for their health by providing them with information, skills, reinforcement, and support. However, Freire purports that knowledge imparted by the collective group is significantly more powerful than information provided by health educators. This learner-centered approach attempts to uncover the social and political aspects of problems and encourages group members to define and develop action strategies. Hence, there is keen recognition that health and behavior changes are multifaceted and usually do not have immediate solutions; therefore the term problem *posing*, rather than problem *solving*, better describes this empowerment process (Wallerstein et al., 2015). As Kark and Steuart (1962) once stated, "health education must achieve its ends through means that leave inviolate the rights of self-determination of the individuals and their community."

The goal of **participatory action research** (PAR) is social change. PAR is also quite consistent with the role and responsibilities of nurses who are engaged in community health (Olshansky et al., 2005) and embraces the use of community-based participatory methods. What this means is that participation and action from stakeholders and knowledge about conditions and issues help facilitate strategies reached collectively (e.g., access to care, access to information). By way of definition, stakeholders are individuals, groups, or organizations that have common and direct interests and concern in a topic, situation, or health outcome. Some examples of the use of PAR include the following projects: Marsh and colleagues (2017) described the use of PAR to inform the creation of a community garden that functioned as a therapeutic place for end-of-life and bereavement support. This work further informed the effective planning of community campus gardens based on input from community and university stakeholders, resulting in greater connections, psycho-social health and wellbeing and social equity in regions (Marsh et al, 2020). In another example, Zehbe and colleagues. (2016) developed a PAR project in collaboration with 11 Ojibwa and Oji-Cree First Nations—Anishinaabe—communities in Northwest Ontario, Canada, to promote cervical cancer screening through education that respectfully depicted female bodies, sexuality, and health behaviors through a First Nations lens.

❓ ACTIVE LEARNING

1. Identify a specific intended group in the community that you are interested in (e.g., people who are medically underserved, residents of rural communities, people who are experiencing homelessness, older adults age 80 and older, teen parents to be, adults who are transgender, children who are deaf, etc.).

a. Describe the group's characteristics, learning needs, and strengths.
b. Identify your methods for obtaining this information.
c. Next, describe the application of Freire's empowerment education model to address health education priorities. How would you engage them in determining learning priorities?

Examples of Empowerment Education and Participatory Methods

To illustrate the use of empowerment principles, consider the following projects: Moya and colleagues (2017) related how photovoice was used as a participatory research method with participants experiencing homelessness in El Paso Texas, referred to as "The Voices and Images of the Residents of the Opportunity Center for the Homeless: A Visual Project on the Identity and Challenges Homeless Adults Face on the Border Region." Four themes that represented their experiences as well as their aspirations were depicted in their pictures: (1) broken systems, (2) invisibility, (3) opportunities and what works, and (4) growth and determination. The photographs were then shown at a gallery along with narratives. Along with the photographs, a "call to action" was formulated that asked the community, policy, and decision makers to commit to change in the current social, economic, and political conditions affecting individuals experiencing homelessness. As such, the use of photovoice offered an important and creative way to facilitate shared knowledge to achieve social change.

Streuli and colleagues (2021) described a community codesign process used to create the educational content for a suitable virtual reality (VR) vaccination education tool for a Somali refugee population. Participatory methods included focus groups, interviews, and surveys among Somali community members and expert advisors. Key to the development of the vaccine (MMR) educational tool (directed toward MMR vaccine series) was involving the Somali community from project inception throughout project development including product testing to ensure cultural and linguistic relevance (i.e., storyline, imagery, use of prompts). The final product was a 4-minute health education 360 degrees video animation (https://youtu.be/NS8GvtxnIk0) available in Somali and English languages—which can be viewed online using a tablet, a smart phone or with VR goggles. Future research is planned to assess the efficacy of the VR.

Ross and Meier (2020) described a nurse-delivered intervention intended to improve older adult's coping with COVID-19. Using a convenience sample of 44 older adults from 14 states residing in the community, three interventions (data-gathering survey, a telehealth teach-back tool, and a telehealth listening tool) were implemented concurrently and studied through Plan—Do—Study—Act QI cycles. The original educational sessions centered on COVID-19 prevention, yet nurses identified new needs during implementation (e.g., loneliness related to social isolation resulting from the pandemic, etc.) and the educational sessions changed over time. Nurses empowered community members during the sessions and used teach-back and active listening to deliver information to community members. A total of 86% of participants reported learning something new, and 100% of participants reported feeling a connection with the nurse implementer. The impact of nurses went beyond information exchange and nurses made a social connection with community members experiencing loneliness.

Overall, these projects emphasize empowering principles that illustrate the wide range of settings, formats, and participatory methods that can be used to implement health education in the community. These papers also highlight the need for nurses to respond to emergent learning needs. Think for a moment how these approaches and methods could be used in your health education outreach activities.

Community Empowerment

Community empowerment is a central tenet of community organization, whereby community members take on greater power to create change. It is based on community cultural strengths and assets. An empowerment continuum acknowledges the value and interdependence of individual and political action strategies aimed at the collective while maintaining the community organization as central (Minkler et al., 2012). As such, community organization reinforces one of the field's underlying premises as outlined by Nyswander (1956): "Start where the people are." Furthermore, Labonte (1994)

states that the community is an engine of health promotion and a vehicle for empowerment. He describes five spheres of an empowerment model, which focus on the following levels of social organization: interpersonal (personal empowerment), intragroup (small-group development), intergroup (community), interorganizational (coalition building), and political action. A multilevel empowerment model allows us to consider both macro-level and micro-level forces that combine to create both health and disease. Therefore it seems that both micro- and macro-viewpoints on health education provide nurses with multiple opportunities for intervention across a broad continuum. In summary, health education activities that respond to McKinlay's (1979) call to study "upstream," that is, to examine the underlying causes of health inequalities through multilevel education and research allow nurses to be informed by critical perspectives from education, anthropology, and public health. For additional information on CBPR; view an excellent resource: *Community-Based Participatory Research for Health: Advancing Social and Health Equity* (Wallerstein et al., 2017).

To effect change at the community level, nurses should become familiar with and knowledgeable about key concepts central to community organization (Table 8.4). This approach is an effective methodological tool that enables nurses to

TABLE 8.4 Community Engagement and Organization Practice

Key Concepts	Application to Health Education (Nursing Actions)
Empowerment Help individuals, families, and groups gain insight and mastery over life situations through problem solving and dialogue.	The nurse works with community members in identifying and defining issues. The nurse creates mechanisms for discussion and problem solving and identifies other factors that have an impact on everyday lives.
Principle of Relevancy Know what issues are important to community members (these may differ from the issues important to nurses).	The nurse holds "town hall meetings" and/or community group discussions to allow members to share concerns, needs, and important issues. The nurse encourages community members to define issues (*what is important to them*). The nurse facilitates communications with community members to help them make decisions about health programs and messages.
Principle of Participation Learn by doing.	The nurse encourages group support. The nurse recognizes that active rather than passive participation results in greater likelihood of attitude and behavior changes.
Issue Selection Identify problems that the community believes are specific, meaningful, and attainable.	The nurse uses problem-solving techniques to help group members identify relevant issues and needs (e.g., group process activities, door-to-door surveys, charlas/talking circles).
Creation of Critical Consciousness Encourage relationships of equality and mutual respect among group members and educators to identify root problems and generate appropriate action plans.	The nurse uses problem-posing dialog (Freire, 2005) to understand root issues and devises creative and innovative methods to transform situations.
Social capital Foster relationships (networks) between community members (i.e., trust, engagement)	The nurse encourages community members to work together to improve social networks and social capital. Community members work together on a particular health gap in their community through partnership and trust-building and capacity building activities.

Modified from Wallerstein N, Minkler M, Carter-Edwards L., et al.: Improving health through community engagement organization and community building. In Glanz K, Rimer BK, Viswanath K, editors: *Health behavior: theory, research, and practice*, ed 5, San Francisco, 2015, Jossey-Bass; Minkler M, editor: *Community organizing and community building for health and welfare*, ed 3, 2012, Rutgers University Press.

partner with the community; identify common goals; develop strategies; and mobilize resources to increase community empowerment, capacity, and community competence. Key concepts inherent in community health education programming are empowerment, principle of participation, issue selection, principle of relevance, social capital, and creation of critical consciousness (Minkler et al., 2012).

The development of LUNA in Tampa, Florida, as described in Clinical Example 8.2, illustrates how the basic tenets of community need and organization fueled the development of a locally initiated group. LUNA represents a grassroots initiative to meet the needs of the growing numbers of Hispanic cancer survivors and serves as a model for nurses, researchers, and community advocates working with cancer survivors.

Clinical Example 8.2

Example of Community Empowerment-Collaboration-Participation: LUNA.

More than a decade ago (2002), a Latina nurse (Melba Martinez, RN, BSN), who had been diagnosed with breast cancer in 1995, started the first grassroots support group for Latinas in West Central Florida. The group began with five members and within the first year had 38 active members who attended monthly meetings. The group was initiated in response to an unmet need in the Tampa Bay area, that is, lack of education services for Latinas who had been diagnosed with breast cancer and who primarily spoke Spanish. Over the years, LUNA has grown and expanded to include Latinos with any type of cancer and incorporated as a nonprofit organization and has created a network of over 500 cancer survivors and partnered with other support programs in the area.

LUNA Inc. (Latinas Unidas por un Nuevo Amanecer, Inc.), mission is to provide emotional support and health education to cancer survivors and their families, friends, and caregivers from Latino/a/x communities of West Central Florida. The organization primarily serves underserved, Latinas with limited English proficiency; assists with navigating the healthcare system; and functions as a community resource. LUNA draws on the tenets of community organization and empowerment fueled by problem-posing education. The three components of the LUNA model are (1) education (e.g., classes and presentations, Spanish cancer information, healthcare navigation, community outreach); (2) support (e.g., peer to peer, home, hospital and phone visits, communications); and (3) social reintegration (e.g., celebration of life events such as birthdays, cancer camps, walks, and other social events), are similar to the features used for the startup of the ALS support group previously described.

Outcomes of LUNA

1. Campamento Alegria: The first-ever Spanish-language oncology camp for Latina cancer survivors. A biennial program designed to provide Latinas in whom cancer has been diagnosed a positive and unforgettable experience through a variety of activities that help sustain them through their cancer journey (Martinez et al., 2008). Campamento Alegria aims to serve 100 women who would otherwise not have the opportunity to participate in such activities. There are no fees for the patients/survivors for a

Clinical Example 8.2—cont'd

3-day/2-night stay at the retreat facility, meals and related activities, orientation, and reunion meeting.
2. Community education and outreach: Attendance at various community events and health fairs to increase breast cancer screening awareness and provide cancer information and resources in Spanish. These events are popular, and attendance increases each year.
3. Ongoing monthly educational support group meetings are in person and virtually via Zoom. Presentations and classes provided by Spanish-speaking health professionals on various survivorship issues and cancer-related topics.
4. Plans to develop a patient navigator program for Latina patients with newly diagnosed cancer.

The process for creating LUNA began with one nurse who, through dedication and dialogue with others in the same situation, began taking charge of the situation based on input from other community members. From both her nursing and personal experiences, she knew how hard it was for Hispanic women in whom cancer was diagnosed to navigate the healthcare system, how difficult it is to take time for self-care, and how challenging it was for Hispanic women to talk about their fears. She recognized that Latinas with breast cancer should reach out to one another with understanding and compassion in their own language to move toward self-education and self-actualization. Since its inception, LUNA has partnered with various community-based organizations, hospitals, academic centers, churches, and other social support services to create a strong web of support. For example, LUNA has a strong partnership with researchers from the TBCCN, a community network program funded by the NCI's Center to Reduce Cancer Health Disparities, as well as with local hospitals. LUNA also has worked with researchers to understand the information needs of women undergoing chemotherapy and to transcreate a stress management program for Latinas undergoing chemotherapy (Hoogland et al., 2018; Martinez et al., 2016), which was evaluated in a multisite clinical trial. LUNA represents a ground-up effort, which got its start because someone (a nurse) listened to the needs of Hispanic cancer survivors. It serves as an excellent model and reminder for nurses, researchers, and community advocates that the best ideas come from the "soul." For more information, view https://www.lunacancerfl.org.

Never doubt that a small group of thoughtful, committed citizens can change the world. Indeed, it is the only thing that ever has.

Margaret Mead.

Acknowledgments: Melba Martinez, RN, BSN, and Dinorah (Dina) Martinez-Tyson, MA, MPH, PhD.

THE NURSE'S ROLE IN HEALTH EDUCATION

Although learning theories and health education models provide a useful framework for planning health interventions, the nurse's ability to facilitate the education process and become a partner with individuals and communities is inherently significant to the method's application for overall population health (Clinical Example 8.3). At the core of health education is the therapeutic relationship between the nurse and individuals, families, and the community. Simply put, nurses hold the process together and are trusted change agents in delivering humanistic care. Nurses activate ideas, offer appropriate interventions, identify resources, and facilitate group empowerment. It is beyond the scope of this chapter to describe multiple communication techniques in detail, but the reader is reminded of the value of establishing "inclusion and trust" before delivering health education content.

Clinical Example 8.3

Mr. Chen is new to the area and starts to visit the local neighborhood community center weekly to play cards and have lunch with his brothers, who have lived in the area for several years. Adjacent to the center (men call it "the club") is a nurse-managed clinic, which was started more than 20 years ago by the college of nursing at the local university. The clinic offers education and free or low-cost screenings on a regular basis. Many community members take advantage of this convenient service for their primary care. Mr. Chen has limited resources, so this community resource provides him with valuable access to healthcare services and information. On his first visit to the clinic, Mr. Chen is seen by a nursing student (Jong) and his blood pressure is 174/92 mm Hg. He states that the public hospital that cared for him in another city treated him for high blood pressure for more than 7 years, that doctors prescribed several medications 6 months earlier, and that he received many written materials to read (they were all in English). Although he reads somewhat in English, he tells the nurse that it would have been nice to see materials in his familiar and native Chinese language.

The nurse's assessment reveals that Mr. Chen takes his medication only when he does not "feel so good." He said his doctor advised him to take his medicines regularly, and he states that he takes them faithfully when he does not feel well. He tells the nurse that he remembers getting some educational booklets about his medications and "blood," but he found them long and tiring to read. Jong's educational assessment reveals that Mr. Chen has completed 8 years of schooling, does not read much, enjoys television over print, and likes to learn from pictures or from other people in groups. He rarely uses a computer except to get email messages from his daughter. He states that he would really like to get his health information in easy English but would mostly prefer to get some easy materials in Chinese. His reading skills have not been verified by health providers and he states that he is not confident in being able to read all the health materials that are given to him. Yet it seems that he has taken the health instruction literally (e.g., he interprets "take regularly" to mean take consistently when "I don't feel right" vs. take the pills on a regular schedule). He states his is interested in learning some basic computer skills.

To facilitate learning, the Park establishes a teaching plan with Mr. Chen's input. Jong also notes that e-health literacy is often low due to several influencing factors such as language, background, and not having been taught (Shi et al., 2021). This patient-centric plan involves communicating health instructions in more relevant ways (e.g., using pictures, drawings, mnemonics, videos), providing word cards for him in Chinese with the help of the local translation services, and putting him in touch with county financial resources to assist in buying his medicines. The nurse also establishes a follow-up plan with a bilingual nurse to verify Mr. Chen's understanding of how to take his medications by asking him to repeat back in his own words when/how he takes them (teach-back method). Jong also plans to develop a series of health education group classes at "the club" about health and wellness, with high blood pressure as one of the topics of discussion; and start a series of classes in collaboration with the neighborhood library to boost computer literacy and teach Internet search skills.

ENHANCING COMMUNICATION

The critical step of *inclusion* establishes the base for possible health action; it "sets" the relationship. What this means is that the nurse needs to be especially cognizant of those first introductory oral exchanges and interactions. Inclusion may simply entail greeting individuals, families, and groups in a warm fashion; offering comfort; and attending to their immediate concerns or worries. Education does not begin with the first instructional word. Rather, education begins with establishing an atmosphere conducive to learning, whereby a therapeutic trusting relationship forms the foundation for a healing and colearning relationship. If the nurse attends to *inclusion* first, individuals, families, and groups next begin to *trust* the nurse and thereby trust the *content* of the health education message. This trust is evident through active engagement in and commitment to the education process.

It is important to note that the ongoing enhancement and refinement of nursing knowledge and skills to provide **culturally effective and responsive care** is critical to community health education. Nurses are fundamental in responding to community members' everyday health concerns with meaningful, understandable, and actionable information. This involves taking time to get to know individuals, their families, and their everyday lived experiences.

Meleis (1999) describes culturally competent care as care that exhibits sensitivity to individuals based on their vast experiences and their responses, which are due to their backgrounds, sexual orientation, gender identity, socioeconomic status, ethnicity, literacy, and cultural background to name a few. She depicts several properties that make up the "essence of health nurses" who deliver culturally competent care. First, they possess an explanatory system that values diversity. This is a system that is not drained by the constant attempt to interpret symbols, but rather is energized by the variations. Second, they show expert assessment skills to discern different and similar patterns of responses that help in planning appropriate educational interventions. Third, culturally competent nurses are aware of the diversity of communication patterns and how language and communication influence "trust within the relationship."

For more information on the provision of CLAS and healthcare standards, view the updated (last modified

Continued

November 2018), enhanced 15 standards (USDHHS OMH, 2018) that represent a comprehensive series of guidelines to improve healthcare quality and advance health equity among the nation's increasingly diverse communities. a (https://www. thinkculturalhealth.hhs.gov/). These standards were created in response to growing concerns about health inequities and the need for healthcare systems to reach increasingly diverse patient populations. The standards reinforce the ability of nurses and organizations to understand and respond well to the cultural and linguistic needs brought by patients and community members to the healthcare setting. Several standards have strong relevance to community nursing. For example, Standard one signifies the importance of providing effective, equitable, understandable, and respectful quality care and services to people who have varied cultural health beliefs and practices, preferred languages, **health literacy**, and other communication preferences. And bear in mind that cultural effectiveness and responsiveness is an ongoing journey that requires an openness to acknowledge what one does not know and the willingness to seek better ways to get the job done. It is a process, not simply a program or an end point. Consider also how **health literacy** is an ethical and pressing issue of concern in the community and how it too contributes to health equity.

ETHICAL INSIGHTS

Ethical Issues Related to Health Education and Health Literacy

Health literacy—Do community members understand the printed, digital, and oral health messages communicated to them in terms of language, ease of reading, and linguistics? Are these communications helpful to their decision making? To address the national problem of health literacy, nurses should assess their roles as educators, information brokers, advocates, facilitators, collaborative problem-solvers, and navigators. Nurses should consider the impact that the multitude of demands of the healthcare system has on client autonomy. To explain, health literacy universal precautions refer to strategies to reduce the complexity of healthcare, increase patient understanding of health information, and enhance support for patients of all health literacy. View the Agency for Healthcare Research and Quality website at https://www.ahrq.gov/health-literacy/improve/precautions/index.html.

Individual versus collective/societal rights and responsibility for health—What communication factors should the nurse consider when balancing the health education needs of the individual against those of the collective (e.g., family and community)? What communication gaps can be bridged by the development and implementation of health information that is relevant culturally, linguistically, and in terms of literacy?

Social justice and equity—Do all community members enjoy equity in their access to health education and information? What types of language-specific materials are available? What strategies, programs, and evidence-based interventions are available to reduce the discovery-to-delivery disconnect? How can nurses play a role in reducing the literacy demands of an organization? How might navigation strategies be useful?

Allocation of resources—In what way do policies promote and/or hinder promotion of health literacy? Do national/local government and corporate/institutional policies affect the availability, accessibility, and equitable distribution of information resources? In what way do current policies

reward and support patient education? How can nurses get involved in shaping and redirecting health policy and moving policy into practice? This includes policies at the institutional, community, local, and national levels.

Cultural effectiveness and responsiveness—What skills, knowledge, and experiences are necessary to the planning and delivery of health education within the context of people's history and everyday realities? How might nurses promote access to nondigital and digital materials/media to support and advance community health? Nurses should assess their health education tasks with confidence, compassion, competence, and cultural humility with a lens on inclusivity (Levin-Zamir and Bertschi, 2018; USDHHS OMH, 2018)

❓ ACTIVE LEARNING

Discuss how you envision the role of the nurse in health education. Outline specific nursing activities and roles that can produce a colearning environment. Share with one another what factors might enhance/impede the cultural and literacy responsiveness of this central role.

FRAMEWORK FOR DEVELOPING HEALTH COMMUNICATIONS

Within the community, the nurse's intended learning audience may be an individual, family, group, or many segments of the community. Using a systematic approach to the development, design, and delivery of health education programs provides the nurse with an organized, user-friendly way to deliver health messages. Although nurses may select and use a variety of educational models, theoretical frameworks, and teaching and learning principles, the "Framework for Developing Health Communications" to create a variety of health education messages and programs may be a particularly helpful tool (USDHHS, 2008: https://www.cancer.gov/publications/health-communication).

This organizing framework has four stages and is depicted by a circular loop that offers the opportunity for continuous assessment, feedback, and improvement. The framework has been used widely by the author to develop cancer education materials and media on such topics as smoking, biobanking, cancer screening, stress management, clinical trials to name a few (Fleming et al., 2018; Hoogland et al., 2018; Meltzer et al., 2021; Meade et al., 2015; Wells et al., 2015). This framework can be easily adapted to the design and development of all types of health education topics, such as diabetes, hypertension, HIV, vaccines, and nutrition.

This framework is based on the principles of social marketing and health education and on mass communication theories, and it relies on intended audience assessment to guide the process. It is highly congruent with Freire's model of empowerment education, which encourages ongoing dialogue with potential consumers and users of health education services. Although this model focuses on communication strategies aimed at the programmatic level, the basic elements are applicable to individual, family, and group systems. Do not expect to apply the model in a linear manner, but rather to move back and forth between the stages. These stages mirror the nursing process (assessment, planning, implementation, and evaluation) and provide a practical, sequential, and organized path for continuous assessment, feedback, and improvement toward achieving a successful health education communication program (Clinical Example 8.4 and Fig. 8.1).

Clinical Example 8.4

The H. Lee Moffitt Cancer Center and Research Institute, or Moffitt, formed a partnership with Suncoast Community Health Centers, Inc., or Suncoast, in rural Hillsborough County, Florida. The partnership initially brought breast cancer education and screening services to Hispanic migrant and seasonal farmworkers, many who experience poverty, via Moffitt's Lifetime Cancer Screening Mobile Unit. Initiated by a cancer center physician who visited Suncoast, a federally funded, community-based center located about 30 miles south of Tampa, he was struck by the center's services and impressed with the clinic's dedication to reaching medically underserved populations. Suncoast consisted of multiple comprehensive federally qualified healthcare clinics in Plant City, Ruskin, Brandon, and Dover, Florida, and offered a wide range of primary healthcare services, yet it did not have mammography facilities. Moffitt was expanding its community outreach initiatives through mobile outreach services and through the addition of nurses and outreach workers. Moffitt, is a freestanding, private, nonprofit NCI-designated comprehensive cancer center, located at the University of South Florida campus in Tampa. After a series of meetings between Suncoast and Moffitt's Cancer Screening Center, the groups formed a partnership based on a mutually shared cancer prevention goal—to improve the breast health of high-risk and medically underserved women. Both parties determined that the goal was to develop and offer community culturally appropriate education, accessible mammography service, and follow-up care.

Description of Health Issue and Intended Audience

Despite progress in the fight against cancer, many communities continue to bear a disproportionate share of the cancer burden. Cancer disparities, like many other health disparities arise from the complex interplay of factors (i.e., determinants of health)—such as economic stability, education access and quality, healthcare access and quality, neighborhood and built environment, and social and community factors) that impede awareness about screening and follow-up care (Healthy People, 2030: https://health.gov/healthypeople/objectives-and-data/social-determinants-health). Together, these factors affect access to care and cancer survival and yield an uneven distribution of cancer morbidity and mortality, which substantially affects disparate populations (American Cancer Society, 2021; Braun et al., 2015; Kuehnert et al., 2021). Thus it is critical to layer on additional levels of understanding of and sensitivity to the myriad social, cultural, environmental, and political conditions of home countries, language and literacy

needs, obstacles to basic healthcare access, cultural significance of gender and age roles, culturally mediated etiologic perceptions of disease, illness experiences, religiosity, and the sociopolitical nature of immigration situations. Such considerations affect the design and meaning of health communication and health education.

Our assessment revealed that many women did not show up for breast screenings because of a "fear of cancer" and uncertainty of how to navigate the healthcare system. Many did not seek preventive healthcare, but rather sought care for episodic acute illnesses. The lack of mammography screening and education for Hillsborough County's medically underserved women living in a rural setting represented a significant health service gap. Educational and communication interventions and tools that address (1) belief and value systems, (2) relevant and specific cultural, literacy and language/linguistic factors, and (3) access issues—as well as that capitalize on the strengths of the women—were needed. Our experiences reminded us that women wanted and needed information about breast health but that they also experienced everyday struggles. As such, peer outreach/navigation was a key strategy to deconstruct those concerns and engage community members in their health.

What was required was the delivery of a culturally relevant health service in a geographically convenient area. Women aged 40 years and older were eligible for this service. The initial intended audience was primarily Hispanic migrant and seasonal farmworkers but also grew to include women from other racial/ethnic backgrounds and from rural settings (i.e., Haitian, white).

Goal: To prevent premature death and disability from breast cancer through early detection, screening, and culturally and linguistically relevant education.

Objectives: To increase education, mammograms, clinical breast examinations, and follow-up programs among medically underserved women in rural Hillsborough County.

Selecting Channels and Methods

A combination of channels to communicate health information about breast cancer, screenings, and early detection methods were examined (e.g., community-based clinics, missions, social service agencies, health events, and fairs). Nurses conducted individual interactions at the mobile or stationary site at the screening center. They also collected a variety of health materials and media about breast cancer from national, state, and local sources. However, many printed materials were geared toward higher reading levels, and few were available in Spanish or Haitian Creole.

Developing Materials

Grants from Avon, National Alliance of Breast Cancer Organizations, Susan G. Komen for the Cure Florida Suncoast Affiliate, and NCI supported the development of English, Spanish, and Haitian Creole materials to educate women about breast health. Additionally, although translators were sporadically present, it became apparent that bilingual/bicultural staff was necessary. Ongoing dialogue with community members and clinics helped refine the screening process, the education component, and follow-up services to ensure

Continued

Clinical Example 8.4—cont'd

effectiveness, efficiency, appropriateness, and timely follow-up.

Implementation

The mass media publicizes the services and disseminates human-interest stories, especially during October—Breast Cancer Awareness Month. The outreach workers posted flyers at a variety of sites (e.g., beauty shops, laundromats, missions, churches, grocery stores, churches, unemployment offices, and community centers). Twice per month, the mobile unit traveled to rural areas. There, staff greeted women and answered questions about the mammography procedure and follow-up.

Assessing Efficiency
Process Evaluation

Newspapers/flyers, television, and radio advertisements publicized the free or low-cost mammography service and highlighted the importance of breast health. Also, several human-interest stories emerged, which communicated the screening services to a wider audience. Since the onset of the program, increases in the number of staff involved in the program, the number of volunteers, and the number of funded projects that supported the program enhanced its breadth and depth and sparked the development of new initiatives.

Notably, this early community partnership provided an exceptional foundation for the establishment of the Tampa Bay Community Cancer Network (TBCCN), a community-academic network established in 2005 (Suncoast was one of the founding members). TBCCN has served as a springboard to address community health concerns about cancer prevention. As a result of community partner needs assessments, Gwede et al. (2010); Simmons et al. (2015) cancer education workshops, health events, cancer services, and research were broadened and evaluated.

For example, funding for a Patient Research Navigation Program augmented outreach efforts. Designed to eliminate barriers to cancer diagnosis and treatment, this project generated new knowledge for the advancement of an evidence-based, culturally and literacy appropriate, lay navigation program for community members who had a breast/colorectal cancer abnormality by evaluating timeliness to resolution of abnormality and enhancing timeliness to diagnosis and delivery of cancer care (Meade et al., 2014; Wells et al., 2011, 2015). Or based on an identified community need for increasing colorectal cancer screening, a series of nurse-led studies were carried out in community clinics and demonstrated increases in CRC screening uptake through the delivery of evidence-based interventions (language-specific education plus provision of a FIT (Christy et al., 2016; Davis et al., 2016; Gwede et al., 2019).

Outcome Evaluation

During the mammography screening program's initial years, fewer than 200 women received mammography screening per year. The number of women screened approached more than 1000 per year in subsequent years. Currently, mammography services are provided at stationary screening sites at the cancer center through the cancer center's

Clinical Example 8.4—cont'd

mammography referral and voucher program)—funding opportunities and institutional support sustain the program. The number of community partners has grown considerably, a reflection of enhanced community capacity and awareness. Regular health events are scheduled; refinement of screening services and follow-up are ongoing.

Feedback

Reports describing process and outcome evaluation and analysis provide a point of reference for continual improvements. Such reports apply knowledge and outline methods to enhance and improve the service's efficiency and effectiveness. The mammography program has incorporated a network of outreach and educational components to reach migrant and seasonal farmworkers and has now extended its efforts to other medically underserved groups within the cancer center's catchment area. Although the program provided desired links to screening services and has formed successful community partnerships, it was important to develop and continually refine community empowerment strategies through outreach and education to sustain and widely disseminate the program. A key lesson learned here is that community outreach, based on trust, respect, and mutual commitment, can fuel community-identified health education and research priorities and lead to the testing and evaluating of evidence-based interventions for community benefit.

- The reader is encouraged to think about how health education messages or outreach programs can be planned in using this model. The exercise in Fig. 8.1 can be helpful to organize your ideas.

Stage I: Planning and Strategy Development

The planning stage provides the foundation for a communication program's planning process and is crucial in setting the stage for creating salient communications. Understanding the intended audience's learning needs and targeting the program or message to the audience are pivotal to activating effective health education. This step reinforces Freire's philosophical tenets of ascertaining an audience's needs and creating open dialogue. This stage also reduces expensive alterations once the program is under way.

Questions to Ask

- Who is the intended audience?
- What is known about the audience and from what sources?
- What are the communication and education objectives and goals?
- What evaluation strategies will the nurse use?
- What are the issues of most concern? (Note: These may not necessarily be health issues but may be important ones to link to the health issue when planning, e.g., safety, transportation).
- What is the health issue of interest?

Instructions: Think about a target group that you are currently working with and planning to deliver/create a health education program or message. Complete the exercise by asking yourself the following questions:

Questions to Ask

Action Plan

• **What is the overall intended message/goal?** (What are my reasons for planning this message? How do I know that it is needed or wanted by the audience?)

• **Who is the intended audience?** (Write a brief statement describing the characteristics of the group.)

• **What are the benefits of this message to the group?**

• **What channels will I use to deliver the message?** (Provide a rationale.)

• **Will I need to create materials?** (Are there available materials that are appropriate for the group?)

• **How will I know if my message gets across to the audience?** (Did the audience respond? How many people were reached? Who responded?)

• **Was there change?** (What are the reasons the message was or was not effective? What can be modified to strengthen the message?)

Fig. 8.1 Planning your health education message.

Collaborative Actions to Take

- Review available data from health statistics, census data, local sources, libraries, newspapers, and local or community leaders/stakeholders.
- Get community partners involved. Form advisory groups.
- Obtain new data (e.g., interviews, talking circles, surveys, and focus groups using problem-posing dialogue format).
- Determine the intended group's needs and perceptions of health problems (i.e., identify audiences).
- Determine the community's assets and strengths:
  - Physical (e.g., gender, age, and health history)
  - Behavioral (e.g., lifestyle characteristics and health-related activities)
  - Demographic (e.g., income, years of schooling, preferred language, and cultural characteristics, place of residence)
  - Psychographics (e.g., beliefs, values, and attitudes)
  - Identify issues behind the issues and identify health knowledge gaps.
  - Establish goals and objectives that are specific, attainable, prioritized, and time specific.
  - Assess resources (e.g., money, staff, and materials).

Stage II: Developing and Pretesting Concepts, Messages, and Materials

The nurse's decisions in stage I can help guide in the selection of appropriate communication channels and producing of effective and relevant materials. Consider how to reach the intended audience and use interesting and engaging supporting materials and media. *Channel* refers to how the nurse reaches communication sites or venues (i.e., churches, clinics, missions, other nurses, or community-based organizations, or digital platforms). *Format* refers to how the nurse communicates the health message (e.g., through individual or group discussion) (Table 8.5). Keep in mind that **materials and media** are the program's tools, not the program itself (Table 8.6). Education is a human activity and should not focus on materials/media exclusively. To ensure that messages are relevant and meaningful, the nurse can employ qualitative research methods (pretesting, learner verification) to obtain feedback about the understandability and acceptability of the materials). Learning now what works and does not work saves a lot of time and money later!

TABLE 8.5 Teaching-Learning Formats

Teaching Format	Application to Health Education
Brainstorming session	Allows participants the freedom to generate ideas and discuss them in a group setting.
	Cultivates creativity.
	Promotes empowerment to allow members to identify health issues and find solutions.
Community-wide programs	Reaches large numbers of community members through a systematic plan.
	Includes individual or group approaches with a defined intended audience.
Demonstration	Effective in learning perceptual motor skills.
	Aids in visual identification.
	Encourages sense of mastery.
Group discussion	Members can learn from each other and receive support. Nurses can personalize teaching content to group needs.
	Ideal for groups combining patients and families. Nurses, health professionals, or lay members can lead the groups.
	Facilitator must be comfortable with group method and familiar with group characteristics.
Lecture	Varying group sizes can use formal oral presentations.
	Group members share expertise and experiences.
	Presenter must be comfortable and possess speaking ability.
	Requires organizational skills and ability to highlight key points in interesting and creative ways.
	A combination of lecture media may enhance learning.
	Audience participation is linked to the presenter's speaking style and ability.
	Audience feedback is limited.
Individual discussion	Allows individual assessment and identification of cultural barriers, physical impairments, learning needs, knowledge and awareness, literacy, and anxiety.
	Promotes the tailoring of health education plans.
	Ideal to capture "teachable moments."
	Does not allow sharing and support from others.
	High cost in terms of staff time.
Role playing	Effective in influencing attitudes and opinions.
	Encourages problem-solving and critical thinking skills.
	Enhances learner participation. Some members may be hesitant to become involved.
Task force committees/community organizing meetings/community advisory groups	Joins individuals with diverse backgrounds and expertise to achieve a goal.
	Represent many interests and perspectives (collective wisdom)
Talking circles/charlas	Engages people in small group discussions (May be held in convenient settings such as missions, homes, or library settings.
Town hall meetings (online or in person)	Offer shared experiences in familiar settings, schools, community sites, gardens. Can connect to technologies.
Citizen science meetings combine project tasks and engagement of participants (scientists, educators, nurses, etc.)	Allows different perspectives and support from others.
(Kloetze et al., 2021)	

Data from Rankin SH, et al.: *Patient education in health and illness*, ed 5, Philadelphia, PA, 2005, Lippincott Williams and Wilkins, etc.; Redman BK: *The practice of patient education: a case study approach*, ed 10, St. Louis, 2007, Elsevier; U.S. Department of Health and Human Services: *Making health communication programs work: a planner's guide, pink book*, Bethesda, MD, 2008, Office of Cancer Communications, National Cancer Institute. Available from: https://www.cancer.gov/publications/health-communication/pink-book.pdf.

Questions to Ask

- What channels are best?
- What formats should be used?
- Are there existing resources?
- How can the nurse present the message?
- How will the audience react to the message?
- Will the audience understand, accept, and use the message?
- What changes/refinements can improve and optimize the message?

Collaborative Actions to Take

- Identify messages and materials.
- Decide whether to use existing materials or produce new ones.
- Select channels and formats.
- Develop relevant materials with the target audience.
- Pretest the message and materials and obtain audience feedback (e.g., through interviews, questionnaires, focus groups, and readability/usability testing). Pretesting helps ensure suitability (attraction, comprehension, cultural acceptability, persuasion, self-efficacy).

Stage III: Implementing the Program

At the third stage, the nurse introduces the health education message and program to the intended audience, reviews and

TABLE 8.6   Materials and Media

Media	Considerations in Health Education Settings
Audio response system (ARS) Web-based personal response systems	Allows high interactivity and participation among audience. Personal response systems offer accessible data collection and assessment tools such as ARSs and web-based interactive live polling platforms (e.g., Mentimeter, poll everywhere, meeting pulse, quizizz, etc.). Helps assess immediate understanding and redirect learning (Leprevost et al., 2021).
Audiotapes	Do not require reading. Portable and small. Individuals can use them at home in a comfortable setting and replay and use them at their own pace. Helpful for individuals with visual difficulties or low literacy skills.
Bulletin boards	Inexpensive and easy to develop. Direct attention to a specific message; use few words.
Demonstrations	Helpful when conveying psychomotor skills; encourage patient involvement and tactile learning (e.g., penis model for condom placement or breast model to show breast self-examination, or "mini" portable toilet to show how to collect a stool specimen using FIT kit). Note: Our team has used this teaching tool at a variety of health fairs/activities and it is widely popular! No reading is needed. Promotes sense of mastery right on the spot.
Digital health technologies (e-health, m-health, telehealth	New communication technologies create opportunities to reach communities virtually and improve experiences of patients, caregivers, and groups while adapting to user of new communication tools. These include collaborative team communication tools (e.g., slack, Microsoft teams, Google docs), engagement platforms and video conferencing apps (Zoom, WebEx, Google meet), collaborative whiteboards (Mural, lucidspark, Miro), and other virtual communication technologies.
Exhibits and displays	Graphics offer appeal. Placement in high-traffic areas (e.g., waiting rooms and examination rooms) reach wide audiences.
Flip charts, chalkboards, and whiteboards	Excellent format to enlarge teaching concepts or cue reader to salient points; graphics and diagrams may be added Chalkboards are reusable; flip charts have replacement pads, so inexpensive. Tech-oriented alternatives (slides or digital interactive whiteboards) are also available in many classroom settings
Games, simulations, animations,	Involve patients in a fun manner; involve the entire family. Highly effective with children.
Graphics Drawings and visuals	Can convey important points in salient and visual fashion. Can aid understanding for low-literacy audiences. Visual messages should be pretested to ensure acceptability and understanding.
Journal clubs (community-academic)	Facilitates understanding of varying concepts in an interactive way (e.g., health disparities, screening, literacy, science, technology). Brings into play perspectives from various stakeholders (e.g., community-academic discussions).
Interactive media, e-health: (Embodied conversational agents (ECAs), tablets, kiosks	A variety of computer programs, talking touch screens, interactive kiosks, conversational agents, computer-assisted instructive media, e-coaching, mobile tablet technology based, etc. Algorithms and branching decisions can aid patients in motivation, decision making, problem solving, and fact acquisition. Brings information directly to people. Consideration of patients' interests and preferences for receiving information, as well as their computer/technology use comfort level is needed.
Models and real objects Storytelling/playback theater/narratives	Bring the teaching concept to the patient in a familiar way. Incorporate models and real objects into teaching. Reading is minimal. Encourages questions and elicits insights (Cueva et al. 2016) helpful in individual and group instruction and can also take shape as digital storytelling (Mojtahedzadeh et al., 2021).
Photographs, picture books, pictographs, and slide series (i.e., PowerPoint slides); photo-essay and photovoice prezi presentations	Help promote understanding and empowerment by showing realistic images and real situations. Help patients make connections to their lives. May help elicit individual, relational, community, organizational, and societal levels of a socioecological model that inform health. Photographs may appear alone or in combination with other photographs, or slides or may be placed in an album, ppt, or digital loop (Leung et al. 2017). PowerPoint slides are easily updated. Helpful for patients with limited literacy skills; offer visual presentation of concepts. Effective with an individual and with small groups (i.e., self-study or reflection). Easily updated and visually appealing.

Continued

TABLE 8.6   Materials and Media—cont'd

Media	Considerations in Health Education Settings
Printed materials (brochures, leaflets, or booklets)	Portable, widely available, and economical.
	Useful in reinforcing health concepts and interactions. Printed text continues to be a convenient and familiar way to send/receive information.
	Patients can set and adjust the pace and refer back to information later and there is still a place for pamphlets (Sium et al., 2017).
	Can be effective with individuals, families, groups, or community-wide dissemination.
	Materials written at simple levels can be effective and acceptable for people of all literacy levels.
	Tailored/targeted materials are a promising strategy for health education that can be developed based on stages of behavioral change.
	Nurses should assess issues of readability, design, layout, cultural relevance, language sensitivities, and appropriateness of content (Baur et al., 2014).
	CDC's clear communication index (2014): http://www.cdc.gov/healthcommunication/ClearCommunicationIndex/.
Programmed materials, self-help guides, workbooks	May involve printed materials combined with visuals to allow self-pacing.
	Helpful for learning facts.
	Nurse should assess individual or group to determine whether independent learning style is preferred.
	Can be easily personalized.
Teaching/flash cards	Portable, use few words, and offer visual interpretations.
	Can be easily personalized.
	The nurse can create them economically and update them easily.
	Effective with individual, small-group, or family instruction.
Television, radio, and newspapers (mass media)	Reach large audiences within the community.
	Effective in conveying general health information in a user-friendly manner.
	Nurses can play an active role in disseminating health information via the local media.
	Effective in influencing attitudes and behaviors.
	Offer a familiar medium for viewers to learn about many health topics.
	Intergenerational reach.
Telephones/smartphones/patient portals Text messaging	Automated phone systems: Reminder phone calls, SMS, patient portals, telenursing, telehealth
Videotapes, digital streaming, telenovela/YouTube	Combine audio and visual media to convey realistic images (digital storytelling tools (e.g., YouTube, VoiceThread, Adobe spark) aid in engaging adult learners and communities).
	Videotapes that incorporate a role-modeling concept can be used to convey a wide variety of health topics. Can offer closed captioning for persons who are deaf.
	Takes time to produce and update; may require access to audiovisual equipment and viewing sites. Computerized digital editing makes updating easier. Telenovela storytelling
Online resources (i.e., Internet, simple dial-up services, information, databases, bulletin board chat services, blogs, and World Wide Web)	Electronic information sources can link individuals, families, and groups to health.
	Can reach large audiences rapidly.
	Websites should be evaluated by nurses/providers for accuracy, credibility, and relevancy.
	Digital technologies and innovations can help consumers find health information, advice, and support.
	Broadband speeds should be considered.
Podcasts	Portable video technology that uses media broadcasts and can be accessed via the Internet and viewed on a personal computer or on a handheld device player. Podcasts can be recorded and edited using free online platforms (e.g., Anchor, synth, etc.) and distributed to a targeted audience or a wider audience using platforms (e.g., google play, iTunes, spotify, etc.).
Social media	Online interactive discussions, blogs, social bookmarking, social news, facebook, Twitter, social networking sites, etc.

Data from U.S. Department of Health and Human Services: *Making health communication programs work: a planner's guide, pink book,* Bethesda, MD, 2008, Office of Cancer Communications, National Cancer Institute. Available from: https://www.cancer.gov/publications/health-communication/pink-book.pdf.

revises necessary components. The nurse also analyzes the program and health message for effectiveness and tracks the mechanisms using process evaluation. This way of organizing the implementation process examines the procedures and tasks involved in the program or message, such as monitoring media, identifying the audience's interim reactions, and addressing internal functioning (e.g., work schedules and expenditures).

Questions to Ask

- How should the health education program/message be launched?
- How do we maintain interest and sustainability?
- How can we use process evaluation?
- What are the strengths of the health program?
- How can we keep on track within the timeline and budget?

- How can we find out whether we have reached the intended audience?
- How well did each step work (i.e., process evaluation)?
- Are we maintaining good relationships with our community partners?

Collaborative Actions to Take

- Work with community organizations, adult education centers, libraries, churches, businesses, media, and other health agencies to enhance effectiveness.
- Monitor and track progress.
- Establish process evaluation measures (e.g., follow-up with users of the service, number of community members who used the service, and expenditures).

Stage IV: Assessing Effectiveness and Making Refinements

Outcome evaluation examines whether changes in knowledge, attitudes, and behavior did or did not occur because of the program. Together with process evaluation, the data inform how well the program is functioning and direct future modifications. The nurse prepares for a new development cycle using information gained from audience feedback, communication channels, and the program's planned effect. This stage refines the health messages and iteratively responds to the intended audience's needs. New information and feedback help validate the program's strengths, allow for necessary revisions, and directs nuanced and improved messages.

Questions to Ask

- What was learned?
- How can outcome evaluation be used to assess effectiveness?
- What worked well, and what did not work well?
- Has anything changed within the intended audience?
- How might we refine the methods, channels, or formats?
- Overall, what lessons were learned, and what modifications could strengthen the health education activity even more?

Collaborative Actions to Take

- Conduct outcome evaluations (e.g., randomized experiment, pilot study, evaluation studies, definition of data needed for data collection).
- Reassess and revise goals and objectives.
- Modify unsuccessful strategies or activities and refresh the evaluation plan.
- Generate continual support from businesses, healthcare agencies, and other community groups for ongoing collaboration and partnerships.

HEALTH EDUCATION RESOURCES

A variety of health education materials, digital media, and community resources are available from local, state, and national organizations and agencies. Such associations also provide helpful information about services, educational materials, and links to support groups or self-help groups. Often, these materials/resources are available for free or for a nominal cost. Nurses can help navigate individuals, families, and groups find and access to language-specific community, state and national resources. Additionally, identifying gaps in services and resources may encourage nurses to create new ones. Some examples are:

- Local and regional hospitals, clinics, libraries, adult education centers, health education centers, media outlets, and businesses
- Local and state governmental sources (e.g., health departments and social service agencies); literacy associations (check the Internet for listings)
- Community-based organizations (i.e., advertised, nonadvertised, and those recommended by community leaders; National Association of Community Health Centers; parish nursing associations; faith-based organizations; social service agencies)
- Universities and colleges, community colleges, and academic nursing centers
- Professional organizations (e.g., American Public Health Association, American Nurses Association, National Association of Hispanic Nurses, National Black Nurses Association, National Student Nurses Association, Society for Behavioral Medicine, etc.)
- Commercial organizations (e.g., pharmaceutical companies, medical supply companies, and patient and health education companies); printed and electronic sources are often available)
- Federal government sources (e.g., National Institutes of Health [NIH]; NCI; National Heart, Lung, and Blood Institute; OMH; CDC; National AIDS Clearinghouse; and Office on Smoking and Health) and related websites
- Voluntary agencies and their local affiliates (e.g., American Cancer Society, American Heart Association, ALS Association, American Diabetes Association, American Council for Drug Disorders, American Dairy Council, Alzheimer's Association, and American Lung Association)
- Internet searches
- Medline Plus Health Information (i.e., a service of the National Library of Medicine [NLM] for patient and consumer information) at medlineplus.gov

Can you think of another organization that you or a family member recently obtained information from relating to a health need? Local libraries often provide information on beginning and advanced search strategies and are one of the most credible and accessible sources of information. The National Library of Medicine (NLM), at www.nlm.nih.gov/hinfo.html, maintains extensive health-related bibliographies and offers links to the databases Medline Plus Health Information (http://www.nlm.nih.gov/medlineplus/), Household Products Database, Office of the Surgeon General, and much more.

The nurse can locate many health resources through a variety of search engines on the Internet. As the World Wide Web continues to evolve as a major and rapid source of information exchange, assessments of the quantity, quality, and credible broad nature of information must be undertaken—NLM offers free continuing education classes throughout the year (http://www.medlib-ed.org/catalogs/nnlm-nlmcourses) as well as consumer tutorials on evaluating Internet health information according to https://medlineplus.gov/webeval/webeval.html.

Also central to the nurse's role in the provision of educational resources and information is prioritizing and addressing literacy (see next section).

Literacy and Health Literacy

In her 1944 text, *The Public Health Nurse in the Community*, Rue stated that "The community's illiteracy level is an important factor in health program planning. This factor remains a significant issue in planning health education programs and materials. It should be noted that the term 'illiteracy' is seldom used today due to its 'deficit' connation and has been replaced more broadly by the term 'health literacy'. Yet, this early textbook is a reminder that health literacy has continued to be a problem of great magnitude and has considerable implications across the continuum of healthcare. It is an influential driver for the improvement of health, well-being, and patient empowerment, and the reduction of disparities in communities.

Consider Clinical Example 8.5.

Clinical Example 8.5

Helena, a 2-year-old, is diagnosed with an inner ear infection and is prescribed an antibiotic at the clinic. Her father understands that his daughter needs the prescribed medication twice a day. After carefully studying the label on the bottle and deciding that it does not tell how to take the medicine, he fills the teaspoon and pours the antibiotic into her ear (Adapted from Parker et al., 2003). What miscommunications happened here?

The nurse in a community setting who sees a sick child at the pediatric clinic might ask the following questions:
- Did the father know the name of the medicine being prescribed for Helena, how it works, and how to give it before leaving the clinic?
- Was the information on the medicine label in his preferred language?
- In what way might have teach-back methods (described later in this chapter) helped the father have a good understanding of how to administer the antibiotic?
- Will the father know what to do if Helena gets a fever?
- Does he know how to read a thermometer? Does the father know whom to call and under what conditions if

Clinical Example 8.5—cont'd

Helena's ear condition worsens? What actions will the father take in case of a very high fever at 1:00 A.M.? Does he have the critical literacy skills to manage similar situations?
- What nursing actions might have enhanced communications?

As background, the conceptual definitions of *health literacy* have evolved greatly over time. At one point, "literacy" was operationally defined as the ability to read and write at the fifth-grade level in any language and was measured on a continuum according to the National Literacy Act, 1991 (Irwin, 1991). In general, literacy has multiple components, namely oral literacy (listening/speaking skills), print literacy (writing/reading skills), numeracy (the ability to understand and work with numbers), and cultural and conceptual knowledge (Nielsen-Bohlman et al., 2004). Health literacy, on the other hand, is about empowerment, that is, having access to information, knowledge, and innovations within the context of health. It is viewed as increasingly important for social, economic, and health development; is a key public health issue in the delivery of effective, safe healthcare; and calls for the development of national policies and programs and intervention tools by community practitioners.

♥ HEALTHY PEOPLE 2030

Healthy People 2030 and Health Literacy
Health literacy is an essential component of *public health goals and* is a central focus of Healthy People 2030. One of the initiative's overarching goals demonstrates this focus: "Eliminate health disparities, achieve health equity, and attain health literacy to improve the health and well-being of all." Also, the specific naming of six developmental research objectives in developed by the HP 2030 Health Communication and Health Information Technology (IT) workgroup focus specifically on health literacy (https://health.gov/healthypeople/objectives-and-data/browse-objectives/health-communication/increase-health-literacy-population-hchit-r01). The objectives in this topic area describe many ways in which health communication and health IT can have a positive impact on health, healthcare, and health equity and these objectives align with the previously developed National Action Plan to Improve Health Literacy (USDHHS, 2010). Examples especially pertinent to health education actions taken by nurses include building partnerships, delivering accurate, accessible, and actionable health information that is targeted or tailored to increasing health literacy skills, providing personalized self-management tools and resources, and following sound principles in the design of programs and interventions that result in healthier behaviors.

So, what is health literacy? Health literacy is a constellation of skills needed to perform basic tasks required to function in the healthcare environment for accessing, understanding, processing, and using information to make health decisions. For example, health literacy skills entail knowing when and where to go for health screenings; reading labels on prescription bottles; understanding public health messages about flu, Ebola, Zika, or COVID-19; recognizing the dangers of text messaging while driving; completing health insurance forms; recognizing how to read food labels for sodium content; and being aware of the day-to-day expectations of a clinical trial. *It might mean being able to understand, make sense, and apply the information contained in this book or chapter to the care of members of your community.*

Healthy People 2030 provides expanded definitions that address both "personal health literacy" and "organizational health literacy."

- **Personal health literacy** is the degree to which individuals have the ability to find, understand, and use information and services to inform health-related decisions and actions for themselves and others.
- **Organizational health literacy (OHL)** is the degree to which organizations equitably enable individuals to find, understand, and use information and services to inform health-related decisions and actions for themselves and others.

These new definitions emphasize people's ability to use health information rather than just understand it, focus on the ability to make *well-informed* decisions rather than *appropriate ones*, incorporate a public health perspective, and most significantly, acknowledge that *organizations* have a responsibility to equitably address health literacy. The inaugural inclusion of health literacy in Healthy People 2030 as a foundational principle sends a clear message that health literacy is key to achieving health and well-being. Importantly, raising health literacy awareness, especially among providers and organizations among is a crucial aspect for helping individuals achieve positive health outcomes (Santana et al., 2021).

A helpful way to view health literacy is from three health literacy levels as posited by Nutbeam (2009). These levels inform interventions that have individual and population benefits: (1) functional/basic health literacy (focus is on increasing basic reading/writing skills to function in a health setting), (2) communicative/interactive health literacy (focus is on enhancing cognitive abilities in social settings to extract information and interact with providers), and (3) critical health literacy (focus is on advancing skills to analyze information critically and use the information to control and manage life situations). Too often, Nutbeam asserts that the provider's focus is on basic literacy rather than on critical literacy. The latter, he asserts, increases community members' empowerment abilities to successfully cope and handle their everyday lives.

Nutbeam (2008) further emphasizes that health literacy from public health and health promotion perspectives should be conceptualized as an "asset." In this manner, strategies to promote literacy move beyond mere transmission of content to the promotion of skills that develop confidence in how to act on the information. This viewpoint regards health literacy as a critical component of empowerment by improving people's access to health information and their capacity to use it. Moreover, Peerson and Saunders (2009) hold that implicit in understanding the broad concepts of health literacy is that motivation and behavioral activation must be considered separate entities. Simply put, having knowledge does not necessarily equate to action. Therefore the quality of provider interactions and a greater awareness of and sensitivity to the possible impact of low literacy on individuals and communities is paramount (Nutbeam, 2008; Rowlands and Nutbeam, 2013). Furthermore, Paakkari and Okan (2020) relate that health literacy should be viewed as a shared responsibility (such as with the case of COVID-19 messaging) by both people in need of information and the providers and educators who make information accessible.

The National Academy of Medicine (NAM), formerly called the Institute of Medicine (IOM) published its landmark report titled *Health Literacy: A Prescription to End Confusion*, which brought to light that millions of U.S. adults were unable to read and act on health instructions and messages (Nielsen-Bohlman et al., 2004). Since, then, there has been a plethora of studies demonstrating that health literacy is an important driver of health and well-being. For example, studies that show that health literacy affects health promoting behaviors of adolescents (Prihanto et al., 2021); parent acquisition of knowledge that in turn affects child health outcomes across disease prevention, acute illness care, and chronic illness care domains (Morrison and Glick 2019); uptake of stop-smoking messages (Stevens et al., 2019); positive associations with physical activity (Buja, 2020); understanding of COVID-19 information about transmission and infection control (McCaffery et al., 2020); efficacy in using patient portals among older adults (Son and Nahm, 2019); reproductive health knowledge (Nahata et al., 2020); insurance use and completion of forms (Villagra et al., 2019); dialysis maintenance (Green, 2013); better diabetic glycemic control (Tefera et al., 2020); and positive cancer clinical, treatment and screening outcomes including safe use of prescription opioid medicine among cancer survivors (Housten, 2021; Samoil et al., 2021; Tyson et al., 2021), to name a few. Health literacy also has been shown to affect better access to healthcare services and utilization of costs (MacLeod et al., 2017); participation in population health and clinical research (National Academies of Sciences, Engineering, and Medicine (NAM), 2020); and uptake and use of e-health interventions (Cheng et al., 2020; Pourrazavi et al., 2020).

The intersection of health literacy and disparities in healthcare represents a key contributor to high-quality, equitable healthcare. Although the exact relational mechanisms between literacy and health are still unclear, it is known that individuals with very low literacy skills are at an increased risk for poor health, which contributes to health disparities. One conceptual causal model that aims to explain associations between limited health literacy and health outcomes centers on three distinct aspects of care: (1) access and utilization of healthcare, (2) patient—provider relationships, and (3) self-care. The relationship of literacy to health outcomes is not necessarily linear—as people exist within a sociocultural network—and it has been suggested that health literacy be viewed as a risk factor to be addressed in clinical care and education (Hasnain-Wynia and Wolf, 2010; Paasche-Orlow and Wolf, 2007).

The greatest gains in health literacy can be realized by moving beyond the individual by including broader system and multi-sectorial engagement, and mobile technologies and digital communications tools to augment health literacy strategies (Christie and Ratzan, 2020). This focus implores "organizations" to improve navigation, understanding, and use of information through greater intersectoral collaboration and stakeholder empowerment to transform the delivery of person-centered care and services. Such changes must be well integrated throughout the organization and viewed as "strategic" implementation strategies to realize the full benefits of improved health outcomes, satisfaction, quality of care, and cost (Farmanova et al., 2021). This paradigm shift offers a promising and transformational approach to improve community literacy whereby the inclusion of community members is a necessary requirement to coproduce a literacy framework that reflects broader societal influences and social ecological perspectives (Jones et al., 2020; McCormack et al., 2017; Nutbeam 2017). Healthy People 2030's expanded definitions of health literacy align well with these aspirations and targets for achieving health equity.

Many health inequities often stem from the fact that people may view and interpret health, disease, and treatment differently (cultural and historical influences), and many people may not have access to information (health literacy influences). Hence, nurses must maintain a strong resolve toward social justice and health equity and consider the many influencing social, historical, economic, and political conditions and factors that give rise to both health and disease. An enhanced focus on transdisciplinary health education and community literacy can help to deconstruct these fundamental influences that affect health literacy (Meade et al., 2020). This being the case, nurses are ideally qualified and skilled to promote health in the community and address health literacy through the implementation of multiple individual and organizational strategies and techniques, as explained in the upcoming sections.

Assessment of Health Literacy and Materials

The Doaks (Leonard and Cecilia), who brought the literacy issue to the forefront in public health, describes the health community as a written culture. Unfortunately, many written instructions are "over the heads" of patients. Too often, there is a serious mismatch between the readability levels of health instructions and the reading skills of patients, but nurses can adapt the literacy levels of their instructions and reduce this mismatch. Techniques to reduce this mismatch are cogently outlined in the book *Teaching Patients with Low Literacy Skills* (Doak et al., 1996), which offers practical suggestions for preparing and evaluating materials. This book is not currently in print, but all chapters can be accessed through the Harvard health literacy website at https://www.hsph.harvard.edu/healthliteracy/resources/teaching-patients-with-low-literacy-skills/. This is a very helpful resource. The author has used the information contained in this book in the development

of educational materials, community-based programs, and research interventions.

What steps can nurses employ to address health literacy in the community setting? Within Stage I of the Framework for Developing Health Communications model, the nurse can use assessment skills to gauge literacy/reading levels of the intended audience using informal and formal assessment measures. Informal measures include asking a series of simple questions to provide a better indication of reading skills. For example, *Do you enjoy reading? What do you read? How often do you read? Where do you get your health information?* Although years of schooling completed can serve as a gauge of literacy, previous studies suggest that a three-to four-grade—level difference often exists between an individual's literacy level and years of education completed. The nurse could ask patients to read a paragraph from a health document aloud. Skilled readers enjoy reading, are fluent readers, understand content, interpret the meaning of words, and look up unfamiliar words. Limited readers read slowly, miss the intended meaning, take words literally, tire quickly from reading, and skip over uncommon words. Also, the nurse should ask patients a few questions about the information they read. Readers should be able to answer questions about the material's content. Although these strategies are especially helpful to individuals with low literacy, people at all literacy levels prefer and better understand simply written, concise materials and are more motivated by materials that are relevant to their learning needs (Doak et al., 1998).

Formal assessment measures. There has been ongoing attention to the development of literacy screening questions, but continued validation studies are needed before they become routine in clinical care (Chin et al., 2011; Mancuso, 2009). Some formal instruments that have been used in healthcare settings to estimate reading skills include the Wide Range Achievement Test, Level 5 (Wilkinson and Robertson, 2017) and the Rapid Estimate of Adult Literacy in Medicine (REALM), which assesses the ability to read common terms in English (e.g., allergic, jaundice, anemia, etc.) and is used as a brief literacy-screening tool that take only a few minutes to administer. Please note that there is now a short form of the REALM (Davis et al., 1991, 1993, 2006).

Another short assessment tool, called the *Newest Vital Sign (NVS),* created by Weiss et al. (2005), is available in English and Spanish as a six-question assessment tool based on an ice cream nutrition label and is a quick (3- to 5-minute) assessment. Another measure, the Test of Functional Health Literacy in Adults, long and short forms (TOFHLA and S-TOFHLA; Parker et al., 1995) (English and Spanish language). (Although many new and translated health literacy measures have been reported, many health literacy measures have not been properly or fully validated for and non—English language speaking groups (Nguyen et al., 2015). Morris et al. (2006) developed the Single Item Literacy Screener: "How often do you need to have someone help when you read instructions, pamphlets, or other written material from your doctor or pharmacy (1 = never; 2 = rarely; 3 = sometimes; 4 = often; 5 = always)?" This item was found to be reasonably successful in detecting health literacy (in comparison with the TOFHLA), but only moderately sensitive. Yet, it focuses on only one aspect of health literacy, which is reading materials. This work has expanded to three BRIEF screening questions: How often do you have problems learning about your medical condition because of difficulty understanding written information? How often do you have someone help you read hospital materials and How confident are you filling out medical forms by yourself? (Chew et al., 2004; Wallace et al., 2006) Recently, an "ability to read item," that is, how would you rate your ability to read? (one to five scale from very poor to very good) performed the best, supporting use as a screening tool in safety-net systems caring for diverse populations among English/Spanish speakers (Bishop et al., 2016). Other efforts in this field have centered on the development of tools that measure Internet-seeking abilities or e-health literacy (Norman and Skinner, 2006); or gauge numeracy skills such as number sense, tables and graphs, probability, and statistics (Jacobs et al., 2016; Schapira et al., 2014; Fagerlin et al., 2007).

If you are interested in this topic, go to the *Health Literacy Toolshed,* an online database of over 200 health literacy measures (description of measures and psychometric properties), which is compiled by the NLM in collaboration with Boston University, https://www.nlm.nih.gov/news/health_literacy_tool_shed.html.

As one can see, there are many formal tools to measure reading level or word recognition, which in turn may be helpful to gauge an individual's health literacy. Yet the time needed to administer them in community-based settings greatly limits their use. Most importantly, these collective findings underscore that formal assessments should be secondary to the nurse's informal and ongoing assessments, which allow for verification of understanding about specific health content within a specific health context. Nurses need to be astute in their assessment of people's skills and to continually monitor the demands of the healthcare environment and make organizational adjustments as needed. Furthermore, Meade and Calvo (2001) continue to suggest asking patients and community members a series of simple questions on the topic of years of schooling and about their reading habits that will help gauge health literacy, followed by ongoing learner verification and teach-back methods.

Nurses play essential roles in community education, outreach and engagement activities for assessing people's literacy skills, conveying knowledge, deciphering motivations, adapting health education messages, making information accessible, promoting health decisions, and facilitating empowering processes to increase the useful uptake of information. Nurses have integral roles to ensure that health literacy is an organizational value integrated into all aspects of community planning and health operations and viewed as a relationship between individuals and their environment (Koh et al., 2013; McCormack et al., 2017). Optimizing the contribution of health literacy for addressing social determinants of health includes enhancing one's professional skills and knowledge development; facilitating transferable

skills so community members to know how to access and use information; and prioritizing the engagement of population groups who are most disproportionately affected by low health literacy (Nutbeam and Lloyd, 2020). Health literacy and community engagement are crucial in addressing health inequities, and strong investments in health and community literacy education are essential to bring together available community knowledge, skills, and resources for improved health (Jones et al., 2020). The nurse is an impactful change agent and catalyst to enhance health literacy for improved community health from both individual and organizational vantage points. More than ever before, there is high attention being placed on the importance of "language and literacy" in healthcare and teaching—these two factors are now prominently named as key issues in the "Education Access and Quality Domain" of Healthy People 2030's Social Determinants of Health organizing framework.

Helpful Tips for Effective Teaching

- Put patients at ease and establish rapport. Focus on inclusion and trust first before delivering "the content."
- Determine what patient/community members want and need to know.
- Identify motivating factors for learning new information and behaviors.
- Assess literacy and comprehension skills using informal and formal methods.
- Identify language preference.
- Stick with the essentials. Limit the number of concepts or key points. Focus on important critical and survival skills.
- Set realistic goals and objectives. Take cues from your patients about what they want to learn and how to help them learn.
- Use clear and concise language. Avoid technical terms, if possible. For example, you might substitute *problem* for *complication.* Use *high blood pressure* instead of *hypertension* or *chance* instead of *possibility.* Do not needlessly simplify if the intended meaning is lost. Although the words *insulin* and *infection* are polysyllabic words, people with diabetes should become familiar with these terms (Box 8.2).
- Consider developing a glossary or vocabulary list for common words on the health topic. For example, in teaching a family about dental health, create a list of common words about the topic and words that might substitute well (e.g., flossing, toothbrush, cavity, decay, check-ups, X-rays). Get input from learners on the best terms to use.
- Verify translations and the meanings of words.
- Space teaching out over time, if possible. Incorporate health education activities into other activities. For example, ask about smoking habits or immunizations at each visit. Relate teaching to people's everyday concerns.
- Personalize health messages. Use the active voice. For example, instead of saying, "It is important that patients read labels if they want to cut down on fat and sodium intake," say, "Read the labels on foods to know what is in

---

BOX 8.2   Patient Communication: Prostate Cancer and Treatment Options

Version A (Harder to Grasp—Passive)	**Version B (Easier to Grasp—Active)**
The doctor has recently communicated to the patient that he has localized prostate cancer, commonly labeled stage II. In addition to managing the anxieties associated with a life-threatening illness, patients with this disease must carefully consider the available treatment modalities and account for the potential effect each one may have on quality of life. Patients must seriously evaluate the benefits and adverse side effects of each treatment modality and determine the most efficacious intervention for their lifestyle.	You have just been told that you have early stage prostate cancer. You may find it hard to choose a treatment. Yet it is important that you learn about your choices. Besides dealing with fears that often go with cancer, get to know about your treatment options: • Learn about each treatment and how it may affect your life and your family. • Get to know the benefits and side effects of each treatment. • Ask questions. Write them down. Talk it over with your family. • Choose the best treatment for you.

Modified from Doak CC, Doak LG, Root JH: *Teaching patients with low literacy skills*, ed 2, Philadelphia, PA, 1996, Lippincott Williams & Wilkins. (Chapter 10 on learner verification can now be accessed at the Harvard health literacy website: http://www.hsph.harvard.edu/healthliteracy/resources/teaching-patients-with-low-literacy-skills/).

---

them. This will help you figure out what is in the food and cut down on your fat and salt intake."

- Incorporate methods of illustration, demonstration, and real-life examples. Connect the health message to everyday events and real-life situations.
- Identify the role of digital technologies in your health education efforts. Find out if patients and community members have access to and use computers, own phones, and what type, and how they use them.
- Give and get. Review information often. Ask the patient questions before, during, and after teaching.
- Summarize often. Provide the patient with feedback. Obtain feedback from the patient.
- Be creative. Use your imagination to convey difficult concepts (e.g., use picture cards, drawings, objects, streaming videos, audiobooks, podcasts, flip charts, multimedia decision aids, photographs, embodied conversational agents, apps, photovoice, storytelling, use of metaphors).
- Use language-specific resources and materials to enhance teaching and convey ideas (e.g., picture cards, models, tablet devices, whiteboards).
- Praise patients, but do not patronize them. Let them know what they are doing right. Focus on their strengths and assets and what they bring to the teaching encounter.
- Be encouraging throughout the educational steps. We all like to be told what we are doing right.
- Allow time for patients and family members to think and ask questions. Silence gives time to reflect on content and formulate questions.
- Remember that comprehension and understanding require time and practice. Giving feedback and verifying understanding helps refocus the teaching encounter and keeps interactions on track.
- Employ "teach-back" methods. This means asking patients to state in their own words (i.e., teach back) key concepts, decisions, or instructions just discussed (Yen and Leasure, 2019).
- Conduct learner verification (a process that checks suitability of information according to the following elements: attraction, comprehension, self-efficacy, cultural acceptability, persuasion) (Table 8.7) (Chavarria et al., 2021).

- Evaluate teaching plans often adding new information to the interaction based on new learning needs.
- When developing materials/media, get an **R.E.A.L.** mindset, that is make information—**R**elatable, **E**ngaging, **A**ctionable and **L**iteracy Friendly (Meade et al., 2019).

TABLE 8.7   Components of Learner Verification (Checks the Suitability of the Message With Learners)

Components	Description
Attraction	Readers should be attracted to the message. For example, the cover should stimulate interest, and when possible, pictures should foster an identification that "tells me that this is important for my situation." Examples: • Is this material attractive/pleasing to you? • Overall, would you be likely to pick up and read this brochure?
Comprehension	Readers should be able to summarize the main points in their own words, not the vocabulary of the instruction. Examples: • What do you feel is the main point? • Are there any words that are not clear?
Acceptability	Readers need to perceive that the information is culturally acceptable for their lifestyle, situation, and background. Examples: • Is there anything that bothers you about this booklet? • In your opinion, who is this booklet for?
Persuasion	Readers need to feel that the instruction is significant for them. Example: • Do you think that the message in this booklet is important for you?
Self-efficacy	Is the message doable, and does the reader feel confident in carrying it out? Example: • Do you think you could do what is suggested in this booklet (e.g., cut down on cigarettes)?

- Consider your environment and carry out a quick checklist to see if your organization/institution is health literate as well (Kowalski et al., 2015; Rudd et al., 2019). If not, play an active role in being a change agent.

Assess Materials: Become a Wise Consumer and User

Materials are collected, stored, and disseminated within community sites. In many instances, nurses distribute pamphlets, but patients either do not read them or review them only superficially.

People of this country have had so much pamphlet materials passed out to them free that some have lost respect for free literature. Health educators may have contributed to this delinquency by passing out health literature carelessly and indiscriminately. The nurse who expects the pamphlet to take the place of the health teacher is employing weak measures in the health education program.

Rue, 1944, p. 215

This statement continues to be true today. Moreover, many of today's pamphlets are even more complex and lengthier because of technological advances and healthcare innovations. Thus it is important that nurses evaluate health materials, including digital materials and websites, before they disseminate them to or share them with individuals, families, or the public. Health materials should strengthen previous teaching and should be used as an adjunct to health instruction.

Assess Relevancy of Health Materials

It is critical that nurses find and use materials, documents, and media that are appropriate for the intended target audience in community health education initiatives. Questions that the nurse should ask include the following:

- Do the materials match the intended audience?
- Are the materials appealing and culturally and linguistically relevant?
- Do they convey accurate and up-to-date information?
- Are the messages clear and understandable?
- Do the messages promote self-efficacy and motivation?

Fig. 8.2 provides an assessment guide for reviewing health materials that the author has used for gauging the appropriateness of materials. The nurse can use this guide in critiquing printed materials. Similarly, the nurse can make slight modifications in the tool and assess other types of health resources (e.g., booklets, videos, websites, digital media, apps, etc.). To use the tool, gather a few materials/media that are commonly used in the clinical setting where you are based. In a group or individually, begin to assess each category and critically assess the suitability for your intended audience. The tool allows the nurse to review health materials systematically for appropriateness for the intended target audience. The material assessment should focus on the following criteria: format/layout, type, verbal content, visual content, and aesthetic quality. This activity probably will take 10 to 15 min. It can also be used as a group activity with patients or community members. Another useful tool is the Patient Education Materials Assessment Tool (PEMAT), described by Shoemaker and colleagues (2014)) and available on the Agency for Healthcare Research and Quality website: https://www.ahrq.gov/health-literacy/patient-education/pemat.html.

CASE STUDY Application of the Nursing Process

Selected Teaching Approaches and Learning Needs

The following case study and teaching plan provide an example of selected teaching approaches and learning needs for the individual, family, and community.

Emma Jackson, aged 33 years, receives ongoing healthcare at her neighborhood's community-based clinic, a federally funded community health center. She visits the nurse practitioner, and the nurse confirms that Mrs. Jackson is 2 months pregnant. She is married and has an 8-year-old son. Emma tells the nurse she smokes and wants to quit but she has been unable to quit since her last pregnancy. She tells the nurse, "I smoke when I get stressed. I have so many things on my mind." Her husband is also a smoker (actually he vapes too) and has tried to quit at times as well. The nurse refers Mrs. Jackson to a community nursing student named Irene Green for counseling, education, and follow-up.

Assessment

Irene recognizes that smoking during pregnancy is detrimental for the unborn infant, unhealthy for Mrs. Jackson, and harmful for the 8-year-old child, who breathes the secondhand smoke—https://www.acog.org/; https://www.acog.org/clinical/clinical-guidance/committee-opinion/articles/2020/05/tobacco-and-nicotine-cessation-during-pregnancy. Irene also knows that smokers often experience stages of readiness in their attempts to quit and that relapse is often part of the process (Prochaska and DiClemente, 1983). She notes that family and community support systems are important.

Irene assesses Mrs. Jackson on an individual level, as follows:
- Smoking history, smoking patterns, and previous attempts to quit
- Support systems (e.g., family, friends, and peers)
- Perceived obstacles to quitting
- Perceived benefits to quitting
- Perceived priority in addressing this health issue versus other everyday stresses
- Perceived effect of smoking behavior on family communication patterns
- Confidence and perceived efficacy in ability to quit

Assessment of other groups includes families, neighborhoods, churches, community organizations, and environmental messages that promote smoking cessation.

Diagnosis
Individual
- Health concerns related to smoking and personal stressors/triggers
- Desire for more information about ways to quit and stay smoke free

Family
- Effect and impact of smoking on family dynamics

Community
- Need for information about community programs and social support resources

Continued

Planning

Individual

Long-Term Goal

• Mrs. Jackson will quit smoking.

Short-Term Goals

• Mrs. Jackson will recognize that continued smoking is unhealthy for herself, her unborn infant, her young child, and her family.
• Mrs. Jackson will become aware of ways to enhance her confidence during smoking cessation.
• Mrs. Jackson will identify situations and stressors that influence her smoking patterns.
• Mrs. Jackson will learn two strategies to cope with stressful situations and will apply those strategies.

Family

Long-Term Goal

• Mr. and Mrs. Jackson will quit smoking and become a smoke-free family.

Short-Term Goals

• Mr. and Mrs. Jackson will acknowledge the benefits of a smoke-free environment.
• Mr. Jackson will recognize the need to quit smoking.
• The couple will recognize the need to support each other in smoking cessation.
• Mr. and Mrs. Jackson will identify and discuss specific supportive actions during the smoking cessation phases. The couple will enlist the support of another person or network (Irene's sister who quit 1 year ago).

Community

Long-Term Goals

• The community will support and endorse a smoke-free environment and publicize these efforts.
• Community agencies and organizations will integrate smoking cessation and relapse programs and messages into their existing health-related activities.
• Cigarette advertising will cease.

Short-Term Goals

• A coalition of community members will develop and implement policies to support smoking cessation and relapse strategies.
• A consortium of healthcare agencies and community-based organizations will recognize the need to develop partnerships in creating smoking cessation strategies for the community and for high-risk groups.

Intervention

Individual

Planning interventions encourage self-expression, promote the use of adaptive coping mechanisms, offer positive reinforcement, disseminate appropriate smoking cessation strategies, and provide culturally and educationally relevant materials and media. The nurse applies the "5 A's" approach to smoking cessation counseling (Ask, Advise, Assess, Assist, and Arrange). Irene offers empowerment strategies to help Mrs. Jackson cope with her smoking cessation attempts and identifies daily hassles and stressors. Irene gives personalized smoking cessation messages and culturally and educationally appropriate materials and initiates a follow-up plan that is acceptable (American College of Obstetrics and Gynecology—https://www.acog.org/womens-health/infographics/tobacco-and-pregnancy).

Family

Planning and interventions recognize the need for strong support systems within families. Irene provided education and counseling to promote family self-care and recognized that she must address and incorporate Mr. Jackson's support,

into the care plan. Irene makes links to community resources (e.g., health classes, support groups, and networking blogs with other expectant mothers who have quit or are attempting to quit) to build Mrs. Jackson's support system.

Community

Planning and interventions implemented on an aggregate level identify key community leaders, agencies, legislators, and lay members who are committed to supporting smoking cessation/relapse initiatives at a sociopolitical level (e.g., creating smoking cessation/relapse initiatives at various community channels). Program initiatives assist community members in defining issues and solutions to the effects of smoking on individuals, families, and community groups. Developing coalitions and partnerships among community-based organizations, healthcare groups, governmental agencies, and intended audience members through dialogue and increased awareness is essential.

Evaluation

Evaluation is systematic and continuous and focuses on the individual, family, and community.

Individual

An evaluation of Mrs. Jackson's smoking habits occurs within the health system and the community (clinics and Women, Infants, and Children Service). These groups address both process (decrease in number of cigarettes smoked) and outcome (quit or not quit) end points. Mrs. Jackson experiences an increase in her coping skills and support system, which is evident in her personalized care plan.

• Irene tailors smoking cessation messages for Mrs. Jackson to fit her everyday life and addresses negative affect, that is, negative emotional smoking triggers.
• Irene provides Mrs. Jackson with follow-up (e.g., telephone, letter, text messages, and follow-up visits).
• Irene introduces Mrs. Jackson to mindfulness techniques that aim increase an individual's awareness of their environment, thoughts, emotions, and physical sensations as related to craving (Vinci, 2020).
• Irene also used a tablet (iPad) to promote knowledge of tobacco risk and cessation resources for pregnant women (Dotson et al., 2017) and is exploring other digital forms of communication (text messaging, evidence-based apps (Kurti et al., 2019; van den Heuvel et al., 2018) that would fit with Mrs. Jackson's learning preferences.
• Irene provides educational resources for Mrs. Jackson (https://smokefree.gov/).

Readers are suggested to visit a virtual tour to enhance your counseling skills. See Smoking Cessation for Pregnancy and Beyond: A Virtual Clinic, a multimedia program that provides counseling guidance:

Family

Care plans include supporting pattern development with family or significant other in smoking cessation initiatives.

• Irene assesses family health patterns and screens for other at-risk behaviors.
• Irene identifies and addresses family support and communication patterns in the care plan.

Community

Irene introduces smoking cessation and relapse programs and smoking prevention initiatives to at least two channels of dissemination (e.g., churches, schools, worksites, community-based clinics, restaurants).

• Smoking cessation/relapse messages are infused throughout the community by means of radio, television, and billboards.
• Community task forces and coalitions demonstrate a collaborative partnership among lay members, community leaders, organizers, and legislators to address smoking-related health issues.

Assessment of Health Education Materials

Name of material/media _____

Author _____

Intended target audience _____

Cost/availability/producer _____

Directions: Assess your printed material using the following tool. Use the rating scale of 1-4 for each item in a major category. *1 = poor 2 = fair 3 = good 4 = very good N/A = not applicable.*

For each category, give it an overall category rating of: *(+) effective* or *(−) not effective, (X) unsure*

Using the tool(s) that you brought to class, begin your review in groups of 2-3. Assess the material carefully to evaluate its suitability for your audience. Following your small group review, share your comments with others.

Category/criteria Comments	Rating 1 = Poor; 2 = Fair; 3 = Good; 4 = Very Good
Format/Layout	
Organizational style	_____
White/black space	_____
Margins	_____
Grouping of elements	_____
Use of headers/advance organizers	_____
Overall category rating of:	
(+) effective ____ (−) not effective ____ (X) unsure ____	
Type	
Size	_____
Style	_____
Spacing	_____
Overall category rating of:	
(+) effective ____ (−) not effective ____ (X) unsure ____	
Verbal Content	
Clarity	_____
Quantity	_____
Relevancy to intended group (e.g., age, gender, race/ethnicity)	_____
Use of active voice	_____
Difficulty/readability level	_____
Grade level	_____
Accuracy	_____
Currency	_____
Overall category rating of:	
(+) effective ____ (−) not effective ____ (X) unsure ____	

Category/criteria	Rating Comments 1 = Poor; 2 = Fair; 3 = Good; 4 = Very Good
Visual Content	
Tone/mood	_____
Clarity	_____
Cueing	_____
Relevancy to intended group (e.g., age, gender, race/ethnicity)	_____
Currency	_____
Accuracy	_____
Detail	_____
Overall category rating of:	
(+) effective ____ (−) not effective ____ (X) unsure ____	
Aesthetic Quality/Appeal	
Attractiveness	_____
Color	_____
Quality of production	_____
Personalized instructions	_____
Overall category rating of:	
(+) effective ____ (−) not effective ____ (X) unsure ____	
Comments:	

Overall, based on your scoring of 1 to 4 and an evaluation of its effectiveness with the intended target audience, how suitable would you rate this educational tool? Circle one.

1 = **poor:** probably won't work with my intended audience. I would probably not ever use it.

2 = **fair:** has a low likelihood of success with my intended audience. I would use it rarely and only in combination with other sources.

3 = **good:** has a good likelihood of being suitable and relevant for about half of my intended audience. I would use it sometimes.

4 = **very good:** has a high likelihood of being suitable and relevant for most of my intended audience. I would most definitely use it!

Fig. 8.2 Assessment of health education materials.

Format/Layout

- Is the information organized clearly? Does it make sense?
- Do headers or advance organizers cue the reader? Headers help the reader visualize what is next.
- Is there a 50%/50% allocation of white and black space? This proportion gives the reader "breathing space."
- Is the information easy to read and uncluttered?

Type

- Is the type or font a readable size? Consider the age of your intended group and whether visual difficulties are likely.

Verbal Content

- Is the information current, accurate, and relevant to the intended group?
- Is the information culturally acceptable?
- Are difficult terms defined?
- Does the text reflect the racial and ethnic diversity and language of the intended audience?
- What is the reading level?

Visual Content

- Are the graphics accurate, current, and relevant and engaging to the intended group?
- Does cueing help the reader connect the printed words and pictures?
- Will the reader understand the intended meanings of the pictures?
- Is the information culturally acceptable?
- Are the pictures on the cover reflective of the material inside?
- Do the pictures reflect the target audience's racial and ethnic diversity?

Aesthetic Quality and Appeal

- Is the material appealing and engaging?
- Are there helpful special features (e.g., glossary, space for notes, and useful telephone numbers or websites)?

Assessment of Reading Level

Part of the written material's assessment is reading level. Many formulas are available to estimate the printed text's readability and grade level, including the SMOG readability formula.

Readability formulas are objective, quantitative tools that measure sentence and word variables. However, they do not consider factors such as motivation, experience, and need for information (Meade and Smith, 1991). Nor do they determine the effects of visuals or design factors that could influence readability and comprehension or address global text characteristics, including fluency, structure, and content of the text (Kauchak and Leroy, 2016). Formulas do estimate reading ease and provide helpful guidelines for assessing and rewriting health information. Two commonly used formulas are the Flesch-Kincaid and the SMOG formulas. The Flesch-Kincaid Formula (Flesch, 1948) is a broad estimate of reading and is programmed into most computer software programs' grammar editing tools. To test a document's readability on your computer using the Flesch-Kincaid formula, search the term "readability statistic." You will be directed to a series of file and option tabs to reach grammar and spelling, and then readability statistics. The SMOG formula is shown in Resource 8D and is frequently used to calculate the readability estimate of health materials (McLaughlin, 1969).

Learner Verification

The best way to identify material suitability is to deliver the materials to the intended audience and obtain feedback. **Learner verification** and revision (LV & R) is a methodological approach that engages learners in dialogue about the overall suitability of the message. It involves evaluating such elements as: attraction, comprehension, self-efficacy, cultural and linguistic acceptability, and persuasion. This technique supports Freirean principles to produce empowering learning products and engages learner participation in the development process. It ensures that the learner is the active subject of the educational experience and allows the learner to define content and outcomes (Doak et al., 1996; Chavarria et al., 2021).

The process of learner verification helps identify the likelihood that the message is well suited to the audience. It involves verifying whether certain elements work well together to result in a good match of information for the learner. See Table 8.7 for a description of the specific elements and sample questions associated with each one.

The author and colleagues have used learner verification processes on many occasions, for example, to develop a series of education toolboxes on breast and cervical cancer and prostate cancer for Hispanic migrant and seasonal farmworkers and African American women and men. After holding a series of focus groups with members of the intended audience to elicit themes about health, illness, cancer, and prevention, we conducted learner verification measures. Through systematic questions and interviewing processes, we were able to collect information in the intended audience's own words to help shape and refocus the cancer issues (breast, cervical, and prostate) from their own perspective (African American men and women and Hispanic men and women farmworkers). Such verifying checks help assess the understanding of words and pictures; the acceptability of music, narrator, and pictures; the efficacy and persuasion of the message; and the overall attractiveness of the materials/media. For example, we found that the word *prevention* was a term many men found difficult to grasp. What we found was that tuning up one's car was a familiar concept that could similarly be used to convey the importance of ongoing check-ups, as in maintaining prostate health. Similarly, the author and her colleagues used this approach to create biobanking education materials for community members (Meade et al., 2015); and develop prostate cancer information for clients in barbershops (Luque et al., 2015). Overall, the process of learner verification fits well within the framework of community-based participatory research methods, as outlined earlier in this chapter, and can be a very helpful qualitative tool for nurses to use in gauging the suitability of their health education efforts.

❓ ACTIVE LEARNING

1. Identify an issue of concern among community members (e.g., obesity, access to care, education of youth). Discuss sociopolitical and environmental issues that affect this issue and how it relates to health. Outline specific community-based participatory activities and roles that the community nurse can take on that can address this health issue. Identify at least two ways to promote community engagement on this topic. What educational resources might the nurse use?
2. Select a health education brochure or health website. Apply the assessment criteria presented to assess its appropriateness for an intended audience. Evaluate the relative strengths of the printed material or website and potential areas for improvement using learner verification questions. Describe how you and your group can make it more relevant for your audience. What can be improved? How could you involve your audience in its assessment?

SOCIAL MEDIA AND DIGITAL TOOLS

Americans today are increasingly connected to the world of digital information. As such, nurses should consider the role of nondigital and digital channels in connecting communities with reliable health information. Nurses should also think about how mobile health and e-health technologies might improve health outcomes of communities. *Social media* refers to interactive Internet-based communication channels that allow users to create, share, comment on, and modify online content. It facilitates engagement and collaboration and has rapidly become a tool for health promotion and education (Alber et al., 2015). Social media platforms might include blogs, online discussion boards, microblogs such as Twitter, and video-sharing sites such as YouTube, Vimeo, and Flickr. In light of the growing number of people (both here in the United States and globally) who have mobile phones and use social media, such platforms are being used to reach diverse community constituents (urban and rural) with important public

health messages (O'Mara, 2012). It is estimated that most Americans (97%) own some type of a cell phone and most send and receive text messages (Pew Research Center, 2021). Ownership of smartphones is now 85%, up from about 35% since Pew Research Center's first survey of smartphone ownership in 2011. Given this widespread use of cell phones, social media text messaging continues to offer a promising way to directly deliver health information.

Social media sites have the potential to facilitate interactive communications, increase the sharing of health information, and personalize and reinforce health messages, all of which in turn can empower community members to make informed health decisions (CDC, 2010). For example, Schier and colleagues (2019) using qualitative netnography sought to describe the food and nutrition messages shared among the transgender community using video blogs (vlogs) on "You Tube," a popular social networking site; or in a study carried out in rural Northern Kenya, Kazi and colleagues (2017) reported phone usage, ownership characteristics, and feasibility of text-based mHealth interventions (short messaging service [SMS]) among patients for enhancing maternal-child health (antenatal care immunizations). Notably, despite remoteness, most pregnant women and caregivers visiting for antenatal care and routine immunizations had some access to mobile phones, liked the idea of text messaging, and stated that they would use it if available. Hence, if designed appropriately, findings suggest that SMS may be an innovative way to engage women in their health and the health of their families; and Miyamoto and colleagues (2021) described the development of community-driven "Sexual Assault Forensic Examination Telehealth" (SAFE-T) Center—a nurse-led model that provides comprehensive, high-quality sexual assault care in rural and underserved communities at three hospitals in rural Pennsylvania.

Nurses in community health education settings are well poised to explore the utility of novel digital technology to connect individuals, families, and groups to communities of learning and to connect them with reliable and credible information, which has meaning for their everyday health concerns and needs. Nonetheless, nurses should be mindful of the increased ethical issues and inherent concerns and cautions that are evolving today relating to the use of social media (privacy, misinformation, social media celebrities, and its effect on behaviors) (Azer, 2017; Turner and Lefevre, 2017; Suarez-Lledo and Alvarez-Galvez et al., 2021).

▌ SUMMARY

Teaching is a significant component of community health nursing, affecting virtually every nursing activity. The goal of health education is to facilitate a process that allows individuals, families, groups, and communities to make well-informed decisions about health practices. An understanding of learning and the theoretical frameworks that explain behaviors and health actions is inherent in community health education. No

single theory explains human behavior; the nurse must apply multiple theories and approaches.

A powerful role of the nurse is being an information broker—one that facilitates multidirectional knowledge exchanges and interactions among knowledge producers and knowledge users (Thompson et al., 2019). Nurses must be knowledgeable about sociopolitical, cultural, environmental, and ecological and planetary forces affecting community health to ensure the success of health education strategies. Furthermore, relevant health education (classes, talking circles, support groups, individual/family instruction, use of digital technologies, health fairs, apps, etc.) is based on the meeting of individual variables and social, structural, political, cultural, and economic factors within the larger community and organizational systems context. To create meaningful and useful health educational interventions, nurses need to assess their audience(s) and their characteristics thoroughly and employ systematic and engaging approaches when delivering health messages and programs.

Implementing social action strategies, such as advocating health-promoting lifestyles, creating an environment for problem-posing dialogue, and providing links to appropriate language and literacy suitable health resources, supports the philosophy of critical consciousness. Nurses as health educators can facilitate the principle of **social justice** toward health equity by mastering health information subject content and committing themselves to creating empowerment strategies that equip individuals, families, and communities with knowledge and navigation skills for healthy lifestyles and environments.

Further, a variety of creative methods, materials, media, and digital technologies can support health education activities. Continual review and evaluation of such resources are essential to ensure cultural, linguistic, language, and literacy suitability. Embracing the notion that health education is an ongoing interactive process influenced by many internal and external factors is strategic to meeting the needs of individuals, families, and communities. As nurses, important contributions to the prevention of disease and the promotion of community health can be realized with an ongoing colearner mindset and a commitment to impactful empowerment and engagement strategies.

EVOLVE WEBSITE

http://evolve.elsevier.com/Nies/community
- NCLEX Review Questions
- Case Studies

BIBLIOGRAPHY AND REFERENCES

Agency for Healthcare Research and Quality: *Health Literacy Universal Precautions Toolkit*, ed 2, Rockville, MD, 2020, Agency for Healthcare Research and Quality. https://www.ahrq.gov/health-literacy/improve/precautions/index.html.

Alber JM, Bernhardt JM, Stellefson M, et al.: Designing and testing an inventory for measuring social media competency of certified health education specialists, *J Med Internet Res* 17(9):e221, 2015. https://doi.org/10.2196/jmir.4943.

Alcaraz KI, Sly J, Ashing K, et al.: The ConNECT framework: a model for advancing behavioral medicine science and practice to foster health equity, *J Behav Med* 40(1):23–38, 2016. https://link.springer.com/content/pdf/10.1007/s10865-016-9780-4.pdf.

American Cancer Society: *Cancer facts and figures*, Atlanta, GA, 2021, American Cancer Society. Available from: https://www.cancer.org/research/cancer-facts-statistics/all-cancer-facts-figures/cancer-facts-figures-2021.html.

American College of Obstetricians and Gynecologists: Nicotine and tobacco during pregnancy, *Obstet Gynecol* 135(5):e221–e229, 2020. Committee opinion No. 807. Available from: www.acog.org/clinical/clinical-guidance/committee-opinion/articles/2020/05/tobacco-and-nicotine-cessation-during-pregnancy.

American College of Obstetricians and Gynecologists: Smoking cessation during pregnancy, *Obstet Gynecol* 116:1241–1244, 2010. Committee Opinion No. 471.

American Nurses Association: *Nursing: scope and standards of practice*, ed 4, Silver Spring, MD, 2021, American Nurses Association. chrome-extension://oemmndcblidboiebfnladdacbdfmadadm/https://www.nursingworld.org/~49d755/globalassets/practiceandpolicy/scope-of-practice/3sc-booklet-2021-june.pdf.

Aranda K, Coleman L, Sherriff NS, et al.: Listening for commissioning: a participatory study exploring young people's experiences, views and preferences of school-based sexual health and school nursing, *J Clin Nurs* 27(1–2):375–385, 2018. https://doi.org/10.1111/jocn.13936.

Azer SA: Social media channels in health care research and rising ethical issues, *AMA J Ethics* 19(11):1061–1069, 2017. https://doi.org/10.1001/journalofethics.2017.19.11.peer1-1711.

Bandura A: Self-efficacy: toward a unifying theory of behavioral change, *Psychol Rev* 84:191–215, 1977a.

Bandura A: *Social learning theory*, Englewood Cliffs, NJ, 1977b, Prentice Hall.

Baur C, Prue C: The CDC clear communication index is a new evidence-based tool to prepare and review health information, *Health Promot Pract* 15(5):629–637, September 2014. https://doi.org/10.1177/1524839914538969.

Becker MH. In *The health belief model and personal health behavior*, Thorofare, NJ, 1974, Health Educ Quart.

Becker MH, Maiman LA, Kirscht JP, et al.: The health belief model and prediction of dietary compliance: a field experiment, *J Health Soc Behav* 18:348–366, 1977.

Bigge ML, Shermis SS. In *Learning theories for teachers*, ed 6, Boston, 2004, Allyn & Bacon Classics.

Bishop WP, Craddock Lee SJ, Skinner CS, et al.: Validity of single-item screening for limited health literacy in English and Spanish speakers, *Am J Public Health* 106(5):889–892, 2016. https://doi.org/10.2105/AJPH.2016.303092.

Braun K, Stewart S, Baquet C, et al.: The National Cancer Institute's community networks program initiative to reduce cancer health disparities: outcomes and lessons learned, *Prog Community Health Partnersh* 9:s21–32, 2015.

Brenner AT, Ko LK, Janz N, et al.: Race/ethnicity and primary language: health beliefs about colorectal cancer screening in a diverse, low-income population, *J Health Care Poor Underserved*, 26(3):824–838. https://doi.org/10.1353/hpu.2015.0075.

Buja A, Rabensteiner A, Sperotto M, et al.: Health literacy and physical activity: a systematic review, *J Phy Act Health* 17(12):1259, October 31, 2020, 74.

Carpenter CJ: A meta-analysis of the effectiveness of health belief model variables in predicting behavior, *Health Commun* 25(8):661—669, 2010. https://doi.org/10.1080/10410236.2010.521906.

Centers for Disease Control and Prevention: What is health literacy? Available from: https://www.cdc.gov/healthliteracy/learn/index.html. Accessed May 19, 2021.

Champion VL, Monahan PO, Springston JK, et al.: Measuring mammography and breast cancer beliefs in African American women, *J Health Psychol* 138:27—37, 2008.

Champion VL, Skinner CS: The health belief model. In Glanz K, Rimer BK, Visnawath K, editors: *Health behavior and education: theory, research, and practice*, ed 4, San Francisco, California, 2008a, Jossey-Bass, pp 45—65.

Champion VL, Skinner CS: The health belief model. In Glanz K, Rimer BK, Viswanath K, editors: *Health behavior and health education: theories, research, and practice*, San Francisco, California, 2008b, Jossey Bass.

Champion VL, Susan M, Rawl SM, et al.: Randomized trial of DVD, telephone, and usual care for increasing mammography adherence, *J Health Psychol* 21(6):916—926, 2016.

Chavarria EA, Christy SM, Simmons VN, et al.: Learner verification: a methodology to create suitable education materials, *Health Lit Res Pract* 5(1):e49—e59, 2021. https://doi.org/10.3928/24748307-20210201-02.

Cheng C, Beauchamp A, Elsworth GR, Osborne RH: Applying the electronic health literacy lens: systematic review of electronic health interventions targeted at socially disadvantaged groups, *J Med Internet Res* 22(8):e18476, 2020.

Chew LD, Bradley KA, Boyko EJ: Brief questions to identify patients with inadequate literacy, *Fam Med* 36:588—594, 2004.

Chin J, Lee EH, Son HJ, et al.: The process-knowledge model of health literacy: evidence from a componential analysis of two commonly used measures, *J Health Communication* 16(Suppl 3):222—241, 2011.

Chinn D: Critical health literacy: a review and critical analyses, *Soc Sci Med* 73:60—67, 2011.

Christie GP, Ratzan SC: Beyond the bench and bedside: health literacy is fundamental to sustainable health and development, *Stud Health Technol Inform* 269:544—560, 2020. https://doi.org/10.3233/SHTI200061.

Christy S, Davis S, Williams K, et al.: A community-based trial of educational interventions with fecal immunochemical test for colorectal cancer screening uptake among blacks in community settings, *Cancer* 122(21):3288—3296, 2016.

Christy SM, Cousin LA, Sutton SK, et al.: Characterizing health literacy among Spanish language-preferring latinos ages 50—75, *Nurs Res* 70:344—353, 2021. https://doi.org/10.1097/NNR.0000000000000519.

Cueva M, Kuhnley R, Lanier A, et al.: Promoting culturally respectful cancer education through digital storytelling, *Int J Circumpolar Health* 11(1):34—49, 2016.

Davis SN, Christy SM, Chavarria E, et al.: A randomized controlled trial of a multi-component targeted low-literacy educational intervention compared with a non-targeted intervention to boost colorectal cancer screening with fecal immunochemical testing in community clinics, 2016, *Cancer*. https://doi.org/10.1002/cncr.30481.

Davis TC, Crouch MA, Long SW, et al.: Rapid assessment of literacy levels of adult primary care patients, *Fam Med* 23(6):433—435, 1991.

Davis TC, Long SW, Jackson RH, et al.: Rapid estimate of adult literacy in medicine: a shortened screening instrument, *Fam Med* 25:56—57, 1993.

Davis TC, Wolf MS, Arnold CL, et al.: Development and validation of the rapid estimate of adolescent literacy in medicine (REALM-Teen): a tool to screen adolescents for below-grade reading in health care settings, *Pediatrics* 118:1707—1714, 2006.

Devia C, Baker EA, Sanchez-Youngman S, et al.: Advancing system and policy changes for social and racial justice: comparing a rural and urban community-based participatory research partnership in the US, *Int J Equity Health* 16(1):17, 2017. https://doi.org/10.1186/s12939-016-0509-3.

Doak CC, Doak LG, Root JH: *Teaching patients with low literacy skills*, ed 2, Philadelphia, 1996, Lippincott Williams & Wilkins. https://www.hsph.harvard.edu/healthliteracy/resources/teaching-patients-with-low-literacy-skills/.

Dotson JAW, Pineda R, Cylkowski H, et al.: Development and evaluation of an iPad application to promote knowledge of tobacco use and cessation by pregnant women, *Nurs Womens Health* 21(3):174—185, 2017. https://doi.org/10.1016/j.nwh.2017.04.005.

Department of Health and Human Services, Public Health Services: Tobacco use and pregnancy. Available from: https://www.cdc.gov/reproductivehealth/maternalinfanthealth/tobaccousepregnancy/index.htm.

Emerson AM, Smith S, Lee J, et al.: Effectiveness of a Kansas city jail-based intervention to improve cervical health literacy and screening, one-year post-intervention, *Am J Health Promot* 34(1):87—90, 2020. https://doi.org/10.1177/0890117119863714.

Fagerlin A, Zikmund-Fisher BJ, Ubel PA, et al.: Measuring numeracy without a math test: development of the subjective numeracy scale (SNS), *Med Decis Making* 27:672—680, 2007.

Farmanova E, Bonneville L, Bouchard L: Organizational health literacy: review of theories, frameworks, guides, and implementation issues, 46958018757848 *Inquiry* 55, 2018. https://doi.org/10.1177/0046958018757848.

Fleming KF, Simmons VN, Christy SM, et al.: Educating hispanic women about cervical cancer prevention: feasibility of a promotora-led charla intervention in a farmworker community, *Ethn Dis* 28(3):169—176, 2018. https://doi.org/10.18865/ed.28.3.169.

Flesch RR: A new readability yardstick, *J Appl Psychol* 32:221—223, 1948.

Freeman HP: Poverty, culture, and social injustice: determinants of cancer disparities, *CA Cancer J Clin* 54:72—77, 2004.

Freire P: *Education for critical consciousness*, New York, 2005, Continuum.

Gardner MS: *Public health nursing*, New York, 1936, Macmillan Co.

Glanz K, Rimer BK, Viswanath K, editors: *Health behavior: theory, research, and practice*, ed 5, San Francisco, 2015, Jossey-Bass.

Green JA, Mor MK, Shields AM, et al.: Associations of Health literacy with dialysis adherence and health resource utilization in patients receiving maintenance hemodialysis, *Am J Kidney Dis* 62(1):73—80, 2013.

Green LW, Kreuter MW: *Health program planning: an educational and ecological approach*, ed 4, New York, 2005, McGraw-Hill. http://www.lgreen.net/hpp/.

Gwede CK, Sutton SK, Chavarria EA, et al.: A culturally and linguistically-salient pilot intervention to promote colorectal cancer screening among Latinos receiving care in a federally qualified health center, *Health Educ Res* 34(3):310—320, 2019. https://doi.org/10.1093/her/cyz010.

Gwede CK, Menard JM, Martinez-Tyson D: Community cancer network community partners. Strategies for Assessing community challenges and strengths for cancer disparities participatory research and outreach, *Health Promot Pract* 11(6):876—887, 2010.

Hasnain-Wynia R, Wolf MS: Promoting health care equity: is health literacy a missing link? *Health Serv Res* 45(4):897—903, 2010. https://doi.org/10.1111/j.1475-6773.2010.01134.x.

Hochbaum GM: *Public participation in medical screening programs: a sociopsychological study*, Washington, DC, 1958, US Public Health Service Pub No 572. Government Printing Office 1589US.

Holliday CE, Wynne M, Katz J, et al.: A CBPR approach to finding community strengths and challenges to prevent youth suicide and substance abuse, *J Transcult Nurs* 29(1):64—73, 2018. https://doi.org/10.1177/1043659616679234.

Holt CL, Roth DL, Huang J, et al.: Longitudinal effects of religious involvement on religious coping and health behaviors in a national sample of African Americans, *Soc Sci Med* 11—19, 2017. https://doi.org/10.1016/j.socscimed.2017.06.014.

Hoogland AI, Lechner SC, Gonzalez BD, et al.: Efficacy of a spanish-language self-administered stress management training intervention for latinas undergoing chemotherapy, *Psycho-Oncology* 27(4):1305—1311, 2018. https://doi.org/10.1002/pon.4673.

Housten AJ, Gunn CM, Paasche-Orlow MK, Basen-Engquist KM: Health literacy interventions in cancer: a systematic review, *J Cancer Educ* 36(2):240—252, 2021.

Irwin, PM. The national literacy act of 1991: major provisions of PL 102—173. CRS Report for Congress. Available from: http://eric.ed.gov/?id=ED341851.

Israel BA, Checkoway B, Schulz A: Health education and community empowerment: conceptualizing and measuring perceptions of individual, organization, and community control, *Health Educ Q* 32:149—170, 1994.

Israel BA, et al.: *Methods for community-based participatory research for health*, ed 2, San Francisco, California, 2013, Jossey-Bass.

Jacobs EA, Walker CM, Miller T, et al.: Development and validation of the Spanish numeracy understanding in medicine instrument, *J Gen Intern Med* 31(11):1345—1352, 2016.

Jemmott JB, Jemmott LS, O'Leary A, et al.: School-based randomized controlled trial of an HIV/STD risk-reduction intervention for South African adolescents, *Arch Pediatr Adolesc Med* 164(10):923—929, 2010. https://doi.org/10.1001/archpediatrics.2010.176.

Jemmott JB, Jemmott LS, O'Leary A, et al.: HIV/STI risk-reduction—intervention efficacy with South African adolescents over 54 months, *Health Psychol* 34(6):610—621, 2015. https://doi.org/10.1037/hea0000140.

Jemmott LS, Jemmott JB, Icard LD, et al.: Effects of church-based parent-child abstinence-only interventions on adolescents' sexual behaviors, *J Adolesc Health* 66(1):107—114, 2020. https://doi.org/10.1016/j.jadohealth.2019.07.021.

Jiao S, Bungay V, Jenkins E: Information and communication technologies in commercial sex work: a double-edged sword for occupational health and safety, *Soc Sci* 10:23, 2021. https://doi.org/10.3390/socsci10010023.

Jones D, Lyle D, McAllister L, et al.: The case for integrated health and community literacy to achieve transformational community engagement and improved health outcomes: an inclusive approach to addressing rural and remote health inequities and community healthcare expectations, *Prim Health Care Res* 21:e57, 2020. https://doi.org/10.1017/S1463423620000481.

Kark S, Steuart GW: *A practice of social medicine, a South African team's experiences in different african communities*, Edinburgh, Scotland, 1962, E. & S. Livinstone.

Kauchak D, Leroy G: Moving beyond readability metrics for health-related text simplification, *IT Prof* 18(3):45—51, 2016. https://doi.org/10.1109/MITP.2016.50.

Kazi AM, Carmichael JL, Hapanna GW, et al.: Assessing mobile phone access and perceptions for texting-based mHealth interventions among expectant mothers and child caregivers in remote regions of Northern Kenya: a survey-based descriptive study, *JMIR Public Health Surveill* 3(1):e5, 2017. https://doi.org/10.2196/publichealth.5386.

Kegeles SS, Kirscht JP, Haefner DP: Survey of beliefs about cancer detection and papanicolaou tests, *Public Health Rep* 80:815—823, 1965.

Kelly PJ, Hunter J, Daily EB, et al.: Challenges to pap smear follow-up among women in the criminal justice system, *J Community Health* 42(1):15—20, 2017. https://doi.org/10.1007/s10900-016-0225-3.

Kleinman A: Concepts and a model for the comparison of medical systems as cultural systems, *Soc Sci Med* 12:85—93, 1978.

Kloetzer L, Lorke J, Roche J, Golumbic Y, Winter S, Jõgeva A: Learning in citizen science. In Vohland K, et al., editors: *The science of citizen science*, Cham, 2021, Springer. https://doi.org/10.1007/978-3-030-58278-4_15.

Knowles MS: *The modern practice of adult education: from pedagogy to andragogy*, Englewood Cliffs, New Jersey, 1988, Cambridge Adult Education.

Knowles MS: *The making of an adult educator: an autobiographical journey*, San Francisco, 1989, Jossey-Bass.

Koh HK, Brach C, Harris LM: A proposed 'health literate care model' would constitute a systems approach to improving patients' engagement in care, *Health Aff (Millwood)* 32:357—367, 2013.

Koskan A, Klasko L, Davis S, et al.: Usage and taxonomy of social media in cancer-related research: a systematic review, *Am J Public Health* 104(7):e20—e37, 2014.

Kowalski C, Lee SY, Schmidt A, et al.: The health literate health care organization 10 item questionnaire (HLHO-10): development and validation, *BMC Health Serv Res* 15(1):1—9, 2015. https://doi.org/10.1186/s12913-015-0707-5.

Kuehnert P, Fawcett J, LePriest K, et al.: *Defining the social determinants of health for nursing action to achieve health equity: a conceptual paper from the American academy of nursing, nursing outlook.*, 2021. Available from: https://doi.org/10.1016/j.outlook.2021.08.003.

Kurti AN, Bunn JY, Nighbor T, et al.: Leveraging technology to address the problem of cigarette smoking among women of reproductive age, *Prev Med* 118:238—242, 2019. https://doi.org/10.1016/j.ypmed.2018.11.004.

Kuwabara A, Su S, Krauss J: Utilizing digital health technologies for patient education in lifestyle medicine, *Am J Lifestyle Med* 14(2):137—142, 2020. https://doi.org/10.1177/1559827619892547.

Labonte R: Health promotion and empowerment: reflections on professional practice, *Health Educ Q* 21:253—268, 1994.

LePrevost CE, Denlea G, Dong L, et al.: Investigating audience response system technology during pesticide training for farmers, *J Agr Edu Ext* 27(1):73—87, 2021.

Leung MM, Agaronov A, Entwistle T, et al.: Voices through cameras: using photovoice to explore food justice issues with minority youth in East Harlem, New York, *Health Promot Pract* 18(2):211—220, 2017. https://doi.org/10.1177/1524839916678404.

Levin-Zamir D, Bertschi I: Media health literacy, eHealth hiteracy, and the role of the social environment in context, *Int J Environ Res Public Health* 15(8):1643, 2018. https://doi.org/10.3390/ijerph15081643.

Lewin K: *The conceptual representation and the measurement of psychological forces*, Durham, North Carolina, 1938, Duke University Press.

Luque JS, Roy S, Tarasenko YN, et al.: Feasibility study of engaging barbershops for prostate cancer education in rural African-American communities, *J Cancer Educ* 30(4):623—628, 2015. https://doi.org/10.1007/s13187-014-0739-2.

MacLeod S, Musich S, Gulyas S, et al.: The impact of inadequate health literacy on patient satisfaction, healthcare utilization, and expenditures among older adults, *Geriatr Nurs* 38(4):334–341, 2017. https://doi.org/10.1016/j.gerinurse.2016.12.003.

Mancuso JM: Assessment and measurement of health literacy: an integrative review of the literature, *Nurs Health Sci* 11:77–89, 2009. https://doi.org/10.1111/j.1442-2018.2008.00408.x.

Marks R: Ethics and patient education: health literacy and cultural dilemmas, *Health Promot Pract* 10:328–332, 2009.

Marmot M, Wilkinson RG: *Social determinants of health*, ed 2, Oxford, United Kingdom, 2005, Oxford University Press. https://doi.org/10.1093/acprof:oso/9780198565895.001.0001.

Marsh P, Gartrell G, Egg G, et al.: End-of-life care in a community garden: findings from a participatory action research project in regional Australia, *Health Place* 45:110–116, 2017. https://doi.org/10.1016/j.healthplace.2017.03.006.

Marsh P, Mallick S, Flies E, et al.: Trust, connection and equity: can understanding context help to establish successful campus community gardens? *Int J Environ Res Public Health* 17(20):7476, 2020. https://doi.org/10.3390/ijerph17207476.

Martinez Tyson DD, Jacobsen P, Meade CD: Understanding the stress management needs and preferences of Latinas undergoing chemotherapy, *J Cancer Educ* 31(4):633–639, 2016.

Maslow AH: *Motivation and personality*, ed 3, New York, 1987, Harper and Row.

Martinez D, Aguado Loi CX, et al.: Development of a cancer camp for adult Spanish-speaking survivors: lessons learned from camp Alegria, *J Cancer Educ* 23(1):4–9, 2008.

McCormack KJ, McCaffery KJ, Dodd RH, Cvejic E, et al.: Health literacy and disparities in COVID-19-related knowledge, attitudes, beliefs and behaviours in Australia, *Public Health Res Pract* 30(4):30342012, 2020. https://doi.org/10.17061/phrp30342012.

McCormack L, Thomas V, Lewis MA, et al.: Improving low health literacy and patient engagement: a social ecological approach, *Patient Educ Couns* 100(1):8–13, 2017. https://doi.org/10.1016/j.pec.2016.07.007.

McLaughlin GH: SMOG grading—a new readability formula of reading, *J Reading* 12(8):639–649, 1969.

McKinlay JB: Epidemiological and political determinants of social policies regarding the public health, *Soc Sci Med* 13A:541–558, 1979.

Meade CD, Christy S, Gwede CK: Improving communications with older cancer patients. In Extermine M, editor: *J Geriatr Oncol*, 2019, Springer Publishing.

Meade CD, Rodriguez EM, Arevalo M, et al.: Introducing biospecimen science to communities: tools from two cities, *Prog Community Health Partnersh*, 2015:51–59, 2015.

Meade CD, Wells KJ, Arevalo M, et al.: Lay navigator model for impacting cancer health disparities, *J Cancer Educ* 29(3):449–457, 2014. https://doi.org/10.1007/s13187-014-0640-z.

Meade CD, Smith CF: Readability formulas: cautions and criteria, *Patient Educ Couns* 17:153–158, 1991.

Meade CD, Menard J, Luque J: Creating community-academic partnerships for cancer disparities research and health promotion, *Health Promotion Pract* 12:456–462, 2011. https://doi.org/10.1177/1524839909341035.

Meade CD, Calvo A, Rivera M: Focus groups in the design of prostate cancer screening information for Hispanic farmworkers and African American men, *Oncol Nurs Forum* 30:967–975, 2003.

Meade CD, Stanley NB, Martinez-Tyson D, et al.: 20 years later: continued relevance of cancer, culture, and literacy in cancer education for social justice and health equity, *J Cancer Educ* 35(4):631–634, 2020. https://doi.org/10.1007/s13187-020-01817-y.

Meleis AI: Culturally competent care, *J Transcult Nurs* 10(12), 1999.

Meltzer LR, Simmons VN, Piñeiro B, et al.: Development of a self-help smoking cessation intervention for dual users of tobacco cigarettes and e-cigarettes, *Int J Environ Res Public Health* 18(5):2328, 2021. https://doi.org/10.3390/ijerph18052328.

Minkler M, Wakimoto P, editors: *Community organizing and community building for health and social equity*, ed 4, New Brunswick, New Jersey, 2012, Rutgers University Press.

Miyamoto S, Thiede E, Dorn L, Perkins DF, Bittner C, Scanlon D: The sexual assault forensic examination telehealth (SAFE-T) center: a comprehensive, nurse-led telehealth model to address disparities in sexual assault care, *J Rural Health* 37(1):92–102, 2021. https://doi.org/10.1111/jrh.12474. Epub 2020 Jun 8. PMID: 32511800; PMCID: PMC7722006.

Mojtahedzadeh R, Mohammadi A, Emami AH, et al.: How digital storytelling applied in health profession education: a systematized review, *J Adv Med Educ Prof* 9(2):63, 2021.

Morris NS, MacLean CD, Chew LD: Single item literacy screener: evaluation of a brief instrument to identify limited reading ability, *BMC Fam Pract* 21, 2006.

Morrison AK, Glick A, Yin HS: Health literacy: implications for child health, *Pediatr Rev* 40(6):263–277, 2019. https://doi.org/10.1542/pir.2018-0027.

Moya EM, Chavez-Baray SM, Loweree J, et al.: Adults experiencing homelessness in the US–Mexico border region: a photovoice project, *Front Public Health* 5:113, 2017. https://doi.org/10.3389/fpubh.2017.00113.

Murdaugh CL, Parsons MA, Pender NJ: *Health promotion in nursing practice*, ed 8, Englewood Cliffs, New Jersey, 2019, Prentice Hall.

National Center for Education Statistics: *Technical report and data file user's manual for 2003*, National Assessment of Adult Literacy. NCES 2009476. 2009. Available from: http://nces.ed.gov/pubsearch/pubsinfo.asp?pubid=2009476.

Nahata L, Anazodo A, Cherven B, Logan S, Meacham LR, Meade CD: Optimizing health literacy to facilitate reproductive health decision-making in adolescent and young adults with cancer, *Pediatr Blood Cancer*, 2020:e28476, 2020. https://doi.org/10.1002/pbc.28476.

National Academies of Sciences, Engineering, and Medicine: *Improving Representation in Clinical Trials and Research: Building Research Equity for Women and Underrepresented Groups*, Washington, DC, 2022, The National Academies Press. https://doi.org/10.17226/26479.

Nielson-Bohlman L, Panzer A, Kindig D, editors: *Health literacy: a prescription to end confusion*, Washington, DC, 2004, National Academies Press. https://doi.org/10.17226/10883.

Nightingale F: *Notes on nursing*, New York, 1859, Appleton-Century-Crofts.

Nguyen TH, Park H, Han HR, et al.: State of the Science of health literacy measures: validity implications for minority populations, *Patient Educ Couns* 98(12):1462–1512, 2015. https://doi.org/10.1016/j.pec.2015.07.013.

Norman C, Skinner HA: eHEALS: The eHealth literacy scale, *J Med Internet Res* 8(4):e27, 2006. https://doi.org/10.2196/jmir.8.4.e27.

Nutbeam D, McGill B, Premkumar P: Improving health literacy in community populations: a review of progress, *Health Promot Int* 33(5):901–911, 2017. https://doi.org/10.1093/heapro/dax015.

Nutbeam D: The evolving concept of health literacy, *Soc Sci Med* 67:2072–2078, 2008.

Nutbeam D: Defining and measuring health literacy: what can we learn from literacy studies? *Int J Public Health* 54(5):303–305, 2009.

Nutbeam D, Lloyd JE: Understanding and responding to health literacy as a social determinant of health, *Annu Rev Public Health* 42:159–173, 2021e. https://doi.org/10.1146/annurev-publhealth-090419-102529.

Nyswander DB: Education for health: some principles and their application, *Health Educ Mono* 14:65—70, 1956.

Olshansky E, Sacco D, Braxter B, et al.: Participatory action research to understand and reduce health disparities, *Nurs Outlook* 53:121—126, 2005.

O'Mara B: Social media, digital video and health promotion in a culturally and linguistically diverse Australia, *Health Promot Int* 28(3):466—476, 2012.

Paakkari L, Okan O: COVID-19: health literacy is an underestimated problem, *Lancet Public Health* 5(5):e249, 2020.

Paasche-Orlow MK, Wolf MS: The causal pathways linking health literacy to health outcomes, *Am J Health Behav* 31(Suppl. l):S19—S26, 2007.

Padden DL, Connors RA, Posey SM, et al.: Factors influencing a health promoting lifestyle in spouses of active duty military, *Health Care Women Int* 34(8):674—693, 2013.

Padilla GV, Bulcavage LM: Theories used in patient/health education, *Semin Oncol Nurs* 7:87—96, 1991.

Parker EA, Israel BA, Williams M, et al.: Community action against asthma: examining the partnership process of a community-based participatory research project, *J Gen Intern Med* 18:558—567, 2003.

Parker RM, Baker DW, Williams MV, et al.: The test of functional health literacy in adults: a new instrument for measuring patients' literacy skills, *J Gen Intern Med* 10:537—541, 1995.

Pavlov IP: *Experimental psychology, and other essays*, New York, 1957, Philosophical Library.

Peerson A, Saunders M: Health literacy revisited: what do we mean and why does it matter? *Health Promot Int* 24:285—296, 2009.

Pender NJ, Murdaugh C, Parsons MA, et al.: *Health promotion in nursing practice*, ed 7, 2015, Pearson.

Pew Research Center: *Internet and technology. Mobile fact sheets.* Available: https://www.pewresearch.org/internet/fact-sheet/mobile/.

Piaget J: *Adaptation and intelligence: organic selection and phenocopy*, Chicago, Illinois, 1980, University of Chicago Press.

Pourrazavi S, Kouzekanani K, Bazargan-Hejazi S, Shaghaghi A, Hashemiparast M, Fathifar Z, Allahverdipour H: Theory-based e-Health literacy interventions in older adults: a systematic review, *Arch Public Health* 78:72, 2020. https://doi.org/10.1186/s13690-020-00455-6.

Prihanto JB, Nurhayati F, Wahjuni ES, et al.: Health literacy and health behavior: associated factors in Surabaya high school students, Indonesia, *Int J Environ Res Public Health* 18(15):8111, 2021. https://doi.org/10.3390/ijerph18158111.

Prochaska JO, DiClemente CC: Stages and processes of self-change of smoking: toward an integrative model of change, *J Consult Clin Psychol* 51(3):390—395, 1983.

Quad Council Coalition Competency Review Task Force. *Community/public health nursing competencies. 2018*, Available from: https://www.cphno.org/wp-content/uploads/2020/08/QCC-C-PHN-COMPETENCIESApproved_2018.05.04_Final-002.pdf. Accessed October 8, 2021.

Quinn GP, Albert AB, Sutter M, et al.: What oncologists should know about treating sexual and gender minority patients with cancer, *JCO Oncol Pract* 16(6):309—316, 2020. https://doi.org/10.1200/OP.20.00036.

Quinn GP, Sanchez JA, Sutton SK, et al.: Cancer and lesbian, gay, bisexual, transgender/transsexual, and queer/questioning populations (LGBTQ), *CA Cancer J Clin* 65(5):384—400, 2015. https://doi.org/10.3322/caac.21288.

Rankin SH, et al.: *Patient education in health and illness*, ed 5, Philadelphia, PA, 2005, Lippincott Williams and Wilkins.

Rawl SM, Christy SM, Monahan PO, et al.: Tailored telephone counseling increases colorectal cancer screening, *Health Educ Res* 30(4):622—637, 2015. https://doi.org/10.1093/her/cyv021.

Rawl SM, Skinner CS, Perkins SM, et al.: Computer-delivered tailored intervention improves colon cancer screening knowledge and health beliefs of African Americans, *Health Educ Res* 5:868—885, 2012. https://doi.org/10.1093/her/cys094.

Redman BK: *The practice of patient education: a case study approach*, ed 10, St. Louis, Missouri, 2007, Elsevier.

Robbins LB, Ling J, Sharma DB, et al.: Intervention effects of "girls on the move" on increasing physical activity: a group randomized trial, *Ann Behav Med* 53(5):493—500, 2019. https://doi.org/10.1093/abm/kay054.

Rogers CR: *A Carl Rogers Reader*, Boston, 1989, Houghton Mifflin.

Rosenstock I: Why people use health services, *Milbank Mem Fund Q* 44:94—127, 1966.

Rosenstock IM, Strecher VJ, Becker MH: Social learning theory and the health belief model, *Health Educ Q* 15(2):175—183, 1988.

Ross L, Meier N: Improving adult coping with social isolation during COVID-19 in the community through nurse-led patient-centered telehealth teaching and listening interventions, *Nurs Forum* 56(2):467—473, 2020. https://doi.org/10.1111/nuf.12552.

Rowlands G, Nutbeam D: Health literacy and the 'inverse information law, *Br J Gen Pract* 63(608):120—121, 2013. https://doi.org/10.3399/bjgp13X664081.

Rudd RE, Oelschlegel S, Grabeel KL, et al.: *The HLE2 assessment tool*, Boston, 2019, Harvard T.H. Chan School of Public Health. Available from: chrome-extension://oemmndcbldboiebfnladdacbdfmadadm/https://cdn1.sph.harvard.edu/wp-content/uploads/sites/135/2019/05/april-30-FINAL_The-Health-Literacy-Environment2_Locked.pdf. Accessed November 19, 2021.

Rue CB: *The public health nurse in the community*, Philadelphia, Pennsylvania, 1944, Saunders.

Sieh P-L: Applying the Pender's health promotion model to identify the factors related to older adults' participation in community-based health promotion activities, *Int J Environ Res Public Health* 18:9985, 2021. https://doi.org/10.3390/ijerph18199985.

Samoil D, Kim J, Fox C, et al.: The importance of health literacy on clinical cancer outcomes: a scoping review, *Annals Cancer Epidemiol* 5, 2021. https://doi.org/10.21037/ace-20-30.

Santana S, Brach C, Harris L, et al.: Updating health literacy for healthy people 2030: defining its importance for a new decade in public health, *J Public Health Manag Practice* (27):S258—S264, 2021. https://doi.org/10.1097/PHH.0000000000001324.

Schapira MM, Meade C, Nattinger AB: Enhanced decision-making: the use of a videotape decision-aid for patients with prostate cancer, *Patient Educ Couns* 30:119—127, 1997.

Schapira MM, Walker CM, Miller T, et al.: Development and validation of the numeracy understanding in medicine instrument short form, *J Health Commun* 19(Suppl 2):240—253, 2014. https://doi.org/10.1080/10810730.2014.933916.

Schier HE, Linsenmeyer WR: Nutrition-related messages shared among the online transgender community: a netnography of youtube vloggers, *Transgend Health* 4(1):340—349, 2019. https://doi.org/10.1089/trgh.2019.0048.

Shoemaker SJ, Wolf MS, Brach C: Development of the patient education materials assessment tool (PEMAT): a new measure of understandability and actionability for print and audiovisual patient information, *Patient Educ Couns* 96(3):395—403, 2014. https://www.ahrq.gov/health-literacy/patient-education/pemat.html.

Shi Y, Ma D, Zhang J, Chen B: In the digital age: a systematic literature review of the E-health literacy and influencing factors among

Chinese older adults, *Z Gesundh Wiss* 4:1—9, 2021. https://doi.org/10.1007/s10389-021-01604-z.

Singh A, Nichols M: Nurse-Led education and engagement for diabetes care in sub-Saharan Africa: protocol for a mixed methods study, *JMIR Res Protoc* 9(6):e15408, 2020. https://doi.org/10.2196/15408.

Simmons VN, Fleming K, Koskan AM, et al.: Participatory evaluation of a community-academic partnership to inform capacity-building and sustainability, *Eval Program Plann* 52:19—26, 2015.

Sium A, Giuliani M, Papadakos J: The persistence of the pamphlet: on the continued relevance of the health information pamphlet in the digital age, *J Canc Educ* 32:483—486, 2017. https://doi.org/10.1007/s13187-015-0948-3.

Skinner BF: About behaviorism. In *Vintage books*, New York, 1976, Random House.

Son H, Nahm ES: Older Adults' experience using patient portals in communities: challenges and opportunities, *Comput Inform Nurs* 37(1):4—10, 2019. https://doi.org/10.1080/10410236.2014.940675.

Stevens EM, Vidrine DJ, Hoover DS, et al.: Enhancing smoking risk communications: the influence of health literacy on need for cognition, *Am J Health Behav* 43(5):950—962, 2019. https://doi.org/10.5993/AJHB.43.5.7.

Strecher VJ, DeVellis BM, Becker MH: The role of self-efficacy in achieving health behavior change, *Health Educ Q* 13:73—92, 1986.

Streuli S, Ibrahim N, Mohamed A, Sharma M, Esmailian M, Sezan I, Farrell C, Sawyer M, Meyer D, El-Maleh K, Thamman R, Marchetti A, Lincoln A, Courchesne E, Sahid A, Bhavnani SP: Development of a culturally and linguistically sensitive virtual reality educational platform to improve vaccine acceptance within a refugee population: the SHIFA community engagement-public health innovation programme, *BMJ Open* 11(9):e051184, 2021. https://doi.org/10.1136/bmjopen-2021-051184.

Suarez-Lledo V, Alvarez-Galvez J: Prevalence of health misinformation on social media, *Systematic Rev J Med Internet Res* 23(1):e17187, 2021. https://doi.org/10.2196/17187.

Tefera YG, Gebresillassie BM, Emiru YK, et al.: Diabetic health literacy and its association with glycemic control among adult patients with type 2 diabetes mellitus attending the outpatient clinic of a University Hospital in Ethiopia, *Plos One* 15(4):e0231291, 2020. https://doi.org/10.1371/journal.pone.0231291.

Teitelman AM, Jemmott AM, Bellamy SL, et al.: Partner violence, power and gender differences in South African adolescents' HIV/STI behaviors, *Health Psychol* 35(7):751—760, 2016. https://doi.org/10.1037/hea0000351.

Thompson MR, Schwartz Barcott D: The role of the nurse scientist as a knowledge broker, *J Nurs Scholarsh* 51(1):26—39, 2019. https://doi.org/10.1111/jnu.12439.

Thorndike EL: *Educational psychology*, New York, 1969, Arno Press.

Thurman W, Pfitzinger-Lippe M: Returning to the profession's roots: social justice in nursing education for the 21st century, *Adv Nurs Sci* 40(4):318, 2017. https://doi.org/10.1097/ANS0000000000000140.

Tucker CM, Wippold GM, Williams JL, Arthur TM, Desmond FF, Robinson KC: A CBPR study to test the impact of a church-based health empowerment program on health behaviors and health outcomes of black adult churchgoers, *J Racial Ethn Health Disparities* 4(1):70—78, 2017. https://doi.org/10.1007/s40615-015-0203-y.

Turner PG, Lefevre CE: Instagram use is linked to increased symptoms of orthorexia nervosa, *Eat Weight Disord* 22(2):277—284, 2017. https://doi.org/10.1007/s40519-017-0364-2.

Tyson DM, Chavez MN, Lubrano B, et al.: Understanding cancer survivors' educational needs about prescription opioid medications: implications for cancer education and health literacy, *J Cancer Educ* 36(2):215—224, 2021. https://doi.org/10.1007/s13187-021-01957-9. Erratum in: *J Cancer Educ.* 36(4):893, 2021.

U.S. Department of Health and Human Services: *Making Health Communication Programs Work: A Planner's Guide*, pink book, Bethesda, MD, 2008, Office of Cancer Communications, National Cancer Institute. Available from: https://www.cancer.gov/publications/health-communication/pink-book.pdf.

U.S. Department of Health and Human Services, Office of Disease Prevention and Health Promotion: *National Action Plan to Improve Health Literacy*, 2010. Available from: https://health.gov/communication/hlactionplan/pdf/Health_Literacy_Action_Plan.pdf.

U.S. Department of Health and Human Services, Centers for Disease Control and Prevention, National Center for Chronic Disease Prevention and Health Promotion: The health consequences of smoking: a report of the Surgeon General. Atlanta, GA, Office on Smoking and Health.

U.S. Department of Health and Human Services, Public Health Services: Healthy People 2030, n.d. Available from: https://health.gov/our-work/national-health-initiatives/healthy-people/healthy-people-2030/health-literacy-healthy-people-2030.

U.S. Department of Health and Human Services: *Public Health Services, Office of Minority Health (OMH): The National Standards for Culturally and Linguistically Appropriate Services in Health and Health Care (The National CLAS Standards)*, 2018. Available from: https://minorityhealth.hhs.gov/omh/browse.aspx?lvl=2&lvlid=53.

U.S. Department of Health and Human Services. SmokeFree.gov. Available from: https://smokefree.gov/.

Vamos CA, Kline N, Lockhart E, et al.: Stakeholders' perspectives on system-level barriers to and facilitators of HPV vaccination among hispanic migrant farmworkers, *Ethn Health*, 2021:1—23, 2021. https://doi.org/10.1080/13557858.2021.1887820.

van den Heuvel JF, Vamos CA, Groenhof TK, Veerbeek JH, et al.: eHealth as the next-generation perinatal care: an overview of the literature, *J Med Internet Res* 20(6):e202, 2018. https://doi.org/10.2196/jmir.9262. PMID: 29871855; PMCID: PMC6008510.

Van Wyk NC: Health education as education of the oppressed, *Curationis* 22:29—34, 1999.

Villagra VG, Bhuva B, Coman E, Smith DO, Fifield J: Health insurance literacy: disparities by race, ethnicity, and language preference, *Am J Manag Care* 25(3):e71—e75, 2019.

Vinci C: Cognitive behavioral and mindfulness-based interventions for smoking cessation: a review of the recent literature, *Curr Oncol Rep* 22(6):58, 2020. https://doi.org/10.1007/s11912-020-00915-w.

Wallace LS, Rogers ES, Roskos SE, et al.: Brief report: screening items to identify patients with limited health literacy skills, *J Gen Intern Med* 21:874—877, 2006.

Wallerstein N, Bernstein E: Empowerment education: Freire's Ideas adapted to health education, *Health Educ Q* 15:379—394, 1988.

Wallerstein N, Duran B, Oetzel J, et al.: *Community-based participatory research for health: advancing social and health equity*, ed 3, San Francisco, CA, 2017, Jossey-Bass.

Ward M, Schulz AJ, Israel BA, et al.: A conceptual framework for evaluating health equity promotion within community-based participatory research partnerships, *Eval Program Plann* 70:25—34, 2018. https://doi.org/10.1016/j.evalprogplan.2018.04.014.

Weiss BD, Mays MZ, Martz W, et al.: Quick assessment of literacy in primary care: the newest vital sign, *Ann Fam Med* 3:514–522, 2005.

Wells KJ, Otero CV, Bredice M, et al.: Acceptability of a virtual patient educator for hispanic women, *Hispanic Health Care Int* 13(4):179–185, 2015. https://doi.org/10.1891/1540-4153.13.4.179.

Wells KJ, Meade CD, Calcano E: Innovative approaches to reducing cancer health disparities: the Moffitt cancer center patient navigator research program, *J Cancer Edu* 26(4):649–657, 2011.

Wertheimer M: *Productive thinking*, New York, 1959, Harper.

Wilkinson GS, Robertson GJ: *Wide range achievement test 5 professional manual*, Lutz, FL, 2017, Psychological Assessment Resources.

World Health Organization Commission on the Social Determinants of Health: *Achieving Health Equity: From Root Causes to Fair Outcomes*, Geneva, Switzerland, 2007, World Health Organization. http://apps.who.int/iris/bitstream/10665/69670/1/interim_statement_eng.pdf.

Yen PH, Leasure AR: Use and Effectiveness of the teach-back method in patient education and health outcomes, *Fed Pract* 36(6):284–289, 2009.

Zehbe I, Wood B, Wakewich P, et al.: Teaching tools to engage Anishinaabek first nations women in cervical cancer screening: report of an educational workshop, *Health Edu J* 75(3):331–342, 2016. https://doi.org/10.1177/0017896915580446.

9

Case Management

Karyn Leavitt Grow and Jean Cozad Lyon

OBJECTIVES

Upon completion of this chapter, the reader will be able to do the following:

1. Define case management, care management, and care coordination and compare the differences.
2. Discuss the guiding principles of case management.
3. Identify the origin and purpose of case management.
4. Identify the case management process.
5. Discuss the roles and characteristics of case management in a reformed healthcare environment.
6. Incorporate case management concepts into clinical practice settings.
7. Identify educational preparation and skills recommended for case managers.

OUTLINE

KEY TERMS

care management
case management
chronic care management
continuum of care
patient-centered medical home
transitional care management
utilization review

OVERVIEW OF CASE MANAGEMENT

Case management is a term that describes a wide variety of patient care coordination programs in acute hospital and community settings. Case management is also referred to as *care management* and *care coordination*. These terms apply to community health settings that include patient-centered medical homes (PCMHs), occupational health, geriatric services, ambulatory care clinics, mental health settings, and outpatient primary care settings. Patient populations of all ages receive case management services.

Since the late 1980s and the 1990s, a variety of case management programs have emerged (Huber, 2002). From 1990 to 2005, case management evolved rapidly in response to changes in the healthcare environment and an increase in the number of managed care programs. Client service use reflects a greater emphasis on healthcare costs. Third-party payers evaluate the appropriate use of healthcare resources such as diagnostic tests, laboratory tests, length of hospital visits, use of emergency services, and duration of home healthcare services. Healthcare providers, interested in close monitoring of resources, introduced various forms of case management programs.

More recently, healthcare evolved from a quantity-driven delivery system to a quality-driven system. In 2001, the National Academy of Medicine (NAM), formerly called the Institute of Medicine (IOM), published a report, *Crossing the Quality Chasm*. It recommended a redesign of the healthcare system to provide care that is safe, efficient, effective, timely, equitable, and patient centered. The report names care coordination as an essential function to reach these goals and improve healthcare quality (IOM, 2001). Case management has emerged as an intervention strategy for quality improvement initiatives. A single definition of case management does not exist. The Case Management Society of America (CMSA) (2016) offers the following definition of case management:

> *Case management is a collaborative process of assessment, planning, facilitation, care coordination, evaluation and advocacy for options and services to meet an individual's and family's comprehensive health care needs through communication and available resources to promote patient safety, quality of care and cost effective outcomes. (p. 11)*

The Commission for Case Management Certification (CCMC) (2021) defines case management as:

> *a collaborative process that assesses, plans, implements, coordinates, monitors and evaluates the options and services required to meet the client's health and human service needs. It is characterized by advocacy, communication, and resource management and promotes quality and cost-effective interventions and outcomes.*

Case management programs, however, aim to provide a service delivery approach to ensure the following: cost-effective care, alternatives to institutionalization, access to care, coordinated services, and patient's improved functional capacity (Lyon, 1993) (Box 9.1). These goals apply to community health and acute care settings. Subsets of case management are care management, care coordination, and transitional care management (TCM).

The case management, care management, care coordination, and TCM programs focus on high-need, high-cost patients.

BOX 9.1   Possible Case Management Functions

- Identifying the target population
- Determining screening and eligibility
- Arranging services
- Monitoring and follow-up
- Assessing
- Planning care
- Reassessing
- Assisting clients through a complex, fragmented healthcare system
- Providing care coordination and continuity

Care Management

Care management consists of programs that apply systems, science, incentives, and information to improve medical practice and to allow clients and their support systems to participate in a collaborative process with a goal of improving medical, psychosocial, and behavioral health conditions more effectively. Care management is a concept that is evidence based, patient centered, and clinical care focused.

The overall goal of care management is to improve the coordination of services provided to clients who are enrolled in a care management program. Examples of groups of people who may be served by care management services are the elderly, children from low-income families who receive Medicaid services, and groups of people with chronic illnesses.

Care Coordination

Care coordination was identified in the NAM report *Crossing the Quality Chasm* as an essential function in improving health quality (IOM, 2001). It has also been recognized as an approach to integrate fragmented healthcare, improve the transitions of care between providers, and decrease the unnecessary utilization of resources and costs. Care coordination programs are those that target chronically ill persons at risk for adverse outcomes and expensive care and that meet their needs by filling the gaps in healthcare. They (1) identify the full range of medical, functional, social, and emotional problems that increase patients' risk of adverse health events; (2) address those needs through education in self-care, optimization of medical treatment, and integration of care fragmented by setting or provider; and (3) monitor patients for progress and early signs of problems. Such programs hold the promise of raising the quality of healthcare, improving health outcomes, and reducing the need for costly hospitalizations and medical care (Chen et al., 2000).

There are many definitions of care coordination. In its 2005 report, *Closing the Quality Gap: A Critical Analysis of Quality Improvement Strategies, Volume 7: Care Coordination*, the Agency for Health Care Research and Quality (AHRQ) defines *care coordination* as follows:

> *The deliberate organization of patient care activities between two or more participants (including the patient) involved in a patient's care to facilitate the appropriate delivery of health care services. Organizing care involves the marshaling of personnel and other resources needed to carry out all required patient care activities, and is often managed by the exchange of information among participants responsible for different aspects of care. Care coordination is a process component and function of case management.*
>
> *McDonald et al. (2005)*

And in the American Nurses Association (ANA) white paper titled *The Value of Nursing Care Coordination*, the term *care coordination* is defined as follows:

> *Care coordination is (a) a function that helps ensure that the patient's needs and preferences are met over time with*

respect to health services and information sharing across people, functions, and sites; and (b) the deliberate organization of patient care activities between two or more participants (including the patient) involved in a patient's care to facilitate the appropriate delivery of health care services. Additionally, the best coordination model is one in which a patient experiences primary care as delivered by an integrated, multidisciplinary team that explicitly includes at least one staff care coordinator.

ANA (2012).

Care coordination and care management are terms that are used interchangeably. In the quality-driven healthcare system where healthcare organizations are responsible for the quality and cost of caring for patients, care management and care coordination programs such as the Medicare Chronic Care Management (CCM) program focus on high-need, high-cost patients; the 5% who account for 50% of healthcare spending (DHHS, 2012).

Transitional Care Management

TCM programs seek to improve communication between healthcare providers and coordination of care and services for patients across healthcare settings. This process is a subset of the case management, care management, and care coordination programs.

There are many transitional care models in practice that have variations in staffing preferences. Two of the most widely implemented and respected models are the Transitional Care Model and the Medicare program Transitional Care Management.

TCM is the process of providing a postdischarge patient with a high or moderate risk of readmission a face-to-face visit with their practitioner within a defined period (7—14 days) and care coordination services to prevent readmissions and improve outcomes. The TCM care coordinator follows a patient post-hospitalization to improve patient/caregiver understanding and self-management of new disease processes, discharge instructions, medication management, coordination of care and resources, and timely access and follow-up with the patient's primary care provider (DHHS and CMS, 2016).

The paper *Continuity of Care: The Transitional Care Model* by foundational authors including Mary Naylor, defines the Transitional Care Model as follows:

A nurse-led intervention targeting older adults at risk for poor outcomes as they move across healthcare settings and between clinicians. The model has nine core components that include screening, staffing, maintaining relationships, engaging patients and caregivers, assessing/managing risks and symptoms, educating/promoting self-management, promoting continuity, and fostering coordination.

The Transitional Care Model uses advanced practice registered nurses (APRNs) to provide patient-centered, comprehensive, holistic care and to provide oversight to other team members (Hirschman et al., 2015).

The transitions of care process is an integral component of all successful case management programs.

ORIGINS OF CASE MANAGEMENT

Case management has a long history with the mentally ill, elderly patients, and the community setting (Steinberg and Carter, 1983). Public health, mental health, and long-term care settings have implemented and studied case management services and have reported them in their literature for many years (Mahn and Spross, 1996).

Case management has evolved with many iterations of the healthcare delivery system including managed care, accountable care organizations, disability management, and value-based purchasing processes.

Public Health

Community service coordination, which was a forerunner of case management, appeared in public health programs in the early 1900s. During this time, healthcare providers reported these community service and case management programs in the nursing literature. Programs focused on community education in sanitation, nutrition, and disease prevention became prevalent. Lillian Wald and Mary Brewster conducted many of these programs at the Henry Street Settlement House in New York City. The Metropolitan Life Insurance Company later expanded nursing services for individuals, families, and the community to include disease prevention and health promotion (Conger, 1999).

The concept of **continuum of care** originated after World War II to describe the long-term services required for discharged psychiatric patients (Grau, 1984). Service coordination evolved into case management, a term that first appeared in social welfare literature during the early 1970s.

Case Management in Behavioral Health

During the late 1960s and early 1970s, mental healthcare emphasized moving patients from mental health institutions back into the community (Crosby, 1987; Pittman, 1989). The Community Mental Health Center Act of 1963 placed federal approbation on deinstitutionalization, which emphasized the importance of community mental health services. Mental health providers began to move patients from large state institutions to the community.

Several problems resulted from the deinstitutionalization of mentally ill patients. In 1977, Congress acknowledged that many disabled people had been deinstitutionalized without basic needs, proper follow-up, or healthcare monitoring. Congress further recognized that a systematic approach to service delivery could have prevented many state hospital readmissions. Case management in community mental health helped avoid client service fragmentation (Pittman, 1989).

Case Management and the Elderly

Specific elderly services recognized that age-generic programs do not adequately assist older people. Many older people have special, population-specific healthcare needs. Thus, case management services frequently target the elderly population, specifically homebound individuals, or those with complex problems. However, not all older people who subscribe to multiple services require a case manager. Older adults may not need a case manager if they possess adequate functional status and can coordinate and access services for themselves, if they have family support, or if they have formal or informal caregivers who provide these functions for them.

With the shift of healthcare from a fragmented, quantity-driven healthcare system to a quality-driven or value-based healthcare system, many more seniors with chronic conditions are accessing case/care management or care coordination services. Payers are realizing the benefits of coordination of care and services, self-management practices, and increased communication between providers and resources as an efficient process to increase quality outcomes and decrease the cost of healthcare services. Thus, payers or insurers (including Medicare) are making case/care management services available at free or low cost to the elderly population with chronic conditions in the community setting.

Disease-Specific Case Management

Case management services are often provided for individuals who are identified as having medical conditions that are high-cost or high-volume acute and chronic illnesses. Examples are asthma, diabetes, chronic obstructive pulmonary disease, and chronic cardiac conditions such as congestive heart failure. The goal of disease-specific case management is to keep the individuals as healthy as possible and stable in their home environments. One particular goal is to decrease the frequency and length of hospital stays and consequently reduce healthcare costs.

PURPOSE OF CASE MANAGEMENT

Case management, care management, and care coordination are patient-centered and system-centered processes. Case management focuses on care coordination, financial management, and the utilization of resources for a patient-centered plan of care.

Patient-centered case management improves self-management of chronic disease; helps the client or patient proceed through a complex, fragmented, and often confusing healthcare delivery system; and achieves specific client-centered goals. System-centered processes recognize that healthcare resources are finite. The upward spiral in healthcare costs leads third-party payers such as Medicare, managed care organizations, and commercial payers to demand cost-effective healthcare. Providers are reimbursed for care provided on the basis of value-based purchasing; this includes hospitals, skilled-nursing facilities, home health organizations, and practitioners. Client consumers insist on cost-effective, efficient, high-quality care. This demand forces healthcare providers to reevaluate the way they administer care, to emphasize quality improvement, and to focus on decreasing cost. Healthcare resources then become

allocated to those populations with the greatest needs. Case management is used to promote and integrate the coordination of clinical services, linking patients to community services and agencies. Case managers monitor resources used by clients, support collaborative practice and continuity of care, and enhance patient satisfaction (Yamamoto and Lucey, 2005).

Care Management

Care management has emerged as a primary means of managing the health of a defined population through coordination of services and self-management care. The purpose of care management is to reduce health risks and cost of care for a defined population (AHRQ, 2015).

In the "Care Management Issue Brief: Implications for Medical Practice, Health Policy and Health Services Research," AHRQ highlights three key strategies to enhance care management for target populations:

(1) Identify population(s) with modifiable risks; (2) Align CM services to the needs of the population(s); and (3) Identify, prepare, and integrate appropriate personnel to deliver the needed services.

Care Coordination

Care coordination is an emerging process. It encompasses collaborating with the patient to develop a plan of care and patient-centered goals, working to develop improved chronic disease self-management skills, and providing coordination of services. It is a subset of the case management process. AHRQ defines care coordination as

the deliberate organization of patient care activities between two or more participants (including the patient) involved in a patient's care to facilitate the appropriate delivery of health care services. Organizing care involves the marshalling of personnel and other resources needed to carry out all required patient care activities, and is often managed by the exchange of information among participants responsible for different aspects of care.

McDonald et al. (2005)

Utilization Review and Managed Care

Equity and cost-effectiveness require management and allocation of available resources in a hospital, community, city, state, or particular health care client population. **Utilization review** (UR), as defined by CMSA, consists of the evaluation of medical appropriateness or medical necessity of care. This review ensures that patients receive the right level of care at the right time to improve clinical outcomes and lower costs.

Case management programs are often motivated by the need to evaluate, use, and allocate healthcare resources. Many case management programs evolved from UR departments. These departments showed that monitoring service use alone is insufficient for managing patient populations with diverse resource needs. Over time, the UR nurses assumed the additional case manager responsibilities.

TRENDS THAT INFLUENCE CASE MANAGEMENT

Numerous trends have influenced case management programs. During the 1970s, hospitals billed Medicare, Medicaid, and other third-party payers for client services and received reimbursement. Healthcare costs skyrocketed and rapidly became the basis for discussion and concern throughout the healthcare industry and the country. In 1983, PL 98-21 of the Social Security Amendments introduced the prospective payment system (PPS) in the acute care setting. Under the PPS, healthcare providers receive a fixed amount of money based on the relative cost of resources they use to treat Medicare patients within each diagnosis-related group. Other third-party payers followed this example and negotiated reimbursement schedules through preferred provider programs or managed care contracts (US Department of Commerce, 1990).

More recently, Medicare's value-based purchasing measures drive healthcare organizations to improve their cost and quality by adjusting reimbursement. This model is now also adopted by commercial payers. This has led to new models of care including the accountable care organization (ACO) model. The ACO relies heavily on case management programs to increase quality outcomes, patient satisfaction, and decreased healthcare costs.

Another recently recognized focus of the case management process is the social determinants of health (SoDH). SoDH have exposed links to disparities in access to care and decreased or poor health outcomes. The SoDH can be defined as the conditions in which people are born, live, work, and age and are shaped by the distribution of money, power, and resources (Lax et al., 2017). These conditions include access to fresh and affordable food, safe housing and reliable transportation, employment, social support, health literacy, education, and personal safety. It is increasingly recognized as an integral piece of the personal healthcare puzzle. While access to quality clinical care contributes about 20% toward overall positive health, social and economic conditions contribute 40%, health behaviors 30%, and physical environment 10% (University of Wisconsin, 2021). Therefore, assessing and coordinating services for the client's social determinants are increasingly becoming an important focus for the case/care management and care coordination programs for comprehensive, positive client outcomes.

Changes in Healthcare Reimbursement

Title III of the Patient Protection and Affordable Care Act (2010) (Public Law 111-148), passed by Congress in March 2010, includes provisions that require improvement in the quality and efficiency of healthcare. The Centers for Medicare and Medicaid (CMS) has established value-based purchasing programs for hospitals, postacute providers, and practitioners. These programs link Medicare payments to quality performance, utilization of evidence-based practices, cost of care, and patient experience scores (CMS.gov, 2017). Providers who participate and exceed in their relative scoring will be eligible for incentive payments; additionally, there are financial penalties for nonparticipating providers (Public Law 111-148, 2010).

To assist practitioners with success in the value-based reimbursement structure, CMS provides reimbursement for chronic care management programs and transitions of care programs.

Access to Healthcare for More Americans

The Patient Protection and Affordable Care Act removes many barriers to healthcare for Americans. With insurance coverage available to people through employers or purchased through healthcare access networks, more Americans have insurance and have access to healthcare. These changes opened up opportunities for nurses working in case manager or care coordination roles. Case managers have developed and expanded their roles in working with diverse patient populations. These issues have influenced, and continue to influence, the expansion of case management services to control costs and distribute healthcare resources in a variety of settings.

EDUCATION AND PREPARATION FOR CASE MANAGERS

It is essential to determine what classification of healthcare provider is best qualified to provide case management services. Traditionally, case managers were social workers (SWs) who assumed the role of discharge planner. Client healthcare needs have become more complex, the need for ongoing patient assessment has emerged, and available resources have become more numerous and diverse; therefore, nurses have become case managers. Several healthcare organizations exclusively employ SWs in case manager roles, others exclusively employ nurses in case management, and others use a combination of SWs and nurses, depending on the client population's needs. Combining the strength and knowledge of the nurse's clinical background with the SW's community service background can efficiently move a client through the complex healthcare system (Lyon et al., 1995).

Nurse Case Managers

Although both nurses and SWs have proved themselves to be excellent case managers, this chapter focuses on the nurse case manager in discussing educational requirements. A nurse case manager's optimum education level is debatable. The basic nursing education for case managers required by employers can vary. Some require a baccalaureate degree, and others do not. In some settings, a master's degree or APRN is required. Some programs are more interested in prior experience, continuing education, and case management certification than in the entry-level nursing degree. Education and experience requirements may vary, depending on the program's geographic location, specific client needs, and available staff.

Online academic education is available and makes undergraduate and graduate nursing education for nurses living in rural areas accessible.

Regardless of the educational requirements in the individual case management program, case managers need a minimum skill level to ensure success in the role. These skills include sound knowledge of reimbursement structures; knowledge of available resources within the institution, organization, or community; working knowledge of the identification and evaluation of quality outcomes; the ability to perform cost–benefit ratios; and an understanding of financial strategies. In addition to the required knowledge, the nurse case manager needs flexibility, creativity, excellent communication skills, and the ability to work autonomously.

Case Manager Certification Options

There are a few options for case managers to become certified. The certifications are offered by the Commission for Case Manager Certification (CCMC), the American Case Management Association (ACMA, 2021), and the American Nurses Credentialing Center (ANCC).

Commission for Case Manager Certification

The Commission for Case Manager Certification offers certification in case management. The certification granted is the Certified Case Manager (CCM) credential. Following are the requirements for applicants (Commission for Case Manager Certification, 2013):

- Licensed healthcare worker or a bachelor's degree in a health or human services field
- Twelve months experience supervised by a CCM, or 24 months as a full-time case manager, or 12 months as a supervisor of individuals who provide case management

American Nurses Credentialing Center

The ANCC offers certification in nursing case management; it is the CMGT-BC. To be eligible to take the certification examination, applicants must

- hold a current, active registered nurse (RN) license within a state or territory of the United States or the professional, legally recognized equivalent in another country;

- have practiced the equivalent of 2 years full time as an RN;
- have a minimum of 2000 h of clinical practice in case management nursing within the past 3 years;
- have completed 30 h of continuing education in case management nursing within the past 3 years.

American Case Management Association

The American Case Management Association offers an Accredited Case Manager (ACM) certification. The details of this certification are as follows:

- Specifically addresses case management in health delivery settings.
- The exam consists of two components: core case management questions that test the knowledge skills and abilities clinical staff in a hospital/health system and discipline-specific clinical simulations.

Other certifications. Several other certifications in specialty case management are available: disability management, healthcare quality, utilization management, managed care, and case management administrator certification. Case management professionals who are interested in obtaining certification should carefully research the options available for certification and should select the credentialing program that fits their work performed, education, and future career goals (CMSA, 2016).

CASE MANAGER SERVICES

Although case management programs differ in structure and design, case managers provide services regardless of the program's location. There is a consensus in the literature that there are six components to case management: client identification and engagement, assessment, care plan development, implementation and coordination of plan of care, monitoring and evaluation, and closure of professional services (CMSA, 2016). The focus of each of these functions varies depending on the case management model.

Examples of care coordination include assisting the client or family member with medical appointments, equipment acquisition, home meal delivery, home follow-up services (e.g., home health or public health nursing), the SDoH (such as housing, transportation, and access to food), and medical insurance or Medicare form completion. The types of services differ depending on the location of the case management program, the population of clients, and the scope of case management services. Some case managers in managed care environments monitor whether the patient keeps medical appointments and follows the prescribed course of treatment.

Depending on the setting, community case management services continue for varying lengths of time. Some programs continue service coordination indefinitely for populations such as the high-risk elderly and the chronically ill. Other programs move clients' case management status from active to inactive when patients no longer require services. However, the status becomes active again if their conditions change. Case management services continue in the home healthcare setting until the client is discharged from the program. Care coordination in the primary healthcare delivery setting is increasingly being provided in PCMHs and primary care clinics. It is widely recognized that early intervention on the part of a case manager and appropriate referrals prevent costly complications and can result in better health outcomes (Thurkettle and Noji, 2003).

CASE MANAGER ROLES AND CHARACTERISTICS

The individual case manager's role will vary depending on the specific program's services. The role functions of case managers are defined by the CMSA as including assessment, planning, facilitation, coordination, monitoring, evaluation, and advocacy, achieved through collaboration with the client and others involved in the client's care (CMSA, 2016).

The ANCC (2009) describes the practice of a nurse case manager as follows:

Nurse case managers actively participate with their clients to identify and facilitate options and services, providing and coordinating comprehensive care to meet patient/client health needs, with the goal of decreasing fragmentation and duplication of care, and enhancing quality, cost-effective clinical outcomes. Nursing case management is a dynamic and systematic collaborative approach to provide and co-ordinate health care services to a defined population. Nurse case managers continually evaluate each individual's health plan and specific challenges and then seek to overcome ob-stacles that affect outcomes. A nurse case manager uses a framework that includes interaction, assessment, planning, implementation, and evaluation. Outcomes are evaluated to determine if additional actions such as reassessment or revision to a plan of care are required to meet clients' health needs. To facilitate patient outcomes, the nurse case man-ager may fulfill the roles of advocate, collaborator, facili-tator, risk manager, educator, mentor, liaison, negotiator, consultant, coordinator, evaluator, and/or researcher.

Nurse case managers must be flexible. The healthcare environment experiences rapid change, and new regulations and reimbursement schedules frequently emerge. The health-care provider must respond to these changes rapidly to remain competitive. It is an ideal job for the self-directed nurse who enjoys being involved in a larger healthcare team within the organization and in the larger community. CMSA (2016) de-fines the standards of case management practice (Box 9.2).

CASE IDENTIFICATION

Identification of case management clients occurs in many ways, and each program should determine the criteria for eligibility for case management services. These criteria depend on the services provided, the service's location, the population served, and whether the service is in an acute care or community

> ### BOX 9.2   CMSA Standards of Case Management Practice
>
> **Client Selection Process for Case Management** demonstrated by consistent use of high-risk screening criteria.
>
> **Client Assessment** using standard tools to assess health history; cognition; spiritual, cultural, and support systems; resources; and other components.
>
> **Care Needs and Opportunities Identification** that would benefit from case management intervention.
>
> **Planning** the identification of short-term, long-term, and ongoing needs and strategies to address those needs.
>
> **Monitoring** the ongoing assessment and documentation to measure the client's response to the plan of care.
>
> **Outcomes** demonstrating the efficacy, quality, and cost-effectiveness of the case manager's intervention.
>
> **Closure of Professional Case Management Services** once established, case-closure guidelines are met.
>
> **Facilitation, Coordination, and Collaboration** between the client and other stakeholders to achieve goals and maximize positive client outcomes.
>
> **Qualifications for Case Managers,** which are maintaining unrestricted licenses and certifications or involve a bachelor's or higher health degree from a nationally accredited school.
>
> **Legal** adherence to all local, state, and federal laws, as well as employer policies and practice.
>
> **Confidentiality and Client Privacy,** including consent for case manage-ment services.
>
> **Ethical Behavior,** including the five basic ethical principles—beneficence, nonmalfeasance, autonomy, justice, and fidelity.
>
> **Advocacy** for the client at the service delivery, benefits administration, and policy-making levels.
>
> **Cultural Competency** of the client's cultural and demographic diversity.
>
> **Resource Management and Stewardship** of the healthcare and finan-cial resources for effective and efficient utilization.
>
> **Professional Responsibilities and Scholarship** to maintain current knowledge, competencies, and evidence-supported innovations.

setting. Some programs are diagnosis based and use many community healthcare resources; for example, clients with chronic obstructive pulmonary disease often require numerous hospitalizations. Programs may focus on a particular popula-tion (e.g., the elderly or chronically ill with a specific chronic condition) and establish criteria to identify which clients to target for services (e.g., the high-risk elderly who are chroni-cally ill, recently discharged from a hospital setting, and would benefit from case management services).

All clients referred for case management must undergo screening to determine their appropriateness for inclusion in the program. Not all referred clients need the services of a nurse case manager. Often, a nurse can arrange community services or instruct the client and family in the most appropriate follow-up based on client need and program design. The screening instrument must be comprehensive enough to determine which clients meet the program's criteria and user friendly enough to allow the screener to evaluate the clients rapidly to determine their appropriateness for the program. The screener should refer clients to more suitable services within the community if they are not appropriate candidates for a particular case management program.

THE REFERRAL PROCESS

The nurse may perform program referrals in a variety of ways. In the acute care hospital setting, referrals are usually based on patient diagnosis, complex care needs, social issues such as homelessness or lack of transportation, extended length of stay, or rehospitalization. Internal mechanisms alert the case manager of the patient's admission (e.g., a computerized list). Patients are also screened at discharge for risk of readmission and referred to the TCM case manager as appropriate.

A variety of tools are used to identify people who would benefit from case management services. They include health risk screening tools; evidence-based criteria; risk stratification through data management; and referrals from hospitals, healthcare providers, and families. Information is collected by the case manager and analyzed to determine whether the individual being referred is a candidate for case management services (CMSA, 2016).

In community settings, referrals originate from a variety of sources, such as a client's family, a primary care provider, and a hospital case manager. These referrals may be written or verbal. Staff in community agencies can also make service referrals; for example, the American Heart Association or American Cancer Society may receive calls from clients and families requesting information and assistance.

APPLICATION OF CASE MANAGEMENT IN COMMUNITY HEALTH

Case management can be used in all community health settings, with interventions at the primary, secondary, and tertiary levels of prevention, according to the community program and population served. Nurses working as case managers in the community setting have diverse roles and responsibilities.

Primary Care
Chronic Care Management

The CMS has recently developed criteria and reimbursement for **chronic care management** (CCM) and TCM in the primary care setting. Patients are referred to the CCM program by a practitioner who has identified the patient as having two or more chronic conditions that put the patient at a high risk of functional decline or death within the next 12 months (CMS.gov, 2021). Care coordinators work with patients and their caregivers to improve self-management of the disease process via support and education and coordinate care to empower patients to access care appropriately and efficiently.

Transitional Care Management

TCM patients are referred by practitioners or hospital staff for follow-up face-to-face visits with the outpatient practitioner

and care coordination services for 30 days postdischarge. Patients are educated about new medications, condition-specific processes, and discharge instructions. As mentioned, care is coordinated for the patient, including a follow-up face-to-face visit with a practitioner. The goal of this program is to improve patient outcomes, increase understanding of condition-specific issues, and decrease hospital readmissions (DHHS and CMS, 2016).

Patient-Centered Medical Home

The **PCMH** is a model of care developed to provide collaborative, quality-driven, safe primary care. The PCMH utilizes care coordination and case management processes to provide comprehensive, patient-centered, cost-effective, high-quality care (Henderson et al., 2012). In 2007, the report *Joint Principles of the Patient-Centered Medical Home*, sponsored by four medical professional organizations, described the seven principles or characteristics of the PCMH, which are listed in Box 9.3 (Patient-Centered Primary Care Collaborative, 2007).

PCMHs are a care delivery model that utilizes the care coordination process as a foundational principle. The five key functions of the PCMH are care that is comprehensive, patient centered, coordinated, accessible, and safe (AHRQ, 2017).

The American Academy of Family Physicians (AAFP, 2008) defines the PCMH as follows:

Transition away from a model of symptom and illness based episodic care to a system of comprehensive coordinated primary care for children, youth and adults. Patient centeredness refers to an ongoing, active partnership with a personal primary care physician who leads a team of professionals dedicated to providing proactive, preventive and chronic care management through all stages of life. These personal physicians are responsible for the patient's coordination of care across all health care systems facilitated by registries, information technology, health information exchanges, and other means to ensure patients receive care when and where they need it. With a commitment to continuous quality improvement, care teams utilize evidence-based medicine and clinical decision support tools that guide decision making as well as ensure that patients and their families have the education and support to

---

BOX 9.3 Principles of a Patient-Centered Medical Home

The patient-centered medical home has the following seven characteristics:
- The patient's relationship with the primary care physician
- The physician-led, team-based care
- The patient as a "whole person" who requires comprehensive care at various stages of life
- Integration and coordination of care
- Quality and safety
- Improved access to care
- A payment system that accurately reflects the efforts and care provided by the team

actively participate in their own care. Payment appropriately recognizes and incorporates the value of the care teams, non-direct patient care, and quality improvement provided in a patient-centered medical home.

High-Risk Clinic Settings

There are many examples of healthcare settings that provide services to high-risk clients in which the nurse serves as case manager. A few examples are diabetic clinics, settings that provide healthcare services to high-risk perinatal clients, clients who have received transplants, dialysis settings, oncology clinics, and infusion centers. The case management services offered by the nurse are determined by the specific needs of the clients seen in these settings. The models of case management are also developed for the needs of the clients.

Public Health Clinic Settings

Depending on the services provided in the public health setting, the nurse has an opportunity to provide education, screening, and referrals as needed to the clients served. Examples of primary prevention include an antepartum clinic, where the nurse interacts with women and can teach about pregnancy, diet, and exercise during pregnancy.

Working with parents in pediatric settings, the nurse case manager can teach nutrition, growth, and development and provide anticipatory guidance (primary level of prevention). The nurse can also screen children for growth and development and make referrals as needed to the Women, Infants, and Children program and other specialty programs available in the area for the clients' needs (secondary prevention).

Nurses can also serve as case managers working with elderly clients, providing nutrition education (primary prevention), screening for hypertension (secondary prevention), and even assisting with medication management and care of chronic diseases (tertiary prevention). The opportunities for community health nurses to provide case management services are vast, depending on the location, the populations served, and the resources available in the community.

Occupational Health Settings

More employers are providing health screening and education to their employees to keep their work forces healthy. Community health nurses who work in occupational health settings are in a position to provide primary prevention in health education classes designed to meet the needs of the employees. These classes can be designed on the basis of the health status of workers and to prevent the types of injuries to which they are prone. The nurse in this setting can also provide primary prevention by offering influenza vaccines and other immunizations to keep the employees healthy.

Secondary prevention can be provided to employees through screening clinics for hypertension and other potential chronic illnesses or health problems to which the employees may be more susceptible because of the nature of work performed. Referrals can be made as needed for follow-up with these employees. The occupational health nurse would continue to

follow these employees and case-manage any health issues that could affect the employees' ability to perform the duties of their jobs.

Case management for tertiary prevention can include keeping in touch with injured employees and monitoring their recovery, therapy, or other services that are provided to the employees in the process of returning to health and their jobs. The occupational health nurse who provides case management services to these employees offers them education, referrals as needed, and assistance in their recovery process.

Home Health and Hospice Settings

The community health nurse working in home health or hospice services is often assigned a case load of clients for whom he or she provides case management services. In both of these settings, the nurse case manager provides primary, secondary, and tertiary prevention to clients. These services are designed on the basis of the individual needs of clients and their families. Coordination of care, referrals, assessment, medication management, patient and family education, and the development of plans of care are just a few of the nursing functions that are provided through a case management model.

RESEARCH IN CASE MANAGEMENT

Case management research is increasing in the last decade, much of it as a result of the quality reforms in health care and the role of case management in these reforms. A literature search in *PubMed* and the *Cumulative Index to Nursing and Allied Health* found many categories of case management research. These include disease management, evidence-based practice, roles and functions, models, transitions of care, and roles in quality improvement initiatives. Specific research evaluating case management and quality improvement examined the roles of case management in transitions of care and readmissions, core measures, hospital-acquired conditions, and patient satisfaction. Other research evaluated the effect of case management on geriatric populations, disabled populations, and end-of-life situations. The documented studies describe the implemented programs and evaluate the program outcomes. An example is given in the Research Highlights box.

RESEARCH HIGHLIGHTS

Geriatric Care Management for Low-Income Seniors: A Randomized Controlled Trial

Counsell et al. (2007) conducted a randomized clinical control study of 951 adults 65 years or older with annual incomes less than 200% of the federal poverty level whose primary care physicians were randomly assigned to the intervention group (474 patients) or usual care (477 patients) in community-based health centers. The intervention consisted of 2 years of home-based care management by a nurse practitioner and SW, who collaborated with the primary care physician and a geriatrics interdisciplinary team and were guided by 12 care protocols for common geriatric conditions. Results of the study showed that integrated and home-based geriatric care management resulted in improved quality of care and reduced acute care utilization among a high-risk group, in comparison with community-based care. Improvements in health-related quality-of-life issues were mixed, and physical function outcomes did not differ between the groups.

Case management programs in all settings require further study. Terms used in case management programs should be defined for comparison in various clinical sites. Programs with similar organizational structures and services can then be compared among settings. Critical to the success of case management programs are the inclusion of costs and cost savings and the evaluation of quality outcomes. The researcher or case manager must report the program's description as well as the case manager's role and professional background. Well-defined patient and program outcomes are essential to the evaluation of case management programs. With the implementation of well-designed research with measurable outcomes, management in healthcare settings across the continuum of care can identify the most cost-effective programs for specific populations served.

CASE STUDY Application of the Nursing Process

Comprehensive Case Management Program

The following case study is an example of a comprehensive case management program. It follows steps utilizing the Case Management Body of Knowledge (CMBOK) case management process. Case management programs and the served populations are diverse; this is only one example of case management implementation.

June Wilson is a 76-year-old recently widowed female with poorly controlled type 2 diabetes, hypertension, and functional decline. She recently had a fall in her apartment and injured her ankle. She sees Kate Newman APRN, a family practitioner at a PCMH clinic.

June's son Mike, who lives nearby, made an appointment with Kate after his mom fell and was having issues with her mobility. In the clinic appointment, Kate identified specific medical and social issues with June including the following:

Type 2 diabetes, poorly controlled with an A1c of 9.8
Hypertension
Mild situation depression
Poor nutrition
Possible diabetic retinopathy
Sprain of left ankle due to ground level fall
Impaired mobility
Risk of institutionalization

Kate referred June to Diana the care manager for case management services. Diana met June and Mike at the visit, and they agreed to care management services. They set up an appointment for an assessment at June's home with Mike present.

Screening

June was screened and referred into the care management program due to her acute ankle injury with functional decline and chronic conditions that put her at risk of loss of independence and/or other poor outcome.

Assessing

Diana met with June and Mike in the patient's home. June lives alone in a small house that is approximately 20 min from her son, who works fulltime and has a family of his own. He indicates that he tries to visit his mother weekly on his day off. June does not drive and uses the bus for transportation. Diana notes fall risks in the home including throw rugs, exposed cords, and poor lighting. Mike indicates that June was independent prior to the death of her husband and has been in a decline since. She is not eating, socializing, or caring for her diabetes. He is worried that she may not be able to continue to live alone. June is temporarily homebound due to her ankle injury.

Diana asks June and Mike what their primary goals are for June and her health. They indicate that they want her to remain safe in independent living and want her to have better control of her diabetes. June indicates that she is sad and lonely and would like companionship too. Diana asks her what her hobbies are and June replies that she used to knit and play cards with friends.

Diana does a thorough assessment that includes physical, mental, cognitive, psychosocial, support system, self-care ability, and financial, functional, and environmental subjects. She also does a medication reconciliation and asks for a demonstration of her glucose monitoring skills. She notes that June has an old meter and has problems reading the results with her sight decline.

Stratifying Risk

June is risk stratified into the high-risk category due to risk of loss of independence due to functional loss (vision and mobility), SDoH issues (transportation, nutrition, and social support), and poor diabetic control. She will initially require more intensive case management and community resources to meet her goals.

Planning

Diana works with June and Mike to develop a care plan utilizing their top goals of keeping June independent, improving her diabetic control, and improving her mood and social isolation. The care plan is patient-centric; they work together to develop it and all agree with the plan and recommendations.

Diana notifies the APN Kate of the assessment, care plan goals, and recommendations. She also notifies Kate that the patient would benefit from physical therapy for mobility training and a home safety evaluation. Due to June's homebound status, they order Home Health PT. Diana makes the referral and updates the Home Health therapy team of the assessment, care plan, and concerns.

Diana also notifies Kate of the patient's difficulty with her blood glucose meter and eyesight. They agree that the patient could benefit from diabetic education. Kate makes a referral to the clinic diabetic class that begins in 2 weeks, and Diana makes arrangements for a new blood glucose meter and ophthalmologist referral.

Implementing/Care Coordination

Diana initially meets weekly with June. She implements the following referrals and resource coordination:

Home Health for PT safety evaluation and mobility training includes the following:
- Coordination of installation of safety equipment including shower bars, stair rail on front steps, removal of tripping hazards, and improved lighting
- Initiation of a falls notification safety device
Referral to Diabetes Education Clinic also requires the following:
- Transportation coordination
- Blood glucose meter and supplies
- Referral to dietician for meal planning and diet education
Referral to ophthalmologist requires the following:
- Transportation to and from appointment
Referral to senior center for the following:
- Meals on Wheels until mobility is improved and she can participate in onsite lunches and socialization
- Knitting club, when mobility improves and she is no longer home bound
- Silver Sneakers when ankle injury and mobility are improved to continue physical strengthening and socialization
- Bingo and card club for socialization

Follow-up

Diana follows up weekly with June and Mike. The physical therapy visits are going well, and June is ambulating without a walker within 4 weeks. The safety features have been completed, and fall hazards have been removed. June has been receiving Meals on Wheels daily for lunch and is maintaining her weight. She continues in the diabetic education classes and demonstrates her ability to use her new glucose meter. She has recently seen the ophthalmologist and has received new glasses; this has improved her mobility and falls risk and her ability to use her blood glucose meter. She is interested in going to the senior center twice weekly for an afternoon to have lunch, socialize, and participate in group activities. She requests Tuesdays and Thursdays as an old friend participates on those days.

Diana makes arrangements for the senior center van to pick June up on Tuesdays and Thursdays at 11 a.m. and return her at 3 p.m. She signs June up for lunch, knitting club, and bingo games. They will defer the Silver Sneaker walking club until June's ankle has completely healed.

Diana continues to check in by phone weekly with June and Mike; they meet monthly for a follow-up visit and care plan modification.

Transitioning (Transitional Care)
Because of the intense case management intervention, June was not admitted to the hospital. Diana provided transitional care in the communication between providers (Home Health PT, Kate APN, and the ophthalmologist).

Communicating Posttransition
After 3 months of case management services, June has progressed very well with her mobility, diabetic management, mood disorder, and socialization. She participates at the senior center three times weekly and is walking with the Silver Sneaker club. Mike, June, and Diana decide that June no longer requires case management services. Diana will check in telephonically every 3 months for follow-up.

Evaluating
To evaluate the case management intervention, Diana reviews June's initial and postintervention biometric numbers. These include the PHQ-9 (indicating depression) that dropped from 13 to 7, her A1c that dropped from 9.8 to 7.1, and her blood pressure that has been consistently lower after medication education and exercise.

Diana will check in quarterly with the patient for follow-up needs and is available for more intensive case management services as needed.

EVOLVE WEBSITE

http://evolve.elsevier.com/Nies/community.
- NCLEX Review Questions
- Case Studies

BIBLIOGRAPHY

Agency for Healthcare Research and Quality (AHRQ), 2017. Available from: https://www.pcmh.ahrq.gov/page/tools-implementing-pcmh.

Agency for Healthcare Research and Quality (AHRQ): *Issue brief: implications for medical practice, health policy and health services research*, 2015. Available from: www.ahrq.gov/sites/default/files/publications/files/caremgmt-brief.pdf.

American Academy of Family Physicians (AAFP), 2008. Available from: AAFP.org.

American Case Management Association: *A certification for health delivery-system case management and transitions of care professionals*, 2021. Available from: https://www.acmaweb.org/acm/.

American Nurses Association: *The value of nursing care coordination, a whitepaper of the American Nurses Association*, 2012. Available from: www.nursingworld.org.

American Nurses Credentialing Center: *Case management nursing*, 2009. Available from: www.nursingworld.org.

Case Management Society of America: *Standards of practice for case management*, Little Rock, AR, 2016, Author.

Chen A, Brown R, Archibald N, et al.: *Best practices in coordinated care*, 2000. Available from: https://innovation.cms.gov/files/reports/cc-full-report.pdf.

CMS.gov: *Value-based programs*, 2017. Available from: https://www.cms.gov/Medicare/Quality-Initiatives-Patient-Assessment-Instruments/Value-Based-Programs/Value-Based-Programs.html.

CMS.gov: *Chronic care management services*, 2021. Available from: https://www.cms.gov/About-CMS/Agency-Information/OMH/equity-initiatives/ccm/hcpresources.

Commission for Case management Certification: *Case management body of knowledge*, 2021. Available from: https://cmbodyofknowledge.com/content/introduction-case-management-body-knowledge.

Commission for Case Manager: *Certification: certified case manager (CCM) certification requirement*, 2021. Available from: www.ccmcertification.org.

Commission for Case Manager Certification: *Definition and policy statement*, 2021. Available from: https://ccmcertification.org/about-ccmc/about-case-management/definition-and-philosophy-case-management#.

Conger MM: Nursing case management: a managed care organizational strategy. In Conger MM, editor: *Managed care: practice strategies for nursing*, Thousand Oaks, CA, 1999, Sage Publications.

Counsell SR, Callahan CM, Clark DO, et al.: Geriatric care management for low-income seniors, *JAMA* 298:2623−2633, 2007.

Crosby RL: Community care of the chronically mentally Ill, *J Psychosocial Nurs* 25(1):33−37, 1987.

Department of Health and Human Services (DHHS), Center for Medicare and Medicaid Services: *Transitional care management services, ICN 908628*, 2016.

Department of Health and Human Services (DHHS): *Statistical Brief #354: the concentration and persistence in the level of health expenditures over time: estimates for the U.S. population, 2008−2009*, 2012. Available from: https://meps.ahrq.gov/data_files/publications/st354/stat354.shtml.

Grau L: Case management and the nurse, *Geriatr Nurs* 5(8):372−375, 1984.

Henderson S, Princell C, Martin CO: The patient centered medical home: this primary care model offers RNs new practice—and reimbursement—opportunities, *Am J Nurs* 112(12):54−59, 2012.

Hirschmann K, Shaid E, McCauley K, Pauly M, Naylor M: Continuity of care: the transitional care model, *Online J Issues Nurs* 20(3), 2015.

Huber DL: The diversity of case management models, *Lippincott's Case Manag* 7(6):212−220, 2002.

Institute of Medicine: *Crossing the quality chasm*, 2001. Available from: http://nationalacademies.org/hmd/reports/2001/crossing-the-quality-chasm-a-new-health-system-for-the-21st-century.aspx.

Lax Y, Martinez M, Brown N: Social determinants of health and hospital readmission, *Pediatrics* 140(5), 2017.

Mahn VA, Spross JA: Nursing case management as an advanced practice role. In Hamric AB, Spross JA, Hanson CM, editors: *Advanced nursing practice: an integrative approach*, Philadelphia, 1996, Saunders.

McDonald K, Sundaram V, Bravata D, et al.: *Closing the quality gap: a critical analysis of quality improvement strategies: care coordination*, AHRQ technical reviews No. 9.7 (vol 7), Rockville, MD, 2005 Agency for Healthcare Research and Quality.

Patient-Centered Primary Care Collaborative: *Joint principles of the patient-centered medical home*, 2007. Available from: https://www.aafp.org/dam/AAFP/documents/practice_management/pcmh/initiatives/PCMHJoint.pdf.

Patient Protection and Affordable Care Act, Title III: *Improving the quality and efficiency of healthcare, 2010, Public Law,* pp 111–148. Available from: www.gpo.gov.

Pittman DC: Nursing case management: holistic care for the deinstitutionalized mentally Ill, *J Psychosoc Nurs* 27(11):23–27, 1989.

Public Law 111-148, 2010. Available from: https://www.govinfo.gov/content/pkg/PLAW-111publ148/pdf/PLAW-111publ148.pdf.

Steinberg RM, Carter GW: *Case management and the elderly*, Lexington, MA, 1983, Lexington Books, DC Health.

Thurkettle MA, Noji A: Shifting the healthcare paradigm: the case manager's opportunity and responsibility, *Lippincott's Case Manag* 8(4):160–165, 2003.

University of Wisconsin: *The other half of health: an introduction to social determinants part 1 family and social support*, 2021. Available from: https://uwphi.pophealth.wisc.edu/wp-content/uploads/sites/316/2018/01/EBHPP-SocialDeterminants_FullEventSlides.pdf. Accessed February 2021.

U.S. Department of Commerce/International Trade Administration: *Health and medical services: US industrial outlook*, Washington, DC, 1990, Author.

Yamamoto L, Lucey C: Case management "within the walls": a glimpse into the future, *Crit Care Nurs Q* 28(2):162–178, 2005.

10

Policy, Politics, Legislation, and Community Health Nursing

Tanna Woods*

OBJECTIVES

Upon completion of this chapter, the reader will be able to do the following:

1. Discuss how the structure of government affects the policy development process.
2. Describe the legislative, judicial, and administrative (executive) processes involved in establishing federal, state, or local health policy.
3. Examine the power of nursing to influence and change health policy.
4. Discuss current health policy issues.
5. Identify the social and political processes that influence health policy development.
6. Discuss the nurse's role in political activities.
7. Discuss nursing's involvement in private health policy.

OUTLINE

KEY TERMS

administrative agencies
Clara Barton
coalition
Florence Nightingale
government
health policy

institutional policies
Lavinia Dock
laws
Lillian Wald
lobby
lobbyist

Mary Breckenridge
nursing policy
organizational policies
organizations
policy
policy analysis

*The author would like to acknowledge the contributions of Cathy Arvidson, who edited this chapter for the previous edition.

political action committee (PAC)
politics
public health law
public policy

Ruth Watson Lubic
social policy
Sojourner Truth
sovereign power

statutes
Susie Walking Bear Yellowtail
Sylvia Trent-Adams

This chapter addresses the interrelationships of the processes through which health policies are determined and instituted. **Politics** and legislation are the routes through which public health policies are established. Policy, politics, and legislation are the forces that determine the direction of health programs at every level of government, as well as the private sector. These programs are crucial to the health and well-being of the nation, the state, the community, and the individual. Nurses influence the maintenance and improvement of the health of individuals, groups, and communities by contributing to policy and legislative advancement.

The healthcare delivery system, including nursing practice and research, is profoundly influenced by policies set by both government and private entities. Nurses who understand the system of health policy development and implementation can effectively interpret and influence policies that affect nursing practice; the health of individuals, families, groups, communities, and populations; and, when required, offer an international health perspective.

OVERVIEW: NURSES' HISTORICAL AND CURRENT ACTIVITY IN HEALTH CARE POLICY

The more a nurse knows about the political process, the more he or she tends to become involved. Individual nurses may become politically active on a local, state, or national level. Nurses may work collectively within a group such as the National Student Nurses Association, the American Nurses Association (ANA), and state boards of nursing to lobby for health causes. There are more than 3.8 million employed registered nurses (RNs) (American Association of Colleges of Nursing [AACN], 2019). Together nurses can be patient advocates, change agents, and policy makers. Lawmakers respect nurses and thus are usually effective as consultants in both the legislative and executive branches at local, state, and federal levels. It is the hallmark of the U.S. system of government that citizens have the right to have an influential voice in the governance of the community. Nurses are able to communicate concerns about conditions and issues in health care, the health care needs of individuals and communities, and the profession of nursing. United, nurses can influence political leaders to make changes to the healthcare system that are beneficial to all. Nurses experienced in the political arena can mentor novices to it.

Many individual nurses in the past and present have been instrumental in working with legislation and politics. A few exemplary nurses who had an impact on public health are

Florence Nightingale was an influential nurse who exerted political pressure on a government (McDonald, 2020). In the 1850s Nightingale was asked to establish the first nurse corps to tend the soldiers in the Crimea War. She transformed military health and knew the value of data in influencing policy. She was a leader who knew how to use the support of followers, colleagues, and policy makers. As discussed in Chapter 2, Nightingale collected and analyzed data about health services and outcomes, an activity that now is a critical element of public health.

Sojourner Truth beginning in the 1840s became an ardent and eloquent advocate for abolishing slavery and supporting women's rights. Her work helped transform the racist and sexist policies that limited the health and well-being of African Americans and women. She fought for human rights and lobbied for federal funds to train nurses and physicians (NurseJournal, 2021).

Clara Barton was responsible for organizing relief efforts during the U.S. Civil War. In 1882, she successfully persuaded Congress to ratify the Treaty of Geneva, which allowed the Red Cross to perform humanitarian efforts in times of peace. This organization has had a lasting influence on national and international policies Kalisch and Kalisch (2004); Davidson, (2021).

Lavinia Dock was a prolific writer and political activist. She waged a campaign for legislation to allow nurses to control the nursing profession instead of physicians. In 1893, with the assistance of Isabel Hampton Robb and Mary Adelaide Nutting, she founded the politically active American Society of Superintendents of Training Schools for Nurses, which later became the National League for Nursing (Kalisch & Kalisch, 2004). She was also active in the suffrage movement, advocating that nurses support the woman's right to vote, encouraged workers to form trade unions, and was an early advocate for birth control (Voda, 2012).

Lillian Wald's political activism and vision were shaped by feminist values. Working in the early 1900s, she recognized the connections between health and social conditions. She was a driving force behind the federal government's development of the Children's Bureau in 1912. Wald appeared frequently at the White House to participate in the development of national and international policy (Voda, 2012).

Mary Breckenridge worked to develop nursing in rural Kentucky in the 1920s, establishing the Frontier Nursing Service. This was a complete healthcare system that provided health care to an underserved, rural area (Voda, 2012).

Susie Walking Bear Yellowtail was a Native American nurse who walked from reservation to reservation, working to improve health services for this population from the 1930s to 1960s. She also established the Native ANA.

Florence Wald was a nursing leader in establishing hospice care in the United States—modeled after similar services offered in the United Kingdom—in the 1970s.

Dr. Ruth Watson Lubic is a nurse-midwife who crusaded for freestanding birth centers in this country, being influential in the opening of New York City's first birthing center in 1975. After developing the birth center model through the Maternity Center Association in New York City, Dr. Lubic expanded the model to Washington, DC, where the infant mortality rate was twice the national average. In 1993, Lubic was awarded the MacArthur Fellowship Grant and, in 2001, the National Academy of Medicine's Lienhard Award (Lyttle, 2000; Rychnovsky, 2011).

DEFINITIONS

Policy denotes a course of action to be followed by a government, business, or institution to obtain a desired effect. *Merriam-Webster's Dictionary* defines policy as "a definite course or method of action selected from among alternatives and in light of given conditions to guide and determine present and future decisions" (Merriam-Webster, 2021). Policy encompasses the choices that a society, segment of society, or organization makes regarding its goals and priorities and the ways it allocates its resources to attain those goals. Policy choices reflect the values, beliefs, and attitudes of those designing the policy (Mason et al., 2007).

Public policy denotes precepts and standards formed by governmental bodies that are of fundamental concern to the state and the whole of the general public. The field of public policy involves the study of specific policy problems and governmental responses to them. Political scientists involved in the study of public policy attempt to devise solutions for problems of public concern. They study issues such as health care, pollution, and the economy. Public policy overlaps comparative politics in the study of comparative public policy with international relations in the study of foreign policy and

national security policy, and with political theory in considering ethics in policy making. See the examples in Table 10.1.

Health policy is a statement of a decision regarding a goal in health care and a plan for achieving that goal. For example, to prevent an epidemic, a program for inoculating a population is developed and implemented, and priorities and values underlying health resource allocation are determined.

Nursing policy specifies nursing leadership that influences and shapes health policy and nursing practice. Nursing, and therefore nursing leadership, is shaped dramatically by the impact of politics and policy. Effective nursing leadership is a vehicle through which both nursing practice and health policy can be influenced and shaped.

Institutional policies are rules that govern worksites and identify the institution's goals, operation, and treatment of employees.

Organizational policies are rules that govern organizations and their positions on issues with which the organization is concerned (Mason et al., 2007).

A **political action committee (PAC)** is a fundraising group usually associated with an organization. Money is raised from the members with the purpose of financially supporting political causes. Organizations are allowed to support candidates, but only PACs are permitted to donate money to candidates or legislation (Mason et al., 2007).

Social policy is policy associated with individuals and communities. In very general terms, social policy can be defined as the branch of public policy that advances social welfare and enhances participation in society. Social safety nets, however, often contribute to social exclusion, especially in urban settings, instead of being universally accessible. In most Western societies, social protection usually depends on contributory social insurance schemes to which only regular job holders have access (either in their own right or as dependents). In the United States, this is particularly evident with respect to the way the health care system and Social Security retirement benefits work. Social justice argues that all individuals and groups receive fair treatment in society as well as impartially share in the benefits of that society (Almgren, 2017).

Administrative agencies are departments of the executive branch with the authority to implement or administer particular legislation.

Laws are rules of conduct or procedure; they result from a *combination* of legislation, judicial decisions, constitutional decisions, and administrative actions.

Public health law focuses on legal issues in public health practice and on the public health effects of legal practice. Public health law typically has three major areas of practice: police power, disease and injury prevention, and the law of populations. Statute, ordinance, or code prescribes sanitary standards and regulation for the purpose of promoting and preserving the community's health. Public health law consists of legislation, regulations, and court decisions enacted by government at the federal, state, and local levels to protect the public's health. This includes case law and treaties.

TABLE 10.1	Terminology Example
Topic	**Example**
Public policy	A local or regional effort to prevent the sale of tobacco or alcohol to minors. Public policy directs that the right to health of the majority must be preserved over individual freedoms and corporate interests.
Public health law	New York State Public Health Law §2164: "Every person in parental (statute) relation to a child in this state shall have administered to such child an adequate dose of an immunizing agent against poliomyelitis, mumps, measles, diphtheria, rubella, varicella, *Haemophilus influenza* type B, and hepatitis B ..."
Common law	The Supreme Court decision in *Roe v. Wade*, making first-trimester abortion legal, is an example of how common law becomes enforceable.
Regulation	Reporting of communicable diseases to state and local health departments, which then report them to the Centers for Disease Control and Prevention.
Treaty	Multilateral treaty: Treaty to eliminate all forms of discrimination against women.

Statutes are any laws passed by a legislative body at the federal, state, or local level.

Organizations are associations that set and enforce standards in a particular area; a group of individuals who voluntarily enter into an agreement to accomplish a purpose.

A *professional association* (also called a *professional body, professional organization,* or *professional society*) is a nonprofit organization seeking to further a particular profession, the interests of individuals engaged in that profession, and the public interest. It is a volunteer group that seeks to join large numbers of individuals who have a significant wealth of knowledge and experience in a particular field such as the Association of Public Health. There are also pooled funds for lobbying purposes (Association of Public Health Nurses [APHN], 2016). The roles of these professional organizations are viewed as maintaining the control and oversight of the professional occupation as well as safeguarding the public trust. There is an element of protecting the interests of the professional practitioners, as in a cartel or labor union. Inherent in these organizations is the promotion of general standards for the performance of its members and the expectation of continued professional development.

Many professional bodies are involved in the development and monitoring of professional educational programs and the updating of skills, and thus they perform professional certification to indicate that a person possesses qualifications in the subject area. Sometimes membership in a professional body is synonymous with certification, though not always. Membership in a professional body, as a legal requirement, can in some professions form the primary formal basis for gaining entry to and setting up practice within the profession. Professional bodies also act as learned societies for the academic disciplines underlying their professions.

A MAJOR PARADIGM SHIFT

Policy is based on values, and the first step in forming policy is identifying the issue. Therefore it would seem rational to define "health" as the starting point for any policy annexed to healthcare issues. Historically, health was defined in the context of infectious diseases. Current definitions encompass prevention and management of chronic conditions. The World Health Organization (WHO) considers health to be the state of complete physical, mental, and social well-being and not merely the absence of disease or infirmity. Despite this broad definition, it is only in the most recent decades that the WHO is refocusing on its initial definition as it attempts to deal with environmental issues such as nuclear contamination and industrial toxins in industrialized nations and the exploration of carcinogenic commercial products such as tobacco products. On a global level, the WHO is working to prevent, treat, and care for communicable diseases such as HIV/AIDS, tuberculosis, malaria, and, most recently, the Zika virus. In addition, WHO focuses on noncommunicable diseases such as heart disease, stroke, cancer, diabetes, and lung diseases, which are responsible for more than 70% of all deaths worldwide. WHO emphasizes promoting health through the life cycle, taking into account environmental risks and social determinants of health. Thus there is a realization that health is a basic human right and that health problems are linked to government actions and, hence, affect human rights.

Human rights violations occur when governments fail to provide their people with the infrastructure, services, and information necessary to promote health, reduce risk, and control disease. For example, for every year of education women have, their infant mortality is decreased by 10%; yet education of women is not a global reality.

On a national level, an example of changing emphasis is the Centers for Disease Control and Prevention (CDC). It is committed to achieving true improvements in people's lives by accelerating health impact and reducing health disparities. Box 10.1 describes this priority for the CDC. All people, and especially those at greater risk of health disparities, will achieve their optimal lifespan with the best possible quality of health in every stage of life. However, a shift in the paradigm of health concepts would necessitate a substantial reallocation of resources, because the vast majority of health spending is directed at medical care and biomedical research and, as such, reflects a viewpoint of health care as a commodity. If one considers that in 2019 32.8 million people in the United States younger than 65 years had no health insurance and 5.1% of children were uninsured, it becomes clear that the health and human rights relationship is not yet reflected in our health policies (CDC, 2021). In addition, many people are underinsured. Their insurance coverage is not at the level it should be to cover full services or longer-term needs. The economics of health care are discussed further in Chapter 12.

The publication of *Healthy People 2000* by U.S. Surgeon General C. Everett Koop in 1990 led to a resurgence of interest by the federal government in the health and welfare of Americans. However, fiscal resources for public health interventions declined, and only marginal progress was made in meeting the goals. In early 2000, *Healthy People 2010* marked the beginning of the new millennium and an enhanced focus on population-based health promotion strategies (U.S. Department of Health and Human Services [USDHHS], 2000). Many *Healthy People 2020* objectives directly or indirectly involved health policy with enhanced focus on the social determinants of health and health policy (Office of the Assistant Secretary for Health [OASH],

---

BOX 10.1   Strategic Plan Priorities for the Center of Disease Control Strategic Framework

Strategic Priority #1	Improve health security at home and around the world.
Strategic Priority #2	Better prevent the leading causes of illness, injury, disability, and death.
Strategic Priority #3	Strengthen public health and health care collaboration.

From Centers for Disease Control and Prevention: CDC strategic framework, 2016. Available from: https://www.cdc.gov/about/organization/strategic-framework/index.html.

2020). Building on previous iterations, the updated 2020 version had four "over-arching goals" for 2020: attain high-quality, longer lives free of preventable disease, disability, injury, and premature death; achieve health equity, eliminate disparities, and improve the health of all age groups; create social and physical environments that promote good health for all; and promote quality of life, health development, and health behaviors across all life stages. Of the 42 Healthy People topic areas, 25 had a 50% or more of the trackable objectives were either improved, met, or exceeded (OASH, 2020). With the Public Health Infrastructure topic area, 75% ($n = 36$), 18.8% ($n = 9$) improved, 4.2% ($n = 2$) had little or no detectable change, and 2.1% ($n = 1$) worsened (OASH, 2020).

As 2020 has passed, there is a fifth iteration, Healthy People 2030, that builds on the knowledge learned during the first 4 decades of the initiative (Office of Disease Prevention and Health Promotion [ODPHP], 2021a). Healthy People 2030 has objectives of three types (core, developmental, or research) across the three main categories of leading health indicators (LHIs), social determinants of health (SDOH), and overall health and well-being measures (OHMs) (ODPHP, 2021a). There are a total of 355 core—or measurable—objectives and other items that are considered developmental and research objectives.

The LHIs category looks at leading health indicators, which can impact the important causes of death and disease in the United States. There are 23 leading health indicators included and include items like adults with hypertension whose blood pressure is under control. That indicator is then tied to an objective. Regarding blood pressure, the related objective of HDS-05 is to increase control of high blood pressure in adults.

In the SDOH category, how personal, social, economic, and environmental factors impact health is the focus. The SDOH are environmental conditions related to where people are born, live, work, play, worship, and age as these can impact a wide range of functioning, health, and quality-of-life outcomes. SODH has five domains where the items are grouped including economic stability, education access and quality, healthcare access and quality, neighborhood and built environment, and social and community context. The SODH relates to one of the overarching goals of Healthy People 2030: "Create social, physical, and economic environments that promote attaining the full potential for health and well being for all" (ODPHP, 2021b). The domain of Health Care Access and Quality includes many important public-health-related items including ECBP-D07: "Increase the number of community organizations that provide prevention services" (ODPHP, 2021c). For more information on improving access and getting screenings, see Healthy People 2030 box.

The OHMs are broad measures with global outcomes that attempt to address the Healthy People 2030 vision (ODPHP, 2021d). There are 8 OHMs that are grouped into three tiers: health life expectancy, well-being, and summary mortality and health. These items do not have targets as the LHIs and core objectives have. An example of this group is item OHM-8: "Respondent-assessed health status — in good or better health (all ages). There is a single question where respondents will answer if their health is poor, fair, good, very good, or excellent. This will provide information related to OHM-8.

♥ HEALTHY PEOPLE 2030

Content Related to Preventative Health Measures

Goal
To increase access to compressive, high-quality health care services.

Overview
Lack of insurance and affordable care affects the ability of people in the United States to get the health care they need. Healthy People 2030 has prioritized improving health via connecting people with timely, high-quality healthcare services. Further, screenings are important in public health settings, and there is an issue of people getting these screenings, which can be related to not having a primary care provider.

Why Are Health Screening Important?
There is a known issue of people not having access to primary healthcare providers and living too far from providers who could provide vital health screenings. Developing interventions to increase access to healthcare professionals and improve communication—via remote or in-person means—can help get people vital care.

These components are necessary to fulfill the following 10 essential public health services:
1. Monitor health status to identify and solve community health problems.
2. Diagnose and investigate health problems and health hazards in the community.
3. Inform, educate, and empower people about health issues.
4. Mobilize community partnerships and action to identify and solve health problems.
5. Develop policies and plans that support individual and community health efforts.
6. Enforce laws and regulations that protect health and ensure safety.
7. Link people to needed personal health services and assure the provision of health care when otherwise unavailable.
8. Ensure competent public and personal healthcare workforces.
9. Evaluate effectiveness, accessibility, and quality of personal and population-based health services.
10. Research for new insights and innovative solutions to health problems.

Sample of Healthcare Access and Quality Objectives
- AHS-08: "Increase the proportion of adults who get recommended evidence-based preventative care."
- AH-01: "Increase the proportion of adolescents who had a preventative health care visit in the past year."
- C-03: "Increase the proportion of adults who get screened for lung cancer."
- C-05: "Increase the proportion of females who get screened for breast cancer."
- ECBP-D07: "Increase the number of community organization that provide prevention services."
- STI-01: "Increase the proportion of sexually active female adolescents and young women who get screen for chlamydia."

From Office of Disease Prevention and Health Promotion: *Healthy People 2030*, 201, Health Care Access and Quality. Available from: https://health.gov/healthypeople/objectives-and-data/browse-objectives/health-care-access-and-quality.

STRUCTURE OF THE GOVERNMENT OF THE UNITED STATES

Government is the structure of principles and rules determining how a state, country, or organization is regulated. Among its purposes are regulation of conditions beyond individual control and provision of individual protection through a population-wide focus. These tasks are accomplished through passage and enforcement of laws. Requirements of childhood immunizations for school attendance, disease vector control, and sewage treatment are examples of regulations to protect the health of the population.

Government can also be viewed as the sovereign power vested in a nation or state. **Sovereign power** is the independent and supreme authority of the nation or state. Historical documents describe the government's responsibility for health in the United States and the subsequent authority to enact laws (including health laws). These documents reflect the values of the country's founders. They give the government the authority to enact laws, but they also limit that power. The earliest of these statements was the Mayflower Compact, through which the Pilgrims committed themselves to making "just and equal laws" for the general good. The Declaration of Independence later established the doctrine of inalienable rights, life, liberty, and the pursuit of happiness. However, it was not until the representatives of the individual states signed the Constitution of the United States that the federal government realized its sovereign power. At the same time that its power was realized, a limit to that power was placed on the federal government. The drafters of the Constitution sought to balance the need to empower the new federal government to "establish Justice, insure domestic Tranquility, provide for the common defense, promote the general Welfare, and secure the Blessings of Liberty" for its people but with limits on that power. That balance is achieved in several important ways.

The federal government is a government of limited powers, which means that for a federal action to be legitimate, it must be authorized. Only those actions that are within the scope of the Constitution, the supreme law of the land, are authorized. The Constitution separates governmental powers among the branches of government (Table 10.2).

Some examples of the separation of powers doctrine that are written into the U.S. Constitution are as follows:

- The legislature is prohibited from interfering with the courts' final judgments.
- The Supreme Court cannot decide a "political question"; the issue must be an actual case or controversy.
- Congress must present a bill to the president before it can become law (Box 10.2).
- The president needs consent of the Senate to appoint Supreme Court justices or to make treaties.
- The president and members of Congress are elected; the judiciary is appointed.

The Constitution not only set forth the responsibilities of the federal government but also provided for the individual citizen's rights and freedoms. These are contained in the first 10 amendments, which were added after the original Articles of the Constitution were ratified in 1787. These 10 amendments, added in 1791, are known as the *Bill of Rights*. The rights guaranteed in the Bill of Rights, such as those of free speech and freedom of religion, applied only to the laws and actions of the federal government. It would take another 72 years for these rights to be guaranteed within the states. "Liberty interests" and "privacy rights" have been found to exist by Supreme Court determinations and have become guiding principles in setting policy and enacting legislation. Note that these rights are applicable only to state or federal government's interaction with people. Violations of restrictions on rights such as free speech do not apply to nongovernmental entities, unless a specific law states otherwise.

The balance of powers is an important concept in the U.S. government. Federalism is the relationship and distribution of power between the national and the state governments. This balance flows directly from the text of the Constitution: "The powers not delegated to the United States by the Constitution, nor prohibited by it to the States, are reserved to the States respectively, or to the people." Box 10.3 highlights one of the changes in the federal government since the Constitution: the development of administrative agencies. This development has had a major impact on government functioning.

TABLE 10.2   Government Branches

Branch of Government	Includes
Executive branch	The president, the vice president, and the administrative agencies
Legislative branch	The Senate and the House of Representatives (Congress)
Judicial branch	At the federal level: district courts, circuit courts, and the Supreme Court At the state level: state and county courts

BOX 10.2   An Example of the President's Response to a House Bill (A President May or May Not Respond to a Bill)

State Children's Health Insurance Program (SCHIP)

H.R. 2 (and related bills H.R. 57, H.R. 72, and S. 275) became Public Law 111–3, The Children's Health Insurance Reauthorization Act of 2009. This was signed into law by President Barack Obama on February 4, 2009. It went into effect on April 1, 2009. This bill:

- Allows certain state plans under Titles XIX (Medicaid) or Title XXI (State Children's Health Insurance Program, referred to in this Act as CHIP) of the Social Security Act that require state legislation to meet additional requirements imposed by this Act additional time to make required plan changes.
- Provides for coordination of CHIP funding for the 2009 fiscal year.
- Amends SSA Title XXI to reauthorize the CHIP program through FY2013 at increased levels.

See http://thomas.loc.gov/home/thomas.php for more information.

BOX 10.3 Administrative Agencies

One of the most dramatic changes in American government since the ratification of the Constitution is the growth of administrative agencies. Federal administrative agencies have broad power. They exercise all of the powers of government: executive, legislative, and judicial.

The U.S. Food and Drug Administration (FDA) is one such administrative agency. Its power is in regulating the pharmaceutical industry as well as the food industry.

States retain powers not delegated to the federal government; therefore much of public health law is under state jurisdiction and, as a result, varies considerably from state to state. These powers to enact laws for the public welfare are referred to as the states' *police powers*. Additionally, states may delegate these powers to local governments. In the United States, legislative activities of the three levels of government (federal, state, and local) may vary greatly in their expectations, actions, and results. The state legislatures, for the most part, are directly involved in health care, yet the federal government influences health policy, directly and indirectly, through the financing of health care for many groups (e.g., Medicare, Medicaid), regulation activities (e.g., approval of drugs), and setting of standards (e.g., air quality).

Decisions affecting the public's health are made not only at every level of government but also in each branch of government. The separation and balance of powers, referred to as *checks and balances*, is as important to health as it is to the economic or military status of the country.

The legislative branch (i.e., Congress at the federal level; legislature, general assembly, or general court at the state level) enacts the statutory laws that are the basis for governance. The executive branch administers and enforces the laws, which are broad in scope, through regulatory agencies. These agencies, in turn, define more specific implementation of the statutes through rules and regulations (i.e., regulatory or administrative law). The judiciary body provides protection against oppressive governance and against professional malpractice, fraud, and abuse. Its function through the courts, both state and federal, is to determine the constitutionality of laws, interpret them, and decide on their legitimacy when they are challenged. Decisions of the U.S. Supreme Court are binding law for the nation. Decisions of an individual state's highest court are binding law within that state alone. The courts also have jurisdiction over specific infractions of laws and regulations.

OVERVIEW OF HEALTH POLICY

Public Health Policy

To review, public policy refers to decisions made by legislative, executive, or judicial branches of one of the three levels of government (local, state, or federal). These decisions are intended to direct or influence actions, behaviors, or decisions of others. Public health policies influence health care through the monitoring, production, provision, and financing of health care services. Everyone, from health care providers to consumers, is affected by health policies. Likewise, health policy influences corporations, employers, insurers, colleges of nursing, hospitals, clinics, producers and retailers of medical technology and equipment, and senior care facilities.

The authority for the protection of the public's health is largely vested with the states, and most state constitutions specifically delineate their responsibility. Municipal subdivisions of states, such as counties, cities, and towns, generally have the power of local control of the services, conferred by the state legislature. The responsibilities of local, state, and federal governments for health services may differ under varying circumstances, sometimes complicating attempts to determine the locus of political decision making. The supremacy of the state prevails in most instances; therefore the state is a critical arena for political action. An example is the state's authority to license health professionals and health care institutions.

Each state establishes policies or standards for goods or services that affect the health of its citizens. However, if the federal government or the local government imposes a higher standard than the state requires, the lower standard is negated by the higher standard. An example would be standardization of pasteurized milk. A state may hold to one standard, whereas interstate commerce, which is under federal jurisdiction, may dictate a higher standard that must be met by that state.

The federal government has a strong influence on the health services available in each state. Constitutionally, this authority is derived from the federal role in interstate commerce and through broad interpretation of the "general welfare" clause (e.g., Medicare and Medicaid). States vary considerably in resources allocated to provide health programs; therefore significant de facto authority derives from the promise of revenues or threats to remove funding (e.g., funds for interstate highway repair are often tied to air quality requirements). Federal funds typically fund most health care programs fully or partially.

Compliance by states with federal program standards is voluntary, but the advantage of the revenue, which is withheld from the states that fail to comply, is seldom ignored. Programs such as a statistical reporting system of sexually transmitted infections and control are standardized across the country in response to the indirect but marked effect of federal funding.

Health Policy and the Private Sector

In addition to the public policy–making sector, health policies can be made through the private sector. For example, an insurance company or an employer can determine some of what illnesses and preventive care is covered by the insurance program, what drugs are included in the formulary, and how much to charge for an insurance policy. The private sector includes employers, professional organizations (e.g., American Hospital Association), nonprofit health care organizations (e.g., American Heart Association), and for-profit corporations that deliver, insure, or fund healthcare services outside government control. In particular, health insurance companies and managed care organizations are increasingly setting policies that affect a large number of individuals.

In the private sector, health policy evolves differently from in the public sector. One difference is that private health policy is largely influenced by theories of economics and business management, as compared to the social and political theories that predominate in the public sector. In the private sector economics is central, whereas in the public sector economics is but one of many factors. In the private sector, decisions can be swift and are often proactive, whereas in the public sector decisions are slow, deliberate, and more reactive. Private-sector needs are determined by consumerism, market trends, and economics. Public-sector needs are determined by voting shifts, electoral realignment, and term limits. Box 10.4 provides the history of several critical examples of government-funded healthcare legislation.

The Legislative Process: How a Bill Becomes a Law

As stated in the previous section, there is a balance of powers within the government at both state and federal levels. The three branches of government, executive, judicial, and legislative, form a three-legged stool that is in equilibrium. Along with a separation of powers of the three branches of government, there is an additional mechanism that balances the power of the Congress: bicameralism (consisting of two houses). Bicameralism ensures that the power to enact laws is shared between the House of Representatives and the Senate. The procedure through which legislation must pass to eventually become law is similar for all legislative bodies in the country. Once a concept has been drafted into legislative language, it becomes a bill, is given a number, and

---

BOX 10.4 **History of Several Examples of Government-Funded Health Care Legislation**

- **1965:** The Social Security Act established both Medicare and Medicaid. Medicare was a responsibility of the SSA, whereas federal assistance to the state Medicaid programs was administered by the Social and Rehabilitation Service (SRS). SSA and SRS were agencies in the Department of Health, Education, and Welfare (HEW).
- **1977:** The Health Care Financing Administration (HCFA) was created under HEW to effectively coordinate Medicare and Medicaid.
- **1980:** HEW was divided into the Department of Education and the Department of Health and Human Services (HHS).
- **2001:** HCFA was renamed the Centers for Medicare and Medicaid Services (CMS). CMS is the federal agency that administers the Medicare and Medicaid programs.
- **2010:** The Patient Protection and Affordable Care Act was a very comprehensive attempt to improve access to care by providing health insurance to most of the nation's uninsured.
- **2012:** The Food and Drug Administration Safety and Innovation Act reauthorizes user fees for the FDA.
- **2016:** Veterans Affairs (VA) Health system rule change granting veterans direct access to care by nurse practitioners, certified nurse midwives, and clinical nurse specialists who work in the VA health system.

---

moves through a series of steps. The bill's passage is sometimes smooth, but, more often than not, the bill is extensively altered through amendments or even "killed" (dropped from or stopped in the process).

In Congress and in the 49 states that have bicameral legislatures, a bill must succeed through the two legislative bodies, that is, the House of Representatives and the Senate (Fig. 10.1). Nebraska, which has a single-house legislature, is the exception. A bill that has moved successfully through the legislative process has one final hurdle, which is the chief executive's approval. The approval may be a clear endorsement, in which case the governor or president signs it. If the executive neither signs nor vetoes it, the bill may become law by default. An explicit veto conclusively kills the bill, which then can be revived only by a substantial vote of the legislature to override the veto. This is another example of the checks and balances of the government process.

Issues that find their way into the legislative arena are commonly controversial, and proponents and opponents quickly align themselves. Defeating a bill is much easier than getting one passed; therefore the opposition always has the advantage.

Health legislation, which usually requires preventive action (e.g., toxic waste management) or creates a new service (e.g., nursing center organizations for Medicare recipients), is at a disadvantage from several standpoints. Few elected officials are knowledgeable about the health care field. Typically, they have staff who have more expertise in this area, and it is the staff who write legislation. Although health is readily recognized as a national resource, it is not easily quantified into the economic terms that make the issue easy to grasp. Health legislation is often costly to implement. As a result even legislation that has large bipartisan support may not pass due to the cost. Other disadvantages are the backgrounds, biases, and ambitions of each legislator. Despite these obstacles, good health laws can be passed when concerned nurses and other healthcare workers understand the legislative process and use it effectively. Nurses have been recognized as one of the most trusted professions. Nurses should educate their elected officials and function as expert tutors for them. In addition, this is yet another mode of intervention that nurses may perform on behalf of clients.

Major Legislative Actions and the Healthcare System

An examination of the major legislative actions that federal and state governments have taken and recognition of their influence on health and healthcare delivery are critical to understanding the evolution of the healthcare system in the United States. Throughout the 20th century, the U.S. Congress enacted bills that had a major influence on the private and public healthcare subsystems. Legislation pertaining to health increased in scope in each decade of the 20th century, with the goal of improving the health of populations and coping with changing healthcare needs. During the last 2 decades, concerns about an increase in

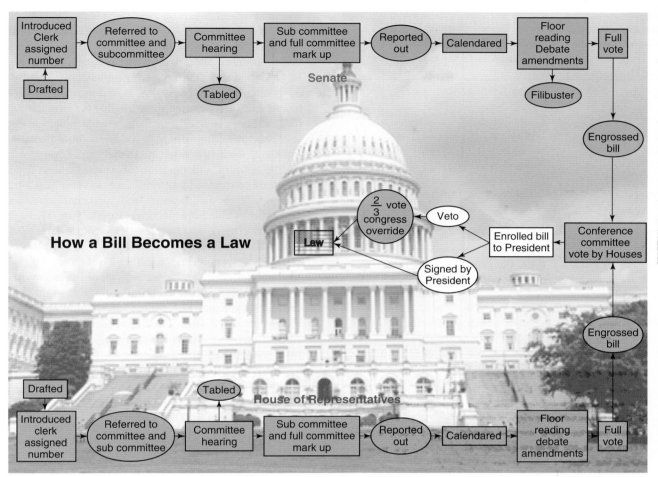

Fig. 10.1 How a bill becomes a law at the federal level. (Available from: http://publicdomainclip-art.blogspot.com/2007_09_01_archive.html.)

health care costs and the growth of managed care stimulated even more legislation. The Patient Protection and Affordable Care Act (ACA) was signed into law in March 2010 with a plan to increase health care coverage to previously uninsured Americans. The ACA had many supporters and opponents, resulting in much debate even after its implementation. Indeed, healthcare reform/health insurance reform was a major issue during both the 2012 and 2016 presidential elections. The Supreme Court also reviewed a major case related to the health care reform legislation, tying all levels of government to this landmark legislation—administrative, legislative, and judicial. The Court decision did not lead to major changes in the health care reform law. At the time of publication, the debate continues on introducing new legislation to repeal and replace the ACA. Issues of affordability, preexisting conditions, requirements for citizens to buy health insurance, and tax credits are being discussed.

Federal Legislation

This section describes some of the landmark federal laws that have influenced health services and health care professionals. They are listed in Table 10.3.

Pure Food and Drugs Act of 1906: This act established a program to supervise and control the manufacture, labeling, and sale of food. Subsequent legislation included meat and dairy products, pharmaceuticals, cosmetics, toys, and household products. Since 1927, the U.S. Food and Drug Administration (FDA) has administered elements of this act.

Children's Bureau Act of 1912: The Children's Bureau was founded to protect children from the unhealthy child labor practices of the time and to enact programs that had a positive effect on children's health. In 1921, the Sheppard-Towner Act extended children's health care programs by providing funds for the health and welfare of infants.

Social Security Act of 1935 and its amendments (1965, 1972): The Social Security Act and its subsequent amendments have had a far-reaching effect on health care for many groups. The Social Security Administration (SSA) provides welfare for high-risk mothers and children. Benefits were later expanded to include health care provisions for older adults and the handicapped. This major governmental action was the enactment of legislation for Medicare and Medicaid.

Medicare, Title XVIII Social Security Amendment (1965): This federal program, administered by the Centers for Medicare

TABLE 10.3 Critical Federal Legislation Related to Health Care

Year(s)	Legislation or Other Government Action
1906	Pure Food and Drugs Act
1912	Children's Bureau Act
1921	Sheppard-Towner Act
1935	Social Security Act
1944	Public Health Act
1945	McCarren-Ferguson Act
1946	Hill—Burton Act
1953	Establishment of the Department of Health, Education and Welfare as a cabinet-status agency; in 1980 establishment of U.S. Department of Education as separate from Department of Health and Human Services
1956	Health Amendments Act
1964	Nurse Training Act
1965	Social Security Act amendments: Title XVIII Medicare, Title XIX Medicaid
1970	Occupational Safety and Health Act
1972	Social Security Act amendments: Professional Standards Review Organization; further benefits under Medicare and Medicaid, including dialysis
1973	Health Maintenance Act
1974	National Health Planning Resources Act
1981, 1987, 1989, 1990	Omnibus Budget Reconciliation Acts
1982	Tax Equity and Fiscal Responsibility Act
1985	Consolidated Omnibus Budget Reconciliation Act
1988	Family Support Act
1990	Health Objectives Planning Act
1996	Health Insurance Portability and Accountability Act
1996	Welfare Act
2003	Nurse reinvestment Act
2004	Medicare reinvestment Act
2008	Mental Health Parity and Addictions Equity Act
2010	Patient Protection and Affordable Care Act

and Medicaid Services (CMS; formerly Health Care Financing Administration [HCFA]), pays specified health care services for all people 65 years of age and older who are eligible to receive Social Security benefits. People with permanent disabilities and those with end-stage renal disease are also covered. The objective of Medicare is to protect older adults and the disabled against large medical outlays. The program is funded through a payroll tax of most working citizens. Individuals or providers may submit payment requests for health care services and are paid according to Medicare regulations. See Chapter 12 for more information on Medicare.

Medicaid, Title XIX Social Security Amendment (1965): This combined federal and state program provides access to care for the poor and medically needy of all ages. Each state is allocated federal dollars on a matching basis (i.e., 50% of costs are paid with federal dollars). Each state has the responsibility and right to determine the services to be provided and the dollar amount allocated to the program. Basic services (e.g., ambulatory and inpatient hospital care, physical therapy, laboratory, radiography, skilled nursing, and home health care) are required to be eligible for matching federal dollars. States may choose from a wide range of optional services, including drugs, eyeglasses, intermediate care, inpatient psychiatric care, and dental care. Limits are placed on the amount and duration of service. Unlike Medicare, Medicaid provides long-term care services (e.g., nursing home and home health) and personal care services (e.g., chores and homemaking). In addition, Medicaid has eligibility criteria based on level of income. Table 10.4 provides the U.S. Department of Health and Human Services (HHS) poverty guidelines for 2020. The Medicaid population has complex needs, and managed care organizations may not always be able to provide optimum services to these beneficiaries. See Chapter 12 for more information on Medicaid.

Public Health Act of 1944: The Public Health Act consolidated all existing public health legislation into one law. Since then, many new pieces of legislation have become amendments. Some of its provisions, either in the original law or in amendments, provided for or established the following:

- Health services for migratory workers
- Family planning services
- Health research facilities
- National Institutes of Health
- Nurse training acts
- Traineeships for graduate students in public health
- Home health services for people with Alzheimer disease
- Prevention and primary care services
- Rural health clinics
- Communicable disease control

McCarren-Ferguson Act of 1945: The McCarren-Ferguson Act has had a major influence on the insurance industry through giving states the exclusive right to regulate health insurance plans (Knight, 1998). No federal government agency is solely responsible for monitoring insurance, as this supervision is in the hands of state governments. Some federal agencies are involved in insurance reimbursement; however, the structure of the benefit program for federal employees and military personnel, Medicare, and Medicaid allows Congress to pass laws that can override state health insurance laws if the laws do not meet certain criteria.

Hill—Burton Act of 1946: The Hill—Burton Act authorized federal assistance in the construction of hospitals and health centers with stipulations about services for the uninsured. As a result, hospitals with obligations to care for the uninsured were built in towns and cities across the United States. Through these measures, hospital care became more accessible, but by the late 1990s, the high cost of health care, combined with decreasing lengths of stay and increasing use of primary care, forced the closure of many of the hospitals built with Hill—Burton funds.

TABLE 10.4 2017 Federal Poverty Guidelines[a] for the 48 Contiguous States and the District of Columbia				
Family Size	Gross Yearly Income ($)	Gross Monthly Income ($)	Approximate Hourly Income ($)
1	12,060	1005	5.81
2	16,240	1353	7.81
3	20,420	1702	9.82
4	24,600	2050	11.83
5	28,780	2398	13.84
6	32,960	2747	15.85
7	37,140	3095	17.86
8	41,320	3344	19.30
Over 8 add per child	+4180	+348	+$

[a]Federal poverty guidelines: Typically, in January or February of each year the federal government releases an official income level for poverty called the Federal Poverty Income Guidelines, often informally referred to as the "federal poverty level." The benefit levels of many low-income assistance programs are based on these poverty guidelines.
From https://aspe.hhs.gov/2017-poverty-guidelines#guidelines.

Health Amendments Act of 1956: The Health Amendments Act, Title II, authorizes funds to aid RNs in full-time study of administration, supervision, or teaching. In 1963, the Surgeon General's Consultant Group on Nursing noted that there were still too few nursing schools, nursing personnel were not put to good use, and there was limited nursing research. As a result, in 1964, the Nurse Training Act provided funds for loans and scholarships for full-time study for nurses and funds for construction of nursing schools. Since this time, additional legislation has funded nursing education; even the Patient Protection and Affordable Care Act of 2010 provides some funding opportunities.

Occupational Safety and Health Act of 1970: The Occupational Safety and Health Act focuses on the health needs and risks in the workplace and environment. It continues to provide critical programs important to the workplace and the community. See Chapter 30 for more information on both the Occupational Safety and Health Act and the Occupational Safety and Health Administration.

Health Maintenance Organization (HMO) Act of 1973: The HMO Act provided grants for HMO development. The act required that employers offer federally qualified HMOs as a healthcare coverage option to employees and established that states were responsible for the oversight of HMOs. Although initially it was not successful in stimulating HMO growth, this legislation has had a long-term effect on the growth of managed care.

National Health Planning and Resources Act of 1974: The National Health Planning and Resources Act assigned the responsibility for health planning to the states and local health systems agencies. In addition, it required health care facilities to obtain prior approval from the state for expansion in the form of a certificate of need.

Omnibus Budget Reconciliation Acts (1981, 1987, 1989, and 1990): The Omnibus Budget Reconciliation Acts were each enacted in response to the huge federal deficit. They have influenced funding for nursing homes, home health agencies, and hospitals and have set up guidelines and regulations about several issues, including a move from process to outcome evaluation, use of restraints, and prescription drugs for Medicaid recipients.

Tax Equity and Fiscal Responsibility Act of 1982: The Tax Equity and Fiscal Responsibility Act was a major amendment to the Social Security Act of 1935, establishing the prospective payment system for Medicare, the diagnosis-related group (DRG) system. This law changed health care radically by introducing a new reimbursement method. See Chapter 12 for more information on DRGs.

Consolidated Omnibus Budget Reconciliation Act of 1985: The Consolidated Omnibus Budget Reconciliation Act (COBRA) is a federal law that affects health care delivery and reimbursement. It requires all hospitals with emergency services that participate in Medicare to treat any client in their emergency services, whether or not that client is covered by Medicare or has the ability to pay. This legislation includes requirements for Medicaid services for prenatal and postnatal care to low-income women in two-parent families in which the primary spouse is unemployed. Another important requirement of COBRA focuses on the problem of the loss of health insurance when a person loses his or her job. With the growing number of unemployed, COBRA is even more important. Employers who terminate an employee must continue benefits for the employee and dependents for a specified period if the employee had health benefits before the termination. COBRA is an example of how a federal law can affect state health care practices. The federal government must determine who receives federal Medicare funds; therefore COBRA provides the opportunity for the federal government to legislate health care delivery at the state level.

Family Support Act of 1988: The Family Support Act expanded coverage for poor women and children and required states to extend Medicaid coverage for 12 months to families who have increased earnings but are no longer receiving cash assistance. This act also required states to expand Aid to

Families with Dependent Children (AFDC) coverage to two-parent families in which the principal wage earner is unemployed.

Health Objectives Planning Act of 1990: The Health Objectives Planning Act was initiated in response to the 1979 report *Healthy People: The Surgeon General's Report on Health Promotion and Disease Prevention.* After that report, the federal government began to take a directive approach in identifying and monitoring national healthcare goals. *Healthy People 2000, Healthy People 2010,* and *Healthy People 2020* are also results of this act.

Health Insurance Portability and Accountability Act of 1996: The Health Insurance Portability and Accountability Act (HIPAA) addressed several issues. The law offered protections for patient privacy and confidentiality. Critical insurance issues were the portability of coverage and limits on the restrictions health plans place on coverage for preexisting conditions. This law established that insurers cannot set limits on coverage of longer than 12 months. This is a complex law, but it has been important for consumers with preexisting conditions. It should be noted that 2010 health care reform legislation has eliminated HIPAA applicability to preexisting conditions, and this change went into effect in 2014.

Welfare Reform Act of 1996: The Welfare Reform Act placed restrictions on eligibility for AFDC, Medicaid, and other federally funded welfare programs. The Welfare Reform law decreased the number of people on welfare and forced many individuals to take low-paying jobs, many of which do not offer health insurance. Between 1994 and March 1999, welfare rolls dropped 47% (DeParle, 1999). Many individuals, particularly underserved women and children, subsequently lost Medicaid coverage. In 2012 this became the Temporary Assistance for Needy Families.

The State Child Health Improvement Act (SCHIP) of 1997: This has been a critical law, providing insurance for children and families who cannot afford health insurance. This law has been very important to children's health. The law was extended several times and then it was not renewed by the Bush administration. The program was renewed by the Obama administration in the Children's Health Insurance Reauthorization Act of 2009. See Box 10.2 (referred to as CHIP or SCHIP if "state" is included).

Balanced Budget Act (BBA) of 1997, as amended by the Omnibus Consolidated and Emergency Supplemental Appropriations Act (OCESSA) of 1999: This act was crucial regarding Medicare payments to home health services and creation of the prospective payment system (PPS) (CMS, 2021). More information can be found in Chapter 34.

Medicare Modernization Act of 2003: The Medicare Modernization Act was the most significant law in 40 years for senior health care. After being implemented in January 2006, the law provided seniors and people living with disabilities some prescription drug benefit coverage, more choices, and better benefits.

Nurse Reinvestment Act of 2003: The Nurse Reinvestment Act is significant because it is a response to the critical nursing shortage that has been present across the country. Funding is provided to increase enrollments and the number of practicing nurses.

Mental Health Parity and Addictions Equity Act of 2008: A similar act was passed in the 1990s, but it was not an effective law. Improving the earlier law, this act mandates that if a group health plan includes medical/surgical benefits and mental health benefits and/or substance use disorder benefits, the financial requirements (e.g., deductibles and copayments) and treatment limitations (e.g., number of visits or days of coverage) that apply to mental health benefits must be no more restrictive than the predominant financial requirements or treatment limitations that apply to substantially all medical/surgical benefits.

Patient Protection and Affordable Care Act of 2010: The Patient Protection and Affordable Care Act of 2010, also called the *Health Care Reform Act,* is an extremely complex and comprehensive piece of legislation. One of the primary intents of the act is to reduce the number of uninsured Americans, and a number of provisions directly address this intent. For example, it requires all U.S. citizens and legal residents to have qualifying health coverage, whether provided through employers, individually purchased, or provided by federal plans (i.e., Medicare, Medicaid, CHIP). It also dramatically changes eligibility requirements for Medicaid, allowing coverage of childless adults with incomes up to 133% of the federal poverty line, and expands CHIP. Furthermore, it subsidizes premiums for lower- and middle-income families and requires coverage of dependent adult children up to age 26 for those with group policies (Kaiser Family Foundation, 2016).

Bipartisan Budget Act of 2018 (BBA of 2018): This act provided home health payment reform that started in January 2020 (CMS, 2021). More information is available in Chapter 34.

Coronavirus Aid, Relief, and Economic Security (CARES) Act of 2020: This bill was created in response to the COVID-19 (coronavirus) outbreak, and it had provisions affected taxes, health care, and education (Congress.gov, 2020). Changes for health care included expanding health insurance coverage of diagnostic testing, requiring coverage for preventative services and vaccines, limiting liability for volunteer health care professionals, and allowing emergence use of certain diagnostic tests that do not have FDA approval.

The Health Care Reform Act included significant insurance changes. For example, it (1) establishes high-risk pools to provide health coverage to individuals with preexisting conditions; (2) prohibits insurers from placing lifetime limits on the dollar value of coverage; (3) prohibits insurers from disallowing coverage for some individuals because of preexisting health conditions and dropping policyholders when they get sick; and (4) requires health plans to provide some types of preventive care and screenings without consumer cost-sharing (i.e., copayments or coinsurance). The legislation creates programs to foster nonprofit, member-run health insurance companies that can offer health insurance; to establish state-based health insurance exchanges through which individuals and small businesses can buy coverage; and to permit states to form compacts that will allow insurers to sell policies in any participating state.

Funds for government-financed elements (i.e., Medicare, Medicaid, CHIP) are to be provided through a combination of new fees and taxes and a variety of cost-saving measures. For example, there will be taxes on indoor tanning and new Medicare taxes for people in high-income brackets. The act requires fees for pharmaceutical companies and medical devices as well as penalties for individuals who do not obtain health insurance. To cut costs, there are significant cuts to the Medicare Advantage program and modifications and reductions in Medicare spending. It also enhances efforts to reduce administrative costs, streamline care, and reduce fraud and abuse.

Until passage of the Patient Protection and Affordable Care Act of 2010, the focus of federal legislation was on either prevention of illness through influencing the environment, such as the Occupational Safety and Health Act of 1970, or provision of funding to support programs that influence health care, as demonstrated in the Social Security Act of 1935. Beginning with the Sheppard-Towner Act of 1921 and continuing to the present, federal grants have increased the involvement of state and local governments in health care. The involvement of the federal government through fiscal allocations to state and local governments provided money for programs not previously available to states and local areas. Similar services became available in all states. Funds supporting these services were accompanied by regulations that applied to all recipients. Many state and local government programs were developed on the basis of availability of federal funds. The involvement of the federal government through funding has served to standardize public health policy in the United States (Pickett and Hanlon, 1990).

The health reform legislation of 2010 was strongly influenced by the rising numbers of uninsured and underinsured U.S. citizens. Since the implementation of the ACA the rate of uninsured citizens fell from 16.6% in 2013 to 10% in 2016 (Kaiser Family Foundation, 2016). However, the unsured rate has since increased since 2016, including a 1.7% increased between 2017 and 2019 (Assistant Secretary for Planning and Evaluation [ASPE], 2021). This change was related to policy changes and coverage options under the ACA and Medicaid (ASPE, 2021). In the first half of 2020, 30 million U.S. residents didn't have health insurance (ASPE, 2021). It is still unclear how the COVID-19 health impact has affected insurance. While early estimates show no significant change, these results could have been affected by a shift in how surveys are conducting due to the pandemic. The surveys were moved from in person to telephone; given the reduced response rates, results may have been affected (ASPE, 2021).

The United States continues to be the only major developed country to not have universal health care coverage. The ACA has not reduced the cost of health care as promised. Medicaid expansion has been rejected by 19 states despite the federal support. Former President Donald Trump pledged in 2016 to repeal the ACA and replace it (Chang & Gnuschke, 2019). There was a failed attempt to repeal the ACA in 2017 by republican-controlled Congress. During the Trump administration, the ACA was reshaped using a series of regulatory, administrative, and budgetary maneuvers. Highlights of some of these changes include reducing the tax penalty to those without insurance to zero and having a shorter window for enrollment (Chang & Gnuschke, 2019).

Role of State Legislatures

State governments are also directly involved in healthcare policy, legislation, and regulation. State governments focus particularly on financing and delivery of services and oversight of insurance. The latter has become important as managed care has grown. The 1988 report titled *Future of Public Health* from the National Academy of Medicine (NAM), formerly called the Institute of Medicine (IOM)—noted that it is the state's responsibility to see that functions and services necessary to address the mission of public health are in place throughout the state. The NAM framed the public health enterprise in terms of three functions: assessment, policy development, and assurance. Further the NAM reported in *The Future of the Public's Health in the 21st Century* (IOM, 1988) six areas of action and change:

1. Adopting a population health approach that considers the multiple determinants of health
2. Strengthening the governmental public health infrastructure, which forms the backbone of the public health system
3. Building a new generation of intersectoral partnerships that also draw on the perspectives and resources of diverse communities and actively engage them in health action
4. Developing systems of accountability to assure the quality and availability of public health services
5. Making evidence the foundation of decision making and the measure of success
6. Enhancing and facilitating communication within the public health system (e.g., among all levels of the governmental public health infrastructure and between public health professionals and community members) (IOM, 1988)

The CDC describes the 10 essential public health services that all communities should have:

- Monitor health status to identify and solve community health problems.
- Diagnose and investigate health problems and health hazards in the community.
- Inform, educate, and empower people about health issues.
- Mobilize community partnerships and action to identify and solve health problems.
- Develop policies and plans that support individual and community health efforts.
- Enforce laws and regulations that protect health and ensure safety.
- Link people to needed personal health services and assure the provision of health care when otherwise unavailable.
- Assure competent public and personal healthcare workforces.

- Evaluate effectiveness, accessibility, and quality of personal and population-based health services.
- Research for new insights and innovative solutions to health problems.

❓ ACTIVE LEARNING EXERCISE

Review your state's legislative agenda. Identify bills that relate to health care, and from those bills, identify any bills that might affect community or public health. Discuss the bills in small groups—their impact in general and how nursing might be involved.

PUBLIC POLICY: BLUEPRINT FOR GOVERNANCE

Policy is directed by values. It articulates the guiding principles of collective endeavors, establishes direction, and sets goals. It influences and, in turn, is influenced by politics. Policy directives may become realized or obstructed at any stage in the political process.

Policy Formulation: The Ideal

In ideal circumstances, authorized authoritative bodies (e.g., state health departments, USDHHS, CMS) rationally determine actions to create, amend, implement, or rescind healthcare policy. These groups decide what is right or best and then develop the political strategies to effect the desired outcomes. Whether a particular policy is advocated or adopted depends on the degree that a group or society as a whole may benefit without harm or detriment to subgroups. Of all the seemingly endless limitless factors that may influence policy formation, group need and group demand should be the strongest determinants. The premises supporting the goals of health policy should be equitable distribution of services and the guarantee that the appropriate care is given to the right people, at the right time, and at a reasonable cost.

Policy Formulation: The Reality

In the real world, policy for healthcare exemplifies both conflict and social change theories. Health policy is the product of continuous interactive processes in which interested professionals, citizens, institutions, industries, and other interested groups compete with one another for healthcare dollars and policy initiatives. They also compete with one another for the attention of various branches of government. The most obvious and prominent among these is the legislative branch, although policy is also made through regulatory mechanisms and court decisions. Health policy may also be derived from the recommendations of fact-finding commissions established by the legislative or executive branch or nongovernmental organizations such as the NAM and may also be influenced by judicial decisions.

Health policy is rarely created through discrete, momentous determinations in relation to single problems or issues. It often evolves slowly because changes in the social beliefs and values

that underlie established policy develop within the context of actual service delivery. Once a direct health care service is offered, especially an official tax-funded service, discontinuing is often difficult. Existing programs create tradition by establishing vested interest and a sense of entitlement on the part of the public. An example is the annual updating of the childhood and adolescent vaccination schedule recommended by the CDC. This is also an example of cooperation between professional organizations and government agencies to promote the well-being of individuals and communities (Box 10.5).

Steps in Policy Formulation and Analysis

The tangible formulation of public policy begins with the most critical step, which is defining the issue or describing the problem and placing it on the legislative agenda. This process includes cost—benefit analysis. Health **policy analysis** determines those who benefit and those who experience a loss as the result of a policy. These considerations are critical in order to develop health policies that are as fair as possible to all who are affected. Then legislation is finalized, typically developed by legislative staff. The bill then winds its way through the process in the legislative body at either the state or federal level. This includes a cost analysis of the bill at the federal level by the Congressional Budget Office. If the bill is passed and is signed by either a governor or the president, it becomes law. The next step is the commitment of resources, most often through the passage of legislation, and the development of regulations, which is done by a governmental agency assigned to ensure implementation of a bill that becomes law. A regulatory schedule for the implementation of the law is formulated. Then, an evaluation process is designed that satisfies regulatory and legislative remedies should they be needed. Analysis of health policy is an objective process that identifies the sources and consequences of policy decisions in the context of the factors that influence them.

A 30-day window of opportunity is typical for public input into the development of regulations. Written comments about a political issue are made part of the public record. To facilitate

BOX 10.5 Recommended Childhood and Adolescent Immunization Schedule: United States

The Advisory Committee on Immunization Practices (ACIP) annually reviews the recommended childhood and adolescent immunization schedule to ensure that the schedule is current with changes in vaccine formulations and reflects revised recommendations for the use of licensed vaccines, including those newly licensed. It is the only federal government body that provides written recommendations for the routine administration of vaccines for children and adults in the civilian population. Recommendations and format of the childhood and adolescent immunization schedule for February 2017 were approved by ACIP, and the American Academy of Family Physicians.

From Centers for Disease Control and Prevention: Recommended immunization schedules for persons 0–18 years—United States, 2017, *Morb & Mort Weekly Rep* 66(5):134–135, 2017. Available from: http://www.cdc.gov/vaccines/schedules/hcp/index.html.

correspondence, websites have been set up to promote contacting agencies, governmental organizations, and political figures. Nurses need to be aware of some of the important websites. furthermore, many legislators may have their own web pages so that the nurse can easily access their offices.

The Internet can provide almost unlimited access to information. However, access to information does not ensure its quality or credibility. The user is responsible for evaluating the information and separating quality information from misinformation. Nurses need to be information and communication technology literate. *Technology literacy* is the ability of an individual, working independently and with others, to responsibly, appropriately, and effectively use technology tools to access, manage, integrate, evaluate, create, and communicate information. Technology fluency builds on technology literacy and is demonstrated when nurses apply technology to real-world experiences, adapt to changing technologies, modify current and create new technologies, and personalize technology to meet personal needs, interests, and learning style.

 ACTIVE LEARNING EXERCISE

Participate in a group organized around a public health issue (e.g., disposable diapers, toxic waste, or fluoride).

THE EFFECTIVE USE OF NURSES: A POLICY ISSUE

The Health Resources and Services Administration (HRSA) provides general resources and information to the public and for use in the development of policy by the government. The nursing workforce development programs administered by the HRSA through Public Health Service Act Title VIII funding provide federal support for nurse workforce development. Title VIII provides the largest source of federal funding for nursing education at the undergraduate and graduate levels and favors institutions that educate nurses for practice in rural and medically underserved communities. These programs provide loans, scholarships, traineeships, and programmatic support for nursing students and for nurses who are continuing their education in graduate programs.

An issue that is vital to effective healthcare delivery relates to nurse staffing. The current nursing shortage has been a topic of concern of nurses for many years and is now a health care crisis. This crisis has taken a strange course as a result of the economic crisis in the United States. Many nurses who were due to retire did not; some nurses who were working part time returned to full-time work; and some nurses who had not been employed in nursing returned to the field. These changes reduced the shortage and have also had a negative impact on new graduates obtaining positions. In addition, in some areas of the country, hospital administrators decided that as there are more new graduates, they could focus on hiring graduates with bachelor's degrees instead of associate-degree graduates—who have therefore had more difficulty obtaining jobs. Compounding the

problem is the fact that nursing colleges and universities across the nation are struggling to expand enrollment to meet the rising demand for nursing care. A shortage of nursing faculty and changing demographics contribute to the concern that all 50 states will experience a shortage of nurses in the next few years. In February 2017 Congress introduced the Title VIII Nursing Workforce Reauthorization Act of 2017, which will reauthorize and improve nursing workforce programs, supporting practice in rural and medically underserved communities, as well as providing support for advanced nursing education, diversity, National Nurse Service Corps, nurse faculty loan forgiveness, and geriatric education (ANA, 2017).

NURSES' ROLES IN POLITICAL ACTIVITIES
The Power of One and Many

RNs are the largest healthcare professional group. There has been a push to involve more nurses in policymaking, leadership, and advocacy in an effort to move nurses from recipients to implementers of health policy decisions (Turale, 2019). With campaigns such as the Nightingale Challenge, Nursing Now, and celebrations of the 200th anniversary of Florence Nightingale, the profession has been in the news more. Organizations like the International Council of Nurses and the WHO are pushing nurses to get involved to use their unique knowledge of patients and health to make contributions to policy.

Why are nurses not more politically active? Taylor (2016) examined nurses' motivation for public policy involvement. Reasons nurses become involved in health policy included becoming engaged in an issue, family history of political activity, connection with other nurses, having an influential mentor, and being part of a professional organization. More effort needs to be given to educate nurses about the importance of being informed on health policy issues and to encourage them to be politically active. Exposure to positive role models is particularly important. Nurses must obtain the tools to overcome factors that impede involvement. Nurses most often identify positive role models as the major influence that assisted them to become politically active in the profession. Professional organizations offer a connectiveness that can support the nurse in engaging in political activities. Therefore, mentorship from the student level up to the expert level is important. Box 10.6 describes responses to a survey used by Winter and Lockhart (1997) about what methods were useful in developing awareness in the profession, policy, and politics.

Nurses as Change Agents

The public, as well as the government, recognizes the nursing profession as indispensable, necessary, and a valuable national resource. In their advocacy role, nurses are seen as professionals whose knowledge, skills, and caring concern are used to promote both the individual's and the community's well-being. Nurses have a unique status in caring for patients; they are interpreters of the healthcare system to the public, and government-funded programs influence their professional

---

BOX 10.6 Responses to Policy Activism Survey

Positive Influences and the Importance of Mentorship

"I became involved in politics through a relationship with a professor who felt strongly about an issue."

"I have found communication among peers to be informative and often inspiring. That has motivated my involvement in health care issues."

"I became aware of the potential role nurses could play related to policy as an undergrad. I had a few dynamic professors who were very inspiring by their involvement and passion related to various issues. At that point I didn't consider myself as someone to get involved but I think it ignited a spark for 'someday' .... "

"My exposure to professors who were actually involved in different 'causes' and not just teaching the course made a huge difference in my perspective on getting involved. The continual role model/mentor is also a huge inspiration."

"....nurses who take an interest in current events and enjoy discussing their opinions regarding public policies."

"I think if you don't get exposed to that 'spark' throughout your career, it goes out. An inspiring speaker at a professional meeting will get me every time!"

"I was inspired by my professor who was past president for [the] New York State Nurses Association."

"It would be great if one of the clinical nurse specialists at my hospital were to ask some nurses in a unit what they thought about something and how we could try to change or fix it. We just need that little nudge and some guidance to kindle that passion."

Negative Experiences Influencing Awareness

"I became more aware of the policies from my institution, from preceptors, and when I had a problem. I was more aware as a novice because I was scared to do something that was going to get me into trouble."

"I became more involved at the institutional level after being 'wronged' by administration in regard to a policy, procedure, or benefit."

"I was usually unaware of a policy until it affected me directly; therefore, the need to know became paramount."

---

activities. The private business sector is also involved. Therefore public health nurses must know how to participate in the political process. To do this effectively, they need a sound knowledge of the community, state, and national government organization and function and a clear understanding of how these bodies collectively interact to influence policy. Nurses must know how to influence the creation of healthcare legislation and how to contribute to the election and appointment of key officials.

Although there are more nurses than physicians, hospital administrators, insurance administrators, or other health care professionals, nursing traditionally has not been seen as having major political influence because of a lack of public policy consensus within the nursing community. Unity within professional organizations, coalitions, and lobbying efforts is changing this perception. Policy is fundamental to governance; therefore nurses need to know about the formation of public policy and the acts of government and its agencies. Tables 10.5 and 10.6 give sources of information on these issues.

Nurses must become invested and competent in health policy. This includes communicating with elected officials at the local, state, and federal levels. This may be done through writing letters, emails, or doing personal visits. Contacting legislators gives the nurse the opportunity to "tell their story" in how the issue affects nursing practice. In addition, belonging to a professional organization, serving on advisory boards, speaking publicly, and contributing to a PAC all engage the nurse in effecting policy change. By engaging others affected by an issue, nurses can bring voice to their concerns (Kostas-Polston et al., 2015).

Nurses and Coalitions

When two or more groups join to maximize resources, increasing their influence and improving their chances of success in achieving a common goal, they have formed a **coalition**. Coalitions of healthcare providers often work on issues such as family violence and fluoridation of water supplies. An outstanding example of such cooperative action is the establishment of rehabilitation programs for health professionals whose practice has been impaired by substance abuse or mental health problems.

Nursing and consumer groups often form coalitions to advance their shared interests in health promotion. The ANA joined 16 other organizations (e.g., American College of Nurse Practitioners, American Red Cross, Department of Veterans Affairs, and Sigma Theta Tau) in the 1990s to form a coalition called Nurses for a Healthier Tomorrow. This organization has grown to a membership of 43 organizations. Responding to concerns about a potentially dangerous shortage of nurses, this coalition hopes to raise funds for a national advertising campaign designed to recruit new nurses and encourage existing ones to remain in the profession. The campaign focuses on the message that nurses are essential to the healthcare team and that they save healthcare dollars. The campaign shows that an increased demand exists for nurses, both in specialty areas and outside the hospital (NHT, 2021).

Nurses as Lobbyists

A **lobbyist** is a person who, voluntarily or for a fee, represents himself or herself, another individual, an organization, or an entity before the legislature. A lobbyist typically represents special-interest groups. The term derives from the fact that lobbyists usually stay in the areas (lobbies) next to the Senate and House chambers, seeking to speak with legislators and their aides as they walk to and from the chambers, or as lobbyists await legislative action that might affect their interests.

To **lobby** is to try to influence legislators; it is an art of persuasion. Influencing lawmakers to pass effective health legislation requires the participation of individual nurses and nursing organizations. There are currently more than 100 national nursing organizations. Many also have state chapters. Professional organizations make advocacy easier for members through the use of the Internet. Policy action centers are now part of many organizations' websites. Email alerts can be sent instantly to members residing in targeted districts to contact their legislators on a particular bill or issue. By entering one's postal zip code and pushing a button, one can sign a template letter and send it to one's legislator.

TABLE 10.5 **Sources for Legislative Information**

Government Level	Information Available	Location
Federal	Background of members of Congress Congressional committee assignments Congressional terms of service Congressional news House/Senate vote tabulations Bills in process or legislated (bill number needed) Health and nursing issues in Congress	Congressional directory Government documents section of selected public or university libraries *Congressional Quarterly Weekly Report* U.S. representative or senator (may have local office) *The American Nurse*, ANA, 600 Maryland Ave SW, Suite 100 Washington, DC 20024 (202) 554—4444
	American Nurses Association Political Action Committee (ANA-PAC) Public health issues in U.S. Congress	*The American Nurse* ANA (see above) *The Nation's Health* American Public Health Association (APHA) 1015 15th St NW Washington, DC 20005 (202) 789—5600
State	Bills in process or legislated (bill number needed) Health and nursing issues in state legislature State political action committees for nursing	State representative or senator (may have local office) State nurses association (SNA) (for location, see April directory issue of the *American Journal of Nursing*) National League for Nursing

TABLE 10.6 **Sources for Electoral Information**

Government Level	Information Available	Location
State	State government operations Political subdivisions Legislative information telephone number State election laws and procedures Campaign finance reports	Secretary of State (state capitol) Office of Lieutenant Governor (state capitol)
County or municipal	Similar to state as appropriate to local government Political jurisdictions for each household address	County clerk (county courthouse) City clerk (city hall)
General	Government information Political jurisdictions for each household address Names of current office holders in local jurisdictions	County clerk (county courthouse) City clerk (city hall)

The goal of the first contact with an official is to establish that the nurse is a concerned constituent as well as a credible source of information on health issues. The image of nurses caring for people is a definite advantage at this point. Nurses are considered the most ethical of all healthcare providers and are considered to be trustworthy (Robert Wood Johnson Foundation, 2012). In communities in which nurses have already established strong political credentials, their colleagues will be more readily accepted. An individual who establishes a reputation as a reliable and accurate resource as a lobbyist has substantial influence.

Legislators rely heavily on lobbyists to educate them on issues, and they usually want to hear from all sides before taking a position on an issue. The official must trust the lobbyists to give accurate, though predictably biased, information. Information needs to be timely and up to date.

Each official represents a constituency with varied needs and interests, and each vote must be weighted within this context. The positions taken by legislators will not always be to an individual or organization's liking. Evaluation of their performance should be based on their overall voting pattern, not just on individual votes. Many organizations regularly tally and publish the records of each federal legislator on all issues related to nursing and health. This information can be helpful in evaluating elected officials. Collective action by nursing and health care organizations is critical to meeting their goals. Professional associations monitor legislative activity related to relevant health issues and link the process to their membership. This continual surveillance of the legislative environment is critical because even seemingly minor amendments can have profound effects on health issues. Thorough legislative surveillance requires the participation of people who are knowledgeable about nursing, health care, and the political intricacies of the legislative process. Some of the nursing organizations that have full-time lobbyists who work in Congress are the ANA, the American Academy of Nursing, and the National League for Nursing. State associations also work with state legislators. State legislative contacts become the eyes, ears, and voices of their professional organizations. These associations can then provide testimony and comment on relevant state and federal issues. However, regardless of the effectiveness of association lobbyists in promoting the interests of nurses and society, they always need grassroots cooperation to truly influence decisions. In the final analysis, a sufficiently high number of communications from individual constituents, via email messages, telephone calls, and letters, has the greatest influence. Lobbying is an ongoing activity for health policy issues influencing nursing and health care delivery. Box 10.7 provides an overview of the lobbying process.

ACTIVE LEARNING EXERCISE

1. With a group of two or three, meet with an elected official for a 15-minute appointment to ask about the official's concerns and priorities. Remember to refer to the "ABCs of Lobbying" prior to meeting with the official.
2. Visit the ANA website and explore its political action section at http://nursingworld.org/MainMenuCategories/Policy-Advocacy. What type of information is available?
3. Visit the American Public Health Association website for information about policy outcome evaluation at https://www.apha.org/policies-and-advocacy. Review the various evaluation programs to gain an understanding of policy outcome evaluation.

Nurses and Political Action Committees

PACs have been important sources of collective political influence since the 1970s. These nonpartisan entities promote the election of candidates believed to be sympathetic to their interests. PACs are established by professional associations, businesses, and labor organizations and are highly regulated by federal and state laws that stipulate how they may contribute financially to campaigns. The advantage of a PAC is that small donations from many members add up to a significant donation to a campaign fund in the name of the organization. This gains the attention of the candidate and earns goodwill for the group.

Valid concern exists about the correlation of major PAC contributions and legislators' votes on special-interest legislation. However, as long as PACs are a reality of political life, nurses need to recognize their power and support those that are committed to electing candidates sympathetic to health care issues.

Most national associations of health care providers, including nursing organizations, have PACs. Among the more powerful are those representing hospitals, nursing homes, health insurers, home health agencies, and pharmaceutical companies. A PAC that makes major political contributions is the American Medical Political Action Committee, sponsored by the American Medical Association. State medical associations also have strong PACs. This means that organized medicine has a powerful influence on national and state elections and on healthcare legislation at both levels.

Nurses and Campaigning

Helping someone win an election is a sure way of gaining influence. All candidates are grateful for campaign assistance and usually remember to thank those who have helped. Although campaign contributions are commonly thought of as financial, they can also take the form of participation in campaign activities. Nurses are frequently unable to contribute much money, but they can provide these invaluable services. For the novice, veteran campaigners are eager to help develop the

BOX 10.7   ABCs of Lobbying on a State Level

Before the Meeting
- Appointments will have been made with your legislator(s) for the lobby cay. Tell the staff that you are a constituent and what issue(s) you would like to discuss with your representative. If your legislator is unavailable, you may have a scheduled appointment with a member of the legislative staff.
- If possible, put together a delegation of nurses to attend the meeting. A number of individuals from the legislator's district who are concerned about the same issue will make a big impression. Take along students from their districts because legislators are impressed with their participation.

Preparing for the Meeting
- Establish your agenda and goals. For example, focus on educating the legislators on the profession of nurse midwifery, the legislation that this group would like them to sponsor, the concerns about the malpractice insurance crisis, and the benefit to women's and children's health. Nurse practitioners (NPs) would focus on the cost—benefit of NPs as primary care providers in all settings, including health care homes.
- Research your legislator's stance before the meeting. It is important that you know your official's position so that you can present your stance more effectively and can have an intelligent discussion.
- Meet with the delegation (e.g., midwives, NPs) that will participate in the lobbying. It is important that you review what each person will say during the meeting. Select someone as the group leader, and make a list of points to be made and questions to be asked by each person.

- Prepare materials. Review the packet of information you will leave with your legislator. It is important to include your name and phone number in the packet so that your legislator will have a contact person for more information. Leaving a business card would be appropriate.

During the Meeting
- Be on time for your meeting.
- Be concise and diplomatic. Keep your presentation short and to the point.
- Be a good listener. Look for indications of your legislator's views, and watch for opportunities to provide useful information in order to strengthen or counter particular views.
- Stress why the issues concern you and others in your district.
- Don't be intimidated. Your legislator is in office to serve you. It is important to have a general knowledge of the issues, but you don't have to know every little detail. If he or she asks a question that you do not know the answer to, simply say that you do not know but are willing to find out. Find out the best way to get the information to him or her (fax, email, or a follow-up phone call).

After the Meeting
- Write a follow-up letter. After your visit, write a letter thanking your legislator for his or her time.
- Stay in contact with your legislator. Remember: Your goal is to strengthen advanced practice nurse relationships with your legislators.

Modified from New York State Association of Licensed Midwives (NYSALM). *The Voice of Midwives* letter.

necessary skills. Initially, a volunteer can address or stuff envelopes for mailings. The volunteer can also invite friends and neighbors for a social gathering to meet the candidate, thereby providing an opportunity to discuss issues of concern with constituents. Telephone banks help a candidate identify supporters, opponents, and the critical undecided voters. This last group can make a difference on Election Day and is courted by all candidates. The telephone interviews are highly structured and easily handled by inexperienced campaign workers. Direct contact with potential voters may occur later in the form of house-to-house block walks or poll work on Election Day. The confidence that this process requires comes with experience and a strong commitment to the candidate and the cause. Hosting a social function to allow nurse colleagues to meet the candidate is a welcome contribution to the campaign. Nurses are substantial in number, and their voting record is humanistic; therefore they are valued as a political force. Government employees may be restricted by policies that limit or disallow political activism. Nurses employed at any level of government should be aware of such prohibitions.

Nurses and Voting Strength

With more than 2.8 million RNs in the United States, nurses comprise a large portion of the overall U.S. workforce and are the largest component of the healthcare workforce (American Association of Colleges of Nursing [AACN], 2021). Therefore, if every RN voted, their influence on health policy would be tremendous. If the nursing profession is to meet the challenges of the 21st century and work as a profession to positively influence the health of populations, political action is necessary, and an understanding of the factors that motivate or impede political action is needed (Winter & Lockhart, 1997).

Nurses in Public Office

President Donald Trump named **Sylvia Trent-Adams**, PhD, RN, on April 20, 2017, as acting surgeon general. Sylvia Trent-Adams is the first nurse to hold the position. The Office of the Surgeon General is within the Office of the Assistant Secretary for Health and is responsible for the Commissioned Corps. In addition, the surgeon general is an advisor on public health and scientific issues. The surgeon general also is a spokesperson for certain focused public health issues.

Other women who have been active in the federal government are Carolyn Davis, who in 2001 served as the administrator of the HCFA (renamed the CMS); Shirley Chater, commissioner of the SSA; and Patricia Montoya, commissioner for Children, Youth, and Families. Virginia Trotter Betts, who served as the president of the ANA, was also the senior advisor on nursing and policy to the secretary of HHS in Washington, DC.

Likewise, Dr. Beverly Malone resigned as president of the ANA in 1999 to assume the position of deputy assistant secretary of the HHS. In this capacity, she advised the assistant secretary for the HHS, Dr. David Satcher, in program and political matters, policy and program development, and setting of legislative priorities. Lastly, Janet Heinrich is associate administrator of the HRSA's Bureau of Health Professions, and

Michele Richardson is the senior advisor for national workforce diversity in the Bureau of Health Professions (NLN, 2010).

In the 114th Congress, the number of nurses serving was three. This is a major achievement for nursing. It provides a direct voice for nursing concerns and nursing expertise—related health care in general. The Congressional Nursing Caucus provides a nonpartisan forum for the discussion of issues that affect the nursing profession. It also allows members of Congress, nurses, and nonnurse members who care about these issues to come together to address them.

In the future, more nurses need to run for public office at all three levels of government. Whether serving as political appointees or career bureaucrats, nurses have much to offer. New nurses should accept the challenge of helping advance the nursing practice and the nation's health.

⍰ ACTIVE LEARNING EXERCISE

1. Serve as a volunteer in a campaign for a candidate who is supportive or potentially supportive of public health or nursing issues, or volunteer for a political party.
2. Invite an elected official who is sympathetic to nurses to speak to the local chapter of the National Student Nurses Association to discuss the political process and health policy.
3. Invite an elected official to spend a day engaging in appropriate activities with a public health nurse or nursing student. Take black-and-white photos for press use.

HEALTH CARE REFORM AND RESTRUCTURING OF THE HEALTH CARE INDUSTRY

Health care reform was a major topic of discussion during the 2016 presidential election. With the election of President Trump and significant Republican majorities in both the Senate and the House, it appears that healthcare reform will continue to be a headline. After the failed attempt at comprehensive reform during the early years of the Clinton presidency, politicians recognized some of the major concerns and issues and addressed them proactively. For example, strong opposition from many health care provider groups (e.g., physicians) and healthcare industry groups (e.g., insurers, pharmaceutical companies, hospitals) led to failure of the Clinton plan. In 2009, congressional leaders early on sought ways to attract leaders of these groups and persuade them to support reform measures, although passage of health care reform was not easy and there continues to be variable support for the initiatives in the legislation.

A great deal of debate on what should be included in reform was evident throughout 2009. Major items of contention included whether to require all Americans to purchase coverage (i.e., a health insurance mandate), whether there would be a "government option" whereby people could elect to be covered by an extension of Medicare (or another similar program sponsored and funded by the government), whether government funds would pay for abortions, and how all of the changes and mandates would eventually be financed. After much public and private debate, in March 2010, the House of Representatives rather reluctantly passed the bill that the Senate had approved in late 2009, and President Obama signed it into law on March 23, 2010.

Although the 2010 Patient Protection and Affordable Care Act remains extremely controversial, healthcare reform is a nursing issue, and few nurses will argue with the statement that reform is needed in the health system in the United States. In virtually every practice arena, nurses see the inequalities and inadequacies that diminish the nation's level of wellness. Recognition of these problems is important to discussions of reform, and changing policies and targeting popular beliefs that create barriers to reform are essential in correcting the inequalities and inadequacies.

These are some of the areas targeted by the Health Care Reform Act. For example, insurers will no longer be able to drop coverage for those who are seriously ill because the act prohibits health insurance plans from placing lifetime limits on coverage and prohibits insurers from rescinding coverage for those who are diagnosed with chronic or life-threatening conditions. Additionally, mechanisms to reduce administrative costs are encouraged (Kaiser Family Foundation, 2016).

Popular sentiments about governmental control over health care have mirrored attitudes concerning the government's role in general; this was very evident during the debates over reform. The politically viable range of cost-control measures available to public programs has been limited to cutbacks in payments to providers rather than limits on the demand for clinical services or limits on individual choice.

At the same time the United States is implementing healthcare reform, the country is also coping with the health problems of today's military veterans. When these soldiers are discharged, they continue to require care, often for complex physical and mental issues. According to the Kaiser Family Foundation (2016):

> Given the growing need for providing health care and related benefits to the nation's service members, policymakers will continue to focus on strengthening both the Department of Defense [DoD] Military Health System and the Department of Veterans Affairs (VA) health care system, which operate in parallel and in conjunction with each other. There is also greater emphasis in policy circles on ensuring a "seamless transition" process for service members moving from active duty into the VA health care system. Areas of focused attention include coordination between health and other benefits offered by the DoD and the VA, improving care for injured service members, and easing the transition from combat service to other military or civilian life.
>
> Nurses encounter veterans in all types of community and public health settings. Knowledge about these problems and health policies changes is important to providing effective care in the community.

On December 4, 2016, the Department of Veterans Affairs published a final ruling giving veterans direct access to care by nurse practitioners, certified nurse midwives, and clinical nurse specialists. Through this ruling these advanced practice RNs are able to have full practice authority when practicing at VA health care centers across the country.

RESEARCH HIGHLIGHTS

National Sample of Registered Nurses

The Division of Nursing, a component of the HRSA, helps direct policy through the National Sample Survey of Registered Nurses. Conducted 10 times since 1977, this survey was done most recently in March 2018. The national survey looks at trends in demographics, employment, education, and compensation among RNs. Here are some of the findings (HRSA et al., 2019):

- Number of licensed RNs in the United States grew by almost 29% between 2008 and 2018, to a new high of more than 3.9 million.
- Average age of RNs climbed to 47.9 years with 47.5% of all RNs aged 50 or older. 1980.
- Men in nursing rose from 7.1% in 2008 to 9.6% in 2018.
- The median earning for a full time RN was $73,929, while a part-time RN had a median income of $39,985.
- The share of RNs whose initial nursing education was a bachelor's degree in nursing rose from 33.7% to 39.2% between 2008 and 2018.
- Nearly two-thirds of RNs or 63.9% have a bachelor degree or higher with 44.6% with a bachelor's degree and 19.3% with a graduate degree.
- An estimated 11.5% of RNs completed training for advanced practice, which is an increase from 8.1% in 2008.

Data from Health Resources and Services Administration: *The RN population: initial findings from the 2008 National Sample Survey of RNs,* Washington, DC, 2010, Author.

NURSES AND LEADERSHIP IN HEALTH POLICY DEVELOPMENT

As the role of nurses in changing healthcare policy increases in importance, more nurses are needed who are equipped for this challenge. A strong cadre of nursing leaders who have the vision for change is essential to promoting nursing's policy agenda. National fellowships and internships are available for nurses who are interested in taking leadership roles.

The Robert Wood Johnson Health Policy Fellowship is a 1-year career development program for midcareer health professionals. The goal of this program is to help its fellows gain an understanding of the health policy process and contribute to the formulation of new policies and programs. Robert Wood Johnson Health Policy fellows are selected from academic faculties from diverse disciplines, including medicine, dentistry, nursing, public health, health services administration, economics, and social services. After an extensive orientation on the legislative and executive branches of government, the fellows work with a member of Congress or on a congressional health committee.

The President's Commission on White House Fellowships offers 20 fellowships each year to professionals, including nurses, early in their careers; the average age of participants is 33 years. The White House fellows participate in an education program that involves working with government officials, scholars, journalists, and private-sector leaders to explore U.S. policy in action. Nurses who have been White House fellows may work at the CMS and the Office of Science and Technology Policy, among others (White House, n.d.). These fellowship programs are competitive, but strong leaders are desperately needed.

Nursing should also incorporate private health policy into its policy agenda. Nurses can influence private health care organizations from internal and external positions. From an internal perspective, nurses hold important management positions in healthcare organizations. This placement allows them to have direct involvement in policy setting. Nurses also support and use nursing research that demonstrates positive clinical and economic outcomes. All of these activities serve to validate the importance of nursing within the health system (Pulcini et al., 2000).

External strategies that nurses can use to influence private health policy include participation in discussions regarding quality care and cost of care (Pulcini et al., 2000). Nurses should monitor the quality ratings of healthcare organizations and suggest changes that would improve care. Nurses also are developing entrepreneurial practices to provide lower-cost services for underserved groups. Nurses need to do more to request that nursing services be reimbursable under all types of health care coverage plans and programs. Interprofessional care is a key topic today, and nurses need to work with other healthcare providers to build teams that can influence private policy.

? ACTIVE LEARNING EXERCISE

Look at a current public health issue that affects your community, including an understanding of the causes, effect on the public, and possible solutions. Influence its resolution through any of the following activities:
1. Write a succinct letter to the editor of a local newspaper.
2. Write a position paper and submit it to the "opinion page" of a local newspaper.
3. Write to elected or appointed officials whose jurisdiction may be influential on the issue.
4. Meet with an elected or appointed official to discuss the issue in groups of two or three. Write a one-page summary of your "talking points" to leave with the official.
5. Call in to a radio talk show about the issue.
6. Volunteer to speak on the issue to appropriate consumer or professional groups.

SUMMARY

Historically, nurses have been able to make significant differences in the quality of life experienced by the members of the communities in which they serve. By understanding how government works, how bills become laws, and how legislators make decisions, nurses can influence policy decisions through individual efforts such as electronic letter writing, social networking, participation in political campaigns, and selection of candidates who support policies conducive to improving the health and welfare of all citizens. When organized in lobbying groups, coalitions, and PACs, or when holding office, nurses can be a powerful force that brings about change in the delivery and quality of the health care of aggregates.

EVOLVE WEBSITE

http://evolve.elsevier.com/Nies/community
- NCLEX Review Questions
- Case Studies

BIBLIOGRAPHY

Almgren G: *Health care, politics, policy and services*, ed 3, New York, 2017, Springer.
American Association of Colleges of Nursing: *Nursing fact sheet*, 2021. Available from: www.aacnnursing.org/News-Information/Fact-Sheets/Nursing-Fact-Sheet#:~:text=Nursing%20is%20the%20nation%27s%20largest%20healthcare%20profession%2C%20with,will%20be%20created%20each%20year%20from%202016-2026.%202.
American Nurses Association: ANA advises on health care reform, *Capital Update* 11(8):1, 1993.
American Nurses Association, 2017. http://nursingworld.org/MainMenuCategories/Policy-Advocacy. www.nursingworld.org/Function/menucategory/aboutANA.aspx.
Assistant Secretary for Planning and Evaluation: *Trends in the U.S. uninsured population, 2010–2020*, 2021. Available from: https://aspe.hhs.gov/system/files/pdf/265041/trends-in-the-us-uninsured.pdf.
Association of Public Health Nurses: *Public health policy advocacy guide book and tool kit*, 2016. Available from: https://www.phnurse.org/assets/docs/APHN%20Public%20Health%20Policy%20Advocacy%20Guide%20Book%20and%20Tool%20Kit%202016.pdf.
Centers for Disease Control and Prevention: *Ten essential services for public health*, 2015. Available from: https://www.cdc.gov/stltpublichealth/hop/pdfs/Ten_Essential_Public_Health_Services_2011-09_508.pdf.
Centers for Disease Control and Prevention: *Health insurance coverage*, 2021. Available from, https://www.cdc.gov/nchs/fastats/health-insurance.htm.
Centers for Medicare and Medicaid Services: *Health Plans: General information*, 2021. Available from, https://www.cms.gov/Medicare/Health-Plans/HealthPlansGenInfo.
Centers for Medicare and Medicaid Services: *Home health PPS*, 2021. Available from: http://www.cms.gov/Medicare/Medicare-Fee-for-Service-Payment/HomeHealthPPS/index.html?redirect=/homehealthpps/.
Chang C, Gnuschke J: *How the Trump administration has reshaped and restructured the affordable care act*, 2019. Available from: https://www.commercialappeal.com/story/opinion/2019/10/31/analyzing-changes-made-obamacare-since-trump-administration/2494976001/.
Congress.gov: *CARES act*, 2020. Available from: https://www.congress.gov/bill/116th-congress/senate-bill/3548.
Davidson A: *Clara Barton: Nurse, activist, and founder of the American Red Cross, NurseJournal*, 2021. Available from, https://nursejournal.org/articles/clara-barton-founder-of-the-american-red-cross/.

DeParle J: *States struggle to use windfall born of shifts in welfare law*, 1999, New York Times.

Hall-Long BA: Nursing's past, present, and future political experiences, *Nurs Health Care Perspect* 16(1):24—28, 1995.

Henry J: *Kaiser family foundation: military and veterans' health care.* http://www.kaiseredu.org/Issue-Modules/Military-and-Veterans-Health-Care/Background-Brief.aspx.

Health Resources and Services Administration, U.S. Department of Health and Human Services, Bureau of Health Workforce: *2018 national sample survey of registered nurses: brief summary of results*, 2019. Available from: https://bhw.hrsa.gov/sites/default/files/bureau-health-workforce/data-research/nssrn-summary-report.pdf.

Institute of Medicine: *Future of public health*, Washington, DC, 1988, The National Academies Press.

Kaiser Family Foundation, 2016. Available from: http://kff.org/.

Kalisch PA, Kalisch BJ: *American nursing: a history*, ed 4, Philadelphia, 2004, Lippincott Williams & Wilkins.

Knight W: *Managed care: what it is and how it works*, Gaithersburg, MD, 1998, Aspen Publishers, Inc.

Kostas-Polston E, Thanavaro J, Arvidson CR, Taub LFM: Advanced practice nursing: shaping health through policy, *J Am Assoc Nurse Pract* 27(1):11—20, 2015.

Lewinson SB: A historical perspective on policy, politics and nursing. In Mason DJ, Leavitt JK, Chaffee MW, editors: *Policy and politics in nursing and health care*, ed 7, Philadelphia, 2007, Saunders.

Litman T: *Health, politics and policy*, ed 5, Albany, NY, Delmar.

Lyttle B: Humanizing childbirth, *Am J Nurs* 100(10):52—53, 2000.

Mason DJ, Leavitt JK, Chaffee MW: Policy and politics: a framework for action. In *Policy and politics in nursing and health care*, St. Louis, 2007, Saunders.

McDonald L. The real goods and the oversell, 2020. https://doi.org/10.1111/1740-9713.01374. Retrieved from https://rss.onlinelibrary.wiley.com/doi/10.1111/1740-9713.01374.

Merriam-Webster: *Merriam-Webster dictionary*, 2014. Available from: http://www.merriam-webster.com/dictionary/policy.

National League for Nursing, 2010. http://www.nln.org/newsletter/aug092010.htm.

Nurses for a healthier tomorrow: mission/purpose, 2021. https://www.nursesource.org/mission.html.

NurseJournal: 10 most influential nurses in history, *NurseJournal*, 2022. Available from https://nursejournal.org/articles/influential-nurses-in-history/.

Office of the Assistant Secretary for Health: *Healthy people: an end of decade snapshot*, 2020. Available from: https://health.gov/sites/default/files/2020-12/HP2020EndofDecadeSnapshot.pdf.

Office of Disease Prevention and Health Promotion: *Healthy People 2030: Building a healthier future for all*, 2021a. Available from, https://health.gov/healthypeople.

Office of Disease Prevention and Health Promotion: *Healthy People 2030: Framework*, 2021b. Available from, https://health.gov/healthypeople/about/healthy-people-2030-framework.

Office of Disease Prevention and Health Promotion: *Health care access and quality*, 2021c. Available from, https://health.gov/healthypeople/objectives-and-data/browse-objectives/health-care-access-and-quality.

Office of Disease Prevention and Health Promotion: *Overall health and well-being measures*, 2021d. Available from, https://health.gov/healthypeople/objectives-and-data/overall-health-and-well-being-measures.

Pickett G, Hanlon JJ: *Public health administration and practice*, ed 9, St. Louis, 1990, Mosby.

Pulcini J, Mason DJ, Cohen SS, et al.: Health policy and the private sector: new vistas for nursing, *Nurs Health Care Perspect* 21(1):22—28, 2000.

Robert Wood Johnson Foundation: *Enduring trust: nurses again top gallup's poll on honesty and ethics*, 2012. Available from: http://www.rwjf.org/en/blogs/human-capital-blog/2012/12/enduring_trust_nurs.html.

Rychnovsky J: Dr. Ruth Lubic, a timeliness and tireless visionary for childbearing families, *J Obstet Gynecol Neonatal Nurs* 40(5):509—511, 2011.

Taylor M: Impact of advocacy initiatives on nurses' motivation to sustain momentum in public policy advocacy, *J Prof Nurs* 32(3):235—245, 2016.

Thomas J: Introduction, *Libr Trends* 46(2), 1997.

Turale S: The contribution of nurses to health policy and advocacy requires leaders to provide training and mentorship, *Nurs Health Pol Perspect* 66(3):204—302, 2019. Available from: https://doi.org/10.1111/inr.12550.

U.S. Department of Health and Human Services: *Healthy people*, Conference ed. Washington, DC, 2010, USDHHS.

U.S. Department of Health and Human Services: Office of Disease Prevention and Health Promotion: *Healthy people 2020*, 2013. http://www.healthypeople.gov/2020/about/history.aspx. (Accessed January 22, 2014).

U.S. Department of Health and Human Services: Centers for Medicare and Medicaid Services, 2017 U.S. Department of Health and Human Services: Centers for Medicare and Medicaid services: FY 2017 budget in brief, 2017. Available from: https://www.hhs.gov/about/budget/fy2017/budget-in-brief/index.html.

U.S. Department of Health and Human Services, Health Resources and Services Administration. (Accessed May 1, 2017).

U.S. Department of Health and Human Services: Secretary's Advisory Committee on National Health Promotion and Disease Prevention for 2020: *Healthy people, phase I report*, 2020. Available from: https://www.healthypeople.gov/sites/default/files/PhaseI_0.pdf.

Voda S: Remembering visionaries in nursing practice, *Nursing* 42(8):1—3, 2012. https://doi.org/10.1097/01.NURSE.0000414875.67606.a1.

White House: White House Fellows. Available from: https://www.whitehouse.gov/participate/fellows.

Winter MK, Lockhart JS: From motivation to action: understanding nurses' political involvement, *Nurs Health Care Perspect* 18(5):244—250, 1997.

11

The Healthcare System

Melanie McEwen

OBJECTIVES

Upon completion of this chapter, the reader will be able to do the following:

1. Describe the organization of the public healthcare subsystem at the federal, state, and local levels.
2. Compare and contrast the scopes of the private healthcare subsystem and the public healthcare subsystem.
3. Describe the roles of the members of the interprofessional healthcare team.
4. Discuss the relationship of critical healthcare issues to the healthcare organization and healthcare providers.
5. Discuss future concerns for the healthcare delivery system.

OUTLINE

KEY TERMS

accreditation
Agency for Healthcare Research and Quality (AHRQ)
client rights
community health center
complementary and alternative therapies
electronic health record/electronic medical record
health disparities

Health Plan Effectiveness Stat Information Set (HEDIS)
managed care
managed care organizations
Medicaid
Medicare
National Committee for Quality Assurance (NCQA)
outcomes measures
patient-centered medical homes

Patient Protection and Affordable Care Act (ACA)
patient rights
public health
quality care
telehealth
The Joint Commission
voluntary agencies

OVERVIEW: THE HEALTHCARE SYSTEM

The healthcare system of the United States is dynamic, multifaceted, and not comparable with any other healthcare system in the world. It is regularly praised for its technological breakthroughs, is frequently criticized for its high costs, continues to experience major problems with its quality, and often is difficult to access for those most in need. This chapter describes the major components of the healthcare system, critical healthcare organization and provider issues, and the role of government in public health and healthcare reform and presents a futuristic perspective.

COMPONENTS OF THE HEALTHCARE SYSTEM

The current healthcare system consists of private and public healthcare subsystems (Fig. 11.1). The private healthcare subsystem includes personal care services from various sources, both nonprofit and profit, and numerous voluntary agencies. The major focus of the public health subsystem is prevention of disease and illness. These subsystems are not always mutually exclusive, and their functions sometimes overlap.

With the rapid growth of technology and increased demands on the private and public healthcare subsystems, healthcare costs have become prohibitive. Cost-effectiveness and cost

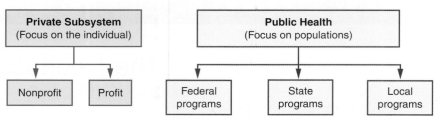

Fig. 11.1 US Healthcare system.

containment have become critical driving forces as healthcare delivery system changes are made; however, cost-effectiveness often conflicts with the provision of quality care. Additionally, considerable attention to "healthcare reform" and subsequent passage of the **Patient Protection and Affordable Care Act (ACA)** in 2010 demonstrated the critical importance of access to healthcare for all Americans, but the enormous challenges that accompany that desire remain. More than a decade following implementation of the ACA, there continues to be a need to apply the resources and tools available and to focus science and information technology in a way that will improve effectiveness and efficiency and produce high-quality, patient-centered healthcare.

Public health nursing requires an understanding of the mission, organization, and role of both the private and the public healthcare subsystems and the contexts within which they function to effectively collaborate with healthcare providers and organizations to reach health goals. An organizational framework in which private and voluntary organizations and the government work collaboratively to prevent disease and promote health is essential. Public health nurses are in a unique position to provide leadership and facilitate change in the healthcare system that will help improve health and safety for all.

Private Healthcare Subsystem

Most personal healthcare services are provided in the private sector. Services in the private subsystem include health promotion, prevention and early detection of disease, diagnosis and treatment of disease with a focus on cure, rehabilitative–restorative care, and custodial care. These services are provided in clinics, physicians' offices, hospitals, hospital ambulatory centers, skilled care facilities, and homes. Increasingly, these private sector services are available through **managed care organizations** (MCOs).

Private healthcare services in the United States began with a simple model. Physicians provided care in their offices and made home visits. Patients were admitted to hospitals for general care if they experienced serious complications during the course of their illness. Currently, a variety of highly skilled healthcare professionals provide comprehensive, preventive, restorative, rehabilitative, and palliative care. Interprofessional teams have become more important. A broad array of services are available, ranging from general to highly specialized, with multiple delivery configurations.

Personal care provided by physicians and other healthcare professionals is delivered under the following five basic models:

1. The solo practice of a physician in an office continues to be present in many communities.
2. The single-specialty group model consists of physicians in the same specialty who pool expenses, income, and offices.
3. Multispecialty group practice provides for interaction among specialty areas.
4. The integrated health maintenance model has prepaid multispecialty physicians.
5. The **community health center**, frequently developed through federal funds, addresses broader inputs into health such as education and housing.

Managed care has become a dominant paradigm in healthcare, affecting many aspects of healthcare delivery. Managed care involves capitated payments for care rather than fee-for-service. Healthcare providers, including physicians, hospitals, community clinics, and home care providers, are integrated in a system such as a health maintenance organization. See Chapter 12 for a more detailed discussion of managed care and reimbursement.

Though change in the configuration of the healthcare system is common, some of the newer changes relate more to the community than in the past. For example, more physician practices are joining together to form multispecialty groups, and hospitals are buying practices to expand their market into the community. The solo practice is fading. In addition, there are more advanced nurse practitioners (ANPs) and physician's assistants (PAs) who are assuming primary practice roles in a variety of settings, including community clinics, retail health clinics, and home health, and many who are opening their own practices. **Patient-centered medical homes** are practices that offer a team approach to assist in coordination of care for positive outcomes, providing comprehensive primary care. This model, which is connected to healthcare reform, is relatively new, and thus, its long-term success is unknown. As healthcare reform legislation continues to be debated and modified, additional changes will likely occur.

Voluntary Agencies

Voluntary or nonofficial agencies refer to the nongovernmental, nonprofit entities that support healthcare provision and sometimes direct health services. **Voluntary agencies** are a part of the private healthcare system that developed in the United States at about the same time that the government was assuming responsibility for public health. During the 1700s and early 1800s, voluntary efforts to improve health were virtually nonexistent, because early settlers from Western Europe were not accustomed to participating in organized charity. Immigration expanded to include slaves from Africa and people from Eastern Europe, and their well-being received little attention.

Toward the end of the 19th century, new immigrants brought a heritage of social protest and reform. Wealthy businesspeople, such as the Rockefellers, Carnegies, and Mellons, responded to the needs of the poor and set up foundations that provided funds for charitable endeavors, including health. District nurses, such as Lillian Wald, established nursing practices in the large cities for the poor and destitute. These services were not exclusively focused on illness, but also on work conditions, health, communicable diseases, living conditions, and language skills. Voluntary initiatives from philanthropically focused families remain an important resource even into the 21st century. An example is the Gates Foundation, which is very active in healthcare concerns, particularly from a global perspective.

Voluntary agencies can be classified into those dealing with the following categories of health (Hanlon & Pickett, 1979):

a. Specific diseases, such as the American Diabetes Association, American Cancer Society, and National Multiple Sclerosis Society
b. Organ or body structures, such as the National Kidney Foundation and the American Heart Association
c. Health and welfare of special groups, such as the National Council on Aging and the March of Dimes
d. Particular phases of health, such as the Planned Parenthood Federation of America

Philanthropic groups also support research and programs. Many professional organizations, such as the American Medical Association, the American Nurses Association, the American Hospital Association, and the American Public Health Association, as well as many other professional organizations, have a significant role in advocacy and in providing professional expertise.

Voluntary organizations are major sources of help in the prevention of disease, promotion of health, treatment of illness, advocacy, consumer education, and research. For example, private and voluntary organizations currently support clients with human immunodeficiency virus (HIV). In many cities, the Chicken Soup Brigade provides meals for clients with HIV who are unable to cook for themselves, and HIV support groups exist in most larger communities. Services for the homeless such as meals, temporary housing and housing during the winter, medical care, and job support are common in most large cities. Overlap of services often occurs among the numerous private, voluntary, and public agencies. The private and public agencies provide a wide array of services, but sometimes duplication causes them to not be cost-effective.

Voluntary agencies and organizations play a very important role in healthcare delivery. Indeed, it is anticipated that the emerging healthcare system will become an amalgam of different public and private forces that will work together to provide integrated, resource-conscious, population-based services. Furthermore, the system needs to become more innovative and diverse in how it responds to health problems and more concerned with disease prevention and promotion of health to address the very significant disparities in healthcare (AHRQ, 2020).

? ACTIVE LEARNING

Identify a voluntary agency or organization and review its website. What services does it offer? How does the agency collaborate with other groups and organizations? How is the agency/organization funded? How does it interface with the local public health agency? What information is available to consumers and professionals? With classmates, set up a site visit.

Public Health Subsystem

Although not explicitly addressing health or healthcare, the US Constitution mandates that the federal government "promote the general welfare of its citizens." The public health subsystem therefore is required by law to address the health of populations by promoting their "general welfare." Legal provisions at the local, state, and federal levels of government direct the establishment, implementation, and evaluation of these activities. At the federal level, Congress enacts laws and writes rules and regulations. The various departments of the executive branch implement and administer them. Interpretations of, and amendments to, the Constitution, as well as Supreme Court decisions over time, have changed and enlarged the role of the federal government in health activities.

Federal policies and practices have had a significant influence on local and state governments in meeting health and social problems, and many laws have been enacted to respond to changing health needs and concerns. Coordination of federal services under several agencies culminated in the establishment of the Department of Health, Education, and Welfare under President Eisenhower in 1953. In 1979, this department was separated into the Department of Education and the Department of Health and Human Services (HHS). Currently, HHS is the second largest department of the federal government; only the Department of Defense is larger.

Public health refers to the efforts organized by society to protect, promote, and restore the people's health. Public health programs, services, and institutions emphasize the prevention of disease and address the health needs of the population as a whole. Public health activities typically respond to changing technology and social values, but the goals remain the same (i.e., to reduce the amount of disease, premature death, and disease-produced discomfort and disability).

The public health subsystem is concerned with the health of the population and a healthy environment. The scope of public health is broad and encompasses activities that promote good health. The public health subsystem is organized into multiple levels (i.e., federal, state, and local) to establish laws, rules, and regulations to protect the public and to more effectively provide services to those who are unable to obtain healthcare without assistance. Fig. 11.2 provides an overview of this system, specifically for the state of Ohio, although the basic organization will be similar across states.

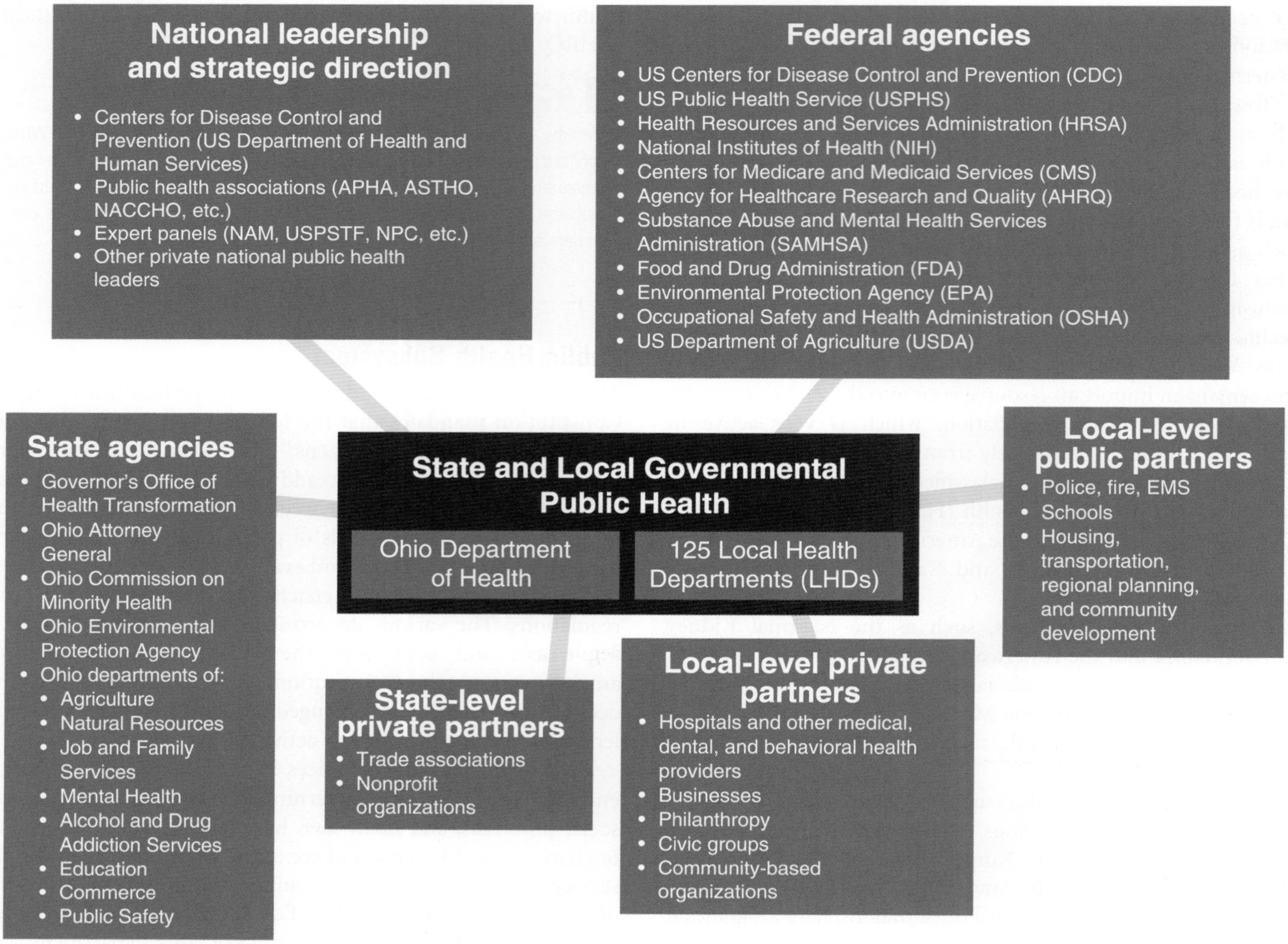

National leadership and strategic direction

- Centers for Disease Control and Prevention (US Department of Health and Human Services)
- Public health associations (APHA, ASTHO, NACCHO, etc.)
- Expert panels (NAM, USPSTF, NPC, etc.)
- Other private national public health leaders

Federal agencies

- US Centers for Disease Control and Prevention (CDC)
- US Public Health Service (USPHS)
- Health Resources and Services Administration (HRSA)
- National Institutes of Health (NIH)
- Centers for Medicare and Medicaid Services (CMS)
- Agency for Healthcare Research and Quality (AHRQ)
- Substance Abuse and Mental Health Services Administration (SAMHSA)
- Food and Drug Administration (FDA)
- Environmental Protection Agency (EPA)
- Occupational Safety and Health Administration (OSHA)
- US Department of Agriculture (USDA)

State agencies

- Governor's Office of Health Transformation
- Ohio Attorney General
- Ohio Commission on Minority Health
- Ohio Environmental Protection Agency
- Ohio departments of:
  - Agriculture
  - Natural Resources
  - Job and Family Services
  - Mental Health
  - Alcohol and Drug Addiction Services
  - Education
  - Commerce
  - Public Safety

State and Local Governmental Public Health

| Ohio Department of Health | 125 Local Health Departments (LHDs) |

Local-level public partners

- Police, fire, EMS
- Schools
- Housing, transportation, regional planning, and community development

State-level private partners

- Trade associations
- Nonprofit organizations

Local-level private partners

- Hospitals and other medical, dental, and behavioral health providers
- Businesses
- Philanthropy
- Civic groups
- Community-based organizations

Fig. 11.2 The public health system in Ohio. *NAM,* National Academy of Medicine. (From Health Policy Institute of Ohio: *Ohio public health basics,* 2012, p. 4. Available from: http://www.healthpolicyohio.org/wp-content/uploads/2014/01/publichealthbasics_final012520131.pdf.)

Federal-Level Subsystem

Most health-related activities at the federal level are implemented and administered by the HHS, which consists of 11 major agencies (Box 11.1). This department is divided into 10 regions and is directed by the secretary of Health and Human Services. The secretary is assisted by numerous undersecretaries and assistant secretaries (USDHHS, 2021a). The surgeon general is the principal deputy to the assistant secretary of HHS, and nurses have fulfilled that role. Indeed, Rear Admiral Susan Orsega (MSN/FNP) serves as "acting" surgeon general in 2021 (USDHHS, 2021b).

In addition to HHS, many federal agencies perform activities related to health. For example, the Department of Education is involved with health education and school health. The Department of Agriculture administers the inspection of meat and milk and provides funds for the Women, Infants, and Children program (WIC) (supplemental nutrition), the food stamp program, and the school-based nutrition program.

Other federal agencies of interest to public health nurses are the US Environmental Protection Agency, the Occupational Safety and Health Administration, the Veterans Administration, and the Federal Emergency Management Agency.

The scope of health services of the federal-level subsystem targets the following major health areas: the general population, special populations, and international health. For the general population, federal activities include protection against hazards, maintenance of vital and health statistics, advancement of scientific knowledge through research, and provision of disaster relief. In recent years, public health efforts have been directed toward changing behaviors by fostering healthy eating habits, encouraging exercise, and preventing or reducing tobacco, drug, and alcohol use. Other programs have provided nutritional food and food stamps to individuals and families to ensure adequate food intake.

Services for special populations include protection of workers against hazardous occupations and work conditions and healthcare for military veterans, Native Americans, Alaska

BOX 11.1 Structure of the US Department of Health and Human Services

The US Department of Health and Human Services (USDHHS) is composed of many agencies that provide different services related to US healthcare. Among them are the following:

- The **Administration for Community Living** combines the Administration on Aging—the agency responsible for coordinating home- and community-based services for older persons and their caregivers—and the Office on Disability and the Administration on Developmental Disabilities in a single agency, with enhanced policy and program support for cross-cutting initiatives to serve these populations.
- The **Centers for Medicare and Medicaid Services** administers Medicare and Medicaid programs.
- The **Administration for Children and Families** provides family assistance (welfare), child support, Head Start, and other programs to strengthen the family unit.
- The **Centers for Disease Control and Prevention (CDC)** conducts and supports programs directed at preventing and controlling infectious diseases; they assist states during epidemics. In addition, they provide services related to health promotion and education and professional development and training. The CDC includes the **Agency for Toxic Substances and Disease Registry**, which serves the public by using the best science, taking responsive public health actions, and providing trusted health information to prevent harmful exposures and diseases related to toxic substances.
- The **Food and Drug Administration** provides surveillance over the safety and efficacy of foods, pharmaceuticals, and other consumer goods.
- The **Healthcare Resources and Services Administration** is concerned with the development of health services programs and facilities. The Division of Nursing is in this unit. A major focus of this agency is funding grants for nursing education and training.
- The **Indian Health Service** provides health services for Native Americans and Alaska Natives.
- The **National Institutes of Health (NIH)** performs and supports research programs. The focus of these efforts is to develop and extend the scientific knowledge base related to their respective areas. The National Institute for Nursing Research, which is part of NIH, focuses on nursing research.
- The **Substance Abuse and Mental Health Services Administration** awards grants and funds research related to problems with substance abuse and mental health.
- The **Agency for Healthcare Quality and Research** works to improve quality, safety, efficiency, and effectiveness of healthcare services for all Americans.

- Protect the health of Americans where they live, learn, work, and play.
- Strengthen the economic and social well-being of Americans across the life span.
- Foster sound, sustained advances in the sciences.
- Promote effective and efficient management and stewardship.

The HHS has been deeply involved in implementation and updating the many facets of the ACA. This has included oversight of the state exchanges, awarding funding to meet the law's requirements; measuring program performance to ensure program integrity; and informing the public of requirements, mandates, and results. Ongoing changes to the ACA will continue to require supervision of the HHS.

State-Level Subsystem

States are responsible for the health of their citizens and are the central authorities in the public healthcare system. The organization and activities of public health services vary widely among the states. A health commissioner or secretary of health is typically appointed by the governor and directs most state health agencies. The health officer is usually a physician with a degree and experience in public health. In some states, the health officer directs the state's health department. Many states have boards of health, which determine policies and priorities for allocation of funds. Staffing of the state agency varies among states; however, in comparison with other state programs, state health programs usually have a large staff.

The state health department does not exist in a vacuum. The United States requires an integrated system so that both federal and state levels work to the benefit of all citizens. Thus, the state health departments are highly dependent on the federal level for resources and guidance. For example, funds contributed by the federal government to **Medicaid**, which is jointly funded by the federal government and states, have been changed over time and vary with respect to beneficiaries and services covered by each state. This has had a major impact on services that states can provide to their most vulnerable citizens.

One of the major provisions of the ACA resulting in large numbers of Americans receiving healthcare coverage was through the expansion of Medicaid; however, each state was allowed to determine whether they would accept this expansion. Ultimately, 39 states and the District of Columbia elected to extend Medicaid coverage through the ACA, 12 chose not to (KFF, 2021a). Pending additional legislative changes involving the ACA, it is possible that more states will chose to expand Medicaid to other beneficiaries with federal assistance.

Cooperation between the state and federal levels of the healthcare system has also been brought to the forefront with efforts to plan for bioterrorism and disasters. According to the scope of health services, the state-level subsystem is responsible for its own public health laws; therefore, state policy varies widely. Factors that affect the level of state services include state-legislated or mandated services; political factors related to division of power between state and local health departments

Natives, federal prisoners, and members of the armed services. In addition, the federal government provides special services for children, older adults, the mentally ill, and the vocationally handicapped.

In the international arena, the federal government works with other countries and international health organizations such as the World Health Organization and the Red Cross. These entities combine efforts to monitor health and diseases and to promote various health programs throughout the world.

The current HHS maintains a strategic plan (USDHHS, 2021c). The goals for 2018–22 are as follows:
- Reform, strengthen, and modernize the Nation's healthcare system.

(LHDs); and competition among officials, providers, and the business community.

As discussed in previous chapters, the three core functions of public health are assessment, policy development, and assurance (IOM, 1988). Assessment activities include the collection of data pertaining to vital statistics, health facilities, and human resources; epidemiological activities, such as communicable disease control, health screening, and laboratory analyses; and participation in research projects. In the area of policy development, states formulate goals, develop health plans, and set standards for local health agencies. Assurance activities involve inspection in a variety of areas, licensing of health professionals and organizations, health education, environmental safety, and resource development.

Local Health Department Subsystems

LHDs are generally responsible for the direct delivery of public health services and protection of the health of citizens, although not all communities/counties have LHDs. State and local (i.e., city and county) governments delegate the authority to conduct these activities. The organization of LHDs varies widely depending on community size, economics, partnerships with the private healthcare system, healthcare facilities, business support, healthcare needs, transportation, and the number of citizens requiring public healthcare. Some LHDs function as district offices of the state health department; others are responsible to local government and the state; and still others—particularly those in large cities—are autonomous. An LHD may be a separate agency or a division within an agency, such as the HHS.

A health officer or administrator appointed by local government directs the LHD. At least half of the states require that the health officer of an LHD have a medical degree. An interdisciplinary team carries out the activities of the department. Public health nurses and health inspectors represent the two largest groups of professional staff members. Other professional staff members include dentists, social workers, epidemiologists, nutritionists, and health educators.

According to the designated scope of services, the LHD subsystem is responsible for monitoring the health status and meeting the health needs of their constituents. This includes identifying unmet needs and taking actions to meet these needs. Most services to groups and individuals are provided at the local level. These services fall into the following four major categories:

Community health services include control of communicable disease such as surveillance and immunizations, maternal–child health programs, nutrition services, and education. Health promotion education is directed toward changing behavior; individuals are encouraged to eat healthy foods; exercise more; and decrease their use of tobacco, drugs, and alcohol. Other programs provide nutritious food and food stamps to individuals and families. A major activity of LHDs is to perform preventive screening for potential problems throughout the life span of their community members.

Environmental health services include food hygiene such as inspection of food-producing and food-processing plants and restaurants; protection from hazardous substances; control of waste, air, noise, and water pollution; and occupational health. The objective of these activities is to provide a safe environment.

Personal health services provide care to individuals and families in clinics, schools, and correctional institutions. In many areas, home healthcare services are provided through the LHD.

Mental health services are provided through LHDs in many communities. These services are supported by funds offered by local and regional mental health and mental retardation facilities and programs. See Chapter 24 for more information on community-based mental healthcare.

LHDs establish local health codes, fund public hospitals such as city and/or county hospitals, and provide services to populations and individuals at risk who often lack health insurance. Programs and services for state health departments and LHDs vary among jurisdictions. The services provided reflect the values of the residents and officials, available resources, and perceived needs of their respective populations within their state and local area. Although the goals of the public health subsystem do not change, the programs and services evolve to meet the changing needs of the public.

Several provisions of the ACA addressed improvement of quality and access to care. For example, the law promoted establishment of local consortiums of healthcare providers to coordinate healthcare services for low-income uninsured and underinsured populations. It also substantially increased funds for community health centers and financed development of school-based health centers and nurse-managed health clinics.

Summary of Public Health's Three Levels

In the preceding description of the three government levels that provide public health services (i.e., local, state, and federal), distinctive and overlapping roles have been discussed. The federal government has been assuming a larger role in the protection of the population through regulation and funding. It finances specific programs such as **Medicare** and categorical programs for mothers and infants and provides direct care to special populations, for example, military veterans. States establish health codes, regulate the insurance industry, and license healthcare facilities and personnel. States also provide funds for services offered through Medicaid. Direct care activities funded by state health departments may include care in mental hospitals, state medical schools, and associated hospitals. LHDs are the primary agencies that provide direct services to communities, families, and individuals.

> ### ? ACTIVE LEARNING
>
> 1. Describe the organization of the state and local health departments.
> 2. Visit the local health department and learn what services are provided. How do these services relate to *Healthy People 2030* objectives?
> 3. Identify regional and state health services and providers.

Healthcare Providers

Providers of healthcare are individuals, groups, and organizations that deliver or support healthcare services. This section describes the different types of healthcare providers, including provider organizations, healthcare professionals, and nontraditional providers.

Provider Organizations

The following are examples of healthcare provider organizations:

- Hospital
- Clinic
- Physician practice
- Ambulatory care center
- Home health agency
- Long-term care facility
- Skilled nursing facility
- Rehabilitation center
- Hospice service
- Public health department
- School health clinic
- Birthing center
- Ambulatory surgical center
- Occupational health clinic
- Crisis clinic
- Community health center
- Retail health clinics located in retail stores, supermarkets, and pharmacies
- Any other type of organization that provides healthcare within the community

Healthcare provider organizations are undergoing tremendous changes. This is particularly true of hospitals, many of which are merging, consolidating, and closing. These changes have an impact on the entire community health system. With the increasing shift to ambulatory and primary care (Box 11.2), hospital stays have shortened, and the patients who are admitted to the hospital are more acutely ill and require more intensive care. Consequently, reduced hospital stays result in more home care admissions or more discharges to long-term care facilities or skilled nursing units for short-term recovery and rehabilitation.

ETHICAL INSIGHTS

Universal Healthcare

Universal healthcare coverage has been a topic of interest in the United States at least since the 1960s. The United States is the only developed country that does not have some form of universal health insurance. Although the ACA significantly reduced the number of uninsured individuals, there were almost 29 million people without healthcare coverage by the end of 2019 (Kaiser Family Foundation, 2021b). Thus, universal health coverage remains elusive. Clients without health coverage have a direct impact on communities, and healthcare providers should consider the following questions: Is healthcare a right of all citizens? Who is responsible for determining the right to healthcare access? What additional reforms will be necessary to resolve these questions? These are difficult questions, particularly in light of the growing problem of healthcare disparities in the United States.

BOX 11.2 Primary Care and Primary Prevention

"*Primary health care* is essential health care based on practical, scientifically sound, and socially acceptable methods and technology made universally accessible to individuals and families in the community through their full participation and at a cost that the community and country can afford to maintain at every stage of their development in the spirit of self-reliance and self-determination... It is the first level of contact of individuals, the family, and the community with the national health system bringing health care as close as possible to where people live and work." (World Health Organization, 1978).

A physician, nurse practitioner, or physician's assistant may provide primary healthcare. Generally, the primary care provider's practice is in family medicine, internal medicine, or pediatrics. The primary care provider is responsible for health maintenance and for treatment of common illnesses and may refer clients to specialists as needed.

Primary prevention is a type of intervention that promotes health and prevents disease. Primary prevention includes immunizations and contraception, as well as promotion of good nutrition, exercise, and healthy lifestyle choices (e.g., avoidance of tobacco, limitation of alcohol).

How do these definitions compare? The WHO definition and the definition of primary care that is usually used in the United States are similar. Primary prevention is an intervention that is used in primary care services.

Healthcare Professionals

The healthcare team has been growing and evolving significantly over the past decade, with members of the team taking on new responsibilities. There is greater emphasis today in all types of healthcare settings on using interprofessional teams to better coordinate care and to promote effective outcomes. The community particularly needs an interprofessional approach, because clients often have complex needs. Interprofessional teams have been recommended by the National Academy of Medicine (NAM), formerly called the Institute of Medicine (IOM) (2015a) and others. Indeed, working on interprofessional teams has been identified as a core competency for healthcare professions.

The following is a brief review of the major types of professional and nonprofessional members of the healthcare team:

- *Registered nurse (RN):* This appears to be a simple designation, but different educational routes (i.e., diploma, associate degree, baccalaureate degree) exist to obtain a license to practice as an RN. In addition, many nurses now obtain master's degrees and doctorates. These advanced degrees provide nurses with the opportunity to do more independent practice, teach, and conduct research. Nurses represent the largest group of professionals providing health services, and they practice in all types of health settings. State legislatures determine licensure requirements and enact nurse practice acts. State boards of nursing are the administrative arm for implementation of these laws and regulations.
- *Advanced nurse practitioner (ANP):* This is a nurse who has obtained education beyond a baccalaureate degree and has

studied content related to primary care or acute care. ANPs specialize in such areas as adult health, pediatrics, neonatology, gerontology, and psychiatric nursing. An ANP may work in a clinic, the community, a private practice, the home, a hospital, or a long-term care facility (i.e., any setting in which healthcare is provided). With healthcare reform raising the demand for primary care, it is expected that ANPs will provide more and more primary care.

- *Clinical nurse leader (CNL):* CNL is a new position that requires a master's degree. The CNL is a provider and manager of care at the point of care for individuals and cohorts, and does not have a clinical specialty in the master's program. The types of positions that CNLs are taking are variable, though many are in acute care settings.
- *Clinical nurse specialist (CNS):* The CNS, who has a master's degree in a specialty area, provides acute care and guides other nursing staff in providing care. There are many fewer CNSs in clinical practice today, as the ANP role has become more common.
- *Nurse-midwife (NM):* An NM is a nurse who has completed an additional educational program focused on midwifery. NMs work in all types of settings in which women's health and obstetrical services are provided, and they may be very active in community health services.
- *Certified registered nurse anesthetist (CRNA):* A CRNA has a master's or doctoral degree (most now are doctorally prepared) that educates them to provide anesthesia, often under a doctor's supervision. They typically work in hospitals, outpatient surgery centers, and physicians' offices.
- *Licensed practical nurse (LPN) or licensed vocational nurse (LVN):* LPNs and LVNs perform some specific nursing functions and play a critical role in providing direct client care. They have high school degrees and additional training (usually 1 year) and work in all types of settings, typically under the direct supervision of an RN or a physician. They may work in hospitals, long-term care facilities, clinics, and homes.
- *Physician (MD or DO):* A physician has a medical degree; most physicians specialize in a specific area of practice (e.g., internal medicine, surgery, pediatrics, gynecology).
- *Physician assistant (PA):* The PA is a "physician extender" who provides medical services under the supervision of a licensed physician. The role was developed in the 1960s in response to a shortage of primary care physicians in certain areas. PAs often work in primary care, but many specialize.
- *Registered dietitian (RD):* This healthcare professional assesses the client's nutritional status and needs. RDs work in hospitals, long-term care facilities, clinics, community health centers, and homes.
- *Social worker (SW):* SWs assist clients and their families with problems related to reimbursement, access to care, housing, care in the home, transportation, and social problems. They are discharge planners, particularly in acute care facilities or hospitals, often as case managers; however, they work in all types of settings. SWs may also have education to specialize in counseling. SWs are employed in many community

agencies to help clients with a variety of needs, such as housing, ensuring that food is accessible, transportation, vocational assistance, medical equipment, and counseling.
- *Occupational therapist (OT):* OTs assist clients with impaired functions or disabilities to reach the clients' maximum level of physical and psychosocial independence. They work in all types of settings, including with clients in their homes through home health agencies.
- *Speech–language pathologist:* Speech–language pathologists assist clients who need rehabilitative services related to speech, hearing, and language/communication disorders, as well as swallowing disorders. They work in all types of settings, including with clients in their homes through home health agencies.
- *Physical therapist (PT):* PTs help clients who are experiencing musculoskeletal problems. These providers focus on maximizing physical functioning and work in all types of settings (e.g., hospitals, long-term care/rehabilitation, home health).
- *Pharmacist:* Pharmacists prepare and dispense medications. Pharmacists have become much more involved in educating clients about medications and in monitoring and evaluating the effects of medications. Many are now prepared at the doctoral level, and they work in all types of settings, including hospitals and community pharmacies.
- *Respiratory therapist (RT):* RTs provide care to clients with respiratory illnesses. They use oxygen therapy, intermittent positive-pressure respirators, artificial mechanical ventilators, and inhalation therapy. Most RTs work in hospitals and long-term care, but they are becoming more common in home healthcare.
- *Chiropractor:* Chiropractors are concerned with improving the function of the clients' nervous system by means of various treatment modalities (e.g., spinal manipulation, diet, exercise, and massage). Chiropractors are mostly community based.
- *Paramedical technologists:* Paramedical technologists work in various medical technology areas (e.g., radiology, nuclear medicine, and other laboratories).
- *Unlicensed assistive personnel (UAP):* Members of the healthcare team known as unlicensed assistive personnel have caused some controversy in the past few years; however, the UAP is a critical member of the team. UAPs provide direct client care, supervised by RNs. The amount of education and training of UAPs is highly variable. UAPs work not only in acute care and long-term care but also for home health agencies.

Nontraditional Healthcare Providers

Nontraditional healthcare providers deliver alternative or complementary therapies. During the two decades, consumers have become more interested in this type of care and have demanded that it be available.

Although many large medical centers are now developing programs and centers that offer complementary therapies, reimbursement for these services is lagging. The National

Institutes of Health (NIH) supports research focused on a wide array of alternative therapies and their effects on health and disease, and in 1998 established the National Center for Complementary and Alternative Medicine to meet the need. The name was recently changed to "National Center for Complementary and Integrative Health" to reflect recognition of the importance of incorporation of nontraditional therapies in healthcare. **Complementary and alternative therapies** provided by a variety of healthcare providers are extremely wide ranging. They include mediation, massage therapy, herbal therapy, healing touch, energetic healing, yoga, acupuncture, and acupressure. Ethnic healers, such as *curanderos,* and folk healers are also found in some communities. Training and licensure requirements for alternative therapists vary but will probably become more standard as their care becomes more accepted. Many nurses have incorporated alternative therapies into their practices and seek educational opportunities on a wide range of associated topics.

CRITICAL ISSUES IN HEALTHCARE DELIVERY

Quality Care

Quality care has been a concern of consumers and providers for decades. Quality care is a difficult concept to define and more difficult to measure. In 1996, President Clinton established the Advisory Commission on Consumer Protection and Quality to address a number of issues that had been identified. This commission produced a report that supported improvement in consumer power and rights, a focus on vulnerable populations, promotion of accountability, reduction in errors, and an increase in healthcare safety. Furthermore, they promoted evidence-based practice and enhanced investment in information systems (President's Advisory Commission on Consumer Protection and Quality in the Health Care Industry, 1999).

This report stimulated a series of more in-depth explorations of the healthcare delivery system. Key among them was the NAM's "Quality Chasm" series. In their series, the NAM defined *quality* as "the degree to which health services for individuals and populations increase the likelihood of desired health outcomes and are consistent with current professional knowledge" (IOM, 2001, p. 232). This series has had a major impact on the US healthcare delivery system, and highlights of a number of the key reports are presented in Table 11.1.

The **Agency for Healthcare Research and Quality (AHRQ)** is the main federal organization that works to improve the safety and quality of the healthcare system. Following the 1999 NAM report "To Err Is Human," AHRQ led the response to improving the safety of healthcare. This was largely through funding research to make care safer and to improve quality by publishing materials to educate healthcare systems and professionals to put research into practice and through generation of measures and data to be used by providers and policymakers (AHRQ, 2021a).

Among their numerous programs and initiatives, AHRQ support efforts for clinicians and providers include clinical guidelines and recommendations, the Team STEPPS program (Strategies and Tools to Enhance Performance and Patient Safety), and evidence-based education and training. With respect to quality and safety reports, AHRQ administers the "Consumer Assessment of Healthcare Providers and Systems" (CAHPS). CAHPS is a survey and reporting entity that collects data and provides reports and detailed information on consumers' experiences with specific aspects of their health plans and providers. This type of survey provides data that help purchasers of plans compare and contrast plans and allows informed consumers to select providers (AHRQ, 2021b). Finally, AHRQ publishes research and reports specifically related to healthcare disparities, quality, and evidence-based practice. These reports can be used by policy-makers and others to make critical decisions about funding and promotion of research endeavors.

Accreditation

Accreditation is one means to assess the quality of services and care of the organization. Specific minimum standards must be met by an organization to obtain accreditation. Indeed, accreditation serves the purpose of instilling public confidence in a program, institution, or organization (NAM, 2016). Purchasers of care, including insurers and MCOs, are concerned about the accreditation status of healthcare organizations when they negotiate reimbursement contracts. Other entities, such as nursing schools and medical schools, which use healthcare organizations for clinical sites, are also concerned with accreditation status.

Many groups provide accreditation for healthcare providers and healthcare organizations. For example, **The Joint Commission** was founded in 1951 to promote healthcare quality through setting and maintaining standards for hospitals. Their work has evolved over the ensuing decades, and The Joint Commission currently accredits and/or certifies more than 22,000 organizations in the United States, including hospitals, home care agencies, long-term care facilities, ambulatory care centers, and laboratories (The Joint Commission, 2021).

The **National Committee for Quality Assurance (NCQA)** began in 1990 and oversees accreditation programs for individual physicians, health plans, and medical groups, including MCOs (NCQA, 2021). During the accreditation process, the NCQA collects data for a widely used set of performance measures, the **Health Plan Effectiveness Data and Information Set (HEDIS)**. HEDIS collects data on about 90% of healthcare plans to measure performance and consumer satisfaction; thus, it allows consumers—including insurers—to compare performance of health plans and providers to regional and national benchmarks (CMS, 2021).

Currently, quality care monitoring focuses on improvement. Quality data are no longer hidden and will continue to be available when new methods are developed to assess improvement on the basis of outcomes. With the improvement approach, **outcomes measures** have moved to the forefront. Accrediting organizations require outcomes data, which they use to assess overall performance. Practitioners use outcomes to identify the treatment goals with the client. "Report cards" are

TABLE 11.1   National Academy of Medicine—Landmark Reports on Quality in Healthcare

Report Title (year)	Major Findings and Recommendations
To Err Is Human: Building a Safer Health System (1999)	Medication errors contribute to 44,000–98,000 deaths each year in the United States (more than motor vehicle accidents or breast cancer). Reported that errors largely result from system failures. Healthcare systems must focus on error prevention and promote changes to improve processes that will promote patient safety.
Crossing the Quality Chasm (2001a)	Among the findings was that the healthcare system is fragmented, poorly organized, does not use resources well, and quality varies considerably. The healthcare system needs improvement because of new technologies, rapid availability of information, and new treatments. Concerns were raised related to the rise in the number of people with multiple chronic conditions. Recommendations included the promotion of evidence-based care, more attention to patients' need for information, and improved access to clinical expertise. Report strongly supported enhanced use of information technology.
Leadership by Example (2003a)	Focused on government-funded programs: Medicare, Medicaid, CHIP, Dept. of Defense's TRICARE, VA program, and Indian Health Services. Report noted that federal leadership is needed to coordinate efforts and promote quality, and there is a notable lack of consistence in performance measurements. Recommended a more systematic approach to promote quality and to use technology in government-funded programs.
Who Will Keep the Public Healthy? (2003b)	Focused on the effects of globalization, travel, and technological advances and demographic changes on public health. Pointed out the need to address public health problems and educate public health professionals to meet current and future needs. Recommendations emphasized informatics, genomics, cultural competence, community-based participatory research, global health, and ethics.
Health Professions Education (2003c)	Education of health professionals is viewed as a bridge to quality care. Identified core competencies for all health professions: provide patient-centered care, work in interprofessional teams, employ evidence-based practice, apply quality improvement strategies, and utilize informatics.
Priority Areas for National Action: Transforming Health Care Quality (2003d)	The IOM identified 20 "priority areas" to be developed and/or addressed through an evidence-based approach to improve quality. Among the processes and issues were care coordination, health literacy, frailty of old age, medication management, and treatment for tobacco dependence. Among the health conditions/diagnoses identified as priority areas were nosocomial infections, obesity, asthma, diabetes, hypertension, stroke, major depression, and pregnancy/childbirth.
Future Directions for the National Healthcare Quality and Disparities Reports (2010)	Updated priority areas focusing on disparities. Areas to include were patient and family engagement, population health, safety, care coordination, palliative care, overuse of care, and improvement of access to care.
Future of Nursing: Leading Change, Advancing Health (2011)	This report addresses barriers that prevent nurses from being effectively used in the rapidly changing healthcare system. Among the main recommendations were that nurses should practice to the full extent of their education and training and that nurses should be encouraged to achieve higher levels of education and training.
Improving Diagnosis in Health Care (2015)	Diagnostic errors affect an estimated 5% of Americans each year; 6%–17% of adverse events in hospitals are the result of diagnostic errors. Reducing diagnostic errors is one of the new efforts to improve quality and safety in healthcare. Recommendations included the following: (1) promote more effective teamwork among healthcare professionals, patients, and family members; (2) ensure that health information technology supports patients and providers during the diagnostic process; (3) establish work systems and culture to support diagnostic processes and improvements; and (4) develop a system that facilitates learning from diagnostic errors and near misses.
Crossing the Global Quality Chasm: Improving Health Care Worldwide (2018)	The report builds on efforts by international health groups to achieve universal health coverage by 2030. It reviews evidence on quality of care worldwide and makes recommendations to improve healthcare quality and expanding access to services. The focus is on low-resources areas with attention to "frontline service delivery" to positively impact outcomes for individual and populations.

IOM, Institute of Medicine.

used to compare and contrast healthcare organizations and healthcare plans. These report cards are available to the consumer, providers, and insurers. Medicare in particular has been increasing the number of its quality initiatives. Among the Medicare quality initiatives are as follows:

- Centers for Medicare and Medicaid Services (CMS) Core Measures
- Quality Payment Program
- Merit-Based Incentive Payment System (MIPS)
- Marketplace Quality Incentives
- ESRD Quality Incentive Program
- Skilled Nursing Facility (SNF) Quality Reporting Program

Managed Care

Managed care refers to any method of healthcare delivery designed to reduce unnecessary use of services, improve cost containment or cost-effectiveness, and ensure high-quality care. Managed care is currently one of the predominant forces in healthcare delivery. It affects healthcare organizations, healthcare providers, and reimbursement and has a direct influence on what care is provided and by whom, where, when, and whether it is to be provided. Chapter 12 provides additional information on managed care and reimbursement.

Information Technology

The development and utilization of information technology (IT) over the past decade has been phenomenal. Clinical staff members use computers and related technologies in all healthcare settings. For example, encouragement of widespread implementation of the **electronic health record (EHR)/electronic medical record (EMR)** was promoted by the Health Information Technology for Economic and Clinical Health, which was a component of the American Recovery and Reinvestment Act of 2009. The EHR/EMR allows for systematization of the collection of patient health information within a digital format that can be shared across healthcare settings and among providers through network-connected information systems. The ACA strongly supported expansion of the EHR, as has the CMS. Although EHR support and usage have climbed exponentially as a result of these efforts, there have been several issues with the widespread implementation. These issues include high associated costs, software deficiencies, difficulties with interfaces between and among systems, privacy concerns, and liability issues. Despite these concerns and issues, the EHR will continue to evolve and should eventually promote better-quality, safer, and more effective and efficient healthcare delivery.

Telehealth is another avenue in which IT is expanding within health care. Use of telehealth means that clients can receive care via technology, such as computer, video, or interactive television. The IOM (2012b) identified "telehealth" as a key component in ensuring access to healthcare services in isolated geographic areas. Furthermore, they suggested that telehealth technologies will enhance the ability to better meet the healthcare needs of those in rural parts of the country, as well as for those in other underserved aggregates.

The Internet has opened doors for consumers and providers, and health information access has expanded rapidly. Although information availability to millions of people has been enhanced, resulting in an explosion of knowledge regarding health and health issues, the quality of this information is sometimes questionable. Providers must address the source and content of information on the Internet.

Social media, likewise, has become a more common source of information and is being widely used to share information about health. This can include health promotion and prevention activities and strategies. Individuals share a great variety of information now through social media, and this venue could be used in more organized efforts to get information out to the public. Finally, smartphones are a rapidly growing resource for engaging the community. Examples include employment of applications (apps) that track weight, exercise, and other health issues (e.g., heart function, blood glucose levels, hypertension).

Consumerism and Patient Rights

The growth of managed care and concerns over cost and value have increased the strength of consumerism. Over the past decade, the Baby Boomer generation has been subsidizing the healthcare system and paying more in premiums than it has taken out in claims. However, growing concern exists that, as this generation ages, it will demand more care than previous generations. Consumers are now critical of the healthcare system and demand changes as they encounter problems. Healthcare organizations, individual providers, and insurers recognize the importance of the consumer voice. *Client-* or *customer-centered healthcare* is a term that has become commonly used in healthcare, and more effort has been made to provide the consumer with information.

Patient or **client rights** are an important healthcare issue that individual states and the federal government have addressed through legislation. Patient rights have evolved over time and include access to medical records and the right to keep them private (through Health Insurance Portability and Accountability Act). In the United States, a number of attempts have been made to enshrine a patients' bill of rights in law, including a bill rejected by Congress in 2001. The ACA included efforts to promote patients' rights, but it was not fully implemented.

Many states have promoted laws or regulations protecting patients. Furthermore, healthcare facilities often have a "patients' bill of rights." Typically, a patients' bill of rights is a list of guarantees or promises for those receiving care at that facility or by providers. Generally included are guarantees of confidentiality, promises of access to information, fair treatment, informed consent, and autonomy over decisions, among other rights. Other patients' rights issues that are vitally important that continue to be discussed and debated are information disclosure, physician and provider choice, direct access to specialists, reimbursement for emergency care, and reimbursement denial.

Coordination and Access to Health Care

Healthcare providers often function in isolation from one another and provide fragmented services. Although multiple services are available for the wellness—illness continuum, coordination is lacking. Services range from office-clinic, home care, adult day care, acute care institutions, and specialized institutions to skilled nursing facilities. The services provided by one agency or one provider do not help the individual transit, or move, across boundaries and receive services offered by others. "Handoffs," when patients are transferred from one provider (e.g., individual provider, unit, agency) to another, are a time of increased risk for errors, reducing the quality of care. In addition, the services tend to be geographically separated, and each agency has different criteria for access. Furthermore, the focus of services has not kept pace with the changing needs of individuals and populations. Millions of Americans lack access to healthcare services, and inadequate financial resources are a deterrent to available health services. Interprofessional teams can address many of these concerns and improve care in the community.

The current healthcare system continues to be pluralistic and competitive, and it provides fragmented and uncoordinated care. Private care agencies and institutions are in competition with one another for clients, health professionals, and resources. Even with recent reforms, two hospitals in the same geographic area may be competing for the same clients, whereas other communities may not have a hospital at all, may have only minimal services, or may lack essential services such as obstetrics. Hospital home care programs are in direct competition with private or public home care agencies. Hospitals diversify services to become economically viable; therefore, they compete with ambulatory care providers for the ambulatory market. Public health services can be viewed as indirectly competing for resources. This fragmentation and duplication must be overcome to provide coordinated, collaborative, and accessible service to all citizens.

Disparity in Healthcare Delivery

Health disparities refer to observable or quantifiable differences in the presence of disease, health outcomes, or access to healthcare among different groups or populations. In the United States, health disparities have long been recognized as particularly problematic among ethnic minorities, including blacks, Native Americans, and Hispanics. Research indicates that often these groups have a higher prevalence of chronic conditions and higher rates of mortality and poorer health outcomes when compared with the white population. Furthermore, it is recognized that in addition to racial or ethnic group, health disparities adversely affect those based on such factors as socioeconomic status; age; mental health; cognitive, sensory, or physical disability; sexual orientation or gender identity; or geographic location.

For example, the Kaiser Family Foundation (2020b) noted that blacks and American Indian and Alaska Native adults have a higher prevalence of asthma, diabetes, and cardiovascular disease than whites. Variations in HIV diagnoses and death

rates from AIDS are very pronounced, with blacks experiencing over 8 to 10 times higher rates of HIV and AIDS diagnoses than whites. Furthermore, infant mortality rates are significantly higher for Blacks and American Indians and Alaska Natives compared with whites; African Americans and Latinos are also approximately twice as likely to develop diabetes. Finally, black males have the shortest life expectancy compared with other groups.

Disparities in healthcare provision have been observed, particularly related to cancer, cardiovascular disease, HIV/AIDS, diabetes, and mental illness. To address this problem, more cross-cultural education for healthcare professionals, including nurses, is needed to improve awareness of cultural and social factors and their impact on healthcare.

ETHICAL INSIGHTS

Limited Healthcare for Some

The healthcare system in the United States is complex, with social policies that favor pluralism, free choice, and free enterprise. The private sector personal care subsystem provides the majority of care to individuals. The private sector includes nonprofit agencies, for-profit agencies, and voluntary organizations. The public health subsystem provides limited personal care services for socially marginalized populations, but, for the most part, subsidizes the private sector through Medicare and Medicaid reimbursement to provide these services.

? ACTIVE LEARNING

1. Review the current National Health Care Quality report and the National Disparities report. They can be accessed at https://www.ahrq.gov/research/findings/nhqrdr/index.html. What frameworks or matrices are used to structure the report? What is the status of healthcare quality and disparities? What can you learn that would affect planning for healthcare services in a community?
2. Discuss how critical health care issues (e.g., managed care, quality care, fraud and abuse, diversity, and disparity) affect healthcare organizations in the community.
3. Cite examples of healthcare consumerism in the local community. What are their histories?
4. Give a personal reaction to healthcare fraud and abuse. How should the principles found in the Code for Nurses apply in practice?
5. Visit the following site on healthcare reform: https://www.hhs.gov/healthcare/about-the-aca/index.html. Review the elements of the law and current status. Discuss implications for nursing in the community. Also review http://www.helpingyoucare.com/21950/hhs-provides-tool-to-find-out-how-the-presidents-health-care-law-benefits-you-your-state. HHS provides this site for comparisons.

FUTURE OF PUBLIC HEALTH AND THE HEALTHCARE SYSTEM

Many changes are occurring in the healthcare system. Following implementation of the ACA, the healthcare system has been required to set limits on the care provided; identify criteria for the use of technology; and determine which conditions will be treated, which interventions are effective, and who should receive the care. The healthcare reform debate, however, is far from over, and additional changes will occur in the near future. Questions that continue to be important are as follows:

- What healthcare services should be provided?
- Who should have access to healthcare services?
- Who should pay for healthcare services?
- How can costs of healthcare be reduced?
- How should healthcare be delivered?
- What is the role of the government?

The importance of health promotion, disease prevention, and a population-based approach to healthcare is becoming increasingly recognized—particularly in the wake of the COVID-19 pandemic. There is recognition of the need for widespread use of the EHR, which, to be effective, must incorporate care provided in the community. The roles of healthcare organizations, practitioners, and the government must address the public health component of the system. There is also the problem of the need to address new and emerging threats such as the problems from the opioid crisis, increasing gang violence, and health conditions such as COVID-19. Finally, local, state, and national political leaders must continue to manage the health of the population and the need to reduce levels of healthcare expenditures.

Futurists rarely identify the public health subsystem as a component of the healthcare system, but this situation is changing. Indeed, the history of the public health subsystem's involvement with the poor and disenfranchised is a major influence on inattention to their problems. Furthermore, focus on environmental influences on the population, such as air quality, is critical for the future health of any nation.

Nursing has also been involved in change. The *Future of Nursing* (IOM, 2011) focused on how the nursing profession might fit into the change process. The key messages in this report were as follows:

1. Nurses should practice to the full extent of their education and training.
2. Nurses should achieve higher levels of education and training through an improved education system that promotes seamless academic progression.
3. Nurses should be full partners with physicians and other health professionals in redesigning health care in the United States.
4. Effective workforce planning and policy-making require better data collection and an improved information infrastructure.

This report offered eight recommendations, many of which are already having a major impact. One of the most significant to date is the drive to increase the number of nurses with bachelor of science nursing (BSN) degrees by developing more RN-BSN opportunities. Public health has been one area of healthcare that often has required a BSN for its entry positions, though with the nursing shortage this situation has been moderated some. Increasing the number of nurses with BSN degrees would help fill empty positions that require a BSN degree. The role of the ANP, as commented on earlier, is also expanding. The IOM report supported significant change, emphasizing these aspects of quality, access, and value:

- The need for patient-centered care
- The need for stronger primary care services
- The need to deliver more care in the community
- The need for seamless, coordinated care
- The need for reconceptualized roles for health professionals
- The need for interprofessional collaboration

Predicting future trends in human values is more difficult than predicting scientific discoveries or the patterns of disease. The past two decades have brought a significant shift in thinking about the future of the healthcare system. Consumer rights and further efforts to control or limit healthcare costs while improving access will be critical issues to be resolved in the future. How these decisions, and implementation of health care reform law, will affect public health is unclear.

SUMMARY

The healthcare system is complex and changes quickly. Federal, state, and local legislation and policies affect the system; and understanding the legislation and its effect on the healthcare delivery system is critical for any nurse. In addition, the implementation and pending changes to the ACA have demonstrated how important it is for healthcare providers to understand the reimbursement system and to learn how to advocate for their clients.

The many different types of healthcare organizations and healthcare providers also affect the healthcare system.

Interprofessional care will be necessary for providers to achieve success in the system and to ensure that the client receives cost-effective, high-quality care. There are many concerns about healthcare, including cost, access, the number of uninsured, quality, and healthcare fraud and abuse. Resolving these problems will not be an easy task, but it must be done. Understanding the system helps as healthcare providers learn to function in the rapidly changing system.

EVOLVE WEBSITE

http://evolve.elsevier.com/Nies/community
- NCLEX Review Questions
- Case Studies

BIBLIOGRAPHY AND REFERENCES

Agency for Healthcare Research and Quality: *2019 National healthcare quality & disparities report*, 2020. Available from: https://www.ahrq.gov/sites/default/files/wysiwyg/research/findings/nhqrdr/2019qdr.pdf.

Agency for Healthcare Research and Quality: *Agency for healthcare research and quality: a profile*, 2021a. Available from: https://www.ahrq.gov/cpi/about/profile/index.html.

Agency for Healthcare Research and Quality: *The CAHPS program*, 2021b. Available from: https://www.ahrq.gov/cahps/about-cahps/cahps-program/index.html.

Centers for Medicare and Medicaid Services (CMS): *Medicare advantage HEDIS public use files*, 2021. Available from: www.cms.gov/Research-Statistics-Data-and-Systems/Statistics-Trends-and-Reports/MCRAdvPartDEnrolData/MA-HEDIS-Public-Use-Files.

Hanlon G, Pickett J: *Public health administration and practice*, ed 9 St. Louis, 1979, Mosby.

Institute of Medicine: *The future of public health*, Washington, DC, 1988, National Academies Press.

Institute of Medicine: *To err is human: building a safer health system*, Washington, DC, 1999, National Academies Press.

Institute of Medicine: *Crossing the quality chasm*, Washington, DC, 2001, National Academies Press.

Institute of Medicine: *Leadership by example*, Washington, DC, 2003a, National Academies Press.

Institute of Medicine: *Who will keep the public healthy?*, Washington, DC, 2003b, National Academies Press.

Institute of Medicine: *Health professions education*, Washington, DC, 2003c, National Academies Press.

Institute of Medicine: *Priority areas for national action: transforming health care quality*, Washington, DC, 2003d, National Academies Press.

Institute of Medicine: *Future directions for the national healthcare quality and disparities reports*, Washington, DC, 2010, National Academies Press.

Institute of Medicine: *The future of nursing: leading change, advancing health*, Washington, DC, 2011, National Academies Press.

Institute of Medicine: *The role of telehealth in an evolving health care environment: workshop summary*, Washington, DC, 2012b, National Academies Press.

Institute of Medicine: *Measuring the impact of interprofessional education on collaborative practice and patient outcomes*, Washington, DC, 2015a, National Academies Press. Available from: https://www.nap.edu/download/21726.

Institute of Medicine: *Improving diagnosis in health care*, Washington, DC, 2015b, National Academics Press.

Kaiser Family Foundation: *Key facts about the uninsured population*, 2020a. Available from: www.kff.org/uninsured/issue-brief/key-facts-about-the-uninsured-population/#:~:text=However%2C%20beginning%20in%202017%2C%20the,2016%20to%2010.9%25%20in%202019.

Kaiser Family Foundation: *Disparities in health and health care: five key questions and answers*, 2020b. Available from: https://www.kff.org/racial-equity-and-health-policy/issue-brief/disparities-in-health-and-health-care-five-key-questions-and-answers/.

Kaiser Family Foundation (KFF): *Status of state medicaid expansion decisions: interactive map*, 2021a. Available from: https://www.kff.org/medicaid/issue-brief/status-of-state-medicaid-expansion-decisions-interactive-map/.

Kaiser Family Foundation: *Health reform*, 2021b. Available from: https://www.kff.org/health-reform/.

National Academy of Sciences: *Engineering, and medicine, health and medicine division: exploring the role of accreditation in enhancing quality and innovation in health professions education*, Washington, DC, 2016, National Academies Press. Available from: https://www.nap.edu/read/23636/chapter/1.

National Academy of Sciences, Engineering and Medicine, Health and Medical division: *Crossing the global quality chasm: improving health care worldwide*, Washington DC, 2018, National Academies Press.

National Committee for Quality Assurance: *About National Committee for Quality Assurance*, 2021. Available from: https://www.ncqa.org/about-ncqa/.

President's Advisory Commission on Consumer Protection and Quality in the Health Care Industry: *Quality first: better health care for all Americans*, Washington, DC, 1999, US Government Printing Office.

The Joint Commission: *About the joint commission*, 2021. Available from: https://www.jointcommission.org/about-us/facts-about-the-joint-commission/history-of-the-joint-commission/.

U.S. Department of Health and Human Services: *HHS Agencies and Offices*, 2021a. Available from: https://www.hhs.gov/about/agencies/hhs-agencies-and-offices/index.html.

U.S. Department of Health and Human Service: *Office of the surgeon general*, 2021b. Available from: https://www.hhs.gov/about/leadership/susan-orsega.html.

U.S. Department of Health and Human Services: *Strategic plan FY 2018-2022*, 2021c. Available from: https://www.hhs.gov/about/strategic-plan/index.html.

U.S. Department of Health and Human Services: *Healthy people 2030*, Washington, DC, 2010, US Government Printing Office.

World Health Organization: *Declaration of Alma Ata*, 1978. Available from: http://www.who.int/publications/almaata_declaration_en.pdf.

FURTHER READING

Institute of Medicine: *Best care at lower costs: the path to continuously learning health care in America*, Washington, DC, 2012a, National Academies Press.

Institute of Medicine: *Envisioning the national health care quality report*, Washington, DC, 2001b, National Academies Press.

12

Economics of Health Care

Melanie McEwen

OBJECTIVES

Upon completion of this chapter, the reader will be able to do the following:

1. Discuss factors that influence the cost of health care.
2. Identify terms used in the financing of health care.
3. Discuss public financing of health care.
4. Discuss private financing of health care.
5. Discuss health insurance plans.
6. Describe trends in healthcare financing.
7. Describe the effects of economics on healthcare access.
8. Identify the future of healthcare economics.

OUTLINE

KEY TERMS

access
actuarial classifications
adverse selection
ambulatory care
capitated reimbursement
carrier
carve-out service
coinsurance
copayment
cost containment
cost shifting
current procedural terminology (CPT) codes

deductible
diagnosis-related group (DRG)
effectiveness
flexible spending account (FSA)
gatekeepers
healthcare providers
health insurance plans
health maintenance organization (HMO)
health savings account (HSA)
high-deductible health plans (HDHP)
indemnity plan

managed care groups
managed care plans
mandates
Medicaid
Medicare
Medigap insurance
outcomes
out-of-pocket expenses
Patient Protection and Affordable Health Care Act (ACA)
point-of-service (POS)
preferred provider organization (PPO)

premiums
primary care provider

prospective payment system (PPS)
surprise billing

transparency

Economics represents the science of allocation of resources. Resources are commonly known as *goods or services*, for example, healthcare services. Economics affects all aspects of health care. Nurses have traditionally avoided the arena of healthcare economics, preferring to focus on the actual, direct care of the client. So strong is the feeling of social justice that some nurses express a reluctance to be informed of the individual client's healthcare financing source for fear that this knowledge will influence their care. Public health nurses who deal with the medically underserved have had more experience in this area. However, even these nurses may have only rudimentary knowledge.

Healthcare costs continue to rise and consume a greater percentage of our nation's resources. Indeed, health care is currently almost 18% of the gross domestic product (GDP) of the United States and is anticipated to rise to 20% in only a few years (CMS, 2020). As a result, nursing can no longer ignore the intricacies of healthcare financing. The health of individuals, families, and aggregates is significantly influenced by economics. Economically disadvantaged individuals who have difficulty obtaining the basics, such as food and shelter, are less likely to have access to health care. Passage of the Patient Protection and Affordable Care Act (AFA) (PL 111-148) in 2010 dramatically influenced health care access, resulting in many more individuals having insurance coverage. Indeed, most citizens have health insurance, whether provided by their employers, through private purchase, or, for those from low-income groups, through state and federal government sources (e.g., Medicare, Medicaid, Children's Health Insurance Plan [CHIP]). This change, however, is not to universal health care coverage—many still remain uninsured.

This chapter focuses on the economics of health care. It specifically discusses factors that influence health care costs, terminology of healthcare financing, and trends in healthcare economics and their impact on population health. This chapter also addresses the future of healthcare financing. Box 12.1 presents terms and definitions that are important to the discussion of these topics.

FACTORS INFLUENCING HEALTHCARE COSTS

Historical Perspective

Until the 1930s, the predominant method of individual healthcare financing in the United States was self-payment. **Healthcare providers** charged a fee for the services they rendered, and the patient paid these **out-of-pocket expenses**. The price of the service was under the control of the provider and generally represented the cost of providing that service. A certain amount of "charity" services was expected. The assumption was that those who could pay would pay and those who could not pay should receive care and pay what they could.

The concept of public financing of health care for a specific aggregate was restricted and varied from geographic area to area until the term *public health* came into common use.

The following types of hospitals existed until the mid-20th century:

Public hospitals, which received public funds and served the healthcare needs of the entire population, regardless of ability to pay

Private hospitals, which cared mainly for those whose ability to pay was greater than that of the general population

For-profit hospitals, which were limited in number, received funds from investors, and cared for those who could definitely pay

Over time there has been growth in private and for-profit hospitals, resulting in large national hospital corporations that then expanded into offering more nonacute services.

This system worked well as long as those who could pay outnumbered those who could not. During the Great Depression, with more than 25% of the population out of work, the number of those capable of paying for health care was greatly reduced. Because public financing of health care was limited, hospitals, physicians, and other providers of health care went bankrupt.

In 1929, schoolteachers in Dallas, Texas, negotiated a prepaid health provision contract with Baylor Hospital. The teachers paid a sum of money each month, which guaranteed them access to health care through the hospital. The concept of insurance for health care proved extremely successful for Baylor Hospital. By 1939, this insurance plan had grown to include other groups and hospitals and became Blue Cross-Blue Shield (Momanyi, 2021).

Health insurance, or the idea of paying a small fee for guaranteed health care, appealed to the public. Societal concerns were mainly focused on sick care and acquisitions of curative therapies whenever needed. A public view that health insurance would provide freedom from fear that illness would impoverish them developed and prevails today. Healthcare providers envisioned guaranteed payment for their services (Higgins, 1997). During World War II, faced with a limited workforce and governmental restrictions on wages, employers began to see health insurance as a means of supplying workers' benefits without granting a wage increase.

To extend this same "insurance" to the general population, the Social Security Act of 1935 was amended in 1965 to create Medicare and Medicaid. **Medicare** provided indemnity insurance to those over the age of 65 years, and **Medicaid**, a state-administered health plan, provided a source for financing health care for some of the poor and the disabled.

As a result of these healthcare resources, a significant majority of the population was protected by indemnity healthcare insurance from various sources. The early indemnity plans lacked an incentive for limitation of use and had few or no provisions for health promotion. The emphasis was placed on illness care, providers received a fee only when a service was

BOX 12.1 Terminology Used in Health Care Financing

The financing of health care has given rise to new terminology. Nurses, as providers of care and consumers of services, need to be knowledgeable about these terms to improve their understanding of healthcare financing.

Terms pertaining to consumers:

Access—Ability to obtain healthcare services in a timely manner, at a reasonable cost, by a qualified practitioner, and at an accessible location.

Carve-out service—A service (e.g., mental health care) provided within a standard benefit package but delivered exclusively by a designated provider or group.

Charges—The posted prices of provider services.

Coinsurance—Cost sharing required by a health plan whereby the individual is responsible for a set percentage of the charge for each service.

Copayment—Cost sharing required by the health plan whereby the individual must pay a fixed dollar amount for each service.

Deductible—Cost sharing whereby the individual pays a specified amount before the health plan pays for covered services.

Fee schedule—List of predetermined payment rates for medical services.

Flexible spending account (FSA) or health savings account (HSA)—A mechanism by which an employee may pay for uncovered healthcare expenses through payroll deductions using pretax dollars.

Gatekeeper—Person in a managed care organization who decides whether a patient will be referred for specialty care. Doctors, nurses, nurse practitioners, and physician assistants function as gatekeepers.

Healthcare provider—An individual or institution that provides medical services (e.g., physicians, hospitals, or laboratories).

Health maintenance organization (HMO)—A managed care plan that acts as an insurer and sometimes a provider for a fixed prepaid premium. HMOs usually employ physicians.

Health plan—An insurance plan that pays a predetermined amount for covered health services.

High-deductible health plans (HDHP)—Insurance plan that uses cost sharing (i.e., high deductibles) to encourage employees to select plans with lower premiums. The intent is to encourage healthcare consumers to become more proactive in healthcare decisions from a financial perspective.

Indemnity plan—A health plan that pays covered services on a fee-for-service basis.

Managed care plan—A health plan that uses financial incentives to encourage enrollees to use selected providers who have contracted with the plan.

Medicaid—Joint federal- and state-funded programs that provide healthcare services for low-income people.

Medicare—A health insurance program for people who are older than 65 years of age, are disabled, or have end-stage renal disease.

Medicare Advantage—Part of Medicare by which recipients may choose to enroll in a coordinated care plan, private fee-for-service, or medical savings account plan created by the Balanced Budget Act of 1997.

Medigap insurance—Privately purchased individual or group health insurance plan designed to supplement Medicare coverage.

Out-of-pocket expenses—Payment made by the individual for medical services.

Point-of-service (POS) plan—A managed care plan that combines prepaid and fee-for-service plans. Enrollees may choose to use the services of an uncontracted provider by paying an increased copayment.

Portability—The guarantee that an individual changing jobs continues to receive healthcare coverage with the new employer without a waiting period or having to meet additional deductible requirements.

Preferred provider organization (PPO)—A health plan that contracts with providers to furnish services to the enrollees of the plan. Usually no insurance copayment is required.

Premium—Amount paid periodically to purchase health insurance benefits.

Primary care provider—A generalist physician, typically a family physician, internist, gynecologist, or pediatrician, who provides comprehensive medical services.

Terms pertaining to providers:

Ambulatory care—Medical services provided on an outpatient basis in a hospital or clinic setting.

Capitation—Payment mechanism that pays healthcare providers a fixed amount per enrollee to cover a defined set of services over a specified period, regardless of actual services provided.

Care management—Process used to improve quality of care by analyzing variations in and outcomes for current practice in the care of specific health conditions.

Cost containment—Reduction of inefficiencies in the consumption, allocation, or production of healthcare services.

Customary charge—Physician payment based on a median charge for a given service within a 12-month period.

Diagnosis-related group (DRG)—A system of payment classification for inpatient hospital services based on the principal diagnosis, procedure, age and gender of the patient, and complications.

Effectiveness—Net health benefit provided by a medical service or technology for a typical patient in community practice.

Full capitation—A stipulated dollar amount established to cover the cost of all healthcare services delivered for a person.

Maximum allowable costs—Specified cost level established by the health plan.

Outcome—The consequences of a medical intervention in a patient.

Physician's current procedural terminology (CPT) codes—A list of codes for medical services and procedures performed by physicians and other healthcare providers that has become the healthcare industry's standard for reporting physician procedures and services.

Practice guidelines—An explicit statement of what is known and believed about the benefits, risks, and costs of particular courses of medical action intended to assist decisions made by practitioners, patients, and others about appropriate health care for specific and clinical conditions.

Utilization review—A formal prospective, concurrent, or retrospective assessment of the medical necessity, efficiency, and appropriateness of healthcare services.

Terms pertaining to third-party payers:

Actuarial classification—Classification of enrollees that is determined by use of the mathematics of insurance, including probabilities, to ensure adequacy of the premium to provide future payment.

Administrative costs—Costs that the insurer incurs for utilization review, marketing, medical underwriting, agents' commissions, premium collection, claims processing, insurer profit, quality assurance activities, medical libraries, and risk management.

Adverse selection—Procedure in which a larger proportion of people with poorer health status enroll in specific plans or options. Plans that enroll a subpopulation with lower-than-average costs are favorably selected.

Capital cost—Depreciation, interest, leases and rentals, taxes, and insurance on tangible assets.

Carrier—An organization that contracts with the Centers for Medicare & Medicaid Services (CMS) to administer claims processing and make Medicare payments to healthcare providers.

Cost contract—Arrangement between a managed healthcare plan and the CMS for reimbursement of the costs of services provided.

Cost shifting—The cost of uncompensated care is passed on to the insured, resulting in higher costs for those with insurance coverage.

Mandate—A state or federal statute or regulation that requires coverage for certain health services.

Risk assessment—Statistical method used to estimate claims costs of enrollees.

rendered, and all costs of services were reimbursed. Insulated from rising healthcare costs, healthcare consumers demanded complex and technologically advanced services whenever illness struck. These demands for costly services represented the major driving force in rising healthcare costs.

By the 1980s, the first efforts to curtail healthcare costs were made by the federal government. With institution of the **prospective payment system (PPS)**, hospital reimbursement for Medicare patients was based on a classification system that identified costs according to diagnosis and client characteristics—**diagnosis-related groups (DRGs)**. The PPS prompted an evolution toward managed care, dramatically altering healthcare financing through the end of the 20th century and into the first decade of the 21st century. Despite containment efforts, however, costs of health care and, consequently, health insurance, have continued to rise.

The spiraling healthcare costs, starting from the mid-1960s and persisting into the 21st century, were fueled by the presence of very rapid technological advances, society's sense of entitlement to these therapies, a guaranteed payer, and the prevailing medical orientation toward curative measures. Prior to implementation of Medicare and Medicaid, national health expenditures represented less than 5% of the GDP. Fifty years later, however, costs have risen exponentially, as described previously.

Use of Health Care

According to economic principles, the existence of a desirable product, the demand for the product, and the availability of financial funding influence the use of the product. Health care is the product, and the demand for this product increases when the need expands and funding is available. In an attempt to reduce unnecessary utilization, insurance plans began to limit coverage for certain services and people; thus the move toward "managed care." Restrictions on use of health care, such as the establishment of a "gatekeeper," limited patient provider choice, requirement of preauthorization for some services, limited coverage for preexisting illnesses, and exclusion of those participants whose use was deemed exorbitant, have been instituted. However, these restrictions had only limited success in curbing healthcare costs. Consumers were activated by these changes made by managed care, protesting them, and in many instances alterations were made.

Despite recognition of the problem of increasing healthcare costs and multiple attempts to address it, spending for health care in the United States is more than double that of many other developed countries (i.e., those in the Organization for Economic Cooperation and Development [OCED]). Indeed, average per capita spending in 2018 was $4200, 8.8% of GDP for OCED countries, compared with $11,071 (17.6% of GDP) in the United States (OCED, 2021). In contrast, Canada, which was 10th highest per capita spending in the OCED, spent $5418 per person, or 10.8% of the GDP on health care. Because the approach in the US. healthcare system is reimbursement with multiple insurers, both private and public, expenses for health care vary according to types of care and sources of funding.

Lack of Preventive Care

Until recently, little to no incentive has existed to prevent illness or promote health. Curative measures have traditionally been the focus of health care. Soaring healthcare costs and an improved knowledge of health have heightened the public's awareness of their obligation to assume responsibility for their health by amending many unhealthy behaviors. As a result, more people are demanding preventive health care from the provider and their healthcare contractors. Public financing of health care has increased funding for such preventive care as screening tests, periodic examinations, and immunizations. Use of these preventive health services has increased, but significant disparities persist in relation to ethnic background and economic status (National Center for Health Statistics [NCHS], 2018). There continues to be a gap between the amount of funding available for preventive treatment modalities and funding for curative treatments.

Lifestyle and Health Behaviors

A healthy lifestyle does not ensure good health but has been shown to contribute to longevity and productivity (Harvard Medical School, 2009). The five leading causes of death and illness can be positively affected by changes in lifestyle. Studies have now found that a low-fat diet, exercise, maintaining of an optimal body weight, smoking cessation, and stress reduction can modify or even prevent many chronic illnesses. Smoking cessation reduces the incidence of lung cancer. Seat belt use decreases the severity of injuries incurred during moving vehicle accidents. Indeed, effective treatment of illness must often be coupled with a change in lifestyle. In the near future, access to expensive and unique medical treatment will probably be influenced less by the patient's ability to pay and more by the person's commitment to compulsory lifestyle changes. For example, legislation has levied "sin taxes" on products whose use has been associated with chronic illnesses. Examples include addition of taxes on cigarettes and other tobacco products, large soft drinks, alcoholic beverages, and certain cooking oils. Income from these taxes is intended to be used to care for, prevent, and conduct research on chronic illnesses.

Significant changes in lifestyle have taken place in the past 30 years. The current "smoke-free" environment appears shocking when contrasted to the nonchalant attitude toward smoking that was pervasive in the 1940s, 1950s, and 1960s. The advent of frameworks and theories such as the Health Belief Model and Pender's Health Prevention Model has given rise to numerous studies into methods of achieving lifestyle changes. The total effects of these changes are just now being seen with dramatic reductions in lung cancer and chronic lung diseases. Meanwhile, the healthcare system must continue to contend with the results of years of unhealthy lifestyles; most striking is the concerning rise in overweight and obesity and the abuse of opioid medications.

Healthcare funding is changing to provide more funding for preventive services. Some insurance plans provide monetary incentives, such as reduction in insurance premiums, for those who participate in behavioral changes toward a healthier lifestyle. Medicare will pay for many screening procedures performed for specific persons at specified times (Centers for Medicare and Medicaid Services [CMS], 2021a,b,c,d). Funding for behavioral changes, however, is often limited, inadequate, or unavailable. Similarly, weight loss programs, support groups for smoking cessation, and participation in relaxation programs are not usually considered reimbursable treatment regimens, but more expensive pharmaceutical interventions are reimbursable.

Societal Beliefs

With the advent of such wonders as penicillin and insulin, society began to believe that the eradication of disease was just a few years away. More and more resources were dedicated to this elusive search. Armed with the belief that disease would soon be eliminated, society had limited interest in preventive care. The general belief was that making more money available for health care would lead to better health care and the greater likelihood that illness would be cured. Society has viewed insurance as an economic shield protecting against all disease and illness. The belief in cure rather than prevention, combined with this financial safety net, encouraged society to become a passive participant in health care. The feeling "I don't have to worry, I have insurance" became the pervasive societal thought (Sloan, 2004).

Healthcare professionals also were slow to embrace preventive care. Most efforts were directed toward curing illness. With what seemed to be an unending source of financing for curative care, illness prevention seemed counterproductive.

As healthcare costs accelerated at an alarming rate and technological advances did not keep up with the increase in illnesses, the health of society had to become a collaborative effort between society itself and the healthcare industry. Although the United States spends more money on health care than any other industrialized country, it ranks significantly behind many other countries in health status indicators (NCHS, 2018; OECD, 2021). People still expect the healthcare system to cure them when they are ill, but there is now an increase in preventive care interest, including interest in health education, health promotion, and behavioral changes. Research into barriers and facilitators to lifestyle changes has increased, but it is not funded at the same level as curative measures (OECD, 2021). As discussed in Chapter 11, the United States continues to spend more money on health care and yet has lower-quality health indicators than many other countries (Fineberg, 2012).

Technological Advances

Modern society has come to expect miraculous technological advances. In response to this expectation, and supplied with funding from various sources, technological advances have become too numerous to mention. The United States leads the world in laboratory and clinical research. People come from all over the world for education and to train in leading American centers for excellence. The United States exceeds other industrialized countries in the availability and use of these technological advances. Such advances can save the lives of people who would otherwise die.

These advances, although remarkable, are expensive. It has been widely suggested that in the United States, 20% of the population consumes 80% of the healthcare resources; the reality is probably closer to one-third of the population consuming two-thirds of the resources (CMS, 2012). As the healthcare dollar shrinks, these advances raise ethical questions involving healthcare access and rationing. Restriction on technology can significantly reduce the cost of health care, but the delays, inconvenience, and limitations to care with rationing would be strongly resisted by most Americans. An example of a growing technology area is telehealth:

> Telehealth has already started to play an even more important role, especially as we move away from the traditional fee for service system and toward new models of care, including accountable care organizations, patient-centered medical homes, and other strategies that focus on outcomes. At the same time, the costs of telehealth technologies are dropping and [they are] becoming even easier to use. These technologies are becoming more widely prevalent in the marketplace, more accessible, and consequently, can be adopted more easily than perhaps 5 or 10 years ago. The pace of technological innovation is accelerating, but the cost of innovation is falling.
>
> **Institute of Medicine (IOM, 2012, p. 7)**

Telehealth has implications for public health as it expands care and access to specialists into the community. A key to success will be the cost factor.

Aging of Society

Healthcare expenditures rise with age, dramatically so at older ages. According to the latest population projections, individuals older than 65 years constituted about 16.3% of the total population in 2016; this proportion is expected to reach more than 22% by the year 2050 (Statista, 2021). As people live longer, the percentage of those older than 85 years is also increasing. Therefore the number of those consuming the greatest amount of healthcare resources will rise more rapidly than the number of those who provide the monetary support for these resources. For example, the cost of care for Alzheimer disease and related dementias is considerable, and the rate of such dementias is expected to rise as Baby Boomers age, with the expectation that cost for this care—which in 2010 was between $159 and $215 billion, depending on what factors were included—is expected to double by 2040 if no effective treatment or cure is found for the diseases (NIH-supported study, 2013).

Pharmaceuticals

A relatively new phenomenon that has influenced healthcare economics is the utilization of drugs, both over-the-counter and prescription drugs. New drugs are improving health outcomes and quality of life. These new drugs and new uses for older drugs are curing some illnesses, preventing or delaying other chronic diseases, and hastening recovery from yet other illnesses. As a result, during the last several decades, costs of prescription drugs have risen dramatically and have become a significant part of health expenditures. Seniors in particular are affected because many have chronic illnesses that require daily medications.

In 2003, to help alleviate the costs of prescriptions for seniors, Medicare added a pharmaceutical benefit for enrollees. With implementation of the Medicare Prescription Drug and Modernization Act (Medicare Part D), all Medicare recipients are eligible to purchase insurance coverage to offset the costs of prescription drugs. As with other healthcare services, once a funding source has been established, utilization and costs increase. One result is that as of 2017, about 9.5% of healthcare expenditures in the United States is for pharmaceuticals, and these expenditures continue to rise (NCHS, 2018).

Shift to For-Profit Health Care

The final contributor to the increase in healthcare costs is a national shift from nonprofit health care to for-profit health care. This has given rise to the term *healthcare industry*. More and more large, for-profit organizations are taking over smaller community organizations. As the emphasis is on profit, mechanisms of achieving higher reimbursement have been developed, which have had an effect on healthcare costs.

Healthcare Fraud and Abuse

Healthcare fraud has been an ongoing problem. The billions of dollars spent on health care and the struggles for control between providers, consumers, and healthcare organizations have increased the risk of fraud and abuse. The Federal Bureau of Investigation (FBI) estimates that healthcare fraud costs the United States tens of billions of dollars annually (FBI, 2021). The FBI is the primary agency that handles this fraud. Though all areas of health care and all payers experience fraud, Medicare and Medicaid have the highest levels (National Health Care Anti-Fraud Association [NHCAA], 2021). A number of actions have been taken to address this problem. Among them are the False Claims Act Amendments of 1986, which allow private citizens to collect a percentage of recovered funds if they report fraudulent Medicare claims and monies are recovered as a result. The Health Insurance Portability and Accountability Act (HIPAA) contains a set of provisions that address fraud, including a Fraud and Abuse Control Program, the Medicare Integrity Program, and the Health Care Fraud and Abuse Data Collection Program. Each of these programs is designed to address concerns over healthcare fraud. In addition, HIPAA legislation dramatically raised funding for fraud enforcement activities (HHS/OIG, 2020).

Major healthcare fraud and abuse incidents have influenced the most vulnerable of the population (i.e., the mentally ill and older adults). For example, overbilling and unnecessary visits in home health care were reported across the United States, resulting in widespread reforms to Medicare reimbursement for home health services (Infante & McAnaney, 2004). Other significant abuses in recent years relate to ambulance/emergency transportation, overbilling/kickbacks, opioid prescription abuse, addiction treatment programs, money laundering, and compounding pharmacies (FBI, 2021).

The Affordable Health Care Act (ACA) included additional provisions to reduce fraud and abuse in public programs. It encouraged screening of providers and enhanced oversight for initial claims for durable medical equipment suppliers. The law required Medicare and Medicaid program providers and suppliers to establish compliance programs and developed a database to share fraud and abuse information among federal and state programs. Finally, it increased penalties for submitting false claims and increases funding for antifraud activities (Kaiser Family Foundation, 2013). Box 12.2 describes consumer tips related to healthcare fraud and abuse.

PUBLIC FINANCING OF HEALTH CARE

As the popularity and benefits of employer-provided insurance plans were recognized during the depression and post-WWII years, it became evident that the health care of some segments of society was being neglected. During the 1960s, a pervasive thrust for social justice in the public and political arenas presented the ideal opportunity for governmental participation in healthcare financing. In 1965, the federal government under President Lyndon Johnson enacted the first movement toward universal healthcare coverage. Titles XVIII and XIX, amendments to the Social Security Act, created Medicare and Medicaid, respectively.

Medicare

Medicare is a federal entitlement program that is totally funded by a combination of payroll taxes, general federal taxes, and beneficiary premiums. This program is intended to help cover the costs of health care for people 65 years of age and older and people who are disabled, have end-stage renal disease, or have been diagnosed with amyotrophic lateral sclerosis. Medicare is divided into four parts. Medicare Part A is basically hospital

---

BOX 12.2   Medicare Fraud

What Is Medicare Fraud?
- Billing Medicare for services not received
- Billing Medicare for services other than those received
- Use of another's Medicare card to obtain services

Be suspicious if providers tell you:
- Medicare wants you to have this service
- They know how to get Medicare to pay for service
- The more services provided, the cheaper they are

Be suspicious if providers:
- Change copayment of Medicare-approved services
- Advertise "free" consultations to those with Medicare
- Claim they represent Medicare
- Use pressure to persuade you of the need for high-priced services
- Use telemarketing as a marketing tool

Whenever you receive a Medicare payment notice, review it for errors. Make sure Medicare was not billed for services not received.

Modified from Centers for Medicare and Medicaid Services: *Help Fight Medicare Fraud.* Available from: https://www.medicare.gov/Pubs/pdf/10111-Protecting-Yourself-and-Medicare.pdf.

insurance. Services covered by Medicare Part A include inpatient care in hospitals and skilled nursing facilities (not unskilled or long-term care). It also covers hospice care and some home health care. Most US residents are eligible for premium-free Medicare Part A benefits when they reach age 65, on the basis of their own or their spouse's employment. Although Medicare Part A is an entitlement program, the enrollee must pay a **deductible** for health services. The Part A deductible is the beneficiary's only cost for up to 60 days of Medicare-covered inpatient hospital care in a benefit period. Beneficiaries have to pay an additional copayment per day for days 61 through 90, and this copayment increases per day for hospital stays beyond the 90th day in a benefit period. The Centers for Medicare & Medicaid Services (CMS) Website (http://www.cms.gov) provides current information on costs for beneficiaries.

Those individuals who are eligible for Medicare Part A may *purchase* Medicare Part B for a monthly fee. Medicare Part B is medical insurance that helps pay for out-of-pocket costs related to physician services, hospital outpatient care, durable medical equipment, and other services, including some home health care. The monthly premium paid by beneficiaries enrolled in Medicare Part B has changed over time. Premiums are now pro-rated, based on income, and in 2021 ranged from a low of $148/month for individuals making $88,000 or less ($176,000 for couples) to a high of $505/month for individuals earning above $500,000 or couples earning above $750,000 per year. In addition to the monthly premium, Part B requires subscribers to pay deductibles and coinsurance (CMS, 2021b). The CMS website provides current information on these costs.

Medicare Part C, also known as the *Medicare Advantage plans,* is optional "gap" coverage provided by private insurance companies that are approved by, and under contract with, Medicare and may include health maintenance organizations (HMOs) and preferred provider organizations (PPOs). Covered services vary by plan and may include vision, hearing, and dental care, as well as other services and supplies not covered by

Medicare Parts A, B, and D. Costs vary by plan, and to be eligible, the individual must have Medicare Parts A and B and must live in the service area of the plan (CMS, 2021a). Enrollment in Medicare Advantage plans has grown steadily, and more than 25% of Medicare beneficiaries are enrolled in these programs.

Medicare Part D was initiated in 2006 to help defray the costs of prescription drugs. Like Parts B and C, Medicare Part D is optional, and if eligible Medicare recipients choose this option, they must enroll in an approved prescription drug plan. Most participants in Medicare Part D pay a monthly premium, a yearly deductible, and copayments, with out-of-pocket costs based on the plan selected and drugs used. In addition to these costs, the enrollee is responsible for cost of prescription drugs once the total costs reach a certain amount in a year, which vary. This is termed the *coverage gap* or *donut hole.* When the enrollee's out-of-pocket total for drugs reaches a particular level, Medicare will pay 95% of the costs of any further prescription drugs. The CMS website provides current information on the amounts to be paid. Fig. 12.1 shows current and projected Medicare costs for each of the four major parts.

Medicaid

Title XIX of the Social Security Act established the Medicaid Program. Medicaid is a public welfare assistance program that was initially designed to finance healthcare coverage for the indigent. Eligibility for this program, a joint venture with state and federal funding, is determined by each state. Initially Medicaid was intended to focus benefits to children, pregnant women, the disabled, and impoverished elders. This changed dramatically, however, with implementation of the ACA, as funds were made available to provide health care for all adults below the poverty line—within states that elected to participate.

The federal government sets baseline eligibility requirements for Medicaid. State governments that wish to provide care to more citizens through this program can alter the eligibility

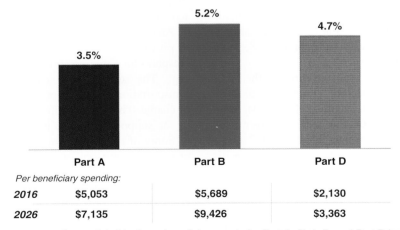

Average Annual Growth in Medicare Beneficiary Costs for Part A, Part B, and Part D Between 2016 and 2026

Per beneficiary spending:	Part A	Part B	Part D
2016	$5,053	$5,689	$2,130
2026	$7,135	$9,426	$3,363

Fig. 12.1 Average annual growth in Medicare beneficiary costs for Part A, Part, B, and Part D between 2016 and 2026. (Adapted from Kaiser Family Foundation: *The facts on Medicare spending and financing,* 2017. Available from: http://www.kff.org/medicare/issue-brief/the-facts-on-medicare-spending-and-financing/.)

requirements. For example, the federal government may set 100% of poverty as an eligibility requirement, but an individual state may set the requirement as 110% of poverty. This means that a family living in that state can have an income slightly above the federal standard and still qualify for Medicaid.

The federal government **mandates** covered services, but state governments may provide more services. Mandated services covered by Medicaid for eligible recipients include inpatient and outpatient hospital care, physician's services, vaccines for children, family planning services, rural health clinic services, home health care, laboratory and radiography services, and Early and Periodic Screening, Diagnosis, and Treatment services for children younger than 21 years. Care provided by pediatric and family nurse practitioners is covered. Optional services that states may elect to provide include optometrist services and glasses, intermediate care facilities for the mentally disabled, rehabilitation, physical therapy, and hospice (CMS, 2021c).

Aside from Medicaid, many children younger than 18 years are eligible for CHIP. Established in 1997, CHIP is a program that provides insurance for children of low-socioeconomic families who do not qualify for Medicaid. Like Medicaid, the program is administered by the states, which share the cost with the national government. The ACA required expansion of Medicaid and CHIP to cover many of those who were previously uninsured.

The final decision as to whether Medicaid would be expanded in a state was determined by each state. The law covered payment of services for newly eligible Medicaid beneficiaries through 2016, and the federal government will pay 90% of the cost for several more years. Ultimately, 39 states and the District of Columbia opted for Medicaid expansion, and 12 states did not (KFF, 2021). It is possible that even more of the "opt-out" states will reconsider and elect to expand Medicaid coverage to more citizens in the near future.

Governmental Grants

Unlike individual healthcare services, governmental grants are directed toward funding large populations and different aggregates. Historically, the bulk of health promotion and disease-preventive measures has been limited to this arena of public health care. All three levels of government provide the major contribution of funding for these programs. On the national level the U.S. Department of Health and Human Services (HHS) administers this funding.

A variety of funding grants are available through the HHS (USDHHS, 2021). The "health-specific" grants are administered through the public health department at each state or community level. A large part of the federal government funding provided to the states is through "block grants." These "blocks" of funds are provided to the states to affect the health of the public as a whole. There are specific restrictions on how these monies can be spent, including limitations on the population that receives the services and what types of programs are to be funded. The states use these monies to provide for the care of the public within these restrictions. Depending on the health needs of the state, these monies may be spent to provide

direct aggregate care, but most often they are used for health promotion activities that are directed at a larger percentage of the population. Each level of government may make funds available for a specific health need of the members of the community.

To ensure that the needs of the community are being addressed, healthcare providers and programs may be required to compete for these funds. Proposals, grant applications, or requests must be submitted, reviewed, and prioritized. Funds are allocated on the basis of need and program merit. This type of funding is directed toward the population in general and not to specific individuals. When the funding is no longer provided, the programs cease, leading to lack of continuity of care. Historically, the funding priorities are closely related to the achievement of the *Healthy People* objectives. Limitations on the amounts provided are related to available governmental resources.

? ACTIVE LEARNING

Interview an official from your local health department about finances. Identify strengths and weaknesses. Consider solutions for one of the weaknesses.

PHILANTHROPIC FINANCING OF HEALTH CARE

A limited amount of the nation's healthcare bill is paid by philanthropic sources, whose priorities are usually capricious and oriented toward research or treatment/interventions related to a specific disease or population aggregate. Eligibility for services through these associations is generally limited to the specific disease or population of interest, as with the American Heart Association, March of Dimes, or Susan Komen Foundation. Few direct services are rendered, and these services are approved on individual case considerations. Ancillary healthcare needs such as transportation, parental housing, or wigs may be addressed. Informational and research activities constitute the majority of services provided by these types of organizations. The organizations fund many educational programs that increase awareness of specific diseases, screening procedures, and preventive measures.

An example of a philanthropic national organization designed to provide care for a specific population group is the Shriners Hospitals for Children (http://www.shrinershospitalsforchildren.org). The services and costs related to this care, including transportation, are often provided to the eligible individual free of charge. The only requirement for care is meeting criteria set by the supporting organization.

Some of the private, nonprofit entities or associations that provide philanthropic services include professional associations such as the American Medical Association, the American Dental Association, and the American Nurses Association. Key groups that support research related to health care, healthcare delivery, and policy making are the Robert Wood Johnson Foundation (http://www.RWJF.org), the Kaiser Family Foundation (http://www.KFF.org), and the Pew Charitable Trusts (http://www.Pewtrusts.org). Examples of disease-specific, philanthropic organizations that provide important, patient-focused education, information, and other resources include the American Cancer Society (http://www.Cancer.org), the Alzheimer's Association (http://www.Alz.org), and the American Diabetes Association (http://www.Diabetes.org).

PRIVATE HEALTHCARE INSURANCE
Historical Perspective

During the 1930s, in an effort to provide care and avoid bankruptcy, healthcare providers began to establish **health insurance plans**. One of the most recognizable of these early plans is Blue Cross and Blue Shield. Blue Cross/Blue Shield was instituted by an agreement between Baylor University Hospital in Dallas and the Dallas area public school teachers. Those enrolled in the plan, called *enrollees,* paid a monthly fee for a guarantee of health care. Baylor providers delivered services to the enrollees and collected payment from the health insurance plan. The insurance plan paid fees plus its administrative costs from money collected from the enrollees (Young & Kroth, 2018).

Throughout the Depression and World War II, when prices and wages were frozen, industries began to offer healthcare insurance as a "fringe benefit" to employees. In 1953, as a further employer incentive to offer healthcare coverage to employees, money spent on health insurance was declared tax-exempt. Over the years, workers' union groups began to negotiate for these benefits. With more available financial resources and the patient largely insulated from the costs, healthcare expenditures increased. Further, reimbursement based on operational expenses represented a strong incentive for healthcare expansion (Higgins, 1997). Private, employer-based insurance became the prevailing model in the United States. This persisted even through implementation of Medicare and Medicaid in the mid-1960s. For the most part, until passage and implementation of the ACA, reasons for lack of healthcare insurance were costs, change in employment, or changes in eligibility such as change in marital status or death of spouse or parent. Even though the United States has an employer-based insurance system, only about half (49.6%) of Americans obtain insurance from their place of employment in 2019 (down from more than 54% in 2008) (Kaiser Family Foundation, 2021). Despite provisions from the ACA, smaller businesses typically find it more costly to provide coverage, and many businesses do not provide coverage for part-time employees. Indeed, despite attempts at controlling them, annual insurance premiums (combined worker and employer contributions) in 2020 averaged more than $21,000 for a family (more than $7400 for an individual) (Kaiser Family Foundation, 2020).

Types of Healthcare Plans
The early Blue Cross and Blue Shield plan was an example of an **indemnity plan**. This plan paid all of the costs of covered services provided to the enrollee. The enrollee enjoyed free choice of provider and services. Indemnity plans preserved the enrollee's right of choice and allowed the person to manage his or her own health care. These plans became very costly because there were no incentives for cost containment. Although indemnity plans are still available, the monthly cost of enrollment has increased to exorbitant amounts, making them cost prohibitive. In an effort to support these plans while preserving freedom of choice, mechanisms of cost sharing were introduced. These cost-sharing methods include **copayment**, deductible amounts, and **coinsurance**. All of these methods represented efforts to have the enrollee share in the cost of health care.

As healthcare costs escalated, variations in healthcare insurance plans were developed. Industries and corporations, the major providers of insurance coverage, began to look for a more economical means of providing health care to their employees. Kaiser Permanente decided to assemble their own healthcare programs. They built hospitals, hired physicians, and provided healthcare services to their employees. In an effort to market this concept, Dr. Paul Elwood coined the phrase **HMO** (Higgins, 1997). HMOs were designed to provide more comprehensive care, but this type of program lacks enrollee freedom of choice. In HMO plans, preventive care is covered and encouraged, but specialty care is somewhat restricted, and HMOs are encouraged to reduce costs by providing only the most necessary services. This loss of choice led to a decrease in the popularity of HMOs. In the United States, the number of HMO plans peaked in the mid-1990s, when about 31% of the population was enrolled in them, and they continue to represent a small portion of the plans. In early years, HMOs were considerably less expensive than other insurance plans, but the difference is now relatively small. In 2010, about 19% of enrollees selected HMO plans, but their popularity has continued to decline, as in 2020 only 13% selected HMOs (Kaiser Family Foundation, 2020).

In an effort to compete with the HMO, physicians and hospitals organized the independent practice model (IPM). The IPM was a separate entity that provided services to enrollees of one insurance company. This model evolved into the **PPO**. These types of insurance plans negotiated with healthcare providers for services at a reduced rate in exchange for a guaranteed increase in consumers. A negotiated reimbursement rate allows the cost of the plan to be somewhat controlled. Plan enrollees are offered cost incentives for choosing health care from within the plan's network of healthcare providers. Because they receive a specific amount of reimbursement, regardless of the rendered services, providers have an incentive to be conscious of the costs of the services provided (Young & Kroth, 2018). PPOs are more flexible than HMOs, but to receive full benefits, the covered individual must use network providers. PPOs are somewhat more expensive than HMO plans (about $90/month on average), but they are the most common type of insurance plan in the United States. Although down from 60% of all plans in 2009, in 2020, almost half (48%) of private insurance plans were PPOs.

Point-of-service (POS) plans combine elements of the HMO and the PPO. In POS plans, the covered individual designates an in-network physician as the primary healthcare provider (PCP). If the individual goes outside the network for care, he or she will be responsible for most of the costs unless referred by the PCP. POS plans were common during the early years of the 21st century (about 12% in 2008), but interest dropped off over time. In 2020, about 8% of all insurance plans were POS plans (Kaiser Family Foundation, 2020).

High-deductible health plans (HDHP) began in the early 2000s as a method to involve the consumer in healthcare decisions. The intent was to encourage employees to select plans with lower premiums but more pronounced up-front cost sharing (i.e., higher deductibles). One incentive is to have the healthcare consumer become more involved in healthcare decisions from an economic standpoint and to "shop around" for lower-cost care. Many HDHPs included **health savings accounts (HSAs),** which are tax-free contributions that employees may make to a fund to cover their healthcare expenses (Young & Kroth, 2018). By 2020, HDHPs have become the second most prevalent insurance plan and represent about 31% of all plans in the United States (Kaiser Family Foundation, 2020).

⚕ GENETICS IN PUBLIC HEALTH

Health Insurance and Genetic Discrimination

The National Library of Medicine (2021) explains that "genetic discrimination occurs when people are treated differently by their employer or insurance company because they have a gene mutation that causes or increases the risk of an inherited disorder." Discrimination with respect to hiring or the ability to get health and life insurance is a common concern of people who seek or are offered genetic testing. These fears may keep them from getting genomics-based tests or participating in research to develop new tests or therapies.

There are federal laws specifically designed to protect people against genetic discrimination. The most comprehensive of these is the Genetic Information Nondiscrimination Act (GINA). GINA has been in effect since 2009 and prohibits genetic discrimination by making it illegal for health insurance providers to use or require genetic information to make decisions about a person's insurance eligibility or coverage. GINA also prevents genetic discrimination in employment, because employers are forbidden to use a person's genetic information in hiring or promotion decisions.

It is important to realize that GINA does not extend to those in the US military or those receiving health benefits through the Veterans Health Administration or Indian Health Service. In addition, it does not protect against genetic discrimination for life, disability, or long-term care insurance.

Portions of other laws are also applicable to the prevention of genetic discrimination. Among them are the Health Insurance Portability and Accountability Act, the ACA, and the Americans with Disabilities Act.

Adapted from National Human Genome Research Institute: *Genetic discrimination,* 2021. Available from: https://www.genome.gov/10002077/; U.S. National Library of Medicine: *What is genetic discrimination?* 2021. Available from: https://ghr.nlm.nih.gov/primer/testing/discrimination.

Private Insurance

Costs of private health insurance are staggering, often prohibitively high, even when sharing the costs with employers. There are, of course, millions of Americans who are self-employed or who do not work for a company that provides health insurance

for all employees. This is the group that has been the focus of the ACA's "health exchanges." The health exchanges are the government-regulated marketplace for health insurance plans. Some of the health exchanges were developed and monitored by the individual state after implementation of the ACA, but most states opted to use the federally designed exchange (Shi & Singh, 2019). In the individual marketplace, through the exchanges, individuals can chose between four tiers of standardized plans: bronze, silver, gold, or platinum. Costs of the plans vary based on cost-sharing levels selected and other actuarial factors. Because of the costs, many plans are subsidized through tax credits or other mechanisms (Young & Kroth, 2018).

Reimbursement Mechanisms of Insurance Plans
Retrospective Reimbursement

When insurance plans were initially offered, the customary method of reimbursement was a fee for the service rendered, or retrospective reimbursement. Calculation of the fee was based on the cost of providing the service. Included in this "umbrella" of costs were such things as salaries, supplies, equipment, building depreciation, utilities, and taxes. Cost-based reimbursement encouraged inflated prices and fraud. Physicians were encouraged to overtreat patients, and participants were encouraged to overuse the healthcare system (Shi & Singh, 2019).

Prospective Reimbursement

Prospective reimbursement, or the PPS, a concept derived from the HMO method of payment, was implemented as a financial alternative to cost-based reimbursement. In the PPS, care, no matter what the provider's cost, is reimbursed to hospitals according to a predetermined amount. The federal government introduced this method of reimbursement for Medicare in 1983, and an immediate savings was noted. The prospective reimbursement rates are based on diagnoses and patient characteristics and are designated by the term DRGs. These factors are represented by codes, following the *International Classification of Diseases, 10th Edition,* or ICD-10 (CDC, 2020).

For determination of the prospective amount, Medicare depends on the DRG to calculate the reimbursement. The amount to be paid to the provider is determined according to the client's primary and secondary diagnoses, age, gender, and complications. This amount is deemed adequate compensation for treatment of the client's health issues. If the provider, at first limited to hospitals but later other types of providers, can provide the treatment for less than this amount, a profit is made. If the required services cost more than this amount, then the provider incurs a loss (Young & Kroth, 2018).

Implementation of the PPS led to a reduction in Medicare costs but did not result in overall healthcare cost savings as intended. Hospitals developed **cost shifting** as a means of supplementing the loss of Medicare funding. Private insurance's reimbursement continued to be cost-based. Therefore, hospitals could include the loss from caring for Medicare patients in their cost. Private insurance companies were paying for the cost of providing care to their enrollees and to Medicare patients.

Only a few years after implementation of the PPS by Medicare, private healthcare plans followed the government's lead. In an effort to ensure appropriate reimbursement, more sophisticated methods of calculating the relative cost of health care were developed. **Actuarial classifications** ensured that adequate **premiums** were charged for the projected healthcare needs of those enrolled, and other means of cost control began to emerge. **Managed care groups** negotiated with healthcare providers to render care for a specified amount of reimbursement based on community ratings modified by group-specific demographics. Prospective reimbursement creates incentives to control costs but also leads to instances of undertreatment and underuse of the system.

Similarly, physician services are given **current procedural terminology (CPT) codes.** Coding of the patient's illness determines reimbursement. Specialists in coding, as well as computer programs, are employed by both third-party payers and service providers. Third-party payers' code specialists scrutinize the claims for the appropriate data to support the code. Service provider code specialists are paid to ensure that the code is as accurate as possible to obtain the higher reimbursement. The appropriateness of services is based on the diagnosis code. For example, spirometry is appropriate (reimbursable) when the patient's diagnosis code indicates a variety of pulmonary and nonpulmonary conditions. Specialists in coding can quickly identify these codes, thus increasing payment for services. Physician visits, or CPT codes, are reimbursed on the basis of the documentation of the degree of "medical decision making" and time spent with the patient. Computerized medical record programs increase the ability to ensure that the visit can be reimbursed at the highest rate possible. This development has changed healthcare practices to the utilization of services that are low in costs and higher in reimbursement. High-cost services are limited or are not offered.

Fig. 12.2 illustrates how the nation's healthcare dollar is spent and the sources of funding for key years.

Covered Services

Until implementation of the ACA, insurance plans designated the types of services for which a plan would be financially responsible. When first developed, health insurance was meant to be a means of protecting an individual or family from economic catastrophe should a serious illness occur. Once an employee's fringe benefits included health insurance coverage, expanded benefit packages were developed. The scope of covered services began to widen to include such things as physician's office visits, medication, and dental costs. Unions began to negotiate for such expansion of covered medical services in lieu of additional wages.

When healthcare costs increased, so did the price of enrollment into the insurance plans. Industries began to refuse to pay these higher premium rates. Workers became disgruntled when their employers passed the cost of increased rates to them. To curtail the escalating premium price, insurance companies began to limit the covered services and dictate the conditions under which these services would be covered. Sites of care delivery changed. More treatments were required to be delivered outside the hospital or in ambulatory care clinics or ambulatory surgical centers. The patient was held financially responsible for "uncovered" services. Providers were pressured to comply with these requirements. Providers began to modify the delivery of health care to accommodate for these changes.

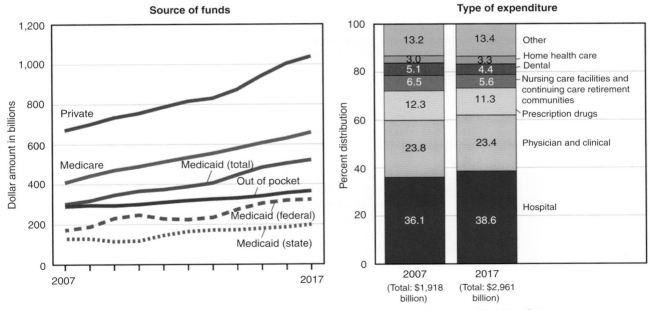

Fig. 12.2 Personal healthcare expenditures: Source of funds/type of expenditure. (Modified from Department of Health and Human Services, Centers for Medicare and Medicaid Services, Office of Actuary, National Health Statistics Group: *Health, United States, 2018—individual charts and tables: spreadsheet, PDF, and PowerPoint files,* 2018. Available from: https://www.cdc.gov/nchs/data/hus/hus18.pdf, p. 23.)

After implementation of the PPS and various managed care options, the rate of hospitalization declined dramatically and the number of outpatient services increased.

All of these changes resulted in conflicts among providers, patients, employers, and the insurance plans, particularly when services deemed necessary by the consumer and provider were denied insurance coverage. Employers looked to the insurance companies to provide healthcare services at a reasonable price. Insurance companies searched for ways to control costs, and providers searched for ways to deliver needed care within the confines of the healthcare policy. Table 12.1 describes some of the advantages and disadvantages of insurance reimbursement plans.

COST CONTAINMENT

Limiting healthcare costs is imperative. All recent presidents have recognized that spiraling healthcare costs have eroded an already suffering economy. The public's increasing demand for care has increased costs, and the costs need to be controlled. This concept is known as **cost containment**. Numerous attempts to control costs have been made over the years, but none has been more than marginally successful.

Historical Perspective of Cost Containment

In addition to implementation of the PPS, health insurers and governmental sources attempted in the mid-1980s to curtail unnecessary proliferation of medical technology by requiring a certificate of need for additions to current healthcare buildings or services. To further reduce use, hospital records were reviewed for the appropriateness of care provided. Admission and treatment of hospitalized patients were reviewed by peer standard review organizations. Physicians and other medical personnel reviewed the hospital records and counseled the attending physician about unnecessary or excessively lengthy stays in the hospital as well as unwarranted services.

ETHICAL INSIGHTS

Cost Containment: How Will You Make Decisions?

You are the gatekeeper meeting with others in your community health organization to determine what services to provide to clients. You have $400,000 to divide among the needs. Who of the following clients will receive the required treatment? Who will not?

- A child with broken leg needs physical therapy (estimated cost: $10,000).
- A 55-year-old man requires knee replacement surgery and physical therapy (estimated cost: $40,000).
- A 76-year-old woman requires hip replacement (estimated cost: $40,000).
- A 32-year-old woman with leukemia requires a bone marrow transplant (estimated cost: $350,000).
- The community clinic needs new equipment for laboratory tests (estimated cost: $60,000).
- There is need for a new nurse who can act as a case manager for patients with complex diseases (estimated cost: $75,000 per year).

Questions to consider:
- How does the American Nurses Association Code of Ethics apply to this case?
- What factors should be considered in the decision?
- How much does the cost of treatment affect the decision?
- How much does the age of the patient affect the decision?
- Is social justice a factor in the decision?

The cost reduction, as a result of prospective payment and other efforts, gave rise to managed care. Unable to shift costs to other entities, and with a predetermined reimbursement rate, providers searched for the most cost-effective mechanism of care provision. Greater ability to predict the cost of care enabled healthcare plans to negotiate the best value for their premiums.

TABLE 12.1 Consumer Advantages and Disadvantages of Insurance Reimbursement Plans

Type	Advantages	Disadvantages
Indemnity	No gatekeeper	High premiums
Fee for service	Unlimited choice of providers	Potential for overuse
	Full access to all services	No incentive for cost containment
Managed care	"Credentialed" providers promote quality assurance	
Health maintenance organization (HMO)	Comprehensive care/primary care provider to oversee all care	Restricted to plan provider except for emergencies
	Lower premium	Potential for lower-quality care to maximize costs
	No or reduced deductibles or copayment	Gatekeeper referral needed to see specialist
Preferred provider organization (PPO)	Greater selection of providers than with HMO	Most expensive premiums
	Expedited provider reimbursement	Additional cost for out-of-plan provider
	Lower premiums	Potential for lower-quality care to maximized costs
Point of service (POS)	More flexibility than HMO	Deductible required
	Comprehensive services with plan	20%–50% copayment for out-of-network services
		Primary care provider referral may be needed for specialized care
High-deductible health plan (HDHP)	Lower deductibles	Higher out of pocket when services are utilized
	Encourages consumer involvement	Must monitor medical expenses to determine when deductible is met
	Often have health savings account to help defray costs	

Current Trends in Cost Containment

The managed care form of healthcare financing changed economic incentives and forced healthcare providers to rethink health management decisions. Treatment recommendations may be tied more to "Can you afford this?" rather than "This is best for you." Costs of the service rendered, rather than enhancement of revenue through service provision, must be considered. These economic or cost-containment incentives can be divided into the following broad categories: **capitated reimbursement**, access limitation, and rationing.

Capitated Reimbursement

The growing visibility of managed care models and their associated success in cost containment through the use of prospective reimbursement to influence provider practice gave rise to various arrangements that link healthcare financing to service delivery such as managed care. Managed care organizations create partnerships with healthcare providers using financial incentives to prevent overuse. Statistical norms, practice parameters, and population data determine the capitated, or maximum, payment for services. This is the maximum reimbursement amount that the healthcare provider will receive for the provision of care. The actual cost of provision of care does not affect the reimbursement. Healthcare providers must provide appropriate medical care while being cognizant of healthcare costs. As a reward for conservative practices, healthcare providers may receive a specified amount of money or a percentage of the agreed reimbursement if services are delivered below the limit set by the third-party payer. Providers whose services are inadequate or exceed this limit may be excluded from the network.

RESEARCH HIGHLIGHTS

Hospital Readmissions From Home Health Care Before and After Change to Prospective Payment System.

In an effort to control the Medicare home health expenditure, home health reimbursement was changed from a fee-for-service system to a PPS. This changed the reimbursement from a per-visit fee to episodes of care. Each episode of care begins on the first billable day and proceeds for a period of 60 days. Reimbursement is based on the diagnosis and type and level of care predicted to be required.

Through the use of a comprehensive evaluative tool, the Outcome and Assessment Information Set, a client is placed in a home health resource group (HHRG). Payment for services is based on the HHRG. Another important factor is that payment is received in two parts: 60% at the start of care and 40% after the episode of care is completed. Adjustments in final payment are made according to changes in the client's condition and may result in more or less than anticipated.

Anderson and colleagues (2005) studied unplanned hospital readmissions, which are an aspect of adverse change in patient condition or outcome. This study was designed to compare characteristics of clients rehospitalized during home health care before and after the institution of PPS.

The researchers determined that it was difficult to conclude whether PPS has any negative effect on home healthcare patient outcomes. Post-PPS clients were judged to be sicker at the time of rehospitalization and were almost twice as likely to be readmitted for another diagnosis. The investigators concluded that, since the institution of PPS, the hospital length of stay has decreased, with the result that clients are sicker at time of discharge.

The study shows that the first 2 weeks after hospital discharge are the most critical. Payments for home health services are suspended at the time of readmission, pending a client's return to home health care after rehospitalization. If the client does not return to home health care and the agency has completed five visits, 60% of the payment will awarded. If the agency has not completed the five visits, only 11% of the amount will be awarded. This arrangement might serve as an incentive for agencies to increase the number of visits after the initial hospital discharge but not after the second discharge.

Data from Anderson MA, Clarke MM, Helms LB, et al: Hospital readmission from home health care before and after prospective payment, *J Nurs Scholarsh* 37(1):73–79, 2005.

Cost Containment Through Access Limitation

All third-party payers, or insurance plans, control access to health care through designation of covered services. Managed care organizations designate the type of covered services and specify the conditions under which the service is covered. Some services may only be accessed upon approval or referral from physicians who are used as **gatekeepers**. The enrollee must choose a **primary care provider** and consult this provider for a referral before seeking specialty services. Without this referral, the enrollee is financially responsible for the service. Even with the referral, choices may be limited to the providers who have contracted with the managed care plan.

Managed care plans may require that less costly healthcare modalities or medications be used. Exceptions to these modalities require justification. More technologically advanced and expensive treatments may be accessed under the most stringent conditions. Preauthorization requirements determine the medical necessity of the service. The process is so complex that the client may not be aware that the service is not covered until the reimbursement for the service is denied.

Cost Containment Through "Transparency"

The major impact of the ACA is directed toward increasing access to health care through promoting health insurance coverage, but the Act has had limited impact on reducing the costs of care. Unlike other goods and services, the costs of health care typically depend on a patients' insurance, deductibles and coinsurance, and whether a hospital and/or physician is in or out of the insurance plan's network. One method to help curtail costs that has been widely proposed and recently accepted is to promote "price transparency." Emphasis on transparency is founded on the reality that healthcare costs—particularly in acute care settings—are negotiated between the institutions and insurance companies, and are "hidden" from consumers. Indeed, until they are billed, patients have very little—if any—access to information related to the cost for their care (Miller et al., 2020; CMS, 2020a,b).

In 2019, President Trump issued an Executive Order (EO 13877) requiring hospitals to disclose charges for procedures, tests, drugs, and other services or items they anticipate will be charged to patients or their insurance companies (Miller et al., 2020). The rule also dictates that information must be posted and available in a format that is easy to access and understand on the hospital's website. Further, the rule mandates that physicians, institutions, and insurers inform patients of anticipated out of pocket costs before providing care (Wilensky, 2019). It is anticipated that when fully implemented in 2023, the rule will provide patients with real-time price information and access to "shopping tools" that will allow them to see negotiated rates and to compare costs for procedures, drugs, and other services and supplies (CMS, 2020a,b).

One of the expected benefits of emphasis on price transparency is that easy access to information will increase competition among providers, and ultimately reduce costs. While potential cost saving benefits and consumer choice can be anticipated, concerns have been mentioned. One such concern is that patients will focus more on cost than on quality when selecting a source for care, or might even forgo care completely when confronted with the anticipated fees. Despite concerns, there is widespread agreement that the initiative will be helpful in both stemming costs and empowering patients in decision-making (Miller et al., 2020).

Cost Containment Through Rationing

Rationing is best described as determining the most appropriate use of health care or directing the health care where it can do the most good. Clinical Example 12.1 dramatizes the problem.

Clinical Example 12.1

A middle-aged woman was diagnosed with ovarian cancer. She was covered by Medicaid, lived alone in subsidized housing, and had a distant relative in another state. After surgery some years ago, she used home health services through the city home health agency. After conventional and high-dose chemotherapy failed, her physician recommended autologous bone marrow transplantation, which was considered experimental at the time. The procedure was approved and performed. Medical costs exceeded $200,000, but the patient died 2 months later.

Was the treatment in the Clinical Example a wise use of medical resources? Health care is not an exact science; too many variables exist. What appears to be the best course of action for one is not the best course of action for another. Making accurate treatment decisions is difficult, and the ramifications of a mistake are great. Complex socioeconomic factors also must be considered. Healthcare providers and third-party payers, including the federal government, are currently investigating the **outcomes** of healthcare practices to determine what methods, if any, can be instituted to improve the accuracy of these choices. Research into the area of treatment outcomes has led to major changes in treatments, many of which are quite costly. This situation presents a dilemma when decisions must be made as to their use.

TRENDS IN HEALTH FINANCING

The public's demand for affordable health care has created a new environment for healthcare financing. The ACA changed a number of things, particularly with respect to eligibility for Medicaid and regarding what is included in health insurance plans. Indeed, one of the significant elements of the ACA was the inclusion of the essential health benefits that must be covered in plans offered in the exchanges. Among the essential benefits are ambulatory care, emergency services, hospitalization, pregnancy/maternity and newborn care, mental health and substance use disorder services, and preventive care (healthcare.gov, 2021). It has been argued that requiring everyone to purchase all of these benefits has resulted in increasing the costs for all, even if the purchaser does not want or need the benefit.

Competition among healthcare providers and third-party payers has led to new and innovative health care. Outpatient services, patient education packages, electronic health records, and telehealth are just a few of these innovations. Increased competition has required insurance plans to be sensitive to the needs of the employee organizations and their enrollees. Individualized plans of covered services can be created. Enrollees can choose the plan that provides them with the services they desire at a selected cost. Healthcare providers advertise to ensure that the consumer selects an insurance plan that includes their services. Some providers, such as hospitals, campaign for inclusion in a plan.

Despite implementation of the ACA, along with the other measures described here, healthcare costs have continued to increase. Major changes are still needed, and indeed inevitable, as the status quo is not sustainable. Although more Americans have health insurance now than before implementation of the ACA, the costs of both insurance and of health care per se have continued to rise (Shi & Singh, 2019; Young & Kroth, 2018). Coupled with concerns over evolving demographics (i.e., aging of the Baby Boomers and resultant expansion of Medicare costs) as well as ongoing issues following the COVID-19 pandemic, it is apparent that more policy changes and interventions need to take place. Some of the more commonly described are mentioned here.

Cost Sharing

Aware of the amount that the employer is willing to contribute for basic coverage, a third-party payer or insurance plan may propose several options, giving the employee freedom to choose services desired. Employees willing to pay may be able to increase the covered services not provided by the basic plan. This arrangement is known as *cost sharing*. Cost sharing may also require the consumer to pay a greater portion of the bill for covered services in return for lower premiums. Enrollees may opt to pay a higher premium for the freedom to choose providers, or elimination of the gatekeeper. This can result in increased consumer control of health care.

Healthcare Alliances

The creation of powerful regional or statewide insurance purchasing pools, or health alliances, is seen as one of the means of reform for the healthcare industry. The alliance would define basic benefits that all insurers would have to offer to everyone at the same price, regardless of health status. These alliances would not regulate insurance prices. Health alliances would collect premiums and help consumers choose among competing insurers and plans. The consumer's choice would be based on published, simple, standard information about benefits and outcomes of the different available plans. Plans would have to compete by offering better outcomes or lower cost. Insurers would have to contract with providers who find ways of delivering cost-efficient care. Medicare is currently participating in healthcare alliances. Enrollees are given a choice between traditional Medicare, Parts A and B, and Medicare Advantage.

Self-Insurance

Many organizations, such as large companies and governmental entities (e.g., school districts or municipalities), have used healthcare information collected by insurance plans to self-insure their employees. This development has enabled industries and other types of organizations to reduce the administrative cost of insurance. Unlike the large industrial HMOs, self-insured status organizations administer their own healthcare plan and purchase healthcare services from an established insurance plan. In these cases, the organizations or businesses are relying on a healthy employee population that will require less health care. The organization or business that uses self-insurance takes a risk and needs to ensure that it can cover any major costs. Healthcare reform will require that there be sufficient funds to cover these costs.

Health Savings Accounts and Flexible Spending Accounts

Another source of funding for uncovered services is the HSA (mentioned earlier) and the **flexible spending account (FSA)**. Both are set up during insurance determination by the employee. With both the HSA and the FSA, the employee determines how much he or she will have to spend for uncovered services and arranges to have this amount deducted from his or her paycheck; these monies are "pretax." When these services are incurred, the employee pays for them with this account. There are some differences between the two types of accounts. First, the HSA is associated with high-deductible health plans (HDHP) and the funds are "owned" by the employee. In contrast, the FSA is set up by the employer through any health insurance plan and is "owned" by the employer. For the FSA, the employee continues to pay into the account until the estimated amount is reached. If the employee overestimates the cost, the remaining amount is forfeited. For HSAs, both the employer and employee contribute to the fund, and the balance does not expire (i.e., unused amounts will remain in the account to be used in subsequent years). Finally, there are limits to the amount of pretaxed funds that can be put into each account. In 2020, FSAs were limited to $2,750; contributions to HSAs were limited to $7,100 for a family with an HDHP.

Reimbursement for Health Promotion and Disease Prevention Initiatives

Unfortunately, until recent years, reimbursement for health promotion and disease prevention has been limited. Whereas, most health insurance plans, both private and public, pay for screening procedures, funding or reimbursement for treatment modalities such as support groups for smoking cessation, home safety evaluation, and relaxation techniques has been sporadic. Obesity is one of this nation's most common health problems, yet the costs of weight loss programs are rarely reimbursed.

Research into barriers and facilitators to changes in lifestyle continues to be funded well below curative treatment research. Lifestyle change interventions are slow to be developed and even more difficult to implement and evaluate. Mandated services required by the ACA include such preventive services as counseling for management of obesity, prevention of sexually transmitted diseases, and tobacco cessation. Until these types of interventions are directly financed, they most likely will not become widely implemented. With the rise in obesity there have been state proposals, and some have been initiated, to incentivize healthy eating habits, such as taxing the sale of sodas and putting calorie counts on restaurant menus. This type of approach relies heavily on policy and subsequent legislation and causes some people to protest because they consider it invasion of their personal decisions. Many businesses, such as restaurants and large fast-food chains, have added calorie and nutritional information to their menus.

Protection from "Surprise" Medical Bills

As mentioned, health insurance plans are typically comprised of a collection of "in network" providers—both physicians and hospitals/clinics—with whom the insurance company has negotiated contracts for reduced rates for services. "**Surprise billing**" occurs when a patient receives a large bill from an "out-of-network" physician, clinic, or hospital. Often this situation occurs with emergencies, when the patient must go to the nearest hospital, or when out-of-network clinicians practice within an in-network facility, but the patient does not have an option for selecting that clinician. For example, if a patient has heart surgery at an insurance-approved hospital, with an in-network surgeon, but the anesthesiologist, surgical assistant, pathologist, or radiologist, is out of network (Colla, 2021). One recent report notes that almost 20% of insured adults received a surprise bill during the last 2 years and two-thirds of adults are worried about being able to afford unexpected medical bills (Politz et al., 2020).

Solutions to surprise billing have been implemented in most states, but wide-spread federal regulations have been lacking. The "No Surprises Act" was signed into law in December of 2020 (H.R. 133—within the Consolidated Appropriations Act), and should be fully implemented by the end of 2021 (KFF, 2021). This law protects consumers from the cost of unanticipated, out-of-network medical bills passed to patients who receive emergency care, including air ambulance services. Per the Act, providers are not allowed to bill patients beyond the applicable in-network cost sharing rates. The No Surprises Act dictates that providers must bill the in-network rate for all charges, whether or not they are treated in an in-network faculty. It also outlines measures for implementation of the provisions and arbitration for disputes.

> ## ❓ ACTIVE LEARNING
>
> 1. Evaluate a family's healthcare coverage. Investigate the type of coverage and the ability of this coverage type to meet the needs of the family. Would another type of insurance coverage meet more of the family's needs? What prohibits their ability to obtain this coverage?
> 2. Interview public health nurses employed in a public health department about their perception of funding for health promotion/disease prevention.

HEALTHCARE FINANCING REFORM

It was estimated that in 2011, before implementation of the ACA, about 44 million (18%) of nonelderly Americans were uninsured (Kaiser Family Foundation, 2019). Underinsurance, likewise, has been a problem, as the underinsured cannot fully cover their health needs. Certain racial/ethnic groups have higher rates for both uninsurance and underinsurance. The ranking of such groups from highest to lowest rate of noninsurance is Hispanic, black/non-Hispanic, Asian, multiracial, and white/non-Hispanic (Kaiser Family Foundation, 2019). After implementation of many provisions of the ACA, by 2016 8 more than 17 million additional people had obtained healthcare coverage, dropping the percentage of uninsured Americans to about 10% (Kaiser Family Foundation, 2019).

Lack of insurance is the major factor associated with lack of access to medical care. Uninsured adults are more than three times as likely as insured adults to go without needed medical care (NCHS, 2018).

The National Academy of Medicine (NAM), formerly called the Institute of Medicine (2012), notes that health literacy and communication will be key factors in success as consumers try to figure out the key elements of the ACA and to use the exchanges to obtain insurance if their employers are not providing this information directly. The success of this process will affect access to health care.

Access to Health Care

Access to health care is a complex situation that is defined by the circumstances of the individual. The primary concern is inadequate access to health care, which leads to unnecessary illness. Most Americans want to believe that the best possible health care will be available for them and their family members at any time, regardless of their age, sex, race, or ability to pay. Anything that obstructs this pursuit can be considered a barrier to health care.

Financial support for health care, through either private insurance coverage or participation in government programs, is the mechanism that is largely responsible for access. Lack of a source for healthcare financing due to lack of insurance coverage, preexisting conditions, unapproved care, and physicians who do not participate in the health plan available to the patient represent the most common factors attributed to difficulty in obtaining care. Other impediments to healthcare access are physical barriers, including structural inaccessibility, lack of appropriate equipment, hours of operation, convenient transportation, inadequate services when needed, and inability to communicate.

Inequality in the distribution of healthcare services represents another type of physical barrier. Even those with insurance coverage may be unable to locate participating healthcare providers. Opportunities to seek health care, especially preventive health care, during work hours is often discouraged by employers, although this situation is gradually changing as some employers recognize that preventive care can reduce overall costs. Rural areas and inner cities have been recognized as medically underserved for many years. Government incentives for increasing available medical services in these areas have not solved the problem.

Sociological barriers to healthcare access exist among poor and ethnic Americans. Poor outpatient diagnosis and treatment, increased use of emergency departments for primary care, and reluctance to hospitalize are possible explanations. Language and fear of reprisals have become important sociological barriers. Many of the poor and uninsured are illegal aliens, and seeking medical attention, even during illnesses, may have severe repercussions. Disparities are discussed later in the text.

Historical Perspective

National health insurance is not a new concept. European countries began a social model of health insurance in the early 1900s. In 1916, President Theodore Roosevelt advocated enactment of a form of national medical coverage. President Franklin Roosevelt wanted national health insurance to be part of the Social Security Act of 1935, but that provision did not pass (Higgins, 1997). During the administration of President Lyndon Johnson, however, a modified form of national health insurance, Medicare and Medicaid, was instituted.

Before the 1930s, most Americans were uninsured. Most healthcare providers considered it their duty to donate time and services to charity. Hospitals and clinics maintained charity wards. Society believed that those who could, and those who could not, should help themselves. The enactment of governmental entitlement programs, coupled with the availability of healthcare insurance as a benefit of one's occupation, helped change this belief. Quickly, the pervasive societal view was that those who could not help themselves should get government assistance or go to work (Higgins, 1997).

As discussed previously, in the 1960s Medicare and Medicaid brought about national health insurance coverage for older adults, the disabled, and those living below the poverty level—particularly children. Expansion of Medicaid with CHIP in the 1990s expanded care coverage for children of the "working poor," or those whose employers did not provide insurance.

Efforts to address access to health care reemerged in the 1990s, when Bill Clinton attempted to reform the healthcare system, ensure coverage, and reduce healthcare costs. The initiative was headed by Hillary Clinton, but after about a year of debate and numerous proposals, the Clinton plan failed to reach a consensus. This was attributed to widespread opposition from various healthcare provider groups and organizations as well as lack of public support. Continuing rising costs combined with eroding access through the early 2000s contributed to the election of Barak Obama and a new mandate to enact healthcare reform. After considerable debate, Congress passed the Patient Protection and Affordable Care Act (PL 111-148), also known as the *Affordable Care Act,* which was signed into law, March 23, 2010. Although the ACA did not ensure "universal coverage," it was originally estimated that when fully implemented, an additional 32 million people would have access to health insurance coverage (Kaiser Family Foundation, 2013).

The ACA was an extremely complex piece of legislation, and the final version of the bill exceeded 2000 pages. Among the law's provisions are mandating that all citizens obtain health insurance, expanding Medicaid eligibility, subsidizing insurance premiums for low-income purchasers, prohibiting denial of coverage for preexisting conditions, and establishing health insurance exchanges. Costs for expansion of coverage and subsidies would be offset by a combination of taxes and fees, reduction in payments for Medicare and Medicaid services and prescription drugs, and enhanced efforts to reduce Medicare fraud and abuse. Box 12.3 outlines some of the major provisions covered in the ACA.

The ACA remains highly controversial, and additional legislative and legal challenges are anticipated. All healthcare providers and consumers should remain alert to both short- and long-term changes. Additional information about the ACA can be found in Chapters 10 and 11.

? ACTIVE LEARNING

1. Learn more about changes in healthcare reimbursement due to healthcare reform by visiting https://www.cms.gov/cciio/index.html. This CMS website is the Center for Consumer Information and Insurance Oversight. What type of information is provided? What is the value of this information to consumers?
2. Investigate the ACA from the points of view of the consumer, healthcare provider, and third-party payer and community health. How has it affected the concerns of each of these constituents? What more needs to be done?
3. Examine the status of healthcare reform implementation in your state. How has the community been informed about changes? Has this been effective? How is it affecting community health in your state?

Societal Perceptions

Health care for all is a concept that most Americans support. Most people state that health care should be one of those necessities available to all without consideration of what it costs; however, when discussion turns to actually doing this, most people become concerned about the implications. Efforts to

---

BOX 12.3 Key Provisions of the Patient Protection and Affordable Care Act (PL 111-148)

Individual Mandate—Requires US citizens and legal residents to have qualifying health coverage.

Employer Requirements—Requires employers with more than 50 employees to offer coverage or vouchers for full-time employees; requires employers with more than 200 employees to enroll employees into health insurance plans offered by the employer.

Expansion of Medicaid—Expands Medicaid to all individuals under age 65 with incomes up to 133% of the federal poverty line.

Expansion of CHIP—Requires states to maintain current income eligibility levels for children enrolled in the Children's Health Insurance Plan (CHIP) until 2019.

Premium and Cost-Sharing Subsidies to Individuals—Creates insurance exchanges to provide premium credits and subsidies to individuals and families with incomes between 133% and 400% of the federal poverty level.

Changes to Private Insurance—Establishes a temporary national high-risk pool to provide health coverage to individuals with preexisting medical conditions; establishes a process for reviewing increases in health plan premiums and requires justification of increases; provides dependent coverage for children up to age 26 years for all individual and group policies; prohibits health plans from placing lifetime limits on the dollar amount of coverage and from rescinding coverage; establishes a website to help residents identify health coverage options; permits states to form healthcare choice compacts and allow insurers to sell policies in any state participating in the compacts.

Cost Containment Provisions—Requires rules to simplify health insurance administration by adopting a single set of rules for payment, verification, and claims status; restructures payments to Medicare Advantage plans; reduces waste, fraud, and abuse in public programs by allowing providers to have screening-enhanced oversight periods for new providers and suppliers; increases penalties for submitting false claims.

Prevention and Wellness—Improves prevention by covering preventive services and eliminating cost sharing for preventive services in Medicare and Medicaid; requires qualified health plans to provide preventive services, recommended immunizations, preventive care for infants, children, and adolescents, and additional preventive care and screening for women; provides grants for small employers who establish wellness programs; requires chain restaurants and foods sold from vending machines to disclose the nutritional content of each item.

Modified from The Henry, J. Kaiser Family Foundation: *Summary of Coverage provisions in the Patient Protection and Affordable Care Act,* 2013. Available from: http://www.kff.org/health-costs/issue-brief/summary-of-coverage-provisions-in-the-patient/.

---

provide universal coverage through increased governmental involvement in health care have failed because of a number of factors, including rejection of much higher taxes, objection to paying for care for noncitizens, concerns over access and availability, and fears of rationing.

The ongoing dilemma is how to provide health care to all Americans in a way that is acceptable and affordable. Other countries provide their citizens with universal health care, but there are aspects of this care that are unpopular with US society. The most concerning or pressing problem relates to funding sources, because significant tax increases would be necessary to provide coverage for all. Furthermore, the United States already spends much more of our resources on health care than any other country; adding more costs is enormously concerning.

Furthermore, waiting several months for nonemergency treatment, lack of choice of treatment, and inaccessibility or unavailability of diagnostic and treatment modalities are not acceptable to most Americans. Indeed, most Americans want assurance that all of the healthcare services that they and their families need, now and in the future, will be available no matter what the condition, age of the patient, job status, or ability to pay. The debate and measures to address the problem of health care financing are ongoing. All nurses—and citizens—need to become familiar with the issues.

ROLES OF THE PUBLIC HEALTH NURSE IN THE ECONOMICS OF HEALTH CARE

Researcher

Nurses need to be engaged in research about the provision of efficient, cost-effective health care. Nurses are in a pivotal role to investigate culturally sensitive treatment modalities, health education, disease prevention, and factors to change behaviors. Health promotion and disease prevention are more cost effective than curative treatment modalities. Public health nurse researchers need to investigate, develop, and evaluate the effectiveness of health promotion and disease prevention. Research on health promotion intervention outcomes, program cost/benefit analysis, and health informatics are just a few of these areas.

Educator

Health education is the foundation of public health nursing practice. Public health nurses agree that knowledge empowers clients to actively participate in their health care. Funding for this education is provided primarily through public, governmental entities (e.g., schools). Educational plans for individuals are rare. In the area of healthcare economics, the nurse needs to demonstrate the value of this education. Outcome measures for health education need to be established.

Provider of Care

Any service delivered by the nurse needs to be appropriate, necessary, and cost effective. Nurses in all areas of practice need to be cost-conscious. Judicious application of the nursing process is imperative. An accurate assessment is the foundation for an appropriate nursing diagnosis. Goals for care, jointly established between members of the community and the community health nurse, will guide the choice of interventions. Evaluation, using previously developed outcome measures, will lead to appropriate modifications of the plan.

Nurses can serve as program service providers, health education providers, and health program participants. Nurses need to participate in the grant proposal process, design, and evaluation for these programs. They need to be familiar with and participate in the statistical information gathering process that serves as the basis for determining community health need.

Advocate

Nurses must become more involved in the economics of health care. Too often, nurses are cognizant of the effects of changes in healthcare economics but feel powerless to act. Increasing knowledge of healthcare funding and policy making will empower nurses to advocate for the type of funding that provides appropriate care to obtain the greatest good. The large number of nurses gives our occupation potential political clout. Nurses need to utilize this political power to influence healthcare funding. Nurses need to advocate for increase in health promotion/disease prevention funding from both public and private sectors. Nurses need to plan programs, seek funding, and evaluate program effectiveness through outcome measures. Nurses need to constantly seek sources of funding for health programs through any available sources.

BEST CARE AT LOWER COST

In 2012, the NAM published a report entitled *Best Care at Lower Cost: The Path to Continuously Learning Health Care in America.* Building on its earlier work in relation to quality care (discussed in Chapter 11), the NAM was asked to examine a critical concern.

> *Health care in America presents a fundamental paradox. The past 50 years have seen an explosion in biomedical knowledge, dramatic innovation in therapies and surgical procedures, and management of conditions that previously were fatal, with ever more exciting clinical capabilities on the horizon. Yet, American health care is falling short on basic dimensions of quality, outcomes, costs, and equity.*
>
> ***IOM (2013, p. 1)***

Among the factors that are pushing this examination is the fact that there is an estimated $750 billion waste of resources in the healthcare system, meaning that the United States loses this amount of money that could be spent on improved healthcare outcomes. We need best care at lower cost, not higher cost. Compared with other countries, the United States is paying more for less poorer outcomes. The system has to manage the complexity that continues to grow and at the same time slow down ever-escalating costs. Citizens want quality care that is evidence based, but the system is not managing this well.

❓ ACTIVE LEARNING

In small groups review, the Institute of Medicine report *U.S. Health in International Perspective: Shorter Lives, Poorer Health* (2013). Divide up the content. Discuss this report from perspectives of the healthcare delivery system, quality care, diversity, and cost of care. The report is fully accessible and can be downloaded from https://www.ncbi.nlm.nih.gov/books/NBK115854/pdf/Bookshelf_NBK115854.pdf https://www.ncbi.nlm.nih.gov/pubmed/24006554 https://www.nap.edu/catalog/13497/us-health-in-international-perspective-shorter-lives-poorer-health.

SUMMARY

Healthcare economics is influencing healthcare practice at all levels. Nurses in the community must become aware of the economics of health care to practice in this new era. Patient outcomes are quickly being seen as a measurement for healthcare financing. As the healthcare system evolves toward health promotion and disease prevention, nursing will play a pivotal role. Public health nurses, whose domain of practice has encompassed these areas, will be in the forefront of this change. This chapter has presented the basics of healthcare economics and its importance in providing effective, quality care in all settings, including the community. An understanding of these elements is essential to the practice of nursing. This is an extremely complex subject with innovations and changes coming every day. To be effective, the nurse must be attentive to these developments.

EVOLVE WEBSITE

http://evolve.elsevier.com/Nies/community
- NCLEX Review Questions
- Case Studies

BIBLIOGRAPHY

Centers for Disease Control and Prevention (CDC): *International classification of diseases, tenth revision, (ICD-10)*, 2020. Available from: https://www.cdc.gov/nchs/icd/icd10.htm.

Centers for Medicare and Medicaid Services (CMS): *Chronic conditions among medicare beneficiaries*, 2012. Available from: https://www.cms.gov/Research-Statistics-Data-and-Systems/Statistics-Trends-and-Reports/Chronic-Conditions/Downloads/2012Chartbook.pdf.

Centers for Medicare and Medicaid Services (CMS): *CMS completes historic price transparency initiative*, 2020a. Available from: https://www.cms.gov/newsroom/press-releases/cms-completes-historic-price-transparency-initiative.

Centers for Medicare and Medicaid Services (CMS): *National health expenditure fact sheet, 2019*, 2020b. https://www.cms.gov/Research-Statistics-Data-and-Systems/Statistics-Trends-and-Reports/NationalHealthExpendData/NHE-Fact-Sheet.

Centers for Medicare and Medicaid Services (CMS): *Medicare and you*, 2021a. Available from: https://www.medicare.gov/sites/default/files/2020-12/10050-Medicare-and-You_0.pdf.

Centers for Medicare and Medicaid Services (CMS): *Part B costs*, 2021b. Available from: https://www.medicare.gov/your-medicare-costs/part-b-costs.

Centers for Medicare and Medicaid Services (CMS): *Medicaid benefits*, 2021c. Available from: https://www.medicaid.gov/medicaid/benefits/index.html.

Centers for Medicare and Medicaid Services: *Medicare fraud: detection and prevention tips*, 2021d. Available from: https://www.medicare.gov/forms-help-resources/help-fight-medicare-fraud/tips-prevent-fraud.

Colla C: Surprise billing—a flashpoint for major policy issues in health care, *JAMA* 325(8):715–716, 2021.

Federal Bureau of Investigation: *Health care fraud*, 2021. Available from: https://www.fbi.gov/investigate/white-collar-crime/health-care-fraud.

Fineberg H: A successful and sustainable health care system—how to get there from here, *N Engl J Med* 366:1020–1027, 2012.

Harvard Medical School: The numbers game: risk factors, lifestyle andlongevity, *Harv Mens Health Watch* 13(8), 2009.

Healthcare.gov: *What marketplace health insurance plans cover*, 2021. Available from: https://www.healthcare.gov/coverage/.

Higgins W: How did we get this way? *Health Care Econ* 11(35), 1997.

Infante M, McAnaney K: Home health agencies can avoid fraud charges with compliance plans, *Hosp Home Health* 21(5):49–51, 2004.

Institute of Medicine: *The role of telehealth in an evolving health care environment: a workshop summary*, Washington, DC, 2012, National Academies Press.

Institute of Medicine: *Best care at lower cost: the path to continuously learning health care in America*, Washington, DC, 2012, National Academies Press. Available from: http://nationalacademies.org/hmd/reports/2012/best-care-at-lower-cost-the-path-to-continuously-learning-health-care-in-america.aspx.

Institute of Medicine (IOM): *Facilitating state health exchange communication through the use of health literate practices: workshop summary*, Washington, DC, 2013, National Academies Press.

Kaiser Family Foundation: *Summary of the affordable care act*, 2013. Available from: http://www.kff.org/health-reform/fact-sheet/summary-of-the-affordable-care-act/.

Kaiser Family Foundation: *The uninsured: a primer*, 2019. Available from: https://www.kff.org/uninsured/report/the-uninsured-and-the-aca-a-primer-key-facts-about-health-insurance-and-the-uninsured-amidst-changes-to-the-affordable-care-act/.

Kaiser Family Foundation: *Employer medical benefits*, 2020. Annual survey. Available from: http://files.kff.org/attachment/Report-Employer-Health-Benefits-2020-Annual-Survey.pdf.

Kaiser Family Foundation: *Health insurance coverage of the total population*, 2021. Available from: www.kff.org/other/state-indicator/total-population/?currentTimeframe=0&sortModel=%7B%22colId%22:%22Location%22,%22sort%22:%22asc%22%7D.

Kaiser Family Foundation (KFF): *Status of state medicaid expansion decisions: interactive map*, 2021a. Available from: https://www.kff.org/medicaid/issue-brief/status-of-state-medicaid-expansion-decisions-interactive-map/.

Kaiser Family Foundation (KFF): *Surprise medical bills: new protections for consumers take effect in 2022*, 2021b. Available from: https://www.kff.org/private-insurance/fact-sheet/surprise-medical-bills-new-protections-for-consumers-take-effect-in-2022/.

Miller BJ, Mandelberg Mc, Griffith NC, Ehrenfeld JM: Price transparency: empowering patient choice and promoting provider competition, *J Med Syst* 44:80, 2020.

Momanyi B: *Blue cross and blue shield of texas handbook of texas online*, 2021, Texas State Historical Association. https://www.tshaonline.org/handbook/entries/blue-cross-and-blue-shield-of-texas; www.tshaonline.org/handbook/online/articles/djbcz. Accessed February 24, 2021.

National Center for Health Statistics: *Health. United States*, 2018. Available from: https://www.cdc.gov/nchs/data/hus/hus18.pdf.

National Health Care Anti-Fraud Association: *Health care fraud: a serious and costly reality for all Americans*, 2021. Available from: https://www.nhcaa.org/tools-insights/about-health-care-fraud/the-challenge-of-health-care-fraud/.

NIH News. NIH-supported study finds U.S. Dementia care costs as high as $215 billion in 2010, April 3, 2013. Available from: http://www.nih.gov/news/health/apr2013/nia-03.htm.

Organization for Economic Co-operation and Development (OECD): *OCED health statistics 2020*, 2021. Available from: http://www.oecd.org/health/health-data.htm.

Politz K, Loopes L, Kearney A, et al.: U.S. statistics on surprise medical billing, *JAMA* 323(6):498, 2020.

Shi L, Singh DA: *Delivering health care in America: a systems approach*, ed 7, Burlington, MA, 2019, Jones & Bartlett Learning.

Sloan T: Consumer-driven to nowhere: study throws cold water on recent efforts to beat health care cost inflation, *Mod Healthcare* 34(49):21, 2004.

Statista: *Share of old age population (65 years and older) in the total U.S. population*, 2021. Available from: https://www.statista.com/statistics/457822/share-of-old-age-population-in-the-total-us-population/

#:∼:text=In%202019%2C%20about%2016.5%20percent,population%20was%2065%20or%20over.

U.S. Department of Health and Human Services (USDHHS): *HHS grants*, 2021. Available from: https://www.hhs.gov/grants/grants/index.html.

U.S. Department of Health and Human Services/Office of Inspector General (HHS/OIG): *Health care fraud and abuse control program report for fiscal year 2019*, 2020. https://oig.hhs.gov/publications/docs/hcfac/FY2019-hcfac.pdf.

Wilensky G: Federal government increases focus on price transparency, *JAMA* 322(1):916–917, 2019.

Young KM, Kroth PJ: *Shultz & Young's health care USA: understanding its organization and delivery*, ed 9, Burlington, MA, 2018, Jones & Bartlett Leaning.

13

Cultural Diversity and Community Health Nursing

Christina N. DesOrmeaux, and Anitra Frederick

OBJECTIVES

Upon completion of this chapter, the reader will be able to do the following:

1. Critically analyze racial and cultural diversity in the United States.
2. Analyze the influence of sociocultural, political, economic, ethical, and religious factors that influence

the health of culturally diverse individuals, groups, and communities.

3. Identify the cultural aspects of nursing care for culturally diverse individuals, groups, and communities.
4. Apply the principles of transcultural nursing to community health nursing practice.

OUTLINE

KEY TERMS

biomedical
cultural competence
cultural imposition
cultural negotiation
cultural stereotyping

culture
culture-bound syndrome
culture shock
culture specific
culture universal

culturological assessment
dominant value orientation
ethnocentrism
Leininger's theory of culture care diversity and universality

magicoreligious
naturalistic
norms
poverty

religion
socioeconomic status
spirituality
subculture

transcultural nursing
value
yin-yang theory

CULTURAL DIVERSITY

Cultural diversity is a multifaceted and complex concept that refers to the differences among people, especially those related to values, attitudes, beliefs, norms, behaviors, customs, and ways of living. It is essential that all nurses understand how cultural groups view life processes, how cultural groups define health and illness, how healers cure and care for members of their respective cultural groups, and how the cultural background of the nurse influences the way in which care is delivered. Nurses in community health settings also need to understand the diversity or differences that occur in families, groups, neighborhoods, communities, and public and community healthcare organizations.

TRANSCULTURAL PERSPECTIVES ON COMMUNITY HEALTH NURSING

Nurses' knowledge of culture and cultural concepts improves the health of the community by enhancing their ability to provide culturally competent care. **Cultural competence** is respecting and understanding the values and beliefs of a certain cultural group so that one can function effectively in caring for members of that cultural group. Culturally competent community health nursing requires that nurses understand the lifestyle, value system, and health and illness behaviors of diverse individuals, families, groups, and communities. Nurses should also understand the culture of institutions that influence the health and well-being of communities. Nurses who have knowledge of, and an ability to work with, diverse cultures are able to devise effective interventions to reduce risks in a manner that is culturally congruent with community, group, and individual values.

The "Standards of Practice for Culturally Competent Nursing Care" established by the Expert Panel on Global Nursing and Health (2010) provides important guidelines to help nurses provide culturally competent care. The 12 standards are:

1. Social justice
2. Critical reflection
3. Knowledge of cultures
4. Culturally competent practice
5. Cultural competence in healthcare systems and organizations
6. Patient advocacy and empowerment
7. Multicultural workforce
8. Education and training in culturally competent care
9. Cross-cultural communication
10. Cross-cultural leadership
11. Policy development
12. Evidence-based practice and research

In the United States, metaphors such as *melting pot* describe the cultural diversity that characterizes the population. Although there is a tendency to identify the federally defined racial and ethnic minority groups when referring to the cultural aspects of community health nursing, all individuals, families, groups, communities, and institutions, including nurses and the nursing profession, have cultural characteristics that influence community health. When planning and implementing healthcare, community health nurses need to balance cultural diversity with the universal human experience and common needs of all people.

POPULATION TRENDS

The population of the United States is becoming increasingly diverse. In recent years, the populations within the federally defined minority groups have grown faster than the population as a whole. In 1970, minority groups accounted for 16% of the population. By 2019, this share had increased to 39.9% (U.S. Census Bureau, 2021). Assuming that current trends continue, the U.S. Census Bureau (2020) projects that by 2060 minorities will account for more than 55% of the total population.

Furthermore, the numbers of certain minority groups, such as Hispanics, are growing considerably faster than those of whites and other groups. In 2019, estimates of population by race and ethnicity were white (non-Hispanic or Latino) 60.1%; Hispanic or Latino, 18.5%; Black/African American, 13.4%; Asian, 5.9%; American Indians and Alaska Natives, 1.3%; other, 3.0% (U.S. Census Bureau, 2021). If current demographic trends continue, the United States will have the following population composition by the year 2060: white, 44.3%; Hispanic or Latino, 27.5%; Black/African American, 15.0%; Asian, 9.1%; American Indians and Alaska Natives, 1.4% and other or combination, 2.7% (U.S. Census Bureau, 2020).

Although the nursing profession has representatives from diverse groups, minorities are generally underrepresented. Currently about 80.8% of registered nurses in the United States are white/non-Hispanic. Estimates for each minority group are as follows: African American, 6.2%; Hispanic, 5.3%; Asian 7.5%; Native Hawaiian/Pacific Islander, 0.5%; and Native American and Alaska Native, 0.4% (American Association of Colleges of Nursing, 2017). Additionally, each minority group is distributed differently around the country. African American nurses are more likely to be found in the South, Hispanics in the West or South (i.e., especially states bordering Mexico), and Asian and Pacific Islanders in the West or Northeast. Native American and Alaska Native nurses are predominantly in states with Native American reservations.

The United States has grown and achieved its success largely through immigration. In 2019 alone 1,031,765 legal immigrants came to the United States (U.S. Department of Homeland Security, 2019). In 2019, the U.S. population according to the American Community Survey included almost 44.9 million foreign-born individuals. Among those foreign born, 50.3% were born in Latin America, 31.4% in Asia, 10.4% in Europe, and the remaining 8% in other regions of the world (U.S. Census Bureau, 2019). The number of immigrants and refugees in the United States is projected to continue to increase.

In addition, people from other countries continue to seek treatment in U.S. hospitals, particularly for cardiovascular, neurological, and cancer care. Furthermore, U.S. nurses have the opportunity to travel abroad to work in a variety of healthcare settings in the international marketplace. In the course of a nursing career, it is possible to encounter foreign visitors, international university faculty members, international high school/university students, family members of foreign diplomats, immigrants, and refugees. Moreover, members of some cultural groups desire culturally relevant healthcare that incorporates their specific beliefs and practices. A growing expectation exists among members of certain cultural groups that healthcare providers will respect their "cultural health rights." However, this expectation frequently conflicts with the monocultural, Western biomedical worldview taught in most U.S. educational programs. Therefore, a serious conceptual problem exists within nursing in that nurses are expected to know, understand, and meet the health needs of culturally diverse individuals, groups, and communities without adequate preparation.

♥ HEALTHY PEOPLE 2030

Foundational Principles

- Health and well-being of all people and communities are essential to a thriving, equitable society.
- Promoting health and well-being and preventing disease are linked efforts that encompass physical, mental, and social health dimensions.
- Investing to achieve the full potential for health and well-being for all provides valuable benefits to society.
- Achieving health and well-being requires eliminating health disparities, achieving health equity, and attaining health literacy.
- Healthy physical, social, and economic environments strengthen the potential to achieve health
- Promoting and achieving the Nation's health and well-being is a shared responsibility that is distributed across the national, state, tribal, and community levels, including the public, private, and not-for-profit sectors.
- Working to attain the full potential for health and well-being of the population is a component of decision-making and policy formulation across all sectors.

From U.S. Department of Health and Human Services: *Healthy people 2030: foundational principles.* Available from: https://health.gov/healthypeople/objectives-and-data/browse-objectives

---

CULTURAL PERSPECTIVES AND *HEALTHY PEOPLE 2030*

Healthy People 2030 identifies priority areas and objectives. By developing a set of national health targets, which includes eliminating racial and ethnic disparities in health, U.S. health officials, together with state and local officials and members of

the private sector, set goals to improve the quality and increase the years of healthy life for all Americans (U.S. Department Health and Human Services (USDHHS), *Healthy People 2030*) objectives embrace and focus on ways to close the gaps in health outcomes. Particularly targeted are racial and ethnic disparities in areas such as diabetes, acquired immunodeficiency syndrome (AIDS), heart disease, infant mortality rates, cancer screening and management, and immunizations. The objectives bring focus on disparities among racial and ethnic minorities, women, youth, older adults, people of low income and education, and people with disabilities (USDHHS, 2020). The *Healthy People 2030* box lists selected objectives from *Healthy People (2030)* specific to a variety of health issues.

The overarching goals of *Healthy People (2030)* are: attain healthy thriving lives, elimination of health disparities, the promotion of healthy behaviors across the life span, promote environments to promote the full potential promotion, and engage key constituents across multiple sector to improve the health and well-being of all (USDHHS, 2020). The initiative is a tool for monitoring and tracking health status, health risks, and use of health services.

Addressing Racial and Ethnic Disparities in Healthcare

As in many nations, people in the United States who come from various racial, ethnic, cultural, and socioeconomic backgrounds often experience marked disparities in healthcare. The occurrence of many diseases, injuries, and other public health problems is disproportionately higher in some groups; access to healthcare may be more restricted and the overall quality of healthcare is deemed inferior, for people from certain racial, ethnic, and cultural populations. Although the overall health of the U.S. population has improved during the past several decades, research reveals that all people have not shared equally in those improvements. For example, 26.8% of Hispanic adults and 21.5% of African American adults report that they are in fair or poor health, compared with 16.4% of non-Hispanic whites (Kaiser Family Foundation, 2019).

Primary care provides the foundation for the healthcare system, and research indicates that having a usual source of care increases the chance that people will receive adequate preventive care and other important health services. Data from the Agency for Healthcare Research and Quality (2017) reveal the following facts:

White Americans are more likely to have health insurance (9% uninsured) than either African Americans (14.6% uninsured) or Hispanics (25.9% uninsured).

Thirty percent of Hispanics and 20% of African Americans lack a usual source of healthcare (compared with fewer than 16% of whites).

Hispanic children are nearly three times as likely as non-Hispanic white children to have no usual source of healthcare.

African Americans (16%) and Hispanic Americans (13%) are more likely to rely on hospitals or clinics for healthcare than are whites (8%).

During the past two decades, health disparities have become the focus of numerous federal, state, and local government studies, and one of the major goals of *Healthy People (2030)* is to achieve health equity, eliminate disparities, and improve the health of all groups (USDHHS, 2020). Therefore, it is essential to look at how to overcome these and other identified factors that contribute to poorer health among members of some minority groups. A survey by the Commonwealth Fund (2007) found that disparities in healthcare can be reduced or even eliminated when adults have healthcare insurance and a medical home, which is defined as "a healthcare setting that provides patients with timely, well-organized care and enhanced access to providers." According to the survey, when adults have insurance and a medical home, "their access to needed care, receipt of routine preventive screenings, and management of chronic conditions improve substantially."

GENETICS IN PUBLIC HEALTH

Genetic Risk Assessment for Cancer: Racial and Ethnic Disparities

Racial and ethnic disparities in deaths attributable to cancer vary considerably for some types of cancer. This is particularly true for breast cancer for African American females, prostate cancer for African American males, and colon cancer for both African American men and women. Despite the widespread recognition of the importance of genetic risk assessment and testing, evidence-based practice guidelines are not followed uniformly in many instances.

Although use of genetic testing and risk assessment among specific populations has increased overall, there are differences based on racial and socioeconomic situations. Underhill and colleagues (2016) pointed out that although African American and Hispanic women have higher rates of hereditary-associated cancers (e.g., breast cancer), they are less likely than white women to be tested for genetic markers. This results in disparities in cancer prevention and early detection. The authors point out that nurses should recognize risk factors for hereditary cancers and refer for genetic testing per established clinical guidelines when appropriate.

Underhill ML, Jones T, Habin K: Disparities in cancer genetic risk assessment and testing, *Oncol Nurs Forum* 43(4):519–523, 2016.

ACTIVE LEARNING

Examine the vital statistics of a community, and compare differences in morbidity and mortality rates for whites and racial and ethnic subgroups. What data are available according to racial and ethnic heritage? What data are missing?

TRANSCULTURAL NURSING

In 1959, Madeleine Leininger, a nurse-anthropologist, used the term **transcultural nursing** to define the philosophical and theoretical similarities between nursing and anthropology. In 1968, Leininger proposed her theory-generated model, and, in 1970, she wrote the first book on transcultural nursing, *Nursing and Anthropology: Two Worlds to Blend* (Leininger, 1970). According to Leininger (1978), transcultural nursing is "a formal area of study and practice focused on a comparative analysis of different cultures and subcultures in the world with respect to

cultural care, health and illness beliefs, values, and practices with the goal of using this knowledge to provide culture-specific and culture-universal nursing care to people" (p. 493). **Culture specific** refers to the "particularistic values, beliefs, and patterning of behavior that tend to be special, 'local,' or unique to a designated culture and which do not tend to be shared with members of other cultures" (Leininger, 1991, p. 491), whereas **culture universal** refers to the commonalities of values, norms of behavior, and life patterns that are similarly held among cultures about human behavior and lifestyles and form the bases for formulating theories for developing cross-cultural laws of human behavior (Leininger, 1991, p. 491).

Although many nurse-scholars have developed theories of nursing, **Leininger's theory of culture care diversity and universality** is the only one that gives precedence to understanding the cultural dimensions of human care and caring. Leininger's theory is concerned with describing, explaining, and projecting nursing similarities and differences focused primarily on human care and caring in human cultures. Leininger used worldview, social structure, language, ethnohistory, environmental context, and the generic or folk and professional systems to provide a comprehensive and holistic view of influences in cultural care and well-being. The following three models of nursing decisions and actions may be useful in providing culturally congruent and competent care (Andrews et al., 2020; Leininger, 1978, 1991, 1995; Leininger et al., 2018):

1. Culture care preservation and maintenance
2. Culture care accommodation and negotiation
3. Culture care repatterning and restructuring

Among the strengths of Leininger's theory is its flexibility for use with individuals, families, groups, communities, and institutions in diverse health systems. Leininger's Sunrise Model depicts the theory of cultural care diversity and universality and provides a visual representation of the key components of the theory and the interrelationships among its components (Fig. 13.1).

The term *cross-cultural nursing* is sometimes used synonymously with *transcultural nursing*. The terms *intercultural nursing* and *multicultural nursing* are also used. Since Leininger's early work, many nurses have contributed significantly to the advancement of nursing care of culturally diverse clients, groups, and communities, and some of their contributions are mentioned in this chapter.

One of the major challenges that community health nurses face in working with clients from culturally diverse backgrounds is overcoming individual **ethnocentrism**, which is a person's tendencies to view his or her own way of life as the most desirable, acceptable, or best and to act in a superior manner toward individuals from another culture. Nurses also must beware of **cultural imposition**, which is a person's tendency to impose his or her own beliefs, values, and patterns of behavior on individuals from another culture. When clients' cultural values and expressions of care differ from those of the nurse, the nurse must exercise caution to ensure that mutual goals have been established.

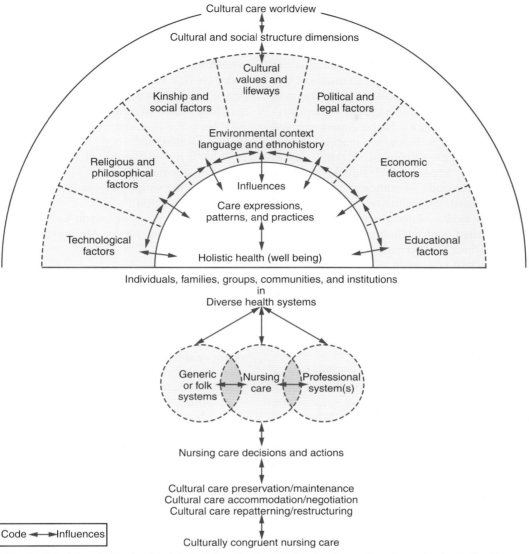

Individuals, families, groups, communities, and institutions
in
Diverse health systems

Nursing care decisions and actions

Cultural care preservation/maintenance
Cultural care accommodation/negotiation
Cultural care repatterning/restructuring

Culturally congruent nursing care

Code ◄──►Influences

Fig. 13.1 Leininger's Sunrise Model, depicting the theory of cultural care diversity and universality. (From Leininger MM: *Culture, care, diversity, and universality: a theory of nursing*, New York, 1991, National League for Nursing Press.)

OVERVIEW OF CULTURE

In 1871, the English anthropologist Sir Edward Tylor was the first to define the term *culture*. According to Tylor (1871), culture is the complex whole, including knowledge, beliefs, art, morals, law, customs, and any other capabilities and habits acquired by virtue of the fact that one is a member of a particular society. Culture represents a person's way of perceiving, evaluating, and behaving within his or her world, and it provides the blueprint for determining his or her values, beliefs, and practices. Culture has four basic characteristics:

1. It is learned from birth through the processes of language acquisition and socialization.
2. It is shared by members of the same cultural group.

3. It is adapted to specific conditions related to environmental and technical factors and to the availability of natural resources.
4. It is dynamic.

Culture is an all-pervasive and universal phenomenon. However, the culture that develops in any given society is always specific and distinctive, encompassing the knowledge, beliefs, customs, and skills acquired by members of that society. Within cultures, groups of individuals share beliefs, values, and attitudes that are different from those of other groups within the same culture. Ethnicity, religion, education, occupation, age, sex, and individual preferences and variations bring differences. When such groups function within a large culture, they are termed *subcultural groups*.

The term **subculture** is used for fairly large aggregates of people who share characteristics that are not common to all members of the culture and that enable them to be a distinguishable subgroup. Ethnicity, religion, occupation, health-related characteristics, age, sex, and geographic location are frequently used to identify subcultural groups. Examples of U.S. subcultures based on ethnicity (e.g., subcultures with common traits such as physical characteristics, language, or ancestry) include African Americans, Hispanics, Native Americans, and Chinese Americans. Subcultures based on religion include members of the more than 1200 recognized religions, such as Catholics, Jews, Mormons, Muslims, and Buddhists. Those based on occupation include healthcare professionals (e.g., nurses and physicians), career military personnel, and farmers. Those based on health-related characteristics include the blind, hearing impaired, and intellectually disabled. Subcultures based on age include adolescents and older adults, and those based on sex or sexual preference include women, men, lesbians, and gay men. Those based on geographic location include Appalachians, Southerners, and New Yorkers. Lastly, military veterans are another very common subculture that shares distinct needs and values (see Chapter 22).

Culture and the Formation of Values

According to Leininger (1995), **value** refers to a desirable or undesirable state of affairs. Values are a universal feature of all cultures, although the types and expressions of values differ widely. **Norms** are the rules by which human behavior is governed and result from the cultural values held by the group. All societies have rules or norms that specify appropriate and inappropriate behavior. Individuals are rewarded or punished as they conform to or deviate from the established norms, respectively. Values and norms, along with the acceptable and unacceptable behaviors associated with them, are learned in childhood.

Every society has a **dominant value orientation**, a basic value orientation that is shared by the majority of its members as a result of early common experiences. In the United States, the dominant value orientation is reflected in the dominant cultural group, which is made up of white, middle-class Protestants, typically those who came to the United States at least two generations ago from Northern Europe. Members of the dominant cultural group are sometimes referred to as *white Anglo-Saxon Protestants*, a term that reflects their ancestry and religious beliefs. In the United States, the dominant cultural group places emphasis on educational achievement, science, technology, individual expression, democracy, experimentation, and informality.

Although an assumption is sometimes made that the term *white* refers to a homogeneous group of Americans, a rich diversity of ethnic variation exists among the many groups that constitute the dominant majority. Countries of origin include those of Eastern and Western Europe (e.g., Ireland, Poland, Italy, France, Sweden, and Russia). The origins of people in Canada, Australia, New Zealand, and South Africa can ultimately be traced to Western Europe. Appalachians, Amish, Cajuns, and other subgroups are also examples of whites who have cultural roots that are recognizably different from those of the dominant cultural group.

Values and norms vary, sometimes significantly, among various cultural groups. According to Kluckhohn and Strodtbeck (1961), several basic human problems exist for which all people must find a solution. They identified the following five questions related to values and norms:

1. What is the character of innate human nature (human nature orientation)?
2. What is the relationship of the human to nature (person—nature orientation)?
3. What is the temporal focus (i.e., time sense) of human life (time orientation)?
4. What is the mode of human activity (activity orientation)?
5. What is the mode of human relationships (social orientation)?

Human Nature Orientation

Innate human nature may be good, evil, or a combination of good and evil. Some believe that life is a struggle to overcome a basically evil nature; they consider human nature to be unalterable or able to be perfected only through great discipline and effort. For others, human nature is perceived as fundamentally good, unalterable, and difficult or impossible to corrupt.

According to Kohls (1984), the dominant U.S. cultural group chooses to believe the best about a person until that person proves otherwise. Concern in the United States for prison reform, social rehabilitation, and the plight of less fortunate people around the world is a reflective perception of the belief in the fundamental goodness of human nature. Recent scientific advances, such as advances in stem cell research and genome studies, have necessitated consideration of ethical quandaries regarding human nature. Questions emerge as to whether science can or should pursue activities that could alter the basic human orientation.

Person—Nature Orientation

The following three perspectives examine the ways in which the person—nature relationship is perceived:
- Destiny, in which people are subjugated to nature in a fatalistic, inevitable manner
- Harmony, in which people and nature exist together as a single entity
- Mastery, in which people are intended to overcome natural forces and to put them to use for the benefit of humankind

Most Americans consider humans and nature clearly separated; this is an incomprehensible perspective for many individuals of Asian heritage. The idea that a person can control his or her own destiny is unfamiliar to many individuals of culturally diverse backgrounds. Some cultures believe that people are driven and controlled by fate and can do very little, if anything, to influence it. The dominant U.S. cultural group, by contrast, has a mastery perspective.

For example, the reader should consider three individuals in whom hypertension has been diagnosed, each of whom embraces one of the values orientations described. The person whose values orientation is destiny may say, "Why should I bother watching my diet, taking medication, and getting regular blood pressure checks? High blood pressure is part of my genetic destiny and there is nothing I can do to change the outcome. There is no need to waste money on prescription drugs and health checkups." The person whose values orientation embraces harmony may say, "If I follow the diet described and use medication to lower my blood pressure, I can restore the balance and harmony that were upset by this illness. The emotional stress I've been feeling indicates an inner lack of harmony that needs to be balanced." The person whose values orientation leads to belief in active mastery may say, "I will overcome this hypertension no matter what. By eating the right foods, working toward stress reduction, and conquering the disease with medication, I will take charge of the situation and influence the course of my disease."

Time Orientation

People can perceive time in the following three ways:
- *The focus may be on the past, with traditions and ancestors playing an important role in the client's life.* For example, many Asians, Native Americans, East Indians, and Africans hold particular beliefs about ancestors and tend to value long-standing traditions. In times of crisis, such as illness, individuals with a values orientation emphasizing the past may consult with ancestors or ask for their guidance or protection during the illness.
- *The focus may be on the present, with little attention paid to the past or the future.* Individuals with this focus are concerned with the current situation, and they perceive the future as vague or unpredictable. Nurses may have difficulty encouraging such individuals to prepare for the future (e.g., to participate in primary prevention measures).
- *The focus may be on the future, with progress and change highly valued.* Individuals with a future focus may express discontent with the past and present. In terms of healthcare, they may inquire about the "latest treatment" and the most advanced equipment available for a particular problem.

The dominant U.S. cultural group is characterized by a belief in progress and a future orientation. This combination implies a strong task or goal focus. The group has an optimistic faith in what the future will bring. Change is often equated with improvement, and a rapid rate of change is usually normal.

Activity Orientation

There are different values orientations concerning activity. Philosophers have suggested the following three perspectives:
Being, in which a spontaneous expression of impulses and desires is largely nondevelopmental in nature
Growing, in which the person is self-contained and has inner control, including the ability to self-actualize
Doing, in which the person actively strives to achieve and accomplish something that is regarded highly

The person with a doing orientation often directs the doing toward achievement of an externally applied standard, such as a code of behavior from a religious or ethical perspective. The 10 Commandments, Pillars of Islam, Hippocratic Oath, and Nightingale Pledge are examples of externally applied standards.

The dominant cultural value is action oriented, with an emphasis on productivity and being busy. As a result of this action orientation, Americans have become proficient at problem solving and decision making. Even during leisure time and vacations, many Americans value activity.

Social Orientation

Variations in cultural values orientation are also related to the relationships that exist with others. Relationships may be categorized in the following three ways:
Lineal relationships: These exist by virtue of heredity and kinship ties. These relationships follow an ordered succession and have continuity through time.
Collateral relationships: The focus is primarily on group goals, and family orientation is important. For example, many Asian clients describe family honor and the importance of working together toward an achievement of the group versus a personal goal.
Individual relationships: These refer to personal autonomy and independence. Individual goals dominate, and group goals become secondary.

The social orientation among the dominant U.S. cultural group is toward the importance of the individual and the equality of all people. Friendly, informal, outgoing, and extroverted members of the dominant cultural group may scorn rank and authority. For example, nursing students may call faculty members by their first names, clients may call nurses by their first names, and employees may fraternize with their employers.

When making health-related decisions, clients from culturally diverse backgrounds rely on relationships with others in various ways. If the cultural values orientation is lineal, the client may seek assistance from other members of the family and allow a relative (e.g., parent, grandparent, or elder brother) to make decisions about important health-related matters. If collateral relationships are valued, decisions about the client may be interrelated with the influence of illness on the entire family or group. For example, among the Amish, the entire community is affected by the illness of a member because the community pays for healthcare from a common fund. Members join together to meet the needs of the client and family for the duration of the illness, and the roles of many in the community are likely to be affected by the illness of a single member.

In another example, there are approximately 11.4 million undocumented residents living in the United States as of January 2015–18 (Baker, 2021). These individuals often create their own social groups which may fear that attempting to access the healthcare system may lead to deportation, and they often have "underground" or private access to home remedies and pharmaceuticals for their healthcare. As a result, they often enter the formal healthcare system via emergency departments when their health status has declined considerably (KFF, 2020).

A values orientation that emphasizes the individual is predominant among the dominant cultural majority in the United States. Decision making about health and illness is often an individual matter, with the client being responsible, although members of the nuclear family may participate to varying degrees.

Culture and the Family

The family remains the basic social unit in the United States. Although various ways exist to categorize families, the following are commonly recognized types of constellations in which people live together in society:

- Nuclear (i.e., husband, wife, and child or children)
- Nuclear dyad (i.e., husband and wife alone, either childless or with no children living at home)
- Single parent (i.e., either mother or father and at least one child)
- Blended (i.e., husband, wife, and children from previous relationships)
- Extended (i.e., nuclear plus other blood relatives)
- Communal (i.e., group of men and women with or without children)
- Cohabitation (i.e., unmarried man and woman sharing a household with or without children)
- Lesbian, gay, bisexual, transgender (i.e., same-gender couples, individuals that identify with another gender, with or without children)

In addition to structural differences in families cross-culturally, accompanying functional diversity may exist. For example, among extended families, kin residence sharing has long been recognized as a viable alternative to managing scarce resources, meeting child care needs, and caring for a handicapped or older family member.

The family constellations associated with teen parenting are unique and provide a special socialization context for infants. For example, Hispanic teen mothers receive more child care help from grandmothers and peers than do white teen mothers. Among African Americans and Puerto Ricans, the presence of the maternal grandmother ameliorates the negative consequences of adolescent childbirth on the infant. In addition, grandmothers are more responsive and less punitive in their interactions with the infant than their daughters (Andrews et al., 2020). Three-generational households can have an influence on the infant's development: by influencing the mother's knowledge about development and providing other more responsive social interactions with the infant.

Families from diverse backgrounds are often characterized as being more conservative in terms of sex roles and parenting values and practices than white families. For example, traditional Japanese American and Mexican American families are family centered, enforce strict gender and age roles, and emphasize children's compliance with authority figures (Giger and Haddad, 2020). Children of culturally diverse backgrounds are involved in family interactions that differ from those of children from the dominant U.S. cultural group. The values of children of immigrants typically evolve, depending on how far removed they are from the country of origin. These children may detach from their cultural traditions, becoming more individually focused or autonomous—often to the dismay of the elders in the family. Often the language of the ancestors is forgotten or, in certain subcultures, forbidden to be spoken, so that the children may assimilate to the dominant culture.

Relationships that may seem apparent sometimes warrant further exploration by nurses interacting with clients from culturally diverse backgrounds. For example, the dominant cultural group defines siblings as two people with the same mother, the same father, the same mother and father, or the same adoptive parents. In some Asian cultures, a sibling relationship is defined as involving infants who are breastfed by the same woman. In other cultures, certain kinship patterns, such as maternal first cousins, are sibling relationships. In some African cultures, anyone from the same village or town may be called "brother" or "sister" (Andrews et al., 2020; Giger and Haddad, 2020).

When providing care for infants and children, the nurse must identify the primary provider of care because this individual may or may not be the biological parent. For example, among some Hispanic groups, female members of the nuclear or extended family (e.g., sisters or aunts) are sometimes the primary providers of care. In some African American families, the grandmother may be the decision maker and primary caregiver of the children (Andrews et al., 2020).

CULTURE AND SOCIOECONOMIC FACTORS

No single indicator can adequately capture all facets of economic status for entire populations, but measures such as median or average annual income, employment rate, poverty rate, and net worth are most often used. The economic status of most individuals, especially children, is better reflected by the pooled resources of family or household members than by their individual earnings or incomes. **Socioeconomic status** (SES) is a composite of the economic status of a family or unrelated individuals based on income, wealth, occupation, educational attainment, and power. It is a means of measuring inequalities based on economic differences and the manner in which families live as a result of their economic well-being. Most families with racially or ethnically diverse backgrounds have a lower SES than the population at large, with a few exceptions (e.g., Cuban Americans and subgroups of Asian Americans).

Poverty is another factor that dramatically influences health and well-being. National poverty data are calculated through the use of the official U.S. Census Bureau definition of poverty, which has remained standard since its initial introduction in the mid-1960s. Under this definition, poverty is determined by comparing pretax cash income with the poverty threshold, which adjusts for family size and composition. Table 13.1 provides an

TABLE 13.1 Poverty Thresholds ($) for 2020 by Size of Family and Number of Related Children Under 18 Years

Size of Family Unit	None	RELATED CHILDREN UNDER 18 YEARS							
		One	Two	Three	Four	Five	Six	Seven	Eight or More
One person under 65 years	13,465								
One person 65 years and over	12,413								
Two people: Householder under 65 years	17,331	17,839							
Two people: Householder 65 years and over	15,644	17,771							
Three people	20,244	20,832	20,852						
Four people	26,695	27,131	26,246	26,338					
Five people	32,193	32,661	31,661	30,887	30,414				
Six people	37,027	37,174	36,408	35,674	34,582	33,935			
Seven people	42,605	42,871	41,954	41,314	40,124	38,734	37,210		
Eight people	47,650	48,071	47,205	46,447	45,371	44,006	42,585	42,224	
Nine people or more	57,319	57,597	56,831	56,188	55,132	53,679	52,366	52,040	50,035

Note: The poverty thresholds are updated each year with the use of the change in the average annual Consumer Price Index for All Urban Consumers (CPI–U). From U.S. Census Bureau: *Poverty thresholds by size of family and number of children, 2020*. Available from: https://www.census.gov/data/tables/time-series/demo/income-poverty/historical-poverty-thresholds.html.

overview of the poverty thresholds according to size of family and number of related children under age 18 years residing in the home. The poverty guidelines are issued each year by the USDHHS. The guidelines are a simplification of the poverty threshold for administrative purposes, such as determining financial eligibility for federal programs (e.g., Head Start, National School Lunch, Medicaid, Aid to Families with Dependent Children) (U.S. Census Bureau, 2020).

According to the U.S. Census Bureau Income and Poverty Report (2020), the poverty rate in 2019 was 10.5%, down 1.3% from 2018, the fifth yearly decline. The distribution of the poor varies considerably on the basis of certain factors such as age, race or ethnicity, and marital status. For example, 9.1% of the White non-Hispanic population, 18.8% of the African American population, 7.3% of the Asian population, and 15.7% of the Hispanic population live in poverty (U.S. Census Bureau, 2020). In addition, children under 6 years of age are particularly vulnerable to poverty, with 21% of all U.S. children in this age group being poor (Colby and Ortman, 2015).

Distribution of Resources

Status, power, and wealth in the United States are not distributed equally throughout society. Rather, a small percentage of the population enjoys most of the nation's resources, primarily through ownership of multibillion-dollar corporations, large pieces of real estate in prime locations, and similar assets. The U.S. population has traditionally been divided into the following three social classes: upper, middle, and lower. SES may be calculated by considering a variety of factors, but it is customarily determined by examining factors such as total family income, occupation, and educational level.

A disproportionate number of individuals from the racially and ethnically diverse subgroups are members of the lower socioeconomic class, whereas a larger percentage of members of the dominant cultural group belong to the upper and middle socioeconomic classes. The United States has socioeconomic stratification; therefore the idealization of America as the land of opportunity often applies more to members of the upper and middle classes than to those of the lower class. The outcome of social stratification is social inequality. For example, school systems, grocery stores, and recreational facilities vary significantly between the inner city, which has a high percentage of minority residents, and the suburbs, where the residents are overwhelmingly of European ancestry.

For many years, healthcare settings and healthcare access have been the subject of study and concern regarding distribution of resources, with members of racial and ethnic minority groups compellingly pointing out the inequalities. Because financing of healthcare in the United States largely relies on a combination of federally funded insurance (i.e., Medicare) and employer-provided health insurance, those from the highest SES groups and elders tend to receive the best healthcare. In contrast, those from low-SES groups (i.e., those without health insurance or with Medicaid) tend to receive less healthcare. Thus, in the United States, SES largely determines access to healthcare as well as the quality of care received.

Education

One of the components considered in determining SES is educational level. Educational attainment is perhaps the single most important factor. In recent years, there has been an improvement in the level of education among those who have historically been less educated (e.g., elders, women, minorities). For example, women now have a higher rate of high school completion than do men. Also, in 2018, dropout rates for both African Americans and Hispanics have reached all-time lows (Child Trends Databank, 2018).

? ACTIVE LEARNING

1. Visit an inner-city grocery store and compare its quality, prices, customer services, and variety of products with those of a suburban grocery store.
2. Watch prime-time television and note the racial and ethnic diversity that is present during the commercials. During the program, note the roles played by racially and ethnically diverse characters. Are they heroes or heroines or the "bad guys"? What are their occupations, SES, religions, and lifestyles?
3. Skim a popular magazine for references to racially and ethnically diverse subgroups. What is being written? Is the nature of the article favorable or unfavorable?

CULTURE AND NUTRITION

Long after assimilation into U.S. culture has occurred, many members of various ethnic groups continue to follow culturally based dietary practices and eat ethnic foods. Often, neighborhood food markets and ethnic restaurants are established soon after the arrival of a new group of immigrants to the United States. The ethnic restaurant is commonly a place for members of a cultural group to meet and mingle, and customers from the dominant cultural group may be of secondary interest. Food is an integral part of cultural identity that extends beyond dietary preferences.

Nutrition Assessment of Culturally Diverse Groups

Factors that must be considered in a nutrition assessment include the cultural definition of food, frequency, and number of meals eaten away from home, form and content of ceremonial meals, amount and types of food eaten, and regularity of food consumption. Twenty-four-hour dietary recalls or 3-day food records traditionally used for assessment may be inadequate when dealing with clients from culturally diverse backgrounds. Standard dietary handbooks may fail to provide culture-specific diet information, because nutritional content and exchange tables are usually based on Western diets. Another source of error may originate from the cultural patterns of eating. For example, among low-income urban African American families, elaborate weekend meals are frequent, whereas weekday dietary patterns are markedly more moderate (Giger and Haddad, 2020).

Although community health nurses may assume that *food* is a culture-universal term, they may need to clarify its meaning with the client. For example, certain Latin American groups do not consider greens, an important source of vitamins, to be food and fail to list intake of these vegetables on daily records. Among Vietnamese refugees, dietary intake of calcium may appear inadequate because low consumption rates of dairy products are common among members of this group. However, they commonly consume pork bones and shells, providing adequate quantities of calcium to meet daily requirements (Giger and Haddad, 2020).

Food is only one part of eating. In some cultures, social contacts during meals are restricted to members of the immediate or extended family. For example, in some Middle Eastern cultures, men and women eat meals separately, or women are permitted to eat with their husbands but not with other males. Among some Hispanic groups, the male breadwinner is served first, then the women and children eat. Etiquette during meals, use of hands, type of eating utensils (e.g., chopsticks or special flatware), and protocols governing the order in which food is consumed during a meal all vary cross-culturally.

Dietary Practices of Selected Cultural Groups

Cultural stereotyping is the tendency to view individuals of common cultural backgrounds similarly and according to a preconceived notion of how they behave. There may be staple foods that may be dominant in a culture such as rice, pasta, or corn-based products. Although aggregate dietary preferences among people from certain groups can be considered, one must never assume that all members of the cultural group eat and like the same things.

Religion and Diet

Cultural food preferences are often interrelated with religious dietary beliefs and practices. As indicated in Table 13.2, many religions have proscriptive dietary practices, and some use food as symbols in celebrations and rituals. Knowing the client's religious practice as it relates to food makes it possible to suggest improvements or modifications that will not conflict with religious dietary laws.

Fasting and other religious observations may limit a person's food or liquid intake during specified times. For example, many Catholics fast or abstain from meat on Ash Wednesday, and

TABLE 13.2 **Dietary Practices of Selected Religious Groups**	
Religion	**Dietary Practice**
Islam	Pork and intoxicating beverages are prohibited.
Judaism	Pork, predatory fowl, shellfish, other water creatures (fish with scales are permissible), and blood by ingestion (e.g., blood sausage and raw meat) are prohibited. Blood by transfusion is acceptable. Foods should be kosher (meaning "properly preserved"). All animals must be ritually slaughtered by a shochet (i.e., quickly with the least pain possible) to be kosher. Mixing dairy and meat dishes at the same meal is prohibited.
Mormonism (Church of Jesus Christ of Latter-day Saints)	Alcohol, tobacco, and beverages containing caffeine (e.g., coffee, tea, colas, and select carbonated soft drinks) are prohibited.
Seventh-Day Adventism	Pork, certain seafood (including shellfish), and fermented beverages are prohibited. A vegetarian diet is encouraged.

each Friday during the season of Lent, Muslims refrain from eating during the daytime hours for the month of Ramadan but are permitted to eat after sunset, and Mormons refrain from ingesting all solid foods and liquids on the first Sunday of each month.

CULTURE AND RELIGION

According to the *2014 U.S. Religious Landscape Study*, 70.6% of U.S. citizens identify with Christian faiths, 5.9% non-Christian faiths, and 22.8% unaffiliated with a faith (atheist, agnostic, and nothing in particular) (Pew Research Center, 2021). Adults who describe themselves as "Christian" have dropped almost eight points since 2007, according to findings by the Pew Research survey. Furthermore, about 66% note that they are members of a church, synagogue, or mosque. The largest religious groups are Protestant, 46.5%; Catholic, 20.8%; Jewish, 1.9%; and Mormon, 1.6% (Pew Research Center, 2021). The largest specific Protestant denominations are the United Methodist Church, American Baptist Church, Evangelical Lutheran Church, Presbyterian Church, and Episcopal Church.

Although the nurse cannot be an expert on each of the estimated 1200 religions practiced in the United States, knowledge of health-related beliefs and practices and general information about religious observances are important in providing culturally competent nursing care. For example, when planning home visits or scheduling clinic visits for members of a specific religious group, the nurse should consult the group's religious calendar and work around designated holy days. The nurse should also know the customary days of religious worship observed by members of the religion. Most Protestants worship on Sundays, whereas Muslims' holy day of worship extends from sunset on Thursday to sunset on Friday, and Jews and Seventh-Day Adventists' holy day extends from sunset on Friday to sunset on Saturday. Roman Catholics may worship in the late afternoon or evening of Saturday or all day Sunday. Some religions may meet more than once weekly.

As an integral component of the individual's culture, religious beliefs may influence the client's explanation of the cause of illness, perception of its severity, and choice of healer. In times of crisis, such as serious illness and impending death, religion may be a source of consolation for the client and family and may influence the course of action believed to be appropriate.

Religion and Spirituality

Religious concerns evolve from, and respond to, the mysteries of life and death, good and evil, and pain and suffering. Nurses frequently encounter clients who find themselves searching for a spiritual meaning to help explain illness or disability. Some nurses find spiritual assessment difficult because the topic is abstract and personal, whereas others feel comfortable discussing spiritual matters. Comfort with personal spiritual beliefs is the foundation for effective assessment of spiritual needs in clients.

Although religions offer various interpretations of many of life's mysteries, most people seek a personal understanding and interpretation at some time in their lives. Ultimately, this personal search becomes a pursuit to discover a supreme being (e.g., Allah, God, Yahweh, or Jehovah) or some unifying truth that will render meaning, purpose, and integrity to existence.

An important distinction must be made between religion and spirituality. **Religion** refers to an organized system of beliefs concerning the cause, nature, and purpose of the universe, especially belief in or the worship of a god or gods. As already stated, more than 1200 religions are practiced in the United States. **Spirituality**, in contrast, is born out of the individual's unique life experience and personal effort to find purpose and meaning in life. Box 13.1 provides suggested guidelines for assessing the spiritual needs of culturally diverse clients. Table 13.3 illustrates a shared belief among various religions.

Religion may influence decisions regarding prolongation of life, euthanasia, autopsy, donation of a body for research,

---

BOX 13.1 Methods of Assessing Spiritual Needs in Culturally Diverse Clients

Environment
- Does the client have religious objects in the environment?
- Does the client wear outer garments or undergarments that have religious significance?
- Are get-well greeting cards religious in nature or from a representative of the client's religious institution?
- Does the client receive flowers or bulletins from a church or other religious institution?

Behavior
- Does the client appear to pray at certain times of the day or before meals?
- Does the client make special dietary requests (e.g., kosher diet; vegetarian diet; or diet free from caffeine, pork, shellfish, or other specific food items)?
- Does the client read religious magazines or books?

Verbalization
- Does the client mention a Supreme Being (e.g., God, Allah, Buddha, or Yahweh), prayer, faith, church, or religious topics?
- Does the client request a visit by a clergy member or other religious representative?
- Does the client express anxiety or fear about pain, suffering, or death?

Interpersonal Relationships
- Who visits the client? How does the client respond to visitors?
- Does a church representative visit?
- How does the client relate to nursing staff and roommates?
- Does the client prefer to interact with others or remain alone?

Data from Andrews MM, Boyle JS, Collins, JW, editors: *Transcultural concepts in nursing care*, ed 8, Philadelphia, PA, 2019, Wolters Kluwer.

TABLE 13.3 Shared Beliefs Among Various Religions: The "Golden Rule"

Religion	Scripture	Source
Buddhism	"Hurt not others in ways that you yourself would find hurtful."	Udana-varga 5:18
Christianity	"Whatsoever you would that men should do to you, do you even so to them."	Matthew 7:12
Confucianism	"Do not do to others what you do not want them to do to you."	Analects 15:23
Hinduism	"One should not behave toward others in a way which is disagreeable to oneself."	Mahabharata 5:1517; Mencius Vii.A.4
Islam	"Not one of you is a believer until he loves for his brother what he loves for himself."	Number 13 of Al-Nawawi's Forty Hadiths
Judaism	"Thou shalt love thy neighbor as thyself."	Leviticus 19:18
Taoism	"Regard your neighbor's gain as your own gain and your neighbor's loss as your own loss."	T'ai Shang Kan Ying P'ien

disposal of a body and body parts including fetus, and type of burial. The nurse should use discretion in asking clients and their families about these issues and gather data only when the clinical situation necessitates that the information be obtained. The nurse should encourage clients and families to discuss these issues with their religious representative when necessary. Before dealing with potentially sensitive issues, the nurse should establish rapport with the client and family by gaining their trust and confidence in less sensitive areas.

Childhood and Spirituality

Serious illness during childhood is especially difficult. Children have spiritual needs that vary according to the child's developmental level and the religious climate that exists in the family. Parental perceptions about the illness of their child may be partially influenced by religious beliefs. For example, some parents may believe that a transgression against a religious law is responsible for a congenital anomaly in their offspring. Other parents may delay seeking medical care because they believe that prayer should be tried first. Certain types of treatment (e.g., administration of blood or medications containing caffeine or other prohibited substances and selected procedures) may be perceived as cultural taboos, which are to be avoided by children and adults.

❓ ACTIVE LEARNING

1. Attend religious services at a church, temple, synagogue, or place of worship for a religion unfamiliar to you.
2. Interview an official representative (e.g., priest, elder, monk, or bishop) of a religion unfamiliar to you. Ask about health-related beliefs and practices, healing rituals, support network for the sick, and dietary practices.

CULTURE AND AGING

Values held by the dominant U.S. culture, such as emphasis on independence, self-reliance, and productivity, influence aging members of society. Americans define people 65 years and older as "old" and limit their work. In some other cultures, people are first recognized as being unable to work and then identified as being old. In some cultures the wisdom, not the productivity, of the older adult is valued; the diminution of one's activity level and the reduction of physical stamina associated with growing old are accepted more readily without loss of status among culture members. Retirement is also culturally defined, with some older adults working as long as physical health continues and others continuing to be active but assuming less physically demanding jobs.

The main task of older adults in the dominant culture is to achieve a sense of integrity in accepting responsibility for their own lives and having a sense of accomplishment. Individuals who achieve integrity consider aging a positive experience, make adjustments in their personal space and social relationships, maintain a sense of usefulness, and begin closure and life review. Not all cultures value accepting responsibility for an individual's own life. For example, among Hispanics, Asians, Arabs, and other groups, older adults are often cared for by family members who welcome them into their homes when they are no longer able to live alone. The concept of placing an older family member in an institutional setting to be cared for by strangers is perceived as an uncaring, impersonal, and culturally unacceptable practice by many cultural groups (Andrews et al., 2019; Giger and Haddad, 2020).

Older adults may develop their own means of coping with illness through self-care, assistance from family members, and social group support systems. Some cultures have developed attitudes and specific behaviors for older adults that include humanistic care and identification of family members as care providers. Older adults may have special family responsibilities (e.g., the older Amish adults provide hospitality to visitors, and older Filipino adults spend considerable time teaching the youth skills learned during a lifetime of experience).

Older adult immigrants who have made major lifestyle adjustments in the move from their homeland to the United States or from a rural to an urban area, or vice versa, may need information about healthcare alternatives, preventive programs, healthcare benefits, and screening programs for which they are eligible. These individuals may also be in various stages of **culture shock**, the state of disorientation or inability to respond to the behavior of a different cultural group because it holds sudden strangeness, unfamiliarity, and incompatibility for the newcomer's perceptions and expectations (Leininger et al., 2018).

Several examples of how being an elderly immigrant influences health can be found in the nursing literature. For example, Wilmoth and Chen (2003) studied living arrangements and symptoms of depression among middle-aged and older immigrants and concluded that immigrants had significantly more depressive symptoms than nonimmigrants.

Furthermore, immigrants who lived alone or with family had more depressive symptoms than those who lived with a spouse.

CROSS-CULTURAL COMMUNICATION

Verbal communication and nonverbal communication are important in community health nursing and are influenced by the cultural background of the nurse and client. *Cross-cultural, or intercultural, communication* refers to the communication process between a nurse and a client with different cultural backgrounds as each attempts to understand the other's point of view from a cultural perspective.

Nurse–Client Relationship

From the introduction of the nurse to the client through termination of the relationship, communication is a continuous process for the community health nurse. First impressions are important in all human relationships; therefore cross-cultural considerations concerning introductions warrant a few brief remarks. To ensure a mutually respectful and trusting relationship, the nurse should introduce himself or herself and indicate how the client should refer to the nurse (i.e., by first name, last name, or title). Having done so, the nurse should ask the client to do the same. This enables the nurse to address the client in a manner that is culturally appropriate, thereby avoiding potential embarrassment. For example, some Asian and European cultures write the last name first; confusion can be avoided in an area of sensitivity (i.e., the client's name).

Space, Distance, and Intimacy

Sense of spatial distance is significant because culturally appropriate distance zones vary widely. For example, the nurse may back away from clients of Hispanic, East Indian, or Middle Eastern origin who invade personal space with regularity in an attempt to bring the nurse closer into the space that is comfortable to them. Although the nurse is uncomfortable with clients' close physical proximity, clients are perplexed by the nurse's distancing behaviors and may perceive the community health nurse as aloof and unfriendly. Table 13.4 summarizes the four distance zones identified for the functional use of space that are embraced by the dominant cultural group in the United States, including most nurses.

Overcoming Communication Barriers

Nurses tend to have stereotypical expectations of the client's behavior. In general, nurses expect behavior to consist of undemanding compliance, an attitude of respect for the healthcare provider, and cooperation with requested behavior throughout the examination. Although clients may ask a few questions for clarification, slight deference to recognized authority figures (e.g., healthcare providers) is expected. However, individuals from culturally diverse backgrounds may have significantly different perceptions about the appropriate role of the individual and family when seeking healthcare. If nurses find themselves becoming annoyed that a client is asking too many

questions, assuming a defensive posture, or otherwise feeling uncomfortable, they may pause for a moment to examine the source of the conflict from a cross-cultural perspective.

During illness, culturally acceptable "sick-role" behavior may range from aggressive, demanding behavior to silent passivity (Cockerham, 2017). Complaining, demanding behavior during illness is may be rewarded with attention in some cultures, whereas others may promote quiet and compliance in clients during illness (Andrews et al., 2020). Furthermore, during an interview, Asian clients may provide the nurse with the answers they think the nurse wants to hear, behavior that is consistent within their cultural value for harmonious relationships with others. The nurse should attempt to phrase questions or statements in a neutral manner that avoids foreshadowing an expected response. Appalachian clients may reject a community health nurse whom they perceive as prying or nosy because a cultural ethic of neutrality mandates that people mind their own business and avoid assertive or argumentative behavior (Giger and Haddad, 2020).

Nonverbal Communication

Unless the nurse makes an effort to understand the client's nonverbal behavior, he or she may overlook important information such as that conveyed by facial expressions, silence, eye contact, touch, and other body language. Communication patterns vary widely cross-culturally, even for seemingly "innocent" behaviors such as smiling and shaking hands. For example, among many Hispanic clients, smiling and shaking hands are considered an integral part of sincere interaction and essential to establishing trust, whereas a Russian client may perceive the same behavior from the nurse as insolent and frivolous (Giger and Haddad, 2020).

TABLE 13.4	Functional Use of Space
Zone	Remarks
Intimate zone (0–1.5 feet)	Visual distortion occurs.
	Best for assessing breath and other body odors.
Personal distance (1.5–4 feet)	Perceived as an extension of the self, similar (1.5–4 feet) to a "bubble."
	Voice is moderate.
	Body odors are inapparent.
	Visual distortion does not occur.
	Much of the physical assessment will occur at this distance.
Social distance (4–12 feet)	Used for impersonal business transactions.
	Perceptual information is much less detailed.
	Much of the interview will occur at this distance.
Public distance (>12 feet)	Interaction with others is impersonal.
	Speaker's voice must be projected.
	Subtle facial expressions are imperceptible.

Data from Hall E: Proxemics: the study of man's spatial relations. In Galdston I, editor, *Man's image in medicine and anthropology*, New York, 1963, International Universities Press.

Gender issues also become significant. For example, among some groups of Middle Eastern origin, men and women do not shake hands or touch each other in any manner outside the marital relationship. However, if the nurse and client are both female, a handshake is usually acceptable (Andrews et al., 2020).

Wide cultural variation exists in the interpretation of silence. Some individuals find silence extremely uncomfortable and make every effort to fill conversational lags with words. In contrast, Native Americans consider silence essential to understanding and respecting the other person. A pause after a question signifies that what the speaker has asked is important enough to be given thoughtful consideration. In traditional Chinese and Japanese cultures, silence may mean that the speaker wishes the listener to consider the content of what has been said before continuing. Arabs and English people may use silence out of respect for another person's privacy, whereas the French, Spanish, and Russians may interpret it as a sign of agreement. Asian cultures often use silence to demonstrate respect for elders (Giger and Haddad, 2020).

Eye contact is among the most culturally variable nonverbal behaviors. Although most nurses have been taught to maintain eye contact while talking with clients, individuals from culturally diverse backgrounds may misconstrue this behavior. Asian, Native American, Indochinese, Arab, and Appalachian clients may consider direct eye contact impolite or aggressive, and they may avert their own eyes during the conversation. Native American clients often stare at the floor when the nurse is talking. This culturally appropriate behavior indicates that the listener is paying close attention to the speaker (Giger and Haddad, 2020; Andrews et al., 2020).

In some cultures, modesty for women is interrelated with eye contact. For a Muslim woman, modesty is achieved in part by avoiding eye contact with men, except for her husband, and keeping the eyes downcast when encountering members of the opposite sex in public situations. In many cultures, the only women who smile and establish eye contact with men in public are prostitutes (Giger and Haddad, 2020). Hasidic Jewish men also have culturally based norms concerning eye contact with women. Such a man may avoid direct eye contact and turn his head in the opposite direction when walking past or speaking to a woman. It is important to understand that the preceding examples are intended to be illustrative and are not exhaustive, nor do they represent values, actions, and beliefs of all members of the cultural groups described.

Language

To assess non—English-speaking clients, the nurse may need the help of an interpreter. Interviewing a non—English-speaking person requires a bilingual interpreter for full communication. Even the person from another culture or country who has a basic command of English may need an interpreter when faced with the anxiety-provoking situation of becoming ill; encountering a strange symptom; or discussing sensitive topics such as birth control, gynecological concerns, and urological problems. The nurse may be

tempted to ask a relative or friend of another client to interpret because this person is readily available and is anxious to help. However, doing so is disadvantageous because it violates confidentiality for the client, who may not want personal information shared with another. Furthermore, the friend or relative, although fluent in ordinary language, is likely to be unfamiliar with medical terminology, clinical procedures, and medical ethics.

Whenever possible, the nurse should use a bilingual team member, trained medical interpreter, and video remote interrupter. This person knows interpreting techniques, has a healthcare background, and understands clients' rights. The trained interpreter is also knowledgeable about cultural beliefs and health practices, can help bridge the cultural gap, and can provide advice concerning the cultural appropriateness of recommendations.

Although the nurse is in charge of the client—nurse interaction, the interpreter is an important member of the healthcare team. Whenever feasible, the nurse should ask the interpreter to meet the client before the visit to establish rapport and learn about the client's age, occupation, educational level, and attitude toward healthcare. This knowledge enables the interpreter to communicate on the client's level.

The nurse should allow more time for visits with culturally diverse clients who require an interpreter. With the third person repeating everything, it can take considerably longer than interviewing English-speaking clients. The nurse will need to focus on the major points and prioritize data.

Line by line and summarization are interpretation styles. Translation line by line ensures accuracy, but it takes more time. The nurse and client should speak only a sentence or two and then allow the interpreter time to interpret. The nurse should use simple language, not medical jargon that the interpreter must simplify before translating. Summary translation is faster and useful for teaching relatively simple health techniques with which the interpreter is already familiar. The nurse should be alert for nonverbal cues as the client talks because they can give valuable data. A good interpreter will also note nonverbal messages and communicate those to the community health nurse. Box 13.2 summarizes suggestions for the selection and use of an interpreter.

Although use of an interpreter is ideal, the nurse may find himself or herself in a situation with a non—English-speaking client in which no interpreter is available. Box 13.3 provides some suggestions for overcoming language barriers when an interpreter is not available.

Touch

Touching the client is a necessary component of a comprehensive assessment. Although benefits exist in establishing rapport with clients through touch, including the promotion of healing through therapeutic touch, physical contact with clients conveys various meanings cross-culturally. In many cultures (e.g., Arab and Hispanic), male healthcare providers may be prohibited from touching or examining all or certain parts of

BOX 13.2 Overcoming Language Barriers: Use of an Interpreter

- Before locating an interpreter, the nurse should know what language the client speaks at home because it may be different from the language spoken publicly (e.g., French is sometimes spoken by aristocratic or well-educated people from certain Asian or Middle Eastern cultures).
- The nurse should avoid interpreters from a rival tribe, state, region, or nation (e.g., a Palestinian who knows Hebrew may not be the best interpreter for a Jewish client).
- The nurse should be aware of the gender difference between the interpreter and client to avoid violation of cultural mores related to modesty.
- The nurse should be aware of the age difference between the interpreter and client.
- The nurse should be aware of socioeconomic differences between the interpreter and client.
- The nurse should ask the interpreter to translate as closely to verbatim as possible.
- An interpreter who is not a relative may seek compensation for services rendered.

BOX 13.3 Overcoming Language Barriers When an Interpreter is Not Available

- The nurse should be polite and formal.
- The nurse should greet the client using his or her last or complete name. The nurse should gesture to himself or herself and say his or her name. The nurse should offer a handshake, nod, or smile.
- The nurse should proceed in an unhurried manner. The nurse should pay attention to efforts by the client or family to communicate.
- The nurse should speak in a low, moderate voice. The nurse should remember that he or she may have a tendency to raise the volume and pitch of his or her voice when the listener appears not to understand, and the listener may perceive that the nurse is shouting or angry.
- The nurse should use words that he or she may know in the client's language. Doing so indicates that the nurse is aware of and respects the client's culture.
- The nurse should use simple words, such as "pain" instead of "discomfort." The nurse should avoid medical jargon and slang. He or she should avoid using contractions such as "don't," "can't," and "won't." The nurse should use nouns repeatedly instead of pronouns. For example, the nurse should say, "Do you take medicine?" instead of "You have been taking your medicine, haven't you?"
- The nurse should pantomime words and simple actions while verbalizing them.
- The nurse should give instructions in the proper sequence. For example, he or she should say, "First, wash the bottle. Second, rinse the bottle," instead of "Before you rinse the bottle, sterilize it."
- The nurse should discuss one topic at a time. He or she should avoid use of conjunctions. For example, the nurse should ask, "Are you cold [while pantomiming]?" and then "Are you in pain?" instead of, "Are you cold and in pain?"
- The nurse should determine whether the client understands by having the client repeat instructions, demonstrate the procedure, or act out the meaning.
- The nurse should write out several short sentences in English and determine the client's ability to read them.
- The nurse should try a third language. Many Indo-Chinese people speak French. Europeans often know three or four languages. The nurse should try Latin words or phrases.
- The nurse should ask who among the client's family and friends could serve as an interpreter.
- The nurse should obtain phrase books from a library or bookstore, make or purchase flash cards, contact hospitals for a list of interpreters, and use both formal and informal networking to locate suitable interpreters.

the female body. During pregnancy, the client may prefer female healthcare providers and may refuse to be examined by a man. The nurse should be aware that the client's significant other also might exert pressure on healthcare providers by enforcing these culturally meaningful norms in the healthcare setting.

Touching children may also have variable meanings cross-culturally. For example, Hispanic clients may believe in *mal ojo* (evil eye), in which an individual becomes ill as a result of excessive admiration by another. Many Asians believe that personal strength resides in the head and consider touching the head disrespectful. The nurse should approach palpation of the fontanelle of an infant of Southeast Asian descent with sensitivity. The nurse may need to rely on alternative sources of information (e.g., assessing for clinical manifestations of increased intracranial pressure or signs of premature fontanelle closure). Although it is the least desirable option, the nurse may need to omit this part of the assessment (Giger and Haddad, 2020).

Gender

Violating norms related to appropriate male–female relationships among various cultures may jeopardize the therapeutic nurse–client relationship. Among Arab Americans, a man is never alone with a woman, except his wife, and is usually accompanied by one or more other men when interacting with women. This behavior is culturally significant, and failure to adhere to the cultural code (i.e., set of rules or norms of behavior used by a cultural group to guide their behavior and interpret situations) is viewed as a serious transgression, often one in which the lone male will be accused of sexual impropriety. The best way to ensure that cultural variables have been considered is to ask the client about culturally relevant aspects of male–female relationships, preferably at the beginning of the

interaction before an opportunity arises to violate culturally based practices.

HEALTH-RELATED BELIEFS AND PRACTICES

One of the major aspects of a comprehensive cultural assessment concerns the collection of data related to culturally based beliefs and practices about health and illness. Before determining whether cultural practices are helpful, harmful, or neutral, the nurse must first understand the logic of the belief system underlying the practice and then be sure to grasp fully the nature and meaning of the practice from the client's cultural perspective.

Health and Culture

The first step in understanding the healthcare needs of clients is to understand personal culturally based values, beliefs, attitudes, and practices. Sometimes this step requires considerable introspection and may necessitate that the nurse confront his or her own biases, preconceptions, and prejudices about specific racial, ethnic, religious, sexual, or socioeconomic groups. The next step is to identify the meaning of health to the client, remembering that concepts are derived, in part, from the way in which members of their cultural group define health.

Considerable research has been conducted on the various definitions of health that may be held by various groups. For example, Jamaicans define health as having a good appetite, feeling strong and energetic, performing activities of daily living without difficulty, and being sexually active and fertile. For traditional Italian women, health means the ability to interact socially and perform routine tasks such as cooking, cleaning, and caring for oneself and others. Individuals may define themselves or others in their group as healthy even though the nurse identifies symptoms of disease (Spector, 2017).

Cross-Cultural Perspectives on Causes of Illness

For clients, symptom labeling and diagnosis depend on the extent of the difference between the individual's behaviors and those the group defines as normal. Other issues that the nurse should consider include the client's beliefs about the causation of illness, level of stigma attached to a particular set of symptoms, prevalence of the disease, and meaning of the illness to the individual and family.

Throughout history, humankind has attempted to understand the cause of illness and disease. Theories of causation have been formulated on the basis of religious beliefs, social circumstances, philosophical perspectives, and level of knowledge. Disease causation may be viewed from the following three major perspectives: biomedical (i.e., sometimes used synonymously with the term *scientific*), naturalistic (i.e., sometimes used synonymously with the term *holistic*), and magicoreligious (i.e., metaphysical or supernatural belief).

Biomedical Perspective

The **biomedical** (i.e., scientific) theory of illness causation is based on the following beliefs:

1. All events in life have a cause and effect.
2. The human body functions more or less mechanically (i.e., the functioning of the human body is analogous to the functioning of an automobile).
3. All life can be reduced or divided into smaller parts (e.g., the human person can be reduced into body, mind, and spirit).
4. All of reality can be observed and measured (e.g., with intelligence tests and psychometric measures of behavior).

Among the biomedical explanations for disease is the germ theory, which posits that microscopic organisms such as bacteria and viruses are responsible for many specific disease conditions. Most educational programs for nurses and other healthcare providers embrace biomedical, or scientific, theories that explain the causes of physical and psychological illnesses.

Naturalistic Perspective

Another way in which clients may explain the cause of illness is from the **naturalistic** (i.e., holistic) perspective. This viewpoint is found most frequently among Native Americans, Asians, and others who believe that human life is only one aspect of nature and a part of the general order of the cosmos. Individuals from these groups believe that the forces of nature must be kept in natural balance or harmony to maintain health and well-being. A combination of worldviews is possible, and many clients are likely to offer more than one explanation for the cause of their illness. As a profession, nursing largely embraces the biomedical-scientific worldview, but some aspects of holism have begun to gain popularity. These include a wide variety of techniques for management of chronic pain (e.g., hypnosis, therapeutic touch, and biofeedback). Many nurses hold a belief in spiritual power and readily credit supernatural forces with various unexplained phenomena related to clients' health and illness states.

Numerous Asians subscribe to the **yin-yang theory**, in which health is believed to exist when all aspects of the person are in perfect balance. Rooted in the ancient Chinese philosophy of Tao, the yin-yang theory states that all organisms and objects in the universe consist of yin or yang energy forces. The origin of the energy forces is within the autonomic nervous system, where balance between the opposing forces is maintained during health. Yin energy represents the female and negative forces (e.g., emptiness, darkness, and cold), whereas yang forces are male and positive, emitting fullness, light, and warmth. Foods are classified as hot and cold in this theory and are transformed into yin and yang energy when metabolized by the body. Yin foods are cold, and yang foods are hot. Cold foods are eaten when one has a hot illness, and hot foods are eaten when one has a cold illness. The yin-yang theory is the basis for Eastern or Chinese medicine.

The naturalistic perspective posits that the laws of nature create imbalance, chaos, and disease. Individuals embracing the naturalistic view use metaphors such as the healing power of nature, and they may call the earth "Mother." For example, from the perspective of the Chinese, illness is seen not as an intruding agent but rather as a part of life's rhythmic course and an outward sign of the disharmony that exists within.

Many Hispanic, Arab, African American, and Asian groups embrace a hot-cold theory of health and illness, an explanatory model with its origin in the ancient Greek humoral theory. Blood, phlegm, black bile, and yellow bile, the four humors of the body, regulate basic bodily functions and are described in terms of temperature, dryness, and moisture. The treatment of disease consists of adding or subtracting cold, heat, dryness, or wetness to restore the balance of the humors.

Beverages, foods, herbs, medicines, and diseases are classified as hot or cold according to their perceived effects on the body, not on their physical characteristics. Illnesses believed to be caused by cold entering the body include earache, chest cramps, paralysis, gastrointestinal discomfort, rheumatism, and tuberculosis. Illnesses believed to be caused by overheating include abscessed teeth, sore throats, rashes, and kidney disorders.

According to the hot-cold theory, the individual as a whole, rather than a specific ailment, is significant. Those who embrace the hot-cold theory maintain that health consists of a positive state of total well-being, including physical, psychological, spiritual, and social aspects of the person. Paradoxically, the language used to describe this artificial dissection of the body into parts is a reflection of the biomedical-scientific perspective, not a naturalistic or holistic one.

Magicoreligious Perspective

Another way in which people explain the causation of illness is from a **magicoreligious** perspective. The basic premise of this explanatory model is that the world is seen as an arena in which supernatural forces dominate. The fate of the world and those in it depends on the action of supernatural forces for good or evil. Examples of magical causes of illness include the belief in voodoo or witchcraft among some African Americans and others from circum-Caribbean countries. Faith healing is based on religious beliefs and is most prevalent among selected Christian religions, including Christian Scientists. Various healing rituals (prayer, anointing, exorcism, laying of hands, etc.) may be found in many religions—Roman Catholicism, Mormonism (i.e., Church of Jesus Christ of Latter-day Saints), and others (Andrews et al., 2020).

Folk Healers

All cultures have their own recognized symptoms of ill health, acceptable sick-role behavior, and treatments. In addition to seeking help from the nurse as a biomedical-scientific healthcare provider, clients from many groups may seek help from folk or religious healers.

Numerous types of folk healers exist, each with a unique scope of practice. Hispanic clients may turn to a *curandero* (male folk healer) or *curandera* (female folk healer), spiritualist, *yerbo* (herbalist), or *sabador* (healer who manipulates muscles and bones). In many instances, people from diverse cultures combine folk healing and biomedicine. Among the main reasons for seeking care from folk healers is the perception that biomedical practitioners (e.g., physicians and nurses) fail to provide holistic care and use medicines that are not natural (Andrews, et al., 2020).

Some African American clients may mention having received assistance from a *hougan* (voodoo priest or priestess), spiritualist, or "old lady" (an older woman who has successfully raised a family and specializes in child care and folk remedies). Likewise, Native American clients may seek assistance from a shaman or a medicine man or woman. Clients of Asian descent may mention that they have visited herbalists, acupuncturists, or bone setters (Giger and Haddad, 2020).

Each culture has its own healers, most of whom speak the native tongue of the client, make house calls, and cost significantly less than healers practicing in the biomedical-scientific healthcare system. In addition to folk healers, many cultures rely on lay midwives (e.g., *parteras* for Hispanic women) or other healthcare providers to meet the needs of pregnant women.

In some religions, spiritual healers may be found among the ranks of the ordained or official religious hierarchy ranks and are called *priest*, *bishop*, *elder*, *deacon*, *rabbi*, *brother*, or *sister*. Other religions have a separate category of healer (e.g., Christian Science "nurses" [not licensed by states] or practitioners) (Andrews et al., 2020).

A comprehensive discussion of the variety of healing beliefs and practices used by the numerous cultural groups is beyond the scope of this chapter. However, the nurse should be aware of alternative practices and folk healers that are used by the groups for which they care. The nurse should also be aware that most indigenous healing practices are innocuous, regardless of whether they are effective.

Cultural Expressions of Illness

A wide cultural variation exists in the manner in which certain symptoms and disease conditions are perceived, diagnosed, labeled, and treated. The disease that is grounds for social ostracism in one culture may be reason for increased status in another.

Bodily symptoms are also perceived and reported in a variety of ways. For example, individuals of Mediterranean descent tend to report common physical symptoms more often than people of Northern European or Asian heritage. To express emotion, East Asian clients sometimes somaticize their symptoms. For example, a client may complain of cardiac symptoms because the center of emotion in the Chinese culture is the heart. If the client has experienced a loss through death or divorce and is grieving, he or she may describe the loss in terms of a pain in the heart. Although some biomedical-scientific clinicians may refer to this pain as a psychosomatic illness, others will recognize it as a culturally acceptable somatic expression of emotional disharmony (Andrews et al., 2020; Giger and Haddad, 2020).

Cultural Expression of Pain

Pain, an extensively studied symptom, is used here to illustrate the manner in which symptom expression may reflect the client's cultural background. Pain is a universally recognized phenomenon and an important aspect of assessment for clients of various ages. It is also a private, subjective experience that is greatly influenced by cultural heritage. Expectations, manifestations, and pain management are all embedded in a cultural context. The definition of pain, like that of health or illness, is culturally determined.

The term *pain* is derived from the Greek word for penalty, a fact that helps explain the long association between pain and punishment in Judeo-Christian thought. The meaning of painful stimuli for individuals, the way people define their situation, and the influence of personal experience combine to determine the experience of pain.

Much cross-cultural research has been conducted on pain (Andrews et al., 2020; Campbell and Edwards, 2012; Zborowski, 1969). Pain has been found to be a highly personal experience that depends on cultural learning, the meaning of the situation, and other factors unique to the individual

(Campbell and Edwards, 2012). Healthcare professionals have identified silent suffering as the most valued response to pain. The majority of nurses have been socialized to believe that in virtually any situation, self-control is better than open displays of strong feelings.

Studies of healthcare providers' attitudes toward pain reveal that the ethnic background of clients is relevant to the assessment of physical and psychological pain (Campbell and Edwards, 2012). Nurses view Jewish and Spanish clients as experiencing suffering the most and Anglo-Saxon Germanic clients as experiencing suffering the least. In addition, nurses who infer relatively greater client pain tended to report their own experiences as more painful. In general, nurses with an Eastern or Southern European or African background tend to infer greater suffering than do nurses of Northern European background. Years of experience, current position, and area of clinical practice are unrelated to inferences of suffering (Andrews et al., 2020).

In addition to expecting variations in pain perception and tolerance, a nurse should expect variations in the expression of pain. Individuals turn to their social environments for validation and comparison. A first important comparison group is the family, which transmits cultural norms to its children.

Culture-Bound Syndromes

Clients may have a condition that is culturally defined, known as a **culture-bound syndrome**. Some of these conditions have no equal from a biomedical or scientific perspective, but others, such as anorexia nervosa and bulimia, are examples of health problems found primarily among members of the dominant U.S. cultural group. Table 13.5 presents selected examples from among more than 150 culture-bound syndromes that have been documented by medical anthropologists.

MANAGEMENT OF HEALTH PROBLEMS: A CULTURAL PERSPECTIVE

After a symptom is identified, the first effort at treatment is often self-care. In the United States, an estimated 70% to 90% of all illness episodes are treated first, or exclusively, through self-care, often with significant success. The availability of over-the-counter medications, a relatively high literacy level, and influence of the mass media/technology in communicating health-related information to the general population have contributed to the high percentage of self-treatment. Home treatments are attractive because of their accessibility in comparison with the inconvenience associated with traveling to a physician, nurse practitioner, and pharmacist, particularly for clients from rural or sparsely populated areas. Furthermore, home treatment may mobilize the client's social support network and provide the sick individual with a caring environment in which to convalesce.

However, the nurse should be aware that not all home remedies are inexpensive. For example, urban African American populations in the Southeast sometimes use medicinal

TABLE 13.5   Selected Culture-Bound Syndromes

Group	Disorder(s)	Remarks
Whites	Anorexia nervosa	Excessive preoccupation with thinness, selfimposed starvation
	Bulimia	Gross overeating, then vomiting or fasting
African Americans	Blackout	Collapse, dizziness, or inability to move
	Low blood	Not enough blood or weakness of the blood that is often treated with diet
	High blood	Blood that is too rich in certain components from ingesting too much red meat or rich foods
	Thin blood	In women, children, and the elderly; renders the individual more susceptible to illness in general
	Diseases of hex, witchcraft, or conjuring	Sense of being doomed by a spell, part of voodoo beliefs
Chinese or Southeast Asians	Koro	Intense anxiety that the penis is retracting into the body
Greeks	Hysteria	Bizarre complaints and behavior because the uterus leaves the pelvis and goes to another part of the body
Hispanics	Empacho	Food forms into a ball and clings to the stomach or intestines, causing pain and cramping
	Fatigue	Asthmalike symptoms
	Mal ojo (evil eye)	Fitful sleep, crying, and diarrhea in children caused by a stranger's attention; sudden onset
	Susto	Anxiety, trembling, and phobias from sudden fright
Native Americans	Ghost	Terror, hallucinations, and sense of danger
Japanese	Wagamama	Apathetic childish behavior with emotional outbursts

potions that cost much more than an equivalent treatment with a biomedical intervention.

Various nontraditional interventions are gaining the recognition of healthcare professionals in the biomedical-scientific healthcare system. Acupuncture, acupressure, therapeutic touch, massage, cupping, biofeedback, relaxation techniques, meditation, hypnosis, distraction, imagery, floating (sensory deprivation), and herbal remedies are interventions that clients may use alone or in combination with other treatments.

Cultural Negotiation

Cultural negotiation refers to the process in which messages, instructions, and belief systems are manipulated, linked, or processed between the professional and lay models of health problems and preferred treatment. In each act, the nurse gives attention to eliciting the client's views regarding a health-related experience (e.g., pregnancy, complications of pregnancy, or illness of an infant).

Katon and Kleinman (1981) describe negotiation as a bilateral arrangement in which two principal parties attempt to work out a solution. The goal of negotiation is to reduce conflict in a way that promotes cooperation. Cultural negotiation is used when conceptual differences exist between the client and the nurse, a situation that may occur for one or more of the following reasons:

- The nurse and client may be using the same words but applying different meanings to them.
- The nurse and client may apply the same term to the same phenomenon but have different notions of its causation.
- The nurse and client may have different memories or emotions associated with the term and its use.

In cultural negotiation, the nurse provides scientific information while acknowledging that the client may hold different views. If the client's perspective indicates that behaviors would be helpful, positive, adaptive, or neutral in effect, the nurse should include them in the plan of care. However, if the client's perspective would result in behaviors that may be harmful, negative, or nonadaptive, the nurse should attempt to shift the client's perspective to that of the practitioner (Spector, 2017).

Pregnancy and childbirth are social, cultural, and physiological experiences; therefore, an approach to culturally sensitive nursing care of childbearing women and their families must focus on the interaction between cultural meaning and biological functions. Childbirth is a time of transition and social celebration that is of central importance in any society; it signals realignment of existing cultural roles and responsibilities, psychological and biological states, and social relationships. Child rearing is also a period during which culturally bound values, attitudes, beliefs, and practices permeate virtually all aspects of life for the parents and child (Andrews et al., 2020). Careful assessment and attention to culturally based practices are particularly important during these occasions.

MANAGEMENT OF HEALTH PROBLEMS IN CULTURALLY DIVERSE POPULATIONS

The factors responsible for the health disparity between minority and white populations are complex and defy simplistic solutions. Health status is influenced by the interaction of physiological, cultural, psychological, and societal factors that are poorly understood for the general population and even less so for minorities. Despite the shared characteristic of economic disadvantage among minorities, common approaches for improving health are not recommended because of the variations in cultural beliefs and practices that exist among the different minority populations. Rather, solving problems among minorities necessitates activities, programs, and data collection that are tailored to meet the unique healthcare needs of many different subgroups. Solutions to healthcare problems among culturally diverse populations include the following recommendations that are the cornerstone of public health nursing (Keller et al., 2011):

- Focus on the health of entire populations
- Reflect community priorities and needs
- Establish caring relationships with the communities, families, and individuals that make up the population
- Remain grounded in social justice, having compassion and respect for the worth of all people, especially the vulnerable
- Provide care for the whole person: mental, physical, emotional, social, spiritual, and environmental aspects
- Promote health through strategies based on epidemiological evidence (evidence-based practice)
- Collaborate with community resources to reach healthcare goals

Providing Health Information and Education

Minority populations need more information about their health risks and treatment options. This is demonstrated by the following facts (American Cancer Society, 2021):

- African Americans have the highest mortality rate and shortest survival rate for many cancers.
- African Americans receive less information about cancer and heart disease than nonminority groups.
- African Americans tend to underestimate the prevalence of cancer, give less credence to the warning signs, obtain fewer screening tests, and receive a diagnosis at later stages of cancer than whites.
- Mexican Americans have a higher incidence of overweight and obesity than non-Hispanic whites, but non-Hispanic Blacks have the highest rates of obesity.

Programs to increase public awareness about health problems have been well received in several areas. For example, the Healthy Mothers, Healthy Babies Coalition, which provides an education program in both English and Spanish, has contributed to greater awareness of measures to improve the health status of mothers and infants. In addition, increased knowledge among African Americans of hypertension as a serious health problem is one of the accomplishments of the National High Blood Pressure Education program. The success of these efforts indicates that carefully planned programs have a beneficial effect, but efforts must continue and must expand to reach even more of the target population and focus on additional health problems.

Planning Health Information Campaigns

Sensitivity to cultural factors is often lacking in the healthcare of minorities. Key concepts for the nurse to consider in designing a health information campaign include meeting the language and cultural needs of each identified minority group, using minority-specific community resources to tailor educational approaches, and developing materials and methods of presentation that are commensurate with the educational level of the target population. Furthermore, the powerful influences of cultural factors over a lifetime in shaping people's attitudes, values, beliefs, and practices concerning health require health information programs to be sustained over a long period. The following are examples of ways in which the nurse can interweave these concepts into health promotion efforts:

- The nurse should involve local community leaders who are members of the targeted cultural group to promote acceptance and reinforcement of the central themes of health promotion messages.
- Health messages are more readily accepted if they do not conflict with existing cultural beliefs and practices. Where appropriate, messages should acknowledge existing cultural beliefs.
- The nurse should involve families, churches, employers, and community organizations as a support system to facilitate and sustain behavioral change to a more healthful lifestyle. For example, although hypertension control in African Americans depends on appropriate treatment (e.g., medication), blood pressure can be improved and maintained by family and community support of activities such as proper diet and exercise.
- Language barriers, cultural differences, and lack of adequate information on access to care complicate prenatal care for Hispanic and Asian women who have recently arrived in the United States. Through the use of lay volunteers to organize community support networks, programs have been developed to disseminate culturally appropriate health information.

Health Education

Although printed materials and other audiovisual aids contribute to the educational process, client education is inherently interpersonal. The success of educational efforts is often determined by the credibility of the source and is highly dependent on the skill and sensitivity of the nurse in communicating information in a culturally appropriate manner. Education programs are particularly critical and necessary for several health problems with the greatest influence on minority health, such as hypertension, obesity, sexually transmittable infection (STI), and diabetes. For example, if patients with diabetes could improve their self-management skills through education, a significant number of complications (e.g., ketoacidosis, blindness, and amputations) could be avoided, saving human misery and healthcare dollars.

Delivering and Financing Health Services

Innovative models for delivering and financing health services for minority populations are needed. According to community health experts, models should increase flexibility of healthcare delivery, facilitate minorities' access to services, and improve efficiency of service and payment systems. One of the most commonly used indicators of the adequacy of health services for a population is the distribution of healthcare providers; however, this is an inadequate measurement. The following observations exemplify the problems associated with health services for minorities:

- The disparities in death rates between minorities and whites remain despite overall increases in healthcare access and use (AHRQ, 2019).
- Language problems hinder refugees and immigrants when they seek healthcare.
- African Americans with cancer postpone seeking diagnosis of their symptoms longer than whites and delay initiation of treatment once diagnosed (American Cancer Society, 2021).
- The infant mortality rate among African American women is more than twice as high as the infant mortality rate among white women (CDC, 2019).

Models of Health Promotion

In most health models, SES is assumed to affect health status through environmental or behavioral factors. These models posit that poor families may not have the economic, social, or community resources needed to remain in good health. For example, poverty is thought to affect children's well-being by affecting health and nutrition, the home environment, caregiver interactions with children, caregiver mental health, and neighborhood conditions. The deficits associated with poverty may lead to an inadequate diet, which results in poor growth and delayed development. Likewise, poor housing raises the risk for exposure to many illnesses and infections; overcrowding results in increased risk for infectious diseases such as tuberculosis, meningitis, influenza, and related conditions; and community violence threatens the safety and well-being of children. The combined effect of these stressors is thought to provide the foundation for a cycle of hopelessness and depression among family members, who in turn may engage in risky health behaviors (e.g., smoking, substance abuse, and poor dietary habits resulting in obesity and high cholesterol levels) and unfavorable family interactions.

Although many Latino children live in poverty, they enjoy relatively good health in comparison with children in other low socioeconomic groups. This finding has been called an epidemiological paradox. The assumption is that if the family promotes beneficial health behaviors among its members, these behaviors will become integrated into the culture. Healthy lifestyle behaviors become an integral component of the family identity, traditions, and history.

Continuity of Care

Continuity of care is associated with improved health outcomes and is presumably greater when a client is able to establish an ongoing relationship with a care provider. Many of the leading causes of death among minorities (e.g., cancer, cardiovascular disease, and diabetes) are chronic rather than acute problems;

therefore they require extended treatment regimens. Consider the following:

- Refugees are eligible for special medical assistance during their first 18 months in the United States. However, after this period, refugees who cannot afford private health insurance and are ineligible for Medicaid or state medical assistance may become medically indigent.
- Illegal immigrants are ineligible for Medicare and Medicaid. They are medically indigent.
- Many Native Americans and Alaska Natives live in areas where the availability of healthcare providers is half the national average.

Healthcare Financing Problems

As mentioned previously, problems associated with financing healthcare tend to be more common in minority groups than in the dominant cultural group. Consider the following National Healthcare Quality and Disparities Report 2018:

- Economic inequalities cause members of minority groups to rely disproportionately on Medicaid for their healthcare needs.
- Older minority people are less likely than whites to supplement Medicare with additional private insurance.
- Proportionately, three times as many Native Americans, African Americans, Hispanics, and certain Asian and Pacific Islander groups as whites live in poverty.
- In 2015, 19.4% of Hispanics lacked insurance coverage, compared with 9.9% of African Americans and 6.2% of whites.

To better manage health problems and reduce the disparity in health indicators, these issues of financing must be addressed. Failure to address them will result not only in continued inequity in access to services but also in continued poor health among minority groups.

Developing Health Professionals From Minority Groups

The need to increase the number of health professionals from minority groups has been recognized for decades. With few exceptions, minorities are underrepresented as students and practitioners of the health professions. Although the number of minority nursing students has been steadily increasing, there still are proportionately more white nursing students.

Differences in the availability of health personnel resources in minority communities are apparent, regardless of the minority group being considered. Communities located in urban-metropolitan areas have significantly more professional resources. Among the factors that contribute to the imbalances in minority representation in health professions are the size of a minority population, number of cultural subgroups, and demographic features. Efforts to encourage more students from minority groups are ongoing, and government and private foundations offer grants, scholarships, internships, and low-cost loans to recruit and retain students from underserved minority groups in nursing and other healthcare professions.

Minority and nonminority health professional organizations, academic institutions, state governments, health departments, and other organizations from the public and private sectors should work together to develop strategies to improve the availability and accessibility of healthcare professionals to minority communities (Sullivan Commission, 2014).

Enhancing Cooperative Efforts With the Nonfederal Sector

Activities to improve minority health should involve participation of organizations at all levels (i.e., community, municipal, state, and national). Community involvement in developing health promotion activities can contribute to their success by providing credibility and visibility to the activities and facilitating their acceptance. Changes in health behavior frequently depend on personal initiative and are most likely to be triggered by efforts from locally based sources.

However, not all minority communities have the ability to identify their own health problems and initiate activities to address them. Support from the state and federal governments and private-sector assistance are needed to assist with identifying and solving health-related problems afflicting the minority community. Assistance may be provided to minority communities in the following ways:

1. The use of technical assistance to identify high-risk groups
2. Assistance with planning, implementing, and evaluating programs to address identified needs
3. Specialized community services (e.g., federally funded projects for infants and frail older adults)
4. Programs supported by businesses and industries (e.g., health promotion programs organized by unions)

The private sector can also serve as an effective channel for programs targeted to minority health projects. National organizations concerned with minorities, such as the National Urban League and the National Alliance for Hispanic Health, include health-related issues in their national agendas and are actively seeking effective ways to improve the health of minorities. Organizations such as these have a powerful potential for effecting change among their constituencies because they have strong community-level, grassroots support.

Promoting a Research Agenda on Minority Health Issues

The National Center on Minority Health and Health Disparities was developed in 2000 and redesignated in 2010 as the National Institute on Minority Health and Health Disparities (NIMHD) (http://www.nimhd.nih.gov) to assist in the investigation of factors affecting minority health (NIMHD, 2020). Its mission is to lead scientific research to improve minority health and to ultimately eliminate health disparities (NIMHD, 2020). The NIMHD conducts and supports research that examines risk factor prevalence and treatment services. It also reviews health education interventions, preventive services interventions, and sociocultural factors that influence health and outcomes of care.

For further information on current research related to culture and community health nursing, the reader should search library databases for reports of completed studies. Electronic bulletin boards also may be valuable when one is searching for research in progress and for communicating with researchers studying a particular phenomenon of interest. An example of recent nursing research related to culturally competent care is described in the Research Highlights box.

⚑ RESEARCH HIGHLIGHTS

Nutritional Patterns of Recent Immigrants

Edmonds (2005) examined the nutritional patterns of 23 women who had recently emigrated from Honduras to assist in understanding health-related nutritional issues in this Hispanic subgroup. She determined that the Honduran women had made both positive and negative changes in their diets since coming to the United States. Rice, beans, natural fruit juices, tortillas, bananas, beef, and eggs were reported as the typical foods eaten every day in Honduras. Positive changes in diets included eating a greater variety of fruits and vegetables, cooking with less grease, baking more frequently than frying, and using vegetable oil rather than lard. The women also ate more meat and dairy products. Negative changes noted were more skipped meals and eating foods high in fat and calories (e.g., fast foods). Research suggests that classes be taught in Women, Infants, and Children programs and other venues that would support the Hondurans' traditional diet and focus on how to eat nutritionally in fast-food restaurants, eat a balanced diet, plan meals and cook ahead, and read food labels.

Data from Edmonds VM: The nutritional patterns of recently immigrated Honduran women, *J Trans Nurs* 16(3):226–235, 2005.

ROLE OF THE COMMUNITY HEALTH NURSE IN IMPROVING HEALTH FOR CULTURALLY DIVERSE PEOPLE

This chapter provides data detailing the healthcare problems of culturally diverse individuals, families, groups, and communities. Given the complexity of the problems and the wide variation in incidence and distribution of these problems within specific subgroups, no simple method exists for providing culturally sensitive community health nursing care to all clients. However, the following strategies may assist the community health nurse when working with culturally diverse clients:

- Conduct a "culturological" assessment.
- Conduct a cultural self-assessment.
- Seek knowledge about local cultures.
- Recognize the political issues of culturally diverse groups.
- Provide culturally competent care.
- Recognize culturally based health problems.

Culturological Assessment

All nursing care is based on a systematic, comprehensive assessment of the client; therefore, the community health nurse must gather cultural data on clients from racially and ethnically diverse backgrounds. A **culturological assessment** refers to a systematic appraisal or examination of individuals, groups, and communities regarding their cultural beliefs, values, and practices to determine explicit nursing needs and intervention practices within the cultural context of the people being evaluated (Leininger, 1995). The term *culturological* is a descriptive reference to cultural phenomena in their broadest sense.

Culturological assessments are as vital as physical and psychological assessments. Culturological assessments tend to be broad and comprehensive because they deal with cultural values, belief systems, and ways of living now and in the recent past. In conducting a culturological assessment, the community health nurse should be involved in determining and appraising the traits, characteristics, or smallest units of cultural behavior as a guide to nursing care. The following sections summarize major data categories pertaining to the culture of clients and offer suggested questions that the nurse may ask to elicit needed information.

Brief History of Ethnic and Racial Origins of the Cultural Group With Which the Client Identifies

- With what ethnic group or groups does the client report affiliation (e.g., Hispanic, Polish, Navajo, or a combination)? To what degree does the client identify with the cultural group (e.g., "we" concept of solidarity or a fringe member)?
- Where has the client lived (i.e., country and city) and when (i.e., during what years)? If the client has recently relocated to the United States, knowledge of prevalent diseases in the country of origin may be helpful.

Values Orientation

- What are the client's attitudes, values, and beliefs about birth, death, health, illness, and healthcare providers?
- Does culture influence the manner in which the client relates to body image change resulting from illness or surgery (e.g., importance of appearance, beauty, strength, and roles in the cultural group)?
- How does the client view work, leisure, and education?
- How does the client perceive change?
- How does the client value privacy; courtesy; touch; and relationships with individuals of different ages, of different social class, or caste, and of the opposite sex?
- How does the client relate to people in a different cultural group (e.g., withdrawal, verbal or nonverbal expression, or negative or positive attitude)?

Cultural Sanctions and Restrictions

- How does the client's cultural group regard expression of emotion and feelings, spirituality, and religious beliefs? How are dying, death, and grieving expressed in a culturally appropriate manner?
- How is modesty expressed by men and women in the client's cultural group? Does the client's cultural group have culturally defined expectations about male–female relationships, including the nurse–client relationship?

- Does the client have restrictions related to sexuality, exposure of body parts, or certain types of surgery (e.g., amputation, vasectomy, or hysterectomy)?
- Does the client have restrictions against discussion of dead relatives or fears related to the unknown?

Communication

- What language does the client speak at home? What other language does the client speak or read? In what language would the client prefer to communicate with you?
- What is the written and spoken English fluency level of the client? Remember that the stress of illness may cause clients to use a more familiar language and temporarily forget some English.
- Does the client need an interpreter? If so, make sure to use an interpreter who is fluent in medical language and is not a relative or friend of the client.
- What are the rules (i.e., linguistics) and modes (i.e., style) of communication?
- Is it necessary to vary the technique of communication during the interview and examination to accommodate the client's cultural background (e.g., tempo of conversation, eye contact, sensitivity to topical taboos, norms of confidentiality, and style of explanation)?
- How does the client's nonverbal communication compare with that of individuals from other cultural backgrounds? How does it affect the client's relationship with the nurse and with other members of the healthcare team?
- How does the client feel about healthcare providers who are not of the same cultural background (e.g., African American, middle-class nurse, or Hispanic of a different social class)? Does the client prefer to receive care from a nurse of the same cultural background, sex, or age?

ETHICAL INSIGHTS

Disclosure of HIV/AIDS Status

Ortiz (2005) examined the experiences of 19 Latinas who disclosed they were living with HIV/AIDS. She described how the women decided to disclose their HIV status to partners, family members, friends, and employers. Four categories emerged: timing of the disclosure, the need to disclose, controlling disclosure, and supportive disclosing. These factors were influenced by the Latinas' relationship with others, the perceived risks to the women and others, the need to disclose, the wish to give support to themselves or others, and the desire to control who should know and when. Ortiz concluded that nurses should be knowledgeable of the realities of Latinas' lives and be able to incorporate that knowledge into comprehensive care plans that will help them maximize the utilization of appropriate resources.

Data from Ortiz CE: Disclosing concerns of Latinas living with HIV/AIDS. *J Trans Nurs* 16(3):210–217, 2005.

Health-Related Beliefs and Practices

- To what cause(s) does the client attribute illness and disease (e.g., divine wrath, imbalance in hot-cold or yin-yang, punishment for moral transgressions, hex, or soul loss)?

- What does the client believe promotes health (e.g., eating certain foods, wearing amulets to bring good luck, exercise, prayer, ancestors, saints, or intermediate deities)?
- What is the client's religious affiliation (e.g., Judaism, Islam, Pentecostalism, West African voodooism, Seventh-Day Adventism, Catholicism, or Mormonism)?
- Does the client rely on cultural healers (e.g., *curandero*, shaman, spiritualist, priest, minister, or monk)? Who determines when the client is sick and when the client is healthy? Who determines the type of healer and treatment that should be sought?
- In what types of cultural healing practices does the client engage (e.g., herbal remedies, potions, massage, wearing talismans or charms to discourage evil spirits, healing rituals, incantations, or prayers)?
- How does the client perceive biomedical-scientific healthcare providers? How do the client and family perceive nurses? What are the expectations of nurses and nursing care?
- What constitutes appropriate "sick-role" behavior? Who determines what symptoms constitute disease and illness? Who decides when the client is no longer sick? Who cares for the client at home?
- How does the client's cultural group view mental disorders? Do they show differences in acceptable behaviors for physical versus psychological illnesses?

Nutrition

- What nutritional factors are influenced by the client's cultural background?
- What meanings does the client attach to food and eating? With whom does the client usually eat? What types of foods does the client usually eat? What does the client define as food? What does the client believe defines a "healthy" versus an "unhealthy" diet?
- How does the client prepare foods at home (e.g., type of food preparation; cooking oils used; length of time foods, especially vegetables, are cooked; amount and type of seasoning added to various foods during preparation)?
- Do religious beliefs and practices influence the client's diet (e.g., amount, type, preparation, or delineation of acceptable food combinations, such as kosher diets)? Does the client abstain from certain foods at regular intervals, on specific dates determined by the religious calendar, or at other times?
- If the client's religion mandates or encourages fasting, what does the term *fast* mean to the client (e.g., refraining from certain types or quantities of foods, eating only during certain times of the day)? For what period of time is the client expected to fast? Does the religion allow exemption from fasting during illness, and, if so, is the client believed to have an exemption?

Socioeconomic Considerations

- Who constitutes the client's social network (i.e., family, peers, and healers)? How do they influence the client's health or illness status?

- How do members of the client's social support network define caring (e.g., being continuously present, doing things for the client, or looking after the client's family)? What are the roles of various family members during health and illness?
- How does the client's family participate in the client's nursing care (e.g., bathing, feeding, touching, and being present)?
- Does the cultural family structure influence the client's response to health or illness (e.g., beliefs, strengths, weaknesses, and social class)? Does a key family member have a role that is significant in health-related decisions (e.g., grandmother in many African American families or eldest adult son in Asian families)?
- Who is the principal wage earner in the client's family? What is the total annual income? This is a potentially sensitive question that should be asked only if necessary. Does the family have more than one wage earner? Does the family have other sources of financial support (e.g., extended family or investments)?
- What influence does economic status have on lifestyle, place of residence, living conditions, ability to obtain healthcare, and discharge planning?

Organizations Providing Cultural Support

- What influence do ethnic and cultural organizations have on the client's receiving healthcare (e.g., National Association for the Advancement of Colored People, African American Political Caucus, churches, schools, Urban League, and community-based healthcare programs and clinics)?

Educational Background

- What is the highest educational level the client has obtained? Does the client's educational background affect the client's knowledge level concerning the healthcare delivery system, how to obtain the care needed, teaching and learning skills, and written material that is distributed in the healthcare setting (e.g., insurance forms, educational literature, information about diagnostic procedures and laboratory tests, and admissions forms)?
- Can the client read and write English, or does he or she prefer another language? If English is the client's second language, are materials available in the client's primary language?
- What learning style is most comfortable or familiar? Does the client prefer to learn through written materials, oral explanation, or demonstration?

Religious Affiliation

- How does the client's religious affiliation influence health and illness (e.g., death, chronic illness, body image alteration, and cause and effect of illness)?

- What is the role of the client's religious beliefs and practices during health and illness?
- What is the role of significant religious representatives during health and illness? Does the client have recognized religious healers (e.g., Islamic imams, Christian Scientist practitioners or nurses, Catholic priests, Mormon elders, and Buddhist monks)?

Cultural Aspects of Disease Incidence

- Does the client have specific genetic or acquired conditions that are more prevalent in a specific cultural group (e.g., hypertension, sickle cell anemia, Tay-Sachs disease, or lactose intolerance)?
- Are any socioenvironmental diseases more prevalent among the client's specific cultural group (e.g., lead poisoning, alcoholism, AIDS, drug abuse, or ear infections)?
- Do diseases exist against which the client has an increased resistance (e.g., skin cancer in a darkly pigmented individual)?

Biocultural Variations

- Does the client have distinctive physical features that are characteristic of a particular racial group (e.g., skin color or hair texture)? Does the client have variations in anatomy that are characteristic of a particular racial or ethnic group (e.g., body structure, height, weight, facial shape and structure [nose, eye shape, and facial contour], or upper and lower extremity shape)?
- How do anatomical and racial variations affect the assessment?

Developmental Considerations

- Does the client have distinct growth and development characteristics that vary with his or her cultural background (e.g., bone density, psychomotor patterns of development, or fat folds)?
- What factors are significant in assessing children from the newborn period through adolescence (e.g., expected growth on standard grid, culturally acceptable age for toilet training, introduction of various types of foods, sex differences, discipline, and socialization to adult roles)?
- What is the cultural perception of aging (e.g., is youthfulness or the wisdom of old age more highly valued)?
- What are cultural practices related to care of older people (e.g., cared for in the home of adult children or placed in institutions for care)? What are culturally acceptable roles for older adults?
- Does the older adult expect family members to provide care, including nurturance and other humanistic aspects of care?
- Is the older adult isolated from culturally relevant supportive people or enmeshed in a caring network of relatives and friends?

- Has a culturally appropriate network replaced family members in performing some caring functions for older adults?

Cultural Self-Assessment

Community health nurses can engage in a cultural self-assessment. Through identification of health-related attitudes, values, beliefs, and practices that are part of the personal cultural meaning brought to the nurse–client interaction, the nurse can better understand the cultural aspects of healthcare from the perspective of the client, family, group, or community. Everyone has ethnocentric tendencies that must be brought to a level of conscious awareness so that efforts can be made to temper ethnocentrism and view reality from the perspective of the client.

Knowledge About Local Cultures

Community health nurses can learn about the cultural diversity characteristics of the subgroup or subgroups that are most prevalent within their communities. The nurse cannot know about all health-related beliefs and practices of the diverse groups served, but he or she can study select ones. The nurse can accomplish this cultural study through a review of nursing, anthropology, sociology, and related literature on culturally diverse groups; in-service programs held at community health agencies, educational institutions in the community, or organizations serving minority groups; enrollment in courses on transcultural or cross-cultural nursing and medical anthropology; and interviews with key members of the subgroups of interest, such as clergy members, nurses, and physicians, to obtain information about the influence of culture on health-related beliefs and practices.

Recognition of Political Issues of Culturally Diverse Groups

Awareness of the political aspects of healthcare for culturally diverse groups and communities can help community health nurses influence legislation and funding priorities aimed at improving healthcare for specific populations. Recognized for their leadership role in community health matters involving culturally diverse groups, community health nurses may be invited by political leaders to participate in political decision making that affects the health of a targeted subgroup. Community health nurses should also be active politically, both individually and collectively, to influence legislation affecting culturally diverse individuals, groups, and communities, and they should offer to serve on key community committees, boards, and advisory councils that affect the health of culturally diverse groups.

Providing Culturally Competent Care

When caring for individuals and families from culturally diverse backgrounds, the community health nurse can assess, diagnose, implement, and evaluate nursing care in a manner that is culturally congruent, competent, relevant, and appropriate. To provide this culturally appropriate nursing care, the nurse must create a relationship of mutual respect by becoming aware of the cultural similarities and differences between herself or himself and the client. A guideline for gathering cultural data has been presented, and the nurse may use this guideline or a similar one to identify significant areas in which the nurse and client differ. Knowledge about biocultural variations in health and illness is particularly important when the nurse is conducting cultural assessments.

Recognition of Culturally Based Health Practices

As discussed previously, the community health nurse should attempt to understand the nature and meaning of culturally based health practices of clients, groups, and communities. Once the practices are understood, the nurse can make a determination regarding their appropriateness in a particular context. Generally, the nurse should decide whether a cultural practice is useful, neutral, or harmful to the client, group, or community. The nurse should encourage or "tolerate" helpful and neutral practices, whereas he or she should discourage harmful practices.

However, the classification of some cultural healing practices is not so easily determined. For example, many Southeast Asians practice coining, which is the rubbing of a coin over body surfaces to expel "bad winds" that are believed to cause illness (Berg et al., 2016; Vitale and Prashad, 2017). Community health nurses are faced with an ethical dilemma when coining is practiced on young children, because it leaves abrasions on the skin and may be viewed by some as child abuse. This practice is not useful, so the nurse must make the decision whether it is neutral or harmful. An argument for the practice's being neutral is that abrasions usually heal quickly, so no harm is done to the child as a result. Furthermore, the practice is meaningful to parents who have much confidence in the healing powers associated with coining (Giger and Haddad, 2020; Vitale and Prashad, 2017).

The argument can also be made that the practice is harmful. The red marks and skin abrasions caused by the coining place the child at increased risk for skin infection. Given that the child may require antibiotics or other medication for a respiratory disorder, encouragement of coining as the only treatment may prevent the child from receiving needed medical intervention and may delay medical treatment. As a solution, the community health nurse may suggest that parents combine traditional treatment with Western biomedicine (i.e., they can use coining in conjunction with a biomedical intervention). Therefore the healing will occur in a manner that has involved the use of both folk and professional healthcare systems (Giger and Haddad, 2020; Vitale and Prashad, 2017).

⚡ ACTIVE LEARNING

1. Select a client from a racially or ethnically diverse background, and conduct a cultural assessment.
2. Interview someone from a racial or ethnic background different from your own to determine beliefs about illness causation, use of the lay and professional healthcare delivery systems, and culturally based treatments.

RESOURCES FOR MINORITY HEALTH

Community health nurses will find federal resources for improving the healthcare of the federally defined minority populations through the USDHHS. Within the USDHHS, the Office of Minority Health (OMH) and the Indian Health Service (IHS) divisions are concerned with health promotion, disease prevention, service delivery, and research for minority groups.

Office of Minority Health

The OMH coordinates federal efforts to improve the health status of racial and ethnic minority populations (i.e., African Americans, Hispanics, Native Americans and Alaska Natives, and Asians and Pacific Islanders). Directed by the deputy assistant secretary for minority health, the OMH was established by the Disadvantaged Minority Health Improvement Act of 1990 (PL 101–527), which was signed by President George H. W. Bush on November 6, 1990. Under the directives of the act, the OMH is charged with duties to:

- Establish short- and long-range goals and objectives relating to disease prevention, health promotion, service delivery, and research on the health of minority people
- Promote increased participation of disadvantaged people, including minorities, in health service and health promotion programs
- Create a national minority health resource center
- Support research, demonstrations, and evaluations of new and innovative models that increase understanding of disease risk factors and support better information dissemination, education, prevention, and service delivery to minority communities
- Promote minority health–related activities in the corporate and voluntary sectors
- Develop minority-focused health information and health promotion materials and teaching programs
- Assist providers of primary care and preventive services in obtaining assistance of bilingual health professionals when appropriate

As the focal point for minority health efforts, the OMH plays a key role in major initiatives launched by the secretary of the USDHHS. Table 13.6 lists some of these initiatives.

Indian Health Service

The IHS is responsible for providing federal health services to Native Americans and Alaska Natives. Federal IHSs are based on a special government-to-government relationship and laws that Congress has passed pursuant to its authority to regulate commerce with the Indian Nations as specified in the Constitution and other documents.

The primary responsibility of the IHS is to elevate the health status of Native Americans and Alaska Natives to the highest level possible. The mission is to ensure quality, availability, and accessibility of a comprehensive, high-quality healthcare delivery system, providing maximum involvement of Native Americans and Alaska Natives in defining their health needs, setting health priorities for their local areas, and managing and controlling their health programs.

The IHS also acts as the principal federal health advocate for Native Americans by ensuring that they have knowledge of, and access to, all federal, state, and local health programs to which they are entitled as American citizens. The IHS carried out its responsibilities through development and operation of a health services delivery system designed to provide a broad-spectrum program of preventive, curative, rehabilitative, and environmental services. This system integrates health services delivered directly through IHS facilities and staff with those purchased by IHS through contractual arrangements. Tribes are also actively involved in program implementation.

The 1975 Indian Self-Determination Act (PL 93–638), as amended, builds on IHS policy by giving tribes the option of staffing and managing IHS programs in their communities and provides funding for improvement of tribal capability to contract under the act. The 1976 Indian Health Care Improvement Act (PL 94–437), as amended, was intended to elevate the healthcare status of Native Americans and Alaska Natives to a level equal to that of the general population through a program of authorized, higher-resource levels in the IHS budget. Appropriated resources

TABLE 13.6 Federally Sponsored Initiatives to Improve the Health of Minority Groups

Initiative	Description
Racial and Ethnic Approaches to Community Health (REACH, 2010)	This program was launched in 1999 to eliminate health disparities in six priority areas: cardiovascular diseases, immunizations, breast and cervical cancer screening and management, diabetes, HIV/AIDS, and infant mortality. REACH 2010 supports community coalitions in designing, implementing, and evaluating community-driven strategies to eliminate health disparities.
National Breast and Cervical Cancer Early Detection Program (NBCCEDP)	NBCCEDP provides breast and cervical cancer screening, diagnosis, and treatment to low-income, medically underserved, and uninsured women (emphasizing recruitment of minority women).
Ryan White Comprehensive AIDS Resources Emergency (CARE) Act B	Ryan White CARE Act provides services to persons living with HIV disease, primarily racial, and ethnic minorities.
National Institute on Minority Health and Health Disparities (NIMHD)	NIMHD mission is to lead scientific research to improve minority health and reduce disparity.

were used to expand health services, build and renovate medical facilities, and step up the construction of safe drinking water and sanitary disposal facilities. It also established programs designed to increase the number of Native American health professionals for Native American needs and to improve healthcare access for Native Americans living in urban areas.

The operation of the IHS healthcare delivery system is managed through local administrative units called *service units*.

A service unit is the basic health organization for a geographic area served by the IHS program, just as a county or city health department is the basic health organization in a state health department. These are defined areas usually centered on a single federal reservation in the continental United States or a population concentration in Alaska. The IHS serves approximately 50% of the total Native American and Alaska Native population in the United States, primarily those residing on reservations.

CASE STUDY Application of the Nursing Process

Asian Family and Cultural Practices

Community health nurse Maria Gonzales visited the home of 5-year-old Nguyen Van Nghi, who was discharged from the hospital on the previous day. The pediatrician had diagnosed pneumonia and "suspected failure to thrive" in the child because the child's growth fell below the third percentile on a standard growth chart for height and weight, and he performed poorly on a screening test used to identify developmental delays for a 5-year-old child.

Residing in the home were the child's parents, four siblings, grandmother, aunt, uncle, and three cousins. Although the child's father and uncle spoke some English, other members of the household communicated in a language unfamiliar to Maria, which "sounded like Chinese." When Maria approached the child, he did not look at her or speak to her, even when she called him Nguyen (pronounced "we'en").

Assessment

In a brief survey of the Nguyens' home, Maria noted that the home and furnishings were modest but very clean. The pantry held a considerable amount of food, including rice and dried noodles. The small refrigerator smelled of fish and contained some vegetables that Maria did not recognize. She did not see any green vegetables, milk, or other dairy products.

During her initial assessment of Nghi, Maria observed multiple tender, ecchymotic areas with petechiae between the ribs on the front and back of the body, resembling strap marks. Suspecting child abuse, Maria told the family that she would return later in the day with an interpreter. She located an interpreter who spoke Mandarin Chinese and briefed him about her concerns with child abuse. When Maria and the interpreter returned to the client's home, she instructed the interpreter to ask the parents for an explanation of the bruises. The interpreter told Maria that the family was Vietnamese and could not understand his Chinese dialect. Both the interpreter and the child's father knew a little French and awkwardly managed to communicate.

The interpreter advised the nurse that in the Vietnamese culture, the person's family name is given first, followed by the middle name and then the first name. Only a few different family names exist among the Vietnamese; therefore it is common practice to call people by their given first name. At this point, Maria also learned that the child was actually 4 years old, because the Vietnamese consider a newborn to be 1 year old at birth.

The interpreter explained that a Vietnamese healer performed cao gio, or coining, to exude the "bad wind" from Nghi. Cao gio is performed by applying a special menthol oil to the painful or symptomatic part of the body and then rubbing a coin over the area with firm, downward strokes. When Nghi's condition seemed to worsen after his hospital discharge, his grandmother persuaded his parents that Western biomedicine had failed and that their son required the stronger power of folk healing.

Diagnosis

- Maria must set priorities and focus on selected cultural data categories because they seem most relevant for the Nguyen family at present.

Individual

- High risk for Nghi's pneumonia to worsen

- Potential for child abuse/neglect
- Possible physical and/or developmental delay (low weight/height for age)

Family

- Increased risk for poor health outcomes related to distrust of Western healthcare practices
- Increased risk for nutritional deficits

Community

- Potential for poor health of area Vietnamese immigrants related to limited knowledge of good nutritional practices and general health promotion

Planning
Individual

Short-Term Goals

- Nghi's pneumonia will resolve.
- Nghi will show no more evidence of the practice of "coining."

Long-Term Goal

- Nghi's height and weight will increase proportionally to at least the 50th percentile for age.

Family

Short-Term Goals

- Family members will cease the practice of "coining."
- Caregivers will recognize the importance of completing the antibiotic therapy as prescribed.

Long-Term Goal

- A family nutritional assessment will be completed, and adjustments will be made to their diet to provide needed nutrients.

Community

Long-Term Goal

- Leaders of the area's Vietnamese community will work with area healthcare providers to promote good nutritional practices.

Intervention
Individual

Through the interpreter, Maria was able to communicate with the Nguyen family that it was vital for Nghi to take all of the prescribed antibiotics. She also attempted to convey the potentially harmful effect of the practice of coining and suggested that procedure be stopped. She set a follow-up appointment for the next day.

Family

Maria was able to bring a Vietnamese interpreter for the follow-up appointment. So in addition to reiterating the importance of taking the medications, she was able to teach about basic nutritional principles and perform additional nutritional assessments. Although Nghi was not as small as initially thought, he was still below the 50th percentile for his age. Maria gave nutritional pamphlets written in Vietnamese to the parents and provided them with information on where to find low-cost foods in the neighborhood.

Community
Working with the health department's social worker and the Vietnamese interpreter, Maria visited several area markets to gather information on diet and nutritional practices of Vietnamese immigrants. They decided that they would seek a small grant to develop more teaching materials on nutrition for this population.

Evaluation
Individual
By the third follow-up visit, Maria determined that although Nghi still had a residual cough, his chest was clearing. In addition, there was no evidence of coining. Furthermore, Maria was shown that the family's refrigerator now contained whole milk and some leafy green vegetables. It was decided that she would return in 6 weeks for a follow-up visit to weigh and measure Nghi.

Family
The presence of the interpreter who spoke Vietnamese and who was familiar with the culture was vital. And by the third visit, most of the family members appeared to be at ease with Maria. Mrs. Nguyen asked a number of questions about nutrition and other health issues and requested that Maria monitor the heights and weights of the other children.

Community
The health department's social worker was able to identify a small grant to develop and purchase teaching materials for the Vietnamese population. The nurse and social worker applied for the funds and are eagerly waiting to hear the outcome.

Levels of Prevention
The following are examples of three levels of prevention as applied to the case study.

Primary Prevention
- Nutritional education for the Nguyen family
- Health education targeted at developing comfort with the U.S. healthcare system and Western medicine
- Education related to potentially harmful practices (e.g., coining)

Secondary Prevention
Monitoring the height and weight of Nghi and his siblings.

Tertiary Prevention
Evaluation of resolution of pneumonia.

SUMMARY

To provide community health nursing for individuals, groups, and communities representing the hundreds of different cultures and subcultures found in the United States, the nurse should include cultural considerations in nursing care. Guidelines for gathering data from clients of culturally diverse backgrounds have been suggested in this chapter and are interwoven throughout the text. Knowledge about culture-specific and culture-universal nursing care is foundational and is an integral component of community health nursing.

EVOLVE WEBSITE

http://evolve.elsevier.com/Nies/community
- NCLEX Review Questions
- Case Studies

BIBLIOGRAPHY

Agency for Healthcare Research and Quality (AHRQ): *2018 National healthcare quality and disparities report*, 2019. Available from: https://www.ahrq.gov/sites/default/files/wysiwyg/research/findings/nhqrdr/2018qdr-final-es.pdf.

American Association of Colleges of Nursing: *Fact sheet: enhancing diversity in the nursing workforce*, 2017. Available from: https://www.aacnnursing.org/Portals/42/News/Factsheets/Enhancing-Diversity-Factsheet.pdf.

American Cancer Society: *Cancer facts & figures for African Americans, 2019–2021*, 2021. Available from: https://www.cancer.org/content/dam/cancer-org/research/cancer-facts-and-statistics/cancer-facts-and-figures-for-african-americans/cancer-facts-and-figures-for-african-americans-2019-2021.pdf.

Andrews MM, Boyle JS, Collins JW: *Transcultural concepts in nursing care*, ed 8 Philadelphia, 2020, Wolters Kluwer.

Baker B: *Estimates of unauthorized immigrant population residing in the United States: January 2015–January 2018*, 2021. Available from: https://www.dhs.gov/sites/default/files/publications/immigration-statistics/Pop_Estimate/UnauthImmigrant/unauthorized_immigrant_population_estimates_2015_-_2018.pdf.

Berg J, Morphew T, Tran J: Prevalence of complimentary and alternative medicine usage in Vietnamese American asthmatic children, *Clin Pediatr* 55(2):157–164, 2016.

Campbell CM, Edwards RR: Ethnic differences in pain and pain management, *Pain Manag* 2(3):219–230, 2012. https://www.ncbi.nlm.nih.gov/pmc/articles/PMC3654683/.

Centers for Disease Control (CDC): Infant mortality statistics from the 2017 period linked birth/infant death data set, National vital statistics reports, 2019. Available from: https://www.cdc.gov/nchs/data/nvsr/nvsr68/nvsr68_10-508.pdf.

Child Trends Databank: *High school dropout rates*, 2018. Available from: https://www.childtrends.org/?indicators=high-school-dropout-rates.

Cockerham WC: *Medical sociology*, ed 14 Upper Saddle River, NJ, 2017, Prentice Hall.

Colby SL, Ortman JM: *Projections of the size and composition of the U.S. population: 2014 to 2060, current population reports, P25-1143*, Washington, DC, 2015, U.S. Census Bureau.

Edmonds VM: The nutritional patterns of recently immigrated Honduran women, *J Transcult Nurs* 16(3):226–235, 2005.

Expert Panel on Global Nursing & Health: *Standards of practice for culturally competent nursing care*, 2010. Available from: http://www.tcns.org/files/Standards_of_Practice_for_Culturally_Compt_Nsg_Care-Revised_.pdf.

Giger JN, Haddad LG: *Transcultural nursing: assessment and intervention*, ed 8, St Louis, 2020, Elsevier.

Kaiser Family Foundation: *Percent of adults reporting fair or poor health status, by race/ethnicity*, 2019. Available from: www.kff.org/other/state-indicator/percent-of-adults-reporting-fair-or-poor-health-status-by-raceethnicity/?currentTimeframe=0&sortModel=%7B%22colId%22:%22Location%22,%22sort%22:%22asc%22%7D.

Kaiser Family Foundation (KFF): *Health coverage of immigrants*, 2020. Available from: https://www.kff.org/racial-equity-and-health-policy/fact-sheet/health-coverage-of-immigrants.

Katon W, Kleinman A: Doctor-patient negotiation and other social science strategies in patient care. In Eisenberg L, Kleinman A, editors: *The relevance of social science for medicine*, Boston, 1981, D. Reidel.

Keller L, Strohschein S, Schaffer M: Cornerstones of public health nursing, *Public Health Nurs* 28(3):249–260, 2011.

Kluckhohn F, Strodtbeck F: *Variations in value orientations*, Evanston, IL, 1961, Row, Peterson.

Kohls LR: *Survival kit for overseas living*, Yarmouth, ME, 1984, Intercultural Press.

Leininger MM: *Nursing and anthropology: two worlds to blend*, New York, 1970, Wiley.

Leininger MM: *Transcultural nursing: concepts, theories, and practice*, New York, 1978, Wiley.

Leininger MM: *Culture, care, diversity, and universality: a theory of nursing*, New York, 1991, National League for Nursing Press.

Leininger MM: *Transcultural nursing: concepts, theories, research and practice*, ed 2, New York, 1995, McGraw-Hill.

Leininger MM, McFarland MR, Wehbe-Alamah HB: *Transcultural nursing: concepts, theories, research and practice*, ed 4, New York, 2018, McGraw-Hill.

National Institute on Minority Health and Health Disparities: National Institute on Minority Health and Health Disparities fact sheet, 2020. Available from: https://www.nimhd.nih.gov/docs/about-nimhd-fact-sheet.pdf.

Ortiz CE: Disclosing concerns of Latinas living with HIV/AIDS, *J Transcult Nurs* 16(3):210–217, 2005.

Pew Research Center: Religious landscape study, 2021. Available from: https://www.pewforum.org/religious-landscape-study/.

Spector RE: *Cultural diversity in health and illness*, ed 9, New York, 2017, Pearson.

Sullivan Commission: *Missing persons: minorities in the health professions*, 2014. Available from: http://campaignforaction.org/wp-content/uploads/2016/04/SullivanReport-Diversity-in-Healthcare-Workforce1.pdf.

The Commonwealth Fund: *Closing the divide: how medical homes promote equity in health care: results from the Commonwealth Fund 2006 healthcare quality survey*, 2007. Available from: www.commonwealthfund.org/Content/Publications/Fund-Reports/2007/Jun/Closing-the-Divide-How-Medical-Homes-Promote-Equity-in-Health-Care-Results-From-The-Commonwealth-F.aspx.

Tylor EB: *Primitive culture*, London, 1871, Murray.

U.S. Census Bureau: *American community survey: selected characteristics of the foreign-born population by period of entry into the United States*, 2019. Available from: https://data.census.gov/cedsci/table?q=foreign%20born&tid=ACSST1Y2019.S0502.

U.S. Census Bureau: *Income and poverty in the United States: 2019*, 2020. Available from: https://www.census.gov/library/publications/2020/demo/p60-270.html.

U.S. Census Bureau: *Current population estimates*, 2021. Available from: https://www.census.gov/quickfacts/fact/table/US.

U.S. Department of Health and Human Services: *Healthy people 2030 framework*, 2020. Available from: https://health.gov/healthypeople/about/healthy-people-2030-framework.

U.S. Department of Homeland Security: *Yearbook of immigration statistics, 2019*, 2020. Available from: https://www.dhs.gov/immigration-statistics/yearbook/2019/table1.

Vitale SA, Prashad T: Cultural awareness: coining and cupping, *Int Arch Nurs Health Care* 3:3, 2017. https://doi.org/10.23937/2469-5823/1510080.

Wilmoth JM, Chen PC: Immigrant status, living arrangements, and depressive symptoms among middle-aged and older adults, *J Gerontol B Psychol Sci Soc Sci* 58B(5):S305–S313, 2003.

Zborowski M: *People in pain*, San Francisco, 1969, Jossey-Bass.

Environmental Health

Tamara Rose[a]

KEY TERMS

air quality index
biosolids
built environment
climate change
critical theory
environmental health
environmental justice

environmental risks to health
food desert
food safety
global warming
Healthy Home
outdoor air quality
participatory action research

population
sick building syndrome
social capital
waste management
water quality
work-related exposures

The World Health Organization (WHO) (2021) refers to environmental health outcomes as "clean air, stable climate, adequate water, sanitation and hygiene, safe use of chemicals, protection from radiation, healthy and safe workplaces, sound agricultural practices, health-supportive cities and built environments as well as the preservation of nature." "As a fundamental component of a comprehensive public health system, environmental health works to advance policies and programs to reduce chemical and other environmental exposures in air,

water, soil, and food to protect residents and provide communities with healthier environments" (National Environmental Health Association, 2016). Fig. 14.1, from the U.S. Department of Health and Human Services *Healthy People 2030* program, demonstrates these factors.

Environmental health experts believe that the purpose of environmental health is to assure the conditions of human health and provide healthy environments for people to live, work, and play. This can be accomplished through risk assessment, prevention, and intervention.

Efforts are made to reduce and eliminate contaminant and contagion threats to human health from air, water, food, and

---

[a]The author would like to acknowledge the contribution of Diane Santa Maria, who wrote this chapter for the previous edition.

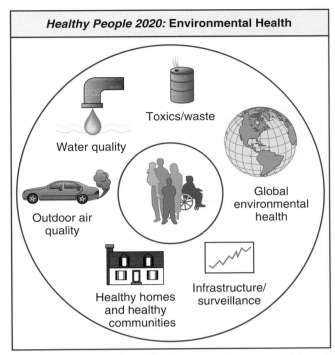

Healthy People 2020: Environmental Health

- Toxics/waste
- Water quality
- Outdoor air quality
- Global environmental health
- Healthy homes and healthy communities
- Infrastructure/surveillance

Fig. 14.1 Healthy People 2020: Elements of environmental health. (From U.S. Department of Health and Human Services: *Healthy People 2010*, ed 2, Washington, DC, 2000, U.S. Government Printing Office.)

the built environment (Lindland and Kendall-Taylor, 2011). Maintaining a healthy environment is vitally important to promoting the health of populations—particular groups or types of people. A healthy environment improves quality of life and increases years of healthy living. Accumulated evidence shows that the environmental changes of the past few decades have profoundly influenced the status of public health. Globally, environmental risk factors, including air, water, and soil pollution, exposure to chemicals, radiation, and climate changes, contribute to nearly 25% of all deaths and increase disease burden (WHO, 2021). The safety, beauty, and life-sustaining capacity of the physical environment are unquestionably of global consequence. Since the beginning of the 21st century, it has become apparent that the world must address urgent environmental difficulties, including extinction of some species, diminishing rainforests, proliferation of toxic waste dumps, progressive destruction of the ozone layer, shortage of landfill sites, consequences of climate change, threats of terrorism, development of deadly chemical and ballistic weapons, adulteration of food by pesticides and herbicides, oceanic contamination through toxic dumping and petroleum spills, overcrowding of urban areas, and traffic congestion.

This chapter uses critical theory to explore the health of communities in relation to the environment. Critical theory is particularly useful in examining environmental health because it offers a framework for discussion and a basis for describing community health nursing practice (Martins and Burbank, 2011; Stevens and Hall, 1992). Applying critical theory is a way of thinking upstream (see Chapter 3). Critical theory is an approach that raises questions about oppressive situations, involves community members in the definition and solution of problems, and facilitates interventions that reduce health-damaging effects of environments. By applying the nursing process in a critical fashion, nurses can be dynamically involved in the design of interventions that alter the precursors of poor health.

Recognition of the gravity and pervasiveness of environmental hazards can be overwhelming. Looking beyond the individual to recognize the environmental determinants of health can be complicated and alarming. Intervening to improve the quality of air, water, housing, food, and waste disposal and reducing the risks of harmful exposures to environmental toxins require individual, social, economic, and political changes. Nurses are powerful change agents who use their assessment, management, and communication skills to promote environmental health locally and nationally. Nurses are becoming increasingly active in efforts to address environmental health issues and to increase awareness of the effects of the environment on well-being.

A CRITICAL THEORY APPROACH TO ENVIRONMENTAL HEALTH

Critical theory suggests that nurses must be aware of environmental threats or factors that might detrimentally affect the safety and well-being of particular populations or deprive them of access to resources necessary in the pursuit of health. This awareness may include recognizing, supporting, and maintaining positive environmental influences. For instance, a nurse must consider the effects of having access to a safe place to walk on one's ability to maintain healthy levels of physical activity. Research studies indicate that access to recreation facilities is an important correlate of physical activity (Kaufman et al., 2019; Troped et al., 2011; Tsunoda et al., 2012). Nurses can help individuals adopt healthy behaviors by considering not only individual-level issues but also those issues in the environment that facilitate or create barriers to healthy living.

Nurses need to ask critical questions about their clients' environments to help discern the contributions of specific hazards to their health. Occupational exposure to environmental hazardous can cause harm to workers as well as their families. For example, farm workers and pesticide applicators who accumulate agricultural chemicals on their skin and clothing take these substances home with them, increasing their children's exposure to toxicants (Thompson et al., 2008). Nurses must provide answers to farm workers who ask questions such as "What do I do if I'm exposed to a pesticide?

How long should I wait until after a pesticide application to go back into the field? How do I find out how toxic a certain pesticide is? Where can I get information on a specific pesticide?" Nurses can take an environmental health history. An environmental health history can benefit the client in the following ways:

- Increase awareness of environmental health concerns
- Improve timelines and accuracy of diagnosis
- Prevent disease and aggravation of conditions
- Identify potential environmental hazards

Environmental health histories should be obtained for both adults and children, although the relationship between the environment and children's health is frequently overlooked. Fig. 14.2 demonstrates common assessment items of an environmental history. When looking at the community from a critical perspective, nurses have the opportunity to promote population health. In identifying environmental sources of health problems, nurses must be involved with the affected communities. Rather than impose their views of the problem, nurses should share their ideas and dialogue with community members. For example, nurses should listen to what the community believes is problematic, help raise consciousness about environmental dangers, and help bring about change. If nurses become involved in conducting community assessments and analyses, they can learn how the community members perceive themselves, their health, and their environmental influences.

From a critical standpoint, helping communities become more aware of the environmental effects on health and helping them make needed changes in their environment are legitimate nursing actions. Collective actions have been instrumental in accomplishing positive environmental changes since the 1980s. Some of the mechanisms have included strategic organization, litigation, public hearing testimony, letter-writing campaigns, legislative lobbying, mass demonstrations, and fundraising. Fundraising for environmental causes such as the 2012 storms that devastated the Northeast United States and the 2010 earthquake in Haiti facilitated rapid availability of resources, minimized loss of life, and helped restore basic necessities such as clean water and shelter. Public response to "acute" environmental disasters needs to be extended to an ongoing, consistent pressure to ensure day-to-day environmental integrity; hence "chronic" environmental problems need to be addressed more effectively.

1. Do you live next to or near an industrial plant, commercial business, dump site, or nonresidential property?
2. Have you been exposed to hazardous materials at work now or in the past?
3. Which of the following do you have in your home?
   __ air conditioner __ air purifier __ central heating (_ gas _ oil)
   __ gas stove __ fireplace __ wood stove
   __ humidifier
4. Have you recently acquired new furniture or carpet, refinished furniture, or remodeled your home?
5. Have you weatherized your home recently?
6. Are pesticides or herbicides (bug or weed killers; flea and tick sprays; collars, powders, shampoos) used in your home, garden, or on your pets?
7. Do you (or any household member) have a hobby or craft?
8. Have you ever changed your residence because of a health problem?
9. Does your drinking water come from a private well?
10. Approximately what year was your home built?
11. Has your routine changed recently?
12. Does anyone in your household smoke?
13. Has your home been tested for radon?

Fig. 14.2 Environmental history assessment.

A critical perspective can help nurses plan and implement population-level interventions by emphasizing collective strategies for change. Acting collectively can empower nurses to affect environmental health. Assessing environmental health problems, planning and implementing interventions, and evaluating the effectiveness of community-based actions need to be based on a wide lens. Community health nurses should be familiar with physical surroundings and their mutual interaction with cultural realities, social relations, economic circumstances, and political conditions of communities, applying a critical perspective to community health.

AREAS OF ENVIRONMENTAL HEALTH

Environmental health hazards are ubiquitous in communities across the United States and place people at risk for disease or injury. This chapter divides the vast field of environmental health into the following subcategories: the built environment, work-related exposures, outdoor air quality, healthy homes, water quality, food safety, and waste management (Table 14.1). A brief discussion introduces nurses to these seven areas of environmental health, describes how they affect health, and demonstrates basic strategies nurses can use to address them. Table 14.2 provides examples of health problems within each area of environmental health.

It should be noted that a critical perspective does not separate the idea of a safe social environment from a safe physical environment. For example, interpersonal violence is a significant and growing risk, with consequences ranging from

bodily injury to psychiatric aftereffects that may last for decades in some individuals. Intergenerational patterns of abuse, hate crimes toward marginalized groups, sexual predators, and hazards of combat might be considered from an environmental health perspective. Issues of violence are discussed in more depth in Chapter 27.

Finally, we must be prepared for the public health effects of terrorism. Terrorism is a word that evokes many images and a range of reactions from rage to grief and loss. Acts of terrorism have drawn the public and political focus to establishing environmental security. Bioterrorism and homeland security are new areas where nurses will have an impact. A critical perspective is needed now more than ever, because security issues are linked to religious imperatives, moral stances, values, profit motives, healthcare systems and information, and cultural differences. These issues are also clearly within the scope

TABLE 14.1 Areas of Environmental Health

Area	Definition
Built environment	Buildings, spaces, and products that are created or modified by people; including homes, schools, workplaces, parks/recreation areas, greenways, business areas, and transportation systems.
Work-related exposure	Occupational exposure to environmental hazards that can cause illness or injury.
Outdoor air quality	The protectiveness of the atmospheric layers, the risks of severe weather, and the purity of the air for breathing purposes.
Healthy home	The availability, safety, structural strength, cleanliness, and location of shelter; including public facilities and family dwellings. This includes indoor air quality.
Water quality	The availability of and accessibility to a clean water supply, the mineral content levels, pollution by toxic chemicals, and the presence of pathogenic microorganisms.
Food safety	The availability, relative costs, variety, safety, and health of animal and plant food sources.
Waste management	The management of waste materials resulting from industrial and municipal processes, human consumption, and efforts to minimize waste production.

TABLE 14.2 Examples of Environmental Health Problems

Area	Problems
Built environment	Drunk driving / Secondhand smoke / Noise exposure / Urban crowding / Technological hazards
Work-related exposure	Asbestos exposure / Agricultural accidents / Excessive exposure to X-rays
Outdoor air quality	Gaseous pollutants / Greenhouse effect / Destruction of the ozone layer / Aerial spraying of herbicides and pesticides / Acid rain / Nuclear facility emissions
Healthy home	Homelessness / Rodent and insect infestation / Presence of lead-based paint / Sick building syndrome / Unsafe neighborhoods / Radon gas seepage in homes and schools
Water quality	Contamination of drinking supply by human waste / Oil spills in the world's waterways / Pesticide or herbicide infiltration of groundwater / Aquifer contamination by industrial pollutants / Heavy metal poisoning of fish
Food safety	Malnutrition / Bacterial food poisoning / Food adulteration / Disruption of food chains by ecosystem destruction / Carcinogenic chemical food additives
Waste management	Use of nonbiodegradable plastics / Poorly designed solid-waste dumps / Inadequate sewage systems / Transport and storage of hazardous waste / Illegal industrial dumping / Radioactive hazardous wastes

TABLE 14.3   A Conceptual Model of How the Built Environment Affects Health

The Built Environment (Underlying Context)	Mediating Factors (Exposure Media)	Downstream Pathways (Human Response)	Health Status (Outcome Indicators)
• Land use patterns • Transportation networks • Infrastructure systems • Public facilities • Buildings	• Environmental toxins • Local climate • Noise level • Crime level • Disasters and accidents • Access to services	• Behavioral (e.g., physical activity, diet behavior, smoking, drinking, taking drugs) • Psychological (e.g., satisfaction, depression/distress, social cohesion) • Physiological (e.g., infection, immune system activation, hormonal response)	• Individual level (e.g., body mass index [BMI], perceived health status, well-being) • Population level (e.g., cause-specific mortality rates, morbidity rates)

Developed by Fan Y, Song Y: Is sprawl associated with a widening urban–suburban mortality gap? *J Urban Health* 86(5):708–728, 2009; adapted from a conceptual model by Klitzman S, Matte TD, Kass DE: The urban physical environment and its effects on health. In Freudenberg N, Galea S, Vlahov D, editors: *Cities and the health of the public*, Nashville, TN, 2006, Vanderbilt University Press, p 364.

of community health nursing and are discussed in more detail in Chapter 28.

The Built Environment

The built environment consists of the connections among people, communities, and their surrounding environments that affect health behaviors and habits, interpersonal relationships, cultural values, and customs. There is growing evidence that the built environment directly and indirectly affects health outcomes and disease rates (Table 14.3). One review of the literature found that neighborhoods that are more walkable are associated with increased physical activity, increased social capital, lower overweight, lower reports of depression, and less reported alcohol abuse (Renalds et al., 2009). Social capital refers to networks and the associated norms and expected collective benefits derived from cooperation between individuals and groups. Structural characteristics of the built environment, such as street condition, neighborhood deterioration, and the proportion of parks and playgrounds, affect levels of physical activity and obesity (Kerr et al., 2010; Schulz et al., 2013) found that women are more likely to increase physical activity if they live in a walkable community compared with men, indicating safety to be an attributing factor. Simply put, having a safe, intact place to walk may encourage exercise among adults.

Many people live within areas that require almost daily contact with potential health risks and threats. These include intoxicated or impaired drivers, secondhand smoke, urban crowding, noise exposure, unabated traffic, and the stress of increased mechanization. The type of area one lives in can greatly affect one's health. For example, a research study found that adolescents living in rural working-class or mixed-race urban neighborhoods were more likely to be overweight than peers in newer suburbs, regardless of their socioeconomic status (SES), age, or race/ethnicity (Nelson et al., 2006). In another study investigating the role of neighborhood characteristics and childhood obesity, neighborhood SES was found to be a greater mediator of childhood obesity than racial or ethnic disparities (Sharifi et al., 2016). Access to equipment and facilities, neighborhood pattern (e.g., rural, exurban,

suburban), walkability, and urban sprawl are also associated with obesity outcomes in adolescents (Ding et al., 2011; Dunton et al., 2009).

Urban sprawl has been defined as the conversion of land to nonagricultural or nonnatural uses at a faster rate than the population growth (Environmental Protection Agency [EPA], 2002). The sprawling development often occurs more rapidly than the expansion of the infrastructure (e.g., schools, sewer systems, water lines) needed for support. The urban sprawl is characterized by four dimensions: "low residential density; rigidly separated homes, shops, and workplaces; roads with large blocks and poor access; and lack of well-defined activity centers" (James et al., 2013, p. 369). Consequences of sprawl include air and water pollution, floods, infrastructure expenses, and a decrease in natural areas and forests (EPA, 2002).

One unfortunately common problem associated with living patterns relates to residing near hazardous facilities (e.g., waste incinerators, sewage treatment plants, landfills, refineries, and some correctional facilities). Molitor et al. (2011) found that higher levels of pollutants are generally associated with higher poverty. Discriminatory land use ensures that many impoverished and marginalized groups, especially minorities, live in close proximity to industrial contamination (Collins, 2011; Nweke, 2011). People who live near such environmental hazards are in danger of becoming victims of illness and injury related to violence, poisonings and exposures, fires, and malignant and nonmalignant diseases. Clinical Example 14.1 provides an example. Though historically outdoor pollution and hazards have been considered the major contributors affecting environmental quality, one must also consider the influence of indoor residential environmental hazards, such as radon, asbestos, lead, insect and pet allergens, chemicals, and other consumer products, as well as secondhand smoke and fungi (Adamkiewicz et al., 2011).

Many communities lack sufficient resources to respond when urban development and technological advances jeopardize the health and well-being of families in affected areas. The environmental movement of the 1960s and 1970s succeeded in building political power capable of passing monumental environmental reforms; however, charges that poor and minority communities are dumping grounds for environmental hazards have been substantiated by governmental agencies (EPA, 2004, 2013c).

Difficulties in alerting state and federal officials about environmental health dangers, as well as in obtaining compensation for environmental toxin—causing disease and death, often result in resident revictimization. Tightly knit social structures and a lack of low-cost housing may hinder the mobility of residents and perpetuate the exposure to health hazards. Residents may be unwilling to disrupt family ties and cultural roots to start over elsewhere, or they may be unable to afford a move. These residents may live with uncertainty and conflict. Long-term, community-wide effects of division, animosity, distrust, cynicism, and despair can abound in these situations, negatively affecting social capital.

In the 1990s, the central issues of equity and justice emerged in environmental health policy. In 1994, President Clinton signed Executive Order (EO) 12898, which required all federal agencies to develop comprehensive strategies for achieving environmental justice. This directive has served to increase public participation and access to information as well as provision of education about multiple risks and cumulative exposures (EPA, 2005, 2013c) (Box 14.1). A recent investigation of the impact of EO 12898 determined the order failed to address an important contributor to environmental justice: poor economic growth in low-income minority communities. In 2008, President Obama signed a memorandum of understanding in regard to EO 12898 to identify and address environmental justice at the program, policy, and initiative level (Geltman et al., 2016). Nurses are part of the interdisciplinary team made up of urban planners, public health practitioners, and policy makers needed to understand and address issues of the built environment that are critical to establishing health equity.

Clinical Example 14.1

In an urban city in the south, the health department is becomingly increasingly concerned about the overweight and obesity rates of young school-age children. At health fairs held around the city, nurses are seeing more children with acanthosis nigricans, elevated blood pressure, high body mass index (BMI), and hypercholesterolemia. Though the public health nurse diligently counsels patients on the benefits of exercise, his patients do not increase their physical activity. When the nurse drives around the neighborhood where many of his patients reside, he realizes there are no recreational parks nearby, the sidewalks are in disrepair, the smokestacks cloud the air, and there appears to be gang-related activity. The nurse considers the impact of the built environment on the ability of his patients to be physically active. In partnership with the school board and neighborhood watch group, the nurse and community members successfully petition for a park to be built within walking distance of the school. Additionally, the partnership is able to establish a "walking school bus," a program where students walk in a group to or from school, as a way for children to increase their physical activity.

Work-Related Exposures

Work-related exposures can happen as a result of poor working conditions and can lead to potential injury or illness. Environmental health problems posed by work-related exposures include such issues as occupational toxic poisoning, machine-operation hazards (e.g., falls, crushing injuries, burns), electrical hazards, repetitive motion injuries, carcinogenic particulate inhalation (e.g., of asbestos, coal dust), and heavy metal poisoning (Centers for Disease Control and Prevention [CDC], 2013; Krieger et al., 2008). Prevention of work-related health problems requires integrated action to improve job safety and the working environment. Occupational and environmental health nurses often collaborate on initiatives to reduce and eliminate work-related exposures, illnesses, and injuries. Nurses can be sure that workers are aware of and know where to access the safety data sheets relevant to their workplace. The U.S. Department of Labor's Occupational Safety and Health Administration (OSHA) (2013) requires chemical manufacturers, distributors, and importers to provide safety data sheets that communicate the hazards of chemical products.

According to the Bureau of Labor Statistics (2015), approximately 2.9 million nonfatal workplace injuries and illnesses were reported by private industry employers in 2015. This rate continues a pattern of decline annually for the past 13 years, apart from 2012, where there was either equal or more days away from work because of injury compared with the previous year (Bureau of Labor and Statistics, 2015). The EPA estimates that 10,000 to 20,000 physician-diagnosed pesticide

BOX 14.1	Landmark Federal Environmental Legislation
Year	**Legislation**
1970	Clean Air Act
	Poison Prevention Packaging Act
	National Environmental Policy Act
1971	Lead-Based Paint Poisoning Prevention Act
1972	Federal Water Pollution Control Act Amendments
	Noise Control Act
	Clean Water Act
1973	Endangered Species Act
1974	Safe Drinking Water Act
1975	Hazardous Materials Transportation Act
1976	Resource Conservation and Recovery Act
	Toxic Substances Control Act
	Surface Mining Control and Reclamation Act
1980	Low-Level Radiation Waste Policy Act
	Comprehensive Environmental Response, Compensation, and Liability Act (i.e., Superfund)
1990	Oil Pollution Act
	Clean Air Act
2003	Healthy Forests Restoration Act
2016	Fuel Economy Standards raised (original legislation: 1975)

EXAMPLES OF ENVIRONMENTAL HEALTH ISSUES AFFECTING COMMUNITIES

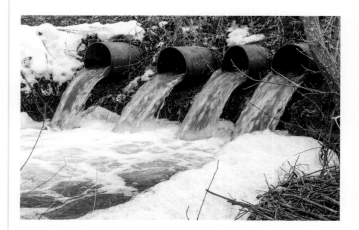

Water pollution from local industry.

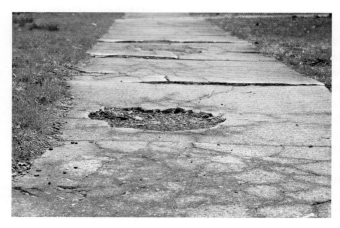

Sidewalks in disrepair.

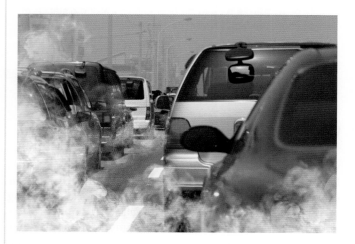

Motor vehicle emissions (primary mobile source of air pollutants).

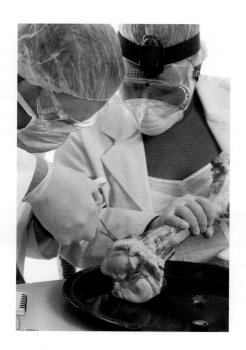

Food safety meat inspection.

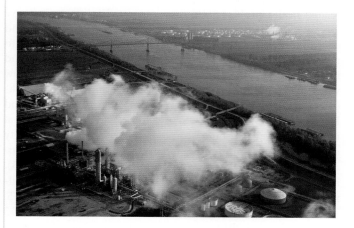

Air pollution from local industry.

poisonings occur each year among the approximately two million US agricultural workers (EPA, 2013). In 1 year (2010), 476 farm workers died from work-related injuries, with tractor overturns being the leading cause of death (CDC, 2013).

These statistics do not reflect unreported health problems. For example, a clerical worker leaves the office every day with back strain and a headache because of ventilation problems in the building. After 5 years on a repetitive hand-movement job task, an employee is diagnosed with carpal tunnel syndrome. An operating room nurse has a miscarriage and recalls that many of her coworkers have also been unable to carry their babies to term. A dry cleaner often leaves work feeling light-headed and dizzy from inhaling solvents at the shop, and 1 day she has a car accident on her way home. Collective problems related to employment or occupation are often perceived as individualized injuries, and no one "connects the dots." Research is ongoing to determine the outcomes of work-related environmental exposures. For example, the GuLF STUDY (Gulf Long-Term Follow-Up Study) is a health study, sponsored by the National Institutes of Health (NIH), for individuals who helped with oil spill clean-up after the 2010 Deepwater Horizon disaster in the Gulf of Mexico (NIH, 2014). Clinical Example 14.2 illustrates another case of work-related exposure.

Clinical Example 14.2

Sanitation workers in an urban area experienced a rising incidence of puncture injuries while transporting hazardous wastes from the public medical center; these puncture injuries caused several cases of hepatitis. When the story became public, members of the city health commission contacted community health nurses and instructed them to politically support the interests of the city and the medical center "at all costs." Subsequently, the sanitation workers' union contacted the community health nursing office and requested information about procedures for safely packaging medical wastes. They also requested that a nurse speak to their membership about immediate measures for preventing further injuries on the job.

The nurses met to resolve the conflict. Most agreed that the sanitation workers had pressing needs for education and support. Despite the city's demand for loyalty, they decided to "choose sides" with the workers and respond to their requests. They collectively drafted a letter to the city health commission and arranged a meeting with the commissioners to discuss their plan to assist the sanitation workers. The health commission held a press conference, which depicted the nurses' actions as mediational efforts that benefited the union and the city. Eventually, the nurses and the commission developed a new medical waste disposal plan, and injured workers received reasonable compensation through an out-of-court settlement.

Outdoor Air Quality

Outdoor air quality refers to the purity of the air and the presence of air pollution. The EPA (2012b) has classified six common air pollutants (Table 14.4). WHO estimates that air pollution contributes to approximately seven million premature deaths annually worldwide (WHO, 2021). Particulate matter, one common pollutant, causes worsening respiratory symptoms, more frequent asthma-related medication use, decreased lung function, recurrent health care utilization, and increased mortality (Anderson et al., 2012).

Air pollution originates from industry (dry cleaning, factories, oil refineries, coal-burning power plants), modes of transportation (cars, buses, trucks, and planes), and naturally occurring events (volcanic eruptions and windstorms). Tornadoes, electrical storms, smog, gaseous pollutants (e.g., carbon monoxide), excessive hydrocarbon levels, aerial herbicide spraying, and acid rain all contribute to air pollution. Under provisions of the Clean Air Act, the EPA sets the national ambient air quality standards for pollutants considered harmful to humans or the environment.

Ozone is the most common pollutant in the United States and is the primary component of smog. Ozone is formed when nitrogen oxides (created by the burning of fossil fuels in power plants, automobiles, and factories) react with oxygen and sunlight (EPA, 2021). Ozone, along with other hazardous atmospheric pollutants, causes and/or contributes to asthma, allergic reactions, bronchitis, lung cancer, chronic respiratory disease, and death and harms animal and plant species (Ciencewicki et al., 2008; Sheffield et al., 2011; EPA, 2021). Furthermore, sulfur dioxide, a by-product of burning coal and other fossil fuels, contributes to acid rain, which affects terrestrial ecosystems by increasing soil acidity, reducing nutrient availability, mobilizing toxic metals, leaching soil chemicals, and altering species composition (EPA, 2021).Two significant issues related to outdoor air quality are of global concern. First, the amount of protection in the atmospheric layers is diminishing (EPA, 2013e). Chemicals such as chlorofluorocarbons, halons, and carbon tetrachloride, which have been in widespread use for refrigeration, air conditioning, and aerosol propellants, remain in the atmosphere. These molecules cause depletion of the atmosphere's protective ozone layer. The resulting "holes" in the ozone layer allow excess ultraviolet radiation to penetrate, which has harmful effects on many organisms. Long-term problems include increases in rates of skin cancer and cataracts, suppression of immune response, and environmental damage.

Second, there is a disruption in the key processes that break down atmospheric carbon dioxide. The ongoing deforestation of the earth's surface, especially the diminishing of tropical rainforests, not only releases the carbon stored in the biomass but also eliminates sources of photosynthesis (i.e., the process by which plants absorb carbon dioxide and release oxygen). The loss of carbon dioxide—consuming resources increases carbon dioxide and traps part of the heat reemitted by the earth. As a result, the earth's surface temperature is rising (i.e., the "greenhouse effect"), with potentially catastrophic ecological consequences. Global climate change, including evidence that glaciers are shrinking, ice on rivers and lakes is breaking up earlier than usual, and a shift in plant and animal ranges, has already been observed (NASA, 2014).

TABLE 14.4   Major Air Pollutants

Pollutant	Sources	Effects
Ground level-Ozone: A colorless gas that is the major constituent of smog at the earth's surface	Ozone is formed in the lower atmosphere as the result of chemical reactions among oxygen, volatile organic compounds, and nitrogen oxides in the presence of sunlight, particularly during hot weather. Sources of this harmful pollutant include vehicles, factories, landfills, lawn equipment, farm equipment, and industrial solvents.	Ozone can irritate the respiratory tract; impair lung function; and cause throat irritation, chest pain, cough, and susceptibility to lung infection. Individuals with asthma and other existing respiratory conditions are particularly vulnerable. Ozone can also reduce agricultural yields and injure forests and other vegetation.
Carbon monoxide: A colorless and odorless gas that is emitted in the exhaust of motor vehicles and other kinds of engines during combustion of fossil fuels	Carbon monoxide is emitted from the engines of cars, buses, trucks, and other small engines and from some industrial processes. High concentrations can be found in confined spaces (e.g., parking garages, poorly ventilated tunnels, or along roadsides during periods of heavy traffic).	Carbon monoxide reduces the ability of the blood to deliver oxygen to vital tissues, affecting primarily the cardiovascular and nervous systems. Lower concentrations have been shown to adversely affect individuals with heart disease and to affect exercise performance. Higher concentrations can cause symptoms such as dizziness, headaches, and fatigue.
Nitrogen dioxides: A light-brown gas at lower concentrations; in higher concentrations, a significant component of brown urban haze	Nitrogen dioxide forms from the burning of fuels in utilities, industrial boilers, and the engines of cars and trucks.	Nitrogen dioxide is a major component of smog and acid rain. When concentrations are high, it can increase respiratory illnesses (e.g., chest colds and coughing) in children. For asthmatic people, it may exacerbate breathing difficulty.
Sulfur dioxide: A colorless gas, odorless at low concentrations but pungent at very high concentrations	Sulfur dioxide is emitted from industrial, institutional, utility, and apartment-house furnaces and boilers as well as petroleum refineries, smelters, paper mills, and chemical plants.	Sulfur dioxide is one of the major components of smog. At high concentrations, it can harm humans; asthmatic people are particularly vulnerable. It can also harm vegetation and metals; and acidify lakes and streams.
Particulate matter: Droplets from smoke, dust, ash, and condensing vapors that can be suspended in the air for long periods	Particulates are emitted from industrial processes, vehicles, wood smoke, dust from paved and unpaved roads, construction, and agriculture.	Particulates can affect breathing and elicit respiratory symptoms, causing increased respiratory disease and lung damage. Children, elders, and people with heart or lung disease are especially at risk. They can also damage paint, soil, and clothing and reduce visibility.
Lead: A metal found in nature as well as a byproduct of industry; can contaminate substances (e.g., soil, dust) that can be directly inhaled	Metals processing is the major source of lead emissions into the air today. Lead is generally found near lead smelters, waste incinerators, utilities, and lead-acid battery manufacturers.	Lead can adversely affect mental development and performance, kidney function, and blood chemistry. Young children are particularly at risk to its effects.

From Environmental Protection Agency: *What are the six common air pollutants?* Retrieved September 2, 2021 from: https://www.epa.gov/criteria-air-pollutants.

In 1968, the National Air Pollution Control Administration developed the **air quality index** (AQI) to increase public awareness of air pollution (Fig. 14.3). The AQI is a number used by government agencies to communicate current and forecasted air pollution conditions to the public. As the AQI rises, a larger percentage of the population, particularly vulnerable populations, may experience adverse health effects. The AQI fluctuates on the basis of the dilution of air pollutants. Air stagnation can lead to high concentrations of pollutants and haze. Although most air contaminants do not have an associated AQI, many countries monitor ground-level ozone, particulates, sulfur dioxide, carbon monoxide, and nitrogen dioxide to calculate the AQI (EPA, 2013g). Nurses need to be aware of the AQI and the corresponding recommendations for the public to limit exposure to outdoor air during peak times of high AQI (Clinical Example 14.3). Additionally, nurses must

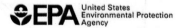

Air Quality Guide for Particle Pollution

Good	0-50	None
Moderate	51-100	Unusually sensitive people should consider reducing prolonged or heavy exertion
Unhealthy for Sensitive Groups	101-150	People with heart or lung disease, older adults, and children should reduce prolonged or heavy exertion.
Unhealthy	151 to 200	People with heart or lung disease, older adults, and children should avoid prolonged or heavy exertion. Everyone else should reduce prolonged or heavy exertion.
Very Unhealthy Alert	201 to 300	People with heart or lung disease, older adults, and children should avoid all physical activity outdoors. Everyone else should avoid prolonged or heavy exertion.

Fig. 14.3 Environmental Protection Agency air quality index. (From Air-Now: *Local air conditions and forecasts*, n.d. Available from: www.airnow.gov.)

consider the AQI when making recommendations for physical activity, particularly for asthmatic patients. One study suggests that population-level health benefits from increased physical activity in high-walkability neighborhoods may be offset by the adverse effects of exposure to air pollution (Hankey et al., 2012). A recent study on the effects of particulate matter for individuals who walk or cycle to work found that the health benefits of active travel far outweighed the health risks from air pollution (Tainio et al., 2016).

Clinical Example 14.3

During a recent summer, a sudden increase occurred in the number of clinic visits from residents of a particular urban neighborhood. The patients were elderly men and women who felt ill after going for a walk and asthmatic children with worsening respiratory symptoms. A nurse at the federally qualified health clinic in the neighborhood suspected that air pollution might be contributing to the increase in health concerns.

The nurse went online to the site www.airnow.gov and searched for the AQI for the region. She discovered that the region was experiencing a very unhealthy level of outdoor air pollution. She immediately alerted the healthcare staff that people with heart or lung disease, older adults, and children should avoid all physical activity outdoors and that everyone should avoid prolonged or heavy exertion outdoors. The nurse contacted the local summer camps and nursing homes in the area to alert them of the recommendation. The clinic quickly decided to move their regularly scheduled outdoor picnic to an indoor venue. One week later, the nurse noticed a drop in the number of patients complaining of respiratory distress.

Healthy Homes

A Healthy Home refers to the availability, safety, structural strength, cleanliness, location, and indoor air quality of shelter. According to the EPA (2017), many of the health concerns related to indoor living are a result of exposure to radon, carbon monoxide, molds and dust, secondhand smoke, cooking vapors, lead paint, and rodents. The CDC and surgeon general have developed a Healthy Home checklist that nurses can use with patients to guide a thorough assessment and develop a care plan to help patients improve the quality of their homes and their indoor air quality (CDC, 2011).

Radon causes an estimated 21,000 lung cancer deaths in the United States every year. It is the second leading cause of lung cancer, after active smoking, and the leading cause among nonsmokers (EPA, 2021). Nine federal agencies in 2011 initiated a plan to reduce radon exposures and illnesses (EPA, 2013d). Four years after implementation of the Federal Radon Action Plan (FRAP), the EPA joined forces with other lead agencies and sectors to develop the National Radon Action Plan (NRAP) with goals to mitigate five million high radon homes

and save 3200 lives annually from death related to lung cancer (EPA, 2021). Carbon monoxide is an odorless, colorless, toxic gas. It can cause mild flulike effects such as headaches, dizziness, disorientation, nausea, and fatigue at lower levels of exposure and death at higher levels (EPA, 2012d). Molds, dust, and secondhand smoke exposure can often exacerbate asthma symptoms.

Other health problems related to housing include fire hazards; lack of accommodations for people with disabilities; illnesses caused by overcrowding; psychological effects of architectural design (e.g., low-cost, high-rise housing projects); injuries sustained from collapsed building structures; and exposure deaths from inadequate indoor heating or cooling (Clinical Example 14.4). Poor housing conditions can contribute to the spread of infectious disease (EPA, 2012e) as well as cardiovascular and respiratory disorders, cancers, allergies, and mental illnesses (Ali et al., 2018; Barton et al., 2007; Jones-Rounds et al., 2013; Rauh et al., 2008). The term sick building syndrome describes a phenomenon in which public structures and homes cause occupants to experience a variety of symptoms, such as headache, fatigue, and exacerbation of allergies. It typically results from poor ventilation and building operations, hazardous building materials, furniture and carpeting substances, and cleaning agents (EPA, 1991). Additionally, volatile organic compounds (VOCs) have been found in soil and soil vapor as a result of industrial spills that contaminate indoor air. One such spill in Endicott, New York, has been linked to congenital cardiac defects, low birth weight, and fetal growth restriction (Farand et al., 2012).

Other problems may arise related to building structures, composition, and settings. For example, commercial buildings with offices near underground parking garages may cause workers to have carbon monoxide intoxication. Formaldehyde, asbestos, and VOCs—which are common components of thermal insulation, cement, flooring, furnishings, and household consumer products—have carcinogenic properties. Additionally, "toxic mold" arising from chronically damp wood and improperly sealed areas in homes and offices has been recognized as contributing to respiratory irritation, allergies, and infections in susceptible individuals (EPA, 2021).

Clinical Example 14.4

In a large, northeastern US city, an economic recession led to large company layoffs, leaving many unemployed or underemployed. Because of the loss of income, many families faced tough decisions during the upcoming winter months. Temperatures often went below zero, requiring constant heating. Unfortunately, many people did not have the money to continue to pay their heating bill, fix leaky windows and doors, or buy warm clothes. Some families began to use space heaters and burned scraps of wood that were discarded. Often, this wood came from old abandoned buildings and homes. Other families took to sleeping in their cars.

Continued

Clinical Example 14.4—cont'd

Soon, hospitals began to see an uptick in patients presenting with respiratory illnesses, carbon monoxide exposure, and burns. The community health nurses in the area met with struggling families to assess their needs and determine a plan to meet their immediate needs. The nurses met with local politicians and church groups to find ways to supply healthy wood for heating, help financially with home utility bills, provide warm clothes for families, and find shelters for homeless families. Within a few months, the local hospitals began to see a decline in home-related injuries and illnesses.

Water Quality

Water quality refers to the water supply's availability, volume, mineral content levels, toxic chemical pollution, and pathogenic microorganism levels. Water quality consists of the balance between water contaminants and the existing capabilities to purify water for human use and plant and wildlife sustenance. Water quality problems include experiencing droughts, dousing reservoirs with chemicals to reduce algae, contaminating aquifers with pesticides and fertilizers (Clinical Example 14.5), leaching lead from water pipes, and oil spilling from transport tankers or leaking offshore wells. Other sources of water pollution are microbial contamination from poorly managed or maintained septic or sewage systems and animal feedlot wastes (EPA, 2013b). Water pollution can be from point sources (a well-defined source, e.g., factory wastewater discharge) or nonpoint sources (urban runoff, domestic lawn care, and air-to-water transfer).

Advances in water treatment technologies in industrialized countries have controlled many water-related diseases, such as cholera, typhoid, dysentery, and hepatitis A. Nevertheless, disease outbreaks resulting from contamination by untreated groundwater and inadequate chlorination are increasing in both urban and rural areas. In addition, more than 45 million Americans (15%) obtain their drinking water from private water supplies (e.g., wells) that have no treatment or monitoring guidelines (CDC, 2021b). Other potential water contaminants include accelerated soil erosion caused by construction, agriculture, and deforestation, which can contribute to high sediment levels in drinking water supplies.

Heavy metal and toxic chemical pollution may also occur during the water treatment process or in the drinking water distribution system. The EPA monitors drinking water for more than 90 organic and inorganic pollutants that have potential health effects in humans, including those who are most vulnerable, such as children and people with weakened immune systems (EPA, 2016). Pesticides, herbicides, and carcinogenic industrial waste infiltrate an increasing amount of groundwater, the underground source of half the US population's drinking water (U.S. Geological Survey, 2005). Additionally, commonly used medications and personal care products that contain endocrine disruptors have been found in water supplies (Wu et al., 2012). This development is particularly tragic because groundwater is uniquely susceptible to long-term contamination. Unlike river or lake water, once groundwater becomes contaminated, it is impossible to cleanse.

Clinical Example 14.5

In a Midwestern farm community, there is growing concern about seepage of agricultural pesticides and herbicides into groundwater. Families obtain water from private wells rather than a central municipal source. The families had heard about potential long-term carcinogenic effects of the chemicals, such as pesticides and herbicides, commonly used on the farms in the community. Although family farmers decreased their use of these chemicals, the large-scale agribusiness companies continued to use large amounts of these chemicals.

A community health nurse from the county health department lobbied local officials to begin a comprehensive program to monitor groundwater pollutants and enforce standards for herbicide and pesticide use. However, the powerful agribusiness companies pressured these officials to stand back. Together, some county farmers and nurses organized grassroots information and support groups for the rural families. The families and nurses, in coalition with environmental activist groups in the state, established several projects. These projects included collecting and testing samples from each family well, forming a local organization called "Water Watch" to coordinate actions and communications, and implementing a research project with a local university to track water contamination and health problems of local residents. The organization also disseminated an emergency plan to families whose wells were found to have toxic levels of pesticides, herbicides, or other pollutants.

Food Safety

Food safety refers to availability, accessibility, and relative cost of healthy food free of contamination by harmful herbicides, pesticides, and bacteria. Food safety concerns include malnutrition, bacterial food poisoning (Clinical Example 14.6), carcinogenic chemical additives (e.g., nitrites, dyes, and cyclamate), improper or fraudulent meat inspection or food labeling, microbial epidemics among livestock (e.g., *Escherichia coli*), food products from diseased animal sources, and disruption of vital natural food chains by ecosystem destruction. Increased mobility and globalized trade also contribute to global contamination of the food supply. Finally, there are significant disparities in access to healthy and fresh food supplies, with poor minority families being more likely to live in a **food desert**—a neighborhood with little to no access to healthy foods (Institute of Medicine [IOM], 2009).

Annually, nearly 60 to 70 million Americans contract gastrointestinal illnesses, accounting for about 10% of all hospitalizations and 15% of in-patient hospital procedures for the treatment of digestive diseases (National Institute of Health [NIH], 2009). Potential microbial contaminants of foods include bacteria (e.g., *Shigella, Salmonella, E. coli, Campylobacter,*

Listeria), parasites (e.g., *Balantidium coli, Cryptosporidium parvum, Entamoeba histolytica, Giardia intestinalis*), and viruses (e.g., calicivirus, rotavirus, hepatitis A virus, enterovirus) (FoodSafety.gov, 2016). The federal government utilizes meat inspectors to prevent misbranded meat and meat products from being sold as food and ensure that meat animals are slaughtered and meat products processed under sanitary and humane conditions. The United States currently depends on the Foodborne Diseases Active Surveillance Network (FoodNet) of the CDC's Emerging Infections Program to collect data on diseases caused by enteric pathogens transmitted through food (CDC, 2020). Public health nurses play a key role in foodborne illness investigations.

Food can also be contaminated by agrichemicals, such as pesticides and fertilizers; materials from mechanical handling devices; detergents; and organic packaging materials. Toxic chemicals from farming and ranching may be introduced into the food chain, increasing risk of reproductive and mutagenic effects in humans (Driehuis et al., 2008; Knobeloch et al., 2009). For instance, farmers spray dioxin-containing weed killers on rangeland. Beef cattle graze on the land, herbicide accumulates in their fatty tissue, and the contaminated meat is sold in markets. The complexity of transfer of these contaminants makes for difficulty in establishing causality and tracing accountability for these health risks.

Unsuitable handling, storage, processing, and transport techniques can damage food and make it unsuitable for consumption. Nurses can council patients on the proper handling of food (Fig. 14.4). Furthermore, additives are often used to improve food properties. For example, vitamins and minerals are used to enhance nutritional content; salt, sugars, and monosodium glutamate are used to improve flavor; dyes are used to enhance color; leavening agents, gums, or thickening agents are used to improve consistency; and various preservatives are used to increase shelf life. Many of these additives are not nutritious, and some may be harmful. Additionally, residues from the overuse of antibiotics in animal husbandry remain in meat and milk products, causing consumers to develop resistance, thus rendering these antibiotics ineffective in treating human infections (Hurd and Malladi, 2008).

Another potential threat related to food quality involves "genetically modified" (GM) or genetically engineered foods. GM foods, which have been in existence since the early 1970s, are created by a process in which scientists splice plant or animal genes with particular traits into the DNA of other organisms. This technology has contributed to crops and livestock that grow faster, are more resistant to disease and insects, and produce higher yields and greater nutritive value. Often GM crops require less water and fertilizer. There is concern that genetic alteration of food is growing despite the fact that the long-term health effects of eating GM food are unknown. Some believe that allergies and other immunity problems may proliferate because unique antigens are present on GM proteins, and GM foods have unpredictable metabolic processes in animals, humans, and plants (Whitney et al.,

CLEAN SEPARATE COOK CHILL

Fig. 14.4 Steps to food safety. (From FoodSafety.gov: *Keep food safe,* n.d. Available from: http://www.foodsafety.gov/keep/basics/index.html.)

2004). Although the US Department of Agriculture and the U.S. Food and Drug Administration set policy for foods produced from new plant varieties and breeding, a number of groups and organizations have called for greater public awareness of the potential risks of genetically engineered foods and are working to require more stringent testing of them. The American Nurses Association was among several professional groups that developed principles of a healthy and sustainable food system (Box 14.2) (American Planning Association, 2010).

Clinical Example 14.6

A southwestern US town with a population of 10,000 has three elementary schools. School nurses at all three schools had an influx of children into their offices one afternoon with complaints of gastrointestinal symptoms. After verifying that this was happening at all three schools, the nurses called the county health department to report possible foodborne illness outbreak. The county health nurse came out to the schools that afternoon to investigate the foodborne outbreak. She interviewed the school nurses, the affected and unaffected students, and the cafeteria staff.

After having all students in the school fill out a form describing what they had eaten for lunch, the county nurse was able to determine that the chicken salad was the likely source of contamination. The nurses sent the chicken salad as well as samples of all the ingredients in the salad for laboratory testing. Within 2 days, the nurse received confirmation that the chicken salad had been the source of the illness, related to the use of contaminated celery. The nurse then alerted federal officials. A warning was issued on www.foodsafety.gov to alert officials across the nation. Food inspectors were sent to the factory that prepared and sold the celery. The source of contamination was isolated to three of the five machines used to slice the prepackaged celery. The factory was temporarily shut down for thorough disinfection. The school and county nurses worked together to assess the outbreak, alert the appropriate officials, and stop the outbreak from spreading. They undoubtedly saved thousands from illness and possibly death.

Waste Management

Waste management entails the handling of waste materials resulting from industry, municipal processes, and human consumption as well as efforts to minimize waste production. Environmental health problems related to waste management include nonbiodegradable plastics, inefficient recycling

BOX 14.2 Healthy and Sustainable Food Systems

Health-Promoting

- Supports the physical and mental health of all farmers, workers, and eaters
- Accounts for the public health impacts throughout the entire lifecycle of how food is produced, processed, packaged, labeled, distributed, marketed, consumed, and disposed

Sustainable

- Conserves, protects, and regenerates natural resources, landscapes, and biodiversity
- Meets our current food and nutrition needs without compromising the ability of the system to meet the needs of future generations

Resilient

- Thrives in the face of challenges, such as unpredictable climate, increased pest resistance, and declining, increasingly expensive water and energy supplies

Diverse In

- Size and scale—includes a variable range of food production, transformation, distribution, marketing, consumption, and disposal practices, occurring at different scales, from local and regional to national and global
- Geography—considers geographic differences in natural resources, climate, customs, and heritage
- Culture—appreciates and supports a diversity of cultures, sociodemographics, and lifestyles
- Choice—provides a variety of health-promoting food choices for all

Fair

- Supports fair and just communities and conditions for all farmers, workers, and eaters
- Provides equitable physical access to affordable food that is health promoting and culturally appropriate

Economically Balanced

- Provides economic opportunities that are balanced across geographic regions of the country and at different scales of activity, from local to global, for a diverse range of food system stakeholders
- Affords farmers and workers in all sectors of the system a living wage

Transparent

- Provides opportunities for farmers, workers, and eaters to gain the knowledge necessary to understand how food is produced, transformed, distributed, marketed, consumed, and disposed
- Empowers farmers, workers, and eaters to actively participate in decision-making in all sectors of the system

---

programs, unlicensed waste dumps, inadequate sewage systems for growing populations, unsafe dumping of industrial toxins, exportation of radioactive medical wastes, illicit dumping (Clinical Example 14.7), and nonenforcement of environmental regulations.

American consumers' increasing trash production and the improper treatment, storage, transport, and disposal of waste are a significant concern. Routinely, commercial and institutional wastes are dumped with household waste in the same municipal incinerator, landfill, or sewer system. These commercial enterprises are generally exempt from the strict waste regulation applied to industry, although they often generate the same hazardous materials. Small businesses such as dry cleaners, photography laboratories, pesticide formulators, construction sites, and car repair shops discard a variety of substances that can cause serious public health problems.

Traditionally, US economic development has produced optimal wealth with the assumption that the environmental health consequences would be minor. This notion of sustainable development has proved inadequate, and cumulative hazardous episodes necessitate tough pollution control technologies. The sustainability paradigm has led to a shift from disposing to recycling of biosolids. Biosolids refers to sewage sludge that has been treated for pathogens to meet the regulatory requirements for land application. This has been a cost-effective practice, but more research needs to be conducted on human health risks of biosolid distribution in the ecosystem.

A number of potential health problems are associated with waste management. For example, solid waste landfills accumulate methane gas, a by-product of decomposing organic wastes. Without proper venting, this volatile gas can move through soil and cause fires and explosions in nearby areas. Waste incineration causes particulate air pollution and is ineffective in the combustion of many materials. Improper design, operation, or location of a waste site causes hazardous substances to spread through air, soil, and water to poison humans, animals, and plant life. Alarmingly, only a small percentage of hazardous waste actually reaches the designated waste sites; much is disposed of in open pits and in bodies of water, with dangerously uncertain long-term effects. New methods are being developed to estimate long-term rates of leaching of materials in various types of waste sites, based on probability principles (Sanchez and Kosson, 2005).

In 1980, Congress passed the Environmental Response Compensation and Liability Act, which established a revolving fund called the *Superfund* to clean up several hundred of the worst abandoned chemical waste disposal sites. One of the most notorious sites is the Love Canal in Niagara Falls, New York. For 40 years before the 1960s, more than 80 different types of chemicals, including benzene, dioxin, trichloroethylene, toluene, and chloroform, were dumped in an abandoned canal. Afterward, the covered area became the site for a school and several hundred homes. In the winters of 1976 and 1977, heavy snowfall and rain caused toxic wastes to reach the surface. Subsequently, the inhabitants experienced elevated miscarriage rates, blood and liver abnormalities, birth defects, and chromosome damage.

Clinical Example 14.7

In a city on the Mississippi River, an outbreak of shigellosis was traced to a group of high school students who had been swimming in a particular area of the river. The local meat-packing plant was releasing waste material, including human and animal feces, directly into the river. After intervening to contain the *Shigella* outbreak, the local community health nurses began to assess the situation. Their research indicated that the meatpacking facility had been in violation of waste control laws for some time. City officials imposed fines, which the company paid, but the dumping continued. Signage placed along the riverbanks prohibited swimming. Frustrated by their attempts to negotiate with the city and the plant, the nurses wrote a letter to the state capital newspaper, which had a large state readership. In the letter, they voiced concern about the community's health and the river's ecological integrity. The paper published their commentary, prompting responses from two local environmental groups, several activist groups, and a national organization concerned with clean water. These groups provided legal support and brought a collective suit against the meatpacking company. Subsequently, the company improved its waste treatment process to avoid legal ramifications.

GENETICS IN PUBLIC HEALTH

The Built Environment

Obesity is a preventable condition, yet worldwide has nearly tripled in the past 4 decades (World Health Organization, 2017). Obesity and weight gain is linked to genetic disposition but not as an isolated factor (Trasande et al., 2009). Lifestyle interactions with the built and natural environments are implicated in obesity risk where access to safe and walkable surroundings is not available (Hruby et al., 2016). Integrating environmental information with genetic characteristics allows for developing better understanding about health outcomes and health behavior (Population Reference Bureau) and identifying risk predictors for obesity and other human conditions (Liu et al., 2012).

EFFECTS OF ENVIRONMENTAL HAZARDS

Environmental hazards are ubiquitous, and their effects on the public's health are complex and generally interconnected. Nurses must understand the multiple and complex sequences leading to health concerns (Fig. 14.5). For example, nuclear power plant emissions may contaminate water and air supplies, affecting water quality, atmospheric quality, and radiation risk. Overcrowded housing may exacerbate problems in managing human waste, which may taint foodstuffs and contribute to the spread of communicable disease. Climate change continues to affect humans, the food chain, vegetation, and wildlife.

Effects of environmental hazards may be general or specific. For example, the ramifications of high unemployment, drought, and extensive smog cover affect the public generally. Other environmental health concerns, such as the housing needs of elderly people who use walkers or canes, the occupational risks of electrical line repair workers, and the mentally incapacitating effects of elevated blood lead values in children, affect the public more specifically.

Environmental health effects can be immediate, long-term, or intergenerational. Burns, gunshot wounds, hurricane

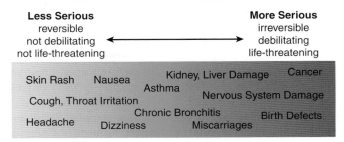

Fig. 14.5 Degrees of health effects from environmental exposures. (From Environmental Protection Agency: *Air pollution and health risk*, 1991. Available from: http://www.epa.gov/ttnatw01/3_90_022.html.)

damage, and outbreaks of gastrointestinal distress among cafeteria customers are examples of immediate effects from health-damaging environments. Examples of long-term health effects include gradual occupational hearing loss, "black lung" in coal miners, and increased rates of thyroid cancer among young victims of the Chernobyl nuclear reactor accident (Ron, 2007). Intergenerational effects will likely occur with climate change by affecting women of childbearing age.

Certain environmental exposures have been found to have a direct relationship with the development of some cancers, chronic diseases, and other health-related problems (Boyd and Genuis, 2008; Crouse et al., 2015). Furthermore, oppressive environments may affect health directly. In one case, an American company dumped dangerous waste material in Mexico rather than pay for proper disposal (Schrieberg, 1991). Poor children who lived nearby and scavenged for food in the dump picked up and played with the shiny, brightly colored radioactive medical waste. The severe burns they suffered and the wine-colored spots on their skin were direct effects of the illegally dumped toxic waste.

Effects of environmental risks may also be indirect, such as in the case of global warming (Akhtar et al., 2009; Pan and Kao, 2009). Global warming is the gradual increase in the average temperature of earth's near-surface air and oceans since the mid-20th century and its projected continuation (Easterling, 2011). Rising global temperatures may enhance the quantity and distribution of parasites, insects, and other disease vectors, potentially increasing the prevalence of a variety of infectious diseases. For example, global warming contributed to the entry and propagation of the West Nile virus in the United States (Epstein, 2001) and is suspected in facilitating the rapid spread of the Zika virus (Chan et al., 2016). Higher air and water temperatures facilitate the spread of vectorborne diseases transmitted by mosquitoes (e.g., West Nile virus). As a result, 2012 saw more cases of West Nile virus infection (5387) than any year since 2003, with a higher proportion of deaths (243) (CDC, 2012); however, between 2012 and 2015 there has been an annual consecutive reduction in both the number of cases and deaths related to West Nile Virus (CDC, 2016).

EFFORTS TO CONTROL ENVIRONMENTAL HEALTH PROBLEMS

The 1970s were the decade of environmental concern. Cynicism toward institutions grew during the years of US involvement in Vietnam, and legislative activism for environmental preservation exploded (Burger, 1989). During the 1970s, Congress created new agencies to regulate environmental conditions on a national level, including the EPA, the Occupational Safety and Health Administration, and the Nuclear Regulatory Commission. The EPA has enormous responsibilities for protecting the environment and minimizing risks to human health. Among its roles are health surveillance and monitoring; setting standards for air and water quality; evaluating environmental risks; acquiring information; screening new chemicals; performing basic research and training; and establishing, evaluating, and enforcing regulatory efforts.

The legislative activism of the 1970s was aimed toward a comprehensive national environmental policy. For example, stricter automobile fuel and emissions standards created improvements in air quality, which caused lead levels in urban air to decrease dramatically over the next decade. The momentum to control environmental pollution in the United States slowed in the 1980s and 1990s, with several policy reversals and the defunding of regulatory mechanisms. In recent years, administrative and legislative activity related to the environment has focused on such issues as climate change, oil spills, hazardous waste, and toxic exposures.

Frequently, laws and regulatory structures are weak or nonexistent with regard to environmental health problems. For example, federal mandates for recycling do not exist, although local communities have made great strides in this area. Comprehensive groundwater legislation, similar to adopted measures to preserve marine and surface waters, also does not exist. Additionally, the EPA tends to set priorities for the reduction of environmental problems but does not allocate the resources necessary to accomplish these goals.

EMERGING ISSUES IN ENVIRONMENTAL HEALTH

Within the past decade, we are beginning to recognize that our environmental public health infrastructure is quite weak and that the United States is susceptible to many of the same problems that burden the rest of the world. For example, the illegal use of pesticides, medical waste incineration, and the increased incidence of asthma related to air pollution are just a few of the challenges facing the United States today. The manufacturing of methamphetamine in home-based and mobile laboratories continues to rise, and the "cooking process" emits dangerous levels of toxic chemicals into the air. Similarly, the abandoned labs also pose a threat (Grant et al., 2010). Finally, natural disasters and climate change affect the entire world.

Natural disasters can disrupt and oftentimes overwhelm private and public health systems. Natural disasters, such as the tsunami that struck the coast of Indonesia in December 2004, Hurricane Katrina in August 2005, the devastating earthquakes in the Sichuan Province of China in 2008 and in Haiti in 2010, and superstorm Sandy in 2012, require mobilization of disaster relief units that offer substantial assistance and expertise. Natural disasters such as hurricanes, tornados, and earthquakes frequently receive notable publicity, but other, more insidious disasters, such as droughts, floods, heat waves, and extreme cold, also pose major public health concerns. All of the aforementioned threats can cause significant mortality and morbidity and therefore have the potential to burden the healthcare delivery system.

Global warming is part of a larger issue called *climate change* that poses significant health hazards. Climate change is the change in weather over a certain period. Weather patterns are greatly affected by atmospheric and oceanic temperature rises. Climate change projections suggest that heat waves and hot weather are likely to increase in frequency, with the overall temperature distribution shifting away from extreme cold

---

◢ RESEARCH HIGHLIGHTS

I PREPARE: Development and Clinical Utility of an Environmental Exposure History Mnemonic

The I PREPARE environmental exposure history mnemonic is a quick reference tool created by Paranzino et al. (2005) for primary care providers. A total of 159 healthcare providers, both students and professionals, were asked to evaluate a prototype of the mnemonic, to suggest new health history questions, and to propose the deletion of less relevant questions. The prototype was formatted as a pocket guide. The goal of this evaluation was to create a practical and clinically relevant mnemonic rather than to obtain quantitative estimates of its validity. This mnemonic is meant to serve as a mental cue to facilitate the collection and documentation of health information in a systematic manner:

I—Investigate Potential Exposures
P—Present Work
R—Residence
E—Environmental Concerns
P—Past Work
A—Activities
R—Referrals and Resources
E—Educate

Questions to ask are presented for each letter in the mnemonic, except for Referrals and Resources, which provides sources of additional information. A checklist of strategies to prevent or minimize exposures can be used by the healthcare provider to help clients identify potential exposures. The sequence of I PREPARE makes intuitive sense by cueing the provider to ask specific questions and then provide educational materials to the client. The final version was reprinted on heavy laminated material. The I PREPARE mnemonic increases the repertoire of tools clinicians have available to elicit an appropriate health history. The national improvements in the quality of environmental exposure history are predicated, in part, on the creation of simple and convenient tools for use in clinical practice.

Most of the US environmental health efforts have aimed for short-term results rather than anticipating future issues and problems. A crucial need exists in the development of human resources in the area of environmental health. Nurses in all areas of practice should be aware of the implications of the environment for their clients and their health. It is for this reason that nurses need to take and record an environmental health history for every client.

Data from Paranzino GK, Butterfield P, Nastoff T, Ranger C: I PREPARE: development and clinical utility of an environmental exposure history mnemonic, *J American Association Occupational Health Nurses* 53(1):37–42, 2005.

(O'Neill and Ebi, 2009). Climate change can have severe adverse health effects, such as health-related illness and death; increases in air pollution; water-, food-, vector-, and rodent-borne diseases; malnutrition; contaminated water supply; and injuries and deaths related to extreme weather and storm surges (Balbus, 2011; Sheffield et al., 2011). There are regional differences in the effects of climate change, although vulnerable populations will be affected the most. For instance, climate change will raise the risks of infant and maternal mortality, birth complications, and poorer reproductive health, especially in developing countries (Rylander et al., 2013).

Nursing Actions

Nurses must work with the public to promote more stringent and actively enforced environmental legislation and regulations. In the 21st century, actions must include not only national but also worldwide environmental policies. Ozone depletion, climate change, fossil fuel burning, marine dumping, abandonment of active land mines in war-torn areas, and destruction of tropical rainforests are among the key global environmental health concerns.

Environmental concerns for clean air, clean water, and freedom from noxious chemicals must become nursing concerns. Community health nurses can be catalysts to neighborhood efforts to produce safe living environments. Community health nursing must expand its theory and practice to incorporate the fact that individual and community health ultimately depends on global environmental integrity. Many organizations work to preserve and protect the environment and could benefit from the active involvement and support of nurses. Box 14.3 lists some of these organizations. Nursing must include an environmental perspective by committing to environmental health promotion initiatives that promote social justice and environmental responsibility.

APPROACHING ENVIRONMENTAL HEALTH AT THE POPULATION LEVEL

In the United States, personal independence and individual responsibility for success and failure are valued. These values can lead nurses to overlook environmental hazards and instead blame individual clients for their health problems. Placing responsibility for the cause and cure of health problems exclusively on the individual reinforces the belief that all individuals are free to exert meaningful control over the quality and length of their lives. Such a perspective absolves society, government, industry, and business from accountability.

Research suggests that changing individual behaviors does not lead to significant reductions in overall morbidity and mortality in the absence of basic social, economic, and political changes (Bhatia and Wernham, 2008). Emphasizing only interventions that address deleterious personal habits through exercise programs, weight loss regimens, smoking cessation classes, and stress reduction tactics fails to take into account the broader environmental origins of disease, injury, and ecological

BOX 14.3 Nongovernmental Environmental Organizations

- Alliance of Nurses for Healthy Environments (http://envirn.org/)
- American Farmland Trust (http://www.farmland.org/)
- Citizens for a Better Environment (http://www.cbezambia.org/)
- Clean Water Action (http://www.cleanwateraction.org/)
- Green America (http://www.greenamerica.org/)
- Environmental Defense Fund (http://www.edf.org/)
- Environmental Working Group (http://www.ewg.org/)
- Greenpeace (http://www.greenpeace.org/usa/en/)
- International Rivers Network (http://www.internationalrivers.org/)
- National Audubon Society (http://www.audubon.org/)
- National Environmental Law Center (http://www.nelconline.org/)
- National Geographic Society (http://www.nationalgeographic.com/about/)
- Natural Resources Defense Council (http://www.nrdc.org/)
- National Wildlife Federation (http://www.nwf.org/)
- Ocean Alliance (http://www.oceanalliance.org/)
- Pesticide Action Network (http://www.panna.org/)
- Rainforest Action Network (http://ran.org/)
- Sierra Club (http://www.sierraclub.org/)
- The Nature Conservancy (http://www.nature.org/)
- Trust for Public Land (http://www.tpl.org/)
- Wilderness Society (http://wilderness.org/)
- World Wildlife Fund (http://worldwildlife.org/)

For further information, see the report by the Institute of Medicine Committee on Enhancing Environmental Health Content in Nursing Practice: *Nursing, health, and the environment*, Washington, DC, 1995, National Academies Press.

degradation. An attempt to build a healthier future for all is the *Healthy People 2030* initiative (USDHHS, 2013). The *Healthy People 2030* box lists selected environmental health objectives of the *Healthy People 2030* initiative.

HEALTHY PEOPLE 2030
Selected Objectives for Environmental Health

EH—1: Reduce the number of days people are exposed to unhealthy air
EH—2: Increase trips to work made by mass transit
EH—3: Increase the proportion of people whose water supply meets Safe Drinking Water Act regulations
EH—4: Reduce blood lead levels in children aged 1—5 years
EH—5: Reduce health and environmental risks from hazardous sites
EH—6: Reduce the amount of toxic pollutants released into the environment
EH—7: Reduce exposure to arsenic
EH—8: Reduce exposure to lead
EH—9: Reduce exposure to mercury in children
EH—10: Reduce exposure to bisphenol A
EH—11: Reduce exposure to perchlorate
EH—D01: Increase the proportion of schools with policies and practices that promote health and safety
EH—D02: Reduce diseases and deaths related to heat

From U.S. Department of Health and Human Services. *Environmental health*, n.d. Available from https://health.gov/healthypeople/about/workgroups/environmental-health-workgroup.

ETHICAL INSIGHTS
Protecting Vulnerable Aggregates

Community health nurses have a mandate to assist vulnerable aggregates who have fewer options in protecting themselves from pollution, inadequate housing, toxic poisoning, unsafe products, and other hazards. Non–English-speaking individuals, children, very low-income women and families, undocumented manual laborers, and people from racial and ethnic minorities are just some of the groups in the United States who hold minimal influence with industry, government, business, and other large institutions for environmental changes and compensations for harm from environmental hazards.

Interventions designed for individuals must consider the environmental determinants of behavior and health outcomes (Bartholomew et al., 2011; Coughenour et al., 2014). Community health nurses who base their practices on theory and evidence are better prepared to respond to collective challenges. These nurses can facilitate community participation in identifying and solving environmental health problems and bringing about changes that improve environments and eliminate hazards.

CRITICAL ENVIRONMENTAL HEALTH NURSING PRACTICE

The National Center for Environmental Health, the CDC, and the American Public Health Association has established three core competencies for environmental health professionals: assessment, management, and communication (Box 14.4). Several clinical examples throughout the chapter illustrate how nurses can focus their efforts by organizing groups of people, taking a stand, and acting as advocates for change. The nurses ask critical questions, stay engaged with the communities they serve, form coalitions, and use various collective strategies. The American Nurses Association highlights 10 critical environmental health principles. In the interest of educating future practitioners about the critical practice of environmental community health nursing, the following sections discuss each of these interventions.

Taking a Stand: Advocating for Change

Nurses must make individual and collective decisions about which interests they want to serve with their specialized knowledge and skills. Nurses may choose to work with vulnerable people or those disproportionally experiencing the consequences of environmental hazards. Vulnerable groups are exposed to more health-damaging effects than less vulnerable groups (Chakraborty and Zandbergen, 2007; EPA, 2013c). Nurses can work toward health equity through the decisions they make, the positions they accept, and the interventions they undertake. Environmental problems are clearly intertwined with social, political, and economic policies; resource barriers; and the interests of those in positions of control. Nurses need to connect the immediate and long-term health problems experienced by particular communities to this larger sphere of influence.

Asking Critical Questions

Community health nurses must also consider the relationships between nonhealth policies and health policies. They should

---

BOX 14.4   Core Environmental Health Competencies

Assessment
Research: The capacity to identify and compile relevant information to solve a problem and the knowledge of where to go to obtain the relevant information.

Data analysis and interpretation: The capacity to analyze data, recognize meaningful test results, interpret findings, and present the results in a meaningful way to different types of audiences.

Evaluation: The capacity to evaluate the effectiveness or performance of procedures, interventions, and programs.

Management
Problem solving: The capacity to understand and solve problems.

Economic and political issues: The capacity to understand and appropriately utilize information concerning the economic and political implications of decisions.

Organizational knowledge and behavior: The capacity to function effectively within the culture of the organization and to be an effective team player.

Managing work: The capacity to plan, implement, and maintain fiscally responsible programs/projects using appropriate skills and to prioritize projects across the employee's entire workload.

Computer/information technology (IT): The capacity to utilize information technology as needed to produce work products.

Reporting, documentation, and record keeping: The capacity to produce reports that document actions, keep records, and inform appropriate parties.

Partnering: The capacity to form partnerships and alliances with other individuals and organizations in order to enhance performance on the job.

Communication
Education: The capacity to use the environmental health practitioner's frontline role to effectively educate the public on environmental health issues.

Communication: The capacity to effectively communicate risk and exchange information with colleagues, other practitioners, clients, policy makers, interest groups, media, and the public through public speaking, print and electronic media, and interpersonal relations.

Conflict resolution: The capacity to facilitate the resolution of conflicts within the agency, in the community, and with regulated parties.

Marketing environmental/public health as a service: The ability to articulate basic concepts of environmental health and public health and convey an understanding of their value and importance to clients and the public.

Data from American Public Health Association: *Environmental Health Competency Project: draft recommendations for non-technical competencies at the local level,* 2013. Available from: http://www.apha.org/programs/standards/healthcompproject/corenontechnicalcompetencies.htm.

---

ask how policies concerning ecological preservation, energy, housing, immigration, civil rights, crime, nutrition, minimum wage, occupational safety, and defense might affect the health and well-being of people. Addressing critical questions such as who has access to resources in this country and whose interests are served in the existing system provides a way to include social, political, and economic factors in environmental nursing assessments. Box 14.5 provides a sample set of questions that are useful in this endeavor. Nurses can ask these critical questions when approaching environmental health problems.

BOX 14.5 Critical Questions About Environmental Health Problems

- What is the problem?
- Who is defining the problem?
- In what terms is the problem described?
- How are others in the situation viewing the problem?
- What is the history of the problem?
- How did things get the way they are?
- What other situations does this problem directly affect?
- Who does the problem affect?
- Whose health is damaged because things are this way?
- Who benefits from the way things are?
- Whose interests do current solutions serve?
- What are the economic inequities in the situation?
- Who has political power in the situation?
- Who knows about the problem?
- Who needs to know more about the problem?
- How effective are current programs, strategies, and policies?
- What are the barriers to solving the problem?
- What strategies may alleviate the problem?
- How successful have these strategies been?
- What existing groups might deal with this problem?
- What resources are needed to solve the problem?
- How accessible are the resources?
- How can nurses evaluate potential solutions?

Facilitating Community Involvement

Approaching community health from a critical perspective requires working to improve health conditions and creating the context in which people can identify health-damaging problems in their environments. One important nursing goal is to help people learn from their own experiences and analyze the world with an intention to change it. It is essential that the affected people participate in the process of identifying and working to solve environmental problems (White et al., 2014). To foster community-based, active participation, nurses must be prepared to take leadership positions and join in mutual exchanges with community members that consider each person's experience. The nurse's role changes from presenting solutions and directing lifestyle changes to providing support, information, and expertise to assist in meeting the group goals. Using critical questions, community health nurses can help community members look beyond immediate environmental problems and explore social, cultural, economic, and political circumstances that contribute to them. Nurses can share their knowledge about the scientific basis for health problems, their insights about the historical origins of particular environmental hazards, their technical skills, and their expertise in communicating and organizing. By addressing people's everyday concerns and targeting the problems they identify, nurses situate their efforts in community struggles.

Forming Coalitions

Another very important nursing task that arises from approaching environmental health from a critical perspective involves forming coalitions to produce social change. By initiating dialogue and building a strong base of collective support, nurses join with communities to eliminate hazards and improve public health. Nurses can approach existing community organizations, churches, and family and friendship networks to help mobilize aggregate members who have not previously socialized or acted together. Nurses can then discuss environmental concerns, assess needs, plan actions, secure appropriate resources, and advocate for legislative changes.

Nurses can be instrumental in these efforts by helping community groups make connections with larger, more powerful organizations. Nurses can organize forums whereby community groups meet with scientific experts who can help them gather evidence about health threats, with business managers whose actions impinge on the economic life of the community, with industry leaders whose companies create ecological hazards, and with legislators who can bring community concerns to lawmaking bodies. Using available institutional resources, skills, and knowledge, nurses can also explore what is happening elsewhere. Making connections with groups in other locales who are struggling for similar environmental changes can enhance collective strength and solidarity. Press releases, media events, interviews, television spots, speeches, newsletters, and leaflets are important means of calling attention to a situation and raising awareness among communities.

Using Collective Strategies

Nurses can use a variety of strategies to intervene at the population level and facilitate improvement in a community's health. Nurses can organize people to change health-damaging environments through combinations of strategies, including building coalitions, providing educational forums, facilitating a community needs assessment, disseminating research, and lobbying for legislative changes.

One collective strategy that is an effective population-level community health nursing intervention is participatory action research (PAR). This form of research calls for nurses, community members, and other resource people to work together in identifying health problems, designing the studies, collecting and analyzing the data, disseminating the results, and posing solutions to the problems (Garwick et al., 2010; Li et al., 2011). In PAR applied to environmental health, community health nurses and community members would gather information on suspected environmental hazards, determine their effects on health, and devise a plan of action to mitigate the threat.

Although nurses have not traditionally used all of these collective strategies to intervene in community health matters, environmental hazards are multiplying geometrically, pushing nurses to expand their skills repertoire. Pioneers such as Hollie Shaner, RN, have embraced that concept and are blazing the path to environmental awareness (Sattler, 2003). In the 1990s, Shaner frequently left her home, where she avidly separated and recycled, to work at a Vermont hospital, where none of the waste was recycled. Shaner was not comfortable throwing everything into a "red bag" and decided that there must be a way to change the environmental unfriendliness of her place of employment. She began voluntarily recycling the hospital's cardboard and then began to recycle the newspapers, glass, and plastics. In addition, she received a grant from the state of Vermont to maximize her efforts in medical waste reduction. The efforts and savings did not go unnoticed by the hospital, as Shaner received a new job title of clinical waste reduction coordinator and saved the hospital $175,000 per year.

Shaner also wrote a book for the American Hospital Association on medical waste management. She quickly realized the negative impact the healthcare industry was having on the environmental health of the communities served. Mercury was being released into the streams from medical waste, and dioxins were being released into the air from medical waste incineration. From this realization, in 1996, Shaner and a small group of other health professionals launched a campaign to lead the health care industry toward environmental stewardship. This campaign, supported by the American Nurses Association, was named Health Care Without Harm. "The goal of the campaign was to reduce the environmental health risks that were being created by the health care industry" (Sattler, 2003, p. 8). The campaign still exists and is building momentum; today there are more than 1000 participating organizations in 52 different countries (Health Care Without Harm, 2021). In 2015 the 2020 Health Care Climate Challenge was launched, aiming to reduce the healthcare carbon footprint, respond with resiliency to the changing patterns of disease, and lead the way for creating a healthier climate (Global Green and Healthy Hospitals, 2020).

RESEARCH HIGHLIGHTS
Participatory Action Research

Asthma is a significant public health problem that disproportionately affects preschool-age, low-income children. Indeed, children from low-income families have significantly higher asthma prevalence rates, hospitalization rates, and emergency department visits than children from middle-income and wealthier families. This problem is even more pronounced among children in urban areas.

A team of public health nurses led by Garwick et al. (2010) used PAR techniques in working with teachers in an urban Head Start program with multiple sites to address asthma management among the children at their sites. In this project, teachers and managers from 16 Head Start centers were identified to participate in three focus groups. During the focus groups, participants identified asthma management issues and challenges, including undiagnosed and unreported asthma, coordination of asthma care with parents, medication administration issues, and variability among asthma action plans. As a result of the PAR, a standardized, comprehensive Head Start asthma action plan was developed that outlined strategies the teachers could use to better manage the problem of asthma among the children.

PAR, Participatory action research. Data from Garwick AW, Seppelt A, Riesgraf M: Addressing asthma management challenges in a multisite, urban Head Start Program, *Public Health Nurs* 27(4):329–336, 2010.

CASE STUDY   Application of the Nursing Process
Air Pollution

In July 2001, the *Metro Pulse* newspaper reported an extensive air pollution problem in the city of Knoxville, Tennessee (Tarr, 2001). The American Lung Association had recently named Knoxville the ninth most polluted city in the country on the basis of the ozone contamination in the air. The following case study expands on some of the reported facts of the situation to construct hypothetical nursing interventions.

Knoxville's community health nurses and the public health department were aware of increasing rates of asthma in particular neighborhoods. In the wake of alarming newspaper and research articles about the dangerous incidence of air pollution and related asthma, the nurses decided to make the health issues a priority. The community health nurses and several nursing students assigned to their department researched the topics and uncovered the following information.

Asthma has long been recognized as a condition in which an acute respiratory response may follow inhalation of a material to which a person is sensitized. Scientists now know that air pollution can lead to nonspecific generalized inflammation. One study found strong evidence that ozone can *cause*, as well as exacerbate, asthma (Sheffield et al., 2011). The study found that days with worse AQI values resulted in significantly higher school absences due to respiratory illness, and asthma was more likely to develop in children living in high-ozone communities who actively participated in several outdoor sports than in children in communities not participating in sports.

Indeed, the nation's leading group of pediatricians, the American Academy of Pediatrics (AAP), revised its policy statement on outdoor air pollution and the health hazards to children (Schwartz, 2004). The AAP's Committee on Environmental Health strengthened its warning about the dangers that air pollution poses to children because of the recent studies correlating air pollution with asthma and negative lung growth and function. Estimates are that more than 25 million Americans have asthma, including six million children under the age of 18 (CDC, 2021b).

An economically depressed neighborhood in Knoxville, hypothetically called Trent Park, is situated near numerous railways, freeways, and industrial yards. High numbers of African American, Latino, and Southeast Asian residents live in the older homes that line the streets of Trent Park. Isolated by language and economic circumstances, many Trent Park residents do not know they are exposed to these environmental health hazards.

Assessment
Elena Garcia, an 8-year-old girl who lives in Trent Park, presented to the pediatric primary clinic at the health department at 8 a.m. in November. Elena had been diagnosed with asthma 2 months ago and was now in mild respiratory distress. Elena explained to the nurse that she had gone trick-or-treating the night before in her neighborhood. It had turned cold that weekend, and she had also played outside in her neighborhood with friends the day before. In addition, the child's mother explained that Elena had recently had a respiratory virus. The nurse realized that Elena and her mother both mentioned several factors, such as her playing outside on a cold afternoon/evening in a polluted neighborhood and a respiratory virus, that could have exacerbated her asthma.

At the clinic visit, the nurse assessed the following:
- Elena's heart rate and cardiovascular status
- Elena's pattern of breathing, which includes rate, rhythm, and effort
- Elena's asthma medication history
- Evidence of diaphoresis, papillary dilation, and fear, which are all features of the adrenergic response to hypoxia
- Elena's global central nervous system function, such as alertness, cooperation, and motor activity
- Elena's environmental health assessment

Diagnosis
Individual
- Ineffective respirations related to environmental exposure to air pollution
- Insufficient knowledge related to precipitating factors that can cause/worsen an asthma attack
- Stress related to ongoing fear of daughter's illness

Continued

CASE STUDY   Application of the Nursing Process—cont'd

Family
- Risk for family crisis related to instability caused by the illness
- Insufficient knowledge related to factors that can cause/worsen an asthma attack

Community
- Risk for increased incidence of asthma due to air pollution
- Inadequate programs for asthma screening

Planning
A plan of care was developed at the individual, family, and community levels. Mutual goal setting and contracting are essential if the outcome is to be optimal.

Individual
Long-Term Goals
- Client will modify outdoor time daily according to the AQI
- Client will reduce exposure to allergy triggers
- Client will avoid secondhand tobacco smoke
- Client will keep pets out of the bedroom
- Client will experience successful maintenance of asthma

Short-Term Goals
- Client will report reduced outdoor time on days with poor AQI values
- Client will keep an asthma diary and identify which allergy triggers are problematic
- Client will remain free of acute asthma attacks

Family
Long-Term Goals
- Family will follow the city's daily AQI
- Family will encourage child to stay indoors on days with high pollution levels
- Family will remove as many allergy triggers from home as possible
- Family will enforce the pets-out-of-the-bedroom policy
- Family will cope effectively with daughter's asthma

Short-Term Goals
- Family will provide encouragement for client to keep an asthma diary

Community
Long-Term Goals
- Citizens will be involved in decision-making process about proposed activities that could pose an environmental hazard
- Citizens will encourage utility companies, government, and industries to reduce air pollution
- Citizens will be encouraged to use mass transit and carpools to reduce vehicle emissions

Short-Term Goals
- Citizens will be alerted about the air pollution problem in the area
- Citizens will be educated about the AQI and its implications for outdoor activity

Intervention
Individual
- Identify Trent Park children with asthma and plan follow-up home visits to provide education on basic pathophysiology, symptoms of distress, and environmental controls needed for successful asthma management
- Add environmental health assessments to child health assessment protocol
- Coordinate with school nurses to ensure they incorporate similar changes into their health assessment protocols
- Prepare and distribute an educational pamphlet with members of Trent Park that details Trent Park residents' air pollution and asthma risks

- Prepare translations of the pamphlet in languages and reading levels appropriate for Trent Park residents, and mail it to individual households

Family
- Facilitate the formation of a support group for families with children who have asthma

Community
- Initiate an asthma awareness program for Trent Park community members.
- Coordinate with school nurses to implement an asthma awareness program in Trent Park schools.
- Develop an asthma action team consisting of Trent Park community members.
- Participate in the action team's development of an intervention to reduce asthma-related illness in Trent Park.
- Encourage nursing students and community health nursing faculty from the local university and college programs to participate.
- Lobby state legislatures, municipal officials, local medical associations, local hospitals, and city clinics regarding the project.
- Form broader coalitions with Knoxville churches, the local nurses association, several preschool and day care centers, and the Knoxville School Board to design a comprehensive, nonduplicative, cost-effective asthma screening program.
- Train action team members on how to conduct Healthy Home assessments.
- Contact state environmental groups for advice on local efforts, and join in their fight for stricter regulation of air pollutants and toxic wastes.
- Contact local media (e.g., television, radio, and newspaper) about running a series of stories about Knoxville air pollutants and related asthma risks; supply information and contacts for interviews and photographs.

Evaluation
Individual
- Evaluate the child's and mother's understanding of asthma treatments at follow-up home visits.
- Facilitate the evaluation of ongoing interventions.
- Track the number of asthma screening tests that Trent Park children receive and their rates of asthma to determine the effectiveness of their efforts in these areas.
- Keep close contact with the school nurses and organize an after-school educational and screening program at schools that are understaffed.
- Ask school nurses to report on the educational sessions' success.

Family
- Document participation levels at educational programs and family training sessions.
- Document ongoing participation in referrals and support groups.

Community
The action team was able to get funding to provide Healthy Home assessments and asthma screening to at-risk youth in Trent Park.

Levels of Prevention
Primary Prevention
Educating the community regarding air pollution and its relationship to asthma.

Secondary Prevention
Screening at-risk populations for asthma.

Tertiary Prevention
Follow-up treatment for people with asthma and reduction of air pollutants in the community environment.

? ACTIVE LEARNING

1. Identify a health-related problem associated with some aspect of the environment. It may be a problem in a nearby community, a problem publicized in the media, or a difficulty experienced by a family. Examine the problem using the sample series of critical questions listed in Box 14.5. Without sharing the results, present the problem to the group and ask them to discuss it by responding to the same questions. Were there differences or similarities in the initial results and the group's answers? On what points did everyone agree? Why? What questions caused the most disagreement? Why? Now repeat the entire activity by involving people other than nursing students in the group discussion. How did this discussion compare with the previous discussion and responses?

2. Attend meetings that hold environmental hazard discussions. If meetings or public forums are not available in the vicinity, write for information about the state's actions to fight environmental hazards. The reference librarians at colleges or public libraries can suggest ways of contacting sources and will supply addresses. Organizations that are likely to sponsor forums and provide information include those listed in Box 14.3, the Environmental Protection Agency, the National Institute for Occupational Safety and Health, state and municipal agencies for environmental protection and occupational health, environmental caucuses of political parties, the American Public Health Association, the local public health department, farmers' organizations, and labor unions.

3. This chapter described how to use participatory research as an intervention in dealing with ecological hazards. In a group, brainstorm about possibilities for participatory action research (PAR) projects in the area. Try to identify examples from a variety of environmental health areas. Be creative in planning. How might a nurse mobilize community support and participation in the research? What groups would be approachable? What critical questions might facilitate dialogue about the problem? What kinds of data could be collected, and how could they be used? How could research results be publicized? What ramifications could the completed study have for community members, other communities in the state, and community health nurses in other locales?

4. Nurses may have to supplement their knowledge of collective strategies by reading books about political action and by learning from community members who are experienced in political organizing. Visit a college or public library to investigate books and journal articles outside the nursing literature. Compile a list of references related to one of these political strategies (e.g., grassroots organizing, legislative lobbying, community education, policy analysis, use of the media, coalition building, citizen surveys, public protest, letter-writing campaigns, or consciousness-raising groups). Exchange reference lists with peers to benefit from their efforts. Then choose one or two books of interest and read them.

■ SUMMARY

This chapter provided a glimpse into the complex world of environmental health from a critical community health nursing perspective. The case study and clinical examples illustrate that nurses must evaluate the broader picture in assessing the environmental health status of communities and the vulnerable aggregates within them. In preventing, minimizing, and resolving environmental health problems, nurses must recognize patterns, detect subtle changes, identify underlying issues, and work collaboratively with a variety of individuals and groups. In the past, environmental threats to health were usually suspected only when other possible causes of illness were ruled out. Nurses can expect this pattern to change dramatically in the 21st century as environmental health moves increasingly to the forefront of the public health agenda.

EVOLVE WEBSITE

http://evolve.elsevier.com/Nies/community
- NCLEX Review Questions
- Case Studies

BIBLIOGRAPHY

Adamkiewicz G, Zota AR, Fabian MP: Moving environmental justice indoors: understanding structural influences on residential exposure patterns in low-income communities, *Am J Publ Health* 101(1):238–245, 2011.

Akhtar AZ, Greger M, Ferdowsian H, et al.: Health professionals' roles in animal agriculture, climate change, and human health, *Am J Prev Med* 36(2):182–187, 2009.

Ali SH, Foster T, Hall NL: The relationship between infectious diseases and housing maintenance in indigenous Australian households, *Int J Environ Res Publ Health* 15(20):2827, 2018. https://doi.org/10.3390/ijerph15122827.

American Planning Association: *Principles of a healthy sustainable food system*, 2010. Available from: http://www.planning.org/nationalcenters/health/foodprinciples.htm.

Anderson JO, Thundiyil JG, Stolbach A: Clearing the air: a review of the effects of particulate matter air pollution on human health, *J Med Toxicol* 8(2):166–175, 2012.

Asthma and Allergy Foundation: *Asthma facts and figures*. Available from: http://aafa.org/display.cfm?id=8&sub=42.

Balbus JM: Health implications. In *Climate change: mastering the public health role, a practical guidebook*, Washington, DC, 2011, American Public Health Association, pp 15–30.

Bartholomew LK, Parcel GS, Kok G, et al.: *Planning health promotion programs: an intervention mapping approach*, Hoboken, NJ, 2011, Jossey-Bass/Wiley.

Barton A, Basham M, Foy C, et al.: The Watcombe housing study: the short term effect of improving housing conditions on the health of residents, *J Epidemiol Community Health* 61:771–777, 2007.

Bhatia R, Wernham A: Integrating human health into environmental impact assessment: an unrealized opportunity for environmental health and justice, *Environ Health Perspect* 116(8):991–1000, 2008.

Boyd DR, Genuis SJ: The environmental burden of disease in Canada: respiratory disease, cardiovascular disease, cancer and congenital affliction, *Environ Res* 106(2):240–249, 2008.

Bureau of Labor Statistics: *Current injury, illness, and fatality data*. Available from: http://data.bls.gov/search/query/results?cx=013

738036195919377644%3A6ih0hfrgl50&q=2008+inurl%3Abls.gov%2Fiif.

Bureau of Labor Statistics: *Employer reported workplace injuries and illnesses*, 2015. Available from: https://www.bls.gov/news.release/pdf/osh.pdf. Accessed March 2017.

Bureau of Labor Statistics: *Workplace injuries and illnesses*, 2011. Available from: http://www.bls.gov/news.release/archives/osh_10252012.pdf.

Burger EJ: Human health: a surrogate for the environment: the evolution of environmental legislation and regulation during the 1970s, *Regul Toxicol Pharmacol* 9:196–206, 1989.

Centers for Disease Control and Prevention: *Asthma*. Available from, https://www.cdc.gov/asthma/asthmadata.htm. Accessed, September 9, 2021.

Center for Disease Control and Prevention: *Asthma*, 2021. Available from: https://www.cdc.gov/asthma/asthmadata.htm.

Center for Disease Control and Prevention: *Drinking water*, 2021. Available from: http://www.cdc.gov/healthywater/drinking/private/wells/.

Centers for Disease Control and Prevention: *Healthy homes*, (2011). Available from: http://www.cdc.gov/healthyhomes.

Center for Disease Control and Prevention: *Preliminary FoodNet data on the incident of infection with pathogens transmitted commonly through food*, 2020. Available from: https://www.cdc.gov/foodnet/index.html.

Centers for Disease Control and Prevention: Novel influenza A (H1N1) virus infection—Mexico, March–May 2009, *MMWR Morb Mortal Wkly Rep* 58(21):585–589, 2009.

Centers for Disease Control and Prevention: Preliminary FoodNet data on the incident of infection with pathogens transmitted commonly through food: 10 sites—United States, 2009, *MMWR Surveill Summ* 59(14):418–422, 2010. Available from: https://www.cdc.gov/foodnet/index.html. Retrieved: September 6, 2021.

Center for Disease Control and Prevention: *West Nile virus*, (2012). Available from: http://www.cdc.gov/ncidod/dvbid/westnile/index.htm.

Center for Disease Control and Prevention: *West Nile virus*, 2016. Available from: http://www.cdc.gov/ncidod/dvbid/westnile/index.htm.

Centers for Disease Control and Prevention: *West Nile virus disease cases and presumptive viremic blood donors by state—United States*, 2015. Available from: https://www.cdc.gov/westnile/.../wnv-disease-cases-and-pvds-by-state-2015_0707201. Accessed March 2017.

Center for Disease Control and Prevention: *Workplace safety and health topics agricultural safety*, 2013. Available from: http://www.cdc.gov/niosh/topics/aginjury/.

Chakraborty C, Zandbergen PA: Children at risk: racial/ethnic disparities in potential exposure to air pollution at school and home, *J Epidemiol Community Health* 61:1074–1079, 2007.

Chan JFW, Choi GKY, Yip CCY, et al.: Zika fever and congenital zika syndrome: an unexpected emerging arboviral disease, *J Infect* 72:507–524, 2016.

Ciencewicki J, Trivedi S, Kleeberger SJ: Oxidants and the pathogenesis of lung disease, *J Allergy Clin Immunol* 3(122):456–468, 2008.

Collins MB: Risk-based targeting: identifying disproportionalities in the sources and effects of industrial pollution, *Am J Publ Health* 101(suppl 1):S231–S237, 2011.

Coughenour C, Coker L, Bungum TJ: Environmental and social determinants of youth physical activity intensity levels at neighborhood parks in Las Vegas, NV, *J Community Health* 39:1092–1096, 2014.

Crouse DL, Peters PA, Hystad P, et al.: Ambient pm$_{2.5}$, O$_3$ and NO$_2$ exposures an associations with mortality over 16 years of follow-up in the Canadian census health and environment (CanCHEC), *Environ Health Perspect* 123(11):1180–1186, 2015.

Ding D, Sallis JF, Kerr J, et al.: Neighborhood environment and physical activity among youth: a review, *Am J Prev Med* 41(4):442–455, 2011.

Driehuis F, Spanjer MC, Scholten JM, et al.: Occurrence of mycotoxins in feedstuffs of dairy cows and estimation of total dietary intakes, *J Dairy Sci* 91(11):4261–4271, 2008.

Dunton GF, Kaplan J, Wolch J, et al.: Physical environmental correlate of childhood obesity: a systematic review, *Obes Rev* 10:393–402, 2009.

Easterling D: Basic Climate change science. In *Climate change: mastering the public health role, a practical guidebook*, Washington, DC, 2011, American Public Health Association, pp 7–14.

Environmental Protection Agency: *Air quality index (AQI): a guide to air quality and your health*, 2013. Available from: http://www.airnow.gov/index.cfm?action=aqibasics.aqi.

Environmental Protection Agency: *An introduction to indoor air quality*. Available from: http://www.epa.gov/iaq/co.html.

Environmental Protection Agency: *Drinking water contaminants*, 2016. Available from: http://water.epa.gov/drink/contaminants/.

Environmental Protection Agency: *Ensuring risk reduction in communities with multiple stressors: environmental justice and cumulative risks/impacts*, Washington, DC, Environmental Protection Agency

Environmental Protection Agency: *Environmental justice*. Available from: http://www.epa.gov/environmentaljustice/.

Environmental Protection Agency: *Federal radon action plan: celebrating success, looking to the future*. Available from: http://www.epa.gov/radon/pdfs/FRAP_2013Accomplishments.pdf.

Environmental Protection Agency: *Food safety*. Available from: http://www2.epa.gov/safepestcontrol.

Environmental Protection Agency: *Ground level ozone pollution*. Available from: https://www.epa.gov/ground-level-ozone-pollution.

Environmental Protection Agency: *Highlighting success: the region 9 environmental justice small grant program, fiscal years 1994–99*, EPA 909-R99–002., Washington, DC, Environmental Protection Agency

Environmental Protection Agency: *Indoors air facts No.4 (revised)*, 2017. Available from: https://www.epa.gov/indoor-air-quality-iaq.

Environmental Protection Agency: *Mold*. Available from: https://www.epa.gov/mold/brief-guide-mold-moisture-and-your-home.

Environmental Protection Agency: *Ozone layer protection*. Available from: http://www.epa.gov/ozone/strathome.html.

Environmental Protection Agency: *Public water systems: laboratories and monitoring*. Available from: http://water.epa.gov/infrastructure/drinkingwater/pws/labmon.cfm.

Environmental Protection Agency: *Radon*. Available from: https://www.epa.gov/radon/health-risk-radon#head; https://www.epa.gov/radon/federal-radon-action-plan-frap#expands.

Environmental Protection Agency: *Radon: health risks*. Available from: http://www.epa.gov/radon/healthrisks.html.

Environmental Protection Agency: *The effects of acid rain*, 2021. Available from: https://www.epa.gov/acidrain/effects-acid-rain.

Environmental Protection Agency: *Urban sprawl modeling, air quality monitoring and risk communication: The Northeast Ohio Project*, n.d.f. EPA/625/R-02/016, Washington, DC, Environmental Protection Agency.

Environmental Protection Agency: *What are the six common air pollutants?* Available from: http://www.epa.gov/airquality/urbanair/.

Environmental Protection Agency: *You're your house and healthy home*. Available from: http://yosemite.epa.gov/ochp/ochpweb.nsf/content/Healthy_Homes_Action_Card_English.htm/$File/Healthy_Homes_Action_Card_English.pdf.

Epstein PR: West Nile virus and the climate, *J Urban Health* 78:367—371, 2001.

Fan Y, Song Y: Is sprawl associated with a widening urban—suburban mortality gap? *J Urban Health* 86(5):708—728, 2009.

Farand SP, Lewis-Michl EL, Gomex MI: Adverse birth outcomes and maternal exposure to trichloroethylene and tetrachloroethylene through soil vapor intrusion in New York State, *Environ Health Perspect* 120(4), 2012.

Food Safety.gov: *Causes of food poisoning*, 2016. Available from: http://www.foodsafety.gov/poisoning/causes/index.html.

Garwick AW, Seppelt A, Riesgraf M: Addressing asthma management challenges in multisite, urban Head Start Program, *Publ Health Nurs* 27(4):329—336, 2010.

Geltman EG, Gill G, Jovanovic M: Beyond baby steps: an empirical study of the impact on environmental justice executive order 12898, *Fam Community Health* 39(3):143—150, 2016.

Global Green and Healthy Hospitals: *health care climate change challenge*, 2020. Available from: https://noharm-global.org/issues/global/2020-health-care-climate-challenge. Accessed March 2017.

Grant P, Bell K, Stewart D, et al.: Evidence of methamphetamine exposure in children removed from clandestine methamphetamine laboratories, *Pedi Emerg Care* 26(1):10—14, 2010.

Hankey S, Marshall JD, Brauer M: Health impacts of the built environment: within-urban variability in physical inactivity, air pollution, and ischemic heart disease mortality, *Environ Health Persp* 120(2):247, 2012.

Health Care Without Harm: *About us*, 2021. Available from: http://noharm.org/us_canada/about/.

Health Care Without Harm: *Environmental health*. Available from: https://noharm-global.org/content/global/mission-and-goals. Accessed September 12, 2021.

Health People 2030: *Environmental health objectives*. Available from: https://www.who.int/health-topics/environmental-health#tab=tab_1.

Hruby A, Manson JE, Qi L, et al.: Determinants and consequences of obesity, *Am J Publ Health* 106(9), 2016.

Hurd HS, Malladi S: A stochastic assessment of the public health risks of the use of macrolide antibiotics in food animals, *Risk Anal* 28(3):695—710, 2008.

Institute of Medicine: *Committee on enhancing environmental health content in nursing practice: nursing, health, and the environment*, Washington, DC, National Academies Press

Institute of Medicine: *The public health effects of food deserts: workshop summary*, 2009. Available from: http://www.iom.edu/Reports/2009/FoodDeserts.aspx.

James P, Troped PJ, Hart JE, et al.: Urban sprawl, physical activity, and body mass index: nurses' health study and nurses' health study II, *Am J Publ Health* 103(2):369—375, 2013.

Jones-Rounds ML, Evans GW, Braubach M: The interactive effects of housing and neighborhood quality on psychological well-being, *J Epidemiol Community Health* 68:171—175, 2014.

Kaufman TK, Rundle A, Neckerman KM, Sheehan DM, Lovasi GS, Hirsch JA: Neighborhood recreation facilities and facility membership are jointly associated with objectively measured physical activity, *J Urban Health* 96(4):570—582, 2019. https://doi.org/10.1007/s11524-019-00357-1.

Kerr J, Norman GJ, Adams MA, et al.: Do neighborhood environments moderate the effect of physical activity lifestyle interventions in adults? *Health Place* 16:903—908, 2010.

Klitzman S, Matte TD, Kass DE: The urban physical environment and its effects on health. In Freudenberg N, Galea S, Vlahov D, editors: *Cities and the health of the public*, Nashville, TN, 2006, Vanderbilt University Press, pp 61—84.

Knobeloch L, Turyk M, Imm P, et al.: Temporal changes in PCB and DDE levels among a cohort of frequent and infrequent consumers of Great Lakes sportfish, *Environ Res* 109:66—72, 2009.

Krieger N, Chen JT, Waterman PD, et al.: The inverse hazard law: blood pressure, sexual harassment, racial discrimination, workplace abuse and occupational exposures in US low-income black, white, and Latino workers, *Soc Sci Med* 67:1970—1981, 2008.

Li IC, Chen YC, Hsu LL, et al.: The effects of an educational training workshop for community leaders on self-efficacy of program planning skills and partnerships, *J Adv Nurs* 68(3):600—613, 2011.

Lindland EH, Kendall-Taylor N: *People, polar bears, and the potato salad: mapping the gaps between expert and public understandings of environmental health*, Washington, DC, 2011, Frame Works Institute.

Liu C, Maity A, Lin X, Wright RO, Christiani DC: Design and analysis issues in gene and environment studies, *Environ Health* 11(93), 2012.

Martins DC, Burbank PM: Critical interactionism: an upstream-downstream approach to health care reform, *Adv Nurs Sci* 34(4):315—329, 2011.

Molitor J, Su JG, Molitor NT, et al.: Identifying vulnerable populations through an examination of the association between multipollutant profiles and poverty, *Environ Sci Technol* 45(18):7754—7760, 2011. Available from: http://dx.org/10.1021/es104017x.

National Aeronautics and Space Administration (NASA): *Global climate change: Vital signs of the planet*, 2014. Available from, https://climate.nasa.gov/. Accessed March 2017.

National Environmental Health Association: *Annual report*, 2016. Available from: https://www.neha.org/. Accessed March 2017.

National Institute of Health: National Institute of Environmental Health Sciences: *GuLF study*, n.d.a. Available from: https://gulfstudy.nih.gov/en/index.html. Accessed January 2014.

National Institute of Health: National Institute of Environmental Health Sciences: *Gulf study*, 2014. Available from: https://gulfstudy.nih.gov/en/index.html.

National Institute of Health (NIH): *Opportunities and challenges in digestive diseases research: recommendations of the national commission on digestive diseases,(2009)*. Available from: https://www.niddk.nih.gov/.../NCDD%20Research%20Plan/NCDD_04272009_Research.Accessed March 2017.

Nelson MC, Gordon-Larsen P, Song Y, et al.: Built and social environments: associations with adolescent overweight and activity, *Am J Prev Med* 31(2), 2006.

Northridge ME, et al.: Environmental equity and health: understanding completely and moving forward, *Am J Publ Health* 93(2):209—213, 2003.

Nweke OC: Achieving environmental justice: perspectives on the path forward through collective action to eliminate health disparities, *Am J Publ Health* 101(S1):S6—S8, 2011.

O'Neill MS, Ebi KL: Temperature extremes and health: impacts of climate variability and change in the United States, *J Occup Environ Med* 51(1):13—25, 2009.

Pan TC, Kao JJ: Inter-generational equity index for assessing environmental sustainability: an example of global warming, *Ecol Indicat* 9(4):725—1721, 2009.

Paranzino GK, Butterfield P, Nastoff T, Ranger C: I PREPARE: Development and clinical utility of an environmental exposure history mnemonic, *J Am Assoc Occup Health Nur* 53(1):37—42, 2005.

Prus-Ustun A, Wolf J, Corvalan C, Bos R, Neira M: *Preventing disease through healthy environments: a global assessment of the burden of disease from environmental risks*. World Health Organization: Available from: www.who.int/quantifying_ehimpacts/publications/preventing-disease/en/. Accessed March 2017.

Rauh VA, Landrigan PJ, Claudio L: Housing and health: intersection of poverty and environmental exposures, *Ann N Y Acad Sci* 1136: 276–288, 2008.

Renalds A, Smith T, Hale P: A systematic review of built environment and health, *Fam Community Health* 33(1):68–78, 2009.

Ron E: Thyroid cancer incidence among people living in areas contaminated by radiation from the Chernobyl accident, *Health Phys* 93(5):502–511, 2007.

Rylander C, Odland JO, Sandanger TM: Climate change and the potential effects on maternal and pregnancy outcomes: an assessment of the most vulnerable—the mother, fetus, and newborn child, *Glob Health Action* 11(6):1–9, 2013.

Sanchez F, Kosson DS: Probabilistic approach for estimating the release of contaminants under field management scenarios, *Waste Manag* 25(4):463–472, 2005.

Sattler B: The greening of health care: environmental policy and advocacy in the health care industry, *Pol Polit Nurs Pract* 4(1):6–13, 2003.

Schrieberg D: Death from a healing machine: radioactive waste goes on Mexican odyssey after sale of medical device, *San Francisco Examiner* 1:2, 1991.

Schulz A, Mentz G, Johnson-Lawrence V, et al.: Independent and joint associations between multiple measures of the built and social environment and physical activity in a multi-ethnic urban community, *J Urban Health*, 2013.

Schwartz J: Air pollution and children's health, *Pediatrics* 113: 1037–1046, 2004.

Sharifi M, Sequist TD, Rifas-Shiman SL: The role of neighborhood characteristics and the built environment in understanding racial/ethnic disparities in childhood obesity, *Prev Med* 91:103–109, 2016.

Sheffield PE, Knowlton K, Carr JL, et al.: Modeling of regional climate change effects on ground-level ozone and childhood asthma, *Am J Prev Med* 41(3):251–257, 2011.

Stevens PE, Hall JM: Applying critical theories to nursing in communities, *Publ Health Nurs* 9:2–9, 1992.

Tainio M, Nazelle AJ, Gotschi T: Can air pollution negate the health benefits of cycling and walking? *Prev Med* 87:233–236, 2016.

Tarr J: Knoxville's pollution rivals that of Los Angeles, Houston and Atlanta, but Green Power might help clear the air, *Metro Pulse* 11(18), 2001.

Thompson B, et al.: Para Ninos Saludables: a community intervention trial to reduce organophosphate pesticide exposure in children of farmworkers, *Environ Health Perspect* 116(5):687–694, 2008.

Trasande L, Cronk C, Durkin M, et al.: Environment and obesity in the national children's study, *Environ Health Perspect* 117(2), 2009.

Troped PJ, Tamura K, Whitcomb HA, et al.: Perceived built environment and physical activity in U.S. women by sprawl and region, *Am J Prev Med* 41(5):473–479, 2011.

Tsunoda K, Tsuji T, Kitano N: Associations of physical activity with neighborhood environments and transportation modes in older Japanese adults, *Prev Med* 55:113–118, 2012.

U.S. Department of Health and Human Services: *Office of Disease Prevention and Health Promotion: Healthy People 2030*, 2013. Available from: https://health.gov/healthypeople/about/workgroups/environmental-health-workgroup. Accessed September 6, 2021.

U.S. Department of Labor: Occupational Safety and Health Administration: *OSHA QUICKCARD: hazard communication safety data sheets*, 2013. Available from: http://www.osha.gov/Publications/HazComm_QuickCard_SafetyData.html.

U.S. Food and Drug Administration: *Food safety for moms-to-be: medical professionals fast facts*. Available from: http://www.fda.gov/Food/FoodborneIllnessContaminants/PeopleAtRisk/ucm091671.htm.

U.S. Geological Survey: *What is ground water?* 2005. Available from: http://pubs.usgs.gov/of/1993/ofr93-643/.

White BM, Hall ES, Johnson C: Environmental health literacy in support of social action: an environmental justice perspective, *J Environ Health* 77(1):24–29, 2014.

Whitney SL, Maltby HJ, Carr JM: "This food may contain…" what nurses should know about genetically engineered foods, *Nurs Outlook* 52:262–266, 2004.

World Health Organization: *Air quality*. Available at: https://www.who.int/teams/environment-climate-change-and-health/air-quality-and-health/ambient-air-pollution; https://www.who.int/health-topics/air-pollution#tab=tab_1.

World Health Organization: *Environmental health*, 2021. Available from: https://www.who.int/health-topics/environmental-health#tab=tab_1.

World Health Organization: *Global alert and response (GAR): Severe acute respiratory syndrome (SARS)*. Available from: www.who.int/csr/sars/guidelines/en/index.html.

World Health Organization: *Influenza A (H1N1) update 46*, Available from: http://www.who.int/csr/disease/swineflu/en/index.html.

World Health Organization: *Ionizing radiation in our environment* Available from: http://www.who.int/ionizing_radiation/env/en/.

World Health Organization: *World day for safety and health at work 2005: a background paper*, Geneva, International Labour Office.

Wu Q, Shi H, Adams CD, et al.: Oxidative removal of selected endocrine-disruptors and pharmaceuticals in drinking water treatment systems, and identification of degradation products of triclosan, *Sci Total Environ* 439:18–25, 2012.

Health in the Global Community

Julie Cowan Novak

Healthcare equity and healthcare reform are subjects of critical political, social, moral, and ethical debate throughout the world. Human health, population health, and their influence on every aspect of life are central to the global agenda. Nurses are the largest segment of the healthcare workforce and most trusted. Nurses assess, plan, evaluate, and develop policy to promote and restore health to individuals, families, and communities across settings and geographic boundaries. Nurses study models of health promotion, community assessment, community empowerment, service learning, sustainability, and innovation to improve healthcare access, create meaningful action, and efficient, effective delivery systems. Community public health nurses must be aware of forces that threaten health in the global community. Our global society, the Internet, and reduction in travel time provide access that was unimaginable several decades ago. **Globalization**, the process of increasing social and economic dependence and integration as capital, goods, persons, concepts, images, ideas, and values cross state boundaries, is inextricably linked to the benefits and challenges of our time.

This chapter highlights population characteristics; international patterns of health and disease, including the COVID-19 pandemic; social, cultural, and economic factors; international healthcare agencies and organizations; healthcare providers; healthcare delivery systems and models; and the community public health nurse's role as a leader in the global community. The chapter presents an International Community Assessment Model (ICAM); a Service-Learning Model for thoughtful community-based service and meaningful, structured reflection; faculty and student discovery, learning, engagement, policy, and system design; and the Integrated Nurse-led Model of Sustainability and Innovation (INMSI) (Novak, 2019a,b) and its evolution to Nurse Practitioner Clinic Sustainability and Innovation (NP–CSI) (Novak, 2020).

Population characteristics, including patterns of growth, demographics, and pandemics, are among the many health issues that merit attention and study as they have global effects that threaten human life on a mass scale. This chapter explores these issues and other environmental factors, including identified stressors and patterns of health and disease.

POPULATION CHARACTERISTICS

Population growth and the most recent pandemic present a threat to the health and economy of most nations. The exponential nature of world population growth is evident. In 1804, the world population was approximately one billion. From 1804 to 1927, the population reached two billion; 1927 to 1960: 3 billion; 1960 to 1974: 4 billion; and 1974 to 1987: 5 billion. In 1999, the world population was about six billion and by 2016 it had grown to 7.4 billion. The population is projected to reach 8 billion by 2025, 9.8 billion by 2050, and 11.2 billion by 2100 (United Nations, 2020). Of utmost concern is that 99% of the growth is expected to occur in resource-poor countries (Population Reference Bureau, 2020).

In any society, large populations create pressure. For example, feeding a population becomes problematic in developing countries when famine, international trade problems, war, and pandemics occur. Malnutrition, disease, and/or death are outcomes. Pressures from population growth are also felt in industrialized nations. Although food may be plentiful for the majority, overcrowding leads to pollution, stress, disease, and violence. Each of these challenges represents a major barrier to economic growth. The poor suffer this burden of excess mortality and morbidity disproportionately. Thus, comprehensive health promotion, a strong public health and environmental infrastructure, and effective healthcare delivery systems will address the origins of poverty, increase productivity, and ultimately improve health and quality of life. The global COVID-19 pandemic has further exposed inequities including inadequate access to and shortages of essential basic and specialized healthcare, vaccines, medications, and even oxygen.

World population distribution is uneven. More than 50% of the population lives in just four countries: China (1.439 billion), India (1.38 billion), Indonesia (274 million) (World Bank, 2021), and the United States (332.5 million) (US Census Bureau, 2020). In 2019, 26% of the world's population consisted of children 0 to 14 (Ritchie and Roser, 2019); 8.5% were aged 65 and older (NIH, 2016).

The COVID-19 pandemic continues to cause significant loss of life, disrupted livelihoods, and undermined well-being throughout the world. The crisis underscored how ill-prepared and inequitable most health systems are and the negative impact this can have toward achieving the United Nations Sustainable Development Goals (SDGs). There is an urgency to invest in health systems, services, and workforce and to "track population health and its determinants in a comprehensive and continuous manner" (World Health Statistics [WHO], 2021). Key messages include: (1) "Life expectancy and healthy life expectancy (HALE) increased by over 8% globally 2000–2016 and remain profoundly influenced by income." The largest gains were due to reducing child mortality and fighting infectious diseases; however, lower-and middle-income countries continue to have the poorest overall health outcomes. There was an emphasis on implementation of health policies and interventions to minimize the potential impact of COVID-19 on life expectancy; (2) Much of the world's population does not have access to essential health services, as coverage in low- and middle-income countries remains well below coverage in wealthier countries. There is a need to build health systems with improved access to quality health services, lowered financial cost, and a strengthened health workforce; (3) While there have been improvements in controlling communicable disease, there has not been similar progress in preventing and controlling noncommunicable diseases (NCDs). Indeed, NCDs accounted for 71% of all global deaths; many occurred in low- and middle-income countries. Improvements in areas such as tobacco use and level of alcohol consumption are overshadowed by the rise of obesity and the numbers of individuals with preexisting NCD conditions such as hypertension and diabetes. Addressing risk factors to prevent NCDs such as obesity and mental health conditions is vital; (4) Country health information systems should be strengthened to improve timeliness of The International Health Regulations monitoring framework, one of the tools for data collection that have demonstrated value in evaluating and building country capacities to prevent, detect, assess, report, and respond to public health emergencies. Objective and comparable data are crucial to determine the effectiveness of different national strategies used to mitigate and suppress, and better prepare; and (5) Over the last 20 years, prevention and treatment have substantially improved for major infectious diseases and maternal, neonatal, and child healthcare leading to a steady decline in incidence and mortality from those diseases. Efforts need to be made to preserve progress and to be vigilant for early detection and continual monitoring to seek solutions for high-risk and resource limited populations (World Health Statistics, 2021).

ENVIRONMENTAL FACTORS

The relationship between humans and their environment is an important component of individual, family, and global health. The fields of environmental health and sustainable resource development have exploded over the past 4 decades. Environmental stressors are categorized into five types: (1) lead poisoning and air pollution directly assault human health; (2) the effects of air pollution on products and structures damage society's goods and services; (3) noise and litter affect QOL; (4) global warming and climate change interfere with the ecological balance; (5) global pandemics such as COVID-19, natural disasters, terrorism, and war affect all aspects of life.

Air pollution, water pollution, and land pollution are among the consequences of environmental stressors. From 2010 to 2020, the percent change in air quality due to carbon monoxide was minus 12% in the United States (EPA, 2021); however, 50% of worldwide air pollution remains attributable to carbon monoxide. Other primary pollutants, such as nitrogen monoxide, sulfur oxides, particulate matter, and hydrocarbons, combine with carbon monoxide to create 90% of the world's pollution.

According to joint World Health Organization (WHO) and United Nations Children's Fund (UNICEF) data (2019), more than half of the world's population lack access to basic sanitation facilities, and one in three people globally do not have access to safe drinking water. Inadequate access to sanitation and clean water contributes to the deaths of 4000 vulnerable children each day. "Closing inequality gaps in the accessibility, quality and availability of water, sanitation and hygiene should be at the heart of government funding and planning strategies. To relent on investment plans for universal coverage is to undermine decades worth of progress at the expense of coming generations." (Naylor, UNICEF; WHO, 2019b).

Agricultural, industrial, residential, and commercial wastes increase land pollution. For example, organic farming is growing in use, popularity, and consumer demand; however, chemical fertilizers, synthetic pesticides, and petrochemical products continue to displace natural, more healthful products. Disposable goods still replace reusable goods, resulting in increased waste. Production technologies contribute to worldwide environmental and ecological stress.

PATTERNS OF HEALTH AND DISEASE

Lifestyles, health and cultural beliefs, infrastructure, economics, and politics affect existing illnesses and society's commitment to prevention. Disease patterns vary throughout the world; therefore primary causes of death differ in developed and developing countries. Racial, ethnic, and access disparities exist within and between countries. For example, of the 56.4 million deaths worldwide in 2020, 54% were due to ischemic heart disease and stroke. This was followed by chronic obstructive pulmonary disease, pneumonia, tracheal and bronchus lung cancers, and diabetes. Deaths from Alzheimer's disease and other dementias doubled between 2000 and 2015, making dementias the seventh leading cause of death globally. In contrast, deaths from diarrheal diseases halved between 2000 and 2015, making it the eighth leading cause of death globally. Finally, deaths from diabetes mellitus and kidney disease rounded out the top 10. Notably, HIV/AIDS is no longer among the world's top 10 causes of death (WHO, 2019b). Tuberculosis (TB) is the eighth leading cause of death globally when the target population is low income. In spring, 2020, the COVID-19 virus rose to be the leading cause of death in the US. Compared with leading causes of death from the same period in 2018, COVID-19 was the third leading cause of death for children and adults (697.5 deaths/million), ranking only behind heart disease (128.7/million) and cancer (121.9/million) (Koh et al., 2021). In the US postvaccine roll out, COVID-19 fell to the seventh leading cause of death by July 2021.

Once plagued with high rates of infectious disease, developed countries significantly reduced such rates through improved sanitation, nutrition, immunization, and improved healthcare. Most developed countries have a more stable economy and a wide range of industrial and technological development. These countries experience an epidemiological transition. For example, the morbidity and mortality profile of a country changes from a lesser developed one to a developed one. Many developed countries experienced an epidemiological transition from having an infectious disease profile to having a chronic disease profile and are now plagued by chronic diseases such as cardiovascular disease, respiratory disease, and cancer secondary to air pollution and the tobacco use pandemic. This altered profile created a demographic transition from traditional societies, in which almost everyone is young, to societies with rapidly growing numbers of middle-aged and elderly people. COVID-19 altered this pattern with the US having the highest case and death rates in the world (Woolf et al., 2020). "The year 2020 ended with COVID-19 massively surging, as it did in the spring (2020), to be the leading cause of death. Ending this crisis will require not only further advances in treatment but also unprecedented commitment to all aspects of prevention, vaccination, and public health. Only by doing so can future years see this illness revert back to the unfamiliar and unknown condition it once was" (Koh et al., 2021).

Other infectious diseases that contribute to higher mortality rates in developing countries are AIDS, TB, malaria, hepatitis B, rheumatic heart disease, parasitic infection, dengue fever, and the COVID-19 pandemic. Although these diseases claim the lives of millions, it is estimated they could be reduced by 50% through effective public health interventions. It is hoped that many of these diseases could join smallpox as a disease known only to history through the development and implementation of immunization and vaccination programs, the most powerful and cost-effective strategies at our disposal for infectious diseases. Efforts to reduce the incidence of TB were included in the "Commission for Africa" report, which called for wealthy nations to double their aid to Africa to rebuild systems to deliver public health services, provide staff training, develop new medicines, and provide better sexual and reproductive health services. The bacille Calmette-Guerin vaccine series, for example, induces active immunity to TB, but it does not reduce the transmission of infectious types of TB. At least one quarter of the world's population is estimated to be infected by the TB bacteria, *Mycobacterium tuberculosis*. Other WHO programs, including COVID-19 2021 Strategic Preparedness and Response plan (SPRP2021); Zika: Then, Today, Tomorrow; Roll Back Malaria; Unite to End TB; HIV/AIDS Control; Tobacco Free Initiative; and Avian Influenza Pandemic Preparedness target key infectious and chronic disease issues of the 21st century.

COVID-19 Vaccine Global Access (COVAX) is a worldwide effort for equitable access to vaccines. Directed by Gavi, the Vaccine Alliance; the Coalition for Epidemic Preparedness Innovation (CEPI); and the WHO. COVAX coordinates international resources to enable low-to-middle-income countries equitable access to COVID-19 tests, therapies, and vaccines (COVAX explained, WHO, February 25, 2021). 100 million doses had been delivered as of July 6, 2021 (WHO, 2021).

Although significant progress has been made, AIDS continues to be a global concern. In 2019, 10.7 million people were living with HIV in eastern and southern Africa with 6.7% adult HIV prevalence (ages 15–49), 730,000 new HIV infections, 300,000 AIDS-related deaths, 73% of adults on antiretroviral treatment of all adults/children living with AIDS, and 58% of children on antiretroviral treatment (UNAIDS Data, 2020). Eastern and southern Africa is the region hardest hit by HIV. Although it has only 6.2% of the world's population, it has over half (54%) of the total number of people living with HIV in the world (20.6 million people). In 2018, there were 800,000 new HIV infections, just under half of the global total (UNAIDS, 2019).

Urbanization and within-country migration play a role in the spread of AIDS. For instance, in Rwanda the HIV seroprevalence is 14 to 20 times higher in urban areas than in rural areas. Annually, HIV threatens more lives as more people migrate to the world's largest cities. In 2020, 56.2% of the global population lived in cities (Buchholz., 2020). This is an increase from 25% in 1970. Over the past 4 decades, significant progress has been made in HIV education, prevention, treatment, social policy, and legislation; however, stigma against people living with HIV persists.

Malaria is a life-threatening parasitic disease transmitted by mosquitoes. Today, approximately 40% of the world's population is at risk for malaria; however, because of improved public health efforts, malaria rates fell 21% between 2010 and 2015. Malaria is found throughout the tropical and subtropical regions of the world and causes more than 212 million acute illnesses and at least 429,000 deaths annually (WHO, 2020). Effective low-cost strategies are available for its prevention,

treatment, and control, including insecticide-treated nets and new-generation medications. Successful administration of antimalarial medications has included a challenge of evolving drug-resistant parasites and the search for new drug formulations. Indeed, resistance to chloroquine has rendered the drug ineffective in many regions. The development of effective, durable vaccines against the human malaria parasites *P. falciparum*, *P. malariae*, *P. ovale*, *P. vivax*, and *P. knowlesi* remain a key priority. *P. falciparum* is the most life threatening (Stanfordhealthcare.org, 2021). The synthesis of rational antigen selection, immunogen design, and immunization strategies offer promise for achieving sustained high-level protection (Draper et al., 2018). The first malaria vaccine was approved in 2015 and reported an efficacy of 25% to 50%. While 2019 clinical trials using the R-21/MM antimalarial vaccine reached the 75% efficacy rate set by WHO (Corbley, 2021).

Globally, tobacco kills more than eight million people annually worldwide (WHO, 2020). Seven million of those deaths are the result of direct tobacco use and 1.2 million are the result of nonsmokers being exposed to secondhand smoke. More than 80% of the world's 1.3 billion tobacco users live in low- and middle-income countries (WHO, 2020). Tobacco control is a critical component of the international healthcare agenda. Including deaths from secondhand smoke, in 2020, an estimated one in seven deaths worldwide was tobacco related. Since 1990, tobacco control and secondhand smoke policies have been implemented at various political levels in the United States and abroad. The magnitude and consequences of the tobacco pandemic were unexpected. Smoking prevention and cessation programs, state and federal mandates, tobacco taxation, the 1998 Tobacco Master Settlement Agreement, antitobacco media campaigns, strict licensing of tobacco retailers, the elimination of tobacco vending machines and point-of-sale advertising, and the elimination of tobacco sales by pharmacies have had a significant impact on tobacco sales in the United States. An increasing number of countries have passed legislation mandating smoke-free laws; 36 US states along with the District of Columbia, American Samoa, Guam, the Northern Mariana Islands, Puerto Rico, and the US Virgin Islands have 100% smoke-free laws (American Non-smokers Rights Foundation, 2021). Because of health concerns and cost, 43 countries, from Ireland to New Zealand, have developed tobacco-free policies and banned tobacco advertising, promotion, and sponsorship. Although American adults have enrolled in cessation programs, there are 480,000 tobacco-related US deaths annually (Smoking and Tobacco Use, Fast Facts, CDC, June 2021). The tobacco industry continues to target youth with e-cigarettes and vaping while significantly increasing international exports.

In 2008, the WHO introduced MPower, which stands for **M**onitor tobacco use and prevention policies; **P**rotect people from tobacco use; **O**ffer help to quit tobacco use; **W**arn about the dangers of tobacco; **E**nforce bans on tobacco advertising, promotion and sponsorship; and **R**aise taxes on tobacco (WHO, 2018).

In summary, a global approach to tobacco control can guide the development of effective interventions based on best evidence and best practice. Countering potential threats to health from economic crises, unhealthful environments, or risky behavior is critical. Promotion of a healthy lifestyle underpins a proactive strategy for risk reduction, tobacco product use prevention and cessation, immunization and vaccination provision, cleaner air and water, adequate sanitation, healthful diets, fitness and exercise programs, and safe transportation.

INTERNATIONAL AGENCIES AND ORGANIZATIONS

Promoting worldwide health is humankind's greatest challenge. Several global agencies, such as the WHO, the Pan American Health Organization (PAHO), the United Nations (UN), UNICEF, the World Bank, the Centers for Disease Control (CDC), and nongovernmental organizations such as foundations, play important roles in improving the health of all nations. Founded on April 7, 1948 (World Health Day), the **WHO** is an international health agency of the UN. With six regional offices and 150 field offices in the United States, Congo, Denmark, Egypt, India, and the Philippines, the WHO's primary role is to direct and coordinate international health efforts, disseminate global health standards and guidelines, and help countries address public health concerns within the UN system. The main areas of work include health systems, promoting health through the life course, communicable diseases, NCD, preparedness, surveillance, response, and corporate services. In 1978, the WHO's goal of **"health for all by the year 2000"** was framed at the conference in Alma-Ata, the former USSR (now known as Almaty, Kazakhstan). The conference defined "health for all" as "the attainment by all citizens of the world by the year 2000 of a level of health that will permit them to lead a socially and economically productive life". Not being met, the target year for achievement of "health for all" was extended to 2010 and 2020.

The Alma-Ata conference on primary healthcare expressed the need for urgent action by all governments. The WHO's statement of beliefs, goals, and objectives is outlined in the **Declaration of Alma-Ata**. The concept of primary healthcare stresses health as a fundamental human right for individuals, families, and communities; the unacceptability of the gross inequities, inequalities, and disparities in health status; the importance of community involvement; and the active role of all WHO sectors.

The program promotes seven elements of primary healthcare: (1) health education regarding disease prevention and cure; (2) proper food supply and nutrition; (3) adequate supply of safe drinking water and sanitation; (4) maternal and child healthcare; (5) immunizations; (6) control of endemic diseases; and (7) the provision of essential drugs. According to the Declaration, a primary healthcare system should provide the entire population with universal coverage; relevant, acceptable, affordable, and effective services; a spectrum of comprehensive services that provide for primary, secondary, and tertiary care and prevention; active community involvement in the planning and delivery of services; and integration of health services with development activities to ensure that complete nutritional, educational, occupational, environmental, and safe housing needs are met (WHO, 2021).

The year 2010, the 10th anniversary of the adoption of the WHO Global Strategy on Diet, Physical Activity, and Health, presented a time for reflection and evaluation of progress. The WHO created an action plan depicting 2020 targets related to the prevalence of unhealthy diets, inactivity, tobacco use, and alcohol.

The PAHO is an international public health agency, located in Washington, DC, with over a century of experience in working to improve the health and living standards of the Americans. It serves as the regional office of WHO and is recognized as part of the UN system. Healthy People 2030 (CDC, 2020) has identified goals for this decade including: attain healthy, thriving lives and well-being, free of preventable disease, disability, injury, and premature death (CDC, 2020).

Founded in 1945 after World War II, the UN now comprises 193 member nations committed to world peace and security through international cooperation. The UN attempts to resolve global conflicts and formulates policies that affect all nations. Regardless of size, wealth, or political system, all member nations have an equal vote in the decision-making process. UN decisions seek to reflect world opinion and the moral authority of the community of nations (United Nations, 2018). In 2000, the **Millennium Development Goals** were developed to coordinate and strengthen global efforts to meet the needs of the poorest of the poor (United Nations, 2000). The SDGs also known as the Global Goals, were adopted by the UN in 2015 as a universal call to action to end poverty, protect the planet, and ensure that by 2030 all people enjoy peace and prosperity. The 17 SDGs are integrated. They recognize that action in one area will affect outcomes in others, and that development must balance social, economic, and environmental sustainability. Countries have committed to prioritize progress for those who are furthest behind. The SDGs are designed to end poverty, hunger, AIDS, and discrimination against women and girls. The creativity, expertise, technology, and financial resources from all of society are necessary to achieve the SDGs in every context (United Nations Development Programme, 2021) and include

1. No poverty
2. Zero hunger
3. Good health and well-being
4. Quality education
5. Gender equality
6. Clean water and sanitation
7. Affordable and clean energy
8. Decent work and economic growth
9. Industry, innovation, and infrastructure
10. Reduced inequalities.
11. Sustainable cities and communities
12. Responsible consumption and production

13. Climate action
14. Life below water
15. Life on land
16. Peace, justice, and strong institutions
17. Partnerships for the goals

The **U.S. Department of Health and Human Services** (USDHHS) created a program titled *Healthy People* that serves as the foundation for efforts throughout the HHS to create a healthier Nation. *Healthy People 2030* is based on the accomplishments of the previous *Healthy People* initiatives which began in 1979. *Healthy People 2030* is the most recent iteration of the initiative. *Healthy People 2030* addresses our most critical public health priorities and challenges and includes hundreds of measurable objectives with ambitious but achievable national targets. Compared with *Healthy People 2020*, the 2030 version has a smaller set of objectives with: (1) More rigorous data standards, (2) New objectives related to e-cigarettes, flavored tobacco use in adolescents, and opioid use disorder, (3) Resources for adapting *Healthy People* to emerging health issues like COVID-19. For the first time *Healthy People 2030* sets 10-year targets for objectives related to social determinants of health with an update of health literacy definition to emphasize how both individuals and organizations can help improve health literacy (USDHHS, 2021).

The **Centers for Disease Control and Prevention** (CDC) located in Atlanta, Georgia, is one of the 11 major operating components of the U.S. Department of Health and Human Services (USDHHS, also called HHS). The CDC is principal agency in the U.S. government for protecting the health and safety of all Americans and for providing essential human services; the CDC was founded in 1946 to help control malaria. The agency has remained at the forefront of public health efforts to prevent and control infectious and chronic diseases, injuries, workplace hazards, disabilities, and environmental health threats and to protect the health of international travelers through advisories and immunization and vaccine recommendations. The CDC is globally recognized for conducting research and investigations and for its action-oriented approach. It applies research and findings to improve people's daily lives and responds to health emergencies, a feature that distinguishes the CDC from many of its peer agencies. The CDC is committed to achieving evidence-based health improvements. Lewis (2021) examined what went wrong and what went right regarding the US COVID-19 pandemic response and CDC and WHO roles. The WHO called COVID-19 a pandemic on March 11, 2020.

In general, the US fared worse than most other countries, with more than 34 million cases and 622,000 deaths. Nearly 99.5% of recent COVID-19 deaths are from unvaccinated individuals and the Delta variant represents over 50% of sequenced samples across the US, an increase of 24% over 3 weeks prior to the briefing (CDC, 2021). Scientists and public health experts have identified key successes as well as mistakes in the US's response to the pandemic. Key successes include the rapid development of two double-dose (Pfizer and Moderna) vaccines that have proven 95% effective in preventing symptomatic COVID-19 and the single-dose Johnson & Johnson COVID-19. These were authorized by the FDA for emergency use in the US in record time. In addition, the healthcare workforce and other essential workers across the service industries risked their own lives to save others. Furthermore, early in the pandemic, the majority of the public wore masks, maintained social distancing, and stayed home. Issues where the public response dropped were that many ultimately, for example, downplayed the danger. Initially, there were slow and flawed testing, slow approval of tests made by private companies, and confusing mask recommendations and misinformation. Furthermore, there was early inadequate PPE for healthcare providers and the general population, inadequate government and hospital stockpiles, and a decentralized response (Lewis, 2021).

Collaborating with the UN are **nongovernmental organizations** (NGOs) such as the Carter Center and the Gates Foundation. Founded in 1982, the **Carter Center** is a nonprofit NGO founded by former President Jimmy Carter and First Lady Rosalynn Carter in partnership with Emory University and based in Atlanta, Georgia. With a fundamental commitment to human rights and the alleviation of human suffering, the Center seeks to prevent and resolve conflicts, enhance freedom and democracy, and improve health. The Center: (1) believes that people can improve their own lives when provided with the necessary skills, knowledge, and access to resources; (2) emphasizes action and measurable results in the lives of the people it seeks to help; (3) values the courage to break new ground, fill vacuums, and address the most difficult problems in the most difficult situations; (4) recognizes that solving difficult problems requires careful analysis, relentless persistence, and the recognition that failure is an acceptable risk; and (5) is nonpartisan and seeks to work collaboratively with other organizations from the highest levels of government to local communities (The Carter Center, 2021).

> *The bond of our common humanity is stronger than the divisiveness of our fears and prejudices. God gives us the capacity for choice. We can choose to alleviate suffering. We can choose to work together for peace. We can make these changes—and we must.*
>
> **Jimmy Carter, Nobel Laureate, Carter Center (2016).**

Founded in 2000, the **Gates Foundation** has local, national, and global objectives guided by the belief that every life has equal value, working to help all people lead healthy, productive lives. In developing countries, it focuses on improving people's health and giving them the chance to lift themselves out of hunger and extreme poverty. In the United States, it seeks to ensure that all people, especially those with the fewest resources have access to the opportunities they need to succeed in school and life. It seeks to achieve Foundation goals by: (1) Spurring innovations that improve the human condition by stepping in where governments and businesses leave gaps, (2) Strengthening global cooperation by bringing together governments, businesses, philanthropies, and communities to save and transform lives around the world, (3) Creating market incentives for lifesaving products by supporting the development and delivery of vaccines, treatments, diagnostics, and other tools for those most in need, (4) Generating high-quality data and evidence that drive progress by showing what is working and what is not (Gates Foundation, 2021). In 2010, the Gates Foundation committed $10 billion over 10 years to help research, develop, and deliver vaccines for the world's poorest countries. Within Africa, the foundation has had a profound effect on improving access to antiretroviral medications, prevention and treatment for HIV, TB, malaria, and providing access to COVID-19 vaccinations. Between January 2020 and June 2021, total funding from all sources to combat COVID-19 has exceeded $21.7 trillion according to the Devex funding platform (Devex.com, 2021). Although COVID-19 began as a health crisis, its rapid and ongoing global spread has meant it became an economic crisis first and foremost for many economies.

Created in 1946, the **United Nations International Children's Emergency Fund (UNICEF)** was founded to assist millions of sick and hungry children in war-ravaged Europe and China. In 1950, the UNICEF mandate was expanded to address the needs of children and women throughout the world. UNICEF works for children's survival, development, and protection by developing and implementing community-based programs with well-documented achievements in child health, nutrition, education, water, sanitation, and women's rights. In 1953 the name was shortened to the UN Children's Fund; however, the UNICEF acronym was retained (WHO, 2020). During the pandemic, UNICEF has helped protect children and their families from exposure to the COVID-19 virus and to minimize mortality. It is noted that this includes providing accurate information through risk communication and community engagement. There are also efforts to promote hygiene and provide essential services and supplies (UNICEF.org, 2021).

Within a dramatically changing world economy, the mission of the **World Bank** is to end extreme poverty by reducing the share of the global population that lives in extreme poverty to 3% by 2030; to promote shared prosperity by increasing the incomes of the poorest 40% of people in every country (World Bank, 2021). The World Bank was established in 1945 to provide low-interest loans and grants to developing countries for education, health initiatives such as education of healthcare providers, disease prevention and control, infrastructure, agriculture, communications, environmental protection, and economic and institutional development (World Bank, 2017). As of 2021 it has 189 member countries. Since 1970, the World Bank has become more focused on health-related initiatives to promote sustainable economic growth. Projects include the alleviation of poverty, safe water, effective sanitation, and affordable housing. The World Bank has been tracking changes in poverty levels related to the COVID-19 pandemic. Globally, the increase in poverty that occurred in 2020 due to COVID-19 lingers, and the COVID-induced poor in 2021 continues to be 97 million people. The World Bank estimates that "there will be a global rebound in poverty due to COVID-19 in 2021 that will not be equal for all." They predict declines in poverty in high- and middle-income countries, particularly in countries in South Asia and East Asia and the Pacific. But, countries in Sub-Saharan Africa and other low-income areas are anticipated to experience further increases in poverty (Mahler et al., 2021). Since the start of the COVID-19 pandemic, the World Bank Group has committed over $150 billion to fight its impact. The World Bank made $20 billion available to help developing countries finance the purchase and distribution of COVID-19 vaccines. The World Bank Group's crisis response has three stages; relief, restructuring, and resilient recovery in four main areas: (1) saving lives, (2) protecting poor and vulnerable people, (3) ensuring sustainable business growth and job creation, (4) strengthening policies, institutions, and investments (World bank, 2021).

Founded in 1899 and representing 20 million nurses in 135 national/international nurses associations, the **International Council of Nurses (ICN)** works to ensure quality nursing care for all; sound health policies; the advancement of nursing knowledge; and the presence of a respected, competent, and satisfied nursing workforce worldwide. Nursing research, advanced practice registered nursing (APRN), doctoral education, socioeconomic welfare, first responders, disaster preparedness, mass casualties, policy, advocacy, and more recently COVID-19 are focus areas. The ICN has five core values: visionary leadership, inclusiveness, flexibility, partnership, and achievement and three goals: (1) To bring nursing together worldwide, (2) To advance nurses and nursing worldwide, (3) To influence health policy. The ICN Code of Ethics for Nurses originally developed in 1953 and last revised in 2012, serves as a critical model for ethical standards in the nursing profession. The ICN Code is currently being revised by an International Steering Committee. Revisions will include nurses' need for cultural sensitivity and proficiency linked to transcultural work, need to maintain professional and practical knowledge generally and specialty related, and the core values of the nursing profession regarding equity, social justice, self-determination, personal responsibility and accountability, as well as emphasis on the advocacy role of nurses in being partners in decision-making with patients and other healthcare staff, and to the right of the nurse to be supported by employers to maintain general and mental health. The revision will also address the nurses' role in achieving the SDGs, adopted by all UNs' Member States in 2015 and the increased role of genomics in healthcare (Stievana and Tschudin, 2019). ICN, WHO, the UN, the World Bank, the International Labor Organization, and a wide range of NGOs are attempting to address the global shortage of nurses and other healthcare providers and complex global healthcare challenges.

INTERNATIONAL HEALTHCARE DELIVERY SYSTEMS

In the comparison of healthcare systems, developed and developing countries can learn much from one another. Although transferring specialized medical technologies from developed to developing countries may not always be appropriate, developing countries are currently learning from healthcare reform policies and the technological revolution. Likewise, developed countries have much to learn about low-technology initiatives, such as oral rehydration therapy for the treatment of diarrhea and the delivery of primary healthcare as defined by the WHO. Participatory approaches to healthcare delivery, such as community involvement in health and education and maternal-newborn interventions such as delayed cord clamping, are also essential. This exchange is important, given the evolving state and complexities of healthcare policy and global challenges.

Even in countries with socialized medicine, medical costs rise annually and citizens are faced with paying supplemental medical fees or copayment. There is a need to expand the knowledge base that made the 20th-century healthcare revolution possible. In the 21st century, it is critical to provide research and development that are relevant to the infectious diseases that overwhelmingly affect the poor. In addition, it is necessary to systematically generate an information base that countries can use to shape the future of their healthcare systems. Misinformation, politization, and inequities of the COVID-19 pandemic have further polarized families, communities, and nations.

The seminal Lalonde Report (1974) on the health of Canadian citizens proposing the "health field concept" is a classic contribution to public health science. It is a useful way to frame the determinants of health including knowledge of human biology, lifestyle, environment, and health services. The report signified a healthcare paradigm shift from the traditional medical model to a more holistic systems-based and environmental perspective.

In the 1980, 1990s, and early 2000s, the rising costs of healthcare were a major catalyst for change, focusing attention on the need to provide alternative models of care. Over the past 4 decades, population-based approaches to health promotion and disease prevention and new nursing degrees such as the Doctor of Nursing Practice (DNP) have been developed to emphasize leadership, health policy, healthcare finance, systems, access, quality, efficiency, effectiveness, and value-based care (Porter, 2016; Wall et al., 2005). Nurse-led and managed clinics, wellness centers, birthing centers, same-day surgery, outpatient services, home care and provide alternatives to hospital-based care. In each of these areas, the nurse plays a prominent role and brings an increased emphasis on health promotion and disease prevention to anyone attempting to navigate a complex healthcare system.

An emphasis on the integration of research/discovery, teaching/learning, and practice/service/engagement with nurse-led innovation and public health principles was foundational to the development of the Integrated Nurse-led Model of Sustainability and Innovation (INMSI) presented in Fig. 15.1.

The earliest iteration of the INMSI was developed by the author in 1994 to address primary healthcare workforce development needs in rural Virginia (Novak and Corbett, 2000). Community assessment, surveys, focus groups, local and state demographic and public health analyses, and direct feedback from patients, family members, community leaders and students guided the earliest and subsequent iterations. The model evolved further during global health projects in Mexico and South Africa, in rural and urban Indiana and Texas with significant clinic development, expansion, and replication. The model development resulted in 12 US nurse-led clinics in a variety of settings, including Head Start, K-12 school systems, a college student health and employee health system, refugee health, rural and urban primary healthcare, and rural and urban clinic development in Mexico and South Africa.

The model was further refined and expanded in California with the development of a nurse-led specialty clinic (Novak, 2019a,b). Creation of the Neonatal Intensive Care Unit Follow-up Clinic was informed by the INMSI. The clinic was subsequently designated as a California Children's Services (**CCS**) High-Risk Infant Follow-up clinic and funded through a variety of foundation grants and billing. Concurrently, the INMSI was used to design a system of care for the Neighborhood House Association Head Start Pre-K Health and Wellness Mobile Van. The program is offered at Head Start Early Childhood Educational sites throughout San Diego County and further deployed through a mobile health van that offers health screenings, developmental assessments, nutrition and activity counseling, behavioral health, parent coaching, and staff education. Childhood vaccines will be offered in 2022. The van provides a safety net for parents and children who face healthcare access and transportation challenges.

Each of the 14 INMSI clinics meet the Institute for Healthcare Improvement (IHI) Triple Aim and Quadruple Aim goals of (1) better healthcare and access, (2) better health with a focus on population health and the patient experience, and (3) lower cost including per capita cost analysis (Berwick, 2014) and joy in work for healthcare providers (Bodenheimer and Sinsky, 2014). In addition, each clinic demonstrates integration of the educational, practice, and engagement mission of the parent institution and achieves sustainability through a diverse financial portfolio that includes billing, philanthropy, and grant funding (Novak, 2020).

The INMSI (Novak, 2007, 2011, 2017, 2019a,b, 2020) consists of 12 **key** elements, illustrated in Fig. 15.1. The first four elements, from 12 o'clock to 3 o'clock, focus on relationship-based communication, building community partnerships, and ensuring cultural humility and proficiency as foundational to clinical enterprise development. The remaining eight components focus on the mosaic of support or diverse portfolio for long-term sustainability and innovation. Signature characteristics of the INMSI appear in Box 15.1.

Before developing the business plan for a nurse-led clinical enterprise, nursing leaders must carefully lay the groundwork through relationship-based communication, careful selection of community partners, and hiring a team of culturally proficient members across all levels of the project, from clinicians to administrators to community outreach to billers and coders to engineering support and facilities management. Each of these individuals contributes to the sustainability, innovation, and

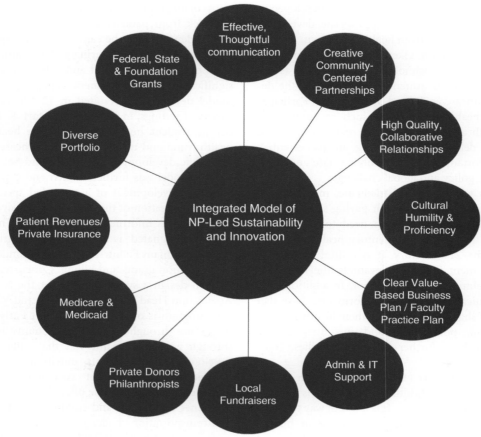

Fig. 15.1 The Integrated Nurse-Led Model of Sustainability and Innovation (INMSI). (From Novak JC: Interdisciplinary and interprofessional collaboration. In Dreher HM, Glasgow EMS, editors: *Role development for doctoral advanced nursing practice*, New York, 2017, Springer, pp 397–414.)

overall success of the clinical enterprise. The INMSI helps to create a diverse and inclusive community of clinical experts, scholars and leaders for value-based healthcare delivery imbedded in a strong public health infrastructure (Novak, 2019a,b).

BEST PRACTICES FOR APPLICATION OF THE INMSI

The evolution of INMSI has led to the development of six training modules (NP Clinic Sustainability and Innovation [NP–CSI]) (Novak, 2020) that are available to guide application of the model to global health projects, academic nursing clinics, faculty practice, or a variety of community/public health settings (Novak, 2019). The six 1-h stand-alone CE modules can be completed separately to meet the needs of busy healthcare team members or in one 6-h period (Fig. 15.2).

Nurses must think more broadly about potential collaborators in solving the complex problems of the healthcare delivery system. Disciplines such as industrial engineering have much to offer nursing and other healthcare professionals as engineering principles are applied to information technology, system design, patient safety, vaccine and medication administration and

reconciliation, simulation, chronic disease management, and hospital and clinic development, design, and renovation. The DNP was developed by nursing leaders and endorsed by the American Association of Colleges of Nursing to reengineer healthcare (Wall et al., 2005). Since 2000 this revolution in nursing education has grown to 357 programs with 106 new DNP programs in the planning phase (AACN Fact Sheet, 2020).

In 2020, US expenditures for healthcare exceeded 18% of the gross domestic product (GDP) and are expected to grow to 19.9% GDP by 2025 (Centers for Medicaid and Medicare Services [CMS], 2020). The Affordable Care Act (ACA) addressed the large number of uninsured Americans. Since its implementation in 2010, the ACA has been repeatedly challenged and modified. Expanding Medicare, removing barriers to full APRN practice authority, and other proposals will augment and strengthen the healthcare delivery system.

Given the two basic healthcare systems, market based and population based, and the fact that countries at different levels of development need to learn from one another, it is evident that a single model of healthcare delivery is not appropriate for every country. For example, in 1985, Cuba was recognized for reaching WHO's goal of "health for all." Cuba began to demonstrate to the world that healthcare could be provided as a

BOX 15.1 Characteristics of the INMSI

- Relationship-based communication, reflective practice, structured reflection, journaling, cultural proficiency, value-based healthcare delivery, and a diverse portfolio/mosaic of support.
- Strong community partnerships that overcome social circumstances and place resources
- Close to those who need them most.
- Optimal use of digital innovation, technology, and data analytics, including: a Customized electronic health record to promote accessibility, efficiency, and effectiveness; support student and faculty research; enhance care continuity and patient safety/quality; facilitate communication with system and community partners; and track the most frequent presenting concerns and clinical outcomes.
- Best practice and education that are evidence-based and integrated into promotion and tenure processes for faculty.
- Interprofessional discovery, learning, and practice/engagement for faculty and students from nursing, engineering, public health, audiology, medicine, pharmacy, PT, OT, and IT (Novak et al., 2016).
- Application and integration of public health and systems engineering principles, including LEAN six sigma to improve performance by systematically removing waste; reducing variation through cross-training for multi-clinic coverage; and using just-in-time purchasing to reduce cost, analyze use, and competitive bidding (Novak in Yih, 2011; Novak, 2020).

basic human right rather than a privilege. In another example, Canada developed a universal healthcare system, and Canadian community health nurses (CHNs) created innovative models for practice focusing on health promotion, fostering public participation in decisions that affect health, strengthening community health service networks with the disadvantaged communities they serve, and coordinating public health policy efforts.

The pressure for change provides the opportunity for reform, and the broad goal of "health for all" should guide this reform. Effective healthcare delivery systems must increase access and efficiency, improve health status through health promotion and disease prevention, eliminate health inequities and disparities, and protect individuals and families from financial loss due to catastrophic illness. Forty years after initiation of "Health for All" programs, inequity in health in Canada is still linked to socioeconomic status. Collective mandates, such as healthy diets and required physical education classes in elementary and middle schools, may be instrumental in changing the social and economic environments in which people live. Effective health and wellness programs reduce disease by providing accessible, culturally proficient, evidence-based programs. Effective health promotion programs are committed to social justice and equity, particularly as seen through the lens of social determinants of health.

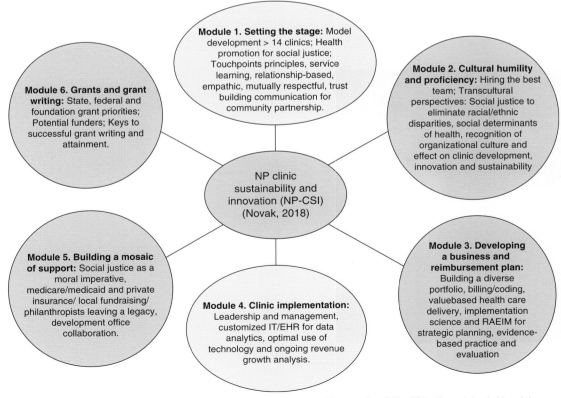

Fig. 15.2 Six training modules for NP Clinic Sustainability and Innovation (NP—CSI). (Copyright J. Novak.)

The Role of the Community Health Nurse in International Health Care

In a rapidly changing healthcare environment, the nursing role is evolving and expanding. The traditional structure of provider roles is challenged as professional disciplines are recruited to provide innovative and diverse healthcare services. The nursing role is reciprocal and collaborative with patients, families, physicians, other healthcare professionals, and community members. The nurse's role expectations and societal expectations are foundational to defining the role of the community and public health nurse in global healthcare.

Florence Nightingale was the first nurse to establish international linkages and networks that moved from her own country of England to nurses throughout the world. As the first woman and first nurse inducted into the Royal Statistics Society, she recognized the importance of evidence-based nursing and healthcare. Every obstacle to health and wellness confronted her. She overcame obstacles systematically, developing the foundation and legacy for modern nursing and for community and public health nursing. Nightingale channeled her energies into all aspects of health, from the care of wounded soldiers at Scutari in the Crimea to broad public policies for the

HEALTH INITIATIVES TAKING PLACE THROUGHOUT THE WORLD

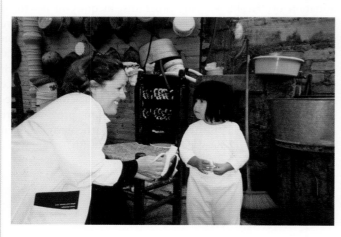

Home health visit, San Luis, Xochimilco, Mexico. (Courtesy Dr. Julie Novak.)

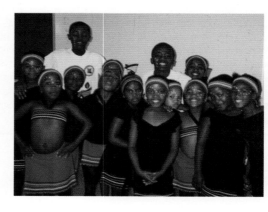

Cape Town, South Africa, school inauguration and health fair. (Courtesy Dr. Julie Novak.)

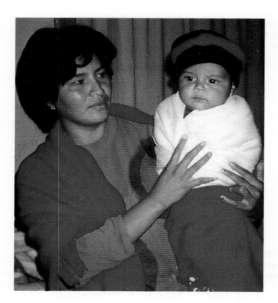

Nurse-managed public health clinic, Universidad Nacional Autonomo de Mexico, San Luis, Xochimilco, Mexico. (Courtesy Dr. Julie Novak.)

British military and the general public, affecting health in her time and beyond.

CHNs seek to ensure the attainment of health for all in a cost-effective, efficient, accessible healthcare system. They must be involved in research, community assessment, planning, implementation, management, evaluation, health services delivery, disaster preparedness, emergency response, health policy, advocacy, and legislation. Nurses in all countries coordinate their work with other healthcare personnel, as well as informal and formal community leaders. The changes in the health environment, such as technological advancements, changes in the morbidity and mortality patterns of the population, and social and political changes, all form the basis for the nursing role and system redesign.

Community health nurses have played a critical role in the response to the COVID-19 pandemic from providing timely information and education resources; screening; testing; case-finding; robust contact tracing; teaching public health principles such as recommendations for proper hand washing, use of hand sanitizers, disinfecting of objects and surfaces, face coverings (masks and shields), isolation, quarantine, staying home when ill, social distancing guidance; hygiene kit distribution; home visits; phone calls, social media; and providing vaccinations and COVID-19 treatment world-wide. These efforts contribute to reducing racial and socioeconomic disparities and how COVID-19 affects various communities. Community health nurses also provide specific information about COVID-19 to businesses, faith organizations, schools, the military, and service providers for people experiencing homelessness.

With the development of the nurse practitioner (NP) role over the past 55 years in the United States and over the past 40 years abroad, nurses with advanced degrees and areas of specialization have strengthened the community-based healthcare system. The development of the DNP degree in the United States and PhDs in nursing in many countries further elevates the knowledge and skill base for nursing's role in reengineering healthcare.

Because primary healthcare and primary care may be practiced differently in other countries, the NP and the CHN face multiple challenges. **Primary healthcare** refers to essential services that support a healthy life. It involves access, availability, service delivery, community participation, and the citizen's right to healthcare. In contrast, **primary care** refers to first-line or point-of-access medical and nursing care controlled by providers and primarily focused on the individual. Primary care may not be the norm, particularly in communities in developing or less developed countries that have overwhelming needs for necessities such as safe drinking water, sanitation, and basic hygiene. In this case, the needs of the group directly represent the needs of the individual.

Nurses can make a difference in solving the existing and emerging health problems in countries throughout the world. The advent of technology has enhanced global communication and facilitated travel. With approximately four million nurses in the United States and 27.9 million worldwide, nurses are the largest cadre of healthcare professionals (ANA, 2020).

Community public health nurses improve access to care for the most vulnerable and hard-to-reach groups. The future demands evidence-based education, practice, engagement, service, growth in information technology/health informatics, and local to global health policy and advocacy. Community/public health nursing experts are critical to solving the challenges of the fragmented, mismanaged, expensive, ineffective, inefficient healthcare delivery system that exists in many parts of our global community.

? ACTIVE LEARNING

1. Compare and contrast the scientific progress for COVID-19, HIV, TB, and malaria. Discuss public health measures and methods of prevention.
2. Conduct research and compare the rates of infant mortality and life expectancy in Africa, India, Mexico, Japan, China, Brazil, and the United States.
3. What factors might account for the similarities and differences in rates between the developing and the developed countries?
4. Discuss six key components of community-based clinic sustainability and innovation.

RESEARCH IN INTERNATIONAL HEALTH

Since 1990, international nursing research has focused predominantly on the following areas: (1) multiple aspects of student and faculty educational exchange programs, (2) diverse clinical conditions and experiences, (3) maternal-child health, (4) the global development of home care or transition from hospital to home, and (5) the global COVID-19 pandemic.

WHO collaborating centers in nursing and midwifery development provide a framework for research, education, practice, and service delivery partnerships in 44 institutions from the six WHO sectors. Purdue University and the University of Virginia, collaborated with Case Western Reserve University and the University of Mexico WHO Collaborating Centers for Team Reach Out Mexico and Team Reach Out South Africa was subsequently developed Case Study 15.2.

CASE STUDY Application of the International Community Assessment

A Collaborative Model for Community Assessment, Education, and Health Care Delivery.

In Mexico and South Africa, the provision of equitable healthcare services to populations that are geographically and educationally disparate is both economically and logistically challenging. Both countries are further challenged by a lack of infrastructure necessary for health promotion, protection, and maintenance. South Africa is challenged by extreme poverty and staggering rates of COVID-19, HIV, and TB. In planning interventions, nurses need a globally diverse assessment tool and methodology to empower communities to achieve healthcare goals and reduce healthcare costs. US nursing students gaining international healthcare experience in a community in rural Mexico and urban South Africa can implement the International Community Assessment Model (ICAM) (Fig. 15.3) before planning targeted programs with local community leaders. The ICAM, tested in rural Mexico and as a component of

Team Reach Out South Africa (see Case Study 15.2), is part of an ongoing project. US nursing students compare and contrast practices in various countries using the ICAM and Service-Learning Models. Service-Learning is community-based, experiential model that relies heavily on community partnerships, meaningful, structured reflection, debriefing, and journaling. The projects were embedded in community/public health, leadership, and APRN course objectives.

THE MODEL

Community Empowerment

A critical element of designing and implementing global healthcare projects is community empowerment. If a community is not fully engaged, the project will be unsustainable. In community empowerment, the community identifies its problems and a plan of action, and nurses remain as partners, consultants, and team members. Working with communities is a dance, and the community leads the dance. This mutually respectful, shared decision-making process helps the community develop interventions that are culturally acceptable, breaking down cultural barriers. In developing countries, health promotion programs that do not involve community participation and education often fail after the so-called experts leave the community.

Assessment

During the assessment phase, the nurse identifies key influential community members and leaders and encourages them to join a board of community partners with the goal of assessing community health. The community partners may choose to use the ICAM for the purpose of providing a globally diverse assessment framework and for data gathering. Assessment of community culture helps identify potential cultural barriers to nursing interventions. The center of the model assesses the heart of the community's culture by identifying individual, family, and community characteristics, including their history, demographics, values, beliefs, rituals, and the effect of these characteristics on social and economic conditions.

The ICAM assesses:

1. *Recreation*: Community cardiovascular fitness; stress management; energy renewal; and relaxation through sports, hobbies, games, fun runs/walks, 5Ks, yoga, and tai chi.
2. *Perceptions*: Community perceptions of health, including community members' physical, social, and mental health and lifestyle choices.
3. *Spirituality*: The community's traditional and nontraditional religious beliefs and practices.
4. *Support systems*: Family support systems, parental support of children and adult children, adult children's support of their parents, and support among extended family members.

The physical environment encompasses the community's infrastructure, including homes, neighborhood, water sources, waste disposal sites, roadways, transportation, buildings for businesses and shops, factories, power lines, and considerations related to occupational health. Nurses must seek a broad range of collaborators in solving diverse and complex problems.

The ICAM also assesses:

(1) *Education*: The concept of education reflects the community's knowledge, skills, level of schooling or training, and literacy rate.
(2) *Transportation*: Defined as how community members travel from point A to point B.
(3) *Safety*: Evaluation of the community's safety includes examining both the potential dangers in the community that could lead to injury or death and the safety measures and plans developed by the community to prevent these problems.
(4) *Government and politics*: How the community is governed or ruled.
(5) *Economy*: The efficacy of economic resources is analyzed in terms of production, dispersal, and expenditure of resources.
(6) *Communication*: Communication is evaluated by examining face-to-face and community-wide information exchange through speech, body language, writing, and drawings. Key components of the community's communication are native languages and forms of communication, such as letters, cellphones, land lines, computer networks, electronic health records, the Internet, fax machines, television, billboards, signs, magazines, newspapers, and telegrams.
(7) *Access*: Healthcare, public sanitation, public water systems, electricity, radio, television, technology, computers, the

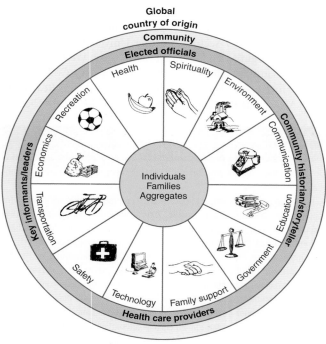

Fig. 15.3 International Community Assessment model. (Courtesy J.C. Novak.)

Internet, fax machines, libraries, industrial machinery, and agricultural practices must be examined.

The ICAM encourages the partners to examine all the public health threats to the community and additional barriers to an effective cultural awareness, sensitivity, proficiency, and humility. It also reflects the importance of assessing the country of origin and global effects on the community. When assessing a community, the nurse must consider external factors. For example, the economy of the community depends on vendors and international purchasing of their main exports.

After the community assessment, the collaborative team develops a program that identifies potential challenges to an educational program or intervention. This program should motivate community partners to identify challenges or problems and then search for effective solutions. As partners become further aware of the healthcare barriers or health hazards, resources should be provided that will aid in their response.

Next, partners should be assisted in completing a survey and offering focus groups related to the needs assessment, identified needs, community priorities, interests resources, and gaps.

The nursing team, local experts, key community informants, and partners need to establish the root cause of problems in a collaborative manner to develop effective interventions.

Planning and Intervention

The board and community identify central issues, challenges, and barriers. The board then enters the planning phase of the intervention campaign. Community board members can collaborate with environmental experts and the nurse to identify individual, family, and community educational and service-learning goals, strategies, and interventions based on best evidence and practice.

The collaborative team subsequently analyzes possible interventions. This body of knowledge allows the community partners to determine which, if any, of the proposed interventions would be relevant and appropriate for their community. In addition, they may be able to apply these ideas in creating their own interventions. When the community partners have selected or developed an intervention for their project, they can be encouraged to create relevant strategies to educate the community.

Implementation

Before the project is implemented, the outcome of the community needs assessment must be analyzed and clarified. The community must be given the opportunity to provide feedback to all collaborators regarding proposed interventions. The partners must be willing to listen and compromise to meet the community's needs. After community-wide education has occurred and necessary consensus and compromise have been achieved, the project can be implemented. At this point, the community members understand and discuss ways to sustain the project. Once the implementation is completed, evaluation of the project can begin to ensure that the goals and objectives of the board and the community are met.

Evaluation

The collaborative team should evaluate the project in a formative and summative manner. In addition, the nurse should conduct community surveys to determine whether members continue to recognize the need to maintain the project; to provide feedback related to progress, facilitators, and barriers; and to identify necessary modifications or innovations.

APPLICATIONS

The ICAM was tested in rural Mexico and South Africa as part of Team Reach Out projects. The targeted communities have a high rate of poverty. As a result, 80% of the communities reside in crowded living conditions. Many factors in the community pose serious health threats, including infectious disease, chronic conditions, tobacco use, secondhand smoke, farm chemicals, and air pollution. Field workers are often powerless and have minimal recourse when exposed to unhealthy environmental contaminants causing increased morbidity and mortality for themselves and their family members through secondary contamination and exposure.

In rural Mexico, the top causes of mortality in the communities are infectious diseases, cardiac disorders, diabetes, and cancer. Motor vehicle accidents, and violence are more common in urban Mexico, border communities and related to drug cartels/trafficking. The leading causes of morbidity are respiratory infections, diabetes, hypertension, and gastrointestinal illnesses. The community's high rate of gastrointestinal illness is related to limited access to potable water. The community historians, community political leaders, key employers, full-time staff at nurse-run public health clinics, local community health faculty, and the *pasantes* (nursing graduates who have completed 1 year of community service at nurse-run clinics and public health agencies) are critical to the success of the project.

A multidisciplinary team of key influential community members, environmental experts, and nurses will further assess the community using the ICAM model. The goal of this assessment is to assist the community members in further diagnosing the community's healthcare needs and other issues as they are identified. Nurses collaborate with community partners to develop culturally proficient interventions. After the interventions are developed, the local partners, clinic staff, and *pasantes* continue to evaluate the effectiveness of these interventions, promoting a sense of ownership of the project within the community and helping ensure improvements in healthcare long after the multidisciplinary team leaves the community (Case Study 15.2).

STUDENT RESPONSES

Team Reach Out South Africa students provided poignant and insightful reflections about their experiences. Community partners indicated that the students were very professional and were able to provide much-needed support, education and healthcare (Richards and Novak, 2010).

CASE STUDY   Application of the International Community Assessment

Team Reach Out South Africa

Team Reach Out started as a student-initiated service-learning project with the goal of providing ongoing assistance to hurricane victims. Team Reach Out later refocused its efforts in Cape Town, South Africa. Senior nursing students and a premed science student integrated their leadership skills with the application of public health knowledge, compassion, and concern as they worked in partnership with several international health agencies. This case reviews the service-learning framework course planning, implementation, and evaluation.

Service learning is a reciprocal partnership that bridges the gap between professional education and societal needs. It is a powerful teaching and learning strategy that engages students in learning while helping communities help themselves. Service-learning provides an experiential, collaborative, discipline-based relationship between students and community members for a reciprocal learning experience and allows an opportunity for reflection. Service learning sets the stage for a lifelong commitment to the development of civic duty, social awareness, and engagement while providing unique learning experiences that focus on building citizenship, cultural diversity, community partnerships, knowledge of community resources, critical thinking skills, and mutual respect. Both students and the community benefit from service-learning. Students benefit from the exposure to real-life dilemmas and firsthand experience of joint team efforts. Communities benefit from the knowledge and creativity available from academia.

The author/faculty team leader/advisor completed an exploratory trip to Johannesburg and Cape Town, South Africa, meeting with prospective community partners. Each of the local healthcare leaders invited the development of a collaboration. Because of the richness of each setting and the overwhelming need for human and financial resources, the choice was extremely difficult. Cape Town was selected as the city site through a comprehensive assessment using the ICAM. Health care and educational partners within the city were selected in collaboration with the school nurse, faculty, and staff of Christel House Academy in Cape Town. Subsequently, students from the School of Nursing and College of Science were invited to apply through notification in their respective student newsletters. Selection was based on the clarity of the student's goals and understanding of cultural humility and service learning. After selection, each student wrote an additional travel grant application to the university's Office of Engagement. Following is a description of the partners involved in this project and the experiences each provided.

Christel House International is a 501(c) (3) public charity that operates learning centers in impoverished neighborhoods with the goal of creating sustainable social and educational impact, breaking the cycle of poverty through a comprehensive holistic approach that transforms the child, family, and community. It provides robust K-12 education, and a strong character-development program complimented with regular healthcare, nutritious meals, guidance counseling, career planning, family assistance, and college and career support. Between 1999 and 2020, Christel House opened eight learning centers in Mexico City, India (2 sites), South Africa, Indianapolis USA (3 sites), and Jamaica. Currently, Christel House serves more than 5662 students, their families, and communities. Christel House K-12 Academy in Cape Town helps children around the world break the cycle of poverty, realize their hopes and dreams, and become self-sufficient, contributing members of society (Christel House, 2021). The academy invited the students to participate in the inaugural celebration of a new school facility and campus. Weekend cultural experiences included a trip to Robben Island, an ecological and historical heritage site where Nelson Mandela was imprisoned from 1963 to 1990; Table Mountain, a protected natural habitat with 1500 plant species; and a game and nature preserve.

The Themba Care Home of Hope provides a safe and compassionate environment for approximately 92 children and 87 families, many of whom are HIV positive. In most cases their parents have died of AIDS; however, some children are placed in the setting by their parents to avoid stigma within their respective communities. The Themba Care Home of Hope is run by an executive director, two registered nurses/"sisters," a teacher, a staff of five nursing assistants, and local volunteers. Team Reach Out worked with volunteers from three different US universities on site. In addition to one older child, 95% of the children at the Home ranged in age from 18 months to 4 years. Students were able to complete Denver Developmental Screenings and health assessments and to work with the sisters in medication dispensation and reconciliation. The majority of the children demonstrated global developmental delay on the screenings. Students played with, fed, and cared for the children in this warm, caring, inviting preschool environment. The students reflected on their difficulty in saying goodbye to the children.

The Tafelsig Community Health Center provides care to approximately 10,000 low-income patients each month. Patients receive health promotion visits throughout the lifespan with services that include: child health, immunizations and vaccines, general HIV care, family planning, STI assessment and treatment, antiretroviral services, drug and alcohol outpatient treatment, basic antenatal care, chronic medication HIV testing postnatal care, and COVID-19 testing. Tafelsig treats one of the largest TB and HIV patient populations in Cape Town. Students were able to complete health assessments and immunize patients under the supervision of a South African RN, specialty clinic coordinators and their faculty advisor.

The student clinical experiences culminated with a presentation of a health fair at the Christel House Academy. The health fair focused on school and family health promotion; prenatal and newborn care and parenting; prevention of TB, HIV, and malaria; healthcare careers; science experiments; and health screenings, including measurements of height, weight, blood pressure, glucose, and cholesterol. The academy ran special bus routes from the school to and from area informal settlements to bring parents and other community members to the school health fair. The students worked with the WHO, the CDC, Johnson & Johnson, and local Cape Town universities to ensure culturally appropriate materials for the health fair. Team Reach Out Christel House Academy Health Fairs were typically attended by more than 600 children and 200 parents.

SUMMARY

Students felt strongly that service learning enhanced their community public health experience while building relationships with community service organizations. Students reported encountering minimal barriers to the implementation of this project and were not reluctant to participate in these activities. Students also agreed that they would continue to participate in service-learning activities in the future. Travel bans and the COVID-19 pandemic prevented travel and resumption of the project, delaying return until 2022. Virtual contact with South African partners has been maintained.

1. Compare population-focused nursing in a developing country with community health nursing in the US. How are they the same, and how do they differ?
2. Test the ICAM in a community. Evaluate its effectiveness.
3. Describe the Service Learning Model and its potential application in global projects.

4. Describe the key elements of an effective healthcare delivery system that emphasizes. Nurse-led innovative, sustainable models of health promotion, disease prevention.

SUMMARY

Community public health nurses face many exciting challenges in healthcare reform and the design of effective systems of healthcare delivery. These include being responsive to emerging needs and health issues in the population, developing multidisciplinary practice models that adhere to the principles of primary healthcare in the context of a reengineered healthcare system, and mobilizing research dissemination and practice implementation strategies to ensure best practice. Using evidence-based models as a framework for local to global community public health partnerships and projects should be tested and evaluated. There is still much to be done to meet the challenge of WHO's goal of "health for all." Studying the progress achieved in other countries is critical; however, success will ultimately depend on societal commitment to addressing complex issues of poverty, social justice, inequity, disparity, healthcare inaccessibility and achievement of Healthy People 2030 goals. The essential role that community public health nurses play in health promotion, disease prevention, and public health crises, underscores the importance and critical need for a sustained workforce, strong public health infrastructure and sustainable and innovative models of care.

BIBLIOGRAPHY

American Association of Colleges of Nursing: *AACN Fact Sheet*, 2020. Available from: www.AACNnursing.org/news- information/factsheets.

American Non-Smokers Rights Foundation, April 2021.

American Nurses Association: *Workforce*. Available from: www.nursingworld.org/practice-policy/workforce/.

Berwick D: *Promising care: how we can rescue healthcare by improving it*, San Francisco, 2014, Jossey-Bass Publishers.

Bodenheimer T, Sinsky C: From triple to quadruple aim: care of the patient requires care of the provider, *Ann Fam Med* 12(6):573–576, 2014. https://doi.org/10.1370/afm.1713.

Buchholz K: *How has the world's urban population changed from 1950 to today? With the collaboration of Statista. weforum.org*, 2020. Available from: https://www.weforum.org/agenda/2020/11/global-continent-urban-population-urbanisation-percent/.

Carter center: *About the center*, 2021. Available from: www.cartercenter.org/about/index.html.

Centers for Disease Control and Prevention. www.cdc.gov/nchs/healthy_people/hp2030, August 18, 2020.

Christel House: *About us*, 2021. Available from: http://www.christelhouse.org/about-us.

Corbley A: *Landmark malaria vaccine is 77% effective, tackling one of the world's biggest killers of young children*. Available from: Goodnewsnetwork.org.

Cornish L: *Interactive: who's funding the COVID-19 responses and what are the priorities? Devex.com*, 2021. Available from: https://www.devex.com/news/interactive.

COVAX: *"COVAX explained" gavi.org. GAVI*, Retrieved 25, February 2021.

Draper SJ, Sack BK, King R, et al.: Malaria vaccines: recent advances and new horizons, *Cell Host Microbe Elsevier* 24(1):43–56, 2018. https://doi.org/10.1016/j.chom.2018.06.008.

EPA. *Air Quality—National Summary*. Available from: EPA.gov.

Gates Foundation: *Our role*. Available from: www.gatesfoundation.org.

Koh HK, Geller AC, VanderWeele TJ: Deaths from COVID-19, *JAMA* 325(2):1330134. https://doi.org/10.1001/Jama.

Lalonde M: *A new perspective on the health of canadians*, Ottawa, 1974, Minister of Supply and Services.

Lewis T: *How the U.S. pandemic response went wrong-and what went right-during a year of COVID*, March 11, 2021, Scientific American, a Division of Springer Nature America, Inc.

Mahler DG, Yonza N, Lakner C, Aguilar RAC, Wu H: Updated estimates of the impact of COVID-19 on global poverty: turning the corner on the pandemic in 2021? Available from: Blogs.worldbank.org.

National Institutes of Health (NIH): *Worlds' older population grows dramatically*, 2016, National Institutes of Health (NIH). Available from: World's older population grows dramatically.

Novak JC, Corbett C: Nurse practitioner education: the Virginia experience. In Novotny J, editor: *Distance education in nursing*, New York, 2000, Springer, pp 152–179.

Novak JC: Designing a nurse-managed healthcare delivery system. In Yih Y, editor: *Handbook of healthcare delivery systems*, Boca Raton, FL, 2011, CRC Press, Taylor & Francis Group, pp 1–9.

Novak JC: Developing a sustainable nurse-led clinical enterprise and faculty practice, Chapter 15. In Robinson JP, Kenner C, Pressler JL, editors: *Nursing deans on leading lessons for novice and aspiring deans and directors*, New York, 2020, Springer Publishing Company LLC.

Novak JC: Interdisciplinary and interprofessional collaboration. In Dreher HM, Smith ME, editors: *Glasgow. Role development for doctoral advanced nursing practice*, New York, 2017, Springer, pp 397–414.

Novak JC: Pioneering an integrated NP-led model of clinic sustainability, innovation, and faculty practice. In *NAPNAP Annual Conference* Workshop, New Orleans March 9, 2019.

Novak JC: *Pioneering an Integrated np-led model of clinic sustainability, innovation, and faculty practice*, 2019b, Rita and Hillman Foundation Annual Report.

Novak R, Cantu A, Champlin C, Zappler A, Coco L, and Novak J: The future of healthcare delivery: IPE/IPP audiology and nursing student/faculty collaboration to deliver hearing aids to vulnerable adults via telehealth. *J Nurs Interprof Leadership Quality Safety.* 1(I), 2016, Article I.

Population Reference Bureau: *World population data sheet*, 2020. Available from: http://www.prb.org/Publications/Datasheets/201506/201506WorldPopulationDataSheet.aspx.

Porter ME: *Value based healthcare delivery*, 2016, Harvard University School of Business.

Richards E, Novak J: From Biloxi to Cape Town: curricular integration of service learning, *J Community Health Nurs* 27(1):46–50, 2010.

Ritchie H, Roser M: *Age structure. Our world in data*, 2019. https://ourworldindata.org/age-structure.

Stievano A, Tschudin V: The ICN code of ethics for nurses: a time for revision, *Int Nurs Rev* 66(2):154–156, 2019. https://doi.org/10.1111/inr.12525. Wiley Online Library, onlinelibrary.wiley.com, First published May 23.

Standordhealthcare.org: *Types of malaria parasites*, 2021. Available from: https://Standordhealthcare.org/medical-conditions/primary-care/malaria/types.html.

UNAIDS: aidsinfo.unaids.org, 2019.

UNAIDS Data 2020, Available from: aidsdatahub.org.

United Nations: *Resolution adopted by the general assembly: United Nations Millennium Declaration*, New York, 2000, United Nations.

United Nations: *About the UN*, 2018. Available from: http://www.un.org/en/about-un/index.html.

United Nations Development Programme: *undp.org*, 2021.

U.S. Census Bureau: *Population of the U.S. Available from*, United States, 2020, U.S. Census Bureau QuickFacts.

U.S. Department of Health and Human Services: *Healthy People 2030*. Office of Disease Prevention and Health Promotion, 2021. Available from: Health.gov.

Wall B, Novak J, Wilkerson S: The doctor of nursing practice: reengineering healthcare, *J Nurs Educ* 44(9):396–403, 2005.

Woolf SM, Chapman DA, Lee JH: COVID-19 as the leading cause of death in the United States, *JAMA*, 2020. https://doi.org/10.1001/jama.2020.24865.

World Bank: How the World Bank Group is helping countries with COVID-19 (coronavirus). Worldbank.org, July 1, 2021.

World Bank: *What we do*, 2017. Available from: http://www.worldbank.org/en/about, http://www.worldbank.org/en/about/what-we-do.

World Health Organization: *1 in 3 people globally do not have access to safe drinking water*, New York, Geneva, June 18, 2019a. News release.

World Health Organization: *Tobacco free initiative*, 2018. Available from: http://www.who.int/tobacco/en/.

World Health Organization: *The top 10 causes of death worldwide*, 2019b, World Health Organization.

World Health Organization: *WHO called to return to the declaration of Alma-Ata*, 2021. Available from: www.who.int/teams/social-determinants-of-health/declaration-of-alma-ata.

World Health Statistics: Monitoring health for the SDGs (Sustainable Developmental Goals). Geneva, 2020, World Health Organization. License: CGBY-NCSA 3.0 IGO.

FURTHER READING

World Health Organization: *Unite to end TB*, 2016. World Health Organization.

Child and Adolescent Health

Melissa Domingeaux Ethington

OBJECTIVES

Upon completion of this chapter, the reader will be able to do the following:

1. Identify major indicators of child and adolescent health status.
2. Describe social determinants of child and adolescent health.
3. Discuss the individual and societal costs of poor child health status.
4. Discuss public programs and prevention strategies targeted to children's health.
5. Apply knowledge of child and adolescent health needs in planning appropriate, comprehensive care at the individual, family, and community levels.

OUTLINE

KEY TERMS

child maltreatment
childbirth educator
childhood immunization
Children's Health Insurance Program (CHIP)

Early and Periodic Screening, Diagnosis, and Treatment (EPSDT)
fetal alcohol spectrum disorders (FASD)
infant mortality
lactation consultant

late preterm birth
lead poisoning
low birth weight
Medicaid
preconception health
prenatal care

preterm birth
Safe to Sleep
Social determinants of health

Special Supplemental Nutrition Program for Women, Infants, and Children (WIC)

teen childbearing
teen dating violence
WIC

A nation's destiny lies with the health, education, and well-being of its children. The United States has made tremendous progress over the past century toward improving children's lives. Advancements in public health measures—such as sanitation, infectious disease control, environmental regulation, health screening, and education—as well as remarkable strides in health care have all contributed to the good health status that most children enjoy. However, these improvements have not equally benefited children of all races and ethnic groups, children at all income levels, or children in all geographic areas of the country. For example, significant disparities persist in the health status of white children versus children of color. Children living in suburban areas and most outer urban areas experience access to healthcare services superior to that of children living in rural areas and inner cities, especially if they are poor.

Although most of the nation's children are healthy and succeed in school, many are not enjoying optimal health and well-being and are not reaching their full potential as contributing members of society. Despite improvements, the mortality and morbidity rates for US children in all age groups are unacceptably high. Consider the following facts (Haider, 2021; Gentzke et al., 2020; Kann et al., 2016; Kochanek et al., 2020; Martin et al., 2019; Wang et al., 2020):

- Each year more than 21,000 infants die before reaching their first birthday. Black infants are more than twice as likely to die as white infants.
- Nearly one-half million babies are born prematurely each year. Prematurity is the second leading cause of infant death while congenital malformations remains the first.
- Fourteen percent of children under age 18 years live in poverty.
- Every day, five children die as the result of child abuse and neglect; most are younger than 4 years. Alarmingly, this is an increase from 1998, when about three children died each day from abuse and neglect.
- More than 179,800 girls aged 15 to 19 years give birth each year.
- While cigarette smoking among high school students decreased (4.6%) in 2020, e-cigarette use was nearly 20%. Additionally, the highest prevalence of current substance use among high school students were alcohol (29.2%) and marijuana (21.7%)
- Well over half of children currently residing in the United States are affected by violence, crime, abuse, or psychological trauma each year.

The health of a child has long-term implications. Health habits adopted by children and youth will profoundly influence their potential to lead healthy, productive lives. The physical and emotional health experienced by a child plays a pivotal role in his or her overall development and the well-being of the entire family. Children who go to school sick or hungry, who cannot see well enough to read, who cannot hear the teacher, who have learning disabilities, who are troubled by abusive parents or disruptive living circumstances, or who fear for their safety at home or in school often do not perform on the level of their counterparts who are healthy, well nourished, well cared for at home, and safe and secure in their world. From fetal life onward, the health and well-being of individuals has a substantial impact on their futures.

In 2019, there were 73 million US children younger than 18 years. Children represent about 22.3% of the country's population, down from a peak of 36% at the end of the mid-1960s baby boom. While the birth rate for children of all races has declined in recent years, the racial and ethnic diversity of children is changing rapidly. For example, by 2050, Hispanic children are expected to account for 32% of the population, up from 25% in 2015. Indeed, the percentage of children who are Hispanic has increased faster than that of any other racial or ethnic group (Federal Interagency Forum on Child and Family Statistics, 2016, 2020) (Fig. 16.1).

Children are a dependent population and rely primarily on parents or other adults to protect and promote their health and well-being. Community health nurses can learn more about this important population group and the positive and negative factors that influence their health. Nurses can use this information to help improve the chances that children will grow up to be healthy, both physically and emotionally.

This chapter focuses on the health status of children and adolescents and the medical, socioeconomic, cultural, environmental, educational, safety, and public health factors that community health nurses must address to improve child and adolescent health. The chapter also discusses the individual and societal costs of poor child health, public programs targeted to children's health, and strategies to improve child and adolescent health at the individual, family, and community levels.

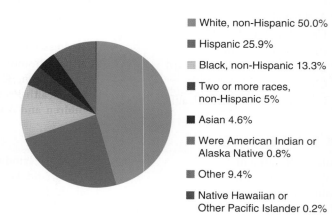

Fig. 16.1 Percentage distribution of US children by race/ethnicity, 2020. (From Federal Interagency Forum on Child and Family Statistics: *America's children in brief: key national indicators of well-being*, 2020. Available from: https://www.childstats.gov/pdf/ac2020/ac_20.pdf.)

ISSUES OF PREGNANCY AND INFANCY

The health of the mother before, during, and after pregnancy has a direct impact on the health and well-being of her child. The conditions that surround a child's fetal development and early years shape his or her life. Adapting healthy lifestyles and obtaining regular medical care before becoming pregnant can help ensure a healthy pregnancy. Unfortunately, many women face barriers to good health throughout their lives, including racism, violence, poverty, and lack of access to health care. A comprehensive approach that helps women identify and treat potential risks and overcome barriers to good health before, between, and beyond their pregnancies will help protect and promote the health of women and children and can help ensure the health of future generations. Consider the following (Moos, 2010; Moos et al., 2010):

1. Women who are not in optimal health before becoming pregnant are at increased risk for poor pregnancy outcomes.
2. Babies whose mothers have uncontrolled health conditions, such as infections, diabetes, hypertension, and obesity, are more likely to be born at low birth weights and with serious medical conditions.
3. A fetus exposed to maternal drug, alcohol, or tobacco exposure or poor nutrition is more likely to have chronic conditions that affect health and well-being.
4. Infants exposed to unsafe environmental conditions, such as secondhand smoke and lead-based paint, are more likely to have chronic conditions throughout childhood and, in some cases, through adolescence and adulthood.
5. Children who do not receive preventive health care and do not obtain all necessary immunizations are more likely to have preventable diseases or chronic conditions that could have been prevented or minimized and controlled.

Infant Mortality

Infant mortality, the deaths of children during the first year of life, is a critical gauge of children's health status. It is an important marker because it is related to several factors, including maternal health, healthcare quality and access, socioeconomic conditions, and public health practices. Infant mortality reflects the health and welfare of an entire community and is used as a broad indicator of health care and health status. Box 16.1 lists some terms and definitions associated with infant health and mortality. The five leading causes of infant death are congenital defects; disorders related to short gestation or low birth weight; unintentional injuries, such as suffocation; sudden infant death syndrome (SIDS; see later in the chapter); and maternal complications of pregnancy. These five factors account for 55% of all infant deaths. The order of the top five leading causes changed slightly from 2018 to 2019. In 2018, maternal complications were the third leading cause, followed by SIDS, whereas in 2019, unintentional injuries was third, SIDS fourth, and maternal complications was fifth (Kochanek et al., 2020). Box 16.2 lists sources of vital statistics birth data.

Surprisingly, the United States ranks a dismal 33rd (out of 43) of economically developed countries in infant mortality,

BOX 16.1 Infant Health Definitions

Infant death: Death of an infant before his or her first birthday.
Infant mortality rate: Number of infant deaths per 1000 live births.
Preterm birth: Birth before 37 completed weeks of gestation.
Very preterm birth: Birth before 32 completed weeks of gestation.
Late preterm birth: Birth from 34 to 36 completed weeks of gestation.
Term birth: Birth from 37 to 41 completed weeks of gestation.

From MacDorman MF, Mathews TJ: *Understanding racial and ethnic disparities in U.S. infant mortality rates, NCHS data brief, no 74,* Hyattsville, MD, 2011, National Center for Health Statistics. Available from: https://www.cdc.gov/nchs/data/databriefs/db74.pdf.

BOX 16.2 Sources of Vital Statistics Data for Children

In the United States, laws require birth certificates to be completed for all babies born. Information concerning an infant's birth, including the total number of the mother's prenatal care visits; the mother's and father's ages and race; mother's marital status and education; and the infant's weight, gestational age, and birth date, appears on a baby's birth certificate.

Information concerning an infant's death, such as the cause(s), date, and other details, appears on the death certificate. In each state, the vital statistics office in the state health department stores these certificates. This agency collects and regularly reports the aggregated data and forwards them to the National Center for Health Statistics.

The National Center for Health Statistics collects, analyzes, and publishes numerous reports on the health and well-being of the nation's infants. These data sources are very important in tracking the health of infants as well as of other population groups; they help determine necessary interventions from various perspectives (e.g., clinical, public health, public policy, and environmental).

From National Institute of Child Health and Human Development: *Safe to Sleep public education campaign,* 2012. https://www1.nichd.nih.gov/sts/Pages/default.aspx.

behind most other industrialized nations, including South Korea, Sweden, Spain, Israel, Italy, France, and Australia (Table 16.1). Fifty years ago, the United States ranked 12th (Organisation for Economic Co-operation and Development [OECD], 2021). The gap in infant mortality between the United States and other nations has occurred in spite of the United States' comparatively high per capita spending on health care and technological advancements.

Despite a poor ranking among other nations in the world, the infant mortality rate in the United States has declined every year since 1940 with the exception of 2002 (Fig. 16.2). The 2018 figure, 5.67 deaths per 1000 live births (CDC, 2020a), was the lowest infant mortality rate ever recorded in this country. This drop can be attributed largely to public health measures and improved standard of living (e.g., better sanitation, a clean milk supply, immunizations against deadly childhood diseases, the increased availability of nutritious food, and enhanced access to maternal health care). Technological advances in neonatal care—for example, the introduction of synthetic lung surfactant—have also contributed to reductions in infant mortality.

TABLE 16.1 International Comparisons of Infant Mortality Rates[a] for Selected Countries and Territories (2015)

World rank	Country	1960	2015
1	Slovenia	N/A	1.6
2	Finland	21.0	1.7
3	Iceland	13.0	2.2
4	Norway	16.0	2.3
5	Czech Republic	20.0	2.5
5	Sweden	16.6	2.5
5	Estonia	N/A	2.5
6	South Korea	N/A	2.7
6	Spain	43.7	2.7
7	Luxembourg	N/A	2.8
8	Italy		2.9
8	Portugal	77.5	2.9
9	Austria	37.5	3.1
9	Israel	N/A	3.1
10	Australia	20.2	3.2
11	Belgium	31.4	3.3
11	Germany	35.0	3.3
11	Netherlands	16.5	3.3
12	Ireland	29.3	3.4
13	Denmark	21.5	3.7
13	France	27.7	3.7
14	Switzerland	21.1	3.9
14	United Kingdom	22.5	3.9
15	Greece	40.1	4.0
15	Poland	54.8	4.0
16	Latvia	N/A	4.1
17	Hungary	47.6	4.2
17	Lithuania	N/A	4.2
18	Slovak Republic	28.6	5.1
19	United States	26.0	5.9
19	Russia	N/A	6.5
20	Costa Rica	N/A	8.5
21	China	N/A	9.2
22	Turkey	189.5	10.7
23	Mexico	92.3	12.5
24	Columbia	89.3	13.6
25	Brazil	129.4	14.6
26	Indonesia	148.4	22.8
27	South Africa	N/A	33.6
28	India	165.1	37.9

[a]Infant mortality rate represents infant deaths per 1000 live births. From Organization for Economic Cooperation and Development: Health: *Key tables from OECD, No. 14: infant mortality*, 2015. Available from: https://data.oecd.org/healthstat/infant-mortality-rates.htm; Centers for Disease Control and Prevention: *Deaths final data 2015*, 2016. Available from: https://www.cdc.gov/nchs/data/nvsr/nvsr65/nvsr65_04.pdf.

Declines in infant mortality have stagnated during the past decade, however, and the gap between black and white infant mortality rates remains stubbornly high, with black infants (10.75 per 1000) dying at a rate of more than two times higher than that of white infants (4.63 per 1000) (CDC, 2020a).

Identifying and remedying the causes of higher infant mortality rates among certain population subgroups remains a vexing societal problem that must be addressed (Fig. 16.3).

The first year of life is the most hazardous a person faces until he or she reaches 65 years. Therefore, it is particularly important for women to be as healthy as possible before becoming pregnant and to receive prenatal care and adopt healthy lifestyle choices, and for infants to receive primary health care to maintain health and prevent or minimize serious, long-lasting health problems.

Preterm Birth and Low Birth Weight

Preterm birth (birth before 37 completed weeks of gestation) and low birth weight (weighing less than 5.5 lb at birth) are the most important predictors of infant health. In 2019, 10.23% of babies in the United States were born preterm; the percentage of low-birth-weight babies rose for the fifth year in a row. Black women are more likely than white women to have a preterm birth and about twice as likely to have babies born at low birth weight (Martin et al., 2020).

Infants born preterm or at a low birth weight have a far greater risk of death as well as of mental and physical disabilities such as cerebral palsy, visual problems such as retinopathy of prematurity, feeding problems, and hearing loss than infants born at term with normal weight. Even babies born late preterm (34—36 completed weeks of gestation) carry a risk for physical problems and developmental delay that is much higher than for babies born at full term. Important growth and development occur even in the last few days of a pregnancy. Factors associated with preterm birth and low birth weight include the following:

1. Minority status
2. Chronic stress
3. Maternal age less than 17 years or more than 35 years
4. Chronic health problems such as diabetes mellitus, hypertension, and some infections
5. Lack of prenatal care
6. Multiple births
7. Certain problems with the uterus or cervix
8. Low socioeconomic status
9. Unhealthy maternal habits (e.g., poor nutrition, obesity, alcohol and drug use, and cigarette smoking)
10. Induced labor before 39 weeks of pregnancy without a medical indication
11. Elective cesarean birth

One reason that infant mortality has declined so slowly in recent years is that the preterm rate rose very quickly from 1990 to 2010. A portion of this rise was due to increases in multiple births, which in turn was due in part to childbearing in later years, which increases the likelihood of multiple conceptions. Also there was an increase in the rate of multiples that resulted from assisted reproductive technology. Yet the rate of preterm births among singleton births also rose during this time. Further, medical management of pregnancy has increased the numbers of labor inductions and elective cesarean births and has helped push the rate of late preterm births upward (Martin

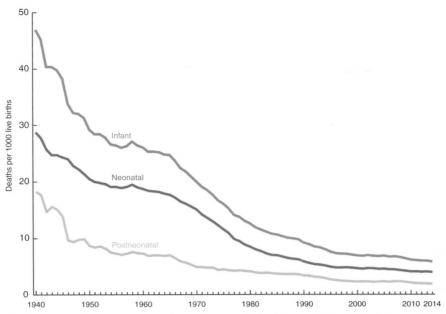

Fig. 16.2 Infant, neonatal, and postneonatal mortality rates: United States, 1940–2014. Rates are infant (under 1 year), neonatal (under 28 days), and postneonatal (28 days–11 months) deaths per 1000 live births in specified group. (From National Center for Health Statistics: Deaths: *Final data for 2014. National vital statistics report* 65[4], 2016. Available from: https://www.cdc.gov/nchs/data/nvsr/nvsr65/nvsr65_04.pdf.)

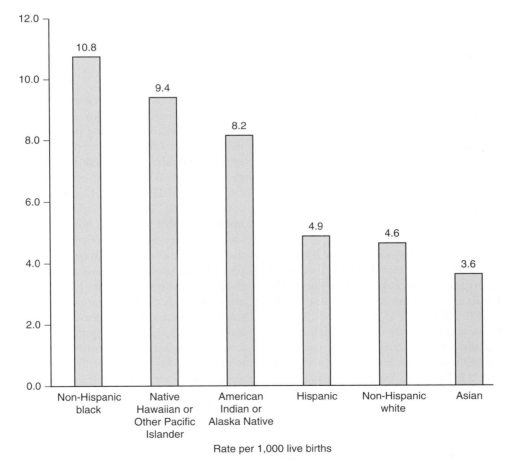

Fig. 16.3 Infant mortality rates by race and ethnicity, 2018. (From https://www.cdc.gov/reproductivehealth/maternalinfanthealth/infantmortality.htm.)

et al., 2020). Success stories of tiny survivors are sensationalized in the news, but the long-term consequences of babies born even a few weeks early are not well publicized. Consequences of preterm and late preterm birth can be long-lasting and costly (Loftin et al., 2010; Waitzman et al., 2021). Because late preterm births account for the majority of preterm births, it is imperative that all possible measures are taken to decrease elective births before 39 weeks of gestation (Oshiro et al., 2009).

Preventing the occurrence of prematurity and low birth weight is a high priority for clinical and public health research and policy. Nurses can play important roles in preventing prematurity through the provision of evidence-based primary care, research, screening, counseling, education, advocacy, referral, and implementation of interventions to reduce risk among target population groups.

Preconception Health

Developing fetal organ systems are highly vulnerable to the effects of poor maternal nutrition, drugs, alcohol, tobacco, chronic maternal diseases, environmental toxins, and other exposures. The fetus can suffer damage very early in pregnancy (3 days after a missed period), even before a woman knows she is pregnant. Although less than half (45%) of the pregnancies in the United States are unintended (Finer and Zolna, 2016), achieving good health for all women throughout their reproductive years—preconception health—can help ensure optimal fetal health and development should pregnancy occur. Healthy lifestyle measures for women (regardless of their intent to become pregnant) include maintaining a healthy weight and good nutrition; tending to chronic medical problems such as diabetes and hypertension; being up to date on vaccinations; avoiding environmental toxins; decreasing stress and eliminating abusive relationships; and avoiding illicit drugs, tobacco, and alcohol. Effective contraception can help women avoid unintended pregnancies and lengthen pregnancy spacing. Close pregnancy spacing (less than 18 months apart) may increase the likelihood of low birth weight, preterm birth, and placental problems (DeFranco et al., 2015). Preconception health focuses on taking steps in the present to ensure the health of future children and considering effective contraception if pregnancy is not desired.

Simple measures such as consuming 400 µg of the B vitamin folic acid every day for at least a month before becoming pregnant and during pregnancy can help decrease the likelihood of defects of the brain and spine, known as *neural tube defects*, by more than 35% (CDC, 2017a). Some foods, such as leafy vegetables, bananas, and beans, are naturally high in folic acid. Other foods, including breads, cereals, flours, cornmeal, pastas, rice, and select grain products, are enriched with folic acid as required by the U.S. Food and Drug Administration.

Prenatal Care

Obtaining early and regular prenatal care enhances a woman's chance of delivering a healthy, term baby. Prenatal care includes client education, risk identification, and monitoring and treatment of symptoms. It also includes referral to health, nutrition, childbirth education, and social service programs that can help a woman optimize her chances for a healthy pregnancy. Until the late 20th century, prenatal care was seen as the best solution for improving birth outcomes. But even with expansions in the Medicaid program to cover health care for increasing numbers of low-income pregnant women and infants and significant federal, state, and local investments, poor pregnancy outcomes have persisted, especially for non-Hispanic black, American Indian, and Puerto Rican women.

Although prenatal care is not the *only* solution to reducing infant mortality, comprehensive prenatal care can improve the identification of specific and treatable causes of infant morbidity and mortality, such as maternal anemia, diabetes, hypertension, urinary tract infections, sexually transmitted infections, and poor nutrition. Ideally, such counseling and treatment of chronic health conditions should begin before a woman becomes pregnant. Optimal health throughout her life, including treatment of chronic health conditions and the adaptation of a healthy lifestyle, will have far more of an impact on healthy pregnancy than prenatal care alone.

Prenatal Substance Use

Tobacco, alcohol, and illicit drug use are social factors that affect the health of women and their children. During pregnancy, substance use profoundly affects the neurological and physical development of the fetus. The use of these substances, in any combination, is dangerous to a woman's health and worsens infant health and development outcomes.

Tobacco

Smoking tobacco during pregnancy is one of the most preventable causes of infant morbidity and mortality. The adverse health effects of tobacco use during pregnancy are well documented; they include low birth weight, prematurity, stillbirth, intrauterine growth retardation, premature rupture of membranes, placenta previa, placental abruption, neurodevelopmental impairment, and SIDS (USDHHS, 2010). Cigarette smoke contains more than 2500 chemicals. The fetal effects of most of these chemicals are unknown. What is known, however, is that when a pregnant woman inhales cigarette smoke, the oxygen supply to her fetus is disrupted by nicotine and carbon monoxide. Nicotine crosses the placenta and becomes concentrated in fetal blood and amniotic fluid. Nicotine concentrations in the fetus of a smoking woman can be as much as 15% higher than maternal levels. Secondhand smoke exposure also is dangerous to the fetus and newborn. It is linked to SIDS, decreased respiratory functioning, and childhood asthma. Pregnant women who are exposed to secondhand smoke have higher odds of giving birth to low-birth-weight babies than women who are not exposed to secondhand smoke during pregnancy (CDC, 2020c).

An estimated 10% of women report smoking during the last 3 months of pregnancy. Teenagers and young women have the highest rates of maternal smoking (Curtin and Mathews, 2016). The elimination of tobacco use among pregnant women would significantly reduce the rates of low-birth-weight infants, preterm delivery, intrauterine growth restriction, and infant mortality. Quitting is very difficult because the nicotine in tobacco is addictive, but quitting is best. Merely reducing cigarette use during pregnancy may not be enough to benefit the fetus because women who cut back tend to inhale more deeply or take more puffs to get an equivalent amount of nicotine.

The need for widespread implementation of smoking cessation programs for women in the childbearing years is clear. Many smoking cessation programs have been developed and implemented by national, state, and local governments and organizations. Because pregnant women who have received even brief smoking cessation counseling are more likely to quit smoking, the nurse should offer evidence-based smoking cessation interventions to the pregnant smoker at the first prenatal visit and throughout the pregnancy.

Alcohol and Illicit Drugs

The use of alcohol and illicit drugs is a major risk factor for poor infant outcomes. Alcohol exposure during pregnancy can lead to fetal alcohol syndrome and other fetal alcohol spectrum disorders (FASDs). FASDs range from mild, subtle learning disabilities to severe learning disabilities. Children with FASDs are at risk for psychiatric problems, criminal behavior, unemployment, and incomplete education. Many children with FASDs also have physical abnormalities, growth deficiencies, and central nervous system disorders. *No level of alcohol intake has been determined to be safe during pregnancy, and there is no safe time to drink during pregnancy.* Women who are pregnant or who may become pregnant should abstain from drinking alcohol (CDC, 2020b).

An estimated 10.2% of pregnant women drink during their pregnancies. Binge drinking, which is defined for women as four or more drinks on an occasion in the past 30 days, is especially harmful to fetal development. About 3.9% of pregnant women report binge drinking (Denny et al., 2019). There is a compelling need for research on intervention strategies that can help prevent alcohol-exposed pregnancies.

Like alcohol, illicit drugs can cause permanent harm to an unborn baby. Current illicit drug use, including marijuana/hashish, cocaine (including crack), heroin, hallucinogens, and inhalants or prescription-type psychotherapeutics used nonmedically among pregnant women has remained constant at 5.9% despite efforts of prevention and education programs (Substance Abuse and Mental Health Services Administration [SAMHSA], 2013). Risks to the baby include prematurity, low birth weight, birth defects, newborn withdrawal symptoms, and learning and behavioral problems. Substance use is often a sign of more complex psychosocial problems, such as depression, poverty, abuse, and violence. Illicit drug use often goes hand in hand with other maternal risks, including tobacco and alcohol use, poor nutrition, intimate partner violence, and risk of sexually transmitted infections. Surveys now indicate that many pregnant women *do* understand the negative impact of substance use during pregnancy and cut back or stop use but then rapidly resume use after pregnancy. Evidence-based public health measures are needed to further reduce substance use during pregnancy and to prevent postpartum resumption.

Because of serious potential risks to the developing fetus, women who are pregnant or who could become pregnant should be asked about substance use and counseled to abstain from alcohol, tobacco, and the use of illicit drugs, through the use of evidence-based practices. For women who already use alcohol, tobacco, and illicit drugs, a comprehensive and long-lasting approach to treatment is required.

Breast-Feeding

Breastfeeding is a natural and beneficial source of nutrition and provides the healthiest start for an infant. In addition to the nutritional benefits, breastfeeding promotes a unique and emotional connection between mother and baby.

American Academy of Pediatrics (2012)

The American Academy of Pediatrics (AAP) recommends exclusive breast-feeding for about the first 6 months of a baby's life, followed by breast-feeding in combination with the introduction of complementary foods until at least 12 months of age, and continuation of breast-feeding for as long as mutually desired by mother and baby. Breast-feeding has many advantages for the mother, for the baby, and for society. The cells, hormones, and antibodies in breast milk protect babies from illness such as infections and lower the childhood risk of asthma, obesity, diabetes, and SIDS. For mothers, breast-feeding is linked to a lower risk of breast and ovarian cancer and type 2 diabetes (Chowdhury et al., 2015). Breast-feeding can save more than $1500 per year in formula and supplies, and even more in the costs of infant illness (Womenshealth.gov, n.d.).

Initiation of breast-feeding occurs in about 77% of hospital births. Maternity practices that discourage separation of mothers and their babies have helped boost these rates, but more attention is required to meet AAP recommendations. The breast-feeding rates have improved in recent years, but vary by race and ethnicity. Current rates for Hispanic infants is 84% compared with 86% for white infants and 74% for black infants. Further, only about 35% of infants are still being breast-fed by 12 months, and the prevalence is lower for black infants, as Black infants have the lowest rates of breast-feeding initiation and duration (CDC, 2021b). This gap points to the need to understand and act upon barriers to breast-feeding that are unique to black women.

The *2011 Surgeon General's Call to Action to Support Breast-feeding* suggests actions aimed at increasing societal support for breast-feeding women. These suggestions call on communities, employers, healthcare providers, governments, and nonprofit organizations to implement strategies to support breast-feeding (U.S. Department of Health and Human Services [USDHHS], Office of the Surgeon General, 2011). There are many community sources of support for breast-feeding mothers, and nurses can play a key role in linking breast-feeding mothers with help if it is needed. In addition to nurses, health professionals such as lactation consultants, childbirth educators, physicians, trained home visitors, and doulas can provide assistance. Peer support groups such as La Leche League and breast-feeding centers can also be helpful. The federally supported Women, Infants, and Children (WIC) program also provides counseling and support for breast-feeding mothers.

Sudden Unexplained Infant Death

Sudden unexplained infant death (SUID) is defined as death in an infant less than 1 year of age that occurs suddenly and unexpectedly, the cause of which is not immediately obvious before investigation. About 3500 infants die each year from SUID. Later investigation may reveal death in infants with SUID to be from poisoning, metabolic disorders, hyperthermia or hypothermia, neglect and homicide, and suffocation. About half of the infants who die from SUID die from SIDS, defined as the sudden death of an infant less than 1 year of age that cannot be explained after a thorough investigation is conducted, including a complete autopsy, examination of the death scene, and review of the clinical history. SIDS is the fourth leading cause of infant mortality. Non-Hispanic black and American Indian/Alaska Native infants are far more likely to die from SIDS than infants of other races (CDC, 2020a).

In 1994, with the recognition that placing infants on their backs for sleep lowered SIDS rates, the federal government, along with private entities, launched the successful Back to Sleep Campaign to heighten awareness of the safety of positioning infants on their backs for sleep. Since 1994, SIDS deaths have declined by more than 50% (CDC, 2017b) (Box 16.3). More has been learned about other factors that can lower the risk of SIDS. In 2016, the AAP released updated guidelines for safe sleeping environments (AAP, 2016). Drawing from the success of Back to Sleep, the Safe to Sleep campaign works to educate parents, caregivers, and healthcare providers about ways to reduce the risk of infant death from SIDS as well as death from known sleep-related causes, such as suffocation.

? ACTIVE LEARNING

1. Examine infant mortality statistics in the community, and compare the rates with state and national averages. Is infant mortality higher for any particular racial or ethnic group within the community?
2. Determine how a non—English-speaking immigrant without finances or available transportation would obtain prenatal care.
3. Accompany a pregnant woman to a local department of social services and observe as she tries to establish Medicaid eligibility for herself and her unborn child.
4. Survey businesses in the community to determine whether they offer maternity health insurance benefits, paid or unpaid maternity or paternity leave, and leave for prenatal care appointments. Is there a location within each worksite where women can pump breast milk? Use this information to develop a strategy to encourage family-friendly policies and practices in the business community.

CHILDHOOD HEALTH ISSUES

At all ages, appropriate and timely medical care plays an important role in children's health status. However, other factors, including parental influences, nutrition, environment, community safety, and the overall quality of home life, exert

BOX 16.3 "Safe to Sleep" Public Education Campaign

Recommendations to reduce the risk of SIDS and sleep-related causes of infant death: Always place a baby on his or her back to sleep, both for naps and at night.

- Use a firm sleep surface, covered by a fitted sheet.
- Your baby should not sleep in an adult bed, on a couch, or on a chair alone, with you, or with anyone else.
- Keep soft objects, toys, and loose bedding out of your baby's sleep area.
- Do not smoke during pregnancy, and do not smoke or allow smoking around your baby.
- Breast-feed your baby.
- Do not let your baby get too hot during sleep.
- Follow healthcare provider guidance on your baby's vaccines and regular health checkups.
- Avoid products that claim to reduce the risk of SIDS and other sleep-related causes of infant death.
- Get regular healthcare during pregnancy, and do not smoke, drink alcohol, or use illegal drugs during pregnancy or after the baby is born.

SIDS, Sudden infant death syndrome.
From National Institute of Child Health and Human Development: *Safe sleep for your baby* (NIH Pub. No. 12—7040), 2013. Available from: https://www.nichd.nih.gov/publications/pubs/Documents/STS_SafeSleepForYourBaby_General_2013.pdf.

even stronger influences over a child's well-being. Childhood is generally a healthy time of life, as evidenced by the improvement in many indicators of child health status over the past century. For example, the incidence of childhood disease has diminished because the majority of children receive a full complement of immunizations during infancy and toddlerhood.

The causes of childhood death vary with age. Parents and the community have important responsibilities in promoting healthy lifestyles, creating safe environments, and ensuring access to medical care. They must take steps to protect children from the leading threats to children's health (i.e., accidental injury and exposure to environmental toxins, abuse, and violence).

⚕ NEWBORN SCREENING

Newborn screening checks for rare but serious health conditions shortly after birth. Often babies with certain health disorders appear healthy at birth; thus all babies are tested for selected conditions that can be treated if they are identified early. Babies can be screened for blood, heart, and hearing conditions.

Screening can be conducted in three ways. Blood screening is conducted by collecting a few drops of blood from the newborn's heel. This sample is tested at a laboratory, and parents are notified of abnormalities. Hearing screening requires that a tiny, soft speaker be placed in the baby's ear to see how the baby responds to sound. Heart screening uses pulse oximetry to evaluate the baby for congenital heart disease.

Newborn screening is state based, and the number of conditions that babies are screened for varies from state to state. All US states and territories currently test for 26 health conditions, including phenylketonuria, galactosemia, congenital hypothyroidism, and sickle cell disease.

Modified from March of Dimes: *Newborn screening,* 2020. Available from Newborn screening tests for your baby (marchofdimes.org) Available from: https://www.marchofdimes.org/baby/newborn-screening-tests-for-your-baby.aspx?gclid=EAIaIQobChMI3cm0g_bB8AIVuf3jBx3ZfQRcEAAYAiAAEgJxtvD_BwE

COMMUNITY HEALTH VISIT

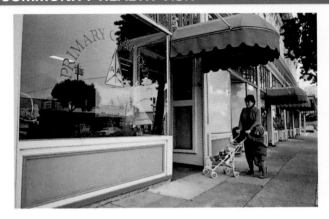

This clinic provides services through the Early and Periodic Screening, Diagnosis, and Treatment (EPSDT) Program, which was developed to provide health care for children in low-income families receiving Medicaid.

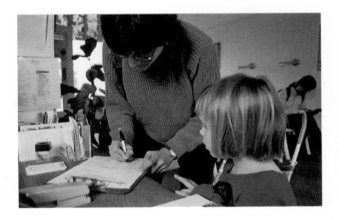

The nurse has an opportunity to observe the client and the family as they register and wait for their appointment. The parent registers the 5-year-old daughter for a school entry health physical examination. Medicaid insurance is verified for the physical.

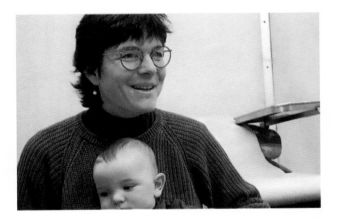

Trust can be established in a short time. The nurse can begin by explaining the steps in the clinic process so that the client knows what is expected. The nurse should always listen to the client attentively and should allow enough time for the client to reflect and respond to questions.

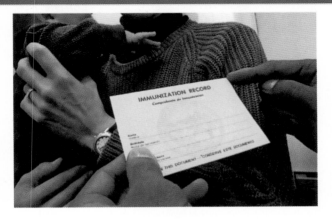

Reviewing immunization records is an important primary prevention role for the community health nurse. This is a teachable opportunity for the nurse to stress the importance of maintaining immunizations for the child. In California, parents are provided with a yellow state immunization record for the child, which they should use to record all immunizations and to show proof of immunizations when needed.

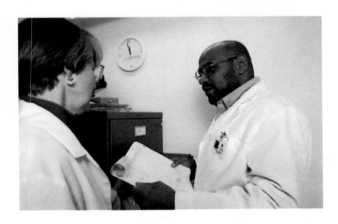

The nurse discusses any concerns about the client with the practitioner before the examination.

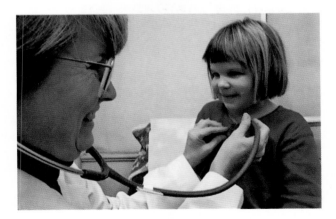

The practitioner performs the physical examination of the child with the help of the parent. The practitioner discusses the result of the vision test with the parent and the need for a follow-up appointment with an ophthalmologist. The child has not undergone a blood lead measurement and requires booster immunizations. The practitioner orders laboratory tests, immunizations, and a referral to an ophthalmologist.

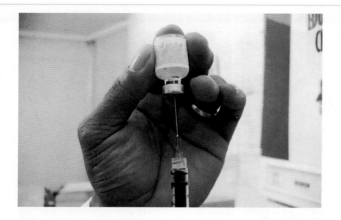

The clinic staff performs the laboratory work: hematocrit, urinary analysis, and lead measurement. The immunization consent forms have been signed by the parent. The nurse administers the immunizations and takes this opportunity to reinforce the importance of immunizations for both children.

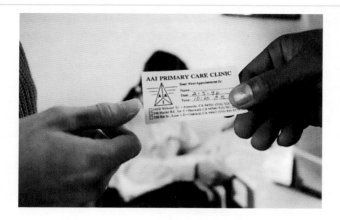

The community health nurse gives the parent a business card with the nurse's name and the agency's address and phone number. The nurse advises the parent to call the nurse if there is anything else that the family may need.

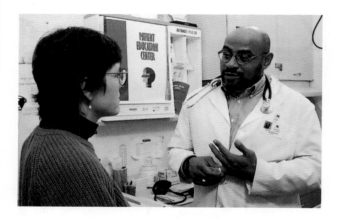

The nurse also offers suggestions to relieve the common side effects of immunizations.

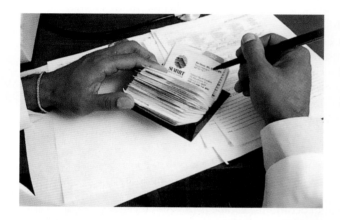

The nurse searches for resources for an ophthalmologist and a family planning clinic that accept Medicaid and a resource for day care providers. The nurse obtains phone numbers for a couple of ophthalmologists, a family planning clinic, and a daycare consortium service.

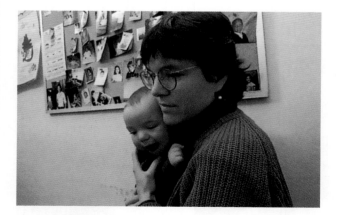

The parent asks about an ophthalmologist who takes Medicaid and about day care facilities in the area for the younger child. The parent also asks about family planning services in the community.

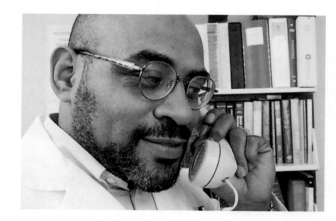

The nurse calls the family with the referrals for an ophthalmologist and a phone number to obtain a list of daycare providers.

Story by Leonard Kaku, RN, MSN. Photography by George Draper.

Accidental Injuries

Infants and young children are at great risk for accidental injuries. They are curious and eager to explore their environments, but they often lack the coordination and cognitive abilities to keep themselves safe from harm. Their small size and developing bones and muscles make them especially susceptible to injury. The leading cause of injury death for children younger than 1 year is accidental suffocation due to choking or strangulation. Unintentional injury is the leading cause of death for children ages 1 to 14. For children younger than 5, drowning is the leading cause of death. From 5 to 14 years, motor vehicle–related injuries are the cause of most deaths (CDC, 2019a). Low-income and minority children suffer disproportionately from accidental injuries. They are more likely to sustain injuries and more likely to die from their injuries. For example, Native American children are more than twice as likely to experience accidental injury as their white counterparts (KidsData.org, 2019).

Many accidents can be avoided by improving the safety of a child's environment. Ensuring a child's safety in a motor vehicle is critical. The most important steps that a parent can take to ensure a child's safety in a motor vehicle is to correctly secure the child into a car seat based on the child's age and size. The safest place for all children younger than 13 years to ride is in the back seat, regardless of weight and height (Durbin et al., 2018). Leaving children unattended in a motor vehicle is another safety concern. In only a few minutes, a car can become hot enough to cause heat stroke in a youngster. Children can also become entrapped in a car trunk or locked in a car. They should never be left alone in a car.

Smoke alarms should be installed on every level of the home and in bedrooms. Escape plans should be practiced often. Small children can drown in as little as an inch of water. Toilets, buckets, bathtubs, and pools are all potential drowning hazards. Storage of medications and hazardous substances and playground safety are also important safety education topics.

Finally, head injury from cycling and other wheeled sports, such as skateboarding, is a leading cause of child death and disability. Without proper head protection, a fall from as little as 2 feet can cause traumatic brain injury. The use of helmets and proper protective equipment can substantially reduce the risk of injuries. Box 16.4 discusses how toys can be another threat to small children.

Low-income parents may have difficulty affording safety equipment such as safety latches for cabinets, smoke alarms, car seats, and helmets. The grassroots coalition Safe Kids Worldwide can help link parents and professionals to child injury prevention advocacy and events in local communities (Safe Kids Worldwide, 2021).

Unhealthy Weight

Childhood obesity has become a health crisis in the United States. The rate of obesity has more than doubled in children and tripled in adolescents since the 1970s, but has leveled off in the past decade. An estimated one-third of children are overweight or obese (Fryar et al., 2016). Children who are overweight are

---

BOX 16.4   Toy-Related Injuries

Although most toys are safe, children are at risk for toy-related injuries and death. Approximately 168,000 children younger than 14 years are treated in hospital emergency departments for toy-related injuries. Though the majority of toy-related injuries are minor, permanent disability can occur. Riding toys, such as nonmotorized scooters and tricycles, are associated with more injuries than any other toy group.

Laws and regulations have been put into place to protect children from toy injuries. An example is the Federal Hazardous Substances Act, which bans children's toys that contain any hazardous substance, such as lead. The Child Safety Protection Act of 1994 was designed to reduce toy-related choking and requires manufacturers to place choking hazard warning labels on balloons, marbles, small balls, and games with small parts intended for use only by children 3 years and older. The act also requires manufacturers, importers, distributors, and retailers to report choking incidents involving such products to the Consumer Product Safety Commission. The U.S. Department of Commerce requires toy guns to be distinguished from real guns. In addition, the toy industry has established voluntary safety standards to minimize risk of injury.

Although regulations and laws are helpful, parents and caretakers must also provide adequate supervision of children and must adopt strategies recommended to prevent toy-related injuries, as follows: use only age-appropriate toys; use Mylar balloons instead of latex (which can cause children to choke or suffocate); purchase a "small parts" tester to determine whether small toys pose choking hazards; check the website of the U.S. Consumer Product Safety Commission (www.cpsc.gov) to obtain information on toy recalls; follow age and safety recommendations on toy labels; and ensure that toys are used in a safe and proper environment.

Data from Safe Kids USA: *Preventing accidental injury: toy safety*. Available from: https://www.safekids.org/safetytips/field_risks/toy-safety?gclid=EAIaIQobChMI16TRze7I2AIVVyOBCh1HPQyXEAAYAiAAEgIWQfD_BwE /.

---

more likely to experience cardiovascular disease, diabetes, bone and joint disease, and sleep apnea and to face social discrimination that can lead to poor self-esteem and depression.

Obesity prevalence is higher among Hispanic (25.8%) and non-Hispanic black (22.0%) children and adolescents than among non-Hispanic white children (14.1%) (Hales et al., 2017). Minority groups, those with less income, and those with lower education levels are more likely to be overweight. The higher cost and unavailability of healthy foods, food insecurity, and the lack of access to safe places to exercise contribute to obesity in lower-income communities (Hilmers et al., 2012; Widome et al., 2009).

The *body mass index* (BMI) is a screening tool calculated from a person's weight and height that can be used to determine whether the person is underweight, of normal weight, overweight, or obese. BMI can be calculated in children from as young as 2 years to teenage with the use of age- and sex-specific growth charts. BMI does not calculate actual body fat percentage, but it is an easy and inexpensive method that can identify weight problems (CDC, 2021a).

A number of factors contribute to childhood obesity. The typical American diet, which is both high in fat and calories and low in nutrients, has resulted in an increase in obesity. Widely available fast food, increasing portion sizes, the presence of vending machines in schools, availability of sugar-sweetened drinks, and the eating of fewer meals at home have contributed to the trend. Modern technologies such as electronic games and television, a lack of safe convenient outdoor exercise areas, and readily accessible transportation have also led to more sedentary lifestyles.

In some urban neighborhoods where high concentrations of people living in poverty are prevalent, there may be little to no access to fresh, nutritious, affordable foods, which also contributes to obesity. Such neighborhoods are called *food deserts*. Residents are limited to obtaining food from convenience stores and fast-food restaurants rather than from grocery stores and fresh food markets; nutritious foods are not available.

Nurses can play a leading role in generating public awareness of factors that contribute to obesity and can focus on preventive measures such as healthy lifestyles and physical activity. For example, breast-feeding provides some protection against later obesity. At least 60 min of moderately strenuous exercise is recommended for children most days of the week. Nurses can design and implement nutrition, healthy eating, and physical activities policies and standards in schools; take part in initiatives that make fresh, healthy foods available to all; and challenge policy makers and industry leaders such as fast-food restaurants to mobilize resources for good nutrition and fitness.

Immunization

Childhood immunization is a benchmark of child health. Maintaining appropriate immunization protects all members of the community, especially immune-compromised individuals and pregnant women, who are particularly vulnerable to certain infectious diseases. Adequate immunization protects children against several diseases that kill or disable many children. Poliomyelitis, a crippling disease of the past, has been eliminated in the United States thanks to the public health effort that made the polio vaccine accessible and affordable. Over the ensuing decades, new vaccines have been developed, and children can now be protected from more than 14 vaccine-preventable diseases. State laws requiring proof of vaccination before entry to school or child care have helped ensure high vaccination levels in the population.

Vaccine-preventable disease levels are at or near record lows, but many children and adolescents remain underimmunized. Concerns about the frequency and timing of vaccines and widespread fears that childhood vaccines are linked to autism have prevented some parents from vaccinating their children (Institute of Medicine, 2013). In 2009, however, the U.S. Court of Federal Claims ruled that childhood vaccines do not cause autism. This ruling was consistent with 18 major scientific studies that failed to show a link between vaccines and autism (U.S. Court of Federal Claims, n.d.). Nurses can help educate community members about the safety of vaccines and recommended vaccination schedules and about the consequences of undervaccination. The following vaccines are recommended for children and adolescents (Wodi et al., 2021):

- Tetanus, diphtheria, acellular pertussis
- Inactivated polio
- Rotavirus
- Influenza
- Measles, mumps, and rubella vaccine
- Hepatitis A vaccine
- Hepatitis B vaccine
- Varicella (chickenpox) vaccine
- *Haemophilus influenzae* type b (Hib)
- Pneumococcal conjugate
- Human papillomavirus vaccine (males and females)
- Meningococcal conjugate
- Pfizer-BioNT COVID-19 vaccination for persons aged ≥12 years

Most insurance plans cover the cost of childhood vaccines, and the ACA required insurance plans to eliminate copays and deductibles for preventive services including vaccinations. Another source of assistance is the Vaccines For Children program, a federally funded program that provides vaccines at no cost to children who might not otherwise be vaccinated because of inability to pay.

Environmental Concerns

Potential threats to the health of children sometimes exist in their living environments. Threats can be found in the air, in the water, and from toxic exposures to chemicals. For example, air pollution, poor indoor air quality, and secondhand smoke can cause or trigger childhood asthma. Asthma is one of the most common chronic childhood disorders, affecting an estimated 5.5 million (7.5%) children in 2018 (CDC, 2021c). Lead—a neurotoxin that can sometimes be found in drinking water (often from lead pipes and fittings), in old paint dust or chips that crumble from walls on older housing units, and in contaminated soil—is a cause of cognitive and behavioral problems, decreased growth, and neurological disabilities. The reduction of childhood blood lead levels is among the greatest public health stories of the latter half of the 20th century, but unfortunately lead is still a threat. Although lead is banned from the manufacture of paint, many millions of housing units in the United States still contain lead-based paint. Most of these units are located in poor, inner-city neighborhoods. Despite dramatic declines in blood lead levels for most US populations, levels remain high among children in low-income families who live in older housing with lead-based paint. Treatment for children with elevated blood lead values is long and difficult and carries risks. Better prevention, elimination of risks in the environment (particularly in older housing units), more efficient tracking, and education of the public are essential to further reduce the menace of lead poisoning.

Exposure to toxic cleaning products, pesticides, medicines, and herbicides is another area of concern. Simple steps can help protect children from accidental exposures, including child-resistant packaging, cabinet safety latches, and careful supervision.

Child Maltreatment

Child maltreatment refers to all types of abuse and neglect of a child under age 18 by a parent, caregiver, or another person in a custodial role (Fortson et al., 2016) and is another indicator of children's physical and emotional health status. Almost five children die every day in the United States from child abuse and neglect. The reported number of child deaths from abuse and neglect increased to 1840 in 2019 1670 in 2017 (CDC, 2021d). Of note, nearly 50% of child abuse victims are under 1 year of age (American Society for the Positive Care of Children, 2021).

Child abuse may be physical, sexual, or emotional. Neglect is by far the most prevalent form of child maltreatment. *Child neglect* is the failure to provide for a child's basic physical, medical, emotional, or educational needs or to protect a child from harm or potential harm. It may include failure to provide affection, warmth, understanding, and supervision adequate for healthy development (CDC, 2021d).

Child maltreatment affects children of all races, ages, and ethnicities. Factors that place children at a higher risk for maltreatment include living in a family that is stressed by drug and alcohol abuse, poverty, chronic health problems, violence in the community or at home, and social isolation (USDHHS Administration for Children and Families, 2017).

There are many long-term effects of child abuse and neglect. The effects may be physical, such as brain damage in shaken baby syndrome; emotional, such as depression and low self-esteem; and behavioral, such as delinquency, promiscuity, eating disorders, poor academic achievement, and drug abuse. Extreme stress caused by abuse and neglect interferes with normal brain development, harming the basic architecture of the brain. Healthy brain development relies on consistent, reciprocal, and appropriate interactions between young children and their caretakers. Chronic deprivation of healthy, reciprocal interactions can lead to the persistent activation of the stress response, leading to poor academic achievement, low self-esteem, depression, promiscuity, drug abuse, and chronic health problems (National Scientific Council on the Developing Child, 2012).

Often, the perpetrators of maltreatment are parents, who themselves were victims, forming a cycle of abuse. The two dominant characteristics of abusive parents are a history of substance abuse and abuse from their own parents. Often, caretakers do not intend to hurt their children. They may be stressed by poverty, illness, or disability, and they may lack social support systems or coping skills. Young and inexperienced parents may not understand the physical, emotional, and behavioral needs of their children.

Children are never responsible for the harm done to them by others, and yet they may feel guilty for causing it. Many professionals, including nurses, social service workers, and teachers, are required by law to report child abuse. Nurses in the community must understand their ethical and legal obligations to report child maltreatment. They can also help create a climate that supports families and provides parents with alternatives to abusive behavior. Programs for parents can take many different forms. Positive parenting skills are at the core of such programs. Positive parenting skills include responsiveness to the emotional and physical needs of children, good communication, and appropriate discipline. This education

may occur in parents' homes, in schools, in medical or mental health clinics, or in other community settings. Nurse home visitors can be key in providing education. The ultimate goal is to prevent child maltreatment before it starts.

Children With Special Healthcare Needs

Children and youth with special healthcare needs are those who are at risk or have chronic physical, developmental, behavioral, or emotional conditions that necessitate health and related services beyond those required by children generally. These conditions include developmental disorders such as Down syndrome and autism spectrum disorder, mental health disorders such as depression and anxiety, seizures, allergies, asthma, and attention-deficit/hyperactivity disorder. Chronic conditions are those expected to last 12 months or more. Often children with special health care needs experience two or more chronic conditions (USDHHS, Health Resources and Services Administration, 2014).

Children with special healthcare needs frequently have multiple service needs, including public health; physical and mental health care; specialized diagnostic services; social services; and educational, vocational, and sometimes corrective services. Families trying to obtain care for children with special needs face challenges in dealing with differing eligibility criteria; duplication and gaps in services; inflexible funding sources; geographic, cultural, and financial barriers; and poor coordination of care. Children with special needs can benefit from a coordinated, comprehensive, integrated system of care—often called a medical home. A *medical home* is not a place, but, rather, an approach to providing care. Having a medical home strengthens the ability of children with multiple service needs to receive comprehensive care for complex conditions (Box 16.5).

The Individuals with Disabilities Education Act (IDEA), enacted by Congress in 1975, is intended to ensure that children with disabilities receive a free, appropriate public education. The law has been amended many times and addresses the needs of babies through school-age children. IDEA is known as

---

BOX 16.5 The Patient-Centered Medical Home

The American Academy of Pediatrics (AAP), as well as other entities the American Academy of Family Physicians (AAFP), and American College of Physicians (ACP), have endorsed the concept of a "medical home." This ideal suggests that every child, including special needs children, should have "accessible, continuous, comprehensive, family-centered, coordinated, and culturally effective" (AAP, 2021).

A medical home should be within a community-based system that has coordinated networks designed to promote the healthy development and well-being of children as they move from adolescence to adulthood. In the medical home, a practice-based care team is responsible for most of the care and refer the child for specialty care as needed. Such a system requires appropriate financing to support and sustain quality care, optimal outcomes, family satisfaction, and cost-efficiency (AAP, 2021).

the nation's "special education law" and is administered through the U.S. Department of Education (2020).

ADOLESCENT HEALTH ISSUES

Adolescence is a time of generally good health. It is a period when preteens and teens form lifelong health habits, including dietary and exercise habits and emotional health skills such as problem solving and coping strategies. Typically, adolescents do not use health services unless they have an underlying chronic condition or an acute illness. They rarely use preventive health services.

In their struggle to gain independence, many adolescents engage in risk-taking behaviors, including alcohol and drug abuse, tobacco use, early and unprotected sexual activity, unsafe driving, and participation in delinquent and violent activities that threaten their health. Such behaviors are influenced by peers, the family, and characteristics of communities in which they live. Risk taking among adolescents is greatly influenced by their ability to control their impulses at this stage of brain development. The part of the brain that is responsible for executive functioning, the prefrontal cortex, is not fully mature until near age 25. Even though a teen may understand that a behavior is risky, he or she may have difficulty "putting on the brakes" because of the immaturity of brain development and connections (USDHHS, Office of Population Affairs, 2020).

Traditional approaches to improving adolescent health have focused on specific risks; however, a collaborative, multipartner approach that centers on the strengths of the whole person in the community, rather than focusing on individual risks, may be more effective in helping adolescents avoid risks and develop social competence. The community health nurse can help parents and communities understand the nonmedical, public health nature of risky behaviors and can assist in the development of community-wide strategies to effectively deal with them. The Youth Risk Behavior Surveillance System (YRBSS), administered by the CDC's Division of Adolescent and School Health, monitors health risk behaviors in ninth through 12th graders that lead to morbidity and mortality (Underwood et al., 2020).

Sexual Risk Behavior

One of many risk-taking adolescent behaviors is sexual intercourse. Adolescent sexual activity is often unprotected and can result in unintended pregnancy, infection with HIV, and other sexually transmitted infections (STIs).

Among students surveyed in 2019, about 38.4% had ever had sexual intercourse. Nearly 27.4% had engaged in sexual intercourse during the 3 months preceding the survey. Of these, 54.3% reported that either they or their partner had used a condom during last sexual intercourse. Another 31.4% used another form of birth control, such as birth control pills, an injectable form of birth control, a birth control ring, an implant, or an intrauterine device to prevent pregnancy. Nearly 11.9% used no method of birth control during the last sexual intercourse. Of consequence, 21.2% had used alcohol or drugs before last sexual intercourse (Szucs et al., 2020).

RESEARCH HIGHLIGHTS

Does a Satisfactory Relationship With Her Mother Influence When a 16-Year-Old Female Begins to Have Sex?

A prospective panel study of more than 1500 female adolescents (not randomly selected) examined whether the dimensions within the mother–daughter relationship during young adolescence influenced sexual initiation prior to age 16 years. Researchers found that three dimensions within the relationship were associated with delayed sexual initiation: positive cohesion, communication, and satisfaction with time spent together. The researchers concluded that efforts in delaying sexual initiation in young adolescents need to be directed toward promoting positive mother–daughter relationships.

Data from Kovar C, Salsberry P: Does a satisfactory relationship with her mother influence when a 16-year-old begins to have sex? *MCN Am J Matern Child Nurs* 37(2):122–129, 2012.

Teen childbearing has been on the decline since the late 1950s, reaching a historic low at 16.7 births per 1000 women aged 15 to 19 years (Martin et al., 2021). In recent years, teens seem to be less sexually active, and more of those who are sexually active seem to be using birth control than in previous years (Szucs et al., 2020). Despite the declines in teen childbearing, the US adolescent birth rate remains one of the highest among industrialized nations (Kann et al., 2018). Large disparities exist among racial and ethnic groups. The teen pregnancy rate is lowest among non-Hispanic Asian and highest among non-Hispanic Native Hawaiian or other Pacific Islander and Black teenagers (Martin et al., 2021).

The consequences of early childbearing on mothers, children, and society are significant. Teen childbearing contributes greatly to high school dropout rates. Only half of teen mothers receive a high school diploma by 22 years of age, compared with approximately 90% of girls who did not give birth during adolescence (Perper et al., 2010). For the infant, having a teenage mother poses serious health risks, including death, prematurity, low birth weight, and social risks, such as lower school achievement, incarceration, teen pregnancy, and adult unemployment. Children born to teenage parents have lower school achievement and are more likely to drop out of high school. They are more likely to be incarcerated at some time during adolescence, father children as teenagers, require public assistance, and face unemployment as young adults. According to an analysis by the National Campaign to Prevent Teen Pregnancy, the estimated national cost of teen childbearing in the United States for taxpayers (federal, state, and local) is at least $9.4 billion per year (National Campaign to Prevent Teen and Unplanned Pregnancy, 2015).

STIs are another consequence of sexual risk behavior. These include human papillomavirus (HPV), *Chlamydia trachomatis*, herpes simplex virus type 2, HIV/AIDS, hepatitis B, gonorrhea, syphilis, and vaginal trichomoniasis. Teenagers are more likely than adults to acquire STIs (CDC, 2019b). For some infections, such as *C. trachomatis*, the difference may be due to a physiological susceptibility. Barriers to health care such as lack of transportation, concerns about confidentiality, and lack of access to preventive health services also contribute to a higher prevalence of STIs among teens. STIs may be asymptomatic in both males and females. Although many STIs clear on their own, others can persist over time, putting women at high risk for cervical cancer, pelvic inflammatory disease, ectopic pregnancy, and infertility. Not only is a woman's health affected, especially if the infections go untreated, but the infant born to a woman with an STI is at risk of infection and can suffer long-term consequences. Routine counseling and voluntary testing for sexually active teens and pregnant women is recommended. The HPV vaccination can protect against related disease and is the best way to prevent many types of cancer. The HPV vaccine is recommended for preteen girls and boys at age 11 or 12 years (CDC, 2019b).

The causes and effects of risky sexual behaviors are complex, and the solutions are multifaceted. One survey found that most parents feel they play an important role in providing guidance to their children about healthy sexual behavior, yet half of children are uncomfortable with these conversations. Parents who were surveyed overwhelmingly support school-based sex education programs, including information about birth control (Planned Parenthood, 2014).

Abstinence from vaginal, anal, and oral intercourse is the only 100% effective way to prevent HIV, other STIs, and pregnancy. Primary prevention models are most successful when they are evidence based and tailored to the community's individual needs. Components of such programs can include the following:
- Abstinence promotion
- Education about contraception and its availability
- Sex education
- Character development
- Problem-solving skill development
- Peer counseling programs
- Strategies for ensuring teenagers' school success
- Job training

Such efforts are more likely to succeed when there are partnerships among parents, adolescents, and agencies for health, education, religion, social service, and government. Nurses working within such organizations can play leadership roles in developing community programs for prevention of adolescent sexual risk behaviors.

Violence

Youth violence can be seen as a reflection of how well parents, schools, and the community are able to supervise and channel youth behavior in positive ways. Children and adolescents can be victims of, aggressors in, or witnesses to violence. For the victims, violence can cause both emotional and physical harm. For too many of the nation's youth, violence is a way of life, a way of coping with challenging and difficult situations, and a significant public health problem.

The rate of serious violent crime against youth ages 12 to 17 years declined 80% between 1995 and 2018. In 2018, male (41.4 victimizations per 1000) and female (25.9 per 1000) youth were equally likely to experience serious violent crime—rape or sexual assault, robbery, and aggravated assault. Black males are the racial group most likely to be victimized (Hullenaar and Ruback, 2020). Homicide is the third leading cause of death for young people ages 15–24 years (National Center for Health Statistics, 2019). Of homicide victims in 2016, 87% were killed with a firearm (Curtin et al., 2018). Handguns are readily accessible to America's youth. Federal law prohibits anyone under age 21 years from purchasing a handgun from a licensed dealer, but it does not prohibit anyone under age 21 years from purchasing a handgun from a nonlicensed dealer (Law Center to Prevent Gun Violence, 2016).

Teen dating violence consists of physical, sexual, or psychological/emotional violence (including stalking) within a dating relationship. In the 2019 Youth Risk Behavior Survey, 8.2% of high school students reported having been hit, slapped, or physically hurt on purpose by their boyfriend or girlfriend in the preceding 12 months (Basile et al., 2020). Teen dating violence can be emotionally and physically traumatizing and can lead to victimization and unhealthy relationships in the future.

Violence among youth is a complex public health problem with multifaceted risk factors. Risk factors include individual factors; influences by families and peers; and social, political, and cultural factors. The home environment is a key to the development of violent behavior in young people. Poor supervision of children and harsh physical punishment are associated with youth violence. Also linked to youth violence is associating with delinquent peers. At the social level, gang involvement, access to firearms, and drug use are more likely to increase youth violence (World Health Organization, 2020).

Teen violence does not have simple remedies. Solutions require community and neighborhood efforts to help young people diffuse anger and frustration before they escalate; to help parents, religious organizations, and schools assist their youth in managing anger and resolving conflicts; and to work with children and teenagers to assure them that they are loved, appreciated, and accepted for who they are. Reducing children's unsupervised exposure to guns (WHO, 2020) and strict firearm legislation may be protective of children even in areas of high gun ownership (Goyal et al., 2019).

Tobacco, Alcohol, and Drug Use

The use of tobacco, alcohol, and illicit drugs has serious and long-lasting consequences for adolescents and for society. The YRBSS (Creamer et al., 2020; Jones et al., 2020) provides a snapshot of behavioral trends. In 2019, the survey revealed the following:
- 6.2% of students had smoked cigarettes in the 30 days before the survey.
- 24.1% of students had ever tried cigarette smoking.
- 32.7% of students had used electronic vapor products in the 30 days before the survey.
- 29.2% of students had had at least one drink of alcohol in the 30 days before the survey.
- 13.7% of students had had five or more drinks of alcohol in a row (i.e., within a couple of hours—also known as binge drinking) in the 30 days before the survey.

- 7% of students had taken prescription opioid without a doctor's prescription in previous 30 days before the survey.
- 14.3% of students had lifetime of prescription opioid misuse.
- 36.8% of students had used marijuana one or more times during their lives (i.e., had ever used marijuana).
- 21.7% of students had used marijuana one or more times during the 30 days before the survey (i.e., current marijuana use).
- 48.8% of students had used synthetic marijuana one or more times during their lives.

Among the findings of the latest YRBSS survey are that smoking rates among teens have continued to decline since peaking in the mid-1990s. In contrast, illicit drug use by youths is constantly evolving as new drugs in new forms are introduced. "Designer drugs" or synthetic cannabinoids (aka "Spice" or "K2") have been banned in most states, but minor changes to the chemical makeup of these substances result in new substances that allow law breakers to circumvent existing drug laws (National Conference of State Legislatures, 2012; Sacco and Finklea, 2016). Also, prescription drugs used outside of medical supervision—for example, OxyContin, Ritalin, and steroids—have become more popular. Vaping prevalence grew rapidly from near-zero prevalence in 2011 to one of the most common forms of adolescent substance use. Despite a decline in 2017, the prevalence of vaping remains substantially higher than the use of any other tobacco product, including cigarettes (Creamer et al., 2020).

According to the Monitoring the Future Project of the University of Michigan, rumors of the supposed benefits of using a drug usually spread much faster than information about the adverse consequences. It generally takes much longer for evidence of adverse consequences, such as death, disease, overdose, and addictive potential, to become widely known, thus contributing to the widespread use of both legal and illegal drugs.

Adolescence is a critical time to prevent substance addiction. Drugs change brains, and early use of drugs increases a person's chances of more serious drug abuse and addiction (National Institute on Drug Abuse, 2020). Broad evidence-based prevention efforts, including addressing the issues of housing, poverty, and crime, are needed.

FACTORS AFFECTING CHILD AND ADOLESCENT HEALTH

As in other age groups, social, nonmedical factors largely determine children's health. Children depend on their families or caregivers for their health and well-being; therefore, the following factors significantly affect children's physical health, mental health, and overall well-being:
- Parents' or caregivers' income, education, and stability
- Security and safety of the home
- Nutritional and environmental issues
- Healthcare access and use

Poverty

Poverty is the greatest threat to child health. Child poverty in the United States is higher than in most other industrialized countries, and the rate is rising. About 11 million (14.4%) of the nation's children live below the federal poverty level (FPL) (Haider, 2021). The official poverty level is calculated by using poverty thresholds that are issued each year by the U.S. Census Bureau. The thresholds represent the annual amount of cash income minimally required to support families of various sizes. The 2021 poverty guideline for a family of three in the 48 contiguous states and the District of Columbia was $21,960 (USDHHS, 2021a,b). Many more children (about 41%) live in low-income families that are close to the poverty level and unable to meet basic living expenses. Children are far more likely than adults to live in poverty. Poverty rates are highest for black, Hispanic, and American Indian children (Koball and Jiang, 2018).

Factors associated with poverty include parental education, employment, and single parenting. Eighty-four percent of children whose parents do not have a high school education live in low-income families. Even if parents have full-time employment, low education levels make their children susceptible to poverty. Likewise, children in households headed by a single parent (usually the mother) are far more likely to live in poverty and thus to have more health risks; 76% of all children with single parents live in low-income families (Koball and Jiang, 2018).

Poverty by itself does not always put a child at risk; however, poor children face the following health and socioeconomic risks that can compound the burdensome influence of poverty (Federal Interagency Forum on Child and Family Statistics, 2020):
- Children in poverty have less access to nutritious food, shelter, and health care.
- Poor children are often deprived of advantages such as good schools, libraries, and other community resources.
- Deaths from unintended injuries, child maltreatment, homicide, STIs, and infectious diseases are more common among poor children.
- Many poor children live in substandard housing, have stressful home lives, may live surrounded by drugs and crime, and lack positive and nurturing adult role models.
- Poor children may feel hopeless about the future.
- Poor children often suffer from low birth weight, asthma, dental decay, high blood lead levels, learning disabilities, and teenage unmarried childbearing.
- Poor children are more likely to move frequently. Residential instability and extreme living conditions of poor children who are homeless or migrants usually compound their health problems.

These social and economic burdens can be overwhelming to parents or caregivers and may cause them to neglect other matters, such as providing a nutritious breakfast before school, taking a child for a well-child appointment, and getting his or her immunizations completed on schedule. They can create a sense of despair and hopelessness among parents and children, which greatly hinders healthy behavior. These factors clearly increase a child's physical and emotional health risks.

Racial and Ethnic Disparities

Although children in the United States are healthier now than in any other time in our nation's history, overall improvements

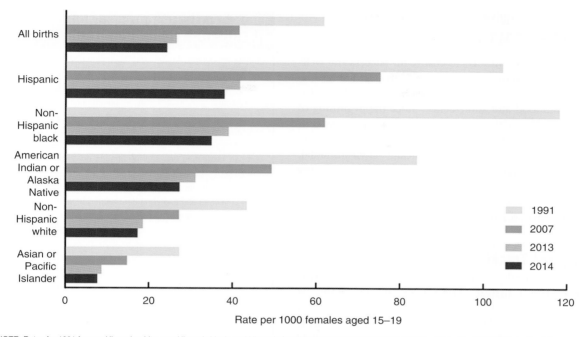

NOTE: Rates for 1991 for non-Hispanic white, non-Hispanic black, and Hispanic females exclude data for New Hampshire, which did not report Hispanic origin.

Fig. 16.4 Birth rates for women aged 15 to 19 in selected years between 1991 and 2019 by ethnicity.

in health mask the poor health of some racial and ethnic subgroups (Fig. 16.4). For example, as mentioned previously, the infant mortality rate has plunged over the past century, yet infants born to non-Hispanic black women are 2.5 times more likely to die in the first year of life than babies born to non-Hispanic white mothers. Native Americans and African Americans account for a disproportionate share of disabilities and deaths due to fetal alcohol exposure. African American youth are at higher risk for gun violence than white youth and are more than four times as likely to die from asthma as non-Hispanic white children. Childhood obesity affects racial and ethnic minority children at much higher rates than non-Hispanic whites, driving up rates of associated diabetes.

Eliminating health disparities is an important national health priority. *Healthy People 2030* (USDHHS, 2020) targets persistent differences in health among children of varying racial and ethnic groups and calls for the elimination of disparities in health. The term "social determinants of health" (SDOH) refers to the conditions within the environment where people live, work, go to school and play (NAS, 2021). The SDOH reflects the circumstances into which children are born, and exert a strong and persistent influence over their lifelong health. A child's ability to be healthy and productive in life is negatively affected by poverty, violence, and a family history of poor health along with systemic inequities such as limited access to quality health care, education, and job opportunities.

Community health nurses can develop an understanding of differences in health based on the SDOH such as race, ethnicity, and economic circumstances. They can translate experiences in the field into evidence-based intervention strategies that incorporate social programs such as education, employment, and housing into solutions for addressing health disparities.

Healthcare Use

Children grow and develop rapidly between infancy and adolescence; therefore, they are extremely vulnerable to the effects of illness and of environmental factors that influence physical and emotional health. Preventive health and dental care offer children and parents a chance to periodically meet with a healthcare provider to do the following:

- Discuss the child's physical and emotional growth and development.
- Learn about good nutrition.
- Address safety issues, such as the use of car seats and seatbelts.
- Receive immunizations and vision and hearing screening.
- Learn about potential environmental threats to the child's health.
- Begin prompt treatment for a condition discovered during the examination.
- Ask other questions or obtain a referral if necessary.

Access to a regular healthcare source can facilitate prompt attention to acute medical problems, which can help prevent chronic, disabling conditions. For example, untreated ear infections can cause hearing loss, which can lead to learning disabilities, school problems, and even school dropout. Resulting low self-esteem can increase the likelihood of depression, behavior problems, early sexual activity, STIs, and unplanned pregnancy. Comprehensive, regular health care helps all children achieve their potential.

STRATEGIES TO IMPROVE CHILD AND ADOLESCENT HEALTH

One of the most important ways to ensure the success and well-being of future generations is for each child to start life healthy and maintain his or her physical and emotional health status throughout childhood and adolescence. Since the beginning of the 20th century, the nation has made remarkable progress in many areas of child and adolescent health, but the results are mixed. Fortunately, scientific, medical, environmental, parenting, and other knowledge can lessen or eliminate many of the problems. It is a matter of making these concerns a priority and taking the necessary steps to elicit change. Box 16.6 lists several resources for monitoring the health and well-being of children.

Monitoring and Tracking

Federal, state, and local governments and many national organizations collect and analyze data to track the well-being of children and adolescents. For example, the Maternal and Child Health Bureau of the Health Resources and Services Administration (HRSA/MCHB, 2020) generates a yearly report, *Child Health USA,* on child population characteristics, health status, and healthcare utilization. Such data are readily accessible online to citizens, health professionals, policy makers, and the media. A number of key indicators are tracked on a regular basis by the federal statistical system so that trends are revealed. State and local data also are used to track the well-being of children.

Healthy People 2030: Child and Adolescent Health

Many professions establish goals and set measurable objectives. Educators use these techniques to organize their teaching materials, measure their students' progress, and evaluate the effectiveness of their teaching strategies and plans. Healthcare professionals use them for similar purposes in client care. The individual community health nurse uses them in working with a family to ensure that the nurse and family are organized and are guided by common purposes. Goals and objectives help the nurse and family evaluate progress and make necessary midcourse corrections.

These strategies are also important at the macrolevel and the programmatic level, where multiple players must collaborate to address complicated statewide or nationwide problems. In 1979, the surgeon general of the United States embarked on an ambitious task of convening hundreds of public health experts, healthcare researchers, health professional organizations, and others to develop the first health goals and objectives for the nation. At each of the intervening decades, these groups have developed a new set of goals and objectives to help bring clear focus to the health concerns of the nation and to set measurable and attainable goals for different age groups and issues across the country.

BOX 16.6   Resources: Monitoring the Health and Well-Being of Children

Centers for Disease Control and Prevention (CDC): Monitors many health and disease prevention efforts, including the Youth Risk Behavior Surveillance System, which monitors youth tobacco, alcohol, and drug use; dietary behaviors; and sexual behaviors contributing to unintended pregnancy and sexually transmitted infections. (www.cdc.gov.)

Federal Interagency Forum on Child and Family Statistics: On an annual basis, produces *America's Children: Key National Indicators of Well-Being,* a report containing detailed information on a set of key indicators of child well-being. (www.childstats.gov.)

National Center for Education Statistics (NCES): The primary federal agency for collecting and analyzing data related to education in the United States. (www.nces.ed.gov.)

National Center for Health Statistics (NCHS): Provides birth and death data, including birth certificate information. (www.cdc.gov/nchs.)

U.S. Bureau of Justice Statistics: Collects information about juvenile offenders. (www.ojp.usdoj.gov/bjs.)

U.S. Bureau of Labor Statistics: Provides a variety of employment data. (http://www.bls.gov/)

U.S. Census Bureau provides current census figures and analysis. (www.census.gov.)

U.S. Department of Health and Human Services (USDHHS): Program *Healthy People 2030* is a framework of goals and objectives for the nation's health. (www.healthypeople.gov.)

Healthy People 2030 (USDHHS, 2021a,b) sets broad national health goals for the third decade of the 21st century. This initiative, like its predecessors, helps define the nation's health agenda and guides policy development. *Healthy People 2030* addresses many challenges facing the country and helps the public and private sectors understand the nation's leading health problems, helps the two sectors develop strategic plans for addressing them, and collaborates to reach common goals. The Healthy People box lists selected objectives from *Healthy People 2030* related to child and adolescent health.

Since the inception of the *Healthy People* initiative in 1979, child and adolescent health has improved. For instance, there have been improvements in infant, child, and adolescent mortality; adolescent smoking; pregnancy; and violence.

♥ HEALTHY PEOPLE 2030

Selected Objectives related to Child and Adolescent Health

AH-05—Increase the proportion of fourth graders with reading skills at or above the proficient level.

AH-08—Increase the proportion of high school students who graduate in 4 years.

EH-09—Reduce exposure to mercury in children.

EMC-02—Increase the proportion of children whose parents red to them at least 4 days per week.

EMC-03—Increase the proportion of children who get sufficient sleep.

EMC-D03—Increase the proportion of children who participate in high-quality early childhood education programs.

EMC-D04—Increase the proportion of children and adolescents who get appropriate treatment for anxiety or depression.

HOSCD-04—Reduce ear infections in children.

IID-02—Reduce the proportion of children who get no recommended vaccines by age 2 years.

IVP-15—Reduce child abuse and neglect deaths.

MHMD-03—Increase the proportion of children with mental health problems who get treatment.

MICH-03—Reduce the rate of deaths in children and adolescents aged 1–19 years.

MICH-17—Increase the proportion of children who receive a developmental screening.

MICH-19—Increase the proportion of children and adolescents who receive care in a medical home.

NWS-04—Reduce the proportion of children and adolescents with obesity.

PA-13—Increase the proportion of children aged 2–5 years who get no more than 1 h of screen time a day.

SDOH-05—Reduce the proportion of children with a parent or guardian who has served time in jail.

V-01—Increase the proportion of children aged 3–5 years who get vision screening.

From U.S. Department of Health and Human Services: *Healthy People 2030*, Washington, DC, 2021, U.S. Government Printing Office. Available from https://health.gov/healthypeople.

Health Promotion and Disease Prevention

Health promotion and disease prevention are more significant and cost-effective for children than for any other age group. Primary health care and early intervention for children and families can help prevent costly problems, suffering, and lost human potential. The following examples illustrate this point:

1. Preterm birth (birth before 37 weeks of pregnancy) is the leading cause of infant death and long-term neurological disabilities in children (CDC, 2020a).
2. Preventing pregnancy among teenagers can reduce the rates of school dropout, welfare dependency, low birth weight, and infant mortality. It has been estimated that teen childbearing costs taxpayers billions of dollars every year in expenses associated with health and foster care, criminal justice, and public assistance (National Campaign to Prevent Teen and Unplanned Pregnancy, 2015).

Health promotion and disease prevention strategies for improving child and adolescent health come in many forms and originate in research institutions, public agencies, private businesses, and community-based organizations. They can include the following:

1. Clinical interventions
2. Public health efforts that identify trends and develop population-based, community-wide, or individual strategies to affect them
3. Philanthropic endeavors that fund initiatives at the community, state, and regional levels
4. Public policy initiatives that create or improve public programs or provide incentives for nongovernmental entities to address identified problems

PUBLIC HEALTH PROGRAMS TARGETED TO CHILDREN AND ADOLESCENTS

A number of public programs address the health needs of children, and many target medically underserved or low-income individuals and families. In addition, local and state public health and social service agencies aim to protect the health of an entire community or state through programs such as water fluoridation, sanitation, and infectious disease control. Furthermore, broad-based strategies such as lead-based paint elimination, mandatory child safety seats in automobiles, bicycle helmet laws, teen pregnancy prevention programs, comprehensive school health clinics, and drug and violence prevention programs serve to improve the health of children using community-wide approaches.

Health Care Coverage Programs

Approximately 5.6% of American children under 18 years of age do not have health insurance. Hispanic children are more likely than children of other races to be uninsured as almost 8% of them were uninsured in 2018 (Tolbert and Orgera, 2020) (Fig. 16.5). Children who do not have health insurance are more likely to lack a source of health care, to have unmet health needs, and to experience worse health outcomes than children with insurance. Efforts to expand health care coverage for pregnant women and children have been successful, and provisions of the ACA helped further ensure affordable preventive services and health care coverage.

Among other provisions, for pregnant women, the ACA expanded options for health care insurance. Job-based health plans and new insurance plans are not allowed to deny or exclude coverage for pregnant women or children on the basis of a preexisting condition, including a disability. The ACA mandated certain preventive services at no cost, such as vaccinations for children and breast-feeding support. Teens and adults younger than 26 years can stay insured under their parent's insurance plan if the plan allows dependent coverage.

Medicaid and the Children's Health Insurance Program

The ability to pay for healthcare greatly influences whether a parent takes a child to see a healthcare provider. Medicaid (Title XIX of the Social Security Act) is a health insurance program for poor and low-income people. It is a federal/state entitlement program that plays an important role in providing health coverage for low-income women and children. The federal government sets the minimum guidelines for Medicaid eligibility, and states can chose to expand eligibility through the Children's Health Insurance Program (CHIP). Depending on the state, the average CHIP income eligibility level for children is 170% to 400% of the FPL. Together, Medicaid and CHIP serve about half of all low-income children (Medicaid and CHIP Payment and Access Commission, 2018).

Within broad national guidelines, each state establishes eligibility standards based on a family's income in comparison with the FPL, determines the type and scope of services, and

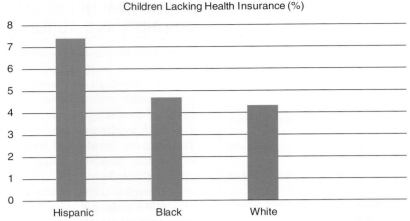

Children Lacking Health Insurance (%)

Fig. 16.5 Children less than 18 years of age and lacking health insurance by race, 2018. (Data from U.S. Census Bureau Current Population Reports: *Health insurance coverage in the United States: 2018 current population reports,* 2020. Available from: https://www.childstats.gov/americaschildren/tables/hc1.asp.)

administers its own Medicaid and CHIP programs. States have some discretion in determining which population groups their programs will cover. Thus a pregnant woman or child who is eligible for the program in one state may not be eligible in another.

Through the Early and Periodic Screening, Diagnosis, and Treatment (EPSDT) program, a child covered by Medicaid can receive a range of health and health-related services beginning in infancy. The program is designed to assure availability and accessibility of health care resources and to help Medicaid recipients and their parents effectively use them. The program's services far exceed those usually covered by private insurance and include the following:

- Health, developmental, and nutritional screening
- Physical examinations
- Immunizations
- Vision and hearing screening
- Certain laboratory tests
- Dental services

Expansions in public healthcare insurance programs have helped many children achieve insurance coverage, but many children still lack insurance or other health care coverage like Medicaid or CHIP for many reasons, some of which are as follows:

- Insurance is too expensive.
- Medicaid has a welfare stigma, and parents do not want to be associated with it.
- Medicaid application forms and processes can be complex and burdensome and can intrude on a family's privacy.
- Parents may be concerned that their illegal immigration status may be revealed.
- Parents may not consider the importance of health insurance.
- Parents may not know their child is eligible for programs such as Medicaid and CHIP.

- Applications and other information may not be available in the family's language.

Although insurance gives a child financial access to health care, some children may not obtain the health care they need for other reasons. Numerous health care or family barriers can still stand in the way. They include the following (Angier et al., 2014; World Health Organization, n.d.):

- Lack of transportation
- Language barriers
- Lack of knowledge and awareness
- Inconveniences associated with provider's office (clinic or office hours that conflict with work or school schedules; overcrowded clinics with delays in the waiting room)
- Competing family or personal priorities that reduce the importance of obtaining care
- Providers' unwillingness to see Medicaid or low-income clients
- Parent's concerns that care providers are either unresponsive to their medical needs or interpersonally disrespectful
- Lack of affordability, such as cost of deductibles, copayments, medications

To successfully meet the health needs of children and adolescents, especially those with known risk factors, the community health nurse must be cognizant of healthcare access issues, family and neighborhood influences, and other social concerns in a child's life. The nurse must be prepared to help the family solve problems, to be their healthcare system advocate, and to address the child's health needs in a culturally competent manner.

Direct Healthcare Delivery Programs

Although Medicaid and CHIP finance health care for their enrollees like private insurance, several other public programs deliver healthcare services directly to underserved populations. Most underserved aggregates live in inner cities or rural areas with few healthcare providers and facilities. Some have Medicaid, CHIP, or other insurance coverage, but many are uninsured.

Maternal and Child Health Block Grant

The Maternal and Child Health (MCH) Block Grant program (also called *Title V,* because it is the fifth section, or title, of the Social Security Act) allocates federal funds to the states, and the states must contribute their own funds for maternal and child health services. It is administered by the Maternal and Child Health Bureau as a part of the USDHHS's Health Resources and Services Administration. Established in 1935, the Title V MCH Block Grant has provided a foundation of healthcare services for mothers, children (including those with special health care needs), and families over the years. States must match every four dollars of federal Title V money with three dollars of state and/or local funding to help ensure the delivery of basic health care to pregnant women and children and help deliver additional services to children with special health care needs. Agencies in state health departments also monitor the health status of mothers and children throughout their respective states and work with other state agencies to develop programs to improve the health of this population.

The Consolidated Health Centers Program, managed by the Health Services Administration (HRSA) within the Department of Health and Human Services (HHS), provides funding to more than 9000 primary healthcare clinics in geographically isolated and economically distressed areas.

These health centers provide comprehensive, culturally competent, primary, and preventive health care to a diverse population, including individuals who are low income, uninsured, and experiencing homelessness. Services are provided to all residents of the service area without regard to an individual's ability to pay. This successful program provides primary care services, including health, dental, mental health, and pharmacy, as well as services that promote access to health care such as language interpretation, case management, and transportation.

School-Based Health Centers

Adolescents are the least likely aggregate to use healthcare services, especially preventive services. Their adolescent healthcare needs are different from their childhood needs, and they may be uncomfortable seeing a pediatrician or their childhood provider. Furthermore, they may or may not be able to discuss sensitive topics such as sexuality, substance use, and peer relationships with their parents. Some may not want their parents to know they have a health problem; therefore, they may not want to see the family's healthcare provider out of concern about privacy and confidentiality. As a result, their healthcare needs may go unmet.

School-based health centers typically provide a combination of screening and preventive services, primary care, mental health and substance abuse counseling, dental health, nutrition education, and other health promotion activities. State dollars,

mostly from general funds and the MCH Block Grant, are the primary sources of funding for school-based health care. A growing number of health centers participate in the Medicaid and CHIP programs, and some provide services within a managed care network. Expansion of school-based health centers has been made possible under the ACA.

Special Supplemental Nutrition Program for Women, Infants, and Children (WIC)

Although it is not a health program exclusively, WIC gives federal grants to states for the purpose of serving nutritionally at-risk, low-income, pregnant and postpartum women, and their children up to 5 years of age. WIC programs provide highly nutritious foods, nutrition education and counseling, and screening and referral to needed services. To be eligible, women and children must meet income guidelines established by each state, and a health professional must determine they are at "nutritional risk." Women and children who participate in Medicaid, the food stamp program, or the Temporary Assistance for Needy Families program are automatically eligible for WIC. Fifty-six percent of all infants born in the United States are served by WIC (U.S. Department of Agriculture Food and Nutrition Service, 2020).

WIC clinics operate in a number of sites, including health clinics, hospitals, schools, public housing sites, and mobile clinics. Women participating in the program are encouraged to obtain prenatal care if they are pregnant. They are also encouraged to maintain healthy diets and obtain preventive health care for themselves and their children, including childhood immunizations.

Established in 1972, WIC is one of the most successful, popular, and cost-effective public health programs. Some of the many benefits attributed to WIC include the following:

- Improvements in birth outcomes and healthcare cost savings
- Improved infant feeding practices, better low-birth-weight rate, and more regular primary care
- Lower rates of childhood obesity

SHARING RESPONSIBILITY FOR IMPROVING CHILD AND ADOLESCENT HEALTH

Most children in the United States are born healthy and remain healthy throughout childhood. However, the protective factors operating in the lives of healthy children and the interventions they receive are not available to all children. Although public-sector programs have attempted to provide a "safety net" for children, these interventions cannot address all the needs of children. For example, the healthcare system may provide emergency care to a 9-year-old child injured by gunfire in a drive-by shooting, but it cannot address the community conditions that perpetuate violence.

Child health is affected by many factors; therefore, the responsibility for improving children's health rests with the entire community. This responsibility begins with parents and includes healthcare professionals, community groups, businesses, and the public sector. When a child is older, he or she can be responsible for practicing healthy behaviors and obtaining proper health care.

Parents' Role

Even before conception, a woman can help ensure the health of her fetus by practicing healthy behaviors herself. Reproductive life planning can help a woman set personal goals and priorities and design strategies to meet these goals. This planning may entail avoiding unwanted pregnancy and/or learning about specific actions she can take to increase her chances for having a healthy baby should she desire a child in the future. If pregnancy is desired, a woman can learn to manage chronic health conditions and to develop healthy behaviors, including proper nutrition with folic acid supplementation and avoidance of tobacco, alcohol, drugs, and other behaviors that could harm a developing baby. It is also important for the mother to receive prenatal care early in pregnancy.

Starting with breast-feeding, parents must give their children nutritious food and ensure that they are immunized, receive needed healthcare services, and acquire healthful lifestyles. Breast-feeding provides many health benefits for mothers and their children (Box 16.7).

Another important task for parents is to ensure that their children have a safe environment at home, in the neighborhood, and at school. They must protect their children from injury, violence, abuse, and neglect. Parents must learn how to nurture, guide, and protect their children effectively through the developmental stages of childhood and adolescence.

Community's Role

Families need support from their community and society to fulfill their roles and responsibilities. This is particularly true for families who live in poverty and for parents who are isolated and disenfranchised. Ensuring access to health care is an important community role, but communities are also responsible for promoting well-being, which goes far beyond the provision of traditional medical care.

Communities should work to create safe neighborhoods and support the development of community-based comprehensive health, education, housing, and social service programs. Collaborative, multipartner approaches that concentrate on helping children and adolescents avoid risks and develop social competence are more likely to be effective than fragmented programs focusing on individual risks, such as teen drug use. Communities are well situated to facilitate the integration of health, education, and social services; to eliminate fragmentation and duplication of services; to provide culturally competent care; and to better organize more comprehensive and streamlined systems of care. Although many health and social service programs exist, they can be poorly coordinated with one another, with little collaboration among the professional disciplines.

The media are part of the community at large and should be involved in promoting child and adolescent health. The media significantly influence children's lives, their perceptions of the world, and their self-images. From developing informational campaigns about prenatal care and immunizations to discouraging violence and explicit sex in advertising and popular television programs, the media can have a profound effect on improving children's health and well-being.

Employer's Role

Business and industry have an enormous stake in the health of the nation's children. A strong, productive workforce is ensured only when the health, social, and educational needs of the next generation of workers are met. Furthermore, health risks cost employers in lost productivity and increased healthcare costs.

The private sector can play a role in improving the health of individual children or the community in general. An employer can make health care more accessible to families with children by offering affordable health insurance that covers employees and dependents. The provision of insurance plans that offer full pregnancy and well-child healthcare benefits is essential to employee health promotion. Employers can meet the requirements of the U.S. Department of Labor (2018) by supporting nursing mothers in the workplace. This includes providing reasonable break time to express milk and a private space other than a bathroom in which to do so.

Maintaining a workplace that allows flexible leave for prenatal and pediatric health care and allows time off to care for newborn and sick children can also contribute to child health improvements. In 1993, the Family and Medical Leave Act (FMLA) mandated that employers with 50 or more employees must allow a total of 12 work weeks of unpaid leave during any 12-month period for the birth, adoption, or foster care of a child or for the care of a seriously ill family member or the employee himself or herself. The Department of Labor issued a Final Rule on February 25, 2015, revising the definition of spouse under the FMLA of 1993. Revision of the definition ensures same-sex married spouses the same ability as all spouses to fully exercise their FMLA rights (U.S. Department of Labor, 2015).

BOX 16.7 Breast-Feeding: The Feeding Method of Choice

Breast-feeding is uniquely superior for infant feeding. The practice imparts many health benefits for mothers and babies.

Benefits for children include the following:
- Decreased incidence and severity of a wide range of infectious diseases
- Decreased infant mortality
- Decreased risk of sudden infant death syndrome (SIDS)
- Reduction in the incidence of diabetes, respiratory infections, and some cancers
- Lower risk of overweight and obesity
- Enhanced cognitive development

Benefits of breast-feeding for mothers include the following:
- Decreased postpartum bleeding
- Earlier return to prepregnancy weight
- Decreased risk of breast and ovarian cancer

The American Academy of Pediatrics (AAP) and many other health organizations recommend exclusive breast-feeding for the first 6 months of life with continuation of breast-feeding for 1 year or longer as mutually desired by mother and infant (AAP, 2021).

In addition, employers can sponsor education opportunities for employees about topics such as healthy diets, healthy pregnancies, substance abuse, and stress management. Businesses can also offer onsite child care and can work with community leaders and public officials to initiate community-wide health promotion projects targeted to children. Finally, employers can be catalysts in their communities for linking health, education, and social services for children.

Government's Role

In the United States, government's role in promoting or ensuring children's health is more limited than in many other countries. Other countries often have defined policies on children's health; the United States does not. Such policies not only indicate that children are a priority of the citizenry but also help shape the operation of programs and their funding.

As discussed earlier, US state and federal governments have several public health programs that provide assistance to children, especially to those at risk from poverty or other disadvantages. Monitoring the health of children is also a governmental role. Although these programs are not a substitute for a family or caregiver's care and concern, they are important in protecting and promoting health and delivering services to those who would otherwise go without. Programs with significant funding exist, but many children with health problems do not receive the services they need for reasons previously discussed.

Managers and front-line workers (e.g., community health nurses, social workers, physicians, and caseworkers) in effective community programs should be encouraged to collaborate and thereby assist children with problems that adversely affect their health. "One-stop shopping" (i.e., user-friendly, accessible services for children and families) is an important concept for public and community programs to embrace to ensure that children easily receive needed services. Outreach and referral efforts should be an integral part of health initiatives to provide children with the services they require. Community health nurses are often an essential part of these efforts.

Community/Public Health Nurse's Role

Public health nurses have always played pivotal roles in improving the health status of pregnant women, children, and adolescents. Within the community, the community health nurse is often most aware of children's health status, any barriers that prevent children from receiving necessary care, and other factors that may adversely affect their health. Armed with this information and knowledge about available health resources in the community, the community health nurse is:

- An advocate for improved individual and community responses to children's needs
- A researcher for effective strategies to serve women and children
- A participant in publicly funded programs
- A promoter of social interventions that enhance the living situations of high-risk families
- A partner with other professionals to improve service collaboration and coordination

One important role of the community health nurse is to help link local health and social services with the school system. Children must be healthy to learn; however, children may come to school with vision, hearing, and other health problems that appropriate education, screening, and treatment could have prevented or alleviated. When children pass the preschool years, the school health nurse is sometimes their only connection to the healthcare system. School health nurses can be important sources of primary health care and health information for students and their families.

Community health nurses can alert the health professional community, business leaders, religious groups, and voluntary organizations to children's and adolescents' needs and to the strategies that can improve their health. Community health nurses can influence the planning and implementation of necessary changes in the healthcare system to ensure improved children's health. Also, they can promote commitment within their own institutions for comprehensive, culturally competent care.

Home visiting is a strategy that connects community health nurses, paraprofessionals, or lay home visitors to families in order to provide education, support, and referrals. One home visiting model, administered through the Nurse–Family Partnership, partners low-income, first-time mothers with maternal and child health nurses. Pregnant women develop trusting relationships with their nurse home visitors and receive the care and support needed for healthy pregnancy and parenting. Financial self-sufficiency is encouraged (Nurse-Family Partnership, 2015).

LEGAL AND ETHICAL ISSUES IN CHILD AND ADOLESCENT HEALTH

Every day, community health nurses are involved in making decisions. In each encounter with a client, the nurse's decisions or the family's choices have the potential to influence the health and well-being of the family or the community at large for better or for worse.

People often assume that healthcare professionals, particularly nurses, are by nature attuned to the ethical implications of their decisions. In addition, the community trusts that nurses are aware of the legal ramifications of their actions and decisions, of their clients' decisions, and of the health care and legal systems' decisions. In reality, the ever-changing pressures of serving the community's healthcare needs leave little time to reflect on the ethical and moral implications of a given situation. In some cases, it may seem easier to avoid tough decisions. An ethical approach to decision making allows the community health nurse to evaluate a client's or a population's needs more honestly and completely and take appropriate action. Understanding the legal environment will help the nurse make informed decisions and effectively assist clients with their decision-making processes.

Ethical Issues

The complex nature of public health and healthcare delivery environments often sets the stage for conflicts of interest and values. Meanwhile, nurses and other health professionals must work within the system to improve child and adolescent health in a country of great differences. Such differences exist between races and cultures, and there are great dichotomies, such as the affluence of some and the poverty of many others. For the perinatal nurse, for example, ethical dilemmas may arise because she is an advocate for two clients: the pregnant woman and her fetus. The scope of ethical and legal dilemmas is broad. The Ethical Insights box lists specific ethical issues related to child and adolescent health.

ETHICAL INSIGHTS

Ethical Issues Related to Child and Adolescent Health

Allocation decisions: Given limited time and resources, what level of care should a nurse offer a child and his or her family?

Maternal-fetal conflict: Sometimes there are opposing ethical concerns for the pregnant woman and her fetus—for example, whether the benefits of prolonging a pregnancy justify the risk of complications for a pregnant woman or whether court-ordered treatment for a substance-abusing pregnant woman overrides the right to autonomy for a pregnant woman.

Client autonomy: In each specific case, who should make healthcare decisions for a young client, especially when opposing opinions arise? The client? The parents or guardian? The nurse or other healthcare professional? At what age does a child become mature enough to participate in such decision making? What laws does any given state have that affect adolescent client autonomy? What should the community health nurse do if he or she believes the client's or parent's decisions are not in the best interest of the client?

Privacy and confidentiality: Is an intervention appropriate if the community health nurse identifies gross noncompliance, neglect, or abuse? Is an intervention appropriate if in making it the nurse must break confidentiality? When and how should the nurse take action?

"Gaming the system": When the health care system's rules appear to impede the nurse's ability to serve the client's best interest, is it acceptable to circumvent the system? If so, what are the moral and legal costs?

Cultural competence: The United States will continue to experience huge demographic changes and greater diversity; nurses will face different cultural definitions of what is and what is not acceptable or ethical. How should the community health nurse respond to a client or population group that does not share the same cultural outlook on health? What is the nurse's legal justification, if any, for responding in a certain way?

Health disparities and access to care: What are the nurses' responsibilities in ensuring that women and children have access to health care? How can nurses influence policy decisions that affect community health care?

Prenatal diagnosis and newborn screening: What are potential long-term consequences of identifying genetic conditions? Are parents fully informed of negative consequences of genetic diagnoses, including stigmatization, discrimination, and psychological effects?

These issues invariably involve value judgments and challenge a nurse's bounds of professional and personal duty. They also require the community health nurse to stay abreast of legislative changes at the local, state, and national levels and participate in professional activities that can help him or her stay current in these important matters. By recognizing the ethical implications of the care and advice they give or the actions they take, nurses can embrace their duty to promote the health and well-being of individual clients and the community more completely, protect their clients from harm, and strive for healthcare fairness and justice for all clients.

Recognizing the value of engaging in a shared dialogue with colleagues regarding ethical decision-making issues and understanding the possible legal implications of their decisions are equally important. The choices can be complex; therefore, receiving the guidance of an ethics board or gaining a second opinion can be critical to making the right choices. On a broader scale, a community health nurse's ethical perspective can enhance any discussion about individual client care and overall community health and also can affect the direction of the country's public health policy.

❓ ACTIVE LEARNING

1. Develop strategies to inform parents whose children are uninsured about the availability of CHIP.
2. Spend a day with a school health nurse and analyze what could help prevent or address the health problems and issues he or she encountered throughout the day.
3. Communicate with those in policy-making positions by writing letters or holding meetings about children's needs.
4. Identify the public health and advocacy organizations in the community that are working to address children's health needs and identify their strategies for promoting child health within the community.
5. If your community has a lay home visitor program, meet with a home visitor and, if possible, accompany him or her during home visits.

CASE STUDY   Application of the Nursing Process

Pregnant Teenager

By applying the principles of the nursing process to the individual, family, and community, the community health nurse can provide services to children and adolescents more systematically and effectively. Most communities offer a range of preventive services and other important programs that children need. The community health nurse must thoroughly understand the needs of the individual child and family and must be aware of available community resources to help meet the child's health needs, as this case study illustrates.

Maria Martinez, a community health nurse working for the county health department, received a call from the high school nurse informing her that a 16-year-old high school student named Kaylah M. would come in that afternoon for a pregnancy test. Kaylah had already missed three menstrual periods and was afraid to talk about it with her family. She had a long discussion with the school nurse and asked her boyfriend, also aged 16, to take her to the health department clinic after school for the pregnancy test.

Assessment

Kaylah's pregnancy test result was positive, and she was an estimated 3-month pregnant. She was upset and would not speak with Maria at the health department. With agreement from Kaylah, Maria arranged to make a home visit the next afternoon.

Knowing that she needed to address a number of issues at the first home visit, Maria prepared by developing a list of possible assessment areas that covered individual, family, and community concerns, as follows:

Individual
- Health risk factors
- Emotional well-being, including concerns about community safety, domestic violence, and sexual abuse
- Cultural beliefs and attitudes toward pregnancy and medical care
- Barriers to communication with providers, such as language, hearing, and sight

CASE STUDY Application of the Nursing Process—cont'd

- Understanding and acceptance of pregnancy
- Health-promoting and risk-taking behaviors
- Understanding the importance of obtaining preventive care services
- Health insurance status
- Access to transportation

Family
- Adequacy of housing structure
- Safety of neighborhood
- Ability of family members to provide emotional support
- Ability of family to provide financial support
- Ability and willingness of the father of the baby to provide support

Community
- Availability of affordable and culturally sensitive prenatal and pediatric care
- Health and social services coordination
- Emotional guidance and counseling
- Educational opportunities for pregnant and parenting teenagers
- Job training
- Nutrition services such as WIC and food stamps
- Pregnancy and parenting education
- Child care availability

Assessment Data
Individual
- Kaylah was already in the early second trimester of pregnancy and had not received prenatal care. She also engaged in risk-taking behaviors (i.e., smoking, alcohol use, unprotected sex, and poor eating habits) potentially detrimental to her baby.
- During the interview, Kaylah seemed quiet and reserved. She said she was excited to have a baby but feared labor and delivery.
- Her boyfriend wanted her to keep the baby but was not committed to supporting Kaylah or the baby. He did not want to involve his own parents.
- Kaylah said she did not think about prenatal care much but would probably visit a health clinic sometime before her delivery. Her family did not have health insurance, and she said they could not afford prenatal care.
- She wanted to keep the baby and remain in school, yet she did not have a realistic understanding of parental responsibilities.

Family
- When Kaylah told her parents she was pregnant, they expressed disappointment. Her mother voiced a willingness to provide emotional support, but her seemingly emotionally distant father expressed anger.
- Both parents expressed concern about how the family would manage financially.
- After a brief review of the family's financial situation, it appeared that Kaylah was eligible for Medicaid and WIC.
- Her parents wanted her to have no further contact with her boyfriend.

Community
- Maria determined that prenatal services were available, but only during school hours. Although the only clinic that accepted Medicaid clients was on the other side of town, a nearby obstetrical practice with a certified nurse-midwife on staff accepted clients with Medicaid coverage. However, their primary clientele consisted of middle-class, married women.
- Applying for Medicaid and the WIC program required Kaylah to go to the welfare office and apply during school hours. However, the hospital outpatient department could make a preliminary Medicaid eligibility determination, which might be more convenient.
- Although Medicaid would pay for some prenatal classes, those nearby were geared to older, married couples.

- Kaylah's school encouraged her to remain in regular classes until her delivery date and participate in home study for a limited time thereafter.
- No parenting classes geared toward adolescents were available.
- Child care was not available at the high school, making a return to school more difficult for Kaylah.
- Although the community has a lay home visitor program that matches mentors with pregnant and parenting teens and provides health information and encouragement, the project does not serve Kaylah's neighborhood.

Diagnosis
Individual
- Unhealthy lifestyle choices related to the lack of prenatal care and the effect of poor nutrition, smoking, and alcohol use on fetal development
- Parenting issues related to unrealistic expectations about parenting responsibilities
- Lack of knowledge related to infant and child safety issues, such as the use of child safety seats, advantages of breast-feeding, safe sleep for infants, and use of preventive health care, including immunizations

Family
- Disrupted family dynamics related to anger and disappointment over daughter's pregnancy
- Altered financial status resulting from the addition of another dependent to the family

Community
- Lack of coordinated, culturally sensitive, accessible prenatal and parenting services for adolescents
- Existing lay home visitor program not available

Planning
To ensure the action plan is complete, realistic, and successfully implemented, Maria must thoroughly identify the factors affecting Kaylah's health and well-being. In addition, Kaylah, her family, and Maria must set mutual goals.

Individual
Long-Term Goals
- Pregnancy outcome will be healthy for mother and infant.
- Kaylah will demonstrate successful parenting behaviors.
- Kaylah will complete high school.

Short-Term Goals
- Kaylah will obtain prenatal care.
- Kaylah will understand the reasons to change nutrition and substance use habits.
- Kaylah and the nurse will plan actions to change poor health habits.
- Kaylah will remain in school throughout her pregnancy and will use the home study program until she returns to school after her baby is born.
- Kaylah will enroll in parenting class. If classes are not available, she will use age-appropriate reading materials, films, CDs, Internet resources, opportunities for group discussion with other teens, or visits with experienced parents.
- Kaylah will breast-feed her baby.
- Kaylah will speak with the community health educator to determine methods to protect the health and safety of her newborn.

Family
Long-Term Goal
- The family's ability to handle crises will improve with their ability to discuss problems and engage in mutual problem solving.

Continued

CASE STUDY Application of the Nursing Process—cont'd

Short-Term Goal

- Kaylah's parents will display supportive behaviors, such as accompanying her to prenatal care appointments, helping her engage in healthy behaviors, and helping her arrange child care so she can remain in school.

Community
Long-Term Goal

- Accessible, comprehensive, culturally sensitive prenatal and other healthcare services will be established, including home visiting and parenting classes targeted to adolescents.

Short-Term Goals

- The health department clinic will extend evening hours to accommodate students and working families.
- A child care facility will open in or near the high school.

Intervention

The nurse, family, and individual must address their immediate, mutual goals to help Kaylah achieve a healthy birth outcome and begin successful parenting. Interdisciplinary planning among Kaylah's school health nurse, caseworker, community health nurse, primary pregnancy care provider, childbirth educator, and family planning nurse is critical. In addition, Maria must be an advocate for community-wide change to ensure that the community is meeting individuals' needs.

Individual

Maria worked with the school nurse and other health professionals to help Kaylah obtain Medicaid and WIC; she was referred to an obstetrician who saw her regularly. Kaylah's pregnancy was also monitored by the school nurse, who had her come to the clinic on a weekly basis to check her weight and blood pressure and to talk with her about pregnancy-related issues.

Working with the school nurse, Maria provided Kaylah with information on childbirth classes and nutrition as well as booklets detailing how to promote a healthy pregnancy. She was counseled to avoid tobacco, alcohol, and all drugs. Near the end of the pregnancy, Kaylah was encouraged to attend parenting classes with her boyfriend.

Family

Maria and the social worker referred Kaylah's parents to other social service agencies that might be able to help financially. In particular, they focused on providers who could assist with utilities, job placement, and child care. The family was also referred to a family counselor who specialized in working with families with adolescent children.

Community

Maria worked with the maternal-child health division of the county health department to help facilitate offering parenting classes at an area high school, targeting the learning needs of pregnant teens. She and the school nurse also met with school district officials and community leaders to stimulate dialogue about the consequences of dropping out of high school and to facilitate action in policies such as child care for parenting teenagers to help them remain in school.

Evaluation

Evaluation strategies must involve both process and outcome measures on the individual, family, and community levels.

Individual

The school nurse was able to monitor Kaylah throughout her pregnancy and was aware that she finished classes for the term. Kaylah's pregnancy was unremarkable, and she delivered a healthy boy. Their healthcare expenses were covered by Medicaid, and the baby was determined to also be eligible for CHIP. A home-based teacher was assigned to work with Kaylah for 1 month after delivery to ensure that she was able to keep up with her coursework. With the assistance of the social worker, Kaylah was able to place the baby in a subsidized day care facility, allowing her to finish school.

Family

Family counseling helped the family resolve some of their issues. Maria observed that Kaylah's parents were proud of their grandson and eager to help with his care.

Community

With the help of the school nurse and other interested parties, Maria was able to initiate a collaborative program in which health department nurses and developmental specialists offered parenting classes in high schools on a regular basis. They were also planning on writing for a Maternal Child Health Block Grant to implement a school-based clinic focusing on the needs of pregnant teens and their infants.

Levels of Prevention
Primary

- Primary prevention depends largely on the child's age. For the youngest children, strategies include encouraging healthy behaviors by girls and women.
- Primary prevention also includes the prevention of unwanted pregnancy, which is especially important for adolescents.

Secondary

- Once pregnant, the woman must receive early and adequate prenatal care, practice healthy behaviors, obtain necessary social and supportive services, and prepare herself for becoming a parent.
- It is incumbent on the community to ensure that adequate preventive health services, such as prenatal care, nutrition and dietary counseling, pregnancy and parent education, and social services, are available.

Tertiary

- Initiate programs and services that prevent future unwanted pregnancy among teenagers and help the parenting teenager provide the best possible care to the child.
- Establish programs such as parenting classes; support services to help adolescents complete their education; coordination of health and social services for the mother and her child; and well-child care, immunizations, and nutrition services.

SUMMARY

Child and adolescent health status remains an important indicator of the nation's health. The health of a child sets the foundation for school readiness and future success. Child and adolescent health problems are reflections of rapidly changing social conditions, not isolated events. Despite generally improving trends in health for most children, community health nurses must address discrepancies that exist between racial and ethnic groups. Poverty is the basis for many continuing health problems among children in this country, and nurses must recognize and treat it as such.

The best way to ensure the success and well-being of future generations is for each child to begin life healthy and maintain that health status throughout childhood. Any health problem (e.g., hunger and poor nutrition, asthma, poor vision or hearing, anemia, dental caries, mental health problems, illicit drug use, or teen pregnancy) can interfere with school attendance, academic success, normal growth and development, learning ability, and life success.

The prevention of health problems is most significant and cost-effective for children. Each dollar spent on the prevention of physical and emotional problems in children is a sound investment. Primary health care and early intervention for children and families can help prevent costly problems, suffering, and the loss of human potential. Community health nurses can use their experience and "inside knowledge" of barriers to child health to educate others. Rather than limiting their approach to caring for the individual and family only, community health nurses can maximize their roles to collaborate and forge necessary alliances to solve children's health problems. Nurses are authority figures in the least expected places. Working on health care's front line is a powerful and very real position to members of Congress, state legislators, mayors, and other leaders. By creatively using this kind of power, community health nurses can contribute greatly to improving the health and well-being of all children.

EVOLVE WEBSITE

http://evolve.elsevier.com/Nies/community
- NCLEX Review Questions
- Case Studies

BIBLIOGRAPHY

American Academy of Pediatrics: Section on breastfeeding: breastfeeding and the use of human milk, *Pediatrics* 129(3):e827—e841, 2012. Also available from: http://pediatrics.aappublications.org/content/early/2012/02/22/peds.2011-3552.

American Academy of Pediatrics: SIDS and other sleep-related infant deaths: updated 2016 recommendations for a safe infant sleeping environment, *Pediatrics* 138(5), 2016. https://doi.org/10.1542/peds.2016-2938.

American Academy of Pediatrics: *What is medical home?*, 2021. Available from: www.aap.org/en-us/professional-resources/practice-transformation/managing-patients/Pages/what-is-medical-home.aspx.

American Society for the Positive care of Children, National child maltreatment statistics. 2021, accessed from: https://americanspcc.org/child-maltreatment-statistics/.

Angier H, Gregg J, Gold R, et al.: Understanding how low-income families prioritize elements of health care access for their children via the optimal care model, *BCH Health Res* 14:585, 2014.

Basile KC, Clayton HB, DeGue S, et al.: Interpersonal violence victimization among high school students—youth risk behavior survey, United States, 2019, *MMWR (Morb Mortal Wkly Rep)* 69(1), 2020. SS 28—37. Accessed March 28, 2021.

Centers for Disease Control and Prevention: *Injury prevention and control*, 2019. Available from: https://www.cdc.gov/injury/wisqars/facts.html.

Centers for Disease Control and Prevention: *Infant mortality in the United States*, 2018. Available from: https://www.cdc.gov/nchs/data/nvsr/nvsr69/NVSR-69-7-508.pdf.

Centers for Disease Control and Prevention: *About BMI for children and teens*, 2021. Available from: https://www.cdc.gov/healthyweight/assessing/bmi/childrens_bmi/about_childrens_bmi.html. Accessed March 26, 2021.

Centers for Disease Control and Prevention: *Sexually transmitted disease surveillance 2018*, Atlanta, 2019b, U.S. Department of Health and Human Services. https://doi.org/10.15620/cdc.79370. Centers for Disease Control and Prevention: HPV vaccine for preteens and teens. Available from: https://www.cdc.gov/vaccines/parents/diseases/teen/hpv-basics-color.pdf.

Centers for Disease Control and Prevention: *Key Findings: folic acid fortification continues to prevent neural tube defects*, 2017. Available from: www.cdc.gov/ncbddd/folicacid/features/folicacid-prevents-ntds.html.

Centers for Disease Control and Prevention: *Facts about fetal alcohol spectrum disorders*, 2020. Available from: https://www.cdc.gov/ncbddd/fasd/facts.html.

Centers for Disease Control and Prevention: *Breastfeeding: key breastfeeding indicators*, 2021. Available from: www.cdc.gov/breastfeeding/data/facts.html#disparities.

Centers for Disease Control and Prevention: *Health effects-smoking during pregnancy*, 2020. Accessed March 24, 2021, https://www.cdc.gov/tobacco/basic_information/health_effects/pregnancy/.

Centers for Disease Control and Prevention: *National Center for Health Statistics: asthma*, 2021c. https://www.cdc.gov/nchs/fastats/asthma.htm.

Centers for Disease Control and Prevention: *Preventing child abuse and neglect*, 2021. Available from: https://www.cdc.gov/violenceprevention/pdf/can/CAN-factsheet_508.pdf.

Centers for Disease Control and Prevention: *Sudden unexplained infant death and sudden infant death syndrome*, 2017. Available from: https://www.cdc.gov/sids/data.htm.

Centers for Disease Control and Prevention: *Reproductive health- preterm birth*, 2020. Available from: https://www.cdc.gov/reproductivehealth/maternalinfanthealth/pretermbirth.htm.

Centers for Medicare and Medicaid Services: *Medicaid & CHIP*, 2018. Available from: https://www.medicaid.gov/medicaid/program-information/downloads/accomplishments-report.pdf.

Chowdhury, et al.: Breastfeeding and maternal health outcomes: a systematic review and meta-analysis, *Acta Paediatr* 105:96—113, 2015.

Creamer MR, Jones SE, Gentzke AS, Jamal A, King BA, et al.: Tobacco product use among high school students—Youth Risk Behavior Survey, United States, 2019, *MMWR* 69(1), 2020. https://www.cdc.gov/healthyyouth/data/yrbs/pdf/2019/su6901-H.pdf.

Cullen KA, Gentzke AS, Sawdey MD, et al.: e-Cigarette use among youth in the United States, *JAMA* 322(21):2095−2103, 2019.

Curtin SC, Heron M, Miniño AM, Warner M: Recent increases in injury mortality among children and adolescents aged 10−19 years in the United States: 1999−2016. In *National Vital Statistics Reports*, Hyattsville, MD, 2018, National Center for Health Statistics, vol 67 no 4.

Curtin SC, Mathews TJ: Smoking prevalence and cessation before and during pregnancy: data from the birth certificate. In *National vital statistics reports*, Hyattsville, MD, 2016, National Center for Health Statistics, vol. 65 no 1.

DeFranco EA, Seske LM, Greenberg JM, Muglia LJ: Influence of interpregnancy interval on neonatal morbidity, *Am J Obstet Gynecol* 212:386, 2015.

Denny CH, Acero CS, Naimi TS, Kim SYC: Alcohol use and binge drinking among women of childbearing age—United States, 2015−2017, *MMWR Morb Mortal Wkly Rep* 68(16):365−369, 2019. Also available from: https://www.cdc.gov/mmwr/volumes/68/wr/pdfs/mm6816a1-H.pdf. https://www.cdc.gov/mmwr/volumes/68/wr/pdfs/mm6816a1-H.pdf.

Durbin DR, Hoffman BD: AAP Council on Injury, Violence, and Poison Prevention. Child Passenger Safety, *Pediatrics* 142(5), 2018. e20182460.

Federal Interagency Forum on Child and Family Statistics: *America's children: key national indicators of well-being*, 2016. Available from March 9, 2017. https://www.childstats.gov/pdf/ac2016/ac_16.pdf.

Federal Interagency Forum on Child and Family Statistics: *America's children in brief: Key national indicators of well-being, 2020*, 2020. Washington, DC: U.S, https://www.childstats.gov/pdf/ac2020/ac_20.pdf.

Finer LB, Zolna MR: Declines in unintended pregnancy in the United States, 2008−2011, *N Engl J Med* 374(9):843−852, 2016. https://doi.org/10.1056/NEJMsa1506575.

Fortson BL, Klevens J, Merrick MT, Gilbert LK, Alexander SP: *Preventing child abuse and neglect: a technical package for policy, norm, and programmatic activities*, Atlanta, GA, 2016, National Center for Injury Prevention and Control, Centers for Disease Control and Prevention. Available from: https://www.cdc.gov/violenceprevention/pdf/CAN-Prevention-Technical-Package.pdf.

Fryar CD, Carroll MD, Ogden CL: *Prevalence of overweight and obesity among children and adolescents aged 2-19 years: United States, 1963−1965 through 2013−2014*, 2016. https://www.cdc.gov/nchs/data/hestat/obesity_child_13_14/obesity_child_13_14.pdf.

Gentzke A, Wang TW, Jamal A, et al.: Tabacco product use among middle and high school students −United States, 2020, *MMWR Morb Mortal Wkly Rep* 69:1881−1888, 2020. https://doi.org/10.15585/mmwr.mm6950a1external icon.

Goyal MK, Badolato GM, Patel SJ, Iqbal SF, Parikh K, McCarter R: State gun laws and pediatric firearm-related mortality, *Pediatrics* 144(2), 2019. https://doi.org/10.1542/peds.2018-3283.

Haider A: *The basic facts about children in poverty*, 2021, Center for American Progression. Available from: https://www.americanprogress.org/issues/poverty/reports/2021/01/12/494506/basic-facts-children-poverty/.

Hales CM, Carroll MD, Fryar CD, Ogden CL: *Prevalence of obesity among adults and youth: United States, 2015−2016. NCHS data brief, no 288*, Hyattsville, MD, 2017, National Center for Health Statistics.

Hamilton BE, Martin JA, Osterman MJK, Rossen LM: *Births: provisional data for 2018. Vital statistics rapid release*, Hyattsville, MD, May 2019, National Center for Health Statistics.

Health Resources and Services Administration/Maternal Child Health Bureau: *Child health USA*, 2020. Available from: https://mchb.hrsa.gov/data-research-epidemiology/research-epidemiology/national-survey-publications-and-chartbooks 2020.

Hilmers A, Hilmers DC, Dave J: Neighborhood disparities in access to healthy foods and their effects on environmental justice, *Am J Publ Health* 102(9), 2012.

Hullenaar K, Ruback B: *Juvenile violent victimization, 1995−2018*, 2020. Available from: https://ojjdp.ojp.gov/juvenile-violent-victimization.pdf.

Institute of Medicine: *The childhood immunization schedule and safety: stakeholder concerns, scientific evidence, and future studies*, Washington, DC, 2013, National Academies Press. https://doi.org/10.17226/13563.

Ip S, Chung M, Raman G, et al.: *Breastfeeding and maternal and infant health outcomes in developed countries* (prepared by Tufts-New England Medical Center Evidence-based Practice Center, under Contract No. 290-02-0022). AHRQ Publication No. 07-E007. *Evidence report/technology assessment No. 153*, Rockville, MD, April 2007, Agency for Healthcare Research and Quality.

Jones CM, Clayton HB, Deputy NP, et al.: Prescription Opioid misuse and use of alcohol and other substances among high school students—Youth Risk Behavior Survey, United States, 2019. *MMWR* 69(1), 2020. https://www.cdc.gov/healthyyouth/data/yrbs/pdf/2019/su6901-H.pdf.

Kann L, McManus T, Harris WA, et al.: Youth risk behavior surveillance—United States, 2017, *MMWR Surveill Summ* 67, 2018. https://doi.org/10.15585/mmwr.ss6708a1. No. SS-8.

Kidsdata.org, California Dept. of Public Health: *Death statistical master files; California Dept. of Finance, Population Estimates by race/ethnicity with age and gender detail 1990−2009; population reference bureau, population estimates 2010−2016; CDC WONDER online database, underlying cause of death 1999−2016*, February 2019. Accessed March 27, 2021.

Koball H, Jiang Y: *Basic facts about low-income children: children under 9 years*, New York, 2018, National Center for Children in Poverty, Columbia University Mailman School of Public Health, 2016.

Kochanek KD, Xu JQ, Arias E: *Mortality in the United States, 2019. NCHS data brief, no 395*, Hyattsville, MD, 2020, National Center for Health Statistics.

Kovar C, Salsberry P: Does a satisfactory relationship with her mother influence when a 16-year-old begins to have sex? MCN, *Am J Matern Child Nurs* 37(2):122−129, 2012.

Law Center to Prevent Gun Violence: *Minimum age*, 2016. Accessed April 1, 2017. Available from: http://smartgunlaws.org/gun-laws/policy-areas/consumer-child-safety/minimum-age/.

Loftin RW, Habli M, Snyder CC, Cormier CM, Lewis DF, DeFranco EA: Late preterm birth, *Rev Obst & Gynecol* (3):1, 2010.

MacDorman MF, Mathews TJ: *Understanding racial and ethnic disparities in U.S. infant mortality rates (NCHS Data Brief no 74)*, Hyattsville, MD, 2011, National Center for Health Statistics. http://www.cdc.gov/nchs/data/databriefs/db74.htm.

Martin JA, Hamilton BE, Osterman MJK: *Births in the United States, 2019. NCHS data brief, no 387*, Hyattsville, MD, 2020, National Center for Health Statistics.

Martin JA, Hamilton BE, Osterman MJK, Driscoll AK: *Births: final data for 2019. National vital statistics reports* (Vol. 70), Hyattsville, MD, 2021, National Center for Health Statistics, p 100472, 2021. https://doi.org/10.15620/cdc.

Martin JA, Hamilton BE, Osterman MJK, Driscoll AK: *Births: dinal data for 2018. National vital statistics reports* (Vol. 68), Hyattsville, MD, 2019, National Center for Health Statistics.

Medicaid and CHIP Payment and Access Commission: *Fact sheet*, 2018. https://www.macpac.gov/wp-content/uploads/2018/02/State-Children%E2%80%99s-Health-Insurance-Program-CHIP.pdf.

Moos MK: From concept to practice: reflections on the preconception health agenda, *J Wom Health* 19(3):561–567, 2010.

Moos MK, Badura M, Posner S, et al.: Quality improvement opportunities in preconception and interconception care. In *March of dimes: toward improving the outcome of pregnancy, III*, White Plains, NY, 2010, March of Dimes Foundation.

National Academy of Sciences: *The future of nursing 2020–2030*, 2021, National Academies.

National Campaign to Prevent Teen and Unplanned Pregnancy: *Annual report-improving the lives and future prospects of children and families*, 2015. Available from: https://thenationalcampaign.org/sites/default/files/resource-primary-download/national-campaign-2015-annual-report.pdf.

National Center for Health Statistics: *Health, United States, 2019*. Table 6. Hyattsville, MD. Available from: https://www.cdc.gov/nchs/hus/contents2019.htm.

National Conference of State Legislatures: *Synthetic drug threats*, 2012. Available from: http://www.ncsl.org/issues-research/justice/synthetic-drug-threats.aspx.

National Institute on Drug Abuse: *Drugs, brains, and behavior: the science of addiction*, 2020. Accessed March 28, 2021, from: https://www.drugabuse.gov/publications/drugs-brains-behavior-science-addiction.

National Scientific Council on the Developing Child: *The science of neglect: the persistent absence of responsive care disrupts the developing brain: working paper 12*, 2012. http://www.developingchild.harvard.edu.

Nurse-Family Partnership: *Nurse-family partnership's, national results of the maternal, infant, and early childhood home visit program*, 2015. Available :2015NFP_MIECHVReport_forprint-1.pdf (nurse familypartnership.org.

Organisation for Economic Co-operation and Development: *Health: infant mortality rates*, 2021. Available from: https://data.oecd.org/healthstat/infant-mortality-rates.htm 2021.

Oshiro BT, Henry E, Wilson J, et al.: Decreasing elective deliveries before 39 weeks of gestation in an integrated health care system, *Obstet Gynecol* 113:804–811, 2009.

Perper K, Peterson K, Manlove J: *Diploma attainment among teen mothers (child trends, fact sheet publication #2010-01)*, Child Trends, 2010. Washington, DC.

Planned Parenthood: Parents and teens talk about sexuality: a national survey 2014. Survey conducted by GfK Custom Research, LLC on behalf of planned parenthood, *Famil Cir Mag and CLAFH*, 2014. Available from: https://www.plannedparenthood.org/uploads/filer_public/ac/50/ac50c2f7-cbc9-46b7-8531-ad3e92712016/nationalpoll_09-14_v2_1.pdf.

Sacco LN, Finklea K: *Synthetic drugs: overview and issues for congress*, 2016, Congressional Research Service. Available from: https://fas.org/sgp/crs/misc/R42066.pdf.

Safe Kids Worldwide: *Safety tips*, 2021. Available from: https://www.safekids.org/safetytips.

Substance Abuse and Mental Health Services Administration: *Key substance use and mental health indicators in the United States: results from the 2019 National Survey on Drug Use and Health*, Rockville, MD, 2020, Center for Behavioral Health Statistics and Quality, Substance Abuse and Mental Health Services Administration (HHS Publication No. PEP20-07-01-001, NSDUH Series H-55). Available from: https://www.samhsa.gov/data/ https://www.samhsa.gov/data/.

Substance Abuse and Mental Health Services Administration: *Results from the 2012 national survey on drug use and health: summary of national findings*, Rockville, MD, 2013, Substance Abuse and Mental Health Services Administration.

Szucs LE, Lowry R, Fasula AM, Pamparti S, Copen CE, et al.: Condom and contraceptive use sexually active among high school students — United States, 2019, *MMWR (Morb Mortal Wkly Rep)* 69(1):11–18, 2020. Accessed March 28, 2021.

Tolbert J, Orgera K: *Key Facts about the uninsured population*, 2020, Kaiser Family Foundation. Available from: https://www.kff.org/uninsured/issue-brief/key-facts-about-the-uninsured-population/.

Underwood MJ, Brener N, Thornton J, et al.: Overview and methods for the youth risk behavior surveillance system—United States, 2019, *MMWR Suppl* 69(1):1–10, 2020.

U.S. Court of Federal Claims: *Autism decisions and background information*, n.d. Available from: http://www.uscfc.uscourts.gov/omnibus-autism-proceeding.

U.S. Department of Agriculture Food and Nutrition Service: *Women, infants, and children (WIC)*, 2020. Available from: www.fns.usda.gov/wic-2017-eligibility-and-coverage-rates#:~:text=In%202017%2C%202.2%20million%20infants,were%20received%20or%20picked%20up.

U.S. Department of Education, U.S. Education: *Department Commemorates 45 years of the IDEA*, 2020. Available from: https://sites.ed.gov/idea/department-commemorates-45-years-idea/.

U.S. Department of Health and Human Services, Health Resources and Services Administration, Maternal and Child Health Bureau: *Child health USA*, Rockville, Maryland, 2014, U.S. Department of Health and Human Services, 2015. Available from: http://mchb.hrsa.gov/chusa14/.

U.S. Department of Health & Human Services: *Administration for Children and Families, Administration on Children, Youth and Families*, 2017, Children's Bureau, Child Maltreatment, 2017. Available from: http://www.acf.hhs.gov/programs/cb/research-data-technology/statistics-research/child-maltreatment.

U.S. Department of Health and Human Services: *A report of the surgeon general: how tobacco smoke causes disease: what it means to you, U.S. Department of Health and Human Services, Centers for Disease Control and Prevention, National Center for Chronic Disease Prevention and Health Promotion, Office on Smoking and Health*, 2010.

U.S. Department of Health and Human Services: *Healthy people 2030*, 2021. Available from: https://health.gov/healthypeople.

U.S. Department of Health and Human Services: *Office of population affairs: title X family planning annual report: 2019 national summary*, 2020. Available from: https://opa.hhs.gov/sites/default/files/2020-09/title-x-fpar-2019-national-summary.pdf.

U.S. Department of Health and Human Services: *Office of the Surgeon General: the surgeon general's call to action to support breastfeeding*, Washington, DC, 2011, Author. https://www.ncbi.nlm.nih.gov/books/NBK52682/pdf/Bookshelf_NBK52682.pdf. https://www.ncbi.nlm.nih.gov/books/NBK52682/pdf/Bookshelf_NBK52682.pdf.

U.S. Department of Health and Human Services: *2021 Poverty guidelines*, Fed Regist (19), 86, 2021, pp 7732–7734.

U.S. Department of Labor: *Wage and hour division: break time for nursing mothers under FLSA*, 2018. Available from: https://www.dol.gov/agencies/whd/fact-sheets/73-flsa-break-time-nursing-mothers.

U.S. Department of Labor: *Wage and hour division: family and medical leave act, final rule to amend the definition of spouse in the family and medical leave act regulations*, February 2015. Available from: https://www.dol.gov/whd/fmla/spouse/.

Ventura SJ, Hamilton BE, Mathews TJ: *National and state patterns of teen births in the United States, 1940-2013, national vital statistics reports* (Vol. 63, no. 4) Hyattsville, MD, 2014, National Center for Health Statistics. Available from https://www.cdc.gov/nchs/data/nvsr/nvsr63/nvsr63_04.pdf.

Waitzman NJ, Jalali A, Grosse SD: *Preterm birth lifetime costs in the United States in 2016: an update*, Available March 24, 2021 from:, 2021 (in press), www.sciencedirect.com.

Wang TW, Gentzke AS, Creamer MR, et al.: Tobacco product use and associated factors among middle and high school students—United States, 2019, *MMWR (Morb Mortal Wkly Rep)* 68(12):SS1—22, 2019. Accessed March 17, 2021.

Widome R, Neumark-Sztainer D, Hannan PJ, et al.: Eating when there is not enough to eat: eating behaviors and perceptions of food among food-insecure youths, *Am J Publ Health* 99:822—828, 2009.

Wodi PA, Ault K, Hunter P, et al.: Advisory committee on immunization practices recommended immunization schedule for children and adolescents aged 18 years of younger—United States, 2021, *MMWR Morb Mortal Wkly Rep* 70:189—192, 2021.

Womenshealth.gov: *Breastfeeding*, n.d. Available from: http://www.womenshealth.gov/breastfeeding/index.html.

World Health Organization-Western Pacific Region: *Barriers to access to child healthcare*, n.d. Available from: www.wpro.who.int/publications.

World Health Organization: *Newsroom. Youth violence key facts*, 2020.

17

Women's Health

Lori A. Glenn

OBJECTIVES

Upon completion of this chapter, the reader will be able to do the following:

1. Identify the major indicators of women's health.
2. Examine prominent health problems among women of all age groups (i.e., from adolescence to old age).
3. Identify barriers to adequate healthcare for women.
4. Discuss issues related to reproductive health.
5. Explain the influence of public policy on women's health.
6. Discuss issues and needs for increased research efforts focused on women's health.
7. Apply the nursing process to women's health concerns across all levels of prevention.

OUTLINE

KEY TERMS

breast cancer
cesarean section
Civil Rights Act
cardiovascular disease
ectopic pregnancy

Family and Medical Leave Act
Title X
Hypertension
intimate partner violence
life expectancy

maternal mortality
multiple family configurations
osteoporosis
pelvic inflammatory disease
sexual harassment

To achieve "health for all," healthcare services must be affordable and available to all. Although adequate healthcare for women is a key to realizing this goal, a significant number of women and their families face barriers to healthcare access and are impacted by the social determinants of health. Additionally, knowledge deficits related to health promotion and disease prevention activities prevent women of all educational and socioeconomic levels from assuming responsibility for their own health and well-being.

Beginning in the 1970s, the women's movement called for the reform of systems affecting women's health. Women were encouraged to become involved as consumers of health services and as establishers of health policy. More women entered professions in which they were previously underrepresented, and those in traditionally female-dominated professions, such as nursing and teaching, became more assertive in their demands to gain recognition for their contributions to society. Healthcare for women has evolved from a focus on the pelvic area and breast to viewing the woman as a holistic being with specialized needs.

In "Preamble to a New Paradigm for Women's Health," Choi (1985) declared that collaboration and an interdisciplinary approach are necessary to meet the healthcare needs of women. She further stated, "[E]ssential to the development of healthcare for women are the concepts of health promotion, disease and accident prevention, education for self-care and responsibility, health risk identification and coordination for illness care when needed" (p. 14). To realize this paradigm, community-based healthcare focuses on health beyond the biophysical, disease-focused approach. Health from a social perspective considers the interaction of individual physiology along with work environment, living conditions, lifestyle choices, and health habits (Ruzek et al., 1997). Community health nurses must work with other healthcare professionals to formulate upstream strategies that modify the factors affecting women's health. Many *Healthy People 2030* objectives address health problems pertaining to women and include specific targets and strategies to improve the health of this aggregate. The *Healthy People 2030* box in this chapter presents a small selection of these objectives, emphasizing the importance of the social determinants of health. This chapter examines the health of women from adolescence to old age. It explores the major indicators of health, including specific health problems and the socioeconomic, sociocultural, and health policy issues surrounding women's health. The chapter also discusses identification of current and future research aimed at improving the health of women. An understanding of these points will enable community health nurses to appropriately apply this expertise in a community setting to help improve women's health.

LEADING HEALTH INDICATORS

In the United States, data collected on major causes of death and illness appraise the health status of aggregates. These data are typically presented in terms of gender, age, or ethnicity and can help us interpret the levels of health in different groups. The primary indicators of health this chapter covers are life expectancy, mortality (i.e., death) rate, and morbidity (i.e., acute and chronic illness) rate.

According to the Census Bureau (2019), there are an estimated 166.6 million women in the United States. Of these women, 13.4% are considered in fair to poor health and 12% have conditions that impair their daily functioning (Centers for Disease Control [CDC], 2019; National Center for Health Statistics [NCHS], 2019). Many factors that lead to death and illness among women are preventable or avoidable. If certain conditions receive early detection and treatment, a significant positive influence on longevity and the quality of life could ensue. Recognition of patterns demonstrated by these indicators can address problems preventively. This section presents an overview of these major indicators of health among women.

LIFE EXPECTANCY

Except in a few countries, such as Bangladesh, Malawi, Niger, Pakistan, Qatar, and Zimbabwe, women typically experience

---

♥ HEALTHY PEOPLE 2030

Selected Objectives for Women's Health

Objective	Baseline (Year)	Target 2020	Final 2020	Target 2030
C-04: Reduce breast cancer death rate. (Deaths per 100,000.)	23 (2007)	20.67	19.7 (2018)	15.3
C-4: Reduce death rate from cervical cancer. (Deaths per 100,000.)	2.4 (2007)	2.2	2.2 (2018)	Not included in *Healthy People 2030*
C-09: Increase the proportion of women 21—65 years who have received a cervical cancer screening	84.5% (2008)	93%	80.5% (2018)	84.3%
C-05: Increase the proportion of women who have received breast cancer screening aged 50—74	73.7% (2008)	81.1%	72.8% (2018)	77.1%
MICH-04: Reduce maternal deaths. (Deaths per 100,000 live births.)	12.7 deaths (2007)	11.4	17.4 (2018)	15.7 This worsened since 1998, when the rate was 9.9, and disparities related to race persist.
MICH-08: Increase the proportion of pregnant women who receive early and adequate prenatal care	75.6% (2016)	83.2%	76.4% (2018)	80.5%
MICH-06: Reduce cesarean births among low-risk women with no prior births	27.4% (2007)	24.7%	25.9% (2018)	23.6%
FP-01: Decrease the proportion of unintended pregnancies	49% (2002)	44%	43%	36.5%
STI 01: Increase the proportion of sexually active adolescent and young females enrolled who are screened for chlamydial infection	52.7% (2008)	70.9%	54.4%	67.5%

Data from U.S. Department of Health and Human Services, Office of Disease Prevention and Health Promotion: *Healthy People 2030*. Available from: https://health.gov/healthypeople/objectives-and-data/browse-objectives.

greater longevity than their male counterparts (World Health Organization [WHO], 2013). For example, women born in the 1970s in the United States have an average life expectancy of 74.7 years, or 7.6 years longer than men born in the same year.

Life expectancy for Americans is at an all-time high, but the discrepancy between males and females remains. Males born in 2019 have a life expectancy of 76 years, compared with 81 years for females. This suggests a trend toward narrowing the gap between male and female life expectancies. Ethnic/racial disparities in life expectancy unfortunately continued into the twenty-first century, as there is considerable variation among races. For example, black females gained an additional 7.1 years, from 69.4 years for those born in 1970 to 78 years for those born beginning in 2005. Although that is a significant gain, it falls behind the 81 years of life expectancy for white females born in 2018 and has not changed since 2005 (Xu et al., 2020) mortality rate.

Table 17.1 lists the seven major causes of death among American women in 2017 (CDC, 2020e). As age increases, the leading causes of death change (Heron, 2019).

In the adolescent to early adulthood years, the leading cause is unintentional injuries (i.e., motor vehicle accidents, drug overdose), followed by cancer and suicide. Suicide is highest in the 20-to-44-year-old group as the fourth leading cause of death. As middle age approaches, chronic diseases are more prominent, with cancer as the number-one cause for women aged 35 to 84 years, followed by heart disease and chronic lung disease. For those over 85 years old, heart disease is the most common cause, followed by Alzheimer's disease.

⬧ RESEARCH HIGHLIGHTS

Nurse Researchers Study the Inclusion of Women in Research

A group of nurse researchers (Crane et al., 2004) examined more than 1000 articles published in nursing journals between 1995 and 2001 to determine whether women had been included in research studies focusing on the leading causes of mortality. They found that 87% of the studies did include women participants. They also noted that there appeared to be a slight increase in inclusion of women from the earlier years to the later years.

Cardiovascular Disease

About one in four Americans has one or more forms of **cardiovascular disease** (CVD) (e.g., high blood pressure, coronary heart disease, stroke, congenital defects, or rheumatic heart disease). In the United States, CVD accounts for one out of every five deaths, making it the leading cause of death (CDC, 2019d, 2021g). One in 16 women under 20 and older has some form of heart disease; the ratio increases to one in three after age 65. In 2015, deaths from heart disease occurred in 276 per 100,000 white women, compared with 236.9 per 100,000 for Black women. Black women are more likely to twice as likely experience a first stroke and have the highest rate of death due to stroke (Vivrani et al., 2020).

TABLE 17.1 Seven Leading Causes of Death Among American Women for All Races by Age Groups in (2017)

Age Group (Years)	Cause of Death (in Rank Order)
1—19	Unintentional injury or accidents (32.7%)
	Cancer (11%)
	Suicide (10.3%)
	Homicide (7.4%)
	Birth defects (6.4%)
	Heart disease (3.4%)
	Influenza and pneumonia (2.0%)
20—44	Unintentional injury or accidents (30.0%)
	Cancer (16.0%)
	Heart disease (9%)
	Suicide (7.6%)
	Homicide (3.8%)
	Chronic liver disease (2.9%)
45—64	Cancer (34.2%)
	Heart disease (16.3%)
	Unintentional injuries (6.9%)
	Chronic lower respiratory disease (5.3%)
	Diabetes (3.8%)
	Stroke (3.6%)
	Chronic liver disease (3.5%)
65—84	Cancer (27%)
	Heart disease (19.9%)
	Chronic lower pulmonary disease (8.5%)
	Stroke (5.8%)
	Alzheimer disease (4.4%)
	Diabetes mellitus (3.3%)
	Unintentional injuries (2.6%)
85+	Heart disease (27.7%)
	Cancer (10.9%)
	Alzheimer disease (8.0%) stroke (8.1%)
	Stroke (8.1%)
	Chronic lower pulmonary disease (4.9%)
	Influenza and pneumonia (2.7%)
	Unintentional injuries (2.6%)

Data from Centers for Disease Control and Prevention: *Leading cause of death by age group, all females—United States*, 2017. Available from: https://www.cdc.gov/women/lcod/2017/all-races-origins/index.htm.

CVD continues to be the number-one overall killer of women. One out of every 5 deaths is from CVD, whereas one out of every 19 deaths is from breast cancer (CDC, 2019d). The overall number of deaths of persons older than 35 due to CVD decreased dramatically from 1034.5 per 100,000 in 1968 to 327.2 per 100,000 in 2015 (Vandyke et al., 2018). Throughout this time period, there were significant differences for black and white persons (1071.6—396.0 per 100,000).

Disparities have improved for women in relation to prevention, diagnosis, and management of heart disease through public awareness campaigns such as "Go Red for Women" and research focusing more on the unique aspects of women and heart disease (American Heart Association [AHA], 2021a). Despite an increased focus, 56% of women do not recognize that heart disease is their number-one cause of death. The number of cardiovascular deaths has decreased, but women were still more likely to die from a first myocardial infarction than men. In part, this phenomenon is due to the subtle or absence of symptoms of coronary artery disease (CDC, 2020a). Women have smaller arteries and higher rates of metabolic syndrome, diabetes, heart failure, and other comorbidities. They tend to be older at their first cardiovascular event, with more urgent and emergency presentations.

Rates of CVD among women can decline further when individuals become more aware of risk factors and accept responsibility for managing their own health and well-being (Pagidipati and Douglas, 2019). Concerned and motivated providers must encourage women to practice heart-healthy behaviors. In 2002, the AHA (2021a) launched the "Go Red" campaign for women and "The Heart Truth" program for healthcare providers, which were designed to educate both groups about the unique features of women and heart disease.

Cancer

Cancer is the second leading cause of death in the United States. For women, one out of five deaths in the United States is due to cancer (Heron, 2020). Cancer rates rose through the early 1990s for a number of reasons, including lifestyle choices (smoking, diet, sun exposure), increasing exposure to environmental carcinogens, and, probably most important, greater life expectancy. Because of improvements in early detection, screening, and treatment of the major cancers, incidence rates have leveled off and, in some cases, decreased. To illustrate, death rates from cancer among women have increased from 136 per 100,000 in 1960 to 167.3 per 100,000 in 2000 (CDC, 2004). Yet there was a decline in the cancer death rate beginning in 2002 to 2004, which was "large enough to overcome the impact of the growth and aging of the population" (American Cancer Society [ACS], 2021c). In 2014–18, the death rate from cancer in women was 133.5 per 100,000 and an estimated 289,150 of women will die as a result of cancer in 2021 (CDC, 2018c).

According to the ACS (2021c, f) in 1987 lung cancer surpassed breast cancer as the leading cause of cancer deaths in women, and death rates from lung cancer increased sharply until about 1990 to 42 per 100,000 women. Lung cancer deaths leveled off and began to decline in 2005 and as of 2018 are less than 30 per 100,000, in due to decreased tobacco use and improvements in treatment (NCI, 2020b).

Other female-specific cancers include ovarian cancer (fourth most common), uterine cancer (sixth most common), and cervical cancer (thirteenth most common) (ACS, 2020c, 2021c; CDC, 2019d, 2020b). Over 90% of women with cervical cancer have evidence of cervical infection with human papillomavirus (HPV). In June 2006, the U.S. Food and Drug Administration (FDA) licensed Gardasil (Merck and Co., Inc.), the first vaccine to prevent HPV infection. Through March 2021, over 120 million doses of HPV vaccines have been given (CDC 2019c, 2021a,b,c,d,e,f,g,h). The vaccines have been shown to be highly effective in preventing the most common types of HPV infection that lead to cervical cancer and is approved for use in females and males between 9 and 26 years of age. Since vaccinations became available, infections with HPV have dropped 86% in teen girls and 71% in adult women, and HPV precancers have dropped 40%.

Five-year survival rates vary according to the type of cancer and stage at diagnosis. For instance, the 5-year survival rate for all clients with lung cancer is 20% and pancreatic cancer had the lowest rate at 10%. For those with breast cancer, 5-year survival is at 90%. Of cancers related to the reproductive tract, ovarian cancer has the lowest survival rate, as only around 48% of women survive for 5 years (ACS, 2021b, c). The 5-year survival rate is 64% for women with colorectal cancer; this rate improves significantly with early detection (ACS, 2021e).

Early diagnosis and prompt treatment are major factors in surviving many types of cancer. Routine cervical cancer screening begins at age 21, at which time a Papanicolaou (Pap) smear should be done every 3 years. Colorectal cancer screenings include annual fecal occult blood tests along with sigmoidoscopy every 5 years or colonoscopy every 10 years (ACS, 2021d).

Certain health choices may reduce an individual's risk of cancer. Women reduce their risk for cancer by never smoking or by quitting if they already use tobacco products. Eating a nutritious, plant-focused, high-fiber diet along with adopting a physically active lifestyle and maintaining a healthy body weight protect against both heart disease and many cancers. Nutrition guidelines include avoiding salt-cured, smoked, nitrite-containing, and charred foods; high-fat foods; and excessive alcohol. Obesity has been associated with an increased risk for cancers of the colon and rectum, endometrium, and breast (ACS, 2021f). Finally, the practice of safe sex has been shown to reduce the spread of cancer associated with sexually transmitted diseases (STDs) such as HPV, hepatitis B and C, and human immunodeficiency virus (HIV) (CDC, 2021h).

Community health nurses must encourage all females (i.e., from childhood to old age) to adopt these healthy lifestyle choices and pursue early cancer detection. Community health nurses play a major role in providing cancer control services that should be culturally sensitive and appropriate to the targeted aggregate. If providers and clients applied everything known about cancer prevention, approximately two thirds of cancer cases would not occur.

Diabetes

According to the CDC (2020d), in 2018 the number of diabetics in the United States reached 34.2 million, which is 10.5% of the population. Seven million persons or 2.8% of the population remained undiagnosed and 88 million or 34.5% are considered prediabetic. Between 1999 and 2016, there was a significant increase in diabetes for all ages, in part attributed to obesity. The highest incidence of diabetes is among those age 45 to 64 (9.9 per 1000) and those over age 65 (8.8 per 1000). Diabetes is more prevalent among Black, Native American, and Indigenous females than their male counterparts.

Diabetes mellitus is a chronic disease that causes the premature death of many women and overall ranks seventh in mortality. Diabetes is the fourth leading cause of death among Native Americans, fifth for Blacks, and Asians, and is sixth Hispanics (Heron, 2017). Women are more likely to be seriously affected by the complications of diabetes, including CVD, stroke, vision loss, and depression (CDC, 2018b).

In addition to being a serious illness in itself, diabetic women are twice as likely to develop CVD; furthermore, it dramatically influences the severity and course of CVD. When comparing men and women with diabetes, of those who suffer a myocardial infarction before age 65, women are more likely to die and suffer long-term health problems. In death certificates from 2004 on which the cause of death was related to diabetes, 68% also listed CVD and 16% also listed stroke (CDC, 2021d). The number of women hospitalized for diabetes and its complications dropped, indicating that better management with tighter control of blood glucose has decreased complications (CDC, 2018b). The community health nurse is an important resource for supporting the tight control of diabetes to prevent its complications. An upstream approach to this problem includes helping women maintain a desirable weight throughout life in an effort to avoid nutrition-related causes of death such as diabetes and CVD.

Maternal Mortality

According to the WHO (2019), 810 women died every day from complications of pregnancy and childbirth in 2017. Complications related to pregnancy and birth are the leading cause of disability and death among women worldwide between the ages of 14 and 49 years. Maternal mortality in developing, low resource countries is 462 per 100,000 live births, whereas it is 11 per 100,000 in developed countries with high incomes. Forty percent of women experience complications during pregnancy, childbirth, and the postpartum period, 15% of which are life threatening. The major complications that account for nearly 75% of all maternal deaths are severe bleeding, infections, hypertensive disorders, delivery complications, and unsafe abortion. See Box 17.1 for information on a group approach to prenatal care.

Reduction of maternal mortality is one of the *Healthy People 2030* objectives for the United States, which has the highest mortality rate of developed countries (Tikkanen et al., 2020). Beginning in the 1950s, maternal mortality rates began to decline in the United States due to the use of blood transfusions, the availability of antimicrobial drugs, and the maintenance of fluid and electrolyte balance during serious complications of pregnancy and birth. The development of obstetrical training programs and obstetrical anesthesia programs was also important.

However, since 1987 the rate of maternal death has increased from 7.2 per 100,000 pregnancies to 17.4 in 2018. Some of this change can be attributed to updated methods for data collection. Before 2003, in the United States, **maternal mortality** was defined as the deaths of women while pregnant or within 42 days after termination of pregnancy. The U.S. Standard Certificate of Death and the 10th revision of WHO's International Statistical Classification of Diseases and Related Health Problems (ICD-10) revised this definition in 2003 to include late causes of maternal death, defined as occurring more than 42 days but less than 1 year after the end of the pregnancy (Hoyert and Xu, 2012; WHO, 2007). Although this change may explain the increase in the mid-2000s, the continued increase in the death rate is still without clear etiology. Researchers cite maternal obesity, older age, and chronic health conditions along with an increasing cesarean section rate as contributing factors (CDC, 2017). In 2020 the leading cause of maternal death was CVD, infection/sepsis, cardiomyopathy, pulmonary embolism, hemorrhage, thrombotic embolism, cerebrovascular accidents, and hypertensive disorders (CDC, n.d.). Data show that from 2011 to 2015, 52% or all maternal deaths occurred after birth, after 7 and up to 42 days postpartum (Tikkanen et al., 2020).

Beginning in the 1950s, maternal mortality rates began to decline in the United States due to the use of blood transfusions, the availability of antimicrobial drugs, and the maintenance of fluid and electrolyte balance during serious complications of pregnancy and birth. The development of obstetrical training programs and obstetrical anesthesia programs was also important.

Racial discrepancy persists, however, in maternal mortality rates as in life expectancy. Table 17.2 illustrates how nonwhite women have a significantly higher incidence of death during pregnancy than white women. The gap in maternal mortality rates between Black and white women has widened over the past several decades. Early in the twentieth century, Black women were two times more likely to die of pregnancy-related complications than white women. Currently, Black women are three times more likely to die (CDC, 2021). Major risk factors for maternal death include lack of antepartum care and family planning services, inadequate health education, and poor nutrition. An additional risk factor of race is advancing age. Black, Native American, and indigenous women four times the risk of dying from a pregnancy-related cause as after the age of 30 (Davis et al.). Intrinsic maternal factors, such as higher frequency of hypertension and greater likelihood of uterine hemorrhage, help explain this increase in the mortality rate among older mothers.

BOX 17.1 Centering Pregnancy: Model for Prenatal Care

Developed in 1993, the Centering Pregnancy model uses a group approach to prenatal care. The prenatal visit occurs with women of similar gestational ages and includes an assessment with the provider along with group learning, facilitated discussion, and support among women. The group dynamic contributes to health-promoting behaviors and to normalizing attitudes to pregnancy. Women report high satisfaction with the care and go on to have fewer preterm births and babies of optimal weight (Centering Health Care Institute, 2021; Manant and Dodgson, 2011).

TABLE 17.2   Maternal Mortality Rate per 100,000 Live Births—Selected Years

Year	Total	Whites	Blacks	Other (Nonwhite)	American Indian/Alaska Native	Asian/Pacific Islander	Hispanic
1992	7.8	5.0	20.8	18.2			
1999	13.2	9.5	32.2	14.5			
2001	14.7	10.2	36.8	9.9			
2003	16.8	11.7	43.5	18.9			
2005	15.4	10.7	38.7	15.9			
2011–15[a]	17.2	13.0	42.8		32.5	14.2	11.4

[a]Davis NL, Goodman D, et al.: Vital signs: pregnancy-related deaths, United States, 2011–15, and strategies for prevention, 13 states, 2013–17. *MMWR Morbidity and Mortality Weekly Report* 68:423–429, 2019. doi:https://doi.org/10.15585/mmwr.mm6818e1.
Data from Berg CJ, Callaghan WM, Syverson C, Henderson Z: Pregnancy-related mortality in the United States, 1998 to 2005, *Obstet Gynecol* 116(6):1302–1309, 2010; and Petersen EE.

Death associated with legal medical or surgical abortion is rare in the United States, at less than one per 100,000 abortions per 5-year time periods (CDC, 2020a). Complications that result in death from legal abortion relate to the woman's age, the type of procedure, the gestational age of the fetus, and general health problems at the time of the abortion.

The medical method of induced abortion includes mifepristone (i.e., RU-486), an antiprogestin medication, together with prostaglandins such as misoprostol has been used in the United States since 2000. It is as effective as surgical abortion and is considered a safe alternative to surgical abortion in pregnancies of less 9 weeks gestation. Use of this method increased 120% between 2009 and 2018 (Kortsmit et al., 2018). In 2018, 38.6% of the legal abortions in the United States employed this method. Curettage is still the most widely used abortion procedure.

Abortion is a controversial issue for providers and for the women in their care. Abortion rates have fallen significantly from 820,151 in 2005 to 619,820 in 2018, as has the rate of complications from this procedure (Kortsmit et al., 2018). Access to free contraception through the Affordable Care Act (ACA) and multiple long-acting methods have contributed to the decreased use of abortion. Nurses must continue to keep abreast of all available pregnancy prevention and termination options to provide the best counsel for women.

Ectopic pregnancy is the leading cause of maternal death in the first trimester. Since the 1980s, the incidence of ectopic pregnancy has decreased from 1.15 to 0.60 per 100,000 live births, the most common cause of death due to hemorrhage (Hoyert, 2020). Racial discrepancy is evident, with rates 6.8 times higher in African Americans. Rates are also 3.5 times higher in women older than 35 years than in those younger than 25 years. The rates are possibly higher because STDs are diagnosed more frequently in this older population and may cause damage and scarring of fallopian tubes, raising the risk of ectopic pregnancy (Creanga et al., 2011).

The most significant risk for ectopic pregnancy is previous pelvic inflammatory disease or salpingitis. Early diagnosis and treatment greatly lower the mortality rate. Prevention interventions for women at risk for acquiring STDs are critical in reducing a woman's risk for an ectopic pregnancy. An important task of healthcare providers is to educate women and men about methods to reduce sexual health risk-taking behaviors. Additional risk factors for ectopic pregnancy include tubal pathology, previous ectopic pregnancy, tubal surgery, and the use of intrauterine contraceptive devices.

Morbidity Rate
Hospitalizations

The 2016 National Hospital Care Survey (NHCS) reported that more women than men are hospitalized each year in the United States (NHCS, 2016). Of the top 10 most common hospital diagnoses five are related to childbirth and pregnancy. Rounding out the top 10 are septicemia, osteoarthritis (OA), heart failure, chronic obstructive pulmonary disease, and urinary tract infections (AHRQ, 2021).

The prospective payment system for hospitalization resulted in a greater demand for skilled nursing services in the home. After community members have been hospitalized for any of several of these conditions, community health nurses may provide ongoing nursing care in the home by referral. Nurses practicing in home environments must be prepared to deliver "high-tech" and "high-touch" services. Chapter 33 discusses home healthcare in detail.

Chronic Conditions and Limitations

Women are more likely than men to be disabled by chronic conditions. Arthritis and rheumatism, hypertension, and impairment of the back or spine decrease women's activity level more often than they affect their male counterparts. The CDC (2019a) reports that prevalence in women is 23.5% as compared to 18.1% of men. Arthritis is often accompanied by comorbidities that contribute to the condition, including obesity, diabetes heart disease. Women are more likely than men to have difficulty performing activities such as walking, bathing or showering, preparing meals, and doing housework (Arthritis Foundation, 2020).

Functional limitations may require home healthcare that community health nurses supervise and deliver. Nurses plan and implement interventions on the basis of functional assessments. Each care plan facilitates optimal resumption of the individual's independence in personal care activities.

Surgery

Women are more likely than men to have surgery. Hysterectomy is the second most frequently performed major surgical procedure among women of reproductive age after cesarean section (CDC, 2019f). Approximately 265,000 hysterectomies were performed in 2016 (Moore, 2016). The overall rate of hysterectomy decreased 12.3% between 2005 and 2013. For women over 50 years old, 36.6% reported having a hysterectomy in 2008, while in 2018 that decreased to 31.7%. Overall, rates of hysterectomy decreased from 5.4 to 5.1 per 1000 in the years 2000 through 2004 (Whiteman et al., 2008).

The most common reason for hysterectomy is uterine fibroids or leiomyoma, which contributes to more than one-third of all such surgeries, but considerably more in blacks (68%) than in whites (33%). White women are more often diagnosed with endometriosis and uterine prolapse, which are the second and third most common reasons for hysterectomy. Hysterectomy rates are the highest in women aged 35 to 54 years (Moore et al., 2016).

Optional procedures are becoming available to women. Myomectomy—removal of only the tumors with repair of the uterus—uterine artery ablation, and the use of a gonadotropin-releasing hormone to shrink the tumors can decrease the need for hysterectomy (American College of Obstetricians and Gynecologists, 2008). Women may not know about these alternatives. Community health nurses function as advocates for women and can provide health education programs related to alternatives to hysterectomy, indications for hysterectomy and oophorectomy (i.e., removal of ovaries), and information regarding the type of surgical approach and the purpose of a second opinion. Second opinions and higher levels of education tend to lower the rate of hysterectomies.

Birth by **cesarean section** (C-section) is the most prevalent surgical procedure experienced by women in the United States and accounts for 31.9% of births (Martin et al., 2019). Several factors contribute to the high rates of C-section, including physician fear of malpractice suits, routine use of early induction of labor, and epidural anesthesia. The technology of fetal monitoring combined with the lack of one on one support in labor has been shown to increase the C-section rate without improving neonatal outcomes (Alfirevic et al., 2017; Chen et al., 2018). Efforts have been underway to decrease the rate of primary C-section in an effort to improve overall maternal morbidity and mortality. Trial of labor after C-section resulting in a vaginal birth has become more common.

Mental Health

The most frequently occurring interruption in women's mental health relates to depression. The WHO (n.d.) reports that women experience depression at a rate of 41.9%, whereas the rate for men is 29.3%. Symptoms of depression include depressed mood, apathy, anxiety, irritability, and thoughts of death and suicide (CDC, 2020e). Unique to women are atypical symptoms including anxiety, increased appetite, weight gain, and somatic complaints along with increased rates of comorbid conditions. Women are more likely to attempt suicide but less likely to be successful (Urbanic, 2009). Women with socioeconomic barriers, such as lower income and lower educational levels, racial/ethnic discrimination, unemployment, poor health, single parenthood, and high-stress jobs, are at greater risk for depression than women with higher educational levels or higher economic status (WHO, n.d.). Other risk factors are childhood negligence and abuse, parental death, negligence, and alcoholism. Nurses practicing in community health settings should be aware of the signs and symptoms of depression and should identify referral sources for professional help within the community.

The community health nurse also plays a vital role in identifying mothers who suffer from perinatal depression specific to pregnancy and postpartum. A mother's depression has significant impact on the health of her pregnancy, as well as her child's development and family functioning. The use of the majority of antidepressant and other psychiatric medications is benefits pregnancy and women should be informed of the risks related to untreated psychiatric disorders (APA, 2018). Nearly one in eight women suffer postpartum depression that interferes with a woman's ability to care for herself, baby, and family and suicide is the second leading cause of death in the postpartum period (CDC, 2020e; Richmond, 2019). A woman experiencing perinatal depression displays a variety of symptoms, including depressed mood, weight changes, sleep disturbances, and fatigue, among others, which can be found in the *Diagnostic and Statistical Manual of Mental Disorders* (APA, 2013).

SOCIAL FACTORS AFFECTING WOMEN'S HEALTH

Healthcare Access

According to the National Center for Health Care Statistics, in 2012 18.2% of the U.S. population, or 48.2 million U.S. citizens, lacked health insurance coverage. With the passing of the ACA in 2012, the number of uninsured citizens had dropped to 28.5 million by 2016. Changes in the requirements for individual mandate and rising costs of premiums led to increased numbers of uninsured increased to 28.9 million people in 2019. The ACA requires all insurers to provide coverage for essential services to women, including preventive screenings (cervical and breast cancer), pregnancy care, breast-feeding support, and. Young adults (i.e., those between ages 16 and 24 years) previously made up approximately 50% of individuals without health insurance, can obtain coverage or stay on their parent's insurance until the age of 26. Women who choose not to enroll in the ACA are not likely to seek healthcare until they or a family member is in acute distress (Kaiser Family Foundation [KFF], 2021). Others may rely on home remedies, over-the-counter drugs, or folk healers

TABLE 17.3 Top 10 Occupations by Decade for Women

Rank	1970	1980	1990	2000	2010	2018
1	Secretary	Secretary	Secretary	Secretary	Teacher	Teacher
2	Teacher	Teacher	Teacher	Teacher	Secretary	Nurse
3	Sales clerk	Bookkeeper	Nurse	Nurse	Nurse	Nurse, psychiatric home health aides
4	Bookkeeper	Nurse	Cashier	Cashier	Cashier	Secretary
5	Nurse	Cashier	Bookkeeper	Retail, sales	Nurse, psychiatric home health aides	Cashier
6	Waiters	Manager, administrator	Manager, administrator	Bookkeeper	Retail, sales	Customer service
7	Typist	Office clerk	Nurse aide, orderly	Nurse, psychiatric home health aides	Customer service	Retail, sales
8	Sewer, stitcher	Waiter	Office clerk	Customer service	Waiter	Waiter
9	Cashier	Sales worker	Supervisor, sales	Childcare worker	Supervisor, retail sales	Supervisor, retail sales
10	Maid, private	Nurse aide, orderly	Sales workers	Waiter	Maids, housekeeping	Managers

for healthcare. Older women on fixed incomes may have difficulty meeting copayments required by Medicare and paying for prescription medications. Many senior citizens have paid hospitalization insurance premiums for policies that fail to meet the gap.

Education and Work

In 1970, 55.4% of all women aged 25 or older were high school graduates, compared with 81.6% in 1995% and 83% in 2016. Of this same age group, 38% completed college, which is nearly four times the 1970 rate of 8.1% (U.S. Census Bureau, 2020). In the workplace, women traditionally predominated as secretaries, administrative assistants, registered nurses (RNs), teachers, cashiers, and retail salespeople. However, in the 1980s, more women began to enter professions traditionally held by men (e.g., lawyers, physicians, and dentists). In 2019, 31% of women were in these professional occupations, with 18.6% in administrative support, 18.2% in management and business, and 16.5% in service (U.S. Bureau of Labor Statistics, 2019). Women make up 38% of lawyers, 36.5% of physicians, and 34.5% of dentists (Cheeseman Day, 2018; KFF, 2020; American Dental Association, 2020). While women have been earning degrees in traditionally male-dominated professions, the top two professions for women have been teacher or secretary since 1970. Trends for employment can be found in Table 17.3.

Employment and Wages

In 2016, 57% of the workforce were women. In addition, more than half (64%) of women with young children (younger than 6 years) were working outside the home (U.S. Department of Labor, 2017). In 1950, only 12% of women were combining these roles (Chadwick and Heaton, 1992).

Several questions concerning women's health and well-being relate to employment issues. A review of female-dominated versus male-dominated jobs discloses inequalities in wage and salary scales; despite the diminishing gap between women's and men's incomes, there is still much room for improvement.

Table 17.4 depicts median annual income by sex and ethnicity for both men and women (Semega et al., 2020). Disparities in income, based on sex and ethnicity, are clear. The Bureau of Labor statistics reports that female full time workers earned 82% of male wages, which is an improvement since 1979 when it was 62% (Bureau of Labor Statistics, 2020).

Women heads of households and their children are the poorest aggregate in the United States. This phenomenon is labeled "the feminization of poverty." In 2019, the poverty rate for single female heads of household was 22.2%, compared with 11.5% for single male heads of households (Semega et al., 2020). Race is a factor in the poverty rate for single head of householders as follows:

- Black 31.7%
- Hispanic 31.1%
- White 17.8% (Creamer and Mohanty, 2019)

The nurse working with impoverished families should be aware of social services, child care programs, emergency services, and other resources for families in need. The community health nurse often needs to act as case manager and advocate for families with social service agencies and other public entities.

WORKING WOMEN AND HOME LIFE

Added to inequalities outside the home are inequalities within the home. A working woman is less likely to have a spouse or partner help with the home and children. Even when a spouse or partner is present, the burdens of housework and child care usually fall more heavily on the woman, regardless of ethnicity. Mothers generally spend more time than fathers preparing meals and training and disciplining their children. These multiple-role demands and conflicting expectations contribute to stress (American Academy of Pediatrics, 2003; Matthews and Power, 2002).

However, men now report spending more time in family activities. Black and Hispanic men tend to spend a little more

TABLE 17.4	Median Annual Earnings by Type of Household in 7 Years Between 1969 and 2011							
Household Type	1969	1979	1989	1999	2003	2007	2011	2018
Married couple with children	41,453	47,793	50,613	56,827	62,405	72,785	74,130	95,351
Female householder No spouse, with children	16,327	18,468	17,651	26,164	29,307	33,370	33,637	45,946
Male householder no spouse, with children	33,749	36,619	34,646	41,830	41,959	49,839	49,567	62,632

From DeNavas-Semega J, Kollar M, Shrider EA, Creamer JF: *Income and poverty in the United States: 2019* (Issued September 2020), 2020. Available from: https://www.census.gov/content/dam/Census/library/publications/2020/demo/p60-270.pdf.

time working at family tasks than white men. Books and articles encourage wives and husbands to make their needs known, encouraging greater communication between partners. Marriage enrichment programs, often offered through churches and synagogues, teach couples how to communicate more effectively with each other, fostering equality between partners.

Family Configuration and Marital Status

Women are members of **multiple family configurations** (e.g., nuclear families, extended family units, single-parent units, families of group marriages, blended family units, adoptive family units, nonlegal heterosexual unions, and lesbian family units). This diversity causes changes in women's roles within families. Whether or not they function in a traditional role, most women do whatever is necessary to maintain the integrity of their families. Early assessment of the strengths of family units by the community health nurse provides a database for positive nursing interventions established on upstream strategies to enhance each family's level of health and well-being.

Many women are delaying marriage, and an increasing number are not marrying. Overall, marriage rates have remained stable, perhaps because the increasing number of remarriages balances the declining rate of first marriages. When a relationship ends in divorce or separation, more women than men have the responsibility of providing for themselves and their children. Single mothers are most often the head of a single-parent family. Even in the face of changing lifestyles, divorce, and increased mobility, which leads to long-distance relationships, most Americans report that they remain connected to their extended families through parents, grandparents, siblings, aunts, and uncles.

One contemporary family configuration involves single women with one or more adopted children. Single-parent adoptions are legal, and a growing number of single women are becoming adoptive parents. An often-ignored family structure is one headed by a lesbian parent. Since the Supreme Court made gay marriage a right in 2015, same-sex couples have made progress in establishing families. Lesbians who become parents have needs similar to those of all mothers. Many cities have lesbian-gay parent groups that provide support, anticipatory guidance, and strategies for coping in society. However, lesbian women often neglect their own health. This selfneglect may be traced to hostile and rejecting attitudes of healthcare providers (Zeidenstein, 2004). However, the parents or guardians must remain healthy to ensure the child's well-being.

 ACTIVE LEARNING

Review county or state health department statistics for leading causes of death among women of varying ethnic or racial groups.

HEALTH PROMOTION STRATEGIES FOR WOMEN

A woman's ability to carry out her important roles can affect her entire family; therefore women should receive services that promote health and detect disease at an early stage. Early detection and improved treatments for disease allow women to return to work or remain working throughout the course of an illness. Although work is essential to the economic and social well-being of many women's families, the workplace itself creates physical and social stress. As more women enter the workforce and face many of the same risks and stressors as men do, it is not surprising that their formerly favorable mortality and morbidity rates have been declining.

Many women seek information that will allow them to be in control of their own health. Since the early 1970s, women have met in selfhelp groups to develop a better understanding of their own health needs. Some of the health behaviors that women learn in these groups are the importance of nutrition and exercise, health maintenance, pregnancy testing and contraceptive awareness; recognition of the early signs of vaginal infections and STDs; and awareness of the variations in female anatomy and physiology.

For women who desire to become more knowledgeable about their own health, books are available in bookstores, in public libraries, and among the holdings of traditional women's groups such as sororities and federated women's clubs. An excellent resource for women is the FDA Consumer (http://www.fda.gov/), the official consumer site of the FDA, which reports on studies that cover a variety of women's health issues such as mammography standards, menopause, treatment for STDs, eating disorders, infertility, cosmetic safety, silicone breast implants, and osteoporosis. Another resource is the U.S. Department of Health and Human Services' Office on Women's Health (www.WomensHealth.gov), which highlights positive health behaviors for women and girls. The community health nurse can use models such as Pender's Health Promotion Model in teaching health behaviors that lead to general health promotion among women. Pender notes that health-promoting behaviors are directed toward sustaining or increasing the level of well-being, selfactualization, and fulfillment of a given individual or group (Pender et al., 2006). However, because many models were developed for the middle class, they may not be useful to community health nurses working with low-income families.

Knowledge deficits related to body awareness prevail among all women, regardless of socioeconomic or educational level. For example, a woman may ask whether she will menstruate after a hysterectomy, whether she should perform a breast selfexamination (BSE), or what she can do to prevent recurrent episodes of vaginitis. Nurses can play an instrumental role in helping women develop a greater sense of selfawareness. Furthermore, community health nurses can remove the mystery surrounding the woman's body and encourage clients to ask previously unmentionable questions.

Chronic Illness

Included among chronic diseases that may affect a woman during her life span are coronary vascular disease and metabolic syndrome, hypertension, diabetes, arthritis, osteoporosis, and cancer.

Coronary Vascular Disease and Metabolic Syndrome

Evidence suggests that CVD and metabolic syndrome in most women are preventable. CVD is caused by atherosclerosis, which results in buildup of plaque that in turn narrows arteries, decreasing blood flow to the heart muscle. Metabolic syndrome is a group of risk factors that have been linked to an increased risk of cardiovascular events. These factors are abdominal obesity (waist circumference more than 35 inches in women), dyslipidemia (elevated triglyceride and low high-density lipoprotein cholesterol values), insulin resistance, and elevated blood pressure. The underlying etiology of metabolic syndrome is related to the combination of inactivity, obesity, and genetics.

At-risk women have nonmodifiable risk factors such as increasing age, race, gender, or family history of CVD and diabetes. Where the greatest impact can be made is with the modifiable risk factors, which are as follows (AHA, 2021b):

- Cigarette smoking
- Obesity
- Diet high in calories, total fats, cholesterol, refined carbohydrates, and sodium
- Glucose intolerance
- Elevated serum lipid values
- Sedentary lifestyle
- Hypertension
- Stress
- Alcohol use

Education by community nurses can assist women in identifying their risk of CVD and metabolic syndrome along with health behaviors that decrease modifiable risk factors.

Hypertension

The latest report of the Joint National Committee on Prevention, Detection, Evaluation, and Treatment of High Blood Pressure defines **hypertension** as blood pressure of 140/90 mm Hg or greater diastolic. If the client is over the age of 60, the threshold is 150/90 mm Hg (Kovell et al., 2015). Essential hypertension is the most common type of chronic hypertensive disorder in women. Approximately one-third of hypertension cases occur during pregnancy as gestational hypertension or preeclampsia. Essential hypertension is the most common type of chronic hypertensive disorder in women, accounting for 85% of such cases. It is also responsible for approximately one-third of all hypertension cases during pregnancy. Hypertension is more common in women than in men and affects more blacks than whites. Hypertension usually starts with an asymptomatic phase; therefore every woman should be screened on an average of every 2 years beginning in her teenage years. Diagnosis is crucial to prevent or modify possible complications of this disease.

Diabetes

According to the CDC (2020a), 34.2 million people (10.5% of the population) have diabetes in the United States, and the number is growing every year. Furthermore, although an estimated 26.8 million have been diagnosed, some 7.3 million people are not aware they have the disease. In previous years, community health nurses have worked to educate women to assume responsibility in their management of diabetes mellitus. More recently, community health nurses have been actively involved in education and screening programs for groups at high risk. Included in these groups are individuals who have a family history of diabetes, those who are obese, and older adults. Nurses who design education programs need to be aware of the ethnic differences in the prevalence of diabetes. African American, Hispanic, American Indian, and Asian women are more likely to have diabetes than their non-Latino white counterparts.

Preexisting diabetes may be may aggravated by pregnancy. Gestational diabetes appears only during pregnancy but increases the risk of developing Type 2 diabetes later in life (ACOG, 2008). Diabetes in pregnancy is linked to other complications. Neonatal complications include macrosomia, hyperbilirubinemia, shoulder dystocia, birth trauma, and stillbirth. Maternal complications include increased risk for cesarean section and preeclampsia. Consequently, screening for diabetes is routine in pregnancy in the second trimester and if diagnosed repeated in the postpartum period (ACOG, 2008). Annual screening for Type 2 diabetes should occur beginning at age 45. Screening methods include the fasting blood glucose, hemoglobin A1C, or 2-hour oral glucose tolerance test. The nurse is involved in explaining the purpose of the screening and how to prepare for the tests that are part of routine and pregnancy screening. In most public health settings, the nurse is responsible for explaining the results.

Arthritis

In 2013—15, 54.4 million people in the United States, or 22% of adults were afflicted with arthritis rheumatoid arthritis (RA), gout, lupus, or fibromyalgia. The incidence of arthritis is higher in women than in men: approximately 26% of women have the condition, compared with 19.1% of men (CDC, 2018a,b; Arthritis Foundation, 2020). In 2018, 15 million adults reported severe pain due to arthritis.

OA is the most common form of the disease, affecting 32.5 million adults and is more common in women over 45 (AF, 2020). It is characterized by degeneration of the joints and is more common with increasing age and in women. OA of the knee is the leading cause of disability in the United States. Modifiable risk factors for OA include excess body mass, joint injury, occupation, and estrogen deficiency (CDC, 2019a).

RA can affect anyone, but for every man affected, two to three women have the disease (CDC, 2020a). Onset usually occurs between 30 and 50 years of age. RA often goes into remission in a pregnant woman, although symptoms tend to increase in intensity after the baby is born, and RA develops more often than expected the year after giving birth. Although women are two to three times more likely to have RA than men, men tend to be more severely affected when they do have it (AF, 2020).

Arthritis is the leading cause of disability in the United States (CDC, 2019a). Nursing interventions focus on healthy diet, joint friendly activities, prevention of joint deformity and modification of lifestyle if necessary.

Osteoporosis

Osteoporosis is a major disorder affecting women, occurring in 25% to 50% of postmenopausal women. Although men may experience osteoporosis, it is four times more common among women. The National Osteoporosis Foundation (2013) estimates that of the 54 million Americans who have osteoporosis and osteopenia. Of those over the age of 50, twice as many women will suffer a fracture caused by osteoporosis. After 65, it increases to five times more for women (24.5%) than men (5.1%) (Looker, 2015). Half of all non-Hispanic white women in the United States will experience an osteoporosis-related fracture during their lifetimes. The most serious complication of osteoporosis is hip fracture, which is experienced by 280,000 Americans annually. Approximately 24% die within a year from complications of hip fracture.

Postmenopausal white women are at highest risk for osteoporosis. Loss of bone begins at an earlier age in women and proceeds twice as rapidly as in men. Guidelines issued by the National Osteoporosis Foundation recommend bone mineral density tests for selected postmenopausal women and the use of oral bisphosphonates as the first-line pharmacological treatment. In light of the results of the Women's Health Initiative Study showing that nonestrogen therapies fail or cause intolerable side effects, hormone replacement therapy is currently considered second-line therapy for the disease (Rosen and Drezner, 2021). Osteoporosis has no cure. Therefore, prevention is especially important early in life. Prevention involves an awareness of dietary practices such as maintaining a correct balance of calcium, vitamin D, and protein throughout life, in addition to regular weight-bearing, muscle-strengthening, and aerobic exercise.

Nurses in ambulatory health practices should encourage women to become more knowledgeable of the strategies to prevent osteoporosis. For women diagnosed with this condition, nurses can assist in various aspects of management (e.g., education regarding prescribed medication, follow-up care, avoidance of complications, and dietary modifications as needed).

Breast Cancer

The incidence of **breast cancer** has been rising since the 1950s. Currently, one out of every eight women will have breast cancer sometime in her life. The chance of dying from breast cancer is about one in 35, and breast cancer is second leading cause of cancer death. In 2016, 250,520 women in the United States were diagnosed with breast cancer and 42,000 died from it (USCS, 2020). The death rate has been decreasing annually by 1% per year, in part due to routine screening, early intervention and improved treatment. Risk factors include aging, personal or family history (especially mother or sister) of breast cancer, early age at menarche, late age at menopause, never having children, and having a first child after age 30. Female gender and aging are the most significant risk factors for breast cancer (ACS, 2021a). An additional risk is a genetic mutation of tumor suppressor genes known as *BRCA1* and *BRCA2*. The lifetime risk for women with this mutation to be diagnosed with breast cancer is 55% to 72%, compared with 13% for the general population. Additional risks are for ovarian cancer, with a 39% to 44% lifetime risk for those who inherit the gene, compared with 1.4% for the general population (ACS, 2020b; NCI, 2020c). Genetic testing is available, and the rights of those tested is protected legally, so insurers and employers cannot use this information to discriminate against those testing positive (Genetic Information Nondiscrimination Act, 2008).

In 2008, United States Preventive Services Task Force, based on a review of scientific evidence, recommended that women not have routine mammography screening between ages 40 and 49 years but should have biennial screenings between the ages 50 and 74 years. This was reaffirmed in 2016, but considered a major shift from the recommendation of annual screening mammograms for women older than 40 years. The researchers cited the reason for this recommended change as improvements in mammography screening films that led to more accurate diagnosing. They also cited the high cost and harmful psychological effect of screening on women related to unnecessary diagnostic testing resulting from the high number of false-positive results. The ACS and American College of Obstetricians and Gynecologists recommend shared decision making with patients between the ages of 40 and 49 recommendation, and annual mammograms after age 50 (CDC, 2020a). Key to mammogram screening is a woman's informed choice based on individual risk factors for development of breast cancer as well as the benefits (early detection and improved survival) and potential harms (false-positive results or missed cancer).

The current position of the U.S. Preventive Services Task Force is that there is insufficient evidence to recommend for or against the teaching of BSE (Thomas et al., 2002). The ACS (2020) also no longer supports the routine use of selfbreast exam or clinical breast examination (CBE) for screening because of this lack of evidence. Instead, women are encouraged to be familiar with the normal look and feel of their breasts and to report changes to a healthcare provider.

For women at low risk who are 40 years and older, the greatest potential to save lives from breast cancer is through early detection with mammography (ACS, 2020a). In addition to annual mammography and CBEs, breast cancer detection may involve ultrasound, MRI, positron emission tomography, and genetic testing for *BRCA1* and *BRCA2* (NCI, 2020a). Box 17.2 lists resources that provide information about breast cancer and early detection.

RESEARCH HIGHLIGHTS

Breast Cancer Study

A study of the data collected in the U.S. National Cancer Institute's Surveillance, Epidemiology, and End Results (SEER) (2021) reports that 2000 to 2017 there was a 0.3% annual increase in this breast cancer, while age adjusted death rates fell 1.4% each year. From 1976 to 2009 there was a 2.07% average compounded increase in the incidence of breast cancer with distant involvement in younger women, age 25–39 years (ACS, 2021c). This increase was highest in Hispanic and African American women (Johnson, 2013).

The CDC monitors United States cancer statistics to determine whether race affects breast cancer outcomes. Trends suggest the incidence of breast cancer diagnosis disparity between black and white women has stabilized, but the disparity in death rate remains (Richardson et al., 2016). Incidence for those over age 60 has decreased in white women while increasing in black women. A combination of health factors like obesity, and health behaviors like participation in screening has caused a shift in the trends. Data from 2005

through 2009 showed that black women had a lower incidence of breast cancer diagnosis and were diagnosed at more advanced stages with a 41% death rate (Cronin et al., 2012). Several initiatives from the federal government have been launched to address the differences for black women that contribute to decreasing the disparity, including:

- Acknowledging the role of family history
- Targeted treatment of the most common type of breast cancer (negative estrogen receptor, progesterone receptor, and HER2 status)
- Public health initiatives to decrease obesity through increased physical activity and improved nutrition
- Increased access to screening mammograms
- Support for follow-up and treatment after diagnosis

Lung Cancer

Although breast cancer is the most common cancer among women after skin cancer, cancer of the lung and bronchus is responsible for more cancer deaths (ACS, 2021c). In 2017, 107,545 women were diagnosed with lung cancer. Between 1990 and 2003, there was a 60% increase in the number of new cases of lung cancer in American women, attributed to increased tobacco use among women (Patel, 2005). Since 2003, the rates of lung cancer diagnosis and death have steadily decreased. Lung cancer is still responsible for more deaths yearly in U.S. women than breast cancer. In 2017, 30.6 of every 100,000 women died from lung cancer, compared with 19.9 per 100,000 from breast cancer (U.S. Cancer Statistics Working Group [USCSWG], 2020). In fact, lung cancer kills more women annually than breast, ovarian, and uterine cancers combined (ACS, 2021c). Of all clients who have lung cancer, 85% to 90% have a history of cigarette smoking. Yet lung cancer develops in only 20% of cigarette smokers, suggesting that the cause of lung cancer is multifactorial.

Widely accepted risk factors for lung cancer include exposure to tobacco through cigarette or cigar smoking, second

BOX 17.2 Resource Materials for Breast Cancer

BCCCP (Breast and Cervical Cancer Control Program)
Website https://bcccp.ncdhhs.gov
Federally funded free breast and cervical cancer screening through state departments of community health

American Cancer Society
Website http://www.cancer.org/acs/groups/cid/documents/webcontent/003165-pdf.pdf
Breast cancer basics
Risk factors for breast cancer
Can breast cancer be found early?
Can breast cancer be prevented?
Imaging tests to find breast cancer
Signs and symptoms of breast cancer

National Cancer Institute
Breast Cancer—Patient Version
https://www.cancer.gov/types/breast.

Breast Cancer Risk in American Women https://www.cancer.gov/types/breast/risk-fact-sheet.
BRCA Gene Mutations https://www.cancer.gov/about-cancer/causes-prevention/genetics/brca-fact-sheet.
Surgery to Reduce the Risk of Breast Cancer https://www.cancer.gov/types/breast/risk-reducing-surgery-fact-sheet.
Reproductive History and Cancer Risk https://www.cancer.gov/about-cancer/causes-prevention/risk/hormones/reproductive-history-fact-sheet.
Breast Cancer Screening https://www.cancer.gov/types/breast/patient/breast-screening-pdq#section/all.
Breast Cancer Treatment https://www.cancer.gov/types/breast/patient/breast-treatment-pdq.

U.S. Department of Health and Human Services, Office on Women's Health
Mammograms https://www.womenshealth.gov/a-z-topics/mammograms.
Medicare.
Mammograms https://www.medicare.gov/coverage/mammograms.

hand tobacco smoke, occupational exposures (radon, asbestos, uranium, arsenic, diesel exhaust), chronic lung disease, air pollution, and a history of tobacco-related cancer or treatment with radiation (ACS, 2019). The possible link between electronic cigarettes (vaping) and smoking marijuana is not yet clear, but some carcinogenic substances are the same as those found in tobacco smoke. Studies have shown that the risks for development of lung cancer are different in women and men and that lung cancer appears to be a biologically different disease in women. Women smokers are more likely than men to have adenocarcinoma of the lung, and women who have never smoked are more likely to have lung cancer than men who have never smoked. These differences are due to hormonal, genetic, and metabolic differences between the sexes (North and Christiani, 2013).

Although medical treatment may be similar for men and women, the symptom distress, quality of life, and demands of illness experienced by women may be different from those in men, because the competing household, child care, and other role-related demands take a toll on many women (Sarna and McCorkle 1996; Sarna et al., 2005). Further, women with advanced lung cancer report more psychological symptoms than men (Hopwood et al. 1995).

Lung cancer is often a fatal illness because it is diagnosed most commonly at an advanced stage; early detection is difficult, and treatment for advanced disease is not as effective. Women appear to have a slight survival advantage over men: the 5-year survival rate is 23.1% for women with lung cancer and 16.5% for men (USCSWG, 2020).

The primary factor in preventing lung cancer is for individuals either to never start smoking or to quit smoking. Nurses must work with other healthcare providers to reverse the morbidity and mortality rates related to this disease. The Agency for Healthcare Research and Quality has developed a useful guideline for healthcare professionals to assist women and their families in smoking cessation efforts plus summaries of more than 400 guidelines on a wide variety of topics, which can be found on their website (http://www.ahrq.gov).

Gynecological Cancers

About 20% of all malignant diseases in women occur in the genital tract. The incidence of invasive cervical cancer has declined dramatically. In 2017, 12,831 women were diagnosed with cervical cancer and 4207 women died from the disease in 2017 (CDC, 2020b). Cervical cancer used to be a leading cause of cancer death, but the use of cytological screening (Pap smears) and routine vaccinations has decreased the mortality rate. One major risk factor is infection with HPV, which is linked to nearly all cervical cancer cases. Other risk factors include coitus at an early age, multiple sexual partners, cigarette smoking, history of *Chlamydia* infection, long-term oral contraceptives, intrauterine device, multiple pregnancies, pregnancy at a young age, HIV, family history, and low socioeconomic status (ACS, 2020b). It is most commonly diagnosed in women between the ages of 30 and 50 years,

because the cellular changes that lead to cancer are caused by chronic infection and inflammation. It is uncommon for women who undergo regular screening to be diagnosed with cancer. Low-income women have access to free or low cost cervical cancer screening through the CDC's National Breast and Cervical Cancer Early Detection Program.

Current guidelines recommend cervical cancer screening to begin at 21 years of age. Screening should then be performed every 3 years until age 65 using liquid-based Pap smear tests. After age 30, cotesting for HPV DNA (CDC, 2021a) is acceptable. Because HPV is a common virus affecting 80 million people, routine screening for HPV is not recommended in women younger than 30. HPV infection is responsible for the majority of these cancers: 91% anal, 75% vaginal and vulvar, 63% penile, and 70% oropharynx (CDC, 2020b). Current recommendations are that girls and boys be vaccinated for HPV beginning at the age of 11 or 12 years. Between 2006 and 2019, more than 120 million doses of HPV vaccine had been administered without serious safety concerns (CDC, 2019c; 2021c). Because of the ACA, vaccinations are covered by private insurers and through the Vaccines for Children Program for eligible children who would otherwise not have access.

The incidence of uterine cancer is highest for black women at 27.5/100,000 and white women at 27.2/100,000 (USCS, 2021). Despite nearly equal rates, mortality is higher among white women. Endometrial cancer is the most common form of uterine cancer. This cancer is commonly found in women during their sixth and seventh decades of life and 80% of women with this condition are postmenopausal. It is estimated that in 2021 66,570 women will be diagnosed with endometrial cancer and 12,940 will die (ACS, 2021b). Factors related to its occurrence are age, obesity, high fat diet and physical inactivity, low parity, family history, diabetes mellitus, breast and ovarian cancer, and endometrial hyperplasia. Conditions or hormonal medications that result in higher circulating estrogen levels and are not countered by adequate progesterone levels put the woman at risk. The most common sign of endometrial cancer, occurring in 90% of women, is abnormal vaginal bleeding. Postmenopausal women experiencing vaginal bleeding should seek immediate gynecological evaluation.

Cancer of the ovary causes more deaths than any other pelvic malignancy, although the mortality rate has fallen 1.6% per year since 2001 (USCS, 2020). The lifetime risk of ovarian cancer is 1.38%. The incidence increases with age, peaking in women 75 to 79 years old at 56.7 per 100,000. Risk factors include increasing age, nulliparity, never having breast-fed, a history of breast cancer, postmenopausal use of hormone replacement therapy, obesity, a family history of breast and ovarian cancer, and testing positive for the *BRCA* mutation. Protective factors against ovarian cancer include use of oral contraceptives, having and breast-feeding children, tubal sterilization, hysterectomy, and prophylactic oophorectomy (NCI, 2020a,d).

Ovarian cancer is a silent cancer. Early-stage detection is difficult; therefore it has usually reached an advanced stage when discovered. The health professional should be alert to ovarian enlargement on pelvic examination with suspicion that ovarian malignancy may be present, especially in a post-menopausal woman. The most common sign a woman experiences is abdominal enlargement. She may complain that her skirts and slacks are getting tighter in the waist. Any woman older than 40 years who experiences vague digestive complaints that persist and are not explained by another cause must have a thorough evaluation for ovarian cancer. According to the ACS (2020c), transvaginal ultrasound, MRI, or computed tomography scan along with a blood test for tumor marker CA-125 may assist in the diagnosis of ovarian cancer. These tests are not recommended for routine screening of all women but are recommended for those with risk factors related to family history (strong family history of ovarian and breast cancer, positive for genetic mutations *BRCA1* and *BRCA2*).

Mental Disorders and Stress

Various circumstances and conditions influence the mental health of women. Women face stressful decisions about career and family, and many express anxieties about these decisions. A woman may feel pressured to make decisions regarding childbearing before she has fulfilled her career goals. Deciding to focus on a career may mean decreased authority and the suffering of stress in the workplace. More women are occupying middle-management positions, which are known for creating stress-related illnesses associated with high demands and little or no power. Women combining motherhood and a career have additional decisions, such as whether to work during pregnancy and choice of child care.

A woman's emotional state can be influenced by ovarian function from the onset of menstruation to the cessation of menstrual periods. Depression may be triggered or worsened by premenstrual hormonal changes. Women with a history of depression are also at increased risk for a recurrent episode of depression during the postpartum period, and they also are at risk for depression during the perimenopausal transition (Blehar, 2003). Depression is more prevalent among women than among men. In all age groups from adolescents through the elderly, approximately two thirds of those affected with depression are women. According to Bhatia and Bhatia (1999), the higher prevalence of depression in women is most likely due to a combination of gender-related differences in cognitive styles, certain biological factors, and a higher incidence of psychosocial and economic stressors.

Mental disorders often go undiagnosed and untreated or undertreated despite the availability of effective treatments. Women may not recognize or correctly identify their symptoms, and even when they do, they may be reluctant to seek care because of stigma associated with mental illness (Blehar, 2003). Community health nurses are in a good position to assess women's moods in diverse aggregates. Being familiar with the symptoms of common mental disorders, nurses can identify these problems and can help women seek and maintain continuity of care.

Reproductive Health

Community health nurses provide a variety of services in the area of women's reproductive health from menarche through postmenopause. Nurses, in collaboration with other healthcare professionals, have identified a persistent group of preventable and correctable problems related to maternal-child health. *Healthy People 2030* (USDHHS, n.d.) provides numerous recommendations. Goals to address the social determinates of health impact the well-being of women significantly. These include improving access to quality healthcare; safe housing, transportation and neighborhoods; nutritious food and physical activity opportunities quality education that enhances literacy; along with economic and job opportunities. Issues surrounding air and water pollution, as well as racism, discrimination and violence are also *Healthy People 2030* goals. There are numerous recommendations for improving maternal and infant health, with objectives that include reduction of cigarette smoking, alcohol and other drug use, and mother-to-child HIV transmission. Objectives also include increased rates of intentional pregnancy, optimal nutrition, and weight gain that includes adequate folic acid; increased maternal TDAP vaccinations to prevent neonatal disease; improved access to early prenatal care and screening for postpartum depression; as well as reduced C-section births and maternal deaths are also priorities.

When looking back at the *Healthy People 2020* initiative, family planning objectives demonstrated progress. While adolescent pregnancy rates are higher than most developed countries, there has been a steady decrease. Between 1991 and 2015, rates decreased 64%, from 61.8 per 1000 to 18.8 per 1000 (CDC, 2019a; Hamilton, 2016). The improvements have been attributed to reduced sexual activity, low-cost and long-acting contraceptives, and condom use. Health disparities remain an issue for Hispanic and black populations who are disproportionality affected by social determinants.

Examples of *Healthy People (2030)* objectives related to family planning are shown in the *Healthy People 2030* box (USDHHS, n.d.).

Dysmenorrhea is painful menstruation that can be diagnosed as a primary disease or as a secondary one with an underlying etiology, peaking in the late adolescence and early 20's. This reproductive health problem affects approximately 50% to 90% of reproductive age women. At least 10% to 20% of women with dysmenorrhea report absenteeism from school and work (Smith and Kaunitz, 2020). Among young women and causes the loss of approximately 140 million working hours annually, therefore the economic influence of this condition is significant (Nelson, 2004).

ETHICAL INSIGHTS

Working With Women's Health

Community health nurses working in the field of women's health will be exposed to ethical dilemmas during their careers. For this reason, nurses must have a working knowledge of the principles of healthcare ethics. The commonly accepted principles include the following:
- Respect for autonomy
- Beneficence
- Nonmaleficence
- Justice

Nursing care revolves around moral values such as compassion, empathy, honesty, trust, and respect. Most encounters will be nonproblematic. Occasionally, nurses may be exposed to clinical situations that challenge their values and beliefs. Clients and family members may, at times, also disagree with the nurse's professional advice/plan. It is important for the nurse to keep his or her personal philosophy, politics, religion, and moral values out of clinical work with individuals and families.

Examples of potential ethical dilemmas related to women's healthcare are emergency contraception, abortion, assisted reproductive technology, and end-of-life issues.

The average age of menopause in the United States is 51 years. *Menopause* is defined as the cessation of menses for at least one full year, but it is characterized by several years of symptoms as the hormonal shifts occur, called perimenopause (Schuiling and Likis, 2017). At this stage, women's health concerns become focused on the symptoms associated with this transition. The most common complaints are related to vasomotor changes causing hot flushes, increased heart rate, insomnia, and night sweats; urogenital atrophy causing incontinence; vaginal dryness and dyspareunia; and mood alterations, including irritability, depression, and anxiety. Treatment with hormone therapy can provide benefits for the woman's quality of life. Depending on the type of hormone, risks include breast cancer (rare), endometrial hyperplasia and cancer, venous thromboembolism, biliary issues, myocardial infarction, stroke, and dementia (North American Menopause Society, 2017). Community health nurses can play a key role in helping women find resources to deal with symptoms, and develop an understanding of the normal processes associated with menopause as well as the risks and benefits of hormone therapy. Also, women in menopause need guidance in promoting a healthy lifestyle because they have an increased risk for development of

chronic conditions such as osteoporosis, coronary heart disease, hypertension, and Type 2 diabetes.

Nutrition

One of the most important factors in a woman's reproductive health is her total life nutritional experience from infancy through childhood and adolescence. Obesity has become a major public health concern. The community health nurse is in an advantageous position to provide nutritional counseling. The U.S. Department of Agriculture (2021) updates the dietary recommendations every 5 years on the basis of current scientific information. The "My Plate" approach to healthy eating is intended to encourage persons to be mindful of the foods they eat in terms of both portion size and proportion to other foods. One-half of the plate should consist of fruits and vegetables, with one-quarter each for meats/proteins and grains, preferably whole grains. Recommendations also include eating less sodium and fewer sugary foods (U.S. Department of Agriculture, 2020).

Pregnancy may provide a motivational factor for developing an awareness of proper nutrition. During the nutritional assessment of a prenatal client, the community health nurse can take the opportunity to determine dietary habits and initiate a referral to the Special Supplemental Food Program for Women, Infants, and Children (USDA, n.d.). This program provides food vouchers for pregnant or breastfeeding women, infants, and children who are at nutritional risk.

Good nutrition must include factors other than kinds and amounts of foods. Elements to consider include age, lifestyle, economic status, and culture. For example, when counseling a pregnant adolescent, the nurse can include the primary person responsible for meal preparation. The nurse should include the adolescent in the planning of her diet, asking her to identify foods that she likes from those recommended. The nurse should make the adolescent aware of the influence of her nutrition on fetal growth and development. This information must be balanced with the young woman's individual needs.

Sexually Transmitted Infections

Sexually transmitted infections (STIs) are commonly found among U.S. women. Community health nurses and other health providers, including physicians, nurse practitioners

♥ HEALTHY PEOPLE 2030

Selected Objectives for Family Planning and Reproductive Health

Objective	Baseline (Year)	Target (2020)	Final (Year)	Target 2030
FP-01: Reduce the proportion of pregnancies that are unintended.	48% (2002)	44%	43% (2013)	36.5%
FP-03: Reduce pregnancies among adolescent females (pregnancies per 1000 females 15—17 years of age).	40.2% (2005)	36.2%	43.4% (2013)	31.4%
FP-11: Increase the proportion of adolescent females at risk for unintended pregnancy who use effective birth control.	45.4% (2011—15)	54.1%	56.3% (2015—17)	70.1%
STD-1: Increase the proportion of sexually active females aged 16—20 screened for *Chlamydia trachomatis* infections.	40.1% (2008)	61.3%	45.8% (2017)	67.5%

Data from U.S. Department of Health and Human Services: *Healthy people 2030*, ed 3, Washington, DC, 2010.

(NPs), nurse midwives, and social workers, must be prepared to provide age-appropriate STD prevention, education, and counseling.

In 2021, the CDC reported there were 26 million new and 68 million total cases in the United States. Half of those affect 15 to 24-year-olds. The 2018 prevalence follows:

- HPV 42.5 million
- Trichomoniasis 2.6 million
- Chlamydia 1.7 million
- HIV 984,000
- Gonorrhea 209,000
- Syphilis (primary, secondary, congenital) 115,045
- Hepatitis B 103,000 (CDC, 2021h)

HPV is the most common STI in the United States. There are 40 types of HPV that can cause infections. While most are asymptomatic and resolve within a few years, persistent infections can lead to anogenital and oropharyngeal warts and even cancer. HPV vaccination has been shown to decrease genital HPV infections, anogenital warts, and high-grade cervical lesions (CDC, 2019g).

Trichomonas vaginalis is a protozoal infection that causes vaginitis and is linked to preterm birth. It affects women 4 times more often than men. Rates have been stable for the past 20 years.

Chlamydia infections increased 14% between 2014 and 2018 and is most common in 14 to 19 year olds. It is diagnosed three times more in women than men, most likely because of the CDC's recommendation for routine screening of any sexually active woman of childbearing age to prevent infertility (CDC, 2019a).

Gonorrhea is diagnosed more often in men, and more likely in 20 to 24-year-olds. Rates for gonorrhea increased 82.6% between 2009 and 2018. The Gonococcal Isolate Surveillance Project (GISP) demonstrated that gonorrhea was becoming resistant to treatment with CDC-recommended fluoroquinolone drugs in 2007. The CDC to revised treatment guidelines with ceftriaxone for first line treatment has remained effective. The GISP is ongoing (CDC, 2019g).

Females are less affected by syphilis. In those aged 25–29 male rates were 55.7 per 100,000 males and women were 10 per 100,000 females. Congenital syphilis contributes to stillbirth and infant death and has increased every year. The rate of the disease from 2013 to 2018 increased by 185%. While syphilis was more common MSM, a heterosexual epidemic has been identified and is affecting childbearing women and their children (CDC, 2019g).

Genital herpes is often an asymptomatic STI and most genital infections are caused by Type 2. Trends indicate decreasing cases of the infection, yet estimates are that 15.7% of the population aged 14–49 is seropositive, but 80% remain asymptomatic. While herpes is not curable, antiviral medications and safer sex practices can decrease the chance or transmission to a partner (CDC, 2019g). The CDC (2021) guidelines for treating STIs are updated regularly and available online (www.cdc.gov/std/tg2015/default.htm). A vital role of the community health nurse is to follow up with the woman's sex partner(s) who require(s) evaluation and treatment. Partner notification and expedited treatment, along with avoidance of sexual activity until treatment/cure, are key to stopping the spread of STIs. In addition to medications, women and their partners need individualized counseling on reducing risky sexual behaviors and correct use of latex condoms.

Human Immunodeficiency Virus and Acquired Immunodeficiency Syndrome (AIDS). Today, the HIV/AIDS epidemic represents a persistent health threat to women in the United States, especially young women and women of color. In 2017, 19% of the 38,739 new HIV diagnoses were women (CDC, 2019b). Among women diagnosed with HIV/AIDS, 59% are Black, 20% White, and 16% Latina. The rate of death for HIV disease decreased 48.4% from 2010–17 (Bosh, 2020). Although, among those with the disease the death rate for women (5.4/1000) is higher than men (4.5/1000). Transmission in women is primarily through heterosexual contact (86%), followed by injection drug use (14%). For all ethnicities, primary transmission in men occurs through sexual contact with other men, whereas in women, the route is high-risk heterosexual contact. As of 2016, HIV diagnoses decreased 21% with the greatest improvement among black women. HIV/AIDS is longer a top 10 cause of death globally, thanks to more available treatment and increased use of safe sex practices (WHO, 2020b). In 2019, the estimated number of people living with HIV around the world was 38 million.

Risk factors for and barriers to prevention of HIV/AIDS for women include the following:

- Young age at sexual initiation
- Lack of awareness regarding disease and condom use
- Sexual inequality in relationships
- Biological vulnerability to STIs
- Substance abuse
- Poverty; dropping out of school
- Stigma surrounding testing and treatment
- Working in the sex trade
- Participants in unprotected sex

The USDHHS (2019) continues to update the *Guidelines for the Use of Antiretroviral Agents in HIV-1 Infected Adults and Adolescents*. Treatment continually evolves with new research and experience. The use of antiretroviral drugs includes using new and combined agents to decrease viral load in those with HIV and prevent transmission for those in high-risk groups. Persons at risk who fear the stigma of testing can easily do selftesting with quick results that connects them with local resources (CDC, 2021b). It is imperative that the community health nurse working with this population stays abreast of the current trends for both counseling and treatment options. Community health nurses also must target at-risk populations and campaign for the use of safer sex practices and routine HIV testing for those at risk.

Other Issues in Women's Health

Unintentional Injury or Accidents and Intimate Partner Violence

Although unintentional injury affects women less commonly than men, several areas of concern still exist for women. For example, older women are at increased risk for accidents such as falls. Falls account for the majority of serious unintentional injuries for older adults. According to the CDC (2017), fall death rates increased 30% between 2007 and 2016. If the rate continues at the same pace there will be seven deaths due to falls every hour in the United States by 2030. Factors that may be responsible for this major cause of injury among older adults are an unsteady gait, reduced vision, and a hazardous environment (Bergen et al., 2016). Older women experience an increasing number of falls; therefore the nurse must identify the preventable factors. Whether working with older adults in the home or in institutional settings, nurses must be knowledgeable about hazards that may be corrected to decrease the incidence of falls.

Intimate partner violence (IPV), sometimes called domestic abuse, is the single largest cause of injury to women between the ages of 15 and 44 in the United States—more common than muggings, car accidents, and rapes combined. IPV is committed by a current or former boyfriend/girlfriend/spouse. In 2015, one in four women were victims of intimate partner violence and the lifetime prevalence is one in 3 (Smith, 2015).

Abuse in women is often explained as accidental injury. Approximately 6% of visits made by women to emergency departments are for injuries that result from physical battering by their husbands, former husbands, boyfriends, or lovers. IPV includes physical, sexual, emotional, economic, and psychological abuse. A subset of IPV is dating violence, which occurs in a romantic relationship. Reports of teen dating abuse indicate that one in 11 females report some sort of abuse and one in eight reports being sexually coerced (CDC, 2021g).

Nurses employed in community health settings need to know how to make assessments, provide support, and make referrals to agencies dealing with IPV (see Boxes 17.3 through 17.5). Understanding the state laws related to reporting known or suspected intimate partner violence is important. The American Medical Association and American Nurses Association advocate that all women be assessed for IPV. Questions should be posed privately in nonjudgmental but specific terms (i.e., "Do you feel safe?" "Have you ever been hit, punched, slapped, or kicked?") with follow-up questions if the woman responds "yes" (Kovach, 2004). Many nurses are past or current victims of abuse; assessing abuse with clients can evoke painful emotions that the nurse may not be ready to confront. Chapter 27 contains additional information about intimate partner violence.

Disability

More women than men have disabilities resulting from acute conditions, but women experience fewer disabilities resulting from chronic conditions because they report their symptoms earlier and receive necessary treatment. Women report proportionately more days of restricted activity than men.

Disabling conditions limit the physical functional abilities of many women, but the healthcare delivery system has often overlooked the unique needs of this aggregate. In planning care for disabled women, community health nurses should focus

---

BOX 17.3 Intimate Partner Violence Strategies for Nurses

It is important not to revictimize the woman who admits to intimate partner violence. Avoid asking the woman "why" or talking negatively about the abuser. Sit down with her, give her time to talk, listen actively. Provide her with privacy and confidentiality as much as you can. It is vital that the nurse believes her story, validates her decision to disclose, and emphasizes that violence is unacceptable. Example responses include:

"I believe what you are telling me."
"What you have told me is very important."
"I am here for you."
"This will only get worse."
"You deserve better."
"I am afraid for your safety."
"You deserve to be treated with respect."
"It is a crime." This approach will empower the victim. Episodes of imminent danger must be reported to the police. An emergency plan should be formulated with the woman. Resources including phone numbers for hotlines and the local women's shelter should be provided in a format that is easy to conceal (such as on a business card).

Adapted from Perry SE, Hockenberry MJ, Lowermilk DL, Wilson D: *Maternal child nursing care*, Maryland Heights, MO, 2018, Mosby; and Power, C. *Domestic violence: What can nurses do?* 2004. Australian Nursing Journal, 12(5), pp. 21–23.

BOX 17.4 Signs of Intimate Partner Violence

- Overuse of health services
- Nonspecific, vague complaints
- Missed appointments
- Injuries without legitimate explanation
- Injuries not matching reported cause
- Untreated serious injuries
- Intimate partner describing the cause of injuries
- Intimate partner refusing to leave the woman's room

Adapted from Perry SE, Hockenberry MJ, Lowermilk DL, Wilson D: *Maternal child nursing care*, Maryland Heights, MO, 2018, Mosby.

BOX 17.5 Resources for Victims of Intimate Partner Violence

National Domestic Violence Hotline: 1-800-799-SAFE (7233) and http://www.thehotline.org
Office on Women's Health. Dating Violence and abuse.: https://www.womenshealth.gov/relationships-and-safety/other-types/dating-violence-and-abuse
National Coalition Against Domestic Violence: http://www.ncadv.org
Office on Violence Against Women: http://www.ovw.usdoj.gov

---

attention on enabling women to strengthen their capabilities. In addition, nurses should be sensitive to barriers in the clinical setting that affect the access of disabled women to healthcare services. Chapter 21 discusses the needs of disabled people in greater detail.

MAJOR LEGISLATION AFFECTING WOMEN'S HEALTH

Several legislative acts have direct or indirect influence on the health of women. Many changes have been made in the past 5 decades that have the potential for improving the health and welfare of all women.

Public Health Service Act

The Public Health Service (PHS) Act, passed in 1944, provides for biomedical and health services research, information dissemination, resource development, technical assistance, and service delivery. In the area of women's health, the PHS Act supports activities related to general health issues, reproductive health, social and behavioral issues, and mental health. Aggregates of women targeted by the PHS Act include those disabled by specific diseases, victims of sexual abuse and intimate partner violence, recent immigrants, and occupational groups.

Title X of the PHS Act is the Family Planning Public Service Act provides funding to state and local health departments to provide family planning services for socioeconomically disadvantaged persons. In 2019, 3.1 million women obtain family planning services, which has decreased from five million since 2008 due to expanded contraceptive coverage under the ACA. Clinics and health departments throughout the country provide access not only to contraception but also to routine preventive health services, education, and counseling. The program is an important part of the public effort to prevent low birth weight through addressing the relationship between lack of family planning and women at greatest risk for low-birth-weight infants (women who are adolescents, single, and/or low income) (Fowler et al., 2020).

Civil Rights Act

Title VII of the **Civil Rights Act** of 1964 prohibits discrimination based on sex, race, color, religion, or national origin in determining employment eligibility or termination, wages, and fringe benefits. The act has been amended to prohibit discrimination against pregnant women and conditions involving childbirth or pregnancy. This landmark legislation makes it unlawful for employers to refuse to hire, employ, or promote a woman because she is pregnant. In addition, employee benefit plans that continue health insurance, income maintenance during disability or illness, or any other income support program for disabled workers must include disabilities resulting from pregnancy, childbirth, and other related conditions. If employers allow disabled employees to assume lighter or medically restricted assignments, the same considerations must extend to pregnant women.

Sexual harassment is unwelcome conduct of a sexual nature severe enough to create intimidating hostile work environment. Sexual harassment is a violation of the Civil Rights Act. Female and male workers may face unwelcome sexual advances or requests for sexual favors or other verbal or physical conduct of a sexual nature. Awareness of sexual harassment in the workplace has increased dramatically over the past decade, but sexual harassment has not been eliminated.

Social Security Act

The Social Security Act provides monthly retirement and disability benefits to workers and survivor benefits to families of workers covered by Social Security. Full retirement benefits are available after 10 years of covered employment, and workers can collect partial benefits beginning at age 62 and full benefits after age 67.

The Social Security Act permits a divorced person to receive benefits based on a former spouse's earning record when that spouse retires, becomes disabled, or dies if the marriage lasted at least 10 years. Since January 1985, a woman who has been divorced for at least 2 years can receive spousal benefits at age 62, if her former husband is eligible for benefits, regardless of whether he is actually receiving them.

Medicare and Medicaid also resulted from the Social Security Act. Medicare is the insurance plan that covers the majority of the healthcare expenses of older adults, including payments for hospital care, physicians, home healthcare, and other services and supplies after copayments and deductibles. Medicaid covers healthcare for indigent and eligible children and includes family planning, obstetrical care, and preventive cancer screening for women, such as mammography and Pap smears. Chapters 10 and 12 describe Medicare and Medicaid in detail, and they are further discussed later in this chapter.

Occupational Safety and Health Act

The Occupational Safety and Health Act, enacted in 1970, helps ensure safe and healthful working conditions for workers throughout the United States. Women experience work related musculoskeletal injuries, job stress, reproductive and cancer hazards, and workplace violence that impacts their overall health (National Institute for Occupational Safety and Health, 2001). For example, little is known about women who work in cottage industries, as domestic workers, as prostitutes, in agriculture, and in the garment industry. Investigations of factors that influence the health of these women workers are needed. Table 17.5 lists specific positions in which a large number of women are employed and the potential for health hazards within these positions. Community health nurses, occupational health nurses, and NPs need to be cognizant of environmental hazards wherever they find women at work. In taking a health history, the nurse should collect data regarding the client's occupational environment to assess the potential risk to emotional, general, and reproductive health. In addition, nurses must work individually and as an aggregate with their legislatures to maintain strong worker health and safety programs to protect the health of all women.

Family and Medical Leave Act

Enacted in 1993, the **Family and Medical Leave Act** (FMLA) allows an employee a minimum provision of 12 weeks unpaid leave each year for family and medical reasons such as personal illness; an ill child, parent, or spouse; and the birth or adoption

TABLE 17.5 Hazardous Occupations in Which Women Are Employed

Occupation	Health hazard
Clerical workers	Organic solvents in stencil machines, correction fluids, and ozone from copying machines
Textile and apparel workers	Cotton dust, skin irritants, and chemicals
Hairdressers and beauticians	Hair, nail, and skin beauty preparations
Launderers and dry cleaners	Heat, heavy lifting, and chemicals
Electronics workers	Solvents and acids
Hospital and other healthcare workers	Infectious diseases, heavy lifting, radiation, skin disorders, and anesthetic gases
Firefighters	Exposure to hazardous materials and rescue environments
Laboratory workers	Biological agents; flammable, explosive, toxic, or carcinogenic substances; exposure to radiation; and bites from and allergic reactions to research animals
Construction workers	Exposure to hazardous materials, dangerous environments
Military personnel	Exposure to hostile persons, hazardous materials, harsh environments, and sexual assault

Data from Centers for Disease Control, *National Institute for Occupational Safety and Health: workplace safety and health topics: industries & occupations*, 2019. Available from: http://www.cdc.gov/niosh/topics/industries.html.

of a child. In 2008, the FMLA was updated to include family providing care to members of the Armed Forces injured in the line of duty. This act guarantees the employee the same or an equivalent job with the same pay and benefits upon the employee's return to work. In addition, health benefits must continue throughout the leave. In 2018, 15% of employees utilized FMLA, the most common reason was for personal illness (51%) followed by care of a new child (25%) and care of a family member (19%). On average, women took longer leaves with an average of 35 days (Brown et al., 2018).

The FMLA is particularly important to female workers because they are more likely to use leave to care for seriously ill family members, whereas male workers more often use leave for personal illness. Employees who must be away from work for family or medical reasons lose income, with the most significant impact on those without job-protected leave. The FMLA is an important step toward equitable leave policies, but more change is needed.

? ACTIVE LEARNING

1. Identify examples from everyday life that support or encourage violence against women (e.g., magazines, books, and television advertisements). Share findings with classmates.
2. Survey lay magazine advertisements and estimate the percentage of total pages that use a woman's image, including aging, menopause, overweight and obesity, and sexuality, to sell products. Share these with classmates.
3. Discuss the need for cancer screening with female relatives; refer to the ACS guidelines.

4. Discuss with female relatives the need for a heart-healthy nutritional plan based on AHA guidelines.
5. Identify resources for mammograms and Pap smears for low-income women.

HEALTH AND SOCIAL SERVICES TO PROMOTE THE HEALTH OF WOMEN

Major changes for women came with the signing of the ACA of 2010 (USDHHS, 2021). Particular to women are protections from being denied coverage by insurance companies or being charged more for healthcare services because of gender. Services include well-woman visits along with screening and counseling for gestational diabetes, HPV, STDs including HIV, contraception, and intimate partner violence. Also included are breastfeeding counseling, support, and supplies. The ACA mandated an expansion of Medicaid to include persons younger than 65 years with income below 133% of the federal poverty level. Medicaid is a health insurance program that was instituted in 1965 for the poor and is funded jointly by the federal and state governments but is administered by individual states. Medicaid is the largest source of funding for medical and health-related services for people with limited income, regardless of age eligibility. Medicaid is classified into five broad coverage groups: children, pregnant women, adults in families with dependent children, individuals with disabilities, and individuals 65 years or older.

Pregnant women who are eligible for Medicaid are at high risk for poor pregnancy outcome, including low birth weight. Ideally, a maternity care provider should examine women with high maternal risk immediately after conception. However, too often these women seek prenatal care late in pregnancy or arrive at the emergency department when delivery is imminent without having previously received prenatal care (see Clinical Example 17.1). Barriers limit access to prenatal care for those most in need. Medicaid allows some access to care. Greater public awareness of facilities and maternity care providers who accept Medicaid are necessary.

Clinical Example 17.1

Anita Rogers, a 16-year-old unemployed single woman, arrived at the Family Services Health Center seeking initial prenatal care at 36 weeks of gestation. She stated that for a few days she noted some brown discharge from her vagina. She told the nurse she knew she should have begun prenatal care earlier, but when she called several health providers' offices, the receptionists told her they were not accepting patients with Medicaid insurance. She reported that the family did not have reliable transportation. Her father was unemployed, and her mother worked at a cafe as a waitress. Anita was sent to the hospital immediately for an ultrasound examination. The sonogram revealed twins, but one of them had died in utero. Anita was hospitalized and began to hemorrhage. She delivered a 3-lb infant.

Women's Health Services

Since the mid-1970s, women have sought health services beyond the conventional mode of care delivery. Women desire a participatory role in their health and have become more assertive. Healthcare facilities have recognized the importance of meeting women's health needs. A notable evolution has occurred in maternity care, in which the demands of women as consumers led to the emergence of freestanding and hospital-based birth centers and family- and sibling-attended births.

The National Women's Health Network has been a strong advocate for women's concerns and has provided testimony at congressional hearings dealing with women's issues. This organization is concerned with women's rights, environmental safety, reproductive rights, warnings about the effects of alcohol and drugs on the developing fetus, and safety in relation to medical devices and to drugs, especially those that may have teratogenic or carcinogenic effects. Examples of the organization's work include recall of the Dalkon Shield intrauterine device, identification of women who may have been exposed to diethylstilbestrol in utero, and promotion of well-woman healthcare.

Other Community Voluntary Services

Networking, the exchange of information among interconnected or cooperating individuals, has been one of the major movements during the past 2 decades. It is a means by which women seek to advance their careers, improve their lifestyles, and increase their income while helping other women become successful. Networking in business, professional support, politics and labor, arts, sports, and health is established throughout the United States enabling women to develop and become empowered to achieve mutual goals.

Many private voluntary organizations spend money, time, and energy in attempting to increase health awareness among its members and provide direct services to the public. Most urban areas have crisis hotline services in which women volunteer to provide counseling to battered women, battering parents, rape victims, those considering suicide, and those with multiple needs. One of the most effective, low-cost, voluntary efforts to assist abused women involves shelters and safe houses scattered throughout the United States. One of the goals of *Healthy People 2030* relates to this issue, as many women needing shelter are often denied emergency housing.

Women's organizations have a long history of voluntary involvement with the community. An increasing number have added activities to their agendas to improve pregnancy outcomes, prevent teen pregnancy, and support older women's rights. Organizations such as the Older Women's League, United Methodist Women, women's groups of other religious denominations, Urban League, sororities, Junior League, Young Women's Christian Association, and the National Association of Colored Women's Clubs, have made women's health a major item on their agendas.

LEVELS OF PREVENTION AND WOMEN'S HEALTH

Primary Prevention

The focus of primary prevention is preventing disease from occurring. Women should recognize the risk of disease and target their healthcare behaviors accordingly. Types of primary prevention include never smoking, following a nutritious diet, practicing safe sex, avoiding drugs, limiting alcohol consumption, and staying physically active.

Consider Jackie, a 39-year-old woman with three first-order relatives diagnosed with breast and/or ovarian cancer. She is at risk for hereditary cancer and should seek genetic counseling and possibly testing. If genetic test results are positive, she should be given information on measures that could prevent cancer from occurring, a process that constitutes primary prevention. These measures include lifestyle choices (early childbearing/breast-feeding); prophylactic surgical procedures (oophorectomy/mastectomy); and medical treatment (contraceptive pills, tamoxifen). Vigilant screenings (pelvic ultrasound with Ca-125 measurement or breast MRI) to detect cancer early would be considered secondary prevention.

Secondary Prevention

The focus of secondary prevention is detecting the disease once it has begun but before it appears clinically. Examples of this level of prevention are routine screening for cervical cancer through Pap smears, tests for chlamydial infections tests on either urine or cervical specimens, and mammogram.

Tertiary Prevention

Tertiary prevention seeks to stop further complications after a disease has become clinically evident. For example, Sandra Smith, a 55-year-old Native American, has had diabetes mellitus for the past 3 years. She attended an urban clinic for monitoring of the diabetes. After the physician examined her, he suggested that she have her annual pelvic examination. She was overdue for one and agreed to be seen by the women's healthcare NP. Ms. Smith described symptoms of a yeast infection (e.g., increase in vaginal discharge and itching) to the nurse. Her examination and a wet mount examination confirmed the diagnosis of *Candida albicans* infection, a common problem among diabetic women. Sandra then learned about the nature of, predisposing factors for, and treatment of the infection.

CASE STUDY Application of the Nursing Process

Pregnant Inmate in a Correctional Facility

John Lawrence, an educator at the state women's correctional center, contacted Donna Williams, a women's healthcare NP and faculty member at the College of Nursing, and expressed concern for the health of an inmate, Lela Marvin. According to Mr. Lawrence, Lela, a 19-year-old pregnant primigravida, was being seen at the state-supported hospital for antepartal care; however, she was not permitted to attend perinatal education classes. He stated that other pregnant women in the facility could benefit from perinatal education. In fact, approximately 4% of female state prison inmates are pregnant when admitted to prison and could benefit from perinatal education (Johns Hopkins, 2019).

Lawrence's call was followed by a call from Herman Martin, an RN who also expressed concern for the other women's needs for information regarding their personal hygiene. Although an RN, Mr. Martin was not knowledgeable of women's health because his primary clinical focus was emergency and trauma care. He indicated that many of the women were overweight, cared little about themselves, and lacked a general knowledge of how to maintain their health.

Assessment

After gaining clearance from the prison officials, Ms. Williams made an assessment of healthcare information needs and started offering classes for the inmates. The immediate need was for perinatal education for women in the last weeks of pregnancy. Lela said she wanted to learn about labor because she had heard only horror stories from other women. Ms. Williams noted that three other women were close to term and they also seemed eager to learn. She knew that students' readiness to learn was key to the course's success. Success of this course would be crucial to future course offerings.

The traditional perinatal education course was designed to promote healthy birth outcomes and an emotionally satisfying birth experience. These goals are also important to pregnant women in a correctional facility; however, perinatal education would have to be modified to meet this group's special needs. For example, information on newborn care is not appropriate because the infant born to an inmate is usually placed with the mother's family or in foster care.

Assessment of nonpregnant women provided opportunities for other health education classes. The next spring and each spring thereafter, junior nursing students under Ms. Williams's guidance were assigned to develop and carry out 1-hour weekly health education and awareness sessions at the correctional facility. Although each student expressed some initial anxiety about the experience, each evaluated it as being worthwhile.

Diagnosis

After assessment, the community health nurse developed community and aggregate diagnoses, which served as the basis for the care plan.

Individual
- Inadequate preparation for childbirth related to lack of resources in prison (Lela).
- Lack of family support related to separation secondary to incarceration (Lela).
- Potential for feelings of loss related to separation from infant after birth (Lela).

Family
- Lela's family visits were rare; therefore she looked for others to provide support during her pregnancy. Lela told Ms. Williams that her cellmate, Julieanna, offered to be her labor support person.
- Lack of knowledge of her role as a labor support person (Julieanna).

Community
- Lack of adequate health-seeking behaviors of women in the correctional facility (i.e., pregnant and nonpregnant women)
- Lack of programs to promote health and prevent diseases among women prisoners.

Planning

After the nursing diagnosis was validated with the individual, family, or community, the plan of care was developed. Examples of long- and short-term goals follow.

Individual
Long-Term Goal
- Individual family members will have a positive birth experience (Lela).

Short-Term Goal
- Family members or friends will help Lela use relaxation techniques to cope with the discomforts of labor.

Family
Long-Term Goal
- The family members will be strengthened through their newly acquired knowledge and skills.

Short-Term Goal
- The family members will demonstrate increased ability to perform their role as labor support people.

Community
Long-Term Goal
- The health and well-being of incarcerated women (i.e., pregnant and nonpregnant) will improve.

Short-Term Goal
- Health education programs will be instituted for individuals, families, and aggregates in the correctional facility.

Intervention

The community health nurse worked with the individual, family, or community to achieve mutually established goals. Intervention was aimed at empowering individuals and groups to take responsibility for themselves and to form links with others to accomplish goals.

Individual
Providing a perinatal education program for Lela was Ms. Williams's first priority. In addition, counseling related to feelings of loss after birth might be appropriate. Referral to a counselor might be necessary, and Ms. Williams had to become familiar with available resources.

Family
Teaching the family the roles and responsibilities of a labor support person was an important intervention. In the correctional facility, interventions must ensure that Lela has a labor support person with whom to practice her relaxation techniques and to be available. In this case, Lela's cellmate, Julieanna, was willing to act in this role, and the nurse had to negotiate with prison officials to allow this arrangement.

Community
Specific interventions with a group of pregnant women in the correctional facility were based on the specific needs of the group. The community health nurse had to identify prison officials who were supportive of health education programs and request their input as to which women should be targeted for such programs. Then the nurse met with targeted women to assess their level of knowledge and skills regarding women's health. For example, the nurse surveyed what each woman perceived as learning needs (e.g., well-woman care, women's anatomy and physiology, self-care in health promotion, health protection, and disease prevention). Then the nurse tailored an intervention that was compatible with the community. Ms. Williams asked each nursing student

Continued

Case Study Application of the Nursing Process—cont'd

to select a topic on the basis of the survey and to develop a teaching plan for presentation to female prisoners (i.e., pregnant and nonpregnant) at least once during the spring semester.

Evaluation

The community health nurse compared the actual and predicted outcomes to determine the efficacy of the plan of care and to make revisions.

Individual

For example, Lela learned necessary relaxation techniques that were useful to her in labor and helped make the birth experience positive. Follow-up of Lela's psychosocial concerns in postpartum was also important.

Family

Evaluation of this nontraditional family would include their level of satisfaction with their role in the birth experience. Evaluation would also include learning how this interaction between family members (i.e., Lela and Julieanna) prepared them for other situations.

Community

The aggregate evaluation focuses on the community. For example, in health education programs designed for pregnant and nonpregnant women in the correctional facility, it was important to do the following:
- Maintain attendance records.
- Seek feedback from women, the referring nurse-educator, and prison officials regarding changes in self-care behavior regarding health.

- Obtain student response to learning experience.
- Make changes in health education programs on the basis of evaluation.

Levels of Prevention

The following are examples of the three levels of prevention as applied to the individual, family, and community.

Primary
- Assessment and teaching perinatal education course to pregnant inmates
- Assessment and teaching health education classes to nonpregnant inmates
- Teaching the family the roles and responsibilities of a labor support person

Secondary
- Screening at the community level (correctional facility) of what is perceived as learning needs
- Educating the family and community of the signs of postpartum depression

Tertiary
- Educating HIV-positive pregnant inmates on the need for antiviral treatment and delivery by cesarean section
- Educating family members and foster parents about the need for neonatal follow-up with regard to HIV status
- Assessing available community resources for counseling and treatment of postpartum depression

ROLES OF THE COMMUNITY HEALTH NURSE

Direct Care

The community health nurse provides direct care in a variety of settings. Often, this care is considered the "hands-on" nursing care given to a client in the home or a clinic.

Educator

The nurse encounters many opportunities for teaching. To be successful with health education, the nurse must attempt to gain the client's trust and must be sensitive to any cultural issues present. The nurse must also be aware of the emotional and physical state of the client. If the client is anxious or in pain, teaching may be ineffective.

Counselor

The counseling role of the nurse occurs in almost every interaction in the area of women's health. Before counseling in the area of reproductive health is begun, it is essential for effective intervention that the nurse becomes aware of his or her value system, including how biases and beliefs about human sexual behavior affect the counseling role.

RESEARCH IN WOMEN'S HEALTH

Women have long been the major users of the healthcare system. Research involving women is beginning to provide information enabling prediction, explanation, or description of phenomena affecting health. In the past, medical treatment for

women was based on findings of research performed with male subjects exclusively, even in conditions that caused more deaths in women. Since the federal mandate regarding women and research was instituted, research efforts to include women in studies have grown. If women are not included in a research project, a rationale must be given for their exclusion.

The National Institutes of Health (NIH) established the Office of Research on Women's Health (ORWH) in 1990. Achievements include women in National Institutes of Health research, increase research in women's health differences, prepare women's health researchers, and focus on interdisciplinary career and gender differences research. Nurse researchers are encouraged to test interventions and question rituals in nursing by conducting research. Following are some of the areas for exploration and research among women:
- Alcohol, tobacco, and other drug use
- Intimate partner violence
- Heart disease
- Health behaviors
- Genetic screening and breast cancer
- Bone and musculoskeletal disorders
- Cancer prevention, screening, diagnosis, and treatment
- Health education at various literacy levels
- Wellness throughout the life cycle
- Differences among women experiencing menopausal symptoms
- Dysmenorrhea
- Safe and effective contraception
- Promotion of breast-feeding

- Infertility
- Coping with chronic illness, such as systemic lupus erythematosus or arthritis
- Discomforts of pregnancy, including morning sickness
- Strengths of single, female heads of households
- Adolescent sexuality
- Multiple-role adaptation
- Menstrual cycle variations
- Control of obesity
- Substance abuse and its effect on pregnancy
- HIV infection and pregnancy
- Influence of diet on osteoporosis
- Effect of socialization on role
- Gender differences in pharmacology
- Maternal morbidity and mortality

The NIH supports research in women's health by the ORWH. Research done by the ORWH (2017) has strengthened knowledge about women's health, including:

- Certain medications affect women differently than men.
- Women have more difficulty in quitting smoking.
- HPV vaccines protect against most cervical cancers.
- HIV transmission between mother and baby can be prevented.
- Chronic pain disorders are more common in women.
- Deployed women are at greater risk of suicide.
- Heart disease and breast cancer can be prevented.
- The overall quality of life can be improved.

With the increased emphasis on community health, community health nurses can make significant contributions to the improvement of women's health through scholarly research, either as principal investigators or through data gathering. Furthermore, they can become consumers of research and develop nursing interventions based on sound research and recommendations.

SUMMARY

Women's healthcare has multiple facets, with many areas for community health nursing intervention. Nurses are advocates and activists for women's health through their involvement in health policy making as a profession. Along with other multidisciplinary and consumer groups, professional nurses are in the forefront of making changes in the healthcare delivery system that will promote an overall quality and research-based health plan for women. Women are at the center of the health of the United States; therefore if better models are developed for improving the health of women, the health of the entire nation will benefit.

EVOLVE WEBSITE

http://evolve.elsevier.com/Nies/community
- NCLEX Review Questions
- Case Studies

BIBLIOGRAPHY

Agency for Healthcare Research and Quality: *Most common diagnoses in hospital inpatient stays—HCUP fast stats*, 2021. Available from: www.hcup-us.ahrq.gov/faststats/NationalDiagnosesServlet?year1=2017.

Alfirevic Z, Gyte GML, Cuthbert A, Devane D: Continuous cardiotocography (CTG) as a form of electronic fetal monitoring (EFM) for fetal assessment during labour, *Cochrane Database Syst Rev* (2). https://doi.org/10.1002/14651858.CD006066.pub3. Art. No.: CD006066.

American Cancer Society: *About breast cancer*, 2021. Available from: https://www.cancer.org/content/dam/CRC/PDF/Public/8577.00.pdf.

American Cancer Society: *American Cancer Society recommendations for early breast cancer detection in women without breast symptoms*, 2020a. Available from: https://www.cancer.org/cancer/breast-cancer/screening-tests-and-early-detection/american-cancer-society-recommendations-for-the-early-detection-of-breast-cancer.html.

American Cancer Society: *Key statistics for endometrial cancer*, 2021a. Available from: https://www.cancer.org/cancer/endometrial-cancer/about/key-statistics.html.

American Cancer Society: *Cancer statistics center*, 2021b. Available from: https://cancerstatisticscenter.cancer.org/?_ga=2.8082290.1535790371.1614724023-595810568.1614724023#!/.

American Cancer Society: *Cancer screening guidelines*, 2021c. Available from: https://www.cancer.org/healthy/find-cancer-early/cancer-screening-guidelines.html.

American Cancer Society: *Cancer type: colorectum*, 2021d. Available from: https://cancerstatisticscenter.cancer.org/?_ga=2.8082290.1535790371.1614724023-595810568.1614724023#!/cancer-site/Colorectum.

American Cancer Society: *Key statistics for lung cancer risk factors*, 2021e. Available from: https://www.cancer.org/cancer/lung-cancer/about/key-statistics.html.

American Cancer Society: *Lung cancer risk factors*, 2019. Available from: https://www.cancer.org/cancer/lung-cancer/causes-risks-prevention/risk-factors.html.

American Cancer Society: *Tests for ovarian cancer*, 2020b. Available from: https://www.cancer.org/cancer/ovarian-cancer/detection-diagnosis-staging/how-diagnosed.html.

American Cancer Society: *What are the risk factors for cervical cancer?*, 2020c. Available from: https://www.cancer.org/cancer/cervical-cancer/causes-risks-prevention/risk-factors.html.

American College of Obstetricians and Gynecologists: *Alternatives to hysterectomy in the management of leiomyomas [Practice Bulletin]*, 2008. Available from: https://www.acog.org/-/media/project/acog/acogorg/clinical/files/practice-bulletin/articles/2008/08/alternatives-to-hysterectomy-in-the-management-of-leiomyomas.pdf.

American Dental Association: *FAQ—dental workforce in the U.S. ADA Health Policy Institute*, 2020. Available from: https://www.ada.org/en/science-research/health-policy-institute/dental-statistics/workforce.

American Heart Association: *Facts about heart disease in women. Go Red for Women*, 2021a. Available from: https://www.goredforwomen.org/en/about-heart-disease-in-women/facts.

American Heart Association: *Understand your risks to prevent a heart attack*, 2021b. Available from: https://www.heart.org/en/health-topics/heart-attack/understand-your-risks-to-prevent-a-heart-attack.

American Psychological Association: *Diagnostic and statistical manual of mental disorders*, ed 5, 2013, Washington, DC, Author.

Arthritis Foundation: *Arthritis by the numbers*, 2020. Available from: https://www.arthritis.org/getmedia/73a9f02d-7f91-4084-91c3-0ed0b11c5814/ABTN-2020-FINAL.pdf.

Association of Women's Health, Obstetric Neonatal Nurses: Intimate partner violence, *J Obstet Gynecol Neonatal Nurs* 48(1):112–116, 2019. https://doi.org/10.1016/j.jogn.2018.11.003.

Bergen G, Stevens MR, Burns ER: Falls and fall injuries among adults aged ≥65 years—United State, 2014, *Morb Mortal Wkly Rep 2016* 65:993–998, 2016. https://doi.org/10.15585/mmwr.mm6537a2.

Bosh KA, Johnson AS, Hernandez AL, et al.: Vital Signs: deaths among persons with diagnosed HIV infection, United States, 2010–2018, *MMWR Morb Mortal Wkly Rep* 69:1717–1724, 2020. https://doi.org/10.15585/mmwr.mm6946a1.

Brown S, Herr J, Roy R, Klerman JA: Employee and worksite perspectives of the family and medical leave act: results from the 2018 surveys, Abt Associates, 2020. Available from: https://www.dol.gov/sites/dolgov/files/OASP/evaluation/pdf/WHD_FMLA2018SurveyResults_FinalReport_Aug2020.pdf.

Bureau of Labor Statistics: *Highlights of women's earnings in 2019 (Report 1089)*, 2020, Available from: https://www.bls.gov/opub/reports/womens-earnings/2019/pdf/home.pdf.

Centering Health Care Institute: *Centering pregnancy*, 2021. Available from: http://www.centeringhealthcare.org/pages/centering-model/pregnancy-overview.php.

Centers for Disease Control and Prevention: *Abortion surveillance system*, 2020. Available from: https://www.cdc.gov/reproductivehealth/data_stats/abortion.htm.

Centers for Disease Control and Prevention: *Arthritis*, 2019. Available from: https://www.cdc.gov/arthritis/data_statistics/national-statistics.html.

Centers for Disease Control and Prevention: *Arthritis-related statistics*, 2018. Available from: https://www.cdc.gov/arthritis/data_statistics/arthritis-related-stats.htm.

Centers for Disease Control and Prevention: *Cervical cancer: what should I know about screening?*, 2021a. Available from: https://www.cdc.gov/cancer/cervical/basic_info/screening.htm.

Centers for Disease Control and Prevention: *Cervical cancer statistics*, 2020a. Available from: http://www.cdc.gov/cancer/cervical/statistics/#2.

Centers for Disease Control and Prevention: *Diabetes and women*, 2018b. Available from: https://www.cdc.gov/diabetes/library/features/diabetes-and-women.html.

Centers for Disease Control and Prevention: *HIV, basics: find self-testing in your state*, 2021b. https://www.cdc.gov/hiv/basics/hiv-testing/hiv-self-tests.html.

Centers for Disease Control and Prevention: *HIV and women*, 2019b. Available from: https://www.cdc.gov/hiv/pdf/group/gender/women/cdc-hiv-women.pdf.

Centers for Disease Control and Prevention: *HPV vaccine safety and effectiveness data*, 2019c. Available from: https://www.cdc.gov/hpv/hcp/vaccine-safety-data.html.

Centers for Disease Control and Prevention: *Human papilloma virus for healthcare professionals*, 2021c. Available from: https://www.cdc.gov/hpv/hcp/index.html.

Centers for Disease Control and Prevention: *Key statistics from the National Survey of Family Growth, Hysterectomy*, 2017. Available from: http://www.cdc.gov/nchs/nsfg/key_statistics/h.htm#hysterectomy.

Centers for Disease Control and Prevention: *Leading causes of death-females-all races/origins 2017*, 2019d. Available from: https://www.cdc.gov/women/lcod/2017/all-races-origins/index.htm.

Centers for Disease Control and Prevention, U.S. Dept of Health and Human Services: *National Diabetes Statistics Report, Atlanta, GA*, 2020d. Available from: https://www.cdc.gov/diabetes/pdfs/data/statistics/national-diabetes-statistics-report.pdf.

Centers for Disease Control and Prevention: *National Diabetes Statistics Report: Estimates of Diabetes and Its Burden in the United States*, Atlanta, GA, 2021d. U.S. Department of Health and Human Services. Available from: https://www.cdc.gov/diabetes/pdfs/data/statistics/national-diabetes-statistics-report.pdf.

Centers for Disease Control and Prevention: *National vital statistics system. Mortality data*, 2021e. Available from: https://www.cdc.gov/nchs/nvss/deaths.htm?CDC_AA_refVal=https://-www.cdc.gov/nchs/deaths.htm.

Centers for Disease Control and Prevention: *Pregnancy mortality surveillance system*, 2021f. Available from: https://www.cdc.gov/reproductivehealth/maternal-mortality/pregnancy-mortality-surveillance-system.htm.

Centers for Disease Control and Prevention: *Preventing Teen Dating Violence*, 2021g. Available from: https://www.cdc.gov/violenceprevention/intimatepartnerviolence/teendatingviolence/fastfact.html.

Centers for Disease Control and Prevention: Quickstats: percentage of women aged 50 years who have had a hysterectomy, by race/ethnicity and year—United States, 2008 and 2018, *Morb Mortal Wkly Rep* 2019 68(935), 2019f. https://doi.org/10.15585/mmwr.mm6841a3.

Centers for Disease Control and Prevention: *Reproductive health. Depression among women*, 2020e. Available from: https://www.cdc.gov/reproductivehealth/depression/index.htm.

Centers for Disease Control and Prevention: *Sexually transmitted infections prevalence, incidence, and cost estimates in the United States*, 2021h. Available from: https://www.cdc.gov/std/statistics/prevalence-2020-at-a-glance.htm.

Centers for Disease Control and Prevention: *Sexually transmitted disease surveillance: national profile, 2018*, 2019g. Available from: https://www.cdc.gov/std/stats18/natoverview.htm.

Centers for Disease Control and Prevention: *Women and heart disease facts*, 2020f. Available from: https://www.cdc.gov/heartdisease/women/facts.htm.

Cheeseman Day J: *Number of women lawyers at record high but men still highest earners*, 2018, The United States Census Bureau. Available from: https://www.census.gov/library/stories/2018/05/women-lawyers.html.

Chen I, Opiyo N, Tavender E, Mortazhejri S, Rader T, Petkovic J, Yogasingam S, Taljaard M, Agarwal S, Laopaiboon M, Wasiak J, Khunpradit S, Lumbiganon P, Gruen RL, Betran AP: Non-clinical interventions for reducing unnecessary caesarean section, *Cochrane Database Syst Rev* (Issue 9). https://doi.org/10.1002/14651858.CD005528.pub3. Art. No.: CD005528.

Choi M: Preamble to a new paradigm for women's health, *Image* 17:14, 1985.

Crane PB, Letvak S, Lewallen, et al.: Inclusion of women in nursing research: 1995-2001, *Nurs Res* 53(4):237–242, 2004.

Cronin KA, Richardson LC, Henley SJ: Vital signs: racial disparities in breast cancer severity—United States, 2005–2009, *Morb Mortal Wkly Rep* 61(45):922–926, 2012. http://www.cdc.gov/mmwr/preview/mmwrhtml/mm6145a5.htm?s_cid=mm6145a5_w.

Fowler CI, Gable J, Lasater B, Asman K: *Family planning annual report: 2019 National Summary. Washington, DC: Office of Population Affairs, Office of the Assistant Secretary for Health, Department of Health and Human Services*, 2020. Available from: https://opa.hhs.gov/sites/default/files/2020-09/title-x-fpar-2019-national-summary.pdf.

Genetic Information Nondiscrimination: *Act of 2008, 493 H.R., § 110,* 2008.

Hamilton BE, Mathews TJ: Continued declines in teen births in the United States, 2015, NCHS data brief, no 259, *Hyattsville, MD: National Center for Health Statistics,* 2016. Available from: https://www.cdc.gov/nchs/data/databriefs/db259.pdf.

Kaiser Family Foundation: *Professionally active physicians by gender,* 2020. Available from: https://www.kff.org/other/state-indicator/physicians-by-gender/?currentTimeframe=0.

Kaiser Family Foundation: *Women's health insurance coverage. Women's Health Policy,* 2021. Available from: https://www.kff.org/womens-health-policy/fact-sheet/womens-health-insurance-coverage.

Kortsmit K, Jatlaoui TC, Mandel MG, et al.: Abortion surveillance—United States, *MMWR Surveill Summ 2020* 69(1—29), 2018. https://doi.org/10.15585/mmwr.ss6907a1external icon.

Kovell LC, Ahmed HM, Misra S, Whelton SP, Prokopowicz GP, Blumenthal RS, McEvoy JW: US hypertension management guidelines: a review of the recent past and recommendations for the future, *J Am Heart Assoc* 4(12), 2015. https://doi.org/10.1161/jaha.115.002315.

Looker AE, Frenk SM: *Percentage of adults aged 65 and over with osteoporosis or low bone mass at the femur neck or lumbar spine: United States, 2005-2010. National Center for Health Statistics,* 2015. Available from: https://www.cdc.gov/nchs/data/hestat/osteoporsis/osteoporosis2005_2010.pdf.

Manant A, Dodgson JE: Centering pregnancy: an integrative literature review, *J Midwifery Wom Health* 56:94—102, 2011.

Martin JA, Hamilton BE, Osterman MJK, Driscoll AK: Births: Final data for 2018, *Natl Vital Stat Rep* 68(13), 2019. Hyattsville, MD: National Center for Health Statistics. Available from: https://www.cdc.gov/nchs/data/nvsr/nvsr68/nvsr68_13-508.pdf.

Moore BJ, Steiner CA, Davis PH, Stocks C, Barrett ML: *Trends in hysterectomies and oophorectomies in hospital inpatient and ambulatory settings, 2005—2013. HCUP Statistical Brief #214,* Rockville, MD, 2016, Agency for Healthcare Research and Quality. Available from: https://www.hcup-us.ahrq.gov/reports/statbriefs/sb214-Hysterectomy-Oophorectomy-Trends.pdf.

National Cancer Institute: *BRCA gene mutations: Cancer risk and genetic testing,* 2020a. Available from: https://www.cancer.gov/about-cancer/causes-prevention/genetics/brca-fact-sheet#how-much-does-an-inherited-harmful-variant-in-brca1-or-brca2-increase-a-womans-risk-of-breast-and-ovarian-cancer.

National Cancer Institute: *New treatments spur sharp reduction in lung cancer mortality rate,* 2020b. Available from: https://www.cancer.gov/news-events/press-releases/2020/lung-cancer-treatments-mortality-drop.

National Cancer Institute: *Surveillance, Epidemiology, and End Results Program: SEER Stat fact sheets: Breast, surveillance epidemiology & end results,* 2020c. Available from: http://seer.cancer.gov/statfacts/html/breast.html.

National Cancer Institute: *Surveillance, epidemiology, and end results program: seer stat fact sheets: Ovarian cancer,* 2020d. Available from: http://seer.cancer.gov/statfacts/html/ovary.html.

National Institute for Occupational Safety and Health: *Women's safety and health issues at work,* 2001. Available from: https://www.cdc.gov/niosh/docs/2001-123/default.html.

National Osteoporosis Foundation: *Who gets osteoporosis: factors that put you at risk,* 2013. Available from: https://cdn.nof.org/wp-content/uploads/2016/02/Who-Gets-Osteoporosis.pdf.

North CM, Christiani DC: Women and lung cancer: what is new? *Semin Thorac Cardiovasc Surg* 25(2):87—94, 2013. https://doi.org/10.1053/j.semtcvs.2013.05.002.

North American Menopause Society: The 2017 hormone therapy position statement of the North American Menopause Society, *Menopause* 24(7):728—753, 2017. https://doi.org/10.1097/GME.0000000000000921.

Pagidipati N, Douglas PS: Clinical features and diagnosis of coronary heart disease in women. In Kaski JC, Pellikka PA, Saperia GM, editors: *UpToDate,* 2019. Available from: https://www.uptodate.com/contents/clinical-features-and-diagnosis-of-coronary-heart-disease-in-women.

Pender N, Murdaugh CL, Parsons MA: *Health promotion in nursing practice,* ed 4 Upper Saddle River, NJ, 2006, Prentice Hall.

Richardson LC, Henley SJ, Miller JW, Massetti G, Thomas CC: Patterns and trends in age-specific black-white differences in breast cancer incidence and mortality—United States, 1999—2014. 2016, *MMWR Morb Mortal Wkly Rep* 65:1093—1098, 2016. https://doi.org/10.15585/mmwr.mm6540a1.

Richmond LM: APA releases new statement on perinatal disorders, *Psychiatr News* 54(6), 2019. https://doi.org/10.1176/appi.pn.2019.3b19.

Rosen HN, Drezner MK: Menopausal hormone therapy in the prevention and treatment of osteoporosis. In Barbieri RL, Crowley WF, Mulder JE, editors: *UpToDate.* Retrieved March 2, 2021, Available from: https://www.uptodate.com/contents/menopausal-hormone-therapy-in-the-prevention-and-treatment-of-osteoporosis.

Ruzek S, Olsen V, Clark A: *Social, biomedical, and feminist models of women's health. Women's health: complexities and differences,* Columbus, OH, 1997, Ohio State University Press.

Sarna L, Brown JK, Cooley ME, Williams RD, Chernecky C, Padilla G, Danao LL: Quality of life and meaning of illness of women with lung cancer, *Oncol Nurs Forum* 32(1):E9—E19, 2005. https://doi.org/10.1188/05.ONF.E9-E19, 19.

Sarna L, McCorkle R: Burden of care and lung cancer, *Cancer Pract* 4:245, 1996.

Schuiling KD: *Likis FE: Women's gynecologic health,* Sudbury, MA, 2017, Jones and Bartlett.

Semega J, Kollar M, Shrider EA, Creamer JF: *Income and poverty in the United States: 2019,* Washington, DC, 2020, United States Census Bureau. U.S. Government Publishing Office. Available from: https://www.census.gov/content/dam/Census/library/publications/2020/demo/p60-270.pdf.

Smith RP, Kaunitz AM: *Dysmenorrhea in adult women: Clinical features and diagnosis,* Up to Date, 2020. Available from: https://www.uptodate.com/contents/dysmenorrhea-in-adult-women-clinical-features-and-diagnosis?search=dysmenorrhea&source=search_result&selectedTitle=2~150&usage_type=default&display_rank=2.

Tikkanen R, Gunja MZ, Fitzgerald M, Zephyrin L: *Maternal mortality and maternity care in the United States compared to 10 other developed countries [Issue Brief],* 2020, The Commonwealth Fund. Available from: https://www.commonwealthfund.org/publications/issue-briefs/2020/nov/maternal-mortality-maternity-care-us-compared-10-countries.

Urbanic JC: Depressive disorders. In Urbanic JC, Groh CJ, editors: *Women's mental health: a clinical guide for primary care providers,* Philadelphia, 2009, Wolters Kluwer.

U.S. Cancer Statistics Working Group: *U.S. Cancer Statistics Data Visualizations Tool, based on 2019 submission data (1999—2017).* U.S. Department of Health and Human Services, Centers for Disease Control and Prevention and National Cancer, 2020. Available from: Institute, www.cdc.gov/cancer/dataviz.

U.S. Census Bureau: *ACS demographic and housing estimates,* 2019, 2021. Available from: https://data.census.gov/cedsci/table?q=women.

U.S. Census Bureau: *Educational Attainment in the United States 2019*, 2020. Available from: https://www.census.gov/data/tables/2016/demo/education-attainment/cps-detailed-tables.html.

U.S. Department of Agriculture: *My plate*, 2020. Available from: https://www.myplate.gov/professionals/toolkits/organizations-and-associations.

U.S. Department of Agriculture: *Special supplemental nutrition program for women, infants, and children (WIC)*, 2021. Available from: https://www.fns.usda.gov/wic.

U.S. Department of Health and Human Services: *Panel on Antiretroviral Guidelines for Adults and Adolescents. guidelines for the use of antiretroviral agents in adults and adolescents with HIV*, 2019, Department of Health and Human Services. Available from: https://clinicalinfo.hiv.gov/sites/default/files/guidelines/documents/AdultandAdolescentGL.pdf.

U.S. Department of Health and Human Services & Office of Disease Prevention and Health Promotion. (n.d.): *Objectives & Data. Healthy People 2030*, 2021. Available from: https://health.gov/healthypeople/objectives-and-data/browse-objectives.

Virani SS, Alonso A, Benjamin EJ, Bittencourt MS, Callaway CW, Carson AP, et al.: Heart disease and stroke statistics—2020 update: a report from the American Heart Association, *Circulation* 141(9):e139—e596, 2020. doi.org/10.1161/CIR.0000000000000757.

World Health Organization: *Trends in maternal mortality 2000 to 2017: estimates by WHO, UNICEF, UNFPA, World Bank Group and the United Nations Population Division. Geneva*, 2019. Available from: https://apps.who.int/iris/handle/10665/327595.

World Health Organization: *Top ten causes of death*, 2020b. Available from: http://www.who.int/mediacentre/factsheets/fs310/en/.

Xu J, Murphy SL, Kochanek KD, Arias E: *Mortality in the United States, 2018 (key findings data from the National Vital Statistics System) [Data Brief]*, U.S. Department of Health and Human Services, Centers for Disease Control and Prevention, National Center for Health Statistics, 2020. Available from: https://www.cdc.gov/nchs/data/databriefs/db355-h.pdf.

Zeidenstein L: Health issues of lesbian and bisexual women. In Varney H, Kriebs J, Gegor C, editors: *Varney's midwifery*, Sudbury, MA, 2004, Jones and Bartlett, pp 299—308.

FURTHER READING

American Cancer Society: *Stay healthy*, 2021g. Available from: https://www.cancer.org/healthy.html.

Arthritis Foundation: *Rheumatoid arthritis*, 2021. Available from: www.arthritis.org/diseases/rheumatoid-arthritis.

Centers for Disease Control and Prevention: *Sexually transmitted diseases treatment*, 2015a. Available from: https://www.cdc.gov/std/tg2015/default.htm Guidelines.

Centers for Disease Control and Prevention: *Birth rates (live births) per 1,000 females aged 15—19 years, by race and hispanic ethnicity, select years*, 2015b. Available from: https://www.cdc.gov/teenpregnancy/about/alt-text/birth-rates-chart-2000-2011-text.htm.

Centers for Disease Control and Prevention: *National Institute for Occupational Safety and Health: workplace safety and health topics: industries & occupations*, 2019e. Available from: http://www.cdc.gov/niosh/topics/industries.html.

Centers for Disease Control and Prevention: *How many cancers are linked with HPV each year?*, 2020c. Available from: https://www.cdc.gov/cancer/hpv/statistics/cases.htm.

Davis NL, Smoots AN, Goodman DA: *Pregnancy-related deaths: data from 14 U.S. Maternal Mortality Review Committees, 2008-2017*. Centers for disease control and prevention, 2019. Available from: https://www.cdc.gov/reproductivehealth/maternal-mortality/erase-mm/MMR-Data-Brief_2019-h.pdf.

National Cancer Institute: *Mammograms*, 2016. Available from: http://www.cancer.gov/cancertopics/factsheet/detection/mammograms.

National Cancer Institute: *HPV and cancer*, 2021. Available from: https://www.cancer.gov/about-cancer/causes-prevention/risk/infectious-agents/hpv-and-cancer.

National Institute of Health: *Women's health research*, 2021. Available from: https://orwh.od.nih.gov/research.

National Center for Health Statistics: *Health insurance coverage*, 2020. Available from: https://www.cdc.gov/nchs/fastats/health-insurance.htm.

PDQ Screening and Prevention Editorial Board: *PDQ ovarian, fallopian tube, and primary peritoneal cancer prevention. Bethesda, MD: National Cancer Institute*, 2020. Available from: https://www.cancer.gov/types/ovarian/hp/ovarian-prevention-pdq.

Power C: Domestic violence: What can nurses do? *Aust Nurs J* 12(5):21—23, 2004.

Smith SG, Zhang X, Basile KC, Merrick MT, Wang J, Kresnow M, Chen J: *The national intimate partner and sexual violence survey (nisvs): 2015 data brief — updated release*, Atlanta, GA, 2018, National Center for Injury Prevention and Control, Centers for Disease Control and Prevention (2015) Available from: https://www.cdc.gov/violenceprevention/pdf/2015data-brief508.pdf.

Sufrin C, Jones RK, Mosher WD, Beal L: Pregnancy prevalence and outcomes in U.S. Jails, *Obstet Gynecol* 135(5):1177—1183, 2020. https://doi.org/10.1097/AOG.0000000000003834.

U.S. Department of Health and Human Services: *Women's health: diabetes*, 2017. Available from: https://www.womenshealth.gov/publications/our-publications/fact-sheet/diabetes.html.

U.S. Preventive Task Service Force: *Breast cancer: screening*, 2016. Available from: https://www.uspreventiveservicestaskforce.org/uspstf/recommendation/breast-cancer-screening.

U.S. Bureau of Labor Statistics: *Highlights of women's earnings in 2019. BLS reports*, 2020. Available from: https://www.bls.gov/opub/reports/womens-earnings/2019/home.htm.

American Psychological Association: *Position statement on screening and treatment of mood and anxiety disorders during pregnancy and postpartum*, 2018. Available from: https://www.psychnews.org/pdfs/Position%20Statement%20Screening_and_Treatment_of_Mood_and_Anxiety_Disorders_During_Pregnancy_and_Postpartum_2019.pdf.

World Health Organization: *Life expectancy by country*, 2020a. Available from: http://apps.who.int/gho/data/node.main.688.

18

Men's Health

Lillian Felicia Jones

OBJECTIVES

Upon completion of this chapter, the reader will be able to do the following:

1. Identify the major indicators of men's health status.
2. Describe physiological and psychosocial factors that have an impact on men's health status.
3. Discuss barriers to improving men's health.
4. Discuss factors that promote men's health.
5. Describe men's health needs.
6. Apply knowledge of men's health needs in planning gender-appropriate nursing care for men at the individual, family, and community levels.

OUTLINE

KEY TERMS

Androgen
chronic condition
illness orientation
life expectancy
medical care
morbidity
mortality

It is common knowledge that women live longer than men and that healthcare use is greater among women than men. Death rates for men are higher than for women in terms of the major causes. Although the overall interest in health promotion and illness prevention has increased, men's health issues remain largely unaddressed (Baerolcher and Verma, 2008). Women's health has become a specialty practice with courses and programs available in many colleges of nursing. At the national level, the Office for Women's Health has existed since 1991, but an "Office for Men's Health" does not exist, and the task of being a men's health specialist has often been delegated to urologists and influenced by the media emphasis on sexual health, pharmaceutical products for enhancing sexual performance, restoring youthful vitality, and curing erectile dysfunction (Quallich et al., 2018).

This chapter focuses on exploring the health needs of men and the implications for community health nursing. Specific areas that are discussed include the current health status of men; physiological and psychological theories that attempt to explain men's health; factors that impede men's health; factors that promote men's health; men's health needs; and planning gender-appropriate care for men at the individual, family, and community levels.

MEN'S HEALTH STATUS

Traditional indicators of health for all persons include rates of longevity, mortality, and morbidity. Reviewing these rates gives nursing students a better understanding of the community aggregate. Box 18.1 lists standardized terminology in the fields of demography and sociology.

Longevity and Mortality

Major gender differences in longevity and mortality rates reveal that men remain disadvantaged despite advances in technology. Although women are more likely to use health services and have higher morbidity rates, mortality rates for men remain higher. Gender differences are generally associated with both physiological and behavioral factors, which place men at greater risk of death. These behavioral factors, together with men's reluctance to seek preventive and health services, have marked implications for community health nursing.

Longevity

Rates of longevity are increasing for both men and women. People can now expect to live more than 20 years longer than their forefathers and foremothers lived at the turn of the 19th century. Infants born in the United States in 1996 can expect to live 77 years, whereas those born in 1900, when the death rate was highest, lived an average of 47.3 years. **Life expectancy** for both males and females has increased, however, the gender gap in longevity continues with women consistently living about 5 years longer than men (Table 18.1). This change in longevity may be attributed to the advances in treatment of heart disease and cancer, which continue to be the major causes of death in United States for males (Table 18.2).

Factors that influence the incongruencies between males and females are race or ethnic origin, socioeconomic status, and education. When reported by race, gender mortality rates show that less advantaged populations in the United States, especially minorities, live significantly fewer years. African American males in general, live about 5 years less than non-Hispanic white males (Arias and Xu, 2020).

Mortality

The United States lags behind several other countries in premature mortality rates for males. In 2018 only six countries had premature mortality rates higher than the United States for males: Estonia, Poland, Hungary, Mexico, Brazil, and Lithuania (Organisation for Economic Co-Operation and Development [OECD], 2020). In the United States, as in most industrialized countries, males lead females in **mortality** rates in each leading cause of death. Although males were the primary source of medical data before the 1970s, and most of the treatment advances have been developed from these data, gender-related disparity in death rates continues. Other factors also account for this mortality gender gap.

In 2019, circulatory diseases remained the leading cause of death causing about one out three deaths across the OECD, with cancer second at one out four deaths in OECD member nations (OECD, 2019). The gender disparity for disease-related deaths has narrowed: since the 1990s, cancer-related deaths in women have declined at a slower rate than those in men. Lifetime risk for lung cancer is estimated to be 9.8% among males and 3.8% among females (Lynch, 2008). However, the death rates for chronic lower respiratory tract disease have increased in females, in 1980 the female death rate was 14.9 deaths per 100,000 population, and in 2017 it was 51.5, while in males, it actually decreased slightly, 49.9 in 1980 to 46.8 in 2017 (Centers for Disease Control and Prevention [CDC], 2018a,b,c). The unintentional injury deaths for the whole population increased to 52.2 per 100,000 compared to 35.9 in 1999 (CDC, 2018a,b,c). Males continue

TABLE 18.1   **Life Expectancy at Birth According to Sex and Race, United States: 1900, 1950, 2000, 2008, and 2018**

YR	ALL RACES			WHITE			BLACK		
	Both Sexes	Male	Female	Both Sexes	Male	Female	Both Sexes	Male	Female
1900	47.3	46.3	48.3	47.6	46.6	48.7	33.0	32.5	33.5
1950	68.2	65.6	71.1	69.1	66.5	72.2	60.8	59.1	62.9
2000	76.8	74.1	79.3	77.3	74.7	79.9	71.8	68.2	75.1
2008	78.1	75.6	80.6	78.5	76.1	80.9	74.0	70.6	77.2
2018	78.7	76.2	81.2	78.6	76.2	81.1	74.7	71.3	78

From Arias E, Xu J: *United States life tables, 2018.* National vital statistics reports vol. 69, no. 12, Washington, DC, 2020, National Center for Health Statistics. http://www.cdc.gov/nchs/products/nvsr.htm.

TABLE 18.2 Leading Causes of Death in Males, United States, 2017

	Percentage
All Males, All Ages	
Heart disease	24.2
Cancer	21.9
Unintentional injuries	7.6
Chronic lower respiratory diseases	5.2
Stroke	4.3
Diabetes	3.2
Suicide	2.6
Alzheimer disease	2.6
Influenza and pneumonia	1.8
Chronic liver disease	1.8
White Males, All Ages	
Heart disease	24.7
Cancer	22.4
Unintentional injuries	7.2
Chronic lower respiratory diseases	5.9
Stroke	4.1
Alzheimer's disease	2.9
Diabetes	2.8
Suicide	2.7
Influenza and pneumonia	1.9
Chronic liver	1.7
Black Males, All Ages	
Heart disease	23.7
Cancer	20.1
Unintentional injuries	7.9
Homicide	5.0
Stroke	4.9
Diabetes	4.3
Chronic lower respiratory diseases	3.2
Kidney disease	2.6
Septicemia	1.7
Hypertension	1.6
Asian or Pacific Islander Males, All Ages	
Cancer	26.8
Heart disease	22.6
Stroke	6.6
Unintentional injuries	5.6
Diabetes	4.3
Chronic lower respiratory diseases	3.2
Influenza and pneumonia	3.1
Suicide	2.7
Alzheimer's disease	2.1
Kidney disease	2.1
Hispanic Males, All Ages	
Heart disease	20.3
Cancer	19.4
Unintentional injuries	11.5
Stroke	4.7
Diabetes	4.7
Chronic liver disease	4.0
Suicide	2.9
Chronic lower respiratory disease	2.5
Homicide	2.4
Alzheimer's disease	2.1

From Centers for Disease Control and Prevention: *Leading causes of death in males, United States*, 2017. http://www.cdc.gov/men/lcod/.

to be at greater risk for death due to unintentional injury with a rate of 68.4 compared with 36.4 for females per 100,000 (CDC, 2018a,b,c). Men are also three to four times more likely to commit suicide, and males older than 85 years are 11 to 12 times more likely than females of the same age to commit suicide (CDC, 2018a,b,c).

Race and ethnic background also are factors to be considered in the evaluation of male mortality rates. African American males are more likely to die of homicides and Hispanic, American Indian and Alaskan natives fare somewhat better but are still more likely to die as a result of homicide than white males (CDC, 2018a,b,c).

More recently, the drug overdose death rate, especially due to opioids, has been recognized as a public health burden and has affected life expectancy statistics (CDC, 2020a,b,c). In the United States, the age-adjusted drug overdose death rates for females increased from 3.9 in 1999 to 14.4 in 2019, for males the increase was from 8.2 in 1999 to 29.6 in 2019 and was higher than the female rate for the entire 10-year period from 1999 to 2019 (Hedegaard et al., 2020).

In 2020, the COVID-19 pandemic added a new component to the statistics on the causes of death. In the United States, male deaths of all ages outnumbered female deaths of all ages, with a difference of almost 28,000 more males dying from COVID-19 than females (CDC, 2021).

Morbidity

Data from the OECD indicates that in member countries, about one in 10 adults consider themselves to be in bad health and almost a third of adults live with two or more chronic conditions (OECD, 2019). In general **morbidity** rates, or rates of illness, are difficult to obtain and have been available usually only in Western industrialized countries. For example, in the United States, reports of analyses of morbidity rates by gender lag several years behind those of analyses of mortality rates by gender. Gender differences in morbidity rates reflect the latest available reports. The following are common indicators of morbidity rate:

- Incidence of acute illness
- Prevalence of chronic conditions
- Use of medical care

Although variations exist, women are more likely to be ill, whereas men are at greater risk for death. Box 18.2 lists several resources for morbidity data in the United States.

Chronic Conditions

A **chronic condition** is a condition that persists for at least 3 months or belongs to a group of conditions classified as chronic, regardless of time of onset, such as tuberculosis, neoplasm, and arthritis. In general, women have higher morbidity rates than men. Women are more likely than men to have a higher prevalence of chronic diseases that cause disability and limitation of activities but do not lead to death. However, men have higher morbidity and mortality rates for conditions that are the leading causes of death.

BOX 18.2   Sources of Data

Health, United States: Submitted by the Secretary of the Department of Health and Human Services, *Health, United States* is an annual report on the health status of the nation. The data are compiled by the National Center for Health Statistics and the Centers for Disease Control and Prevention. The National Committee on Health and Vital Statistics reviews the report (http://www.cdc.gov/nchs/hus.htm).

National Center for Health Statistics (NCHS): Through the National Vital Statistics System, the NCHS collects data from each state, New York City, the District of Columbia, the U.S. Virgin Islands, Guam, and Puerto Rico on births, deaths, marriages, and divorces in the United States (http://www.cdc.gov/nchs/).

National Health Interview Survey: Directed by the National Center for Health Statistics, the National Health Interview Survey is an annual and continuing nationwide sample survey in which data are collected by personal interviews about household members' illnesses, injuries, chronic conditions, disabilities, and use of health services (www.cdc.gov/nchs/nhis.htm).

? ACTIVE LEARNING

1. Examine the vital statistics in the community and compare the gender-specific differences in mortality rates.
2. During a 1-week period, determine the frequency of newspaper articles in the local major newspaper that identify the top 12 causes of death for men.
3. Review major nursing texts (e.g., medical-surgical); examine the tables of contents and the indexes for content on men's health versus women's health.

USE OF MEDICAL CARE

The use of **medical care**—the use of ambulatory care, hospital care, preventive care, or other health services—in the United States also illustrates different gender patterns.

Use of Ambulatory Care

Men seek ambulatory care less often than women. According to the 2010 National Health Interview Survey (NHIS) (Schiller et al., 2012), the physician's office is the primary setting for ambulatory care for both men and women. Responses to the survey indicated that men visited physician offices and clinics or health centers less often than women and emergency rooms more frequently. Additionally, 27% of men, compared with 14% women, had made no office visits to a healthcare provider in the past 12 months. Men were likely to visit a physician only if they experienced a specific health-related symptom (Brown and Bond, 2008; Quallich et al., 2018). Injury-related visits to hospital emergency departments are higher for males than females. Males aged 18 to 24 years are twice as likely to visit hospital emergency departments for unintentional injuries as females in the same age range. Even though gender differences in ambulatory care utilization are lessening, males continue to delay medical treatment, so they are sicker when they do seek healthcare and therefore require more intensive medical care.

Use of Hospital Care

The literature indicates that hospitalization rates also vary by sex. In 2014, rates of hospital stays were lower for males than for females. Hospital stays increase for both men and women after 45 years of age; however, rates for men increase more rapidly. After 65 years of age, men's discharge rates continue to be higher than women's rates (National Center for Health Statistics [NCHS], 2016).

Use of Preventive Care

Preventive examinations and appropriate health-protective behavior are necessary for health promotion and early diagnosis of health problems. Men do not engage in these health-protective behaviors at the same frequency as do females (Brown and Bond, 2008; Quallich et al., 2018). Most men do not have routine checkups. National health surveys indicate that women overall are more likely than men to have visits to various healthcare providers (CDC, 2019a,b). Men are twice as likely to report no usual source of care, although eligibility for primary care in males exceeds that in females (Lynch, 2008).

Use of Other Health Services

Overall, the number of visits to healthcare provider offices and outpatient sites is lower for men aged 18 to 64 than for women in the same age span. Men 18 to 64 tend to have fewer dental healthcare visits (61.1) than do women (66,8) as a percentage of persons with a dental visit in the past year for 2017 (CDC, 2019a,b). In a research study conducted by Frisbee et al. (2010), findings supported the importance of oral hygiene as it relates to the overall health of the individual.

THEORIES THAT EXPLAIN MEN'S HEALTH

As discussed previously, a gender gap exists in health. The data reviewed raise many questions for community health nurses to explore regarding gender differences in health and illness. Although men have shorter life expectancies and higher rates of mortality for all leading causes of death, women have higher rates of morbidity, including rates of acute illness and chronic disease and use of medical and preventive care services. Verbrugge and Wingard (1987) asked why "females are sicker, but males die sooner." Several explanations exist for this paradox.

Nurses traditionally use developmental theories to explain individual behavior. Erickson's model was not gender specific; Levinson focused somewhat on male development. There remains a need for literature detailing the factors and combinations of factors that influence gender differences in the health and illness of populations.

The following explanations proposed by Waldron (1995d) and Verbrugge and Wingard (1987) attempt to account for gender differences in this important area:

- Biological factors, including genetics, effects of sex hormones, and physiological differences, which may be influenced by genetics, hormones, and environment
- Socialization

- Orientations toward illness and prevention
- Data collection of health behavior

Biological Factors

Several biological factors influence sex differences in mortality and morbidity rates, including genetics, effects of sex hormones, and physiological differences, which may be influenced by genetics, hormones, and environmental factors (Waldron, 1995a,b,c,d). The embryo is unisexual until the seventh week of gestation. **Androgen**, a hormone from the Y chromosome, coupled with the maternal androgen sources, results in the development of the male sex. More male births occur than female births. In 2008, 1048 male births occurred for every 1000 female births (Martin et al., 2010). However, during this period, infant mortality rates for males were 21% higher than for females, thus reducing this ratio (Mathews and MacDorman, 2012). Sex ratios at birth appear to be lower for births to American Indian and black fathers (Martin et al., 2010).

Whether sex ratios at birth are influenced by sex ratios at conception or sex differentials in mortality rates before birth is unknown. Current evidence suggests that more than two of every three prenatal deaths occur before clinical recognition of the pregnancy. Embryonic research shows excess male fetuses in early pregnancy and fewer males delivered at term. Males' experience of higher mortality rates for perinatal conditions is attributed to biological disadvantages such as males' greater risk of premature birth, higher rates of respiratory distress syndrome, and higher rates of infectious disease in infancy resulting from the influence of male hormones on the developing lungs, brain, and possibly the immune system of the male fetus (Heron et al., 2009). Sex chromosome—linked diseases, such as hemophilia and certain types of muscular dystrophy, are more common among males than females (Waldron, 1995b).

Biological advantages for females may also exist later in life because of the estrogen-related mechanism that protects against heart disease. Some evidence supports the hypothesis that men's higher testosterone levels contribute to their lower high-density lipoprotein cholesterol levels. Body fat distribution, specifically the tendency for men in Western countries to accumulate abdominal body fat versus the tendency for women to accumulate fat on the buttocks and thighs, may also contribute to sex differences in the development of metabolic syndrome (Kirby et al., 2006). Men's higher levels of stored iron also may contribute to risk for ischemic heart disease. Additional physiological gender differences are as follows (Tanne, 1997):

- During the process of aging, men's brain cells die faster than women's brain cells. This finding may explain why men are more often hospitalized for serious mental disease.
- Male immune systems are weaker than women's.

Socialization

A second theory for explaining sex differences in health is socialization, especially in the area of masculinity. Society emphasizes assertiveness, restricted emotional display, concern for power, and reckless behavior in males (Box 18.3). Pursuit of these attributes results in higher risks in work, leisure, and

BOX 18.3 Four Dimensions of Stereotyped Male Gender-Role Behavior

- *No sissy stuff:* the need to be different from women
- *The big wheel:* the need to be superior to others
- *The sturdy oak:* the need to be independent and selfreliant
- *Give 'em hell:* the need to be more powerful than others, through violence if necessary

Modified from David DS, Brannon R: The male sex role: our culture's blueprint of manhood, and what it's done for us lately. In David DS, Brannon R, editors: *The 49 percent majority: the male sex role*, Reading, MA, Addison-Wesley, 1976.

lifestyle. Internalization of these norms of masculinity reduces the likelihood of engaging in health promotion behaviors for fear these behaviors might be interpreted as a sign of weakness. Gender-role socialization may influence these differences. Peer pressure plays an important role in the adherence to masculine norms. Many men enculturate their sons to believe that risking personal injury demonstrates masculinity (Brown and Bond, 2008). For men psychological factors such as the need for emotional control, fear, embarrassment, and anxiety related to using healthcare services can act as barriers to getting needed care (Quallich et al., 2018). The expectations of employers and other work-related demands may also lead to little time for taking care of personal health and may limited access (Quallich et al., 2018).

According to the CDC's (2020a,b,c) National Institute for Occupational Safety and Health (NIOSH) Workers Health Charts, 53% of U.S. workers are male. Male workers account for 94.3% of the reported severe occupational illnesses and injuries, and for 92.1% of work-related fatalities (CDC, 2020a,b,c). Men's higher exposure to carcinogens at the worksite is associated with high rates of mesothelioma and coal worker's pneumoconiosis. In the United States, men score higher than women on measures of hostility and lack of trust of others, which may place them at higher risk of ischemic heart disease. However, women have different work-related stressors. Statistics indicate that females tended to report more incidence of psychological occupational exposures than men did, specifically in the categories of high job demands, low job control, hostile environment, low supervisory support, and a poor safety climate. Men had a higher incidence in only three categories: work-life interference, perceiving the workplace as unsafe, and worry about job loss (CDC, 2020a,b,c).

Popular male leisure, sports, and play activities place men at high risk for injury. Statistics show that men drive faster than women, receive more traffic violations, and are less likely to wear seat belts, all of which contribute to a greater number of motor vehicle fatalities. Although the prevalence of smoking is decreasing, 28.62% of males over 18 used tobacco products in 2017 (CDC, 2018a,b,c). A current public health concern is the rapidly increasing popularity of electronic or e-cigarettes, which in 2018, 20.8% in 9 to 12 age group reported using (CDC, 2020a,b,c). The concern is that e-cigarettes contain often contain nicotine and other substances which can be addictive and harmful to developing brains (CDC, 2020a,b,c). According to 2017 statistics, 55.5% of men consume alcohol land are twice as likely than women to drink heavily; and, males overall have a greater use of illegal substances and greater nonmedical use of psychotherapeutic drugs (CDC, 2018a,b,c).

Men are more likely to be involved in violent crimes, and violence is a typical precursor to homicide. Men are victims of homicide more often than women (CDC, 2019a,b). For black males, the fifth leading cause of death is homicide. However, for white males, homicide is not one of the top 10 causes of death (CDC, 2019a,b).

Many barriers exist that prohibit positive changes in male health behavior, but female family members were seen as facilitators. Cheatham et al. (2008) reported that several studies show males to be more likely to change health behaviors when these changes are suggested and supported by female family members who the males thought were concerned about their well-being.

Orientation Toward Illness and Prevention

Illness orientation, or the ability to note symptoms and take appropriate action, also may differ between the sexes. Most diseases, injuries, and deaths prevalent among men are preventable. However, the stereotypical view of men as strong and invulnerable is incongruent with health promotion. Boys are socialized to ignore symptoms and "toughen up." Surveys done by the magazine Men's Health reveal that nine million men have not seen a healthcare provider in 5 years. Men may be aware of being ill, but they make a conscious decision not to seek healthcare to avoid being labeled "sick."

Brown and Bond (2008) suggest that men lack the somatic awareness and are less likely to interpret symptoms as indicators of illness. A desire to rationalize symptoms and denial of susceptibility to disease may contribute to the delay in treatment (Brown and Bond, 2008). Men also spend less time at doctor's appointments and get less health advice then women resulting in barriers to appropriate and adequate care (Quallich et al., 2018).

Health-protective behavior, or the ability to take action to prevent disease or injury, also may vary between the sexes. Perhaps as a result of the contraceptive developments of the 1970s, women are more likely to seek preventive examinations. Routine reproductive health screening (e.g., the Papanicolaou smear test and breast examination) has been expanded to include some general screening, such as testing of blood pressure, urine, and blood for signs of chronic problems. Men do not have routine reproductive health checkups that include screening, which would detect other health problems at an early stage. Among respondents to the NHIS, more women than men reported contacting a dentist and a healthcare provider within the previous 6 months, and 22% of men were without a usual place of healthcare, compared with 13% of women (Schiller et al., 2012). Men reported spending more time in leisure activities and muscle-strengthening activities that met the federal physical activity guidelines. However, 41% of men were considered overweight, compared with 28% of women (Schiller et al., 2012).

Gender differences in preventive health behavior are a fertile ground for continued research. Meryn (2009) reported that 21% of research was devoted to men's health, compared with 53% for female health. He suggests that large-scale research in this area would add to the small evidence bases of health promotion behaviors among men. Specific national health objectives have only recently addressed the healthcare needs of this aggregate. Uniformly recognized preventive screening programs for males have only recently been developed. With the advent of managed care and initiatives for healthcare reform, men who are eligible for healthcare coverage will have access to these routine health screenings. For men coverage would be available for immunizations, colonoscopies, nutritional education, obesity screenings, cholesterol and blood pressure screenings, screenings for HIV, depression screenings, and tobacco counseling (Sommers and Wilson, 2012). However, whether men will take advantage of these programs is undetermined. Box 18.4 discusses matters related to men's reproductive health needs.

Reporting of Health Behavior

Data regarding health behaviors are collected from a variety of sources, such as interviews, surveys, questionnaires, and reports. Data from these sources may not be accurate because males are less likely than females to participate in such a data collection process. Men may be less willing to talk, may not recall health problems, and may lack a health vocabulary. Men may be more hesitant to talk about their illnesses. Not only do women participate more in the data collection process, but also they are often solicited in health surveys to report the health behavior of men. In this manner, women are proxies, and proxies have a tendency to underreport behavior. The accuracy of the data does increase with male participation, but men may not want to participate in the socialization of sickness and tend to make light of health problems. Males with an extreme conception of masculinity are less likely to admit their health problems and may conceal or suppress pain in an effort to appear strong (Naslindh-Ylispangar et al., 2008). Men are far less likely than women to seek counseling. Male socialization to suppress expressiveness may represent the explanation for gender differences in reporting health behaviors.

Discussion of the Theories of Men's Health
Interpreting the Data

Community health nurses should be aware of gender disparity when collecting and interpreting data. To avoid bias, the community health nurse should consider the following issues:

Gender-specific interview techniques may be necessary to obtain the most accurate health history. Men respond better to direct questions than to open-ended questions.

How do data obtained by male nurses differ from those obtained by female nurses? Is there personal gender bias in data collection?

BOX 18.4   Men's Reproductive Health Needs

Reproductive health needs are beginning to be recognized as important to both men's health and women's health. Usually the term *reproductive health* is applied to women of childbearing age. Used here, the term applies to the health of reproductive organs, which develop in utero and with which a person is born, either male or female, regardless of whether he or she has sex or reproduces. Males may have reproductive health needs whether child or adult, straight or gay, or virgin or sexually experienced.

Many STDs are at epidemic proportions in the United States and are a major health hazard for many men and women. AIDS is twice as likely to occur in males as in females in the United States. In 2017, death due to HIV in males was 2.4 per 100,000, and for females it was 0.8 per 100,000 (Centers for Disease and Prevention [CDC], 2018a,b,c). Less well known, perhaps, is that many STDs are considered intrinsically "sexist" because clinical evidence, more overt in men, is more likely to facilitate a correct diagnosis in men than in women. These STDs are easier to detect in men because men are more likely to be symptomatic; laboratory tests are more reliable in men; efficiency of transmission is greater from male to female; and men are more likely to seek care for STDs that are symptomatic. For example, the overall incidence rate for *Chlamydia* infection in 2015 for males was 305.2 per 100,000; for females, the rate was 645.5 per 100,000. The rate of gonorrhea was slightly higher among men (140.9 per 100,000 population) than among women (107.2 per 100,000 population). Syphilis was also more common in men than in women (13.7 per 100,000 males; 1.4 per 100,000 females) (CDC, 2012).

Testicular cancer represents only 1% of cancers in males and is the most common cancer to affect young men between the ages of 15 and 35 years. Cancer of the prostate is a leading cause of death from cancer in men, was estimated to account for 18.7 deaths per 100,000 population in 2017 (CDC, 2018a,b,c). The increase in the incidence of prostate cancer has been attributed to factors such as improved methods of detection and greater exposure to environmental carcinogens. Mortality rates for all cancers remain high, especially in males in the 65–84 year range which have the highest rate of cancer deaths (CDC, 2019a,b).

Many occupational and environmental agents associated with adverse sexual and reproductive outcomes in men have been identified, including pesticides; anesthetic gases in the operating room and dental office; inorganic lead from smelters, paint, printing materials, carbon disulfide from vulcanization of rubber, inorganic mercury manufacturing, and dental work; and ionizing radiation from X-rays (Whorton, 1984). Nonchemical agents have also been identified as hazardous in men; for example, hyperthermia experienced by firefighters has been linked to male infertility.

Many pharmacological agents, including prescription, over-the-counter, and recreational drugs, have been found to affect the reproductive outcomes or sexual functioning of men. Examples are drugs from the following categories: antihypertensives, antipsychotics, antidepressants, hormones, sedatives, hypnotics, stimulants, chemotherapy agents used in cancer treatment, amphetamines, opiates, alcohol, marijuana, cocaine, barbiturates, and lysergic acid diethylamide (LSD). Erectile dysfunction has become a "socially acceptable" topic of discussion since many high-profile men, such as U.S. Senator Bob Dole, former National Football League coach Mike Ditka, and retired General Norman Schwarzkopf, have openly discussed their problem. Pharmaceutical companies market their products for treatment of this disorder via mass media. Controversy has arisen as to the use of public funding for these products.

A focus on homosexual men's health has come about largely through the advent of AIDS. Today, homosexuality encompasses not only the male but also the entire family. The community health nurse should develop nonjudgmental assessment skills that foster honest and open expression for all members of the community. Nurses may need specialized skills to work with these individuals.

The accuracy of secondary sources of information is skewed toward the interpretation of the source. How do the data provided by women about male health behavior compare with the data collected from men regarding these same behaviors?

Men are not enculturated to be caregivers. They need assistance to learn how to provide support to a caregiver or to develop a caregiver role.

In response to the question why "females are sicker, but males die sooner," several reasons can be provided. Conditions that affect morbidity rates (e.g., arthritis and gout) do not significantly affect mortality rates. Conditions that affect mortality rates may not significantly affect day-to-day activity until the conditions are advanced. Men tend to delay seeking healthcare until their conditions are advanced. Although mortality rates are, in large part, the outcome of inherited or acquired risks, gender differences in illness and health promotion behaviors, as well as in the reporting of health behaviors, suggest that social and psychological factors also affect morbidity rates. Although males have higher prevalence and death rates for "killer" chronic diseases, injuries, and accidents, females have higher prevalence rates for a greater number of nonfatal chronic conditions.

Gender-Linked Behavior

The largest gender differences in mortality rates occur for causes of death associated with gender-linked behavior and suggest that gender-linked behavior, which is more prevalent and encouraged in men, correlates with the following major categories of death:

- *Tobacco use:* Lung cancer, bronchitis, emphysema, and asthma
- *Substance abuse:* Cirrhosis, accidents, and homicide
- *Poor preventive health habits and stress:* Heart disease
- *Lack of other emotional channels:* Cirrhosis, suicide, homicide, and accidents

Physical conditions can be seriously affected by social and environmental conditions, such as occupational hazards (e.g., carcinogens and stress), unemployment, and massive advertising campaigns that use gender and gender roles to sell alcohol and tobacco. These lifestyle factors are compounded by men's lack of willingness to seek preventive care such as screening and to seek healthcare when a symptom arises. To counter these types of factors, research is needed to determine gender-specific methods of data collection, education, and practice that are aimed at health promotion, illness prevention, and political processes for males.

RESEARCH HIGHLIGHTS

Health Education and Health Screening in a Sample of Older Men: A Descriptive Survey.

Two nurse researchers (Dallas and Neville, 2012) conducted a study to describe the health education and health screening practices of older men living in an area of New Zealand and the perceived barriers to and benefits of healthy lifestyle choices. Data were collected using a self-reported instrument. The sample consisted of 59 men ranging in age from 65 to 91 years. The majority of the men in this sample (66%) reported no barriers to making a healthy lifestyle choice. However, of those men who did report barriers, the most common reason was lack of motivation (12%), followed by lack of knowledge related to availability of programs and screenings (8%). Reported external barriers included lack of programs, associated costs, and transportation challenges. The most common reported benefits of a healthy lifestyle choice were getting to be with other people (62%), having fun (56%), feeling healthier (54%), and feeling better about self (52%). The majority of the men reported their health as good (67%), and healthy lifestyle as always (43%) or frequently healthy (43%). Dallas and Neville (2012) contend that nurses can have a pivotal role in conducting future research endeavors aimed at understanding the health needs of older men that will ultimately improve their health outcomes.

Data from Dallas J, Neville S: Health education and health screening in a sample of older men: a descriptive survey, *Nurs Prax N Z* 28(1):6—16, 2012.

ACTIVE LEARNING

Survey the billboards in the community and determine the frequency of those that depict gender-linked behaviors of men that are associated with risk taking.

FACTORS THAT IMPEDE MEN'S HEALTH

Many factors function as barriers to men's health, including their risk-taking behaviors and infrequent use of the healthcare system. In addition, gaps in preventive health behavior and differences in illness and health orientations and reporting of health behavior all contribute to a diminished health status for men. Several other barriers have been proposed, including the patterns of medical care provided in the United States, access to care, and lack of health promotion.

Medical Care Patterns

Although the data that serve as a foundation for medical treatment were collected from males, the concept of a healthcare provider that specializes in men's health is a relatively new phenomenon. Many health professionals provide care for men with complex health needs in a wide variety of settings. A specialist to which a male could go to for care that "feels right" for him has not been developed. Little effort has been made to create a male-specific healthcare climate (Haines and Wender, 2006). Urologists, who may see men for genital abnormalities or diseases of the prostate, became the proxy "male health specialists." The medical specialty andrology, which originated in Europe to treat problems of fertility and sterility, is considered too narrow in focus to treat "the whole man." Without a primary

care specialty that focuses specifically on men's needs and gender-role influences on health and lifestyle, the gender disparity will continue. Currently, male health concerns are addressed by specialists and generalists who have not received gender-specific training that would enable them to focus on men's health needs. In the current era of managed care and healthcare reform, men will still be left without gender-specific primary care providers who have training focused specifically on men's needs.

Access to Care
Mission Orientation

Historically, society's interest in men's health has focused on efforts necessary to maintain an effective workforce. Men are socialized to view health as a commodity or resource that enables the body to work. Mission-oriented healthcare is a priority for large industries and organized sports. Industries provide workers with preventive healthcare to maintain workplace productivity. Mission-oriented healthcare in the sports arena has given birth to the specialty of sports medicine. Insurance programs such as health maintenance organizations (HMOs) may provide more comprehensive healthcare to men. Perhaps the most complete care is currently offered by the military; however, marked deficiencies exist there in the lack of a focus on prevention and health promotion at the individual and aggregate levels and inattention to policy regarding environmental hazards.

Financial Considerations

Another barrier to healthcare for men is financial ability. A man may receive an annual physical examination if he belongs to an HMO or if he is an executive or an airline pilot, but many private insurance companies reimburse more fully for a diagnosed condition (e.g., for pathology) and less fully for preventive care. A man is more likely to be insured for acute or chronic illness conditions than for health education, counseling, or other types of preventive healthcare. Women have annual gynecological examinations that include screening for other conditions and allow a woman to express other physical or psychological needs; however, men have lacked entrance into the healthcare system for a physical examination on a routine basis. With the advent of managed care and societal interest in preventive health focus, gender differences in routine physical examinations for preventive reasons have narrowed. However, socialization has a marked influence on behavior, and current trends may prevail despite attitudinal changes in healthcare delivery. Men must become advocates for programs that meet their own healthcare needs (Porche, 2009).

Time Factors

Historically, medical care could be accessed between the hours of 9:00 A.M. and 5:00 P.M. Monday through Friday. Men were reluctant to take time from work for a medical visit, especially for reasons other than illness. Fear of loss of income or the stigmatization of being "weak," "ill," or "less of a man" inhibited medical care access for males. Men in the lower socioeconomic group may be too exhausted from working to access healthcare, especially preventive healthcare (Haines and Wender, 2006). Variety in the times and locations of care delivery clinics should improve male access. More walk-in primary care clinics that provide evening and weekend appointments have appeared. These clinics may be housed in occupational settings, malls, and even grocery stores. Data must be collected regarding male utilization of these additional healthcare sites.

Lack of Health Promotion

Limiting the concept of health to being merely absence of disease eliminates health promotion. Using traditional mortality and morbidity rates as reflective of the state of "health" of a population represents only a biological basis of health. To provide the community health nurse with a clearer picture of male health, the presence of behavioral risk factors such as smoking, alcohol consumption, obesity, and sedentary lifestyle should be considered. When asked, men describe "healthy" people as those with proportional body weight and height who do not engage excessively in behaviors detrimental to health. Physical recovery after impairment, illness, or injury is also considered a factor in men's definition of "healthy." Disease prevention and health promotion are not often reflected in a man's perception of health. Addressing and limiting the precursors of death is a recent healthcare phenomenon (Box 18.5). Interventions by many disciplines are needed to prevent current health problems. Nursing can play a pivotal role in the contribution to practice and research in this area of concern.

BOX 18.5 Precursors of Death

The following precursors of death are frequently unaddressed by the present healthcare system:

- Heart disease and stroke
- Hypercholesterolemia
- Hypertension
- Diabetes mellitus
- Obesity
- Type A personality
- Family history
- Lack of exercise
- Cigarette smoking
- Cancer
- Sunlight
- Radiation
- Occupational hazards
- Water pollution
- Air pollution
- Dietary patterns
- Alcohol
- Heredity

The continued focus on disease cure in the present healthcare system reinforces men's perception of health. Coronary heart disease, cancer, and stroke are three conditions that account for two thirds of all deaths and require the greatest use of healthcare resources. The increase in life expectancy exhibits the effect these medical advances have had on mortality rates from these diseases. These advances have resulted in an increase in years of disability, which may account for the rise in suicide among men older than 65 years (NCHS, 2016). An increase in healthcare costs has also resulted.

ETHICAL INSIGHTS

Social Justice Versus Market Justice Ethics

Community health nurses should be involved in political activities that develop health policies that will make a difference in the health of males and the entire population. Such activities are congruent with the philosophy of public health as "health for all" and a commitment to a social justice ethic of healthcare rather than a market justice ethic of healthcare. Examining men's health gives the community health nurse an opportunity to observe the market justice ethic of healthcare's influence on men's health in the United States and how this affects their traditional roles in the family and within the community. The community health nurse can play a vital role in contributing to a social justice ethic of healthcare, particularly in relation to promoting men's health. Nurses must focus on health promotion and prevention at the aggregate and population levels rather than on treatment and cure.

Financial resources are invested in traditional disease-curative care rather than health promotion action. An inordinate amount of funding is poured into the healthcare system each year, with only minimal amounts allotted to public health promotion, as discussed in earlier chapters. According to the World Bank, in 2018 in the United States, the total national health expenditure accounted for 16.8% of the gross domestic product. Of every dollar spent on healthcare in 2017, more than half went to hospital care and physician services (World Bank, 2018), which are in large part curative in focus. The current healthcare system is making limited advances in addressing the precursors of death. It is questionable whether medical care, or another medical specialty, is the answer to men's health needs when social, occupational, environmental, and lifestyle factors continue to place men at risk.

Healthy lifestyles are not a matter of free choice but rather a result of opportunities that are not always equally available to people. Although available, prevention and health promotion are not uniformly applied at the aggregate and population levels. Health policies shape these opportunities for a healthy lifestyle for individuals and aggregates. Policies related to environmental and occupational changes beyond an individual's control are required to significantly affect the health of the population (Meryn, 2009).

ACTIVE LEARNING

Survey local businesses and industries in the community to determine what health promotion and prevention programs are available and used by men and women.

MEN'S HEALTHCARE NEEDS

Lynch (2008) delineated men's healthcare needs that draw from the biological and psychosocial causes of men's distinctive health situation, and these healthcare needs continue today. According to these writers, men need the following:

- Permission to have concerns about health and to talk openly to others about their concerns
- Support for the consideration of gender-role and lifestyle influences on their physical and mental health
- Attention from professionals regarding factors that may result in illness or influence a man's expression of illness, including such things as occupational factors, leisure patterns, and interpersonal relationships
- Information about how their bodies function, what is normal, what is abnormal, what action to take, and the contributions of proper nutrition and exercise
- Self-care instruction, including testicular and genital selfexamination
- Physical examination and history taking that include sexual and reproductive health and illness throughout the lifespan
- Treatment for problems of couples, including interpersonal problems, infertility, family planning, sexual concerns, and sexually transmitted diseases (STDs)
- Help with fathering (i.e., being included as a parent in child care)
- Help with fathering as a single parent, in particular with a child of the opposite sex, in addressing the child's sexual development and concerns
- Recognition that feelings of confusion and uncertainty in a time of rapid social change are normal and that they may mark the onset of healthy adaptation to change
- Adjustment of the healthcare system to men's occupational constraints regarding time and location of healthcare sources
- Financial ways to obtain these goals

Additional healthcare needs of men are for primary prevention and for secondary and tertiary prevention at the individual, family, and community levels to address the precursors of death that influence males so greatly. Men are less likely than women to be consumers in the healthcare system; therefore, alternative approaches must be developed that address their health needs.

The most significant approaches in the future will be those that reach men in the community, schools, the workplace, and public settings. These approaches call for political processes that set policy, for health marketing techniques, and for advocacy (Meryn, 2009).

COMMUNITY HEALTH NURSING SERVICES FOR MEN

A male can be seen by a community health nurse in a well-baby clinic, by a school nurse, by an occupational health nurse, and by a community health nurse or home health nurse on a home visit for follow-up of a chronic disease. However, men are less likely than women to be seen by a community health nurse. Not only is maternal and child health a major focus of many health departments, but neither a medical nor a nursing specialty within a health department routinely exists to specifically

address men's health. Preventive reproductive healthcare (e.g., family planning, prenatal care, and cancer screening) and associated general screening are not routinely available for men. The community health nurse's commitment to health for all requires an increased awareness of men's health issues in their social and cultural context as well as individual and group actions that will improve men's physical, psychological, and social well-being.

Meeting men's healthcare needs can be viewed in a traditional public fashion. By viewing the problem from a primary, secondary, and tertiary intervention method, the nurse can look at the problem in a holistic manner. Factors that promote men's health are in the community, including interest groups in men and men's health, men's growing interest in physical fitness and lifestyle, policy related to men's health, and health services for men.

Gaining Skills Necessary to Address Men's Health Needs

Assessment skills necessary to carry out screening activities with men to detect reproductive health needs may be lacking in nursing education. One community health nurse who worked in a rural health department felt unqualified to respond to male partners' requests for genital examinations when couples came to seek family planning services. This community health nurse requested to work for specified periods with a urologist and in an STD clinic in a large urban area to gain the necessary skills. On return to the rural health department, she felt comfortable with male patients and taught the skills she had learned to nurse colleagues. Cheatham et al. (2008) suggest that providers make efforts to establish a positive patient–provider relationship using nonjudgmental verbal and nonverbal communication techniques. The nurse should engage the male and the female significant other in a manner that is easily understood.

Primary Preventive Measures
Health Education

Healthcare professionals, including the community health nurse, find that health education is the cornerstone of prevention. Although criticized by some as too narrow, health education can be a means of empowerment that helps individuals make behavioral changes. Education about male health issues should begin early. At school, boys should learn the anatomical and physiological aspects of their bodies and the social aspects of taking responsibility for their health. Coeducational discussion classes that cover a variety of social and personal topics can be a venue to encourage boys to talk about their bodies and their feelings. Adolescent males are shown to lack the use of language in comparison with their female counterparts. This may lead to a less selfconscious attitude to health seeking when boys reach adulthood.

Access to health education should follow males into the workplace. Many employers have experienced benefits such as lower healthcare costs when their employees receive health education programs coupled with health screening. Government and private insurance incentives given to employers who provide such programs would provide further impetus. Men who are not in the workplace can access health education in other areas, such as shopping malls, barbershops, and local senior centers. Some healthcare professionals are concerned about such informal dispersion of health literature, citing possible issues with the literacy level of the population. Government benefits programs can function as a medium for health education by including it in their benefit mailings. More control over the readability and the information included can be exerted over this material. Educational material should be written in the context of male interests and should focus on making healthy living relevant to the male (Cheatham et al., 2008).

The use of world-wide web resources is a promising tool for health education dissemination. However, in a recent study by Teh et al. (2019) a review of websites concerning men's health found that 35% of the 357 sites screened from four English-speaking countries were of the nonhealth, nonmedical, or e-commerce type and that only 28% were government, health organization, or educational institution websites. As recent healthcare trends call for the increasing use of the internet by consumers for e-registration, e-appointments and virtual visits, as well as obtaining health information, this study points out that consumers should monitor their internet resources for sponsoring commercial sites and healthcare sites for the most up to date, reliable, accessible, and accurate information (Teh et al., 2019). Regardless, concerning men's health, a variety of strategies by healthcare providers may be needed and nontraditional settings used to increase positive health outcomes in men (Quallich et al., 2017).

Interest Groups for Men and Men's Health

The consumer movement that occurred on behalf of women's health in the 1960s and early 1970s has no counterpart for advocation of men's health. However, a viable men's consumer movement is forming. The National Organization for Men Against Sexism is interested in redefining the male role, particularly those aspects of it that are detrimental to health and growth. The American Assembly for Men in Nursing sponsors annual meetings that address issues such as men's health, men's work environments, research on men's health, and networking and support among male nurses. Researchers are beginning to define and study men's health beyond men's occupational role (e.g., reproductive health). Marketing has changed to include male health promotion public service announcements. Peer-reviewed journals such as *International Journal of Men's Health* and *American Journal of Men's Health* are providing scholars with avenues to disseminate men's health concerns.

Men's Growing Interest in Physical Fitness and Lifestyle

Although cardiovascular diseases (CVDs) are a major health hazard for men, research on the validity and usefulness of preventive and treatment modalities is an issue of considerable debate (Harvard Men's Health Watch, 2009). Men's interest in altering behavior that places them at risk for cardiovascular and other major diseases is increasing, especially among older males (Shapiro and Yarborough-Hayes, 2008). For example, men's smoking behavior has changed dramatically. In 1965, more than 50% of males smoked compared with 21% in 2010%; and, 52.1% of men reported engaging in aerobic activity three times a week or more, compared with 42.7% of females (Schiller et al., 2012). However on the downside, 2017 national statistics indicate that only 29% of men met the physical activity guidelines for Americans set in 2008, and even less women (20%) met these guidelines (CDC, 2018a,b,c).

The health behaviors that have shown the greatest change in a positive direction have been those most influenced by legislative action (e.g., seat belt use, use of smoke detectors, and drunk driving). Even with these legislative actions, males remain three times less likely to use seat belts as females of the same age. In the Southeast, use of seat belts in pickup trucks was 25%, compared with more than 75% in other vehicles. The states of Alabama, Florida, Georgia, Kentucky, Mississippi, North Carolina, South Carolina, and Tennessee have engaged in a campaign called "Buckle Up in Your Truck." The campaign's centerpiece is the use of targeted television and radio advertisements to encourage seat belt use. Intensive enforcement mobilizations in the form of Selective Traffic Enforcement Programs, like Click It or Ticket, have followed periods of pickup truck advertisements. According to Tison and Williams (2010), the Click It or Ticket program has been an important factor in the improved usage of seat belts across the nation. On the basis of data from this report, seat belt use increased by 20 percentage points from 1991 through 2007.

Policy Related to Men's Health

Policies related to any group of people should include the opinions and perceptions of those directly affected. Policy related to men's health should include the male perception of health. Community health nurses can encourage and help males be advocates for policies regarding their healthcare. Male nurses can be extremely instrumental in this endeavor. Liaisons between male consumers and policy planners should be formed.

Secondary Preventive Measures
Health Services for Men

Fewer healthcare clinics are tailored to men's special needs than to women's special needs. The "well-man clinics" set up in the 1980s were designed to identify lifestyle risk factors, not to provide screening clinics like the women's clinics. Once they are identified, a method or resolution for these lifestyle risk factors is formulated. Although many well-man clinics exist in the United Kingdom, male use of these clinics is far below female use of women's clinics (Roberts and Gerber, 2003). Although not based on the medical model, the Men's Shed movement in

Australia has provided men with the socialization needed to make positive health behavior changes. Male screening methods typically have been limited to detecting high blood cholesterol levels and cancers such as prostate cancer, skin cancer, and testicular lumps. The era of managed care and healthcare reform may not encourage the concept of gender-specific care, as men and women receive primary care from the same health services.

Screening Services for Men

- The U.S. Preventive Services Task Force (USPSTF) provides an outline for the kinds of screening tests the adult male population should receive (American Family Physician, 2019):
- Depression screening
- Suicide screening
- Blood pressure check along with a yearly physical.
- Blood cholesterol check yearly for adults 35 and over.
- Prostate cancer screening 55 to 69 (American Cancer Society recommends high risk individuals with relatives who have had cancer, and black males get screened yearly starting at age 45)
- Hepatitis B screening for persons at increased risk
- Hepatitis C screening for persons 18 to 79 years
- HIV screening for persons 15 to 65 years
- Latent tuberculosis screening for adults at increased risk
- Lung cancer screening for adults 55 to 80 with a history of smoking
- Colorectal screening 60 to 75 years old (American Cancer Society recommends a Colonoscopy every 10 years or CT colonography ever 5 years after age 50)
- Syphilis screening for adults at increased risk
- Tobacco use and cessation information
- Blood glucose and Type II Diabetes for adults 40 to 70 years old who are overweight or obese
- One-time screening for abdominal aortic aneurysm for any man 65 to 75 years old who has smoked

Unhealthy drug use screening: adults over 18. Unhealthy alcohol use screening and behavioral counseling interventions: adults 18 and over. Additionally, The Advisory Committee on Immunizations (ACIP) recommends the yearly influenza vaccine, the high-dose vaccine for those over 65 and the Tdap vaccine booster (Heidelbaugh, 2018). For men over 40 years, it is also recommended to have eye exams every 2 to 4 years, increasing to 1 to 3 years for ages 55 to 64, and more frequently if you have diabetes or a family history of eye disease and a yearly dental exams (U.S. National Library of Medicine, 2021). Community health nurses should be familiar with these recommended screening test frequencies and should take every opportunity to encourage men to have these screenings. Through the institution of male healthcare fairs and other organized screenings, nurses are able to work with other healthcare providers to ensure that screenings are performed.

Information can also be provided about simple health examinations that men can be taught to perform themselves to maintain optimal health, some of these include: height and weight monitoring for BMI, heart rate checks, blood pressure checks, testicular cancer self-exams, and skin checks. In a study about attending a specific men's health clinic, by Vincent et al. (2018), suggested that it did not matter if the clinic was exclusively male or female and that men preferred to monitor their own health in order to make decisions on when to seek help for their specific problem. This finding reinforces the need to educate and make available information about self-examinations that men can do.

Tertiary Preventive Measures
Sex-Role and Lifestyle Rehabilitation

Traditional health services for males are available in both private and governmental arenas. The emphasis of these services is on diagnosis and treatment. The traditional male role may change dramatically from treatment modalities. Rehabilitation services for males must include counseling on lifestyle, role changes, and job retraining. Men must be given permission to express their emotions, such as fear and anxiety, over the resultant change (Cheatham et al., 2008).

Goal setting and possible methods for achievement must be acceptable to the man. For example, after a heart attack, a man may be told to stop smoking and begin an exercise program. For the plan to be successful, the male must be an active partner in its formation. (He may be able to exercise, e.g., by walking to the nearest automotive shop to talk with friends rather than spending time on a stationary bicycle at a local gym.)

Time taken away from work because of occupational injuries should be kept to a minimum. Males should be encouraged to return to work in an altered capacity rather than remaining away from work until injuries are completely healed. Occupational accommodation for the treatment regimen will help ensure compliance. Provision of medical care, supportive physical and occupational therapies, and "light-duty" jobs at the worksite help preserve the masculine persona. Box 18.6 lists some ways to address men about their health.

❓ ACTIVE LEARNING

1. Select a family that has a man in the household who is accessible. Select two "door openers" appropriate to initiate discussion of health concerns with this man. Devise a gender-appropriate nursing care plan that includes primary, secondary, and tertiary prevention for this man as an individual, for his family, and for his community.
2. Select a family that has a man in the household who is not readily accessible. Interview the female caregiver in the household and obtain information by proxy about the man's health. If possible, arrange to meet the man for lunch, at work, or after work and obtain information about his health. Compare the information obtained by proxy with that obtained from the client.

BOX 18.6 Door Openers: Ways to Address Men About Health Concerns

Strategies to address men about health concerns include the following:

Ask a man to talk about the last time he had a physical examination, what was done, why it was done, where it was done, and what the recommendations were.

Ask a man how he feels about his health insurance coverage. If he lacks health insurance, ask about the resources he used to obtain medical care for himself and for his family.

Ask a man about how he spends his leisure time, what he is doing to take care of himself, and what his usual physical activities are.

Observe a man for signs of stress such as moist palms, nail biting, posture (e.g., stooped with lack of eye contact), and nervous movements. If signs of stress are present, ask how he is coping with an identified health problem, family problem, or being unemployed.

Observe a man for difficulty clearing the airway (e.g., from smoking) and flushing of the face (e.g., from alcohol). Inquire as to habits of smoking and drinking and whether these habits have increased since the occurrence of the particular health or social problem.

Involve the man in decision making about healthcare to instill a sense of control over events.

NEW CONCEPTS OF COMMUNITY CARE

Specific services for men within health departments continue to be lacking in the United States. With the exception of STD clinics and selected family planning service models, male health concerns remain unaddressed. Two male health visitors (the British term for public health nurses) from the National Health Service (NHS) started an innovative public health nursing program directed at men in Glasgow, Scotland. Health visitors Bill Deans and Bob Hoskins established a nurse-run well-man clinic with the help of the NHS and the Scottish Council for Health Education. During home visits with mothers and infants, Deans and Hoskins observed that fathers excused themselves and went to the local pub when they arrived.

Any intervention regarding men's health needs must include men as willing participants (Lynch, 2008). Noting the characteristics of the male population in their community (e.g., overweight, heavy smoking, drinking, and high unemployment), Deans and Hoskins decided to modify their practice to serve their clients' needs. One afternoon per week, the clinic, which is based on a nursing model rather than a medical model, offers health screening, health education, and primary prevention to men. Marketing is important, and men are referred from general practitioners' and specialists' practices and recruited through newspaper advertisements. Clients with clinical signs and symptoms are referred back to their physicians. Lifestyle counseling and education are offered in areas such as fat and fiber content in diet, smoking, alcohol use, and exercise.

Deans and Hoskins consider the clinic a way to extend the health visitor's role in the NHS's efforts in health education with an aim to "nip potential diseases in the bud." Deans and Hoskins are concerned that the NHS does not provide male

services and are clear that "the unemployed chain-smoking husband needs as much care and health education from the health visitor as do his wife and baby" (Sadler, 1979, p. 18). The well-man clinic and well-woman clinic models can now be found in several communities throughout Great Britain and have been expanded to serve inmates in prison (Ballinger et al., 2009; Woodland and Hunt, 1994). After 10 years in existence, the well-man clinics in Great Britain are only sporadically used by males. Even when the services were expanded to the home, nurses found that men were purposely absent at the appointment time. Usage was highest with informal evening clinics directed by male nurses (Roberts and Gerber, 2003). An attempt to evaluate these nationally funded clinics was undertaken in 2003. It was suggested from the data that a collaborative approach to these interventions is a slow process and that adequate time should be provided before the evaluation (Reid et al., 2009).

In Australia, Men's Shed is a community-based health promotion initiative in men's health. Based on the social rather than medical model, the sheds promote well-being among older males by providing them with accepted and respected activities as well as a male-friendly space for socialization. Ballinger et al. (2009) found that participants in these activities reported an increase in recognition of the importance of health determinants and a sense of well-being.

Public health nurses working in the Benton County Health Department in Corvallis, Oregon, responded to the challenge of teen pregnancy in the 1970s by launching a community-wide effort that included developing a men's health clinic and marketing reproductive health services directly to teenage boys and men. An early effort established an advisory committee that included people from churches, schools, and healthcare facilities. A public health nurse health educator launched an extensive education program in the high school, which focused on decision-making processes and services available in the community. Later efforts involved the establishment of a clinic for men. Teenage boys were members of a consumer advisory committee established by the nurses that recommended the wording and format for advertisements about the clinic that ran in the high school newspaper. The advisory committee also recommended a flyer format that would be attractive to males. Specifically, they requested a card with information about the clinic and how to use condoms that would discreetly fit into their wallets and be available to share with peers.

The nurses have expanded their focus to create inclusive service environments in which teenage girls and boys and adult men and women will feel accepted and comfortable. Particular attention is given to the clinic decor and advertising, reading materials, and posters to transmit a message that includes offering healthcare for males and females. Clinic staff will see males or females at any time; however, a room in which staff members see men has decor geared toward men (e.g., no gynecological stirrups on the examining table) and pamphlets available for men on topics such as testicular cancer and chewing tobacco. Integrated services exist in the areas of family planning, STDs, and HIV counseling and testing.

CASE STUDY   Application of the Nursing Process

Gender-Appropriate Care for Men

Community health nurses are in an ideal position to address the health needs of men at individual, family, and community levels. The community health nurse may promote selfcare in male members of the family, facilitate men's health by addressing needed changes at the family level, buttress women's roles as caregivers of the family's health, and bring about change that influences policies that affect men at the community level.

Planning gender-appropriate care for males is outlined in the following case study, which is an application of the nursing process at the individual, family, and aggregate levels initiated in a home visit, and applies the previous discussions about the levels of prevention, roles of the community health nurse, research, and men's health.

Application of the nursing process to aggregates is facilitated by the use of systems theory, in which the nurse identifies the system and subsystems involved. The nurse may use a deductive or an inductive approach. A deductive approach would involve carrying out a community assessment and identifying an area or areas, such as a program needed by the community. Planning, implementation, and evaluation of the program would be carried out at the family or group level. An inductive approach would involve entering the community system through a person or client via a referral about a problem or concern. Assessment of the individual would be followed by identification of those groups to which the client belongs, such as family and community, and assessment of those groups.

Beth Lockwood, a community health nursing student at a health department, received a referral from the high school nurse to visit the Connors family to assess Richard Connors' mental health status. Richard was a 16-year-old sophomore whose academic work in school had declined rapidly after the premature death of his 46-year-old father. The father had died of a myocardial infarction, which he had while cleaning the garage with Richard one evening after school. Richard and the neighbors failed to revive Mr. Connors, and Richard carries feelings of guilt. Household members include Mrs. Connors, age 44 years, and Richard's sister Yvonne, age 12 years.

Assessment

The referral to assess the Connors family called for an inductive approach to assessment. Beth used a deductive approach later, when her experience with the Connors family piqued her concern about the status of men's health in her community. Beth assessed Richard, his mother, and his sister as household members of the family. However, she could not stop with the immediate family; she had to continue to identify the other groups within the community to which each individual family member belonged. Viewing the community as a system and focusing on systems and subsystems helped Beth organize the data she collected during assessment. Knowing that "the whole is greater than the sum of its parts," Beth prepared for her visit by reviewing adolescent theories of development and family theory. Beyond individual assessment, she noted factors related to the development of sex role—related behavior that may influence health. Examples of assessment areas include the following:

Family Configuration, Traditional, or Nontraditional
- Sex role—related behavior of parents, including work patterns in and out of the home, division of household labor, and decision-making patterns
- Patterns of parenting: mothering, fathering, and substitute father figure(s)
- Ability of male children to disclose feelings to family members and others
- Degree of assertiveness in female children
- Ability of family members to give emotional and physical support during crises and noncrises
- Ability of family members to trade off role-related behavior during crises and noncrises
- Risk-taking health behaviors
- Processing of stress and grief

- Communal lifestyle patterns that place the individual or family at risk (e.g., lack of exercise, poor diet, smoking, and drinking)
- Family history of death and illness
- Healthcare—taking patterns of family members
- Preventive health behaviors
- Leisure activities

Assessment of other groups includes neighborhood and other peer groups, school environments, sports, and church and civic activities.

Diagnosis

Through induction, the nurse makes a diagnosis for each individual and each system component, including family and the community. The following are examples of diagnoses.

Individual
- Loss of interest or involvement in an activity related to conflicting stages of grief process secondary to premature death of father (Richard)
- Expressed dissatisfaction with parenting role related to feelings of helplessness and sadness secondary to premature death of husband (Mrs. Connors)
- Risk of interpersonal conflict resulting from prolonged, unrelieved family stress secondary to premature death of father (Yvonne)

Family
- Decreased ability to communicate related to family stress secondary to premature death of father
- Risk of family crisis related to disequilibrium

Community
- Inadequate systematic programs for linking families in crisis to community resources
- Inadequate systematic programs for populations at risk of premature death related to inadequate planning among community systems

Planning

Planning involves contracting and mutual goal setting and is an outcome of mutually derived assessment and diagnosis. A contract with the family alone is shortsighted and may provide little community benefit over time. The following are examples of other aggregates with which a contract may be established:
- The school subsystem that does not provide ongoing counseling but will meet periodically with family members to evaluate pupil progression
- The school subsystem that provides physical education in football, basketball, and baseball (i.e., nonaerobic, nonlifetime sports) but offers extramural aerobic, lifetime sports such as swimming, tennis, golf, and track after school hours
- The American Red Cross, which does not offer cardiovascular pulmonary resuscitation (CPR) courses on evenings or weekends but offers to consider doing so for a defined minimum-size community

Mutual goal setting requires collaboration regarding long- and short-term goals. Again, mutually defined needs and diagnoses are important to this process. Regardless of the diagnosis, each individual in the family and the subsystem must participate in development of a care plan. The following are examples of goals.

Individual
Long-Term Goal
- Individual family members will be able to trade off role-related behavior.

Short-Term Goal
- Individual family members will express feelings related to abandonment and loss.

CASE STUDY   Application of the Nursing Process

Family

Long-Term Goal

- The family will exhibit an increased ability to handle crisis, as evidenced by ability to discuss roles and interdependencies.

Short-Term Goal

- The family will identify specific ways to recognize and use support services.

Community

Long-Term Goal

- Systematic programs, with ongoing program evaluation, will be established for populations at risk of premature death from coronary heart disease, as evidenced by local planning bodies.

Short-Term Goals

- Information is disseminated to individuals, families, groups, and planning bodies in the community about the incidence of coronary heart disease.
- Existing programs are identified that address coronary heart disease.
- Existing programs are coordinated to bridge gaps and avoid duplication of effort.

Intervention

The nurse, family, and other aggregates carry out interventions contracted during the planning phase to meet the mutually derived goals. Most important, the nurse empowers the family and community to develop the networks and linkages necessary to care for themselves.

Individual

Individual counseling regarding loss and grief may be beneficial to each family member, but options may need to be explored and referrals may need to be reevaluated for members of the rural family. Education regarding preventive measures that combat risk factors for heart disease include those aimed at individual family members and those that address areas such as diet, exercise, smoking, alcohol use, and stress management.

Family

Examples of interventions with the family include counseling, education, and referral aimed at family self-care promotion. For example, Beth's interventions with the Connors family depended on the family's ability to solve problems, investigate community resources, and create linkages between the family and resources. Periodic family conferences at school and more inclusive family therapy may enable the family to work through the death of Mr. Connors; this process results in the development of new roles and the communication necessary to maintain family equilibrium. Education regarding preventive measures to combat risk factors for heart disease may need discussion at the family and individual levels (e.g., diet, exercise, smoking, alcohol use, and stress management).

Community

The nurse must also carry out interventions with other aggregates. These may involve activities such as educating, facilitating program expansion, and tailoring programs to meet community needs. Intervention at the aggregate level calls for group and community work. The nurse carries out interventions at this level in several ways (e.g., by communicating community statistics from a community analysis, relating anecdotes from families served, or linking family experience to program needs by acting as an advocate and bringing family members to board meetings or hearings on community health issues).

Education regarding preventive measures to combat risk factors for heart disease also includes those interventions aimed at the community. A rationale for the development of lifetime aerobic sports is needed not only by Richard but also by school districts. Exploration of options with the school nurse and review of the school district health education curriculum would be beneficial. A community assessment of heart disease awareness, including determination of the availability of resources such as emergency response and CPR courses, is an aggregate intervention. Taking the outcome of the assessment in the form of statistics and the anonymous anecdotal story of the Connors family to planning bodies in the community is also intervention at the aggregate level. Creative programs other communities used (e.g., teaching CPR within the school system) should be investigated and proposed.

Evaluation

Evaluation is multidimensional and ongoing. Using a systems approach to evaluation, the nurse evaluates each component of the system, from individual family member to family and community, in terms of goal achievement. Evaluation consists of noting degrees of equilibrium established, extent of change, how the system handles change, whether the system is open or closed, and patterns of networking. Ongoing evaluation includes noting referrals and follow-up of the individual, the family, and other aggregates in resource use.

Individual

Use of resources such as support groups by the individual family member may be noted. These resources may include a teen support group, a women's support group, support groups for those experiencing the loss of a spouse or other family member, reentry programs for women at a local junior college or university, and Parents Without Partners.

Family

Evaluation of the Connors family would include follow-up of their use of support services specifically for the family, such as counseling options for the family as a unit. Evaluation would also focus on the family's ability to handle crises in the future.

Community

Aggregate evaluation would focus on the community. For example, to what extent do school programs encourage sports options that promote lifetime aerobic activities and prevent premature death from heart disease? Are programs systematically planned in the community for populations that are at risk of premature death from heart disease?

Levels of Prevention

Society's expectations of men and women are in transition. Application of levels of prevention by the community health nurse must take into account men's health status, men's socialization, men's use of healthcare services, men's primary needs for prevention and health promotion, and the role of women as caregivers in family health.

Primary

Men are more likely to engage in risk-taking behavior than women and are less likely to engage in preventive behaviors; therefore primary prevention must be marketed specifically to men. Examples of primary prevention for the Connors family are applied at the following individual, family, and community levels.

Individual

- Assessment, teaching, and referral related to diet and exercise behaviors

Family

- Assessment and teaching related to food selection and preparation at home and food selection at fast-food restaurants
- Teaching and role-modeling gender roles that allow male members of the family to use alternative expressions of emotion

Community

- Provision of CPR courses for members of the community; consultation with schools regarding need for aerobic activities in physical education and sports programs

Continued

CASE STUDY Application of the Nursing Process

- The nurse must pull men from the family, workplace, or other aggregates into involvement with family planning, education, antepartum and postpartum care, parenting, dental prophylaxis, and accident prevention. In addition, assessment of need for immunizations and classes (e.g., retirement preparation) is considered action aimed at primary prevention.

Secondary

Men have higher mortality, morbidity, and healthcare use rates for many of the leading causes of death, but they are second to women in overall use of healthcare services, including preventive physical examinations and screening; therefore early diagnosis and prompt intervention must also meet men's needs. Examples of secondary prevention regarding the Connors family include the following:

Individual

- Screen for risk factors related to CVD in the individual, such as how the individual handles stress.

Family

- Screen for risk factors related to CVD in the family, such as how the family processes stress.

Community

- Organize screening programs for the community, such as health fairs.
- The nurse must screen individuals and aggregates of men according to lifestyle risk factors, mortality rates at different age levels, morbidity rates, and occupational health risks.

Tertiary

Activities that rehabilitate individuals and aggregates and restore them to their highest level of functioning are aimed at tertiary prevention. The nurse in the community is ideally situated to locate people in need of rehabilitation services. The nurse may provide evaluation and physical, mental, and social restoration services. Men in need of rehabilitation may have special needs because their disabilities influence them, their families, and ultimately their communities. Financial assistance and vocational counseling, training, and placement may be priorities for the well-being of the family. Socialization causes men to have difficulty admitting they need help. Community health nurses who teach men with chronic disease to rest at specified periods during the day or to continue with medical regimens or speech or occupational therapy are providing tertiary prevention. Working with couples as a unit is also important because caregiving patterns may shift as a result of chronic disease and disability. Encouraging men to express their concerns about their health, families, and jobs and their frustration with themselves is important. The following are examples of tertiary prevention with the Connors family.

Individual

- Assist individual family members in dealing with grief from the loss of the father and husband.

Family

- Assist family in dealing with grief and assuming alternative roles.

Community

- Assist the community in dealing with loss of a fully functioning family by providing grief support services that include males or target males and females.

SUMMARY

As the information within this chapter shows, there is gender disparity in all areas of disease and all health entities. Health initiatives and programs are changing as more and more attention is given to the healthcare of men.

EVOLVE WEBSITE

http://evolve.elsevier.com/Nies/community
- NCLEX Review Questions
- Case Studies

BIBLIOGRAPHY

American Family Physician: *Adult preventive healthcare schedule: recommendations from the USPSTF (as of August 16, 2019)*, 2019. Available from: https://www.aafp.org/dam/AAFP/documents/journals/afp/USPSTFHealthCareSchedule2019.pdf.

Arias E, Xu J: *United States life tables*, (National Vital Statistics Reports vol. 69, no. 12) Washington, DC, 2020, National Center for Health Statistics. Available from: http://www.cdc.gov/nchs/products/nvsr.htm.

Baerolcher MO, Verma S: Men's health research: under researched and under appreciated, *Med Sci Monit* 14(3), 2008.

Ballinger M, Talbot L, Verrinder G: More than a place to do woodwork: a case study of a community-based Men's Shed, *J Mens Health* 6(1):20—27, 2009.

Brown L, Bond M: An examination of influences on health protective behaviors among Australian men, *Int J Men's Health* 3(7):274—287, 2008.

Centers for Disease Control and Prevention: *Sexually transmitted disease surveillance 2015*, Atlanta, 2012, U.S. Department of health and Human Services.

Centers for Disease Control and Prevention: *Age-adjusted death rates for selected causes of death by sex, by race and Hispanic origin, United States selected years 1950—2017*, 2018. Available from: https://www.cdc.gov/nchs/data/hus/2018/005.pdf.

Centers for Disease Control and Prevention: *Leading causes of death and numbers of deaths, by sex, race, and Hispanic origin: United States, 1980 and 2017*, 2018. Available from: https://www.cdc.gov/nchs/data/hus/2018/006.pdf.

Centers for Disease Control and Prevention: *Use of selected substances in the past month among persons aged 12 years and over, by age, sex, race, and Hispanic origin: United States, selected years 2002—2017*, 2018. Available from: https://www.cdc.gov/nchs/data/hus/2018/020.pdf.

Centers for Disease Control and Prevention: *At a glance table. Health, United States, 2018*, 2019. Available from: https://www.cdc.gov/nchs/hus/ataglance.htm.

Centers for Disease Control and Prevention: *Leading causes of death in males United States*, 2019. Available from: http://www.cdc.gov/men/lcod/.

Centers for Disease Control and Prevention: *Cigarette smoking and electronic cigarette use*, 2020. Available from: www.cdc.gov/nchs/fastats/smoking.htm.

Centers for Disease Control and Prevention: *NIOSH worker health charts*, 2020. Available from: https://wwwn.cdc.gov/NIOSH-WHC/topic.

Centers for Disease Control and Prevention: *Quick facts on the risks of e-cigarettes for kids, teens, and young adults*, 2020. Available from: https://www.cdc.gov/tobacco/basic_information/e-cigarettes/Quick-Facts-on-the-Risks-of-E-cigarettes-for-Kids-Teens-and-Young-Adults.html.

Centers for Disease Control and Prevention: *COVID-19 death data and resources*, 2021. Available from: https://www.cdc.gov/nchs/nvss/vsrr/covid_weekly/index.htm#AgeAndSex.

Cheatham C, Barksdale D, Rodgers S: Barriers to healthcare and health seeking behaviors faced by black men, *J Am Acad Nurse Pract* 20:555—562, 2008.

Dallas J, Neville S: Health education and health screening in a sample of older men: a descriptive survey, *Nurs Prax N Z* 28(1):6—16, 2012.

Frisbee S, Chambers C, Frisbee J: Associations between dental hygiene, cardiovascular disease risk factors and systemic inflammation in rural adults, *J Dent Hyg* 84(4):177—184, 2010.

Haines C, Wender R: Men's health, *Prim Care* 33(1):xiii—xv, 2006.

Harvard Men's Health Watch: *Volume* 13:8, 2009.

Hedegaard H, Miniño AM, Warner M: *Drug overdose deaths in the United States, 1999 to 2019*, 2020. Available from: https://www.cdc.gov/nchs/products/databriefs/db394.htm.

Heron M, Hoyert DL, Murphy SL, et al: *Deaths: final data for 2006.* (National Vital Statistics Reports vol. 57, no. 14) Washington, DC, 2009, National Center for Vital Statistics. https://www.ncbi.nlm.nih.gov/pubmed/19788058

Heidelbaugh J: The adult well-male examination, *Am Fam Phys* 98(12):729—737, 2018.

Kirby R, Kirby M, Aoroso P: Steps by which better overall health for men could be achieved, *BJU Int* 98(2):285—288, 2006. Available from: www.bjui.org/ContentFullItem.aspx?id=81&SectionType=5.

Lynch L: Men's health, *Ir Med J* 101(1):5—6, 2008.

Martin JA, Hamilton BE, Sutton PD, et al. *Births: final data for 2008* (National Vital Statistics Reports vol. 59 no. 1). Hyattsville, MD, 2010, National Center for Health Statistics.

Mathews TJ, MacDorman MF: *Infant mortality statistics from the 2008 period linked birth/infant death data set* (National Vital Statistics Reports vol. 60, no. 5). Hyattsville, MD, 2012, National Center for Health Statistics (5).

Meryn S: Global man and health, *J Mens Health* 6(1):2—3, 2009.

Naslindh-Ylispangar A, Sihvonen M, Kekki P: Health, utilization of health services, "core" information and reasons for non-participation: a triangulation study among non-respondents, *J Clin Nurs* 17:2972—2978, 2008.

National Center for Health Statistics: *Health, United States, 2015: with special feature on racial and ethnic health disparities*, Hyattsville, MD, 2016. Author.

Organisation for Economic Co-Operation and Development (OECD): *Health at a glance: OECD indicators*, 2019, Author.

Organisation for Economic Co-Operation and Development (OECD): *Health status: potential years of life lost*, 2020. Available from: https://stats.oecd.org//Index.aspx?ThemeTreeId=9.

Porche D: Men's health: building the science, *Am J Men's Health* 3(2):92, 2009.

Quallich SA, Lajiness M, Mitchell K: *Manual of men's health: a practice guide for APRNs and PAs*, NY, 2018, Springer.

Reid G, van Teijlingen E, Douglas F, et al.: The reality of partnership working when undertaking an evaluation of national well men's service, *J Mens Health* 1(6):36—49, 2009.

Roberts A, Gerber L: *Nursing perspective on public health programming in Nunavut*. Iqaluit, Nunavut, Canada, 2003, Department of Health and Social Services. www.gov.nu.ca/health/Report%20on%20Nursing%20Perspectives%20on%20Public%20Heatlh%20Programming%20in%20Nunavut.pdf.

Sadler C: DIY male maintenance, *Nurs Mirror* 160(16), 1979.

Schiller JS, Lucas JW, Ward BW, et al.: Summary health statistics for U.S. adults: national health interview survey, 2010, *Vital Health Stat* 10(252):1—217, 2012.

Shapiro A, Yarborough-Hayes R: Retirement and older men's health, generations, *J Am Soc Aging* 32(1):49—53, 2008.

Skelton R: Man's role in society and its effect on health, *Nursing* 26:953, 1988.

Sommers B, Wilson L: *Fifty-four million additional Americans are receiving preventive services coverage without cost-sharing under the Affordable Care Act*, 2012. Available from: http://aspe.hhs.gov/health/reports/2012/PreventiveServices/ib.shtml.

Tanne JH: Medicine's new motto: one sex does not fit all, *Am Health Women* 16(5):54—58, 1997.

Teh J, Wei J, Chiang G, Nzenza TC, Bolton D, Lawrentschuk N: Men's health on the web: an analysis of current resources, *World J Urol* 37(6):1043—1047, 2019.

Tison J, Williams A: *Analyzing the first years of the ticket or click it mobilizations (DOT HS 811 232)*, 2010. Available from: www.nhtsa.gov/staticfiles/nti/pdf/811232.pdf.

U.S. National Library of Medicine: *Health screenings for men ages 40 to 64*, 2021. Available from: https://medlineplus.gov/ency/article/007465.htm.

Verbrugge LM, Wingard DL: Sex differentials in health and mortality, *Women's Health* 12:103, 1987.

Vincent AD, Drioli-Phillips PG, Le J, et al.: Health behaviours of Australian men and the likelihood of attending a dedicated men's health service, *BMC Pub Health* 18(1):1078, 2018.

Waldron I: Changing gender roles and gender differences in health behavior. In Gochman DS, editor: *Handbook of health behavior research*, New York, 1995a, Plenum.

Waldron I: Contributions of changing gender differences in behavior and social roles to changing gender differences in mortality. In Sabo D, Gochman DS, editors: *Men's health and illness: gender, power and the body*, Thousand Oaks, CA, 1995b, Sage.

Waldron I: Contributions of biological and behavioral factors in changing sex differences in ischaemic heart disease mortality. In Lopez A, Caselli G, Valkonen T, editors: *Adult mortality in developed countries: from description to explanation*, New York, 1995c, Oxford University Press.

Waldron I: Factors determining the sex ratio at birth. In *Sex differentials in infant and child mortality*, New York, 1995d, United Nations.

Whorton MD: Environmental and occupational reproductive hazards. In Swanson J, Forrest K, editors: *Men's reproductive health*, New York, 1984, Springer.

Woodland A, Hunt C: Healthy convictions well-man clinic for the inmates of Lindholme prison, *Nurs Times* 90:32, 1994.

World Bank: *Current health expenditure*, 2018. Available from: https://data.worldbank.org/indicator/SH.XPD.CHEX.GD.ZS.

19

Senior Health

Mary Ellen Trail Ross

OBJECTIVES

Upon completion of this chapter, the reader will be able to do the following:

1. Discuss the aging process.
2. Discuss the demographic characteristics of the elderly population.
3. Describe psychosocial issues related to aging.
4. Describe physiological changes due to aging.
5. Recognize *Healthy People 2030* wellness goals and objectives for older adults.
6. Describe health/illness concerns common to the elderly population.
7. Identify nursing actions that address the needs of older adults.
8. Identify resources available to older adults.

OUTLINE

KEY TERMS

activities of daily living (ADLs)
advance directives
aging
alternative housing options
Alzheimer's disease
anxiety disorder
cataract
crime
depression
do-not-resuscitate (DNR)

durable power of attorney for health care
elder abuse
falls
generalized anxiety disorder
glaucoma
guardianship
instrumental activities of daily living (IADLs)
living will

macular degeneration
Medicaid
physician orders for life sustaining treatment (POLST)
Medicare
Social Security
suicide
traumatic brain injury (TBI)

In America, the number of individuals aged 65 years or older grew from three million in 1900 to 52 million in 2018 (Federal Interagency Forum on Aging-Related Statistics [FIFARS], 2020). Life expectancy is increasing; thus larger numbers of people are reaching 65 years and beyond. In view of the increasing number of seniors who potentially will remain living in the community, the role of the nurse becomes very important in helping these seniors continue to live independently and to increase their years of healthy life. For nurses to assist older adults, they must be familiar with the characteristics of seniors, their socioeconomic situations, their health behaviors, health status, health risks, and available community resources. This chapter discusses these issues and gives suggestions as to how nurses might address them.

CONCEPT OF AGING

Aging is a natural process that affects all living organisms. The concept of aging is most often defined chronologically. *Chronological age* refers to the number of years a person has lived. In the United States, an older adult is generally defined as one who is 65 years or older. However, it is important to remember that older adults cannot be grouped collectively as just one segment of the population. The older adult population is a heterogeneous group. Older adults are often categorized as young-old, middle-old, old-old, and oldest-old (Miller, 2019).

Functional age, on the other hand, refers to functioning and the ability to perform **activities of daily living (ADLs),** such as bathing and grooming, and **instrumental activities of daily living (IADLs),** such as cooking, shopping, and managing finances. This definition of aging is a better measure of age than chronological age. After all, most older adults are more concerned with their functional ability than their chronological age. Helping older adults remain independent and functional is a major focus of nursing care.

THEORIES OF AGING

Since early times, scientists have attempted to explain why humans age. There are many biological and psychosocial theories of aging. Biological theories answer questions such as "How do cells age?" and "What triggers the actual aging process?" (Miller, 2019). The biological theories can be subdivided into two main divisions: stochastic and nonstochastic. Stochastic theories explain aging as events that occur randomly and accumulate over time, whereas nonstochastic theories view aging as predetermined. Some of the popular biological theories are summarized in Box 19.1.

The three classic psychosocial theories of aging are behavioristic and examine how humans experience late life. The disengagement theory, proposed by Cumming and Henry (1961), asserts that aging is inevitable, with mutual withdrawal or disengagement from society and decreased interaction between the aging person and others. The activity theory posits that remaining active and involved is necessary to maintain life satisfaction (Havighurst et al., 1963). The continuity theory suggests that a person continues through life in a similar fashion as in previous years (Havighurst et al., 1968).

Concepts gleaned from the various theories are useful to nurses as they care for older adults. For example, knowledge that the immune system is affected by aging implies the need for nurses to be vigilant about preventing infections. Psychosocial theories of aging point out the uniqueness of older individuals as they age and make life adjustments. Knowledge of these theories may help nurses dispel common myths of aging.

DEMOGRAPHIC CHARACTERISTICS

Population

Americans are living longer than ever before, and it is expected that the older population will continue to grow. Currently, people who survive to age 65 years can expect to live an average of 19.5 more years. In 2018, the life expectancy of people who survive to age 85 years is 7 more years for women and 6 more years for men. Life expectancy varies by race, but the difference decreases with age. In 1900, people aged 65 years and older made up 4% of the population. In 2018, 52 million people aged 65 years and over lived in the United States, accounting for 16% of the total population. The oldest-old population (those 85 years and older) grew from just over 100,000 in 1900 to seven million in 2018 (FIFARS, 2020). Lastly, in 2020, there were 93,927 centenarians in the United States (U.S. Census Bureau, 2020). The baby boomers (individuals born between 1946 and 1964) started turning 65 years old in 2011. The older population in 2030 is projected to be more than twice as large as in 2000, growing from 35 million to 73 million and representing 21% of the total U.S. population (FIFARS, 2020).

Racial and Ethnic Composition

In addition to growing larger, the older population is becoming more diverse, as is the rest of the population in general. In 2018, 77% of the population was non-Hispanic white, 9% non-Hispanic black, 5% non-Hispanic Asian, and 8% Hispanic (of any race). The older population will grow among all racial and ethnic groups; however, the older Hispanic population is projected to grow the fastest (FIFARS, 2020).

Geographic Location

The proportion of the population aged 65 years and over varies by state. In 2019, Florida and Maine had the highest proportion of people aged 65 years and over (21% each), followed by West Virginia and Vermont (20% each). More than half (51%) of persons 65 years or older lived in nine states: California, Florida, Texas, New York, Pennsylvania,

---

BOX 19.1   Biological Theories of Aging

Stochastic Theories
Error Theory
The error theory proposes that an accumulation of errors in protein synthesis occurs over time, resulting in impairment of cellular function. Defective cells are produced, which eventually interfere with biological function (Orgel, 1963).

Somatic Mutation Theory
Similar to the error theory, somatic mutation theory also suggests that when cells are exposed to X-ray irradiation or chemicals, alteration of DNA occurs, increasing the incidence of chromosomal abnormalities and decreasing cellular and organ function. The deleterious effects appear in later life (Morley, 1995).

Free Radical Theory
Free radicals are highly reactive molecules that possess an extra electric charge (free electron) that can damage protein membranes, enzymes, and DNA. The body produces antioxidants that scavenge the free radicals (Hayflick, 1996).

Cross-Linkage Theory
The cross-linkage theory posits that aging causes body chemicals (proteins, lipids, nucleic acid, and carbohydrates) to become cross-linked. The cross-linking causes abnormal metabolic activity and waste products to accumulate in the cells. The result is poor functioning of body tissues and structures (Hayflick, 1996).

Wear-and-Tear Theory
Cells and organs wear out after years of use. Proponents of the wear-and-tear theory view the human body as similar to a machine that eventually wears out because of decline in cellular function, death of cells, and mechanical injury and use (Hayflick, 1996).

Nonstochastic Theories
Programmed Theory
The programmed theory postulates that normal cells divide a specific number of times. The number of cell divisions is proportional to the lifespan of the species. Human cells double 40–60 times before the ability to replicate is lost and cellular death occurs (Hayflick, 1996).

Immunological Theory
According to immunological theory, alteration of the B and T cells causes a loss of a self-regulatory pattern between the body and the cells. Autoaggression occurs when cells normal to the body are misidentified as alien and are attacked by the body's immune system (Miller, 1996).

Neuroendocrine Control or Pacemaker Theory
Aging is described in neuroendocrine control theory or pacemaker theory as a programmed decline in the functioning of the nervous, endocrine, and immune systems. Cells lose their ability to reproduce, a process known as *replicative senescence* (De la Fuente, 2008).

Ohio, Illinois, Michigan, and North Carolina (Administration on Aging, 2021).

Gender

Older women outnumber older men in the United States. In 2014, women accounted for 56% of the population 65 years and older and 66% of the population 85 years and older (FIFARS, 2020).

Marital Status

Older men are more likely than older women to be married. In 2018, about 73% of men aged 65 to 74 years were married, compared with 57% of women in the same age group. The proportion married was lower at older ages: 41% of women ages 75% to 84% and 16% of women 85 years and older were married. Widowhood is more common among older women than older men. Women aged 65 years and over were more likely than men of the same age to be widowed: 32% compared with 11%. Nearly 70% of women aged 85 years and over were widowed, compared with 35% of men. Relatively small proportions of older men (12%) and women (16%) were divorced in 2018, and a small proportion (almost 6%) of older men and older women have never married (FIFARS, 2020).

Education

Educational attainment has increased among older adults. In 2018, 86% of older adults were high school graduates (compared with 24% in 1965). Ninety percent of non-Hispanic whites aged 65 and over had completed high school. The percentages of older Asians and blacks who had completed high school (74% and 76%, respectively) were not statistically different. In contrast, 54% of older Hispanics have completed high school. In 2018, 29% of older adults had a bachelor's degree or higher (compared with 5% in 1965). Older Asians had the highest proportion with a bachelor's degree or higher, at 38%; compared with 31% for non-Hispanic whites, 17% for blacks, and 12% for Hispanics. Older men had attained a bachelor's degree more often than older women (33% compared with 24%) (FIFARS, 2020).

Living Arrangements

As age increases and widowhood rates rise, the percentage of the population living alone increases accordingly. In 2018, 67% of older men lived with their spouse, whereas less than half (47%) of older women did. In contrast, older women were more likely than older men to live alone (31% vs. 19%). Older Hispanic (28%), black (31%), and Asian (19%) women were more likely than non-Hispanic white women (11%) to live with relatives other than a spouse. Older non-Hispanic white and black women were more likely than women of other races to live alone (33% of white and 35% of black women lived alone compared with 16% for Asian and 22% for Hispanic women). The percentage of older black men (26%) living alone was three times as high as the percentage of older Asian men (8%). Older Hispanic and black men were more likely (13% and 14%, respectively) than non-Hispanic white men (6%) to live with relatives other than a spouse (FIFARS, 2020).

Housing and Residential Services

Older adults typically prefer to "age in place," or live in their own homes for as long as possible. In 2017, 95% of the

Medicare population aged 65 years and older resided in traditional community settings. Two percent of the Medicare population aged 65 years and over resided in community housing with at least one service available, such as meal preparation, housekeeping, laundry, and assistance with medication. Approximately 3% resided in long-term care facilities. The percentage of people residing in community housing with services and in long-term care facilities was higher for the older age groups. For example, among adults 85 years and older, 81% resided in traditional housing, whereas 8% resided in community housing with services and 12% resided in long-term care facilities (FIFARS, 2020). It is important to make services needed for independent living, such as meal preparation, medication assistance, and housekeeping, accessible to older adults who prefer this type of living arrangement.

Alternative Housing Options for Older Adults

The significant majority (95%) of adults aged 65 years and older resides in the traditional, single-family home; however, some choose to downsize to smaller housing, such as townhouses or condominiums, where maintenance needs are eliminated or minimized. The types of **alternative housing options** included retirement communities or apartments, continuing care retirement facilities, assisted-living facilities, and board and care homes. Services at these facilities include meal preparation, housekeeping, laundry, and medication administration. Approximately 3% of older adults reside in long-term care facilities that provide personal and/or skilled care 24 h a day, 7 days a week. The percentage of people residing in community housing with services and in long-term care facilities is higher for individuals 85 years and older. These older adults generally have more functional limitations (FIFARS, 2020). It is important to note that many older adults who would like to change their current living arrangements find that organized senior housing is too expensive for middle-class and lower-middle-class citizens. On the other hand, these individuals often have too many assets to qualify for subsidized housing.

Although not considered a housing option, adult day care provides a safe and supportive environment during the day for adults who cannot or choose not to stay alone. This service is often needed for caregivers who work during regular hours or need respite. Socialization, recreational activities, medication supervision, and meals are provided on-site. Often transportation to and from the facility is provided.

Income

In 2019, 39% of men and 30% of women aged 65 to 69 years remained in the labor force whereas at age 70 and older 17% of men and 10% of women did so. The median income of older adults was $27,398. Men had a higher median income overall: $36,921 compared to $21, 815 for women. Social security is an important source of income for older adults. It was designed to serve as a supplement to other sources of income. A minimum of 10 years of covered earnings is required to receive benefits (FIFARS, 2020). With aging, a good percentage of income is spent on health care. Most older adults have **Medicare**, which provides health insurance for those who are 65 years or older, are disabled, or have end-stage renal disease. Medicare is funded, in part, by Social Security contributions from employers, employees, and the self-employed. Medicare Part A is a hospital insurance plan that covers inpatient hospital, skilled nursing facility, and some home health care services. For 2021, the Part A inpatient hospital deductible is $1484 for the first 60 days of a hospital stay per benefit period. The coinsurance is $371 per day for the 61st through 90th day of a hospitalization in a benefit period and $742 per day for lifetime reserve days. Medicare Part A will pay 100% of the first 20 days in a skilled nursing facility with a $185.50 daily copay for days 21 to 100 of each benefit period and no coverage after that (U.S. Centers for Medicare and Medicaid Services [U.S. CMS], 2020b).

Medicare Part B covers the costs for physician and nurse practitioner services; outpatient hospital services, such as diagnostic procedures (e.g., laboratory and X-ray); qualified physical, speech, and occupational therapy; ambulance services; durable medical equipment; and some home health care services. For 2021, the Medicare Part B monthly premium is $148.50. There is an annual Part B deductible of $203. This amount is generally deducted directly from the monthly Social Security check. Most Medicare enrollees have a supplemental insurance policy to pay for services not covered by Medicare. A Medicare Advantage Plan (sometimes called *Part C*) is another Medicare health plan choice. This plan is offered by private companies approved by Medicare. There is usually a monthly premium for the Medicare Advantage Plan that varies according to the plan (U.S. CMS, 2020b).

The newest component of Medicare is the prescription drug coverage (Part D). The prescription drug plan is designed to help lower prescription drug costs. The individual chooses the drug plan and pays a monthly premium, and most plans have an annual deductible. Most Medicare prescription drug plans have a coverage gap (also called the *donut hole*). This refers to a temporary limit on what the drug plan will cover. In 2021, once a member and his or her plan have spent $4130 on covered drugs (the combined amount plus the deductible), the member is in the coverage gap and will pay no more than 25% of the cost for the plan's covered prescription drugs (U.S. CMS, 2020a).

For older adults with low income, **Medicaid** may be available to offset the Medicare deductibles and copays and to provide additional health benefits. Each state establishes its own eligibility criteria within the broad guidelines established by the federal government. Medicaid generally covers more services than Medicare, including custodial care in nursing homes, without deductibles or copays. A very significant portion of Medicaid funds are used to offset the cost of long-term care for poor elders.

Poverty and Health Education

To determine who is considered poor, the U.S. Census Bureau compares family income (or an unrelated individual's income) with a set of poverty thresholds that vary by family size and composition and are updated annually for inflation. Since 2000, the poverty rate among the older population (65 years and older) has remained relatively stable at around 9% or 10% compared with 30% in the 1960s. Older women (11%) were more likely than older men (8%) to live in poverty. Older people who live alone have higher rates of poverty than those who are married. Race and ethnicity are also related to poverty among the older population. In 2018, older whites were less likely than older blacks, Hispanics, and Asians to be living in poverty (FIFARS, 2020).

Community nurses will be increasingly called upon to care for older adults of diverse backgrounds who have various living arrangements. Although educational attainment has increased among the elderly population, many older adults have less than a high school education; therefore nurses must be sensitive and creative when providing instruction and teaching. Nurses cannot assume that an older adult has had a formal education. In addition, instructions may need to be given at a slower pace. It may also be imperative to include family or significant others when providing instruction. Also, written information may be sent home for further reference.

On the other hand, increased educational levels of current and future elders also provide a challenge for the community health nurse. These elders are, and will be, more informed and will make greater demands for current and scientifically based information, thus requiring the nurse to be knowledgeable about the latest developments in health care.

Nurses Improving Care for Healthsystem Elders (NICHE) is a program developed by the Hartford Geriatric Institute in 1992 that assists hospitals and health care organizations improve the way in which care is provided to older adults. NICHE provides resources for nurses and other providers who care for older adults. The Geriatric Resource Nurse (GRN) model stems from this program. The GRN model guides nurses in addressing common concerns and complications related to aging using evidence-based practices (www.nicheprogram.org).

The Age-Friendly Health Systems is an initiative of The John A. Hartford Foundation and the Institute for Healthcare Improvement in partnership with the American Hospital Association (AHA) and the Catholic Health Association of the United States. The goal is to have the care of older adults guided by an essential set of evidence-based practices, the 4Ms. The 4Ms include "what matters most, mobility, medication, mentation, and multi-complexity." It is important for health care providers to address the 4Ms with healthy and frail older adults across the continuum of care (AHA Center for Health Innovation, 2021). Geriatrics experts later identified "multi-complexity," the need to manage multiple health conditions at once, as another critical part of person-centered

care for older individuals. Together, these components are referred to as the "Geriatrics 5Ms" (American Geriatrics Society [AGS] Health in Aging Foundation, 2021).

 ACTIVE LEARNING

Your 80-year-old client has become very frail and needs assistance with several ADLs. No family members are able or willing to take care of him full-time. The family has asked you for advice. What information would you share with them about alternative housing options?

PSYCHOSOCIAL ISSUES

In addition to adjusting to physiological changes related to aging and health concerns (discussed later in this chapter), older adults must cope with psychosocial and role changes such as retirement, relocation, widowhood, loss of family and friends, and possibly raising their grandchildren. Retirement may be a happy occasion when voluntary; however, the opposite may be true if it is involuntary. When older adults retire, they inevitably must cope with a change in social status and possibly income level; this may be especially difficult for people whose self-concept is related to job status. For retirees who are married, the spouse must also adjust to the changes related to retirement. Indeed, the adjustment may be more difficult for the spouse than the retiree as the retiree's leisure time will be increased. For elders who have no hobbies or interests, this extra leisure time may be a source of boredom. Nurses should encourage older retirees to pursue old hobbies and interests or establish new ones.

Relocation is another psychosocial issue that many older adults must manage. Often, relocation occurs as a result of health and functional impairment, lack of ability to maintain one's home, unsafe neighborhoods, and lack of assistance with ADLs or IADLs. The relocation may be prompted by the older adult's desire to be closer to family or medical care, or interest in moving to a new location or more supportive housing (as discussed in the section "Alternative Housing Options for Older Adults").

Widowhood is an event experienced by most older adults, especially elderly women. According to Miller (2019), common consequences of widowhood are loss of companionship and intimacy; loss of one's sexual partner; feelings of grief, loneliness, and emptiness; increased responsibilities and dependency on others; loss of income and less efficient financial management; and changes in relationships with children, married friends, and other family members. Widowhood may be especially traumatic for elders who have been married for many decades. In addition to the loss of a spouse, older adults must cope with loss of family members (sometimes their own children) and friends.

On the other hand, many older adults are faced with the responsibility of raising their grandchildren (Fig. 19.1). Substantial increases have occurred in the number of children under age 18 years living in households maintained by their

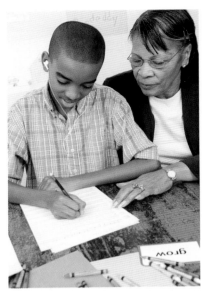

Fig. 19.1 A custodial grandmother doing homework with her grandson. (© 2013 Photos.com, a division of Getty Images. All rights reserved. Image # 86535689.)

grandparents, often without the presence of the grandchildren's parents (Clinical Example 19.1). Antecedents to children being raised by grandparents include neglect related to parental substance abuse, abandonment, emotional and physical abuse, parental death, mental and physical illness, incarceration, teen pregnancy, and grandparents assisting adult children who work or attend school. Although there may be rewards to raising grandchildren, such as satisfaction for keeping the family together, sense of purpose in life, and the opportunity to have a close relationship with one's grandchildren, this arrangement may contribute to both physical and psychological problems, such as stress, depression, and poorer health (Taylor et al., 2017; Trail Ross et al., 2015).

Clinical Example 19.1

Ms. Thomas, age 62, is divorced and has been raising her three grandchildren, aged 11 to 13, for the past 10 years. She was forced to retire from full-time teaching to assume this role. Her daughter, the children's mother, is bipolar and schizophrenic, and has tested positive for HIV. All of the grandchildren have medical problems and/or special needs, including asthma, attention-deficit hyperactivity disorder, and emotional/behavioral concerns. Ms. Thomas is very organized and keeps track of their many medications via a written schedule containing the name of each medication, dose, and time of administration. Ms. Thomas expressed increased stress, tension, and anxiety as a result of caregiving responsibilities and neglect of her own needs. She has hypertension, a "thyroid condition," asthma, gastroesophageal reflux disease, and allergies. She admits to occasionally forgetting to take her own medications because of her busy schedule. She rates her health as "fair" overall and "somewhat worse" in comparison with that of other people her age.

Continued

She reports significantly less time for herself and leisure activities. Nonetheless, Ms. Thomas is determined to raise her grandchildren as well as possible. Despite her circumstances, she is very positive and optimistic that her grandchildren will grow up to be successful and respectable citizens.

Intimacy and Sexuality

Intimacy includes the need for close friendships and relationships, as well as feeling important to and wanted by another person. Expressing love and care, as well as exchanging intimate words and touch with another person, increases intimacy and expresses sexuality. Sexual expression tends to be consistent throughout life (Eliopoulos, 2022). Normal physiological changes of aging discussed in Table 19.1 may decrease older adults' frequency of sexual activity. For example, estrogen level in women decreases after menopause, which may lead to vaginal dryness and thinning and may make sexual intercourse uncomfortable. Effective treatments for vaginal dryness may range from over-the-counter moisturizers and lubricants to estrogen creams, tablets, and rings that are inserted vaginally. In men, testosterone levels decrease causing erections to be less firm and not last as long. Erectile dysfunction (ED) is the most common cause of sexual difficulty in men and increases with age. It is often due to underlying medical or emotional problems such as heart disease or diabetes, medication side effects, or anxiety. Some men who are impotent or have ED have taken advantage of the availability of medications like Viagra to remain sexually active. Medical conditions, medications, chronic pain, and surgical procedures may also affect sexual performance and have a negative impact on sexual response, including a decrease in arousal and interest (HealthinAging.org, 2021).

The main reason many older adults experience a decrease in sexual activity is loss of a spouse or partner. Sexual desires may be unfulfilled because of lack of opportunity, belief that sex is only appropriate in marriage, fear of repercussion from children and society, or attitudes from early teachings about appropriate sexual behavior (Eliopoulos, 2022). On the other hand, with more "open attitudes toward sexuality, internet dating, and the availability of medications like Viagra and estrogen products, some older adults are remaining sexually active" (HealthinAging.org, 2021). It is important to note that older adults are particularly vulnerable to sexually transmitted diseases (STDs). Sexually active older adults who have sex with new or multiple partners may not consider using a condom, because pregnancy is no longer a risk. It is very important for older adults to practice safe sex. Methods might include knowing a partner's sexual background and sharing sexual histories, as well as getting tested—along with their partner—for HIV/AIDS and other STDs before having sex. Using a condom and water-based lubricant until test results are revealed is also advisable to decrease the risk of STDs (HealthinAging.org, 2021). If they do become symptomatic, older adults may be embarrassed to seek medical attention or may attribute the symptoms to normal aging (Clinical Example 19.2).

TABLE 19.1   Normal Physiological Changes Associated With Aging

Physiological Changes	Nursing Intervention(s) and Patient Instructions
Sensory Changes	
Vision	
Decreased visual acuity	Encourage use of corrective lenses as prescribed
Decreased visual accommodation	Use large print for teaching
Yellowing of lens	Encourage adequate lighting and night lights
	Avoid using shades of green, blue, and violet together
Hearing	
Decreased ability to hear (presbycusis)	Decrease extraneous sounds
Decreased ability to hear consonants with high-frequency sounds	Use concise sentences and speak slowly and distinctly in a low-pitched voice
	Encourage hearing examination and use of hearing aids, if needed
Taste	
Diminished taste sensation	Encourage well-balanced meals
Decreased saliva production	Advise to drink plenty of fluids
Decreased sensitivity to sweetness and saltiness	Observe for overconsumption of sweets and salt
	Give options for seasoning other than salt
Smell	
Decreased smell acuity	Advise to use other senses and other people to assist with monitoring the environment for safety (e.g., spoiled food and gas fumes)
Touch	
Decreased sensitivity to touch	Monitor for extreme temperature changes in the environment (e.g., water temperature); maintain adequate room temperature
Reduced capacity to sense pressure and pain	Ensure position changes frequently; monitor for pain
Nervous System	
Reduction in neurons and cerebral blood flow	Assess neurological status
	Ensure frequent position changes
Slower autonomic and voluntary reflexes	Assess for pain and unique responses to pain
Reduced capacity to sense pain and pressure	
Increase in amount of senile plaque and neurofibrillary tangles	
Cognitive Changes and Changes in Balance	
Slower response and reaction time	Allow adequate time for response, information processing, and performance of tasks
Slower learning time	Break instructions into small units
Memory: Long-term memory better than short-term memory	Use shorter teaching sessions; use cues and gestures
Personality consistent with earlier years	Relate education to prior experience
Sleep	
Decrease in stages 3 and 4 sleep patterns	Assess quantity and quality of sleep
Increase in arousals during the night	Allow naps as needed
Slight reduction in total sleep time	Educate about effects of stimulants and caffeine
	Decrease interventions at night and avoid sleep medication use if possible
Cardiovascular System	
Decrease in tone and elasticity of aorta and great vessels	Pace activities and allow rest periods
Thicker and stiffer heart valves	Monitor for activity intolerance
Slowing down of heart's conduction system	Encourage use of ambulation aids when appropriate
Slower recovery of myocardial contractility and irritability	Encourage regular exercise program
Decreased cardiac reserve and output	Prevent or eliminate stressors
Decreased ability to increase heart rate when stress occurs	Monitor heart rate and blood pressure
Increased systolic blood pressure	
Respiratory System	
Reduced size of lungs, lung expansion, activity, and recoil	Encourage influenza and pneumococcal vaccinations
Increased rigidity of lungs and thoracic cage	Encourage regular exercise
Decreased cough response	Encourage adequate fluid intake
Decreased number of alveoli and gas exchange	Monitor oxygen administration

Musculoskeletal System

Atrophy and decrease in muscle fibers	Prevent immobility
Decreased muscle mass and strength	Encourage regular exercise program
Reduced bone minerals and mass, causing porous and brittle bones	Teach safety precautions to prevent falls
Shortening of vertebra	Encourage adequate calcium and vitamin D intake

Gastrointestinal System

Brittle teeth	Encourage dental health (i.e., brushing, flossing)
Decreased esophageal/colonic peristalsis	Encourage diet that is well balanced and has adequate protein and vitamins
Decreased stomach motility	Encourage adequate fluids and fiber intake
Decreased production of saliva, HCl, and digestive enzymes	Monitor diet for deficiencies
Decreased absorption of fat and vitamins B_1 and B_{12}	
Decrease in thirst response	

Renal System

Decreased size of kidneys	Monitor drugs—smaller doses may be needed
Decreased number of nephrons	Observe for adverse responses to drugs
Reduced renal blood flow and tubular function	Monitor electrolytes and laboratory values
Decreased glomerular filtration rate	Prevent dehydration

Genitourinary System

Weakening of bladder muscle, causing increased urinary frequency, urgency, and nocturia	Assess bladder function and assist with frequent toileting
Decreased bladder capacity	Encourage bladder training program, exercises, and medication when needed
Increased retention	Observe for signs of urinary tract infection
Increased nocturia	Ensure safety to bathroom at night

Reproductive System

Women

Atrophy of vulva and flattening of labia	Differentiate between changes due to normal aging and those due to disease or medications
Vaginal dryness and thinning	
Atrophy of cervix, ovaries, and uterus	Advise about use of lubricants for comfort during intercourse
Decreased amount and elasticity of breast tissue	Recommend breast examinations and mammograms

Men

Atrophy of testes and decreased elasticity of scrotal skin	Differentiate between changes due to normal aging and those due to disease or medications
Prostatic enlargement	
Erection takes longer to achieve and is not as firm	Recommend prostate examination

Endocrine System

Increased fibrosis and nodularity of thyroid gland	Recommend pneumococcal, influenza, and tetanus vaccinations
Shrinkage of pituitary gland	Monitor laboratory values and glucose
Decrease in adrenal gland secretion of glucocorticoid	Prevent infection
Decreased levels of aldosterone	Encourage good nutrition
Delayed insulin release	Observe for hypoglycemia or hyperglycemia
Reduced ability to metabolize glucose	
Decrease in testosterone, estrogen, and progesterone	

Immune System

Shrinkage of thymus gland	Prevent infections and exposure to infectious diseases
Decreased production of thymic hormones	Encourage good hand washing
Decreased production of antibodies	Monitor laboratory values
Response to antigens diminishes	

Integumentary System

Decreased skin elasticity	Encourage frequent position changes and inspect skin
Generalized thinning and dryness	Be careful of skin tears, bruising, and pressure ulcers
Atrophy of sweat glands and diminished sweating	Assess body and environmental temperatures to prevent hypothermia and hyperthermia
Altered thermoregulation	Ensure adequate clothing and comfortable room temperature
Variation in pigmentation (age spots)	

Adapted from Eliopoulos C: *Gerontological nursing*, ed 10, Philadelphia, 2022, Wolters Kluwer.

Clinical Example 19.2

It is very important that nurses educate their older adult clients/patients about normal physiological changes, safe sex practices, and STDs. An open approach to discussing sexuality will be very helpful to elders who are embarrassed about bringing these topics up.

"It is estimated that there are over three million lesbian, gay, bisexual, or transgender (LGBT) adults aged 55 and older in the United States, 1.5 million of whom are 65 and older" (Diverse Elders Coalition, 2021). LGBTQ individuals face societal discrimination and many age without proper community support, experience poor health, and financial insecurity. These individuals are more likely to be single, particularly because legal marriages are fairly new, and are less likely to have children compared with heterosexual older adults. Thus they may have less support and fewer caregivers if assistance is needed. Gay and bisexual men have a higher risk of HIV and STDs (Diverse Elders Coalition, 2021). Nurses must recognize and address the health needs of these individuals by providing education and referral to appropriate community resources. In addition, the nurse should provide information about various community resources and make referrals to agencies that might be helpful.

Physiological Changes

Normal physiological changes occur in all body systems in response to aging. However, it is important to note that the rate and degree of these changes are highly individualized. These changes are influenced by genetic factors, diet, exercise, the environment, health status, stress, lifestyle choices, and many other elements. Table 19.1 depicts common physiological changes that occur with aging.

WELLNESS AND HEALTH PROMOTION

Wellness is different from "good health." Wellness exists at one end of a continuum with illness at the other end. Health promotion programs focus on helping individuals maintain their wellness, prevent illness, and manage any chronic illnesses that they may have. Preventive health services are valuable in improving the health status of individuals to their maximum wellness potential.

♥ HEALTHY PEOPLE 2030

- The USDHHS's program *Healthy People 2030* establishes national objectives for health promotion and disease prevention. In one of the defined areas, it "focuses on reducing health problems and improving quality of life for older adults.

  This is critical as while people are living longer, many older adults have two or more chronic illnesses that interfere with their quality of life. *Healthy People 2030* has incorporated specific objectives related to older adults that are designed to promote healthy outcomes for this population.

From U.S. Department of Health and Human Services: *Healthy People 2020 summary of objectives: Older adults*, n.d. Available from: https://health.gov/healthypeople/objectives-and-data/browse-objectives/older-adults http://healthypeople.gov/2020/topics-objectives/topic/older-adults/objectives/Healthy-People/2030.

EXAMPLES OF OBJECTIVES FOR OLDER ADULTS

OA—02: Reduce the proportion of older adults who use inappropriate medications

OA—04: Reduce the rate of pressure ulcer-related hospital admissions among older adults

OA—05: Reduce the rate of hospital admissions for diabetes among older adults

OA—06: Reduce the rate of hospital admissions for pneumonia among older adults

OA—07: Reduce the rate of hospital admissions for urinary tract infections among older adults

DIA- 01- Increase the proportion of older adults with dementia, or their caregivers, who know they have it

IVP-08 - Reduce fall-related deaths among older adults

O- 02 - Reduce hip fractures among older adults

Recommended Healthcare Screenings and Examinations

Many organizations, such as the American Cancer Society, the American Heart Association, the U.S. Preventive Services Task Force, and the Agency for Healthcare Research & Quality, have established guidelines for health promotion screenings and examinations. Box 19.2 depicts some of the more widely agreed-on screenings and examinations for older adults. These recommendations are very useful to community nurses educating older adults about the benefits of screening and early detection of disease. Frequently, earlier detection of disease allows better treatment, lower health care costs, and the possibility of cure.

Physical Activity and Fitness

Physical activity is beneficial for the health of people of all ages (Fig. 19.2). Older adults should do at least 30 min of moderate intensity aerobic activity (gardening, bicycling, dancing, raking leaves, water aerobics) at least 5 days each week (150 min/week) or at least 75 min a week of high intensity aerobic activity (speed walking, jogging, jumping rope, playing tennis, zumba). Adults should also do muscle-strengthening (yoga, lifting weights, working with resistance band, squats, wall push-ups) at least 2 days a week for 20 to 30 min and balance training (marching in place, dancing, leg raises, yoga, tai chi) at least 3 times a week (HealthinAging.org, 2020). Regular exercise improves functional status, reduces blood pressure and serum cholesterol level, decreases insulin resistance, prevents obesity, strengthens bones, and reduces falls. Barriers to exercising include lack of access to safe areas to exercise, pain, fatigue, and impairment in sensory function and mobility.

Objective OA-6 of *Healthy People 2020* reads "increase the proportion of older adults with reduced physical or cognitive function who engage in light, moderate, or vigorous leisure-time physical activities" (https://www.healthypeople.gov/2020/topics-objectives/topic/older-adults/objectives). Nurses may help older adults accomplish this goal by assessing their understanding of the beneficial effects of exercise and identifying barriers that prevent exercise. Nurses should also educate,

BOX 19.2 Recommended Screenings and Examinations for Health Promotion and Disease Prevention in Older Adults

Examinations and Tests

For All Older Adults

Complete physical: Annually

Blood pressure: Annually; more frequently if hypertensive or at risk

Blood glucose: Annually; more frequently if diabetic or at risk

Serum cholesterol: Every 5 years; more frequently if at high risk

Fecal occult blood test: Annually

Sigmoidoscopy: Every 5 years
 OR
Colonoscopy: Every 10 years; more frequently if at high risk

Visual acuity and glaucoma screening: Annually

Dental examination: Annually for those with teeth with cleaning every 6 months; cleaning every 2 years for denture wearers

Hearing test: Every 2–5 years

For Women

Breast self-examination: Monthly

Clinical breast examination: Annually

Mammogram: Every 1–2 years if aged 40 years or older; check with health care provider after age 75, or screening decision may be an individual one.

Pelvic examination and Papanicolaou smear: Annually; may check with health care provider about discontinuation at 66+ years or after three consecutive negative Pap test results or >2 consecutive negative human papilloma virus (HPV) and Pap tests, no abnormal results in previous 10 years and not otherwise at risk, or have had a total hysterectomy

Digital rectal examination: Annually with pelvic examination

Bone density: Once after menopause and more frequently if at risk

For Men

Digital rectal examination and prostate examination: Annually

Prostate-specific antigen (PSA) blood test: Annually, may not be recommended in men 70 years and older, check with health care provider.

Immunizations for All Older Adults

Tetanus, diphtheria, pertussis: Every 10 years

Influenza/flu vaccine: Annually

Pneumonia vaccine: Once after age 65 years; ask physician about booster every 5 years

Hepatitis A and B: For those at risk, two to three doses depending on vaccine

Hepatitis C: Once

Herpes zoster (shingles): Two doses 2–6 months apart

Varicella: If evidence of lack of immunity, never had chickenpox or received the vaccine, and at significant risk for exposure

Data from Centers for Disease Control and Prevention (CDC). *Immunization schedules*, 2021. https://www.cdc.gov/vaccines/schedules/hcp/imz/adult.html; *Adult preventive health guidelines*, 2021 https://www.healthnet.com/content/dam/centene/healthnet/pdfs/general/ca/policies/2021AdultPreventiveHealthGuidelines.pdf; and American Cancer Society: Cancer facts: prevention and screening, 2021. https://www.cancer.org/healthy/cancer-facts/cancer-facts-for-women.html and https://www.cancer.org/healthy/cancer-facts/cancer-facts-for-men.html.

encourage, and assist older adults with exercise. When applicable, antiinflammatory medications may be administered before physical activity to address accompanying pain.

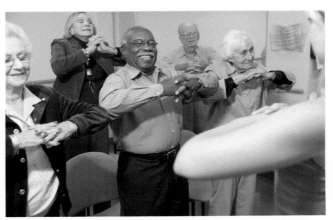

Fig. 19.2 Older adults participate in an exercise class. (© 2013 Photos.com, a division of Getty Images. All rights reserved. Image # 12555 7433.)

Nutrition

The U.S. Department of Agriculture (USDA) and U.S. Department of Health and Human Services (USDHHS) provide authoritative advice on what constitutes a healthy diet. The USDA recommends using *MyPlate* as a means to consuming a healthy diet (MyPlate.gov). The plate picture helps an individual make smart choices from every food group, find balance between food and physical activity, get the most nutrition out of calories, and stay within caloric needs. Food groups emphasized are fruits, vegetables, grains, protein foods, and dairy.

In *Healthy People 2030*, nutrition was identified as a priority area for health promotion for people of all ages. Similar to patterns among other age groups, poor nutrition in the elderly population is common. Older adults require the same or higher levels of nutrients for optimal health outcomes, but poor diet quality is associated with cardiovascular disease, hypertension, type 2 diabetes, osteoporosis, and some types of cancer, as well as conditions related to changes in bone and muscle mass, such as osteoporosis and sarcopenia. Special nutrition considerations for older adults are underconsumption of dietary protein, vitamin B_{12}, and adequate fluids for proper hydration, as well as inadequate calcium, vitamin D, potassium, and dietary fiber (USDA and USDHHS, 2020).

An inappropriate diet may be related to constipation, dental disease, physical inactivity, and depression. Normal physiological changes such as a diminished sense of smell may reduce the enjoyment of eating. Gastrointestinal changes can interfere with absorption of vitamin B_{12} and folic acid, leading to anemia. A diminished thirst sensation may lead to dehydration. Other factors that can affect the nutritional status of the elderly are income, functional status, taking multiple medications, social isolation, lack of transportation, and dependence on others for grocery shopping and cooking. The nutrition checklist presented in Table 19.2 lists warning signs of and risk factors for poor nutritional health described by the mnemonic DETERMINE. The nurse should use this tool to identify the elderly who need help with their dietary intake. The benefits of good nutrition are an important factor in helping maintain independence and quality of life.

TABLE 19.2 Nutrition Checklist for Older Adults: Warning Signs of Poor Nutritional Health

Possible Problem	Question to Answer	Score for "Yes" Answer (Circle if "Yes")
Disease	Do you have an illness or condition that makes you change the kind and/or amount of food you eat?	2
Eating poorly	Do you eat fewer than two meals per day?	3
	Do you eat few fruits, vegetables, or milk products?	2
	Do you have three or more drinks of beer, liquor, or wine almost every day?	2
Tooth loss/ mouth pain	Do you have tooth or mouth problems that make it hard for you to eat?	2
Economic hardship	Do you sometimes have trouble affording the food you need?	4
Reduced social contact	Do you eat alone most of the time?	1
Multiple medications	Do you take three or more prescribed or over-the-counter drugs a day?	1
Involuntary weight loss/ gain	Have you lost or gained 10 pounds in the last 6 months without trying?	2
Needs assistance in self-care	Are you sometimes physically not able to shop, cook, or feed yourself?	1
Elder years >80 years	Are you over 80 years old?	1
	Total:	_____

Scoring:

0–2: Good! recheck your nutritional score in 6 months.

3–5: You are at moderate nutritional risk. See what can be done to improve your eating habits and lifestyle. Your office on aging, senior nutrition program, senior citizens center, or health department can help. Recheck your nutritional score in 3 months.

6 or more: You are at high nutritional risk. Bring this checklist the next time you see your doctor, dietitian, or other qualified health or social service professional. Talk with them about any problems you may have. Ask for help to improve your nutritional health.

http://www.dhs.gov.vi/home/documents/DetermineNutritionChecklist.pdf.

❓ ACTIVE LEARNING

1. Interview an elderly person you know to assess his or her physical activity level and nutritional status using the nutrition checklist and food pyramid. Review the results with the person and help him or her plan a nutritious menu for 1 day. What factors hindered or enhanced your interaction with the person?

2. Find the names, addresses, and phone numbers of local resources for someone interested in, for example, exercise programs for the elderly and smoking cessation programs.

COMMON HEALTH CONCERNS

Chronic Illness

About 80% of older adults have at least one chronic disease, and 68% have at least two chronic conditions, such as diabetes, arthritis, hypertension, and lung disease, that seriously compromise the quality of life of older adults (National Council on Aging, 2021a). The prevalence of chronic diseases rises with age, and chronic illnesses are a major cause of disability and may cause limitations with ADLs and IADLs. The most common conditions are arthritis, hypertension, and diabetes. Chronic diseases are the leading causes of death among persons 65 years and older (Table 19.3).

Medication Use by Elders

The high prevalence of chronic diseases in the elderly population causes this group to use a large number of medications. More than half (54%) of adults 65 and older report taking four or more prescription medications (Kaiser Family Foundation, 2019). Older adults also consume many over-the-counter medications as well as "folk" or herbal remedies. The elderly population is vulnerable to the effects of drugs because of normal aging changes (see Table 19.1) and age-related differences in pharmacokinetics and pharmacodynamics. Polypharmacy may also make older adults vulnerable to drug interactions and dangerous adverse reactions.

🔷 RESEARCH HIGHLIGHTS

Beers Criteria for Adverse Drug Events

Shehab et al. (2016) found that 34.5% of emergency department (ED) visits for adverse drug events occurred among older adults 65 or older. According to the Beers Criteria, medications that should always be avoided in older adults were associated with 1.8% of the ED visits, whereas medications that are potentially inappropriate in older adults were responsible for 3.4% of the ED visits for adverse drug events. Anticoagulants, diabetes agents, and opioids were the cause of 59.9% of older adult visits to the ED for adverse drug events. More efforts are needed among physicians and other health professionals to improve safety and prevent adverse drug events.

The "Beers Criteria" catalogs medications that cause adverse drug events in older adults because of the drugs' pharmacological properties and the physiological changes of aging. An updated version of the Beers Criteria for potentially inappropriate medications in older adults has been published by the American Geriatrics Society (AGS, 2019). A printable copy of the Beers Criteria pocket card is available at http://files.hgsitebuilder.com/hostgator257222/file/ags_2019_beers_pocket_printable_rh.pdf.

Nurses should closely monitor medication use in the home to ensure safety. An easy-to-use pill organizer may be helpful for older adults. In addition, such clients should be educated about potential adverse reactions as well as drug–drug and drug–food interactions. Pharmacists can be very helpful in answering questions about prescriptions and over-the-counter medications.

TABLE 19.3 Leading Causes of Death for Persons 65 Years of Age and Older by Race/Ethnicity

		White	Black	American Indian or Alaska Native	Asian or Pacific Islander	Hispanic
1.	65–84 years	Cancer	Cancer	Heart disease	Cancer	Cancer
	85+ years	Heart disease	Heart disease	Heart disease	Heart disease	Heart disease
2.	65–84 years	Heart disease	Heart disease	Cancer	Heart disease	Heart disease
	85+ years	Cancer	Cancer	Cancer	Cancer	Cancer
3.	65–84 years	Chronic lower respiratory diseases	Stroke	Diabetes	Stroke	Diabetes
	85+ years	Alzheimer's disease	Stroke	Chronic lower respiratory diseases	Stroke	Alzheimer's disease
4.	65–84 years	Stroke	Diabetes	Chronic lower respiratory diseases	Diabetes	Stroke
	85+ years	Stroke	Alzheimer's disease	Stroke	Alzheimer's disease	Stroke
5.	65–84 years	Diabetes	Chronic lower respiratory diseases	Stroke	Chronic lower respiratory diseases	Chronic lower respiratory diseases
	85+ years	Chronic lower respiratory diseases	Chronic lower respiratory diseases	Alzheimer's disease	Influenza and pneumonia	Chronic lower respiratory dis

From Centers for Disease Control and Prevention, 2017. https://www.cdc.gov/healthequity/lcod/men/2017/hispanic/index.htm.

ADDITIONAL HEALTH CONCERNS

Sensory Impairment

Sensory disabilities increase with age and may seriously affect an older person's quality of life and ability to carry out routine daily activities. In 2018, 3% of people aged 65 and older reported a "vision" disability, defined as "cannot do/unable to do" when asked about difficulty with seeing, even if wearing glasses (FIFARS, 2020). Vision loss will likely increase with the country's aging population. The four leading eye diseases affecting older individuals are age-related cataracts, macular degeneration, diabetic retinopathy, and glaucoma.

Cataracts

Cataracts are the leading cause, as well as the most reversible cause, of visual impairment in older adults. A **cataract** is a clouding of the normally clear lens of the eye. Risk factors that increase a person's chances of cataracts include increasing age, diabetes, excessive exposure to sunlight, smoking, obesity, hypertension, previous eye injury, inflammation, surgery, prolonged use of corticosteroids, and drinking excessive amounts of alcohol. Older adults should have annual eye examinations, which allow early detection of cataracts. The only effective treatment for a cataract is surgical removal of the clouded lens and replacement with a clear lens implant. Interventions that may be able to reduce risks are cessation of smoking, wearing of sunglasses, maintaining a healthy weight, choosing a healthy diet, and taking care of other coexisting health problems (Mayo Clinic Staff, 2021a).

Macular Degeneration

There are two types of **macular degeneration:** dry and wet. Dry macular degeneration is more common and less severe. It causes blurred or reduced central vision due to thinning of the macula. It may affect one or both eyes (Mayo Clinic Staff, 2021b). With wet macular degeneration, caused by abnormal blood vessels that leak fluid or blood into the macula, symptoms appear suddenly and progress rapidly, and objects appear smaller or farther away than they really are (Mayo Clinic Staff, 2021d). Any changes in central vision and the ability to see colors and fine details indicate that the individual should be seen by an eye doctor. Treatment differs for the two conditions. Wet macular degeneration cannot be cured, but if treated early, it may slow down its progression. Dry macular degeneration usually progresses slowly, and many people with it can live relatively normal, productive lives. Nurses can recommend the following ways to cope with changing vision: use magnifiers, use alternative options for books, use brighter lights, join a support group, and make arrangements for traveling.

Glaucoma

Glaucoma is one of the leading causes of blindness in America. The condition causes damage to the optic nerve, often caused by an abnormally high pressure in the eye. The most common form of glaucoma, primary or chronic open-angle glaucoma, develops gradually without warning and progresses with few or no symptoms until the condition reaches an advanced stage. The drainage angle formed by the cornea and the iris remains open; however, the aqueous humor drains too slowly. This leads to fluid backup and a gradual buildup of pressure within the eye. Increased eye pressure continues to damage the optic nerve, and more and more peripheral vision is lost. Glaucoma cannot be cured, and its damage cannot be reversed, but treatment and regular eye examinations can prevent vision loss if the disease is found early, or can slow the disease or prevent further vision loss. Treatment consists of prescribed eyedrops or, if medications are ineffective, surgery (Mayo Clinic Staff, 2021c).

Nurses should educate clients about recommended vision screening. To determine the influence of visual impairment, the nurse should inquire about activity limitations associated with poor vision. Determining whether the client is using visual assistive devices such as glasses, contact lenses, magnifying lenses, or large-print books can be beneficial in recognizing the degree of adaptation. The nurse should know about resources that help older adults with eye care and assistive devices. Organizations that provide information include the National Eye Institute, the American Foundation for the Blind, and Lighthouse International.

ACTIVE LEARNING

Devise a nursing care plan for an elder with a visual disturbance (e.g., cataracts, glaucoma, or macular degeneration).

Hearing Loss

Hearing loss is one of the most common conditions affecting older adults. One in three adults 65 to 74 years of age and nearly half of adults 75 years old or older have difficulty hearing (National Institute on Deafness and Other Communication Disorders [NIDCD], 2018). There are three basic types of hearing loss: sensorineural hearing loss occurs when there is damage to the inner ear or the auditory nerve. This type of hearing loss is usually permanent. Presbycusis is the most common type of sensorineural hearing loss and is caused by gradual changes in the middle ear due to aging, loud noises, heredity, head injury, infection, illness, certain prescription drugs, and circulation problems. Conductive hearing loss occurs when sound waves cannot reach the inner ear. The cause may be ear wax buildup, fluid, or a punctured eardrum. Medical treatment or surgery can usually restore conductive hearing loss. A combination of both is known as mixed hearing loss. An example would be if one has hearing loss due to working around loud noises and has fluid in the middle ear simultaneously. The two together might make hearing worse (American Speech-Language-Hearing Association [ASHA], n.d.).

Nurses should assess older adults for hearing impairment. The nurse should ask the individual whether he or she is having trouble hearing over the telephone, finds it hard to follow conversation when two or more people are talking, often asks people to repeat what they are saying, needs to turn up the volume of the radio or TV, or thinks that others are mumbling. If an individual is experiencing hearing problems, a qualified health professional such as an otolaryngologist or ear, nose, and throat specialist or an audiologist should be consulted. Box 19.3 contains tips for healthcare providers who work with older adults who have hearing difficulties.

Dental Concerns

Age brings a host of dental problems that are often neglected because of inadequate dental care, limited mobility and transportation, poor nutrition, the myth that it is natural for older adults to become edentulous, and lack of finances and reimbursement. With proper care it is possible to retain one's natural teeth if one adheres to good dental hygiene and has regular dental

BOX 19.3   Working With the Older Adult Who Has Hearing Difficulties

- Include the person with hearing loss in the conversation.
- Find a quiet place to talk to help reduce background noise, especially in restaurants and social gatherings.
- Stand in good lighting and use facial expressions or gestures to give clues.
- Face the person and talk clearly.
- Speak a little more loudly than normal, but do not shout.
- Speak at a reasonable speed; do not hide your mouth, eat, or chew gum.
- Repeat yourself if necessary, using different words.
- Try to make sure only one person talks at a time.
- Be patient. Stay positive and relaxed.
- Ask how you can help.

From National Institute on Aging: *Age page: hearing loss,* 2018. https://www.nia.nih.gov/health/hearing-loss-common-problem-older-adults

checkups. Common dental problems of the elderly are dry mouth, receding gums, tooth cavities, hypersensitivity of the teeth, and tooth discoloration. Full or partial dentures may be needed to replace missing or badly damaged teeth. Regular dental visits for cleaning and dental evaluation are essential prevention strategies. The National Institute on Aging (NIA, 2020) Age Page "Taking Care of Your Teeth and Mouth" may be very useful in educating patients on proper dental and mouth care.

Incontinence

Aging does not cause incontinence; however, this condition is present in more than half of the nursing home population, and 25% to 45% of community-based older adults experience some degree of urinary incontinence (Milson and Gyhagen, 2018). Urinary incontinence can occur for many reasons. Urinary tract infections, vaginal infection or irritation, constipation, and certain medicines can cause short-term bladder control problems. Weak bladder muscles, overactive bladder muscles, blockage from an enlarged prostate, and damage to nerves that control the bladder may cause longer-lasting incontinence. However, in most cases, urinary incontinence can be treated or controlled, if not cured.

Types of urinary incontinence are stress incontinence, urge incontinence, and overflow incontinence or functional incontinence. The choice of treatment depends on the type of bladder control problem. One of the treatments that health care providers may suggest is Kegel exercises. Other treatment options are biofeedback, timed voiding, lifestyle changes such as losing weight, decrease in caffeine intake, medications, nerve stimulation, and surgery (NIA, 2017). Loss of control of the bowels, or fecal incontinence, leads to leakage of stool from the large intestine. Medical evaluation to determine the cause should be recommended. Treatment varies, depending on the cause.

ELDER SAFETY AND SECURITY NEEDS

Each year, many elderly are injured in and around their homes. Older people are often targets for robbery, purse snatching, pickpocketing, car theft, and home repair scams. There are safety measures that the individual can take to avoid crime and to stay safe.

Falls

The risk of falling rises with age. **Falls** are the number one cause of fractures, hospital admissions for trauma, loss of independence, and injury deaths. Each year, three million older adults are treated in EDs because of falls. Over 800,000 patients a year are hospitalized because of a fall injury, most often because of a hip fracture or head injury (Centers for Disease Control and Prevention [CDC], 2016). Many of the physiological changes that normally occur with aging, as well as a variety of chronic illnesses, can affect balance and make falls more likely. Medications such as blood pressure pills, heart medicines, diuretics, and tranquilizers may increase the risk of falling. Osteoporosis, a disease that causes a gradual loss of bone tissue or bone density, makes bones more susceptible to breaking. There is a link between osteoporosis and broken bones from falls. A person who falls and sustains a fracture may become afraid of falling again and thus will limit his or her activities. Seniors living independently before a fall may be institutionalized for as long as a year after a fracture. Loss of footing and loss of traction are factors that can lead to a fall. Uneven surfaces such as sidewalks, curbs, and floor elevations; wet or slippery ground; and climbing up on household items not intended for climbing can result in loss of footing or loss of traction. In addition, drinking alcoholic beverages increases the risk of falling, because alcohol slows reflexes and response time and may cause dizziness, sleepiness, lightheadedness, and poor balance.

Steps can be taken to reduce the chance of falls. Simple exercises that strengthen leg muscles and exercises that can improve balance are recommended (Box 19.4). Seniors can also improve their environment in order to reduce their risk of falling by checking floor surfaces and curb heights; identifying weather-related problems before venturing outside; wearing supportive, low-heeled shoes; making sure that rooms are well lit; and ensuring that safety equipment is installed in bathrooms and stairwells. Another factor older adults should consider is having a cellular phone with them at all times to call for help directly. Telephone systems providing personal emergency response services may be available on a subscription basis, thus allowing seniors to be monitored; if such a service receives no answer to the call, help can be sent.

Traumatic Brain Injury

Traumatic brain injury (TBI) is a major cause of death and disability. In 2019, there were nearly 61,000 TBI-related deaths (CDC, 2020). TBI is a result of a bump, blow, or jolt to the head or a penetrating head injury, often after a fall, that disrupts the normal function of the brain TBI symptoms may be mild, moderate, or severe. Mild symptoms include headache, confusion, lightheadedness, dizziness, blurred vision or tired eyes, ringing in the ears, bad taste in the mouth, fatigue or

---

BOX 19.4   Improving Balance

Focus on the Following Areas

Perform muscle-strengthening exercises.

Obtain maximum vision correction.

When using bifocal or trifocal glasses, practice looking straight ahead and lowering the head.

Practice balance exercises daily.

Balance Exercises

While holding onto a stable item like a chair or counter, practice standing on one leg at a time for a minute. Gradually increase time, try balancing with eyes closed, and try balancing without holding onto anything.

Practice standing on toes, then rock back to balance on heels. Hold each position for count of 10.

Hold onto a stable item with both hands and then make a big circle to the left with hips. Repeat to the right. Do not move the shoulders or feet. Repeat five times.

Modified from National Institutes of Health Osteoporosis and Related Bone Diseases, National Resource Center: *Preventing falls and related fractures*, 2018. Available from: www.niams.nih.gov/Health_Info/Bone/Osteoporosis/Fracture/prevent_falls.asp.

---

lethargy, and a change in sleep patterns or thinking. Moderate or severe TBI may cause the same symptoms as mild TBI plus a headache that gets worse or does not go away; repeated vomiting or nausea; convulsions or seizures; an inability to awaken from sleep; dilation of one or both pupils of the eyes; slurred speech; weakness or numbness in the extremities; loss of coordination; and increased confusion, restlessness, or agitation (CDC, 2021c). Medical attention should be sought for monitoring and treatment of symptoms. Referral for rehabilitation may be required for persons with disabilities resulting from TBI.

Driver Safety

One of the quality-of-life factors that is important to most seniors is the ability to drive. Many older adults depend on driving in order to maintain independence and personal mobility. Seniors overwhelmingly prefer to drive as their means of transportation, with being a passenger their second preferred option. The number of elderly drivers will be increasing with the extension of life expectancy.

Age alone should not be the determining factor of whether or not a senior can drive safely. Driving skills vary from one elderly person to another. Age-related declines in vision, hearing, and other abilities, as well as certain medical conditions and medications, can affect driving skills (NIA, 2018a). Most older drivers monitor their own driving ability and gradually limit or stop driving, whereas others risk personal injury rather than give up their driver's license. The nurse should be alert to signs of driving impairment in older clients and should offer practical advice so that the driver may either continue to drive safely or be encouraged to find alternative transportation (Box 19.5). The nurse can discuss issues with the senior driver, family, or friends such as drifting out of a lane, becoming confused when entering or exiting a highway, getting

- Physical challenges or limitations
  1. Increasing vision and hearing difficulties
  2. Physical limitations or difficulties including moving foot between pedals, difficulty turning head
- Cognitive problems
  3. Decreasing confidence while driving
  4. Getting lost in familiar places
  5. Becoming easily distracted or confused while driving
  6. Failing to recognize dangerous situations
- Diminishing driving skills
  7. Improper use of turn signals
  8. Difficulty making turns or maintaining correct lane of traffic
  9. Difficulty judging distance between vehicles in traffic
  10. Poor parking abilities
- Potentially hazardous driving
  11. Driving too slowly or too fast for road conditions,
  12. Failing to stop at traffic lights or stop signs,
  13. Frequent "close calls,"
  14. Damage (scrapes or dents) to vehicle or surroundings
  15. Warnings or tickets for moving violations
  16. Multiple accidents

Adapted from https://www.aarp.org/auto/driver-safety/info-2013/warning-signs-unsafe-driving.html?intcmp=AE-ATO-ADS-ASSESS-ROW1-SPOT3.

lost in familiar places, stopping inappropriately, failing to yield the right of way, and speeding or driving too slowly.

Some interventions that older adults could implement are limiting their driving to daylight hours and good weather conditions, planning their trips to avoid rush hour, not listening to the radio, and avoiding talking with passengers while driving. The driver should also be encouraged to find other methods of transportation, such as family and friends, public transportation, taxis, and other private transportation options available in the community.

When the question of driving safely becomes personal, elderly drivers might become very defensive. Therefore, it is important that elderly persons, if at all possible, be involved in the decision-making process of evaluating their ability and deciding what should be done. However, if the individual is greatly impaired and therefore is dangerous to self or others, it may be necessary to involve the family, family physician, or department of motor vehicles in determining whether to suspend or revoke an older person's license. In addition, it may be necessary to take the keys, disable the car, or move it to a location beyond the individual's control to protect the senior and others from injury or accidents.

Residential Fire-Related Injuries

Older adults and people with limited physical and cognitive abilities are at a higher risk of death from fire. In 2018, the risk of dying in a fire for older adults aged 65 or older was 2.6 times higher than for the population as a whole. For older adults aged 85 and older, the risk was 3.8 times higher than that for the general population (U.S. Fire Administration [USFA], 2020).

With the increasing number of older adults, there is likely to be an increase in fire deaths and injuries. This risk of fire-related injuries may be attributed to reduced sensory abilities such as smell, touch, vision, and hearing; diminished mental faculties; slower reaction time; increased disabilities; and economic and social concerns that may prevent necessary home improvements that could reduce fire risk. The predominant causes of fires that result in injuries to older adults are cooking, open flames, smoking, and heating (USFA, 2020). Nurses making home visits can assess their elderly client's home for fire risk and teach fire safety, including the importance of home smoke detectors and fire extinguishers. In many communities, the fire department installs free smoke detectors for older adults. In addition to the U.S. Fire Administration's public information campaign, A Fire Safety Campaign for People 50-Plus, organizations such as the National Fire Protection Association and the American Burn Association have active fire prevention and education programs for older adults.

Cold and Heat Stress
Cold Stress Disorders

Hypothermia is the most serious of the cold stress—related disorders and is the one older individual might experience in the home because of failure of the heating systems or lack of financial resources to pay for sufficient heat. For an older adult, a body temperature of 95°F or lower can cause health problems such as a heart attack, kidney problems, or liver damage (NIA, 2018c). Factors that contribute to the development of hypothermia are age, health, nutrition, exhaustion, exposure and duration of exposure, wind, temperature, wetness, and medications that may decrease heat production, increase heat loss, or interfere with thermostability. Signs of hypothermia are confusion or sleepiness; slowed, slurred speech; weak pulse; a lot of shivering; and poor control over body movements (NIA, 2018c).

Initial management is to prevent further loss of heat. Rewarming of the core temperature at a safe, slow rate is important in order to avoid lethal side effects. The reason for rewarming the core first is to prevent vasodilation that would put the individual into ventricular fibrillation (NIA, 2018c). Measures that can be taken are (1) remove the individual from the cold area as soon as possible; (2) add more clothing, especially to the head (e.g., use a hat or scarf); (3) provide a warm sweetened drink (no coffee or tea); and (4) apply mild heat to the head, neck, chest, and groin areas using hot water bottles or warm moist towels. Emergency care is imperative, and hospitalization may be needed, depending on the stage of hypothermia.

Heat Stress Disorders

The heat stress disorders are heatstroke, heat syncope, heat exhaustion, and heat cramps. As the environment becomes warmer, all methods of heat elimination become less effective, especially for older adults, who may have altered thermoregulation, diminished sweating, and decreased thirst sensation.

These conditions should be taken seriously, and they require immediate attention; heatstroke is life threatening. Heat cramps are painful spasms of muscles of the arms, legs, or abdomen that occur during or after work. Signs and symptoms of heat exhaustion are fatigue, nausea, headache, and giddiness. The skin is clammy and moist, and the complexion may be pale or flushed. The individual may faint on standing, with a rapid, thready pulse and low blood pressure. Signs and symptoms of heatstroke include hot, dry skin that is usually red, mottled, or cyanotic; confusion, loss of consciousness, or convulsions might occur (NIA, 2018b). All of these heat stress disorders may occur in the home without fans or air conditioning, or from being in the sun for prolonged periods, either in recreation or working in extremely hot temperatures and high humidity. In all instances, the individual should be moved to a cooler environment and encouraged to lie down and rest. With heatstroke, immediate and rapid cooling with chilled water or by wrapping in a wet sheet, as well as being moved to a cooler area, should be done while immediate emergency care is being sought (NIA, 2018b).

Elder Abuse

Elder abuse is a serious problem throughout the United States. It is important to remember that abuse is not only a health concern but also a legal problem. States have laws defining abuse and identifying who is required to report abuse to the local Adult Protective Services. *Abuse* is generally defined as the willful infliction of pain, injury, or debilitating mental anguish; unreasonable confinement; or deprivation by a caretaker of services that are necessary to maintain mental and physical health. The categories of abuse are domestic, institutional, and from self-neglect. Domestic abuse is abuse that occurs in the home. Institutional abuse is abuse that occurs in a nursing home or other residential care facility. Self-neglect is defined as abuse that occurs when a person living alone threatens his or her own health or safety.

There are five common types of elder abuse: physical abuse, sexual abuse, psychological/emotional abuse, financial or material exploitation, and neglect. Physical abuse involves slapping, pushing, pinching, and beating or use of physical restraint that results in broken bones, sprains, dislocations, bruises, black eyes, cuts, and rope marks, or sexual assault. Psychological or emotional abuse includes humiliation, intimidation, threats, and destruction of belongings (e.g., glasses). Financial or material exploitation refers to the improper or illegal use of the resources of an older person without consent (e.g., use of automated teller machine card). The most common type of abuse is neglect, which may be self-imposed or caused by another person, such as a caregiver. Signs of neglect include dehydration, malnutrition, untreated health problems, bedsores, unclean or inappropriate clothing, and weight loss.

Approximately one in 10 Americans 60 years of age or older have experienced some form of elder abuse. It is estimated that five million older adults are abused each year; however, only one in 24 cases of abuse are reported (National Council on Aging, 2021b). This problem will steadily increase as more and more elderly are living longer and remaining in their homes. Abuse of the elderly is underreported for a number of reasons, including denial, fear of retaliation and further abuse, no other place to go, love of the abuser and not wanting him or her arrested, dependence on an abuser, shame and embarrassment that a loved one could act in an abusive manner, and lack of physical and/or cognitive ability to report the abuse. In addition, elder abuse may be missed by professionals working with older adults because of lack of training on detecting abuse.

Diagnosis is very difficult because many of the signs and symptoms may truly be the result of normal physiological aging. Ways to tell the difference include conflicting stories about how physical injuries were obtained, "physician shopping," clusters of signs and symptoms, increasing depression of the elder, new poverty, poor personal care, malnutrition, unresponsiveness, hostility, anxiety, confusion, new health problems, improper medication, dehydration, and longing for death.

The abuser is frequently the spouse, adult child, sibling, friend, or caregiver. The family member profile of an abuser is an individual who is middle-aged or older, a daughter or son of the elder, someone with low self-esteem and impaired impulse control. Caregiver behavior to look for includes aggression, defensive or increasingly resentful attitude toward the elder, blaming of the victim for an injury, and treating the elder like a child. Alternatively, the caregiver may show new affluence while withholding food or medication from the elder. Factors that lead to abuse are a lack of knowledge about normal aging, caregiver exhaustion, anger and frustration with the elder, financial problems, and drug and alcohol use by the caregiver. The elders who are most vulnerable are women who are widows or single and more than 75 years of age; those dependent on a caregiver for their shelter and food; and individuals who are frail, ill, incontinent, or mentally disabled.

Prevention activities include professional training of health care personnel, public education about elder abuse and its seriousness, and use of reliable assessment tools for the detection of abuse. The Elder Mistreatment Assessment developed by Fulmer is one accessible assessment for reviewing signs, symptoms, and subjective complaints of elder abuse, neglect, exploitation, and abandonment and is appropriate in all clinical settings (see http://consultgeri.org/ for access to the tool). Nurses and other healthcare providers have an obligation to report suspected abuse to Adult Protective Services and possibly to legal authorities (Ross et al., 2019). Suggestions the community health nurse can give to the elder are to stay sociable, maintain friendships, and participate in senior citizen activities; have pension and Social Security checks deposited directly into bank accounts and obtain a durable power of attorney when no longer able to manage property and assets; consider coguardians so more than one person knows the elder's situation and can act on the elder's behalf; ask for help if needed; keep records, property, and a will in order; and plan ahead for possible disability. Community health nurses also should advise elders to avoid leaving cash, jewelry, and other valuables lying around visible; refuse to sign a document unless someone the elder trusts reviews it first; and resist letting anyone isolate them from others. Educational resources from the National Center on Elder Abuse (ncea.acl.gov/) may be useful.

Crime

Older adults experience the same crimes as the rest of the population; however, older adults may be less likely to recover from their victimization, and are often sought out because of their age, perceived vulnerability, and decreased likelihood of reporting (Office for Victims of Crime, 2018). In addition to the various types of elder abuse mentioned earlier, other crimes consist of robbery, purse snatching, pocket picking, car theft, and various scams (e.g., home repair, credit card fraud).

The key to crime prevention for the senior is to be careful and alert to what is going on in the environment and to the types of crimes to which elders are vulnerable. The elderly person can take measures to lessen the risk of experiencing crime. In the home, safety measures include making sure that door and window locks are strong. Bars on doors and windows need to be installed with caution because they may increase the risk of harm in the event that public officials need to access the home during a fire or to assist the elderly person who may be ill or injured from a fall. The use of a safe deposit box should be recommended to store a list and pictures of expensive belongings and other important documents, such as a copy of the individual's will. Installation of a monitored alarm system with its accompanying outdoor security sign would also help deter criminals. Caution should always be used before answering the door.

Measures that elderly people should observe when out in the community are to stay away from unsafe places, to keep car doors locked and windows up at all times, and to park in well-lit areas. Inside pockets of clothing should be used for valuables such as a wallet, money, and credit cards. A purse should be carried close to the body and kept closed. In addition, the elderly person should be advised not to resist a thief, but to hand over immediately what the person is requesting.

Fraud is the crime that is frequently mentioned in the media as happening to elders. Older people are vulnerable to con games, insurance scams, home repair scams, and telephone scams. Types of Internet fraud include auction fraud, non-delivery of products ordered, securities fraud, credit card fraud, identity theft, bogus business opportunities, and unnecessary professional services. One strategy that can be recommended to seniors to prevent fraud from happening to them is to hang up the phone on telephone salespeople. The elder should request caller identification for the telephone; if no number or individual is identified, the elder may choose not to answer the call. No personal or financial information should be given over the phone unless the elder made the phone call. When in doubt about an inquiry or opportunity, the elder should be encouraged to say "no." The elder should check the references of anyone seeking to do home repairs and should be sure to obtain, in writing, the details of the work to be completed as well as the cost. A job should never be paid for in advance.

Identity theft is on the increase, and elderly individuals are particularly vulnerable. To avoid this problem, Social Security and monthly pension checks should be deposited directly into a bank account. Any information that is sent to the home with credit card offers, personal information, and so forth should be shredded so that the information cannot be used illegally. The elder should check bank statements and credit card account statements carefully for any discrepancies and report them immediately to the respective business. Caution should be used in using the Internet to buy products or pay bills because of websites without security (Federal Bureau of Investigation, n.d.).

> **❓ ACTIVE LEARNING**
>
> 1. Speak with police officers in a local community about elder abuse and crimes against elders. Identify community strengths and weaknesses. Discuss needs and solutions.
> 2. The family of your elderly client is considering taking his car keys from him. They asked you how to decide whether their loved one should stop driving. How would you respond?

PSYCHOSOCIAL DISORDERS

Psychosocial disorders account for a significant number of suicides, especially among older men. Depression is often likely to lead to suicide. The rate of Alzheimer's disease (AD) increases with age. Alcohol and drug abuse are less common in older individuals but are still a concern. Depression and abuse of drugs and alcohol can coexist with one or more anxiety disorders. These conditions are discussed in the following sections.

Anxiety Disorders

Anxiety is a normal human emotion that everyone experiences at one time or another. For elderly individuals, normal age-related worries experienced are financial concerns, health problems, and reduced social interactions due to loss of friends through death and relocation, but these do not mean that the individual has an anxiety disorder. **Anxiety disorders** cause people to have feelings of intense fear and distress that prevent one from doing everyday tasks. Between 10% and 20% of older adults are affected by anxiety disorders in a given year (WebMD, 2021). Anxiety disorders often occur with other mental or physical illnesses, including alcohol or substance abuse, depression, heart disease, diabetes, and other medical problems. The three most common types of anxiety disorders are generalized anxiety disorder, phobia, and panic disorder. **Generalized anxiety disorder** is characterized by excessive, exaggerated anxiety and worry about everyday events and is accompanied by physiological problems, including headaches, insomnia, reduced concentration, muscle tension, feeling tired, irritable, nauseous, and out of breath. The worry is often unrealistic or out of proportion to the real situation, because anxiety dominates the individual's thinking to such a point that it interferes with daily activities. Phobias cause intense fear of a place, thing, or event. Often the fears are irrational and are about things that do not pose a real threat. Common phobias for older adults are fear of death, disaster, and danger to the family. These fears may cause dizziness, shortness of breath, chest pain, or heart palpitations. Panic disorder involves sudden unexplainable feelings of terror often accompanied by a racing heart, chest pain, weakness, nausea, and feeling faint or dizzy (WebMD, 2021).

Anxiety disorders cannot be prevented. Some things that can be suggested to control or lessen symptoms are good diet, adequate sleep, regular exercise, a social support network of family, and friends. Effective treatment for anxiety disorders includes a combination of counseling or psychotherapy, medications, and relaxation techniques (WebMD, 2021). The nurse can help elders realize that what they are experiencing does not need to interfere with their lives if they seek medical help.

Depression

Depression is a condition that interferes with daily life such as ability to work, sleep, concentrate, eat, and enjoy life (National Institute of Mental Illness [NIMH], n.d.). It is a common problem among older adults, but it is not a normal part of aging. It may be overlooked as older adults experience death of loved ones, retirement, stressful life events, or medical problems. The risk of depression in the elderly increases with other illnesses and when ability to function becomes limited. Estimates of major depression in older people living in the community range from less than 1% to about 5% but rises to 13.5% in those who require home health care and to 11.5% in hospitalized elders (CDC, 2021a). Depression may last for days, weeks, months, or even years without treatment. It is a serious condition that increases the risk of death in the elderly population and may even lead to suicide. People with depression may experience several or all of the following symptoms: persistent sad, anxious, or "empty" mood; loss of interest or pleasure in hobbies or activities; feelings of hopelessness; pessimism; decreased energy; fatigue; difficulty concentrating or remembering; difficulty sleeping or oversleeping; appetite and/or unintended weight changes; thoughts of death or suicide; irritability; aches or pain; headaches; or digestive problems (NIMH, n.d.). If any of these symptoms exist, the client should be referred to his or her healthcare provider for diagnosis and treatment. Treatment consists of medication alone or medication with psychotherapy. How long depression lasts depends a great deal on identifying the condition and seeking treatment early. Depression is often undiagnosed or underdiagnosed. Delay in treatment in the elderly can be very dangerous.

Thus the community health nurse can play an important part in recognizing individuals who may be experiencing depression and who need to be referred for medical diagnosis and supervision. Short assessment tools such as the Geriatric Depression Scale—Short Form (Box 19.6) may be used to assess for this problem and assist the nurse in recognizing those at risk.

BOX 19.6 Geriatric Depression Scale—Short Form

Choose the best answer for how you have felt over the past week:
1. Are you basically satisfied with your life? YES/**NO**
2. Have you dropped many of your activities and interests? **YES**/NO
3. Do you feel that your life is empty? **YES**/NO
4. Do you often get bored? **YES**/NO
5. Are you in good spirits most of the time? YES/**NO**
6. Are you afraid that something bad is going to happen to you? **YES**/NO
7. Do you feel happy most of the time? YES/**NO**
8. Do you often feel helpless? **YES**/NO
9. Do you prefer to stay at home, rather than going out and doing new things? **YES**/NO
10. Do you feel you have more problems with memory than most? **YES**/NO
11. Do you think it is wonderful to be alive now? YES/**NO**
12. Do you feel pretty worthless the way you are now? **YES**/NO
13. Do you feel full of energy? YES/**NO**
14. Do you feel that your situation is hopeless? **YES**/NO
15. Do you think that most people are better off than you are? **YES**/NO

Answers in **bold** indicate depression. Score 1 point for each bolded answer.
A score >5 points is suggestive of depression and should warrant a follow-up comprehensive assessment.
A score ≥10 points is almost always indicative of depression.

From Yesavage JA, Sheikh JI: Geriatric Depression Scale (GDS): recent evidence and development of a shorter version, *Clin Gerontol* 5(1/2):165–173, 1986; Yesavage JA: Geriatric Depression Scale, *Psychopharmacol Bull* 24(4):709–711, 1988; and Yesavage JA, et al.: Development and validation of a geriatric depression screening scale: a preliminary report, *J Psychiatr Res* 17(1):37–49, 1982–83. Also available at: http://consultgeri.org/uploads/File/trythis/try_this_4.pdf.

Substance Abuse

Data from the 2018 National Survey on Drug Use & Health sponsored by the Substance Abuse and Mental Health Services Administration (SAMHSA, 2018) revealed that nearly one million adults 65 years or older reported a substance use disorder during the past year. Alcohol and prescription opioids are the two most commonly abused substances among older adults. Other results from the survey about older adults were: 10.7% reported binge drinking in the last month and 1.3% reported misuse of opioids during the past year (SAMHSA, 2018). According to the "Dietary Guidelines for Americans 2020–25," drinking in moderation is limiting alcohol intake to two drinks or less in a day for men and one drink or less in a day for women (USDA and USDHHS, 2020).

Many older adults with substance abuse problems are continuing a pattern of behavior or addiction that began earlier in life. Substance abuse that begins in later life may be due to losses associated with aging such as loss of family and friends, a job, retirement, failing health, or relocation. The warning signs of abuse are less obvious in older adults (WebMD, 2021). For example, many older adults are retired and drink alone at home so they are less likely to be noticed or get into trouble. Also, many of the diseases caused by substance misuse (e.g., hypertension, stroke, dementia, or ulcers) are common disorders in later life, so health care providers and family members may not recognize substance abuse as an underlying cause.

As a result of normal physiological changes discussed earlier in this chapter, older adults generally experience increased sensitivity and decreased tolerance to alcohol and drugs. Because of loss of body mass, reduced absorption rate in the gastrointestinal system, slower kidney function, and slower metabolism, drugs and alcohol remain in the body longer and at higher concentrations, thus prolonging and increasing their effects. The problem is compounded when alcohol and illicit drugs interact with prescribed or over-the-counter medications. This situation may be dangerous because the medications may have a stronger or weaker effect on the body.

Careful screening for such problems must include a thorough review of factors that may be directly affecting substance use and abuse. Several instruments have been utilized with the elderly population, including the CAGE, the Short Michigan Alcohol Screening Test—Geriatric Version (SMAST-G), and the Alcohol Use Disorders Identification Test (AUDIT). The CAGE is an easy-to-use, four-question interview (Box 19.7). The SMAST-G (10 questions) and AUDIT (10 items) are screening instruments that provide a more detailed description of alcohol use. All three of these instruments rely on client self-report.

If substance abuse is identified, the nurse should provide education about the increased health risks. Referral to addiction support groups, counseling or behavioral therapists, or addiction rehabilitation may be useful. Alcoholics Anonymous is a community peer self-help group that may be very beneficial; however, elderly individuals may believe that they do not fit into the group or may have differing concerns from those of younger members. In addition, they may have age-related mobility or hearing problems that prevent participation in peer self-help groups.

Suicide

Suicide, the act of intentionally taking one's own life, is a serious health concern that may be underreported among older adults. Omitted are "silent suicides," for example, deaths from medical noncompliance or overdoses, self-starvation or dehydration, and "accidents." The suicide rate is highest among men aged 75 and over (39.9 per 100,000), especially among white males (CDC, 2021b). Elderly individuals have a high success rate for suicide because they use firearms, hanging, and drowning. "Double suicides" involving spouses or partners occur frequently among the aged.

Elder suicide is associated with depression, chronic illness, physical impairment, and medical conditions that significantly limit functioning or life expectancy, unrelieved pain, financial stress, loss and grief, social isolation, and alcoholism. Warning signs to watch for in the elderly are loss of interest in things or activities that are usually found enjoyable; social isolation; self-care neglect; not following medical regimens (e.g., going off diets, not taking prescriptions); experiencing or expecting a significant personal loss (e.g., spouse or friend); feeling hopeless or worthless; putting affairs in order; giving things away; making changes

BOX 19.7   CAGE Alcohol Screening Instrument

The CAGE screening test is short and simple to administer. Two or more positive answers are correlated with alcohol dependence in 90% of cases.

This screening instrument may not pick up problems in those who are fearful of negative consequences of disclosure, such as those looking for accommodation, people who are fearful of child protection agency staff, and those with mental health problems.

A short questionnaire about your alcohol use:

C: Have you ever thought you should **CUT DOWN** on your drinking?

A: Have you ever felt **ANNOYED** by others' criticism of your drinking?

G: Have you ever felt **GUILTY** about your drinking?

E: Do you have a morning **EYE OPENER**?

From National Institute on Alcohol Abuse and Alcoholism: *Assessing alcohol problems: a guide for clinicians and researchers,* ed 2 (NIH Pub. No. 03–3745), 2003. Available from: http://pubs.niaaa.nih.gov/publications/arh28-2/78-79.htm.

in a will; and stockpiling medications or obtaining other lethal means of committing suicide. The most significant warning sign is any expression of intent. Risk factors that should also be considered in determining whether an elder might be at risk are previous suicide attempts, history of mental disorders, alcohol and substance abuse, family history of suicide, and local epidemics of suicide (Mental Health America, 2021).

Prevention activities include dispelling any myths that exist relating to suicide. Myths that need to be discussed and debunked are that those who kill themselves must be crazy, asking someone about suicide can lead to suicide, and if someone is determined to kill himself or herself, no one can stop that person. Other prevention concepts are to promote awareness, develop broad-based support, reduce stigma associated with aging and being a consumer of mental health, urge use of psychiatric and mental health resources and suicide prevention services, develop community-based suicide prevention programs if none exist, reduce access to lethal means of self-harm, promote participation in education programs related to recognition of at-risk behaviors, and, lastly, promote and support research. The National Suicide Prevention Lifeline is available 24 h/day, 7 days/week; 1-800-273-TALK (8255) and www.suicidepreventionlifeline.org.

Alzheimer's Disease

AD is a slowly progressive brain disorder that begins with mild memory loss and progresses through stages to total incapacitation and eventually death. It is the sixth leading cause of death in the United States and the fifth leading cause of death among those 65 or older. More than six million Americans, mostly older adults, are living with AD (Alzheimer's Association, 2021a). The number of new cases of AD and other dementias is expected to increase as people are living longer. Diagnosing whether an individual has AD is very difficult, because the disease mimics conditions such as depression and other types of dementia. Usually, a tentative diagnosis is reached after all other conditions have been ruled out. The only sure way to diagnose AD is by autopsy, although cerebrospinal fluid analysis and magnetic resonance imaging are being investigated for their diagnostic accuracy. There is no cure, and limited treatment options are available.

A number of screening tools to assess for cognitive impairment have been developed. The clock drawing test (CDT) has become one of the most widely used cognitive screening instruments in clinical and research settings. It has been found to be an effective and easy-to-administer tool to screen for dementia. The CDT has also been incorporated into other widely used cognitive screening instruments such as the Mini Cog (Box 19.8). In addition to the CDT, the Mini Cog assesses for a three-item recall. The Mini-Mental State Examination is another tool used to assess for cognitive impairment. These tools may be accessed from www.consultgeri.org.

Research is ongoing for development of a diagnostic test that could improve recognition of the disease in early stages, resulting in better management using available drugs and therapies. The U.S. Food and Drug Administration has approved five different drugs for treatment of AD. Aricept (donepezil), Exelon (rivastigmine), and Razadyne (galantamine) are cholinesterase inhibitors and are used to treat mild to moderate stages of the disease. Namenda (memantine) and Namzaric are used for moderate to severe cases. *Namzaric* is made from a combination of Aricept and Namenda (Alzheimer's Association, 2021c). These drugs appear to slow down memory loss, confusion, and problems with thinking and reasoning, but they do not stop the progression of the disease. Research regarding etiology, risk factors, diagnosis, treatment, and care issues related to Alzheimer's disease continues.

The behavioral and physical changes due to AD create many challenges for caregivers, family, and friends. Some of the behavioral symptoms are agitation, aggression, wandering, and sleep disturbances. For the individual living alone, inadequate self-care, social isolation, falls, unattended wandering, and injuries occur in addition to problems such as fires from leaving the stove on and having the electricity turned off because bills have not been paid. Communication with a person with AD requires patience, understanding, and good listening skills. The Alzheimer's Association (2021b) provides useful communication strategies for the early, middle, or late stage of AD.

Management strategies for caring for the individual with AD include appropriate use of available treatment options, effective management of coexisting conditions, coordination of care among healthcare professionals and lay caregivers, participation in activities and adult day care programs, and taking part in support groups and support service such as counseling. Caregivers should contact the Alzheimer's Association for their many publications, experts, and local chapter programs. Medical supervision of the physical condition and medications (if clinically indicated) is essential. In addition, AD centers throughout the country offer diagnosis and treatment; provide information about the disease, services, and resources; and give volunteers an opportunity to participate in drug trials and other research projects. A number of resources are available for respite for the caregiver, support groups for both client and family, and day care facilities for the client. For the patient with AD who wanders, the local police should be informed of the potential problem, current pictures of the individual should be available, and safety measures such as installing locks and bells on doors should be taken.

BOX 19.8 The Mini-Cog

Administration
1. Instruct the patient to listen carefully to and remember three unrelated words and then to repeat the words. The same three words may be repeated to the patient up to three tries to register all three words.
2. Instruct the patient to draw the face of a clock, either on a blank sheet of paper or on a sheet with the clock circle already drawn on the page. After the patient puts the numbers on the clock face, ask him or her to draw the hands of the clock to read a specific time. The time 11:10 has demonstrated increased sensitivity.
3. Ask the patient to repeat the three previously stated words.

Scoring (Out of Total of 5 Points)
Give one point for each recalled word after the clock drawing test (CDT) distractor. Recall is scored 0—3.
The CDT distractor is scored 2 if normal and 0 if abnormal.
(Note: The CDT is considered normal if all numbers are present in the correct sequence and position and the hands readably display the requested time. Length of hands is not considered in the score.)

Interpretation of Results
0—2: Positive screen for dementia.
3—5: Negative screen for dementia.

From Borson S, et al.: The Mini-Cog: a cognitive "vital signs" measure for dementia screening in multi-lingual elderly, *Int J Geriatr Psychiatry* 15(11):1021—27, 2000; Borson S, et al.: Improving identification of cognitive impairment in primary care, *Int J Geriatr Psychiatry* 21(4):349—355, 2006; and Lessig M, et al.: Time that tells: critical clock-drawing errors for dementia screening, *Int Psychogeriatr* 20(3):459—470, 2008. Copyright S. Borson. All rights reserved. Reprinted with permission.

? ACTIVE LEARNING

You are asked to lead a 1-hour discussion (see following topic list) for a group of 10 seniors at a senior citizens' center. What would be your goal? What physiological aspects would you include? What psychosocial aspects would you consider?
- Issues related to urine control
- Fall prevention
- Prevention of influenza and pneumonia
- Medications and aging
- Normal aging changes

SPIRITUALITY

As people age and face life's challenges, such as loss of loved ones, declining physical health, and a realization that life's end may be near, spirituality may become more important (Ebersole and Touhy, 2020). Spirituality is a broader concept than religion, encompassing a person's values or beliefs; search for meaning, relationship with God or a higher power, nature, and other people. It includes religion, which is defined as a social institution that unites people in a faith in God, a higher power, and in common rituals and worshipful acts (Ebersole and Touhy, 2020). More than 90% of older adults in the United States consider themselves religious or spiritual (Kaplan and Berkman, 2021).

RESEARCH HIGHLIGHTS

Spirituality and Depression

In a 2-year prospective study of 1992 depressed and 5740 nondepressed older adults (mean age 68.12), Ronneberg et al. (2016) found that religiosity both protected against and helped individuals recover from depression. The older adults who were depressed at the beginning of the study were more likely to be depression-free at follow-up if they had been engaging in frequent private prayer. Those who were depression-free at the beginning of the study were more likely to remain depression-free at the end of the study if they attended religious services frequently.

Addressing the spiritual needs and concerns of a client is part of providing holistic nursing care. If nurses are comfortable with their own spirituality, they will be more attentive to the spiritual needs of their clients. Visible cues, such as the wearing of a religious article or the presence of religious symbols (e.g., Bible, Koran, rosary beads, prayer, or inspirational books), can provide useful insights and a means to open discussion about spiritual needs (Eliopoulos, 2022). Furthermore, use of open-ended questions to begin dialogue about spiritual concerns and use of established spiritual assessments such as the FICA Spiritual History Tool (available at www.consultgeri.org) are helpful. The FICA, which stands for faith, importance/influence, community, and address, provides nurses with a quick and simple means to conduct a spiritual assessment.

Nursing interventions that may be helpful in addressing spiritual needs include the nurse's presence, active listening, caring touch, reminiscence, prayer, hope, conveying a nonjudgmental attitude, facilitation of religious practices, and referral to spiritual care experts (Eliopoulos, 2022).

END-OF-LIFE ISSUES
Advance Directives

Decision making at the end of life is complex. Older adults often experience multiple chronic illnesses, some life threatening; therefore it is especially imperative that this population have advance directives. An older person who is approaching death may not be able to make end-of-life decisions. For such a person, confusion as to how to provide appropriate care may develop.

The Patient Self-Determination Act is a federal law enacted in 1990 that requires health care facilities that receive Medicare and Medicaid funds to ask patients on admission whether they possess an **advance directive** (Miller, 2019). There are three types of advance directives: the living will, do-not-resuscitate order, and durable power of attorney for health care. A **living**

will is a legal document that allows individuals to specify what type of medical treatment they would or would not want if they became incapacitated or had an irreversible terminal illness. Living wills can direct physicians to withhold life-sustaining procedures and can assist family members in making decisions when they are unable to consult a comatose or medically incompetent relative. An individual must be competent to initiate a living will, and he or she can revoke or change it at any time (Miller, 2019).

A **do-not-resuscitate (DNR)** order alerts medical personnel that the individual does not wish to have cardiopulmonary resuscitation in the event the person stops breathing and has no heartbeat. Individuals should place their requests on advance directive forms and inform their physicians. Afterward, a DNR order is written in the medical chart by the physician.

The **physician orders for life sustaining treatment (POLST)** paradigm is a nationally recognized program that promotes discussions about end-of-life care between patients and their health care professionals. The POLST paradigm is intended to support the medically-related wishes of patients who are frail or seriously ill and expected to die within a year. It specifically focuses on decisions made when patients are transitioning between facilities or for patients who live outside of facilities. It differs from the DNR in that POLST forms are a physician's orders in a standardized format which communicates the patient's treatment wishes to emergency personnel. For more information on this program, see http://polst.org/.

A **durable power of attorney for health care** allows a competent individual to designate a health care proxy or surrogate to make decisions about medical care if the person becomes incapacitated. When an individual has no advance directive, is incompetent, or is unable to handle his or her affairs adequately, a guardian may be appointed by the court to direct the individual's medical treatment, housing, personal needs, finances, and property. Because the guardian manages all the individual's affairs and assumes legal rights, a **guardianship** is generally considered a last resort (Miller, 2019).

Advance directives not only make a person's wishes known but may also decrease the stress of decision making experienced by family members at the end of a loved one's life. State-specific advance directives may be ordered from the national organization Caring Info, a program of the National Hospice and Palliative Care Organization, or information may be downloaded from its website (https://www.caringinfo.org).

ETHICAL INSIGHTS

Making End-of-Life Decisions

Al Smith is 76 years old, lives alone, and suffered a massive stroke in his home. He was found by his older brother, Joe, who had come to visit him. Joe immediately called 911, and Al was rushed to a nearby hospital. Joe informed the health care providers at the hospital that he wanted everything done for his brother.

Complications from the stroke included irregular breathing, paralysis on one side of the body, aphasia, severe confusion, and problems with vision. Because of subsequent worsening of his breathing and nonresponsiveness, Al was started on ventilation therapy.

Joe called to inform their sister, Rose, who lives out of town, about the incident and condition of their brother. Rose was very upset with Joe for allowing Al to be connected to a ventilator. She claimed that Al would not have wanted this.

Questions

- What should Al Smith have done to make his wishes known?
- What discussion should his siblings have had to prevent disagreement?
- What are the ethical principles involved in this case?
- What are the legal implications?

The Nurse's Role in End-of-Life Issues

The nurse is encouraged to discuss and educate clients about end-of-life issues. These issues include advance directives and prefuneral considerations when death is imminent. When a client enters a healthcare facility with an advance directive,

nurses should ensure that it is current and reflects the client's wishes. The nurse should inform other members of the health care team and make sure that the document is visible and accessible in the client's chart. The nurse should also encourage clients to discuss their wishes regarding the decisions in these documents with their families. Clients should provide copies of advance directives such as living wills to their family members in case of emergency. Furthermore, clients should discuss their living wills with their physicians so that the documents are made part of their medical records. A copy of advance directives should also be kept in the individual's automobile.

 ACTIVE LEARNING

Your elderly client has a terminal illness. You note that she does not have an advance directive. What issues surrounding this topic would you discuss with her?

CASE STUDY Application of the Nursing Process

75-Year-Old Widow

Mrs. Darren, a 75-year-old widow, was referred to the community health nurse by her physician, who did not believe she could care for herself sufficiently. Her diagnoses were hypertension, mild congestive heart failure, arthritis, and occasional confusion after transient ischemic attacks.

During the initial home visit, the nurse observed that Mrs. Darren lived in a run-down house in an inner-city neighborhood. The roof leaked, and the house had no functioning heat unit. Mrs. Darren told the nurse that she did not have children and her only relative was a sister who lived with her family in another state. She was used to the neighborhood and knew her neighbors, but she was frightened of the teenagers who lingered when she took the bus to the supermarket.

Mrs. Darren received Supplemental Security Income, Medicare, Medicaid, and food stamps. She ate mostly bread and butter and drank coffee, but she enjoyed fried chicken and oranges after going to the supermarket. Constipation was sometimes a problem, and she took a laxative every night. She said she did not always remember whether she took her medication and held out a small bottle containing an assortment of pills of different colors, shapes, and sizes.

Assessment

With Mrs. Darren as the system, or central planning focus, the nurse identified her strengths and weaknesses and looked for actual or potential connections to her family and community. Considering aging theories, the nurse believed Mrs. Darren was undergoing disengagement from her physical and social circumstances and decided that this process might be reversed if her health could be maintained and her links to the community strengthened. On a practical level, the nurse also checked with Mrs. Darren's physician regarding the prescriptions and identified the assortment of pills by taking them to the pharmacist who filled them.

The nurse used a problem-solving approach to data gathering and identified Mrs. Darren's assets as the following:
- Being basically able to care for herself
  - Receiving medical treatment
  - Receiving income from various sources
  - Being accustomed to the neighborhood and knowing her neighbors

Her liabilities were more extensive:
- Inadequate nutrition
- Confusion with medications and improper use of laxatives
- Condition of the house, which was not supportive of health
- Threat of violence in neighborhood
- Physical impairment resulting from age and illness
- No children or other family living nearby

- Probable progression of confusion
- Possibility of a health episode at home while unattended

Diagnoses

Diagnoses and related short- and long-term goals address Mrs. Darren's situation. The nurse wrote plans at the three levels of prevention for the diagnoses and included suggestions for intervention with families.

Individual
- Inadequate nutrition, which was related to difficulty or inability to procure food
- Risk for exploitation due to possibility of theft, or fraud, aging, and progression of disease

Family
Potential for social isolation related to unanticipated loss of interaction with only relative who lives a distance away and Mrs. Darren's declining health.

Community
- Lack of knowledge regarding community resources for nutritional services and financial assistance
- Lack of support programs for medication consistency related to unrecognized need

Planning
Individual
Long-Term Goals
- Mrs. Darren will maintain a nutritionally adequate diet through self-care and use of community programs as evidenced by a steady weight and normal results on tests for nutritional status.
- In her medication regimen related to forgetfulness and mild confusion.
- Mrs. Darren will continue to take medications as ordered, as evidenced by stabilization of disease processes and intermittent demonstration to a nurse.
- Mrs. Darren will explore sheltered housing for older adults and continue contact neighborhood friends.

Short-Term Goals
- Mrs. Darren will improve her diet to include a recommended daily allowance of nutrients, including fiber and fluids, as evidenced by diet recall, and she will report regular bowel habits without use of laxatives.
- Mrs. Darren will utilize memory aids for a consistent medication regimen.

CASE STUDY Application of the Nursing Process—cont'd

- Mrs. Darren will identify medications and know when to take them, as evidenced by demonstration to a nurse.
- Mrs. Darren will improve her home to allow healthy habitation, avoid victimization, expand her social network, and maintain healthcare appointments.

Family
Long-Term Goal
- Mrs. Darren will maintain family contact by mail, telephone, or possible visits.

Short-Term Goal
- Family members' addresses are included in Mrs. Darren's record to facilitate emergency contact.

Community
Long-Term Goals
- Promote publicity campaign to advertise nutritional services for older adults in the community.
- Support community pharmacists in the campaign to increase public awareness of the need to take medications as prescribed.
- Identify and support programs that will assist with provision of prescribed medications for people who have difficulty obtaining prescriptions because of a lack of insurance, money, transportation, or other problems.
- Have community groups work together to maximize use of resources.

Short-Term Goal
- Identify existing programs for older adults in the community.

Intervention
Individual
When the nurse discussed the nursing diagnoses and plans with Mrs. Darren, Mrs. Darren agreed with the short-term goals, but she was not sure that she wanted to leave her home for other housing and agreed to try to meet other people through community activities. During the next few visits, the nurse explained basic nutritional principles and helped make a shopping list and menus for 1 week. Together, they developed a plan to assist with medication scheduling.

The nurse encouraged Mrs. Darren to talk about her earlier life. She had been widowed soon after her marriage, and she had never remarried. She lived in the neighborhood where she grew up, although it had deteriorated over the years. She had worked as a secretary until her retirement; there was no pension plan.

Family
Because Mrs. Darren's family did not live close by, the nurse worked to increase Mrs. Darren's social contacts by introducing her to a group that met frequently and offered several activities she might enjoy. If she were unexpectedly absent, the group would check on her. A neighbor invited her to a senior center, where she became involved in a domino-playing group.

Community
Referrals initiated by the nurse resulted in a greatly improved living situation. A home health aide from the same program came for half a day each week to assist with shopping and cleaning. A local area agency on aging fixed her roof, and a church-sponsored group painted the house and cleaned the yard. A small heater was purchased from the Salvation Army store, and application was made to the utility company for help with bills during the winter months.

Evaluation
Individual
With the nurse as intermediary for and coordinator of community services, Mrs. Darren easily accepted help with the problems related to security. When her home improvements were completed, Mrs. Darren was able to maintain herself more comfortably with the help of the weekly visit from the home health aide.

Family
In the absence of family support, the establishment of an orderly routine, and safer financial arrangements increased Mrs. Darren's feelings of belonging and self-esteem. The nurse reduced her home visits but maintained contact with Mrs. Darren during her visits to the health clinic for blood pressure checks and preventive health care.

Community
Discussion with the home health aide informed the nurse of proposed funding cuts to the city's Supportive Services to the Elderly program, which would result in reduced services. The nurse spoke to the president of the district branch of the Professional Nurses' Association. The association assisted the nurse in working with other local agencies for older adults to establish a publicity campaign against funding cuts through writing letters, speaking at public hearings on the city budget, and speaking at city council meetings. Although funds were reduced, the cuts were less severe than they would have been without the campaign, and most services were able to continue.

Levels of Prevention
Primary Prevention
Goal: Promote good nutrition.

Individual
- Instruct about nutritional needs.
- Plan a shopping list and menus incorporating a prescribed diet for health problems.

Primary Prevention
Goal: Promote safety and prevention of injury.

Individual
- Provide immunizations as appropriate.
- Provide community services for assistance to maintain property and prevent deterioration.
- Encourage a network of friends and family members.

Family
- Provide services of community health nurse or case manager.
- Provide counseling.
- Provide respite care.

Community
- Provide community education programs for older adults.
- Be aware of potential hazards for older adult residents and provide intervention as needed.

Secondary Prevention
Goal: Assess and treat nutrition-related disorders.

Individual
- Provide referral for assessment of possible nutrition-related disorders.
- Provide hospitalization or prescribed nutritional supplements for illness resulting from inadequate nutrition.

Family
- Provide referral for nutritional assessment and counseling.

Community
- Encourage emergency food supplies.

Continued

CASE STUDY   Application of the Nursing Process—cont'd

Secondary Prevention
Goal: Diagnose and treat medication-related injuries.

Individual
- Provide referral for apparent overmedication or undermedication symptoms.
- Diagnose and treat drug or food reactions.

Family
- Reassess the client's understanding of medications.

Community
- Provide a 24-hour poison hotline.
- Provide an ED with 24-hour response.
- Provide medical services.

Tertiary Prevention
Goal: Maintain improved nutrition.

Individual
- Encourage use of community services.

Family
- Encourage exchange of family recipes.
- Encourage attendance at home economics classes.

Community
- Provide campaigns for nutritional awareness and healthy eating.
- Encourage healthy snacks in food machines.
- Encourage use of funding of community food services for emergencies.
- Encourage use of services providing access to food (e.g., food banks, Meals on Wheels, and food stamps).
- Encourage use of transportation to grocery stores or nutrition services.

Tertiary Prevention
Goal: Be consistent with prescribed medications and prevent medication error.

Individual
- When medications are dispensed, provide written and oral instructions at the level of understanding and in the language of the client.
- Have the client repeat instructions to the healthcare provider.

Family
- Have the client repeat instructions to family members.

Community
- Provide a community education program about understanding medications.

SUMMARY

Increasing life expectancy, coupled with the aging of the baby boomer generation, will cause a dramatic rise in the number of older adults. In addition to successful aging, older adults desire to function independently for as long as possible. This chapter has described aging, demographic characteristics, normal aging changes, health promotion and illness prevention interventions, common health and psychosocial concerns, end-of-life issues, and various resources that may assist older adults. Community health nurses have a pivotal role in addressing these issues and concerns so that they may assist older adults have a better quality of life.

EVOLVE WEBSITE

http://evolve.elsevier.com/Nies/community
- NCLEX Review Questions
- Case Studies

BIBLIOGRAPHY

Administration on Aging: *2020 profile of older Americans*, Washington, DC, 2021, U.S. Department of Health & Human Services. Available from: https://acl.gov/sites/default/files/Aging%20and%20Disability%20in%20America/2020ProfileOlderAmericans.Final_.pdf.

Alzheimer's Association: *Alzheimer's and dementia facts and figures*, 2021a. Available from: www.alz.org/facts/.

Alzheimer's Association: *Communication and Alzheimer's*, 2021b. Available from: www.alz.org/care/dementia-communication-tips.asp#early.

Alzheimer's Association: *Medications for memory, cognition and dementia-related behaviors*, 2021c. Available from: www.alz.org/alzheimers_disease_standard_prescriptions.asp.

American Geriatrics Society: AGS 2019 Updated AGS Beers Criteria for potentially inappropriate medication use in older adults, *J Am Geriatr Soc* 67(4):674–694, 2019. Available from: https://pubmed.ncbi.nlm.nih.gov/30693946/.

American Geriatrics Society Health in Aging Foundation: *Age-friendly healthcare & you*, 2021. Available from: https://www.healthinaging.org/age-friendly-healthcare-you.

American Hospital Association Center for Health Innovation: *Age-friendly health systems*, 2021. Available from: https://www.aha.org/center/age-friendly-health-systems.

American Speech-Language-Hearing Association: *Types of hearing loss*, n.d. Available from: https://www.asha.org/public/hearing/types-of-hearing-loss/.

Centers for Disease Control and Prevention (CDC): *Depression is not a normal part of growing older*, 2021a, National Center for Chronic Disease Prevention and Health Promotion. Available from: https://www.cdc.gov/aging/depression/.

Centers for Disease Control and Prevention (CDC): *National Center for Health Statistics: Mortality Data on CDC WONDER*, 2020. Available from: https://wonder.cdc.gov/mcd.html.

Centers for Disease Control and Prevention (CDC): *Suicide mortality in the U.S., 1999–2019*, 2021b, National Center for Health Statistics. Available from: https://www.cdc.gov/nchs/products/databriefs/db398.htm.

Centers for Disease Control and Prevention (CDC): *Traumatic brain injury and concussion*, 2021c, National Center for Injury Prevention and Control. Available from: https://www.cdc.gov/traumaticbraininjury/concussion/symptoms.html.

Centers for Disease Control and Prevention (CDC): *Web-based injury statistics query and reporting system (WISQARS)*, 2016, National Center for Injury Prevention and Control.

Cumming E, Henry W: *Growing old*, New York, 1961, Basic Books.

De la Fuente M: Role of Neuroimmunomodulation in aging, *Neuroimmunomodulation* 15:213, 2008.

Diverse Elders Coalition: *Who we are*, 2021. Available from: https://www.diverseelders.org/who-we-are/.

Ebersole P, Touhy T: Self-actualization, spirituality, & transcendence. In *Ebersole & Hess' toward healthy aging: human needs & nursing response*, St. Louis, 2020, Elsevier, pp 497–498.

Eliopoulos C: *Gerontological nursing*, ed 10, Philadelphia, 2022, Wolters Kluwer.

Federal Bureau of Investigation: *Elder fraud*, n.d. Available from: https://www.fbi.gov/scams-and-safety/common-scams-and-crimes/elder-fraud.

Federal Interagency Forum on Aging-Related Statistics: *Older Americans 2020: key indicators of well-being*, Washington, DC, 2020, U.S. Government Printing Office. Available from: https://agingstats.gov.

Havighurst RL, Neugarten BL, Tobin SS: Disengagement and patterns of aging. In Neugarten BL, editor: *Middle age and aging*, Chicago, 1968, University of Chicago Press.

Havighurst RL, Neugarten BL, Tobin SS: Disengagement, personality, and life satisfaction in the later years. In Hansen PF, editor: *Age with a future*, Copenhagen, 1963, Munksgaard.

Hayflick L: *How and why we age*, New York, 1996, Ballantine Books.

HealthinAging.org: *Physical activity*, 2020. Available from: https://www.healthinaging.org/a-z-topic/physical-activity/basic-facts.

HealthinAging.org: *Sexual health*, 2021. Available from: http://www.healthinaging.org/aging-and-health-a-to-z/topic:sexual-health/.

Kaiser Family Foundation (KFF) Tracking Poll: *Data note: prescription drugs and older adults*, 2019. Available from: https://www.kff.org/health-reform/issue-brief/data-note-prescription-drugs-and-older-adults/.

Kaplan DB, Berkman BJ: *Religion and spirituality in the elderly*, 2021. Available from: https://www.merckmanuals.com/home/older-people%E2%80%99s-health-issues/social-issues-affecting-older-people/religion-and-spirituality-in-older-people.

Mayo Clinic Staff: *Cataracts*, 2021a. Available from: www.mayoclinic.org/diseases-conditions/cataracts/symptoms-causes/syc-20353790.

Mayo Clinic Staff: *Dry macular degeneration*, 2021b. Available from: http://www.mayoclinic.org/diseases-conditions/dry-macular-degeneration/home/ovc-20164874.

Mayo Clinic Staff: *Glaucoma*, 2021c. Available from: https://www.mayoclinic.org/diseases-conditions/glaucoma/symptoms-causes/syc-20372839.

Mayo Clinic Staff: *Wet macular degeneration*, 2021d. Available from: http://www.mayoclinic.org/diseases-conditions/wet-macular-degeneration/home/ovc-20164274.

Mental Health America: *Preventing suicide in older adults*, 2021. Available from: www.mentalhealthamerica.net/preventing-suicide-older-adults.

Miller CA: *Nursing for wellness in older adults*, ed 8, Philadelphia, 2019, Wolters Kluwer.

Miller RA: The aging immune system: primer and prospectus, *Science* 273:70, 1996.

Milson I, Gyhagen M: The prevalence of urinary incontinence, *Climacteric* 22(3):217–222, 2018.

Morley A: The somatic mutation theory of aging, *Mutat Res* 338(1–6):19–23, 1995.

National Council on Aging: *The top 10 most common chronic conditions in older adults*, 2021a. Available from: https://www.ncoa.org/article/the-top-10-most-common-chronic-conditions-in-older-adults.

National Council on Aging: *Get the facts on elder abuse*, 2021b. Available from: https://www.ncoa.org/article/get-the-facts-on-elder-abuse.

National Institute on Aging (NIA): *Age page: taking care of your teeth and mouth*, 2020. Available from: https://www.nia.nih.gov/health/publication/taking-care-your-teeth-and-mouth.

National Institute on Aging (NIA): *Older drivers*, 2018a. Available from: https://www.nia.nih.gov/health/older-drivers#besafe.

National Institute on Aging (NIA): *Hot weather safety for older adults*, 2018b. Available from: https://www.nia.nih.gov/health/hot-weather-safety-older-adults.

National Institute on Aging (NIA): *Cold weather safety for older adults*, 2018c. Available from: https://www.nia.nih.gov/health/cold-weather-safety-older-adults.

National Institute on Aging (NIA): *Urinary incontinence in older adults*, 2017. Available from: https://www.nia.nih.gov/health/urinary-incontinence-older-adults.

National Institute of Mental Illness (NIMH): *Older adults and depression*. Available from: https://www.nimh.nih.gov/health/publications/older-adults-and-depression.

National Institute on Deafness and Other Communication Disorders (NIDCD): *Hearing loss and older adults*, 2018. Available from: https://www.nidcd.nih.gov/health/hearing-loss-older-adults.

Nurses Improving Care for Healthsystem Elders (NICHE), n.d. Available from: www.nicheprogram.org.

Nutrition Screening Initiative: *Determine your nutritional health*, Washington, DC, Author.

Office for Victims of Crime: Crimes against older adults. In *2018 National crime victims' rights week resource guide: crime and victimization fact sheets*. Available from: https://ovc.ojp.gov/sites/g/files/xyckuh226/files/ncvrw2018/info_flyers/fact_sheets/2018NCVRW_OlderAdults_508_QC.pdf.

Orgel LE: The maintenance of the accuracy of protein synthesis and its relevance to aging, *Proc Natl Acad Sci USA* 49:517–521, 1963.

Ronneberg CR, Miller EA, Dugan E, et al.: The protective effects of religiosity on depression: a 2-year prospective study, *Gerontol* 56(3):421–431, 2016.

Ross MET, Thomas KL, Pickens S, Bryan J, Asghar-Ali AA: Elder Abuse. In Balasubramaniam M, Gupta A, Tampi R, editors: *Psychiatric ethics in late-life patients: medicolegal and forensic aspects at the interface of mental health*, ed 1, 2019, Springer, pp 165–181.

Shehab N, Lovegrove M, Geller A, et al.: U.S. Emergency department visits for outpatient adverse drug events, 2013–2014, *JAMA* 316(20):2115–2125, 2016.

Substance Abuse and Mental Health Services Administration, Center for Behavioral Health Statistics and Quality: *National Survey on Drug Use & Health, 2017 and 2018*. Available from: https://www.

samhsa.gov/data/sites/default/files/cbhsq-reports/NSDUHDetailedTabs2018R2/NSDUHDetTabsSect1pe2018.htm.

Taylor MF, Marquis R, Coall DA, et al.: The physical health dilemmas facing custodial grandparent caregivers: policy considerations, *Cogent Med* 4(1), 2017.

Touhy T, Jett K: *Ebersole & Hess' toward healthy aging: human needs & nursing response*, St. Louis, 2020, Elsevier.

Trail Ross ME, Kang DK, Cron S: Psychological profile, salivary cortisol, C-reactive protein, and perceived health of grandmothers with childrearing responsibility, *J Fam Issues* 36(14):1904–1927, 2015.

United States Census Bureau: *National population by characteristics: 2010–2019 tables, median age and age by sex, annual estimates of the resident population by single year of age and sex: April 1, 2010 to July 1, 2018*, 2020.

U.S. Centers for Medicare and Medicaid Services (CMS): *Costs in the coverage gap*, 2020a. Available from: https://www.medicare.gov/drug-coverage-part-d/costs-for-medicare-drug-coverage/costs-in-the-coverage-gap.

U.S. Center for Medicare and Medicaid Services (CMS): *Medicare costs at a glance*, 2020b. Available from: https://www.medicare.gov/your-medicare-costs/medicare-costs-at-a-glance.

U.S. Department of Agriculture: *My plate*, n.d. Available from: https://www.myplate.gov.

U.S. Department of Agriculture & U.S. Department of Health and Human Services: *Dietary Guidelines for Americans, 2020–2025*, ed 9, 2020. Available from: DietaryGuidelines.gov.

U.S. Department of Health and Human Services, Office of Disease Prevention & Health Promotion: *Healthy People 2020: leading health indicators*, n.d. Washington, DC, Author. Available from: https://www.healthypeople.gov/2020/Leading-Health-Indicators.

U.S. Department of Health and Human Services, Office of Disease Prevention & *Health Promotion: Healthy People 2030: Older adults*, Washington, DC, 2021, Author. Available from: https://health.gov/healthypeople/objectives-and-data/browse-objectives/older-adults, https://www.healthypeople.gov/2020/topics-objectives/topic/older-adults/objectives.

U.S. Fire Administration (USFA): *U.S. fire deaths, fire death rates, and risk of dying in a fire*, 2020. Available from: https://www.usfa.fema.gov/data/statistics/fire_death_rates.htmlWebMD.

WebMD. *Substance abuse in older adults*, 2021. Available from: https://www.webmd.com/mental-health/addiction/ss/slideshow-substance-abuse-older-people.

WebMD: *What to know about anxiety in older adults*, 2021. Available from: https://www.webmd.com/healthy-aging/what-to-know-about-anxiety-in-older-adults#1.

20

Family Health

Tonya Bragg-Underwood

> *Family is not an important thing, it's everything.*
> **Michael J. Fox**

OBJECTIVES

Upon completion of this chapter, the reader will be able to do the following:

1. Give a definition of *family*.
2. Identify characteristics of the family that have implications for community health nursing practice.
3. Describe strategies for moving from intervention at the individual level to intervention at the family level.
4. Describe strategies for moving from intervention at the family level to intervention at the aggregate level.
5. Discuss a model of care for families.
6. Apply the steps of the nursing process to individuals within the family, the family as a whole, and the family's aggregate.

OUTLINE

KEY TERMS

cohabitation
ecological framework
ecomap
expressive functioning
external structure
family
family health assessment
family health tree
family interviewing
general systems theory
genogram
instrumental functioning
internal structure
nuclear family
sandwich generation
social network framework
transactional model

To understand changing American families, many sociologists suggest that one needs to only view television and movies. Stereotypical television families have allowed American families to identify with developmental landmarks and to understand changing family demographics and structure. Whether one's view of families is parallel with *All in the Family*, *Family Ties*, or *Modern Family*, television shows illustrate that definitions of American families are unique, diverse, and ever changing. Legal definitions of family have tended not to keep current with modern representations of American families because the definitions have more to do with statistics. For example, the U.S. Census Bureau (2020)

TABLE 20.1   A Comparison of Families by Type in the United States 2014–18

	2014	2018
Married-couple households	47,963,000 (65%)	48,499,000 (66%)
Father-only households	5,825,000 (8%)	5,852,000 (8%)
Mother-only households	19,006,000 (26%)	18,275,000 (25%)
Children in care of grandparents	2,882,000 (4%)	2,787,000 (4%)
Children living with cohabiting domestic partners	5,901,000 (8%)	5,903,000 (8%)
Children living with neither parent	3,631,000 (5%)	4,020,000 (6%)
Children living in married-couple immigrant families	13,525,000 (75%)	13,767,000 (76%)
Children living in single-parent immigrant families	4,549,000 (25%)	4,430,000 (24%)
Children living in single-parent immigrant families (US-born children)	19,895,000 (38%)	19,550,000 (38%)

From Annie E. Casey Foundation: *National kids county key indicators*, 2021. http://www.kidscount.org.

definition of family has remained basically unchanged since 1930:

> *A family includes a householder and one or more people living in the same household who are related to the householder by birth, marriage, or adoption …*

Although these definitions are important, is enough direction provided to healthcare providers who work with many families in many situations? In reality, modern families may be much more complex than families defined by statute or on television because of chronic health issues and the changing societal forces that are affecting the family in ways never before imagined by healthcare professionals. Table 20.1 provides a summary of the changes in family type by year.

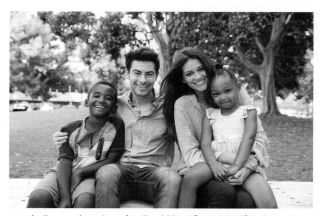

A diverse American family, 2021. (Copyright iStock.com.)

CHALLENGES FACING US FAMILIES

The dynamic forces affecting families are not new, but when combined result in new challenges to families and family nurses. For example, it is well documented that the increase in the number of aging Americans is expected to present new challenges to families and society. "Older American's or persons 65 years or older have increased from 38.8 million in 2008 to 54.2 million in 2018 and is projected to reach 94.7 million in 2060." (U.S. Dept. of Health and Human Services [DHHS], 2020). The oldest

subgroup in this population is the "oldest-old," or those over 80 years of age, "is expected to triple between 2015 and 2050, growing from 126.5 million to 446.6 million" (NIH, 2016). It should be noted that the older population comprises 23.1% of the total disease burden worldwide (World Health Organization [WHO], 2010). In the over-65 age group, approximately 80% have one chronic disease and 68% have two or more (National Council on Aging [NCOA], 2021). The top five occurring chronic diseases in the over-65 age group are hypertension (58%), high cholesterol (47%), arthritis (31%), ischemic/coronary heart disease (29%), and diabetes (27%) (NCOA, 2021). When combined with the declining economy, the increasing population of aging persons has resulted in challenging living arrangements, draining economic resources, and growing numbers of families without sufficient healthcare coverage. Increasing numbers of elderly have created a **sandwich generation** or sandwich family structure, in which adults care for elderly parent(s) either in their homes or by providing financial support (Parker and Patten, 2013). Added to this financial burden is the number of adults also providing financial support to adult children. The primary caregiver of the sandwich family also requires attention by healthcare providers. The increased stressors of caregiving, financial concerns, and related family and marital conflicts has resulted in reports of depression for the caregiver, indicating a potential area of concern for healthcare providers (Abramson, 2015).

The financial burden of the cost of health care is a major challenge for families. The Patient Protection and Affordable Care Act (ACA), when implemented in 2010, made sweeping changes resulting in large numbers of families receiving health insurance either through expanded Medicaid programs or the availability of insurance markets offering lower insurance rates (Cantor et al., 2012). One popular change allowed families to insure dependent adult children up to the age of 26 on the family policy. Table 20.2 lists the changes implemented by the ACA by year.

One study found that the number of young adults (aged 19–25 years) who received health insurance increased by 2.5 million (Sommers and Schwartz as cited in Cantor et al., 2012). For non–income-eligible families purchasing insurance through the health markets, the benefits included limits on cost, including out-of-pocket maximums (Abramowitz and O'Hara, 2014). Healthcare researchers are currently

TABLE 20.2 ACA Provision Timeline, 2010–15

Year	Provision
2010	• Dependents up to age 26 covered by parents • Patient-Centered Outcomes Research Institute (PCORI) created • Expansion of 340B drug discount • Health plans provide certain preventive services without cost sharing • Consumer protections take effect (no preexisting condition exclusions for children, lifetime limits, or rescinding coverage)
2011	• Prescription drug discounts • Free preventive care for senior citizens • Increased access to services at home and in the community
2012	• Incentives for physicians to form Medicare accountable care organizations • Medicare advantage plan payment reductions and bonuses • Annual fees imposed on pharmaceutical manufacturers • Medicare value-based purchasing program established • Medicare hospital readmissions penalties
2013	• Medicare bundled payment pilot program established • Temporary Medicaid payment increase for primary care • Medical device tax takes effect • Reduction in Medicare and Medicaid • Disproportionate Share hospital payments • Medicaid expansion • Individual mandate takes effect • Essential health benefits package created • First individual exchange open enrollment period closes with approximately 8 million signed up • Additional consumer protections (no preexisting condition exclusions, no annual limits)
2015	• Physician payment based on value, not volume • Delayed employer mandate takes effect
2016	• Medicaid expansion—Alaska, Indiana, Pennsylvania
2017	• Medicaid expansion—Louisiana, Montana
2019	• Medicaid expansion—Maine, Virginia

ACA, Affordable Care Act. Data from Reisman M: The Affordable Care Act, 5 years later: policies, progress, and politics, *Pharm Ther* 40(9):575–600, 2015; Levy H, Ying A, Bagley N: What's left of the Affordable Care Act? A progress report, *RSF: The Russell Sage Foundation J Soc Sci*, 6(2):42–66, 2020.

evaluating the possible impact of loss of healthcare insurance should current lawmakers repeal the ACA without new legislation. Eighty-one percent of those losing healthcare coverage will be in working families; 40% will be young adults; and 50% will be non-Hispanic white families. Family nurses must beware of the impact of not only the burden of the cost of health care but the impact of the loss of healthcare coverage (GI, 2016).

Globalization has also affected the family. In many areas manufacturing has replaced agriculture as primary employment. Loss of jobs results in financial decline, personal bankruptcies, and downward social mobility. All of these forces impact individual and family health.

The families described in Clinical Examples 20.1 through 20.4 depict broad contemporary definitions of family and are the kinds of families carried in caseloads by undergraduate community health nursing students. Assessments made by students during home, office, and hospital visits with these families triggered interventions that linked the families to resources provided by the community and, in turn, led to questions about health needs of groups of families or larger aggregates living in the same communities.

Clinical Example 20.1

Rebecca Martin is a 72-year-old widow of 10 years who lives in a rural town in Tennessee. She resides in the home that she and her husband purchased before his death. Her primary source of income is her deceased husband's Social Security benefits, and she also receives a small income from providing childcare for infants at her church. Medicare benefits are her only source of payment for health care. Her only child, a daughter from whom she has been estranged for many years, recently died. The daughter was a never-married, single mother of an 8 years old, medically fragile child with asthma. As the only surviving relative, Rebecca has become the custodial parent for her granddaughter.

Clinical Example 20.2

Joe Hudson is a 74-year-old alcoholic who is being treated at an outpatient department in a large medical center. He lives in a hotel room in downtown Salt Lake City, Utah. He has one living relative, a 76-year-old brother. Mr. Hudson states, "I had a falling out with my brother 20 years ago. I never hear from him. I reckon he's still in Boston, if he's alive at all." Mr. Hudson frequently falls out of bed, dislodging the telephone that the desk clerk has placed precariously close to the bed, which signals the desk clerk that something is amiss. The clerk then goes to Mr. Hudson's room and puts him back in bed. Mr. Hudson's source of income is a check sent to him the first day of each month by a minister who lives in a town 75 miles away. The desk clerk cashes Mr. Hudson's check and helps him pay his bill from the hotel, which provides congregate dining facilities.

Clinical Example 20.3

Lyn Nguyen is a refugee from Vietnam who moved with her family to San Francisco 3 months ago. Mrs. Nguyen is a single parent; Mr. Chan died in an automobile accident shortly after arriving in the United States. Mrs. Nguyen has two children, an 11-year-old son and a 5-year-old daughter. The family resides in a one-room efficiency apartment in the Tenderloin district in downtown San Francisco.

Clinical Example 20.4

Jaime Gutierrez, a 72-year-old Mexican American man, lives with his 36-year-old son, Roberto; his 34-year-old daughter-in-law, Patricia; and his three grandchildren, who are 14, 13, and 12 years of age. Mr. Gutierrez was in good health until he fell from a tree while helping his son make roof repairs on the

Clinical Example 20.4—cont'd

house in 1995. He suffered a concussion, right hemothorax, and fracture of vertebrae T11 and T12. Confined to bed, he is receiving home health care. He requires intermittent catheterization but feels uncomfortable when the nurse suggests that his daughter-in-law is willing to carry out this procedure for him; therefore, Roberto quit work to provide this personal care to his father. Consequently, the family of six lives on Mr. Gutierrez's retirement income, which consists of $239 from Social Security and $244 from a pension plan per month. Roberto would like to improve his job skills while at home. He has finished the fourth grade and has failed the Graduate Equivalency Degree examination twice. Patricia also would like to return to school and pursue job training. Although agreeable to Patricia's interests, Roberto is hesitant to support active steps taken by Patricia to initiate her plan.

Working with families has never been more complex or rewarding than now. Nurses understand the actual and potential impact that families have in changing the health status of individual family members, communities, and society as a whole. Additionally, families have challenging healthcare needs that are not usually addressed by the healthcare system. Instead, the healthcare system most frequently addresses the individual. This holds true for nursing interventions within the healthcare system. This chapter helps the nurse understand and address complex issues that affect family health and suggests methods to improve family health.

UNDERSTANDING FAMILY NURSING

Family nursing is not a new concept and has been taught in schools of nursing since Nightingale's "district nursing" concept (Cook, 1913) and Lillian Wald's (1904) principles on how to nurse families in the home.

The family is composed of many subsystems and, in turn, is tied to many formal and informal systems outside it. The family is embedded in social systems that have an influence on health (e.g., education, employment, and housing). The International Family Nursing Association provides family characteristics that explain "why family nursing?" (2015):

Families have inherent competencies, strengths, and unique interactional processes that influence family health beliefs, goals, and actions. All families have the capacity for transforming their quality of life and family health. All verbal & non-verbal family communication is meaningful. All families possess a cultural heritage that is integral to family health and family life.

p. 1

These competencies explain the importance of including families as a population of interest for nurses. Many disciplines are interested in the study of families; interdisciplinary perspectives and strategies are necessary to understand the influence of the family on health and the influence of the broader social system on the family. This chapter addresses how community health nurses (CHNs) work with families within communities to bring about healthy conditions for families at the family, social, and policy levels. It focuses on the following five areas:

- The changing family
- Approaches to meeting the health needs of families
- The family theory approach to meeting the health needs of families
- Extending family health interventions to larger aggregates and social action
- An example of the nursing process applied to a family

THE CHANGING FAMILY

Definition of Family

Many definitions of **family** exist and vary by professional discipline and the type of family described. For example, psychologists may define family in terms of personal development and intrapersonal dynamics; the sociologist has used a classic definition of family in terms of a "social unit interacting with the larger society." Other professionals have classically defined family in terms of kinship, marriage, and choice: "a family is characterized by people together because of birth, marriage, adoption, or choice" (Allen et al., 2000, p. 7). Friedman et al. (2003) incorporate the idea of many nontraditional definitions: "a family is two or more persons who are joined together by bonds of sharing and emotional closeness and who identify themselves as being part of the family" (p. 10). This definition supports the idea of letting the family define their composition and relationships (Shajani and Snell, 2019).

Wright and Leahey (2012, 2019) state "the family is who they say they are" (p. 70). Current advocacy groups find these definitions even too narrow. The Human Rights Campaign (2020a) urges that health professions acknowledge all types of families. The Human Rights Campaign (2020b) urges that health professions acknowledge all types of families, including lesbian, gay, bisexual, transgender, queer/questioning, and others (LGBTQ+) and even grandparents as heads of family by using this definition:

"Family" means any person(s) who plays a significant role in an individual's life. This may include a person(s) not legally related to the individual. Members of "family" include spouses, domestic partners, and both different-sex and same-sex significant others. "Family" includes a minor patient's parents, regardless of the gender of either parent. Solely for purposes of visitation policy, the concept of parenthood is to be liberally construed without limitation as encompassing legal parents, foster parents, same-sex parent, step-parents, those serving in loco parentis, and other persons operating in caretaker roles.

Human Rights Campaign (2020b), Inclusive definition of family.

In the past, the dominant American definition focused on the intact **nuclear family**. African American families focus on a wide network of kin and community. The "nuclear" family does not exist for Italian families. To them, family means a strong, tightly knit, three- or four-generational group that includes godparents and old friends. Some families of early (e.g., first- or second-) generation Chinese Americans go beyond this and include in their definition of family multigenerational family members and ancestors (Li et al., 2009).

The CHN interacts with communities made up of many types of families. When faced with great diversity in the community, the CHN must formulate a personal definition of family and must be aware of the changing definition of family held by other disciplines, professionals, and family groups. The CHN who interacts with Mr. Hudson, the alcoholic described in Clinical Example 20.2 who lives in a hotel, must have a broad conceptualization of the family. That is, the group of people that the patient deems as significant for his or her well-being.

Regardless of the accepted definition of family, what is evident is the importance of the family unit to society. The family fulfills two important purposes. The first is to meet the needs of society, and the second is to meet the needs of individual family members (Friedman et al., 2003). The family meets the needs of society through procreation and socialization of family members. "The basic unit (family) so strongly influences the development of an individual that it may determine the success or failure of that person's life" (Friedman et al., 2003, p. 4). The family is the "buffer" between individuals and society. The family meets individual needs through provision of basic needs (food, shelter, clothing, affection). The family supports spouses or partners by meeting affective, sexual, and socioeconomic needs. For children, the family is the "first teacher," instructing the children in societal rules and providing values needed for growth and development.

Characteristics of the Changing Family

The characteristics of the US family continue to change. According to a report from the Pew Research Center (PRC) (2018), "in 2016, a record 64 million people, or 20% of the U.S. population, lived with multiple generations under one roof." Facts About the Modern American Family:

- Americans are putting off life's big milestones. The median age for first marriage is 29 for men and 27 for women. Less adults are married today with 53% of adults being married compared to 58% in 1995. Cohabitation rates have risen to 7% from 3% in 1995 (Horowitz et al., 2019).
- More young adults, about half, age 18 to 29 years-old are living with their parents (Fry et al., 2020).
- Today, an American woman is expected to have 1.9 children. This is below what is considered "replacement rate" of 2.1 children per woman.
- Three million (37% of lesbian, gay, bisexual, and transgender [LGBT]) will have a child at some point in their life.
- Families are more blended today and constructed differently. Nearly 44% of young people aged 18 to 29 years have a stepsibling. More babies are born to unmarried women than ever before (5% in 1960).
- Intermarriage among people of different races is increasingly common. In 1980 there were only 7% of people who married a spouse of another race, and in 2015 this had percentage risen to 17%. (U.S. Census Bureau, 2019a,b).

The rate of **cohabitation** or living with a partner in an unmarried arrangement, has also increased over time and was more prevalent than living with a spouse in 2018 among those aged 18 to 24 years old (Gurrentz, 2018). The U.S. Census Bureau (2019a,b) reported the number of cohabitating families has almost tripled in the past 2 decades accounts for 7% of the total adult population. This increase has significantly changed the family structure. Adults aged 65 and older have increased in cohabiting from 2% in 1996 to 6% in 2017. Previous households were likely to include a partner holding a bachelor's degree or higher in 1996 (16%); whereas, in 2017, 28% of cohabitating partners held a bachelor's degree or higher (U.S. Census Bureau, 2019a,b; Horowitz et al., 2019). The nurse should be aware of the potential need for additional support and intervention with such families.

The birth rate among teenagers is the lowest it has ever been at 18 births per 1000 girls aged 15 to 19 (Livingston & Thomas, 2019). During the years 1980 to 2006, the birth rate for unmarried women 15 to 17 years of age increased from 21 to 41.9 per 1000 in the United States, before dropping back 23% in 2012, resulting in a rate of 31.3 births per 1000 teens (Guttmacher Institute, 2016). The Annie E. Casey Foundation (2016) reports that the incidence of single teen parenting continues to rise in all ethnic groups. Single parenting is associated with greater risks because of reduced social, emotional, and financial resources, which affect the general well-being of children and families. In 2019, 23% of all US children lived in single-parent homes. Single parenting is a key indicator of risk for well-being in children (Annie E. Casey Foundation, 2013; Kramer, 2019). Fig. 20.1 provides an overview of the declining birth rate by age of mother.

The proportion of children younger than 18 years who are living with their grandparents has increased since 2007 (American Association for Marriage and Family Therapy [AAMFT], 2016). In 2007, grandparent-headed families accounted for 5% of all families; in 2016 census data document that 2.4 million grandparents are raising 4.5 million children (AAMFT, 2016). The American Academy of Child & Adolescent Psychiatry (2016) suggests that parenting by grandparents may be "due to serious societal issues and problems including increasing numbers of single parent families, the high rate of divorce, teenage pregnancies, AIDS, incarcerations of parents, substance abuse by parents, death or disability of parents, parental abuse and neglect" (p. 3).

The gay or lesbian family is made up of a cohabiting couple of the same sex who have a sexual relationship. In 2019, the U.S. Census Bureau reported 1.1 million same-sex couple households, married or cohabiting. Approximately 15% of same-sex couples are raising at least one child. Same-sex couples are more likely to adopt or foster children compared to opposite-sex couples (Taylor, 2020).

APPROACHES TO MEETING THE HEALTH NEEDS OF FAMILIES

Community health nursing has long viewed the family as an important unit of health care, with awareness that the individual can be best understood within the social context of the family.

U.S. teen birth rate has fallen dramatically over time

Births per 1,000 females ages 15–19, 1940–2019

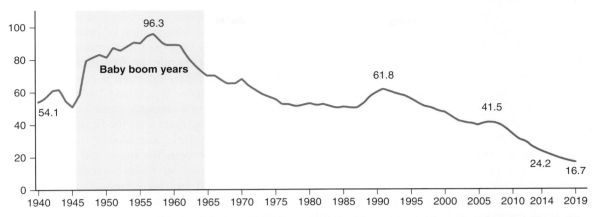

Note: Data labels shown are for 1940, 1957, 1991, 2007, 2014, and 2019. Teens younger than 15 not included. These data only account for live births and do not include miscarriages, stillbirths, or abortions.

Fig. 20.1 US teen birth rate has fallen. (From CDC National Center for Health Statistics: *Births and natality,* 2016. https://www.cdc.gov/nchs/fastats/births.htm.)

Observing and inquiring about family interaction enables the nurse in the community to assess the influence of family members on one another. However, direct intervention at the family rather than the individual client level is a new frontier for many nursing students, most of whom have experience in acute care settings before the community setting. A family model, largely a community health nursing or psychiatric–mental health intervention model, also includes the areas of birthing and parent–child interventions, adult day care, chronic illness, and home care. Nursing assessment and intervention must not stop with the immediate social context of the family; it must also consider the broader social context of the community and society. Friedman and Colleagues (2003, pp. 5–6) suggest reasons why it is important for nurses to work with families:

The family is a critical resource: The importance of the family in providing care for its members has already been established. In this caregiver role, the family can also improve individual members' health through health promotion and wellness activities.

In a family unit any dysfunction (illness, injury, separation) that affects one or more family members will affect the members and unit as a whole: Also referred to as the *ripple effect*, changes in one member cause changes in the entire family unit. The nurse must assess each individual and the family unit.

Case finding is another reason to work with families: As the nurse assesses an individual and family, he or she may identify a health problem that necessitates identifying risks for the entire family.

Improving nursing care: The nurse can provide better and more holistic care by understanding the family and its members.

Moving From Individual to Family

The rationale of Friedman and colleagues (2003) for the importance of moving to family nursing is still relevant.

Community health and home care nurses have traditionally focused on the family as the unit of service. With healthcare system changes throughout the United States, many CHNs continue to focus their practices on individuals residing in the home. As a result of the current era of cost containment, constraints on the CHN and on nurses working within hospitals and in other settings will increase. For example, reimbursement, which is almost entirely calculated for services rendered to the individual, is a major constraint against moving toward planning care for the family as a unit. However, current methods of reimbursing hospitals depend on keeping patients at home, so all nurses must consider the importance of not only the entire healthcare team but also the patient's family unit in meeting health and rehabilitation goals. Moving from individual to family nursing becomes more important than ever. Various creative approaches to meeting the health needs of families are needed, also reflecting interventions appropriate to the needs of the population as a whole.

Family Interviewing

Approaches to the care of families are needed and must be creative, flexible, and transferable from one setting to another. CHNs are generalists who bring previous preparation in communication concepts and interviewing to the family arena. Wright and Leahey (2012) proposed the realm of **family interviewing** rather than family therapy as an appropriate model. In this model, the CHN uses general systems and communication concepts to conceptualize the health needs of families and a family assessment model to assess families' responses to "normative" events such as birth and retirement or to "paranormative" events such as chronic illness and divorce. Intervention is straightforward, as in helping parents educate prepubescent teenage family members about sex by providing appropriate educational materials, or consists of making a referral to another health professional if the level of intervention is beyond the preparation of the nurse. For the purposes of this text, the model is extended to include intervention at the level of the larger aggregate. For example, the index of suspicion based on the health needs of a particular family would prompt the CHN to assess the need for similar information and the resources for intervention with other families in the community, schools, churches, or other institutions. Family interviewing requires thinking "interactionally," not only in terms of the family system, but also in terms of larger social systems.

Wright and Leahey (2005, 2012) identify the following critical components of the family interview: manners, therapeutic conservation and questions, family genogram (and ecomap when indicated), and commendations. Family theorists and practitioners suggest that, with experience, the nurse can accomplish the family interview in 15 min (Bell, 2012; Martinez et al., 2007; Wright and Leahey, 2012).

Manners. Manners are common social behaviors that set the tone for the interview and begin the development of a therapeutic relationship. Wright and Leahey (2012) believe that erosion of these social skills prevents the family nurse from collecting essential data. Many nurses argue that too much formality establishes artificial barriers to communication; however, studies have shown that the essentials of a therapeutic relationship begin with manners. The nurse introduces himself or herself by name and title, always addresses the client (and family members) by name and title (i.e., Mr., Mrs., or Ms., unless otherwise directed by client), keeps appointments, explains the reason for the interview or visit, and brings a positive attitude. Other behaviors (manners) that invite rapport include being honest with the client and checking attitude (the nurse's) before each client encounter.

Therapeutic Conversations. The second key element in the interview is the therapeutic conversation. This type of conversation is focused and planned and engages the family. The nurse must listen and must remember that even one sentence has the potential to heal or help a family member. The nurse encourages questions, engages the family in the interview and assessment process, and commends the family when strengths are identified. Every encounter, whether brief or extended, has "healing potential." Therapeutic conversation may initiate further discussion that brings the family together on issues (Wright and Leahey, 2012). Bell (2016) suggests that therapeutic conversations are "contextually sensitive to language, culture, setting, time available, and theoretical orientation" (p. 442) and are practiced and intentional.

Genogram and Ecomap. The genogram and ecomap constitute the third element and are described in detail later in this chapter. These tools provide essential information on family structure and together are an efficient way to gather information such as family composition, background, and basic health status in a way that engages the family in the interview process.

Therapeutic Questions. Therapeutic questions are key questions that the nurse uses to facilitate the interview. The questions are specific for the context or family situation but have the following basic themes (Wright and Leahey, 2012): family expectations of the interview or home visit; challenges, concerns, and problems encountered by the family at the time of the interview; and sharing of information (e.g., who will relate the family history or information).

Commending Family or Individual Strengths. The fifth element of the family interview is commending the family or individual strengths. Wright and Leahy (2012) suggest identifying at least two strength areas and, during each family interview, sharing them with the family or individual. Sharing strengths reinforces immediate and long-term positive relationships between the nurse and family. Interviews that identify and build on family strengths tend to progress to more open and trusting relationships and often allow the family to reframe problems, thereby increasing problem solving and healing (Wright and Leahey, 2012).

Issues in Family Interviewing. Creative family interviewing requires interviewing families in many types of settings. The prediction of decreased hospitalization, supplemented by a wide variety of healthcare settings ranging from acute to ambulatory to community centers, calls for flexible, transferable approaches. Clinical settings for family interviewing are reviewed by Wright and Leahey (2012) and include inpatient and outpatient ambulatory care and clinical settings in maternity, pediatrics, medicine, surgery, critical care, and mental health. According to Wright and Leahey, CHNs have many opportunities besides the traditional home visit to engage the family in a family interview. CHNs are employed in ambulatory care centers, occupational health and school sites, housing complexes, day care programs, residential treatment and substance abuse programs, and other official and nonofficial agencies. At each of these sites, CHNs meet families and can assess and intervene at the family and community levels.

The family interview assists the nurse in identifying family health risks because the family experiences similar risk factors (i.e., physiological, behavioral, and environmental). Studies have documented the familial predisposition to the three major diseases resulting in morbidity and mortality in the United States: cardiac disease, cancer, and diabetes. Family health practices also influence lifestyle habits among family members. Recognizing the importance of a family health history related to individual and public health, the U.S. Surgeon General initiated the National Family History Initiative in 2003 with a goal to educate individuals about inherited predispositions to disease (McNeill et al., 2008). This website has proved to be successful in engaging American families in learning about their family history and familial and genetic health risk for family members. The project was renamed "My Family Health Portrait Tool" and has been redesigned to be more user friendly for individuals (USDHHS, 2017). Another example would be a Hispanic American family in which a family member has diabetes; the nurse could implement a family health promotion plan based on the needs of the individual within an at-risk family. The family plan for diabetes prevention is based on the nurse's understanding that the National Institutes of Health (NIH, 2015) reports that this group has the second highest rate of diabetes among a nonwhite ethnic group in the United States (Spanakis and Golden, 2013) (Table 20.3).

Involving family members in newborn assessments can aid the CHN in determining the family's adjustment to the newborn and parenthood. The nurse can do this in the home, clinic, or other healthcare center. Family members should be involved during the first contact or visit, and, if they do not attend, a telephone call explaining the nurse's interest in them should take place (Wright and Leahey, 2012).

Children and parents in these families need a chance to express their concerns; the family interview is important and may provide the nurse with necessary information needed to care for these families.

Intervention in Cases of Chronic Illness

The Centers for Disease Control and Prevention (CDC) (2017) reports that as many as 90% of families are dealing with chronic illness in a family member. Chronic disease is responsible for 7 to 10 deaths, and the care of chronic disease uses 86% of the nation's healthcare costs (CDC, 2017). For the family with a member who has a chronic illness, it is important to the individual's and family's adjustment, as well as to the patient's symptom management, that the family is prepared to be emotionally and physically supportive. The CHN can intervene to assist the family coping with related stressors. Also significant is the fact that a resource such as third-party reimbursement forces most families to learn to manage the chronic problems with limited or infrequent intervention from health professionals. The CHN working with families coping with chronic illness in a child, adult, or older adult is aided by the family interview. As Glaser and Strauss (1975) stated, chronic illness injects change into various areas of family life:

Sex and intimacy can be affected. Everyday mood and interpersonal relations can be affected. Visiting friends and engaging in other leisure time activities can be affected. Conflicts can be engendered by increased expenses stemming from unemployment and the medical treatment ... [D]ifferent illnesses may have different kinds of impact on such areas of family life, just as they probably will call for different kinds of helpful agents.

(p. 67)

Changes in family patterns, fears, emotional responses, and expectations of individual family members can be assessed in the family interview. Special needs of the primary caretaker (i.e., often the spouse, daughter, or daughter-in-law) can be assessed. The CHN making family visits to older adults and the terminally ill is able to assess intergenerational conflict and stress and positively influence family interaction (Wright and Leahey, 2012).

Moving From Family to Community

The health of families can affect the health of society as a whole, in both positive and negative ways. The health of a community is measured by the well-being of its people and families.

TABLE 20.3 Age-Adjusted Prevalence of Diabetes Mellitus in the United States by Race/Ethnicity in Adults >18 Years of Age, 2017–18	
Race/Ethnic Group	**Age-Adjusted Prevalence**
Non-Hispanic whites	7.5
Asian Americans	9.2
Hispanic Americans overall	12.5
Non-Hispanic Blacks	11.7
American Indian/Alaskan Natives	14.7

CDC: *National diabetes statistics report,* 2020. Available from: https://www.cdc.gov/diabetes/pdfs/data/statistics/national-diabetes-statistics-report.pdf.

Circumstances such as low-birth-weight infants, lack of health insurance, homelessness, violence, poverty, and low employment rates provide a description of families and nations. CHNs provide family nursing to improve individual and family health; however, the potential result may be improving the health of society. The care of entire populations is the major focus, as stated by Freeman (1963) in her classic work, *Public Health Nursing Practice:*

The selection of those to be served ... must rest on the comparative impact on community health rather than solely on the needs of the individual or family being served ... The public health nurse cannot elect to care for a small number of people intensely while ignoring the needs of many others. She must be concerned with the population as a whole, with those in her caseload, with the need of a particular family as compared to the needs of others in the community.

(p. 35)

The challenge to the CHN is to provide care to communities and populations and not to focus only on the levels of the individual and the family. The CHN, who traditionally carries a caseload of families, extends his or her practice to the community. To do so, an aggregate, community, and population focus must serve as a backdrop to the entire practice.

For example, families must be viewed as components of communities. The CHN must know the community. As stated in previous chapters, a thorough community assessment is necessary to practice in the community. By way of review, the nurse must remember that communities must be compared not only in terms of different health needs but also in terms of different resources to effect interventions that influence policies and redistribute resources to ensure that community and family health needs are met.

CHNs must then compare city data with county data and then county data with state data and national data. In addition, they may need to compare local census tract data and areas of a city or county with other areas of the city or county. For example, community health nursing students in San Antonio, Texas, who were planning home visits to families of pregnant adolescents attending a special high school compared local, state, and national statistics on infant mortality rates as part of a community assessment. They found higher rates of infant mortality in San Antonio in census tracts on the south side of the city, in which the population was predominantly Mexican American. They also found this population to be younger, to have a higher rate of functional illiteracy among adults, to be less educated, to be more likely to drop out of high school, to have higher fertility rates, to have higher birth rates among adolescents, and to be more likely to be unemployed. They found that specific health needs varied among census tracts. Common major health needs of this subpopulation were identified from the community assessment, which helped the students plan care for these families. For example, their goals were broadened from carrying out interventions at the individual level to interventions at the family and community levels. In addition to targeting good perinatal outcomes for the individual teenage parent, nursing students planned to include assessments of functional literacy at the individual and family levels and arranged for group sessions in clinic waiting rooms that offered information about and referral of individuals and family members to alternative resources to enable teenage parents to complete school, take classes in English as a second language, and use resources for family planning and employment at the community level.

In addition to the cross-comparison of communities, the CHN cross compares the needs of the families within the communities and sets priorities. The nurse in the community finds that specific health needs vary among families. The nurse must account for time spent with families and choose those families on the basis of their needs in comparison with the needs of others in the community.

♥ HEALTHY PEOPLE 2030

Access to Health Care

In relation to improving family health, all of the leading health indicators listed as priorities in *Healthy People 2030* can serve as a guide for family nursing interventions. Access to quality healthcare affects every aspect of family nursing because it affects prevention of disease and disability, quality of life, preventable death, and overall life expectancy. The objectives for measurement of this goal include the following:
- Increase the proportion of persons with health insurance.
- Increase the proportion of insured persons with coverage for clinical preventive services.
- Increase the proportion of persons with a usual primary care provider.
- Increase the proportion of persons who have a specific ongoing care.

Data from U.S. Department of Health and Human Services: *Healthy People 2020: objectives.* Available from: https://health.gov/healthypeople/objectives-and-data/browse-objectives/health-care-access-and-quality. (Accessed September 18, 2021).

This chapter has discussed the disparities that exist among families and populations with regard to healthcare access. The community nurse should use political skills, advocacy, and education to influence policy that will result in increased access to health care. The nurse can educate families about available resources and help communities develop resources to improve healthcare access.

Delegation of Scarce Resources

Although the CHN serves the community or population as a whole, fiscal constraints hold the nurse accountable for the best delegation of scarce resources. Time spent on home visits has traditionally allowed the CHN to assess the environmental, social, and biological determinants of health status among the population and the resources available to them. Fiscal accountability, nevertheless, means setting priorities. In 1985, Anderson and colleagues listed the factors that influence public health nursing practice, especially home visits, as "the need to justify personnel costs in a time of fiscal constraint, the increasing number of medically indigent who turn to local public health services for primary care, and the change in reimbursement mechanisms by the federal government and some states" (p. 146). These observations still hold true. In 2010 the number of uninsured rose to 49.9 million, or 16.3% of the US population; however, by 2018 there was a drop to 27.5 million, or 8.5% (Berchick et al., 2018) This drop is attributed to the increase in the number of young adults ages 19 to 26 who could for the first time remain on their parent's primary insurance following graduation from college. The Children's Health Insurance Program (CHIP) of 1997 has greatly increased access to health care for many low-income children. When the CHIP program was initiated, there were 10 million children in the United States and 14% were uninsured; in 2008, 7.4 million children were enrolled in state CHIP plans (Centers for Medicare and Medicaid Services, 2015). The majority of these children lived in families with working, low-income parents. On February 4, 2009, President Obama signed the Children's Health Insurance Program Reauthorization Act, which renewed and expanded coverage of CHIP from 7 million children to 11 million children. The Affordable Care Act of 2010 keeps the CHIP program in place until 2019 (Medicaid.gov, n.d.).

? ACTIVE LEARNING

Define the term *family* with a group of three colleagues. Compare definitions and list similarities and differences. Develop a list of criteria for being a member of a family.

APPROACHES TO FAMILY HEALTH

Many schools of thought regarding the approaches to meeting family health needs exist among community health, community mental health, and public health nursing professionals. Dreher (1982) wrote that the traditional basis for community health nursing intervention has a focus that has long endorsed psychological and social-psychological theories to explain variations in health and patterns of health care, such as those set forth by Erikson (1963), Maslow (1970), and Duvall (1977). Dreher (1982) stated that what is needed are "more encompassing theories which explain the relationship between society and health [and] the policies which will be most effective in assuring health and health care" (p. 508). To help bridge this gap, four frameworks for meeting family health needs are presented here: family theory, systems theory, structural-functional conceptual framework, and developmental theory.

Family Theory

Many reasons exist for why the CHN should work with families. Friedman (1998) listed the following six reasons:

- Any "dysfunction" (e.g., separation, disease, or injury) that affects one or more family members probably affects other family members and the family as a whole (Clinical Example 20.5).
- The wellness of the family is highly dependent on the role of the family in every aspect of health care, from prevention to rehabilitation.
- The level of wellness of the whole family can be raised through care that reduces lifestyle and environmental risks by emphasizing "health promotion, 'self-care,' health education, and family counseling" (p. 5).
- Commonalities in risk factors and diseases shared by family members can lead to case finding within the family.
- A clear understanding of the functioning of the individual can be gained only when the individual is assessed within the larger context of the family.
- The family as a vital support system to the individual member needs to be incorporated into treatment plans.

Nurses have relied heavily on the social and behavioral sciences for approaches to working with families. These approaches include psychoanalytical, anthropological, systems or cybernetic, structural-functional, developmental, and interactional frameworks (for reviews, see Friedman et al., 2003; and Wright and Leahey, 2012). The use of a framework for assessing a family helps the nurse understand the health potential for the family. Three conceptual frameworks (systems, structural-functional, and developmental), often used by nurses in providing health care to families, are described here. These models help the nurse empower the family in the process of family health promotion.

Clinical Example 20.5

Ten-year-old Jean Wilkie was referred by her teacher to the school nurse. She was withdrawn, had no school friends, and was dropping behind in her schoolwork. The school nurse talked to Jean in her office. Jean said that she had no friends because the other girls stayed overnight with one another "all the time" and that she did not want to bring her friends home because her father "drank all the time." The school nurse decided that Jean's problems needed assessment within the context of the family and arranged to visit the family at home. The father refused to participate in the family interview, but Jean's mother, her 13-year-old brother Peter, and Jean expressed concerns that the father had changed jobs several times in the past year, was frequently absent from work, and had been in two recent car accidents while "drinking." The school nurse was able to verify the family context as the basis of Jean's "problems," continue her family assessment, and plan for intervention at the family level. In addition, she was prompted to assess the community's preventive efforts directed toward drinking and the ability to provide ongoing care for families of alcoholics.

Systems Theory

The systems approach has been used in such diverse areas as education, computer science, engineering, and communication. **General systems theory** (Minuchin, 2002; von Bertalanffy, 1968, 1972, 1974) has been applied to the study of families. General systems theory is a way to explain how the family as a unit interacts with larger units outside the family and with smaller units inside the family (Friedman et al., 2003). The family may be affected by any disrupting force acting on a system outside the family (i.e., suprasystem) or on a system within the family (i.e., subsystem). Parke (2002) stated that there are three subsystems of the family that are most important: parent–child subsystem, marital subsystem, and sibling–sibling subsystem. Dunst and Trivette (2009) reviewed 20 years of systems theory and its importance to early childhood interventions, adding that systems theory provides direction for understanding how healthcare providers can expand family capacity by changing parenting and therefore changing child behaviors. Table 20.4 presents definitions of the major terms used in the systems approach.

The past 2 decades have resulted in what many sociologists identify as imposing community subsystems with actual or potential negative influence on the family system. These include communities where violence has become the norm, dangers related to community-acquired diseases—both manmade and natural, disasters, biohazards, and so on. These subsystems have the potential to complicate the care planned by the CHN and require interventions from several subsystems interacting with the family system and community. It is important that the CHN understand systems theory as a tool for both assessing families and communities and identifying resources and support services for families.

Characteristics of Healthy Families

Otto (1973) and Pratt (1976) characterized healthy families as "energized families" and provided descriptions of healthy families to guide the assessment of strengths and coping. DeFrain (1999) and Montalvo (2004) helped identify healthy families. These writers suggest the following traits of a healthy family:

- Members interact with one another; they communicate and listen repeatedly in many contexts.
- Healthy families can establish priorities. Members understand that family needs are priority.
- Healthy families affirm, support, and respect each other.
- The members engage in flexible role relationships, share power, respond to change, support the growth and autonomy of others, and engage in decision making that affects them.
- The family teaches family and societal values and beliefs and shares a religious core.
- Healthy families foster responsibility and value service to others.
- Healthy families have a sense of play and humor and share leisure time.

TABLE 20.4 Major Definitions From Systems Theory

Term	Definition
System	"A goal-directed unit made up of interdependent, interacting parts which endure over a period of time" (Friedman et al., 1992, p. 115). A family system is not concrete. It is made up of suprasystems and subsystems and must be viewed in a hierarchy of systems. The system under study at any given time is called the focal, or target, system. In this chapter, the family system is the focal system.
Suprasystem	The larger system of which the family is a part, such as the larger environment or the community (e.g., churches, schools, clubs, businesses, neighborhood organizations, and gangs).
Subsystem	Smaller unit within the family, such as the relationship between spouses, parent and child, sibling and sibling, or extended family.
Hierarchy of systems	The levels of units within the system and its environment, which, in their totality, make up the universe. Higher-level units are composed of lower-level units (e.g., the biosphere is made up of communities, which are made up of families). Families are made up of family subsystems, and, in turn, family subsystems are made up of individuals, who are made up of organs, which are made of cells, which are made of atoms.
Boundary	An imaginary definitive line that forms a circle around each system and delineates the system from its environment. Auger (1976) conceptualized the boundary of a system as a "filter" that permits the constant exchange of elements, information, or energy between the system and its environments. "The more porous the filter, the greater the degree of interaction possible between the system and its environment" (p. 24). Families with rigid boundaries may lack information necessary and resources pertinent to maintaining family health or wellness.
Open system	A system that interacts with its surrounding environment and gives outputs and receives inputs necessary to survival. An exchange of energy occurs. All living systems are open systems. However, if a boundary is too permeable, the system may be too open to input of new ideas from the outside and may be unable to make decisions on its own (Wright and Leahey, 1994).
Closed system	A system that theoretically does not interact with the environment. This is a self-sufficient system; no energy exchange occurs. Although no system has been found that exists in a totally closed state, if a family's boundaries are impermeable (i.e., less open as a system), needed input or interaction cannot occur. An example is a refugee family from Vietnam living in San Francisco; they may remain a closed family for some time because of their differences in culture and language.
Input	Information, matter, or energy that the open system receives from its environment that is necessary for survival.
Output	Information, matter, or energy dispensed into the environment as a result of receiving and processing the input.
Flow and transformation	The system's use of input may occur in two forms. Some input may be used in its original state, and some input may have to be transformed before it is used. Both original and transformed input must be processed and flow through the system before being released as output (Friedman et al., 1992).
Feedback	"The process by which a system monitors the internal and environmental responses to its behavior (i.e., output) and accommodates or adjusts itself" (Friedman et al., 1992, p. 117). The system controls and modifies inputs and outputs by "receiving and responding to the return of its own output" (Friedman et al., 1992, p. 117). Internally, the system adjusts by making changes in its subsystems. Externally, the system adjusts by making boundary changes.
Equilibrium	A state of balance or steady state that results from self-regulation or adaptation. As with the concept of a system as a mobile in the wind, balance is dynamic and, with change, is always reestablishing itself.
Differentiation	The tendency for a system to actively grow and "advance to a higher order of complexity and organization" (Friedman et al., 1992, p. 117). Energy inputs into the system make this growth possible.
Energy	Energy is needed to meet a system's demands. Open systems require more input through porous boundaries to meet the high energy levels necessary to maintain high levels of activity.

- Healthy families have the ability to cope with stress and crisis and to grow as a result of positive coping. They know when to seek help from professionals.

Structural-Functional Conceptual Framework

With the structural-functional conceptual framework approach, the family is viewed according to its structure, or the parts of the system, and according to its functions, or how the family fulfills its roles.

Structural

Wright and Leahey (2005, 2012) stated that three aspects of family structure can be examined (internal structure, external structure, and context). **Internal structure** of the family refers to the following five categories:

- Family composition, the family members, and changes in family constellation
- Gender
- Rank order, or positions of family members by age and sex
- Subsystem, or labeling of the subgroups or dyads (e.g., spouse, parental, and interest) through which the family carries out its functions
- Boundary, or who participates in the family system and how he or she participates (e.g., a single-parent mother who does not allow her 17-year-old son to have his girlfriend spend the night in their home)

External structure refers to the extended family and larger systems (Wright and Leahey, 2005). It consists of the following two categories:

- Extended family, including family of origin and family of procreation

- Larger systems, such as work, health, and welfare

Context refers to the background or situation relevant to an event or personality in which the family system is nested (Wright and Leahey, 2005, 2012). It comprises the following five categories:

- Ethnicity
- Race
- Social class
- Religion
- Environment

Functional

Wright and Leahey (2005, 2012) also dichotomized family functional assessment, or how family members behave toward one another, into two categories: instrumental functioning and expressive functioning. **Instrumental functioning** refers to routine activities of daily living (e.g., elimination, sleeping, eating, giving insulin injections) (Box 20.1). This area takes on important meaning for the family when one member of the family becomes ill or disabled, is unable to carry out daily functions, and must rely on other members of the family for assistance (Clinical Example 20.6). For example, an older adult may need assistance getting into the bathtub, or a child may need to have medications measured and administered.

The second type of family functional assessment is **expressive functioning**, or affective or emotional aspects. This aspect has the following nine categories:

- *Emotional communication*: Is the family able to express a range of emotions, including happiness, sadness, and anger?
- *Verbal communication* focuses on the meaning of words. Do messages have clear meanings rather than distorted meanings? Wright and Leahey (2005, 2012) gave the example of masked criticism when a father states to his child, "Children who cry when they get needles are babies."
- *Nonverbal communication*, which includes sounds, gestures, eye contact, touch, or inaction. An example is a husband remaining silent and staring out the window while his wife is talking to him.
- *Circular communication* is commonly observed between dyads in families. A common example is the blaming, nagging wife and the guilty, withdrawn husband.
- *Problem solving* refers to how the family solves problems. Who identifies problems? Someone inside or outside the family? What kinds of problems are solved? What patterns are used to solve and evaluate tried solutions?
- *Roles* refers to established patterns of behavior for family members (Wright and Leahey, 2000, 2012). Roles may be developed, delegated, negotiated, and renegotiated within the family. It takes other family members to keep a person in a particular role. Formal roles, with which the larger community agrees, may come into conflict with roles set by family members and influenced by religious, cultural, and other belief systems.
- *Influence* refers to methods used to affect the behavior of another. Instrumental influence is the use of reinforcement

BOX 20.1 Summary of Family Functional Assessment

Instrumental functioning (i.e., activities of daily living)
Expressive functioning
   Emotional communication
   Verbal communication
   Nonverbal communication
   Circular communication
   Problem-solving
   Roles
   Influence
   Beliefs
   Alliances and coalitions

Data from Wright LM, Leahey M: *Nurses and families: a guide to family assessment and intervention*, ed 2, Philadelphia, 1994, FA Davis.

via objects or privileges (e.g., money or use of technology tools). Psychological influence is the influence of behavior through the use of communication or feelings. Corporeal control is the use of body contact (e.g., hugging and spanking).

- *Beliefs* refer to assumptions, ideas, and opinions that are held by family members and the family as a whole. Beliefs shape the way families react to chronic or life-threatening illness. For example, if a family of a person with colon cancer believes in alternative treatments, then acupuncture may be a viable option.
- *Alliances and coalitions* are important within the family. What dyads or triads appear to occur repeatedly in the family? Who starts arguments between dyads? Who stops arguments or fighting between dyads? Is there evidence of mother and father against child? When does this change to parent and child against the other parent? The balance and intensity of relationships between subsystems within the family are important. Questions may be asked regarding the permeability of the boundary. Does it cross generations?

Clinical Example 20.6

When Edna Smith, a 64-year-old client with severe arthritis, received a diagnosis of diabetes, her longtime friend, Frank Gardens, a widower of several years, moved in with her and assumed a caregiver role. The CHN assessed the dietary habits of Mr. Gardens and Mrs. Smith and found that Mr. Gardens did the shopping and the cooking because Mrs. Smith's mobility was severely restricted by her arthritis. Mr. Gardens did the cooking; therefore, he purchased canned fruits and vegetables rather than fresh or frozen. Mr. Gardens perceived cooking, which was a new role for him, as demanding. After several visits, he disclosed to the nurse that his resistance to preparing fresh or frozen fruits and vegetables came from "the time it takes to clean the darn things, cook 'em, store 'em, and clean up the fridge when they go bad on ya." He stated unequivocally that it was stressful caring for Mrs. Smith and that he wanted to do it, but it was "much easier" to just "open a can" and "heat it in a pan" than to take the time and energy that preparation of fresh or frozen foods would require. The shift in roles that is often

Continued

Clinical Example 20.6—cont'd

required of couples when a chronic illness is diagnosed in one can have an influence on the health of the family. Lubkin and Larsen (2013) provide additional reading about how couples manage with chronic illness.

Developmental Theory

Nurses are familiar with developmental states of individuals from prenatal through adult. Duvall, a noted sociologist, is the forerunner of a focus on family development (Duvall and Miller, 1985). In her classic work, she identified stages that normal families traverse from marriage to death (Box 20.2).

To assess the family, the CHN must comprehend these phases and the struggles that families experience while going through them. Wright and Leahey (2005, 2012) called attention to the need to distinguish between "family development" and "family life cycle." They stated that the former is the individual, unique path that a family goes through, whereas the latter is the typical path many families go through.

The developmental categories listed in Box 20.3 outline the six stages of the middle-class North American family life cycle (Carter and McGoldrick, 1988; Wright and Leahey, 2005) and the tasks necessary for the family's resolution of each stage. Nurses may use the stages to delineate family strengths and weaknesses.

⚡ RESEARCH HIGHLIGHTS

Work Hours and Perceived Time Barriers to Healthful Eating Among Young Adults.

Young adults, though identified as underinsured and having limited access to primary care, are also identified as a group knowledgeable about the benefits of healthy eating. This age group (20—31 years) has been confirmed in numerous national surveys as not regularly engaging in healthy eating habits, especially eating fewer than the recommended daily servings of fruits and vegetables and consuming a diet high in fast foods. Earlier studies among college students identified the following barriers: cost, stress, lack of knowledge related to food preparation, peer influence, and lack of time to balance busy lives.

A population study survey involved responses from 2287 individuals who were originally among a population of 4776 high school juniors and seniors participating in a program called Project EAT-III (Eating and Activity in Teens and Young Adults), a program that looked at dietary intake, weight control, and weight control behaviors during 1998 and 1999. Ten years later, the original participants were mailed letters asking them to participate in a new questionnaire, to which 1030 men and 1257 women agreed. Information was collected on time-related beliefs and behaviors about healthful eating, their fast-food intake, fruit and vegetable intake, work hours, and sociodemographics.

This group reported time-related beliefs such as being too rushed to eat breakfast, eating on the run, and no time to eat healthy. They reported eating fast food weekly. Working at least 40 h per week was associated with an increase in time-related poor eating habits for men but not for women. Recommendations included workplace programs—free fruit and vegetables for break, flex time, and other interventions.

Data from Escoto KH, et al.: Work hours and perceived time barriers to healthful eating among young adults. *Am J Health Behav* 36(3): 786—789, 2012.

BOX 20.2 Family Life Cycle

1. Leaving home
2. Beginning family through marriage or commitment as a couple relationship
3. Parenting the first child
4. Living with adolescent(s)
5. Launching family (youngest child leaves home)
6. Middle-aged family (remaining marital dyad to retirement)
7. Aging family (from retirement to death of both spouses)

Adapted from Duvall EM, Miller BC: *Marriage and family development*, ed 6, New York, 1985, Harper and Row; and Carter B, McGoldrick M: *The expanded family life cycle: individual, family, and social perspectives*, Boston, 2005, Pearson Allyn & Bacon.

BOX 20.3 Stages and Tasks of Middle-Class North American Family Life Cycle

I. Launching: single young adult leaves home
 A. Coming to terms with the family of origin
 B. Development of intimate relationships with peers
 C. Establishment of self: career and finances
II. Marriage: joining of families
 A. Formation of identity as a couple
 B. Inclusion of spouse in realignment of relationships with extended families
 C. Parenthood: making decisions
III. Families with young children
 A. Integration of children into family unit
 B. Adjustment of tasks: child rearing, financial, and household
 C. Accommodation of new parenting and grandparenting roles
IV. Families with adolescents
 A. Development of increasing autonomy for adolescents
 B. Midlife reexamination of marital and career issues
 C. Initial shift toward concern for the older generation
V. Families as launching centers
 A. Establishment of independent identities for parents and grown children
 B. Renegotiation of marital relationship
 C. Readjustment of relationships to include in-laws and grandchildren
 D. Dealing with disabilities and death of older generation
VI. Aging families
 A. Maintenance of couple and individual functioning while adapting to the aging process
 B. Support role of middle generation
 C. Support and autonomy of older generation
 D. Preparation for own death and dealing with the loss of spouse and/or siblings and other peers

Data from Wright LM, Leahey M: *Nurses and families: a guide to family assessment and intervention*, ed 2, Philadelphia, 1994, FA Davis.

ASSESSMENT TOOLS

There are many tools for the CHN to use in assessing the family (Butler, 2008; Friedman et al., 2003; Wright and Leahey, 2005, 2012). Reviewed here are the genogram, family health tree, and ecomap. The nurse can use these tools for assessment with families in every healthcare setting. They help increase the nurse's awareness of the family within the community and help guide the nurse and the family in the assessment and planning phases of care.

Genogram

The **genogram** is a tool that helps the nurse outline the family's structure. It is a way to diagram the family. Generally, three generations of family members are included in a family tree, with symbols (Fig. 20.2) denoting genealogy. Children are pictured from left to right, beginning with the oldest child.

The CHN may use the genogram during an early family interview, starting with a blank sheet of paper and drawing a circle or a square for the person initially interviewed. The nurse tells the family that he or she will ask several background questions to gain a general picture of the family. The nurse may draw circles around family members living in separate households.

For example, as depicted in the Case Study at the end of the chapter, family order across generations can be illustrated and specific personal characteristics can be noted in the drawing (Fig. 20.3). Mr. and Mrs. Garcia do not speak English, a factor that will be of importance to the nurse as he or she plans nursing interventions. At times, the usefulness of the genogram is limited by how freely the family member relates significant information such as divorces and remarriages and family health concerns. Other families may be sensitive to the sharing of such information, particularly when it is shown to recur with each generation. For example, a family history of alcohol or substance abuse or depression may be a sensitive issue. For other families, the development of the genogram is an excellent

opening to the discussion of family history or hereditary health problems, or highlights the need for health education and promotion.

Family Health Tree

The **family health tree** is another tool that is helpful to the CHN. Based on the genogram, the family health tree provides a mechanism for recording the family's medical and health histories (Butler, 2008; Friedman, 2003, 1992; USDHHS, 2017). The nurse should note the following information on the family health tree:

- Causes of death of deceased family members
- Genetically linked diseases, including heart disease, cancer, diabetes, hypertension, sickle cell anemia, allergies, asthma, and mental retardation
- Environmental and occupational diseases
- Psychosocial problems, such as mental illness and obesity
- Infectious diseases
- Familial risk factors from health problems
- Risk factors associated with the family's methods of illness prevention, such as having periodic physical examinations, Papanicolaou smears, and immunizations
- Lifestyle-related risk factors (elicited by asking what family members do to "handle stress" and "keep in shape")

The family health tree can be used in planning positive familial influences on risk factors such as diet, exercise, coping with stress, and the pressure to have a physical examination. The USDHHS (2017), under the direction of U.S. Surgeon General Richard Carmona, launched the Family History

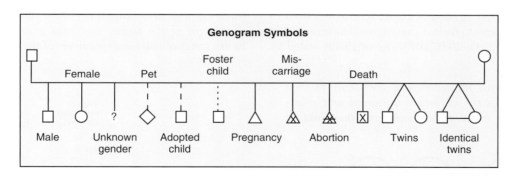

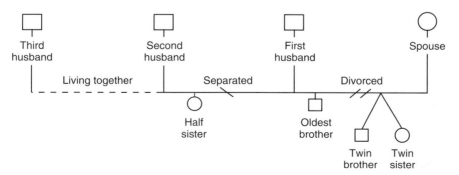

Fig. 20.2 Commonly used genogram symbols. (Redrawn from Genopro Software: *Symbols used in genograms, 2016.* www.genopro.com.)

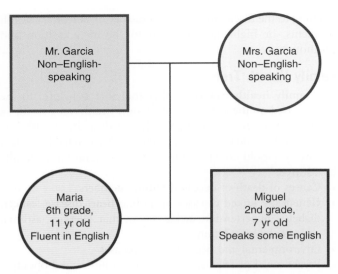

Fig. 20.3 Sample genogram of the Garcia family (see Case Study).

Initiative. Included in this initiative is an online interactive tool, My Family Health Portrait, to help families learn about their risk for disease (https://phgkb.cdc.gov/FHH/html/index.html). Included are questions to ask family members about common diseases, questions that suggest health promotion activities, and goals as established in *Healthy People 2030*. When completed, the "family tree" can be printed. This tool could be incorporated into the family assessment and utilized by the nurse to plan family interventions to improve health.

Ecomap

The **ecomap** (Fig. 20.4) is another classic tool that is used to depict a family's linkages to their suprasystems (Hartman, 1979; Wright and Leahey, 2000, 2005, 2012). As originally stated by Hartman (1979),

> The ecomap portrays an overview of the family in their situation; it depicts the important nurturant or conflict-laden connections between the family and the world. It

demonstrates the flow of resources, or the lacks and depri-vations. This mapping procedure highlights the nature of the interfaces and points to conflicts to be mediated, bridges to be built, and resources to be sought and mobilized.

(p. 467)

As with the genogram, the nurse can fill out the ecomap during an early family interview, noting people, institutions, and agencies significant to the family. The nurse can employ symbols used in attachment diagrams (see Fig. 20.2) to denote the nature of the ties that exist. For example, in Fig. 20.5, the sample ecomap of the Garcia family suggests that few contacts occur between the family and the suprasystems. The community health nursing student was able to use the ecomap to discuss with the Garcia family the types of resources available in the community and the types of relationships they wanted to establish with them.

❓ ACTIVE LEARNING

Complete a personal genogram. What are the high-risk factors in the family history? Current risk factors? Categorize current risk factors into physical, interpersonal, and environmental. Identify needed health education and determine who needs the education. Identify sources of appropriate screening in the community for the identified risk factors.

Complete a personal ecomap. Is the family an "open" or "closed" family system? What resources do families currently use for mental, physical, emotional, social, and community health? What referrals are needed?

FAMILY HEALTH ASSESSMENT

Many agencies in the community have developed guidelines for assessment of the family that help practitioners identify the health status of individual members of the family and aspects of

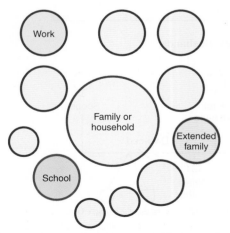

Fig. 20.4 Ecomap. (Redrawn from Hartman A: Diagrammatic assessment of family relationships, *Soc Casework* 59:496, 1978.)

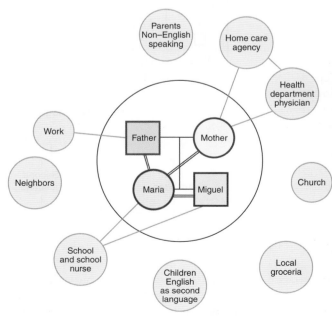

Fig. 20.5 Sample ecomap of the Garcia family (see Case Study).

family composition, function, and process. Often included in family health assessment guidelines is information about the environment, or community context, and information about family. A **family health assessment** form can be used as a guide to help the nurse with both collection of data and organization of the data collected from families over time.

The nurse can obtain information for the family health assessment through interviews with one or more family members individually, or with interviews of subsystems within the family, for example, mother–child, parent–parent, and sibling–sibling dyads. The nurse can also obtain information through observing the environment in which the family lives, including housing, the neighborhood, and the larger community.

Family assessment tools are used with many health disciplines and are useful to assess a range of dimensions of the family, such as marital satisfaction, parental coping abilities, and family dysfunction.

The family health assessment addresses family characteristics, including structure and process and family environment (i.e., residence, neighborhood, and community). Not all dimensions of the family health assessment will be appropriate for every family; therefore, the nurse should modify content of the assessment guidelines and adapt it as necessary to fit the individual family. The guidelines are a means to record pertinent information about the family that will assist the nurse in working with them. The nurse should gather information in the assessment spontaneously over several contacts with the family and various members and dyads within the family. It should also include multiple forays into the community, neighborhood, and home in which the family resides. Several contacts with the family will be required to complete the family health assessment.

Social and Structural Constraints

In addition to the tools just reviewed, an important aspect of family assessment and planning for intervention is the need to make note of the social and structural constraints that prevent families from receiving needed health care or achieving a state of health. These constraints explain why some families differ in mortality rates, ability to achieve "integrity" rather than "despair," or ability to "self-actualize." Social and structural constraints are usually based on social and economic causes, which affect a wide range of conditions (e.g., literacy, education, and employment) associated with major health indicators (i.e., mortality and morbidity rates). Families frequently served by the CHN are disadvantaged in that they lack the financial resources to purchase health care. However, constraints to obtaining needed health and social services are well documented and may come from characteristics of health and social services rather than individual family limitations. The nurse can note these constraints on the ecomap because they influence each family's ability to interact with a specific agency. For example, in addition to noting the strength of the relationship between family and agency or institution, the nurse should note those constraints that prevent use of the resource. Constraints include hours of service, transportation, availability of

interpreters, and criteria for receiving services (e.g., age, sex, and income barriers). Specific examples are the different guidelines posed by each state for Medicaid and by each community for home-delivered meals to the homebound.

Helping families understand constraints and linking them to accessible resources is necessary, but intervention at the family level is not sufficient. The common basic human needs of families in a community add up, and the CHN must tally structural constraints faced repeatedly by families and compare them with those faced by families in other communities. The nurse can then plan and implement interventions at the aggregate level. The following section is an overview of how CHNs can extend intervention at the family level to larger aggregates and social action.

> **? ACTIVE LEARNING**
>
> Identify family types or situations (e.g., families of different cultures, gay or lesbian families, or never-married-mother families) that elicit "discomfort" in working situations. Identify ways to overcome barriers in working with these types of families.

EXTENDING FAMILY HEALTH INTERVENTION TO LARGER AGGREGATES AND SOCIAL ACTION

Institutional Context of Family Therapists

Many theories exist to help bridge the gap between the application of nursing and family theory to the family and broader social action on behalf of communities of families. Most family theorists view the family as a system that interfaces with outside suprasystems or institutions only when a problem is to be addressed, such as in the school or a courtroom. The following three approaches go beyond the family as a system to address the interaction between the family and the larger social system:
- Ecological framework
- Network therapy
- Transactional model

Ecological Framework

The **ecological framework** is a blend of systems and developmental theory that focuses on the interaction and interdependence of humans (families) as biological and social beings with the environment. Using this framework the CHN would assess the family as a system within the context of its environment. Bronfenbrenner (2005) identified four basic systems that make up our ecological environment. The microsystem is our immediate environment that supports our development—the family, school, church, etc. The environment interacts with "age, health, sex, [and] genetic predispositions." The mesosystem recognizes the links between two or more microsystems and the individual. The exosystem includes those settings or institutions that may not directly come in contact with an

FAMILY HEALTH ASSESSMENT: THE GARCIA FAMILY

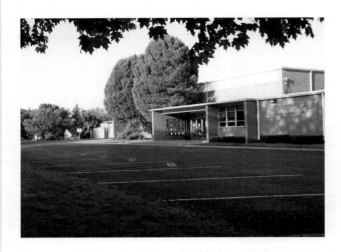

The school nurse, Jana, works with multiple city schools, including this inner-city school, which has a low-income, ethnically diverse population.

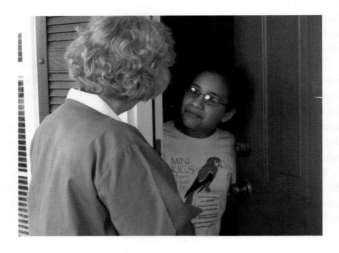

Jana arrives at the Garcia's' home. Maria answers the door and invites Jana in.

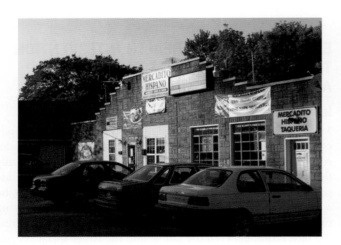

Jana assesses the community as she drives to the Garcia's' home, noting the availability of resources such as the local groceria.

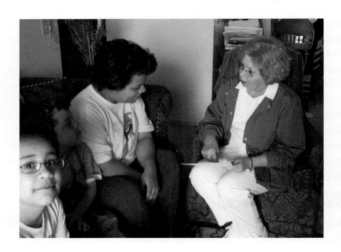

Jana completes the family assessment of the Garcia family with the help of Maria as interpreter for Mrs. Garcia. Mrs. Garcia listens intently as Jana asks questions about the family's health needs.

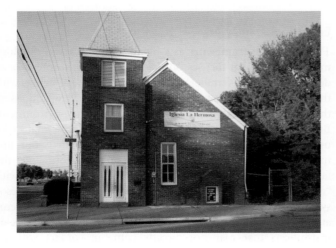

Local churches are a community resource, offering socialization and spiritual support for immigrant families such as the Garcia family.

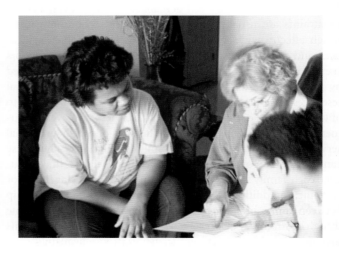

Jana reviews the plan of care and confirms the family's commitment to the plan of care they developed with her.

individual but still influence development in less direct ways, such as government agencies, what is happening in the world, and the media. Lastly, there is the chronosystem, or the future development. This takes into account the notion of time. What happens to the individual and family over time depending on events, and so on (Smith and Harmon, 2011)?

This approach explains the results of healthcare specialization and fragmentation of care based on Western concepts of time and space. It focuses on providing a more complex and flexible structure. For example, Kogan and colleagues (2004) investigated parent—healthcare provider discussions of family and community health risks during well-child examinations. Additionally, they studied the gaps between the issues discussed by the practitioner and the information the parent desired. On the basis of the results of the National Survey of Early Childhood Health, health topics for discussion were identified, including family financial difficulties, the presence of a support partner, parent's emotional support, alcohol, and/or drug use in the home, cigarette smoking in the home, the parent's physical health, and community violence. Cigarette smoking was discussed nearly 80% of the time, and alcohol and drug use was discussed 45% of the time; however, community violence was discussed less than 10% of the time, and financial needs 12%. The results indicate the need for better communication and education between healthcare providers and clients.

Social Network Framework

The **social network framework** (Christakis and Fowler, 2009) is based on earlier network therapy work involving all the connections and ties within a group. In network theory, an identified family member feels marginalized and seeks to replace the family network with others from the wider system to provide more support, hoping to enhance his or her role or functioning in the family. The concept of social network in this instance is related to social support. "Social network refers to a weblike structure comprising one's relationships and social support focuses on the nature of the interactions taking place within social relationships" (Friedman et al., 2003, p. 462). A family's social network includes friends, community groups, church, and agencies. Social network also can be explained as the structure of relationships, and social support as the function of relationships. Examples of network therapy are drawn from community mental health. In the social network framework, a *group* is defined as a collection of individuals with a common attribute. A social network is composed of connected groups. A network has structure (also called *typology*); contagion that flows across connections (e.g., money, violence, fashion, organs, obesity, etc.); connection, who is connected to whom (e.g., family, friends, colleagues); and homophily, or the tendency we have to be with those who are similar to ourselves. To some extent individuals and families control the density of our connectedness, our centrality to the group, and how we are viewed by others. This model has been used to explain health-related issues, such as the spread of sexually transmitted diseases and the obesity epidemic in the United States. It has also

been used to understand the issue of hyperconnectivity and technology. The PRC (2021) states that seven-in-ten U. S. adults have used Facebook and about half use it several times per day. The majority of 18- to 29-year-olds report using Instagram, Snapchat, or TikTok (Gramlich, 2021; Auxier and Anderson, 2021).

Perhaps then, using the research on social marketing, the CHN needs to become familiar with the use of social networks and other technology to ensure individuals and families have accurate health information. Researchers have found that individuals with the following demographics are more likely to seek medical answers online: women, younger, white, income of $75,000 or more, and a college degree. Fifty-nine percent of Americans looked online for health information in 2012 (Parker and Patten, 2013), and the majority began with a search engine, such as Google, Bing, or Yahoo, instead of a website that a CHN might identify as a reliable source such as the NIH or the CDC. Nearly one half of this group was seeking a diagnosis; these individuals are called *online diagnosers*. Thirty-eight percent of this group believed that they could take care of the problem at home and did not seek the advice of a health professional (Parker and Patten, 2013). This presents new issues for the CHN, such as teaching families how to evaluate appropriate online sites.

Transactional Model

In the **transactional model**, the term *transaction* refers to a system that focuses on family processes. The family as an institution, along with other institutions (e.g., religious, educational, recreational, or governmental), is culturally anchored (i.e., each holds a distinct set of beliefs and values about the nature of the world and human existence). An awareness of culture (e.g., beliefs and values) as it is expressed in each system is important (i.e., as it is expressed in mainstream US values vs. the value patterns of the family).

VanderValk and Colleagues (2007) used a transactional model to explore the relationship between parental marital distress and adolescent emotional adjustment. In a 6-year prospective study of 531 parent—adolescent dyads, they found such a relationship, especially for late adolescent and young adult girls and less so for males. The findings suggest that "girls' greater sensitivity to interpersonal problems may be reciprocal and that the parental marriage is still associated with adjustment for girls in late adolescence and early adulthood" (p. 130).

Models of Care for Communities of Families

Models exist to guide the CHN in providing care to communities of families in special need of services that improve access, equality between consumer and provider, and sensitivity to human need. There is generally an increase in the number and type of models that emerge as traditional public and private models of health care decline due to shrinking funding and resources. Many of the programs develop as the result of community efforts or partnerships with existing healthcare providers. The following are examples of such models.

The Kentucky Partnership for Farm Family Health and Safety

The Kentucky Partnership is a community coalition, originally funded by the W. K. Kellogg Foundation, involving farm families, universities, and various community-based organizations. The coalition was originally established to improve the health of farm families in rural Kentucky. Farming is identified as one of the most dangerous occupations in the United States, and few resources have been developed to support the unique needs of farm families. The Partnership identified farm women as the primary "health officers" for farm families. The farm women were provided with opportunities to develop skills in leadership, conflict resolution, and team building. Nurse educators and nursing students provided health education and assisted the farm women in developing a self-sustaining structure to support their efforts to improve family health. Cardiopulmonary resuscitation and first aid classes, the development of unique emergency medical subsystems, and other activities helped improve the health of the farm families. The local members reported an increase in personal knowledge, self-esteem, and personal satisfaction through the Partnership efforts. The Kentucky Partnership for Farm Family Health and Safety continues to affect the health of farm families in south-central Kentucky (Palermo and Ehlers, 2001).

The Health Access Nurturing Development Services Program

The Health Access Nurturing Development Services (HANDS) program is a voluntary home visitation program for any new parent targeting at-risk families that include first-time parents. Implemented through interdisciplinary teams consisting of social workers, nurses, and parent resource persons, the program serves first-time pregnant mothers and their families. HANDS was originally funded through tobacco settlement monies allocated through the state legislature to the Kentucky Cabinet for Health and Family Services. The program services are provided through district health departments and currently are available throughout the Commonwealth of Kentucky. Counseling, education, and support services are provided until the child reaches 2 years of age. On the basis of a systems approach, home visits are made for the purpose of screening, assessment, referrals, care coordination, case management, and policy advocacy. The program implements the "Growing Great Kids" and evidence-based curriculum (https://www.greatkidsinc.org/new-to-great-kids/growing-great-kids-next-generation-p-36/p-36-curriculum-series/) based on building family strengths through parenting, child safety, and connecting families with many resources. Initially the program focused on teen and first-time mothers, but data collected have revealed that at-risk mothers include individuals with previous children but poor support and parenting skills (Kentucky Cabinet for Health and Family Services, 2017).

Programs such as HANDS require time in order to show outcomes. Ten years after the inception of the program the Kentucky Cabinet for Health and Family Services documented the positive impact of HANDS services, which can be seen in decreases in the number of preterm births, emergency department uses, rates of child abuse and neglect, and infant mortality rates in Kentucky as well as a cost savings to the Kentucky Medicaid program (Pew Center on the States, 2012) (Table 20.5). Currently, services have been expanded in eight counties targeting mothers identified as at risk or diagnosed with depression or other mental illness. Home visitors have been taught to use Home Cognitive Behavior Therapy to integrate into the HANDS curriculum for these families (Kentucky Cabinet for Health and Family Services, 2017; Pew Center on the States, 2012).

These alternative health programs are strategies to change the structural barriers that prevent low-income families' access to care. Professional role functions changed as nurses, rather than physicians, provided health care. Active self-care was promoted, and health and medical knowledge was shared. Assistance by family and social networks was encouraged. Both of these programs address aspects of the health needs of populations at risk, but they do not address the social determinants of disease. Neither program addresses the health-damaging conditions that poor people face, such as poor housing, malnutrition, and environmental hazards at the workplace and in the community. Although these programs represent steps in the right direction, changes in access to

TABLE 20.5   Health Access Nurturing Development Services (HANDS) Program: Outcomes and Potential Related Medical Cost Savings

Outcome	Estimated Cost Per Case[a]	Hands Impact	Estimated Annual Cost Savings
Preterm birth	$49,000	32% reduction	$16,900,000
Emergency department use	$420	50% reduction	$5,700,000
Child abuse	$10,400	N/A	$685,940
Child neglect	$1900	33% reduction	$90,900
Infant mortality	N/A	70% reduction	N/A

[a]The original calculations used estimated costs per case drawn from the Children's Safety Network. The estimated cost per case for child abuse and child neglect are hospitalization costs only and do not consider costs associated with child protective services or other expenditures.
Source: Kentucky Cabinet and Family Services and Department for Public Health: *Home visiting: a healthy return on investment—a presentation for the Prichard committee*, 2011; table reprinted from The Pew Center on the States: *Home visiting issue brief, Kentucky: joining HANDS for a comprehensive system of care*, 2012, page 8. Available from: https://www.pewtrusts.org/~/media/legacy/uploadedfiles/pcs_assets/2012/02012home20kentucky20briefwebpdf.pdf © 2012. The Pew Charitable Trusts.

medical and health services are not enough. Social changes also are necessary.

APPLYING THE NURSING PROCESS
Home Visit

The case study presents the application of the nursing process to a family on a home visit. The example notes the use of the home visit to identify health needs of the family within the community and programs planned to meet those needs, which ultimately will benefit a population of families in the future.

The home visit is a crucial experience for the nursing student and family (Friedman et al., 2003). Important factors that may influence the home visit include the family's background experience with the healthcare system, the agency in which the nursing student is working, the family's experience with previous nursing students who have visited the family, and the student's background. For example, nursing student characteristics may vary; students bring differing levels of knowledge of medical and nursing practice, self, and the community.

The nursing student brings previous learning about families, family-related theory, the growth and development of members of different ages within a family, disease processes, and access to the healthcare system. Curricula within schools of nursing vary; therefore, some students will also bring preparation in all specialties—medical-surgical nursing, childbearing, parent—child nursing, and psychiatric and mental health nursing—to the experience. Others may be taking basic clinical courses, such as pediatrics and psychiatric—mental health nursing, concurrently with community health. Thus, the need for review of appropriate theory, health education, and standard assessment tools for individuals and families will vary.

The nursing student's knowledge of self, previous life experiences, and values also are important in planning for home visits. Nursing students must recognize their strengths and weaknesses in preparation for entering a new community and working with families. Additional preparation by all nursing students is necessary before the first home visit, depending on the content of the referral. The student should gather referral information, review assessment forms, and intervention tools (e.g., screening materials, supplies) before going to the home. Flexibility is important in working with families, because the nursing student will not know the family's priority needs until the home visit.

CASE STUDY   Application of the Nursing Process

Student Absenteeism
Jana Parks is a CHN employed by the district health department. She is a school health nurse, providing services for six schools in a moderately sized community. After receiving a referral from school officials related to a student's absenteeism, Jana plans to assess the student and family. (See the photo novella in this chapter for photos that depict this case study.)

Assessment
Jana knows that the school is located in the inner city where 75% of the children come from families with a median family income at or below the federal poverty level. English is the second language for approximately 25% of the students, and 5% are not fluent in spoken or written English. Each year, more than 20% of the student body moves into or out of the school district.

She reviews the school records for the student, Maria Garcia, and learns that this is the first year of enrollment for the sixth grader and her second-grade brother, Miguel. Maria's family moved to the area 6 months ago from the Dominican Republic. School records note that the girl is adequately fluent in spoken English but that the parents do not speak English. The student's father works part-time at a local furniture manufacturer. There has been a noticeable decline in grades over the previous quarter, there have been no disciplinary actions, and teacher comments are positive regarding the student's classroom performance. The health record indicates that she is up to date with required immunizations; no chronic illnesses are noted on the school physical examination record. Jana notes that Maria's brother does not have the same school absence pattern.

Jana contacts the family and identifies her role as the school health nurse. She explains the need for a meeting with the student and family to discuss concerns about Maria's school attendance. A time is scheduled when both parents and the student are available. She confirms the home address and directions.

Jana notes that the house is in need of paint and some windows have been replaced with cardboard; however, the yard is free of clutter, and there are containers of blooming plants on the small porch. Maria Garcia opens the door,

and Jana enters a small, dimly lit room. As the student makes introductions, Mr. Garcia stands and greets Jana with a nod and handshake while Mrs. Garcia remains recumbent on the sofa but raises her hand in greeting. Mrs. Garcia's appearance surprises Jana, as she appears much older than Mr. Garcia. Her skin is pale, her eyes are sunken, and she appears frail, with a distended abdomen and generalized muscle wasting.

Jana is aware that the exchange of social conversation is important in establishing a relationship with Hispanic clients. She mentions the beautiful picture in the room and learns that a family member painted it as a wedding gift for the Garcias. Jana learns that the family has no other relatives in the community and moved to the city through the work of a refugee assistance organization. In this interview, Jana plans to collect information related to individual, family, and/or community functioning.

Throughout the conversation, Jana has noted that both Maria and Mr. Garcia appear tense; Mrs. Garcia is quiet and rarely speaks or smiles. Maria has translated throughout the conversation, although Jana senses that the parents may have limited understanding of spoken English. To lessen anxiety, Jana begins the interview by saying, "I am here because the school and I are concerned about Maria's absences. I want to learn why Maria misses school and to see if there are ways that the school can help."

Through the interview process, Jana learns that Maria likes school and has made friends there. She observes that Miguel stays close to Maria and frequently hides his face into her shoulder when Jana speaks to him. She also notes that Mr. and Mrs. Garcia rarely look at each other, and Mr. Garcia chooses a seat on the opposite side of the room. The family rents the home, and the father has been able to supplement his part-time income by working as a day laborer for a lawn service. The family was beginning to establish connections at a local church and with neighbors when Mrs. Garcia was diagnosed with an abdominal tumor that has required numerous operations over the past 3 months. She is still receiving home care visits for a surgical wound that has not healed. Although Medicaid has covered most physician and hospital expenses, the family has experienced out-of-pocket expenses for noncovered medications. These problems have contributed to family financial stress. Mr. Garcia has to

Continued

CASE STUDY **Application of the Nursing Process—cont'd**

drive his wife to medical appointments; as a result, he is in danger of losing his job. Maria also attends these appointments to serve as the interpreter, resulting in her frequent school absences.

In addition, Jana learns that Maria has assumed responsibility for the household cooking, cleaning, and laundry since her mother's illness. Mr. Garcia shops at a small neighborhood groceria. Jana determines that with food stamps the family has adequate resources to purchase food, although Maria admits that she is still learning to cook. The family eats the evening meal together, frequently rice and beans. Maria and Miguel are eligible for subsidized breakfast and lunch at school. Maria believes that it is her responsibility to help Miguel complete his homework, get to bed on time, and attend school regularly. Mr. Garcia disciplines both children. Jana asks questions regarding family health practices and learns that they see a provider at the health department only when ill or for school requirements and do not seek dental care. She observes a number of medication bottles on a table near the sofa.

Diagnosis
Individual
- Risk for excessive stress related to time-consuming activities, insufficient finances, and insufficient recreation (Mr. Garcia and Maria)
- Risk for personal injury related to improperly stored medications (Miguel)
- Ineffective health promotion related to language and cultural differences and lack of routine dental hygiene (Mr. and Mrs. Garcia, Maria, and Miguel)

Family
Risk for poor parenting and family crisis related to change in Mrs. Garcia's ability to function, financial burden of treatments for ill family member, and disruption of family routines, mother's illness, and mother's prolonged illness.

Community
Inadequate systematic programs for linking Hispanic families to community resources.

Planning
A plan of care is developed to meet the needs of the individuals, family, and community. Planning involves mutual goal setting between the nurse and family; mutual setting of objectives to meet goals, prioritizing, or setting short- and long-term goals with the family, contracting or establishing the division of labor between nurse and family that will meet the objectives, and evaluating the process and outcome.

Individual
Long-Term Goals
- Mr. Garcia will recognize appropriate roles and responsibilities for Maria. He will identify and use resources to allow her to resume suitable educational, social, and family duties.
- Mr. Garcia will identify and use community resources to assist with transportation needs and medication costs.
- Jana noted a long-term need to discuss dental care.
- Mr. and Mrs. Garcia will improve their English comprehension and speaking skills.

Short-Term Goals
- Relieve Maria of interpreting at medical appointments by identifying alternative interpretive resources.
- Store medications in a secure location.

Family
Long-Term Goal
- The family will be able to find and use appropriate services for physical and social support.

Short-Term Goal
- The family will learn to appropriately express their feelings related to the mother's illness, social isolation, role strain, and/or fear.

Community
Long-Term Goal
- The community will establish programs to support immigrant family needs for transportation, interpretation, and enculturation to the American medical system.

Short-Term Goal
- Mr. Garcia will identify existing programs available to support Hispanic immigrants.

Intervention
- Jana recognizes that many interventions must be carried out at the individual, family, and community levels.

Individual
- Education regarding safe medication storage.
- Referral to the Refugee Assistance Society or local churches for interpretive assistance.

Family
Direct nursing interventions aimed at family functioning include the following levels:
- *Cognitive*: New information is provided to the family that promotes problem solving. An example is referring the Garcias to the community free clinic for medical and dental care.
- *Affective*: Families are encouraged to express their feelings, which may be blocking their efforts at problem solving. An example would be Jana's planned validation of Mr. Garcia's concerns regarding finances and the threat of losing employment.
- *Behavioral*: Tasks are negotiated to be carried out either during the family interview or as homework between visits. An example is Mr. Garcia's planned call to the Refugee Assistance Society.

Community
Jana recognizes that her referral of Mr. Garcia to the Refugee Assistance Society to obtain support through existing programs is also an intervention at the community level. She engages in ongoing parafamily work to identify how the community can be mobilized to provide physical, mental, and social support to immigrant families. Does anyone at the community free clinic speak Spanish? Are interpreters available at healthcare facilities? Where do most immigrant families receive health care and social support? Are classes on English as a second language free of charge for Hispanic families? Are job skill training programs available for Mr. Garcia? Questions such as these bring up many areas of assessment that Jana will need to make with the Garcia family and the community in the future.

Evaluation
Individual/Family
Jana helps the Garcias obtain a small lockable box in which to store medications. Mr. Garcia establishes contact with a local church, which provides a volunteer interpreter and driver for medical visits and twice-weekly delivery of meals. Mr. Garcia takes Maria and Miguel to the free clinic, where dental sealants are applied to their molars. The social worker at the community's free clinic meets with Mr. Garcia to offer him assistance in obtaining low-cost medications. Through this conversation, Jana identifies his reluctance to ask for financial assistance. He states that he should provide for his family and that Maria should not have to assume the role of mother for Miguel. However, he

CASE STUDY Application of the Nursing Process—cont'd

does not see any other options at this time. She identifies that Mr. Garcia may be in need of ongoing support and suggests that he talk with a counselor about his concerns. Mr. Garcia refuses to see a counselor but agrees that he will talk to the pastor of his church. Maria and Miguel meet with the school counselor as needed to discuss feelings related to their mother's illness and the resulting family strain.

Community

Jana identified that many community resources are available to immigrant families; however, information about them is limited and not readily accessible. She contacts the director of the Refugee Assistance Society, and together they initiate a community coalition to address this issue.

Levels of Prevention

Society's expectations of the family are in transition. Application of the levels of prevention to families by the community nurse must take into account the changing family configuration; the financial, emotional, and physical burdens often compounded in the single-parent family; and the lack of resources, such as nonexistent or inadequate health insurance.

Primary Prevention

This chapter has established the importance of the family to individuals and society. Primary prevention with families becomes an essential element of any comprehensive family health plan. From the family perspective, health education must address actual and potential challenges to health, such as immunizations of all family members, educating about resources to support the family financially and emotionally, encouraging exercise and activity, and empowering the family to build on strengths. An example is using the family genogram to teach the family about predisposition to diseases and helping the family develop a health prevention plan.

Secondary Prevention

The focus of secondary prevention for the family includes ensuring that the family has continued access to health care and resources for individual and family health problems. The changing economy in the United States has "closed the door" to regular health providers for some families. The challenge to the nurse is helping the family locate and access continued care and teaching the family to move through the system of government assistance, which may be new and unacceptable for the family. The nurse must be politically active in lobbying legislators for continued resources to support families.

Tertiary Prevention

Tertiary prevention for family includes assuring that the needed resources are available to support long-term care of each family member. An example of a community-based organization established and funded solely by volunteers is the Kelly Autism Program (KAP). KAP is "designed to provide services to adolescents and young adults diagnosed along the Autism Spectrum Continuum, as well as their families, while serving as a training opportunity for future professionals in a variety of disciplines. KAP has programs for middle school, high school and post-secondary participants including higher education, vocational training, and job support" (Western Kentucky University, 2016, p. 1). It includes a comprehensive screening program and one-on-one support for young adults with autism capable of living and studying on a university campus.

Developed by Mary Kovar, RN, MSN; and Barbara Minix, RN, MSN.

▮ SUMMARY

This chapter highlights the CHN's work with families and identifies the major family-related healthcare needs that the healthcare system has not adequately addressed. The nature of the family is changing and challenging traditional definitions and configurations. Approaches to meeting the health needs of families must go beyond that of the traditional healthcare system, which addresses the individual as the unit of care. Strategies are given in this chapter for expanding notions of care from the individual to the family and from the family to the community. To guide intervention with families, nurses have traditionally relied on common theoretical frameworks from the disciplines of psychology and social psychology. These frameworks often target individuals; frameworks are needed that go beyond the individual to the family and community and that address social and policy changes needed to alter the social, economic, and environmental conditions under which families must function. This chapter provides tools for assessing the family and the family within the community and gives examples of the extension of family health intervention to larger aggregates, which involves social action to overcome constraints to accessing health services. Nonnursing and community health nursing models of care provided for communities of families are presented and critiqued. The nursing process is applied in a case study at individual, family, and community levels on a home visit. Examples of interventions by the CHN at individual, family, and community levels are presented.

Families remain the core of society, with diversity as the constant for families in the United States. Family nursing must be understood and practiced by CHNs. An understanding of family theory provides a mechanism for assessing and intervening with families to improve their level of wellness and increase the health of the community as a whole.

EVOLVE WEBSITE

http://evolve.elsevier.com/Nies/community
- NCLEX Review Questions
- Case Studies

BIBLIOGRAPHY

Abramowitz J, O'Hara B: The financial burden of medical spending, *Med Care Res Rev* 72(2):187–199, 2014. https://doi.org/10.1177/1077558714563173.

Abramson TA: Older adults: the "Panini Sandwich" generation, *Clin Gerontol* 38(4):251–267, 2015. https://doi.org/10.1080/07317115.2015.1032466.

Allen DR, Fine MA, Demo HD: An overview of family diversity: controversies, questions, and values. In Demo DH, Allen KR, Fine MA, editors: *Handbook of family diversity*, New York, 2000, Oxford Press.

American Academy of Child & Adolescent Psychiatry: *Grandparents raising grandchildren*, 2016. Available from: https://www.aacap.org/AACAP/Families_and_Youth/Facts_for_Families/FFF-Guide/Grandparents-Raising-Grandchildren-077.aspx.

American Association for Marriage and Family Therapy: *Grandparents raising grandchildren*, 2016. Available from: https://aamft.org/Consumer_Updates/grandparents.aspx?WebsiteKey=8e8c9bd6-0b71-4cd1-a5ab-013b5f855b01.

Anderson MP, O'Grady RS, Anderson IL: Public health nursing in primary care: impact on home visits, *Publ Health Nurs* 145(2), 1985.

Annie E: Casey Foundation: *Kids count faststats data book online*, 2016. Available from: http://www.aecf.org/resources/the-2016-kids-count-data-book/.

Auger JR: Behavioral systems and nursing, *AJN* 77(11):1856–1857, 1976.

Auxier B, Anderson M: *PEW: Social media use in 2021*, 2021. Available from: https://www.pewresearch.org/internet/2021/04/07/social-media-use-in-2021/.

Beard M: Home nursing, *Public Health Nurse Q* 7:44–51, 1999.

Bell J: The central importance of therapeutic conversations in nursing: can talking be healing? *J Fam Nurs* 22(4):439–448, 2016. https://doi.org/10.1177/107480716680837.

Bell JM: Making ideas "stick": the 15-minute family interview, *J Fam Nurs* 18:171, 2012.

Berchick ER, Barnett JC, Upton RD: U.S. Census Bureau: *Health Insurance coverage in the United Stated*, 2018. Available from: https://www.census.gov/library/publications/2019/demo/p60-267.html.

Bronfenbrenner U: *Making human beings human: bioecological perspectives on human development*, Thousand Oaks, CA, 2005, Sage Publications.

Butler JF: The family diagram and genogram: comparisons and contrast, *Am J Fam Ther* 36:169–180, 2008.

Cantor J, Monheit AC, Delia D: Early impact of the Affordable Care Act on health insurance coverage of young adults, *Health Serv J* 47(5):1773–1790, 2012. https://doi.org/10.1111/j.1475-6773.2012.01458.x.

Carter E, McGoldrick M: *The changing family life cycle: a framework for family therapy*, ed 2, New York, 1998, Gardner Press.

Centers for Disease Control and Prevention: *Faststats: teen births*. Available from: http://www.cdc.gov/nchs/fastats/teen-births.htm.

CDC: National Center for Health Statistics (NCHC): *Births and natality*, 2016. Available from: https://www.cdc.gov/nchs/fastats/births.htm.

CDC: *Chronic disease prevention and health promotion*, 2017. Available from: https://www.cdc.gov/chronicdisease/.

Centers for Medicare and Medicaid Services: *The children's health insurance program*, 2015. Available from: https://www.cms.gov/Outreach-and-Education/American-Indian-Alaska-Native/AIAN/CHIP-Grantees/Overview.html.

Christakis NA, Fowler JA: *Connected: the surprising power of our social networks and how they shape our lives*, Boston, 2009, Little, Brown & Company.

Cook E: *The life of Florence Nightingale* (vol 2). London, 1913, Macmillan.

DeFrain J: Strong families, *Family Matters* 53:6–13, 1999.

Dreher MC: The conflict of conservatism in public health nursing education, *Nurs Outlook* 30:504, 1982.

Dunst CJ, Trivette CM: Capacity-building family-systems intervention practices, *J Fam Soc Work* 12(2):119–143, 2009.

Duvall EM: *Marriage and family relationships*, ed 5, Philadelphia, 1977, JB Lippincott.

Duvall EM, Miller BC: *Marriage and family development*, ed 6, New York, 1985, Harper and Row.

Erikson E: *Childhood and society*, ed 2, New York, 1963, WW Norton.

Escoto KH, Laska MN, Larson N, et al.: Work hours and perceived time barriers to healthful eating among young adults, *Am J Health Behav* 36(3):786–789, 2012.

Freeman R: *Public health nursing practice*, ed 3, Philadelphia, 1963, WB Saunders.

Friedman MM: *Family nursing: theory and assessment*, ed 3, East Norwalk, CT, 1998, Appleton-Lange.

Friedman MM, Bowden VB, Jones EG: *Family nursing: research, theory and practice*, ed 2, Upper Saddle River, NJ, 1992, Prentice Hall.

Friedman MM, Bowden VB, Jones EG: *Family nursing: research, theory and practice*, ed 3, Upper Saddle River, NJ, 2003, Prentice Hall.

Fry R, Passel JS, Cohn D: *PEW: A majority of young adults in the U. S. live with their parents for the first time since the Great Depression*, 2020. Available from: https://www.pewresearch.org/fact-tank/2020/09/04/a-majority-of-young-adults-in-the-u-s-live-with-their-parents-for-the-first-time-since-the-great-depression/.

Glaser B, Strauss AL: *Chronic illness and the quality of life*, St. Louis, 1975, Mosby.

Gramlich J: *PEW: 10 facts about Americans and Facebook*, 2021. Available from: https://www.pewresearch.org/fact-tank/2021/06/01/facts-about-americans-and-facebook/.

Gurrentz B, U.S. Census Bureau: *Living with an unmarried partner now common for young adults*, 2018. Available from: https://www.census.gov/library/stories/2018/11/cohabitation-is-up-marriage-is-down-for-young-adults.html.

Guttmacher Institute (GI): *Disparities in health coverage persist, despite the affordable care act*, 2016. Available from: https://www.guttmacher.org/infographic/2016/disparities-health-coverage-persist-despite-affordable-care-act.

Hartman A: *Finding families: an ecological approach to family assessment in adoption*, Beverly Hills, CA, 1979, Sage.

Horowitz JM, Graf N, Livingston G: *PEW: marriage and cohabitation in U.S*, 2019. Available from: https://www.pewresearch.org/social-trends/2019/11/06/the-landscape-of-marriage-and-cohabitation-in-the-u-s/.

Human Rights Campaign: *Healthcare equality index 2020*, 2020. Available from: https://reports.hrc.org/healthcare-equality-index-2020?_ga=2.183364846.992314994.1632254234-620565174.1632254234.

Human Rights Campaign: *LGBTQ+ inclusive definition of family*, 2020. Available from: https://www.thehrcfoundation.org/professional-resources/lgbtq–inclusive-definitions-of-family.

Kentucky Cabinet for Health and Family Services: *HANDS program*, 2017. Available from: https://chfs.ky.gov/agencies/dph/dmch/ecdb/Pages/hands.aspx.

Kogan MD, Schuster MA, Yu SM, et al.: Routine assessment of family and community health risks: parent views and what they receive, *Pediatrics* 113:1934–1943, 2004.

Kramer S: *PEW: U.S. has world's highest rate of children living in single-parent households*, 2019. Available from: https://www.pewresearch.org/fact-tank/2019/12/12/u-s-children-more-likely-than-children-in-other-countries-to-live-with-just-one-parent/.

Levy H, Ying A, Bagley N: What's left of the Affordable Care Act? A progress report, *RSF: The Russell Sage Foundation J Soc Sci* 6(2):42–66, 2020.

Li L, Lin C, Cao H: Intergenerational and urban-rural health habits in Chinese families, *Am J Health Behav* 33(2):172–180, 2009.

Livingston G, Thomas D: *PEW: Why is the teen birth rate falling?*, 2019. Available from: https://www.pewresearch.org/fact-tank/2019/08/02/why-is-the-teen-birth-rate-falling/.

Lubkin IM, Larsen PD: *Chronic illness: impact & intervention*, ed 8 Burlington, MA, 2013, Jones & Bartlett.

Martinez AM, D'Arois D, Rennick JE: Does the 15-minute or less family interview influence family nursing practice? *J Fam Nurs* 31(2):157–178, 2007.

Maslow A: *Motivation and personality*, ed 2, New York, 1970, Harper and Row.

McNeill JA, Cook J, Mahon M, et al.: Family history: value-added information in assessing cardiac health, *AAOHN* 56(7):297–305, 2008.

Medicaidgov: *Children's health insurance program reauthorization act*, n.d. Available from: https://www.medicaid.gov/chip/chip-program-information.html.

Minuchin P: Looking toward horizon: present and future in study of family systems. In McHale JP, Grolnick WS, editors: *Psychological study of families*, Mahwah, NJ, 2002, Lawrence Erlbaum.

Montalvo B: Useful coincidences and family strengths, *Contemp Fam Ther* 26(2):117–119, 2004.

National Council on Aging: *The top 10 most common chronic conditions in older adults*, 2021. Available from: www.ncoa.org/article/the-top-10-most-common-chronic-conditions-in-older-adults.

National Institute of Health: *Diabetes in the U.S. population*, 2015. Available from: https://www.nih.gov/news-events/nih-research-matters/diabetes-us-population.

National Institute of Health: *World's older population grows dramatically: NIH-funded census bureau report offers details of global aging phenomenon*, 2016. Available from: https://www.nih.gov/news-events/news-releases/worlds-older-population-grows-dramatically.

Otto H: A framework for assessing family strengths. In Reinhard A, Quinn M, editors: *Family-centered community health nursing*, St. Louis, 1973, Mosby.

Palermo T, Ehlers J: *Coalitions: building partnerships to promote agricultural health and safety*, Washington, DC, 2001, National Institutes for Occupational Health and Safety.

Parke RP: Family & peer systems, *Psychol Bull* 128(4):596–601, 2002.

Parker K, Patten E: *The sandwich generation: rising financial burden for middle-aged Americans (Pew Research Social & Demographic Trends)*, 2013. Available from: http://www.pewsocialtrends.org/2013/01/30/the-sandwich-generation/.

Pew Center on the States: Home visiting issue brief, Kentucky: *Joining HANDS for a comprehensive system of care*, 2012. Available from: http://www.prichardcommittee.org/wp-content/uploads/2015/03/02012HOME20Kentucky20Briefwebpdf.pdf.

Pratt LV: *Family structure and effective health behavior: the energized family*, Boston, 1976, Houghton Mifflin.

Reisman M: The Affordable Care Act, five years later: policies, progress, and politics, *Pharmacol Ther* 40(9):575–600, 2015.

Shajani Z, Snell D: *Wright & Leahey's Nurses and family: a guide to family assessment and intervention*, ed 7, Philadelphia, 2019, FA Davis.

Smith SR, Harmon RR: *Exploring family theories*, New York, 2011, Oxford University Press.

Spanakis E, Golden SH: Race/ethnic differences in diabetes and diabetes complications, *Curr Diabetes Rep* 13(6), 2013. https://doi.org/10.1007/s11892-013-0421-9CDC.

Taylor D, U.S. Census Bureau: *Same-sex couples are more likely to adopt or foster children*, 2020. Available from: https://www.census.gov/library/stories/2020/09/fifteen-percent-of-same-sex-couples-have-children-in-their-household.html.

U.S. Census Bureau: *Cohabiting partners older, more racially diverse, more educated, higher earners*, 2019. Available from: https://www.census.gov/library/stories/2019/09/unmarried-partners-more-diverse-than-20-years-ago.html.

U.S. Census Bureau: *Families and living arrangements*, 2020. Available from: https://www.census.gov/programs-surveys/cps/technical-documentation/subject-definitions.html.

U.S. Census Bureau: *U.S. Census Bureau releases CPS estimates of same-sex households*, 2019. Available from: https://www.census.gov/newsroom/press-releases/2019/same-sex-households.html.

U.S. Department of Health and Human Services (DHHS): *Administration for Community Living: 2019 profile of older Americans*, 2020. Available from: https://acl.gov/sites/default/files/Aging%20and%20Disability%20in%20America/2019ProfileOlderAmericans508.pdf.

U.S. Department of Health and Human Services: *My family health portrait: A tool from the US Surgeon General*, 2017. Available from: https://phgkb.cdc.gov/FHH/html/index.html.

VanderValk I, de Goede M, Spruijt E, et al.: A longitudinal study on transactional relations between parental marital distress and adolescent emotional adjustment, *Adolescence* 42(165):116–136, 2007.

von Bertalanffy L: *General systems theory: foundations, development, applications*, New York, 1968, George Braziller.

von Bertalanffy L: The history and status of general systems theory. In Klir G, editor: *Trends in general systems theory*, New York, 1972, Wiley.

von Bertalanffy L: General systems theory and psychiatry. In Arieti S, editor: *American handbook of psychiatry*, New York, 1974, Basic Books.

Wald L: The family as a unit of care: a historical review, *Publ Health Nurs* 3:427–428, 1904, 515–519.

Western Kentucky University: *Kelly Autism Program*, 2016. Available from: http://www.wku.edu/kellyautismprogram/index.php.

World Health Organization (WHO): *2010 The World Health Report: health systems financing: the path to universal coverage*, Geneva, 2012, World Health Organization.

Wright LM, Leahey M: *Nurses and families: a guide to family assessment and intervention*, Philadelphia, 1994, FA Davis.

Wright LM, Leahey M: *Nurses and families: a guide to family assessment and intervention*, ed 4, Philadelphia, 2000, FA Davis.

Wright LM, Leahey M: *Nurses and families: a guide to family assessment and intervention*, ed 5, Philadelphia, 2005, FA Davis.

Wright LM, Leahey M: *Nurses and family: a guide to family assessment and intervention*, ed 6, Philadelphia, 2012, FA Davis.

21

Populations Affected by Disabilities

Allison P. Edwards, Lisa W. Thomas, and Meredith Troutman-Jordan

OBJECTIVES

Upon completion of this chapter, the reader will be able to do the following:

1. Differentiate among the definitions, models, and social constructs of disability.
2. Describe historical attitudes and perspectives surrounding disability that have contributed to treatment of people with disabilities.
3. Summarize the prevalence of various disabilities.
4. Outline federal legislation that supports the rights of people with disabilities.
5. Identify the unique living experiences of disabled persons and their families.
6. Provide evidence-based interventions to promote function and health management for persons with disabilities and/or chronic illnesses.
7. Identify ethical issues related to the care of people with disabilities.

OUTLINE

KEY TERMS

activity limitation
activities of daily living (ADL)
Americans With Disabilities Act
child(ren) with disabilities (CWD)
developmental disability
disability
fatal five

functional activities
impairment
independent living
Individuals with Disabilities Education Act (IDEA)
instrumental activities of daily living (IADL)

intellectual and developmental disabilities (IDD)
Patient Self-Determination Act (PSDA) of 1990
people/person with disabilities (PWD)
quality of life

Rehabilitation Act of 1973
reasonable accommodations

Social Security Disability Insurance
(SSDI)

SELFASSESSMENT: PERCEPTION OF DISABILITY

Picture what it's like to be born with a disability. Envision yourself unable to use your arms or legs or being confined to a wheelchair and dependent on the assistance of others. Imagine not being able to view anything above chair height. Consider having to prepare yourself for the day with the use of only one arm, from a wheelchair. What might seem like a simple task, like dressing or grooming, may take hours of preparation and assistance for an individual with a physical or cognitive disability. To further complicate the situation, imagine that the person with a disability has a significant health concern such as high blood pressure or diabetes that requires close monitoring or medications.

Now consider individuals who were healthy since birth but became disabled by a disease or accident. How do they adapt to living in their old environment with new physical challenges? How would their employment be affected? Will financial resources and personal and emotional support systems be available?

Finally, think about living in a family affected by disability. Consider the impact of a child with a disability (CWD) on parental activities, family roles, and siblings. Imagine dilemmas encountered by parents faced with the possibility of having a CWD who may not survive without extensive surgeries and, even then, a good and productive quality of life is not guaranteed. These are examples of some of the many different situations experienced by persons with disabilities (PWD).

This chapter discusses general information about the various types of disabling conditions encountered in the community. It summarizes some of the more commonly occurring comorbidities and presents basic information on public policy and legislation that affect PWD. Last, it suggests some interventions that may be used by public health nurses to help care for this vulnerable population.

DEFINITIONS AND MODELS FOR DISABILITY

Disability is an umbrella term describing impairments, activity limitations, and participation restrictions. The Americans with Disabilities Act of 1990 and the Rehabilitation Act of 1973 define having a disability by how it limits carrying out a major life activity, such as the ability to breathe, walk, see, hear, speak, work, care for oneself, perform manual tasks, and learn. The International Classification of Functioning, Disability and Health (ICF) (World Health Organization [WHO], 2002) proposes the scope of disability encompasses impairments, activity limitations, and participation restrictions. These definitions frame the evolution of policy as it pertains to disabilities

and are often used to facilitate eligibility determination for federal or state financial assistance.

Disability affects people irrespective of class, culture, race, and economic level. Depending on the term's definition, disability affects nearly one out of every five Americans. Disability increases with age, often influencing a person's ability to maintain self-care, which is essential to remaining in one's preferred living environment. A physical disability may be readily apparent, as with someone who uses a wheelchair or an individual who is visually impaired, or it may be less obvious, such as an individual's intellectual, sensory, or neurologic deficit.

People who are born with a disability describe their experience somewhat differently from those who acquire a disability. For example, people with a sensory disability, a physical disability, or an intellectual disability (ID) from birth adapt to the world as they know it. Compare this situation with that of a 20-year-old who becomes blind, deaf, or paralyzed because of an accident. In this case, adaptation is likely necessary and lengthy, and the loss may never be fully grieved. If an 80-year-old becomes blind because of diabetes-induced retinopathy, the loss of sight was chronic, progressive, and predictable. There will be loss and grief, but the blindness occurs as part of the aging process. Thus, rather than viewing PWD as "all the same," nurses must be able to see each person as unique, with different goals, knowledge, and experiences.

Physical disabilities, sensory disabilities, intellectual disabilities, serious emotional disturbances, learning disabilities, amputations, spinal cord injuries, and health problems such as asthma or diabetes are examples of disabilities that may substantially limit at least one major life activity. Current nomenclature categorizes disabilities in different ways. Developmental disabilities encompass those conditions that are manifested by limitation before the legal age of adulthood, which is 18. This includes issues that limit or present challenges to the performance of activities of daily living (ADLs). Developmental disabilities encompass those lifelong conditions that are chronic in nature and may incorporate either or both intellectual and physical disabilities. Developmental disabilities are often the result of maternal illness or infection, genetic disorders, or trauma. Examples include fetal alcohol syndrome, fragile X syndrome, spina bifida (SB), Down syndrome (DS), or cerebral palsy (CP), among others.

Disabilities are often categorized according to their onset. They may be conditions from birth, such as DS or CP; conditions diagnosed during early childhood, such as autism spectrum disorder (ASD) or attention-deficit disorder/attention-deficit hyperactivity disorder (ADD/ADHD); conditions acquired as a result of an injury, such as spinal cord injury or traumatic brain injury (TBI); conditions that are progressive with age, such as cognitive decline/dementia and Alzheimer disease; or conditions associated with chronic illness, such as multiple sclerosis or diabetic neuropathy or retinopathy.

In comparison to the term *disability*, an impairment is a problem in body function or structure; an activity limitation is a difficulty encountered by an individual in executing a task or action (WHO, 2002). A disability resulting from an impairment involves a restriction or an inability to perform an activity in a normal manner or within the normal range resulting from a loss or abnormality of psychological, physiological, or anatomical structure or function.

Measurement of Disability

Healthy People 2030, the Affordable Care Act (ACA), and the U.S. Department of Health and Human Services (HHS) helped establish a framework for accurately surveying the extent of disabilities among the U.S. population by mandating that data collection include race or ethnicity, sex, primary language, and disability status. In 2011, HHS established standard questions required for all public health surveys. If a respondent replied positively to any of these:

- Deafness or difficulty hearing
- Blindness or difficulty seeing
- Difficulty concentrating, remembering, or making decisions due to physical, mental, or emotional issues among those 5 years and older
- Difficulty walking, climbing stairs, dressing, or bathing among those 5 years and older
- Difficulty doing errands independently, such as grocery shopping or going to a doctor's appointment, secondary to a physical, mental, or emotional condition among those 15 years and older

Then the respondent was deemed to have a disability. Collecting data to determine the type and prevalence of disabilities continues to be an issue to the extent that Healthy People 2030 has identified establishing collection of this data a "high priority public health issue" secondary to potentially absent baseline data availability (healthypeople.gov).

Other measures of disability emanate from efforts conducted by the Census Bureau and two other federal surveys. The US Census Bureau administers the Survey of Income and Program Participation (SIPP), which examines the confluence of income, employment, health insurance, and government transfer programs. The SIPP is a longitudinal survey that is administered over a 4-year period among the same respondents. It contains a broad but extensive set of disability questions that inquire about limitations in functional activities (e.g., seeing, hearing, speaking, walking, using stairs, lifting, and carrying items), activities of daily living (ADLs) (e.g., getting around inside the home, bathing, dressing, eating, or toileting), and instrumental activities of daily living (IADLs) (e.g., going outside the home, shopping, light house cleaning, preparing meals). Disability prevalence estimates using current SIPP data indicated a dramatic increase since 2008, especially in the age group 40 to 64 from approximately 15% of the population reporting a disability to over 20% (U.S. Census Bureau, 2018).

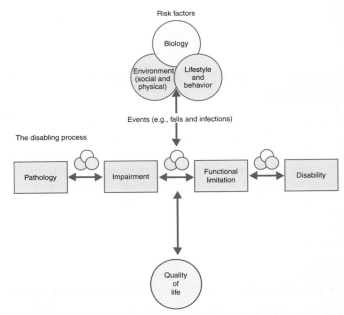

Fig. 21.1 Model of disability. (Reprinted with permission from Pope AM, Tarlov AR, editors: *Disability in America: toward a national agenda for prevention*, Washington, DC, 1991, National Academy Press. Copyright 1991 by the National Academy of Sciences. Courtesy National Academy Press, Washington, DC.)

National Agenda for Disability Model

The Committee on a National Agenda for the Prevention of Disabilities (NAPD) conceptualized a model for disability (Fig. 21.1). The NAPD model complements the concepts defined in the WHO/ICF model, in that disability is noted by the NAPD to be any condition of the body or mind (impairment) that makes it more difficult for the person with the condition to do certain activities (activity limitation) and interact with the world around them; this will in turn influence quality of life (Centers for Disease Control and Prevention [CDC], 2021). The NAPD model provides an alternative framework for viewing four related and distinct stages in the disabling process. Pathology at the cellular and tissue levels may produce impairment in structure or function at the organ level. An individual with an impairment may experience a functional limitation, which restricts their ability to perform an action within the normal range. The functional limitation may result in a disability when certain socially defined activities and roles cannot be performed. Although the model appears to indicate unidirectional progression from pathology to impairment, to functional limitation, to disability, stepwise or linear progression may not occur. Disability prevention efforts can limit or reduce many of the risk factors or stages in the disabling process.

Perceptions of disability influence the opportunities for full inclusion of PWD in society. Four models have been discussed in the literature (Table 21.1), with social and medical models gaining the most attention but the interface model is most often preferred by disability advocates.

TABLE 21.1 Models of Disability

Disability Model	Description
Medical model	PWD is dependent upon medical professionals for care; this model frames the PWD as it relates to their underlying condition, and diagnosis. Disability advocates claim this is "dehumanizing" and promotes prejudice of PWD because the PWD's condition is viewed as unfortunate and cannot be changed (Dirth and Branscombe, 2017).
Rehabilitation model	PWD's disability requires the intervention of rehabilitation health care providers and PWD is viewed as not successful if they are unable to overcome their disability.
Social model	PWD's disability is perceived as a difficulty secondary to the social constructs within the environment such as physical barriers that limit accessibility, policies that inhibit inclusion in society and other impediments such as societal attitudes; utilizing this model is capable of "combatting" marginalization (Dirth and Branscombe, 2017).
Interface model	Considers the PWD's perspective, meets the person "where they are," considers their needs irrespective of disability diagnosis as primary condition, but instead evaluates the intersection or "interface" of the medical diagnosis of the disability and environmental barriers (Smeltzer et al., 2005).

PWD, People/person with disabilities.
Adapted from Smeltzer SC, Dolen MA, Robinson-Smith G, Zimmerman V: Integration of disability-related content in nursing curricula. *Nurs Educ Perspect*, 26(4):210–216, 2005.

RESEARCH HIGHLIGHTS

Disparities in access, care, and outcomes were amplified during the COVID-19 pandemic. PWD often do not have the autonomy or ability to enjoy the same opportunities to practice social distancing secondary to necessary care providers, homes or settings where they reside. Often they are dependent on support services that may be disrupted during times of disaster. Moreover, PWD may have difficulty understanding the rationale for consistent mask wearing, social distancing or other infection control practices. In a recent study of developmental disability (DD) nurses, Desroches et al. (2021) discovered that DD nurses were excluded from COVID-19 planning, and there was an absence of public health guidelines, such as those for residential and day habituation settings, despite PWD/PWID's high risk status. Moreover, in an examination of health records of 42 academic centers, there was a higher case fatality rate among younger PWD/PWID than their non-disabled peers and a higher prevalence of PWD/PWID comorbid conditions associated with poor COVID 19 outcomes (Turk et al., 2020). Other research (Landes et al., 2020; Ne'eman, 2020) reached similar conclusions as PWD/PWID had relatively limited opportunity to utilize medical resources during times of disaster and scarcity.

ACTIVE LEARNING

Ask an experienced nurse about their medical encounters with PWD. Listen to their language and perceptions of disability when assessing care needs for PWD/PWID. Is there evidence of diagnostic overshadowing bias (practice of attributing medical issues to the underlying developmental or ID) on the part of healthcare providers? Can they describe a change in the PWD/PWID's environment, care provider, family structure?

A HISTORICAL CONTEXT FOR DISABILITY

Current models and definitions for disability cannot be understood apart from their historical-sociopolitical context. As cultures have changed, and with them images of beauty and value, *exceptional* people have experienced a wide range of treatment. They have sometimes been viewed as mascots and fascinating freaks. In other cases, people with disabilities have been isolated, ridiculed, and discriminated against or, worse, marked for extermination.

Early Attitudes Toward People With Disabilities

Since the beginning of recorded history, people with disabilities have been set apart from others and viewed as different or unusual. Early Greek and Roman cultures emphasized bodily and intellectual perfection, and babies who were sick, weak, or born with obvious disabilities were commonly killed or left to die (Barnes, 1996). In biblical times, people with disabilities were often viewed as unclean and/or sinful, though Jewish culture prohibited infanticide on the basis of belief in the sanctity of life. Jesus facilitated an expansion of Christian acceptance of individuals with disabilities. Many of the Bible's accounts of miracles performed by Jesus involved him listening, accepting, embracing, and healing those shunned by society.

In early European history, people with disabilities sometimes served as entertainers, circus performers, and sideshow exhibitions. Historically, appearing disabled has often been a matter of risking censure or hostility. The hostility was often linked to the suspicion of malingering or an attempt to profit from the sympathy of others.

Attitudes Toward People With Disabilities: 18th Through 20th Centuries

In the absence of a scientific model for understanding and treating disability, people saw disability as an irreparable condition caused by supernatural agency (Longmore, 1987). People with disabilities were viewed as sick and helpless. They were expected to participate in whatever treatment was deemed necessary to cure or produce a reasonable level of social or vocational performance. During the 19th century, the Industrial Revolution stimulated a societal need for better education. People who were unable to achieve the equivalent of a contemporary third-grade education (e.g., those with ID) were labeled "feebleminded" (Pfeiffer, 1993). Soon, the label was applied to people with vision, hearing, speech, and mobility impairments. Schools for people who were deaf and blind were established in the early 1800s. Although these early efforts demonstrated that people with disabilities could be educated and integrated into society, institutionalization, and segregation of people with disabilities were the norm.

Disability in the 20th Century

Special-interest groups for PWD began to develop later in the 20th century. The first federal vocational rehabilitation legislation, passed in the early 1920s, focused on limitations in the amount or type of work that people with disabilities could perform (Longmore, 1987). In the early 1900s, social Darwinism and the eugenics movement conducted involuntary sterilization of many people with intellectual disabilities (Pfeiffer, 1993). The eugenics philosophy was first advanced by Francis Galton, a relative of Charles Darwin. The root of the word *eugenics* relates to "good birth" or "well born." This movement was characterized by selective genetic breeding meant to advance desirable hereditary traits to improve a culture's intellect. The eugenics philosophy was adopted in the United States in the 1920 to 1930s and advanced by biologist Charles Davenport (Norrgard, 2008). The focus of the U.S. movement was to inhibit individuals with any malady or disability from procreation. This was evident in several published papers and interviews by Margaret Sanger, a birth control advocate, trained nurse and writer. Sanger was the well-known founder of the Birth Control League (later known as Planned Parenthood) and opened the first birth control clinic in the United States. What is less well known is that she also was in favor of compulsory sterilization and targeted PWD (Sanger, 1932). Ultimately, legislation was enacted in over 28 states that mandated forced sterilization of individuals who were "mentally handicapped."

The atrocities of Adolf Hitler's decrees, which ordered euthanasia of mentally ill and disabled individuals, helped reverse these civil rights abuses. Hitler empowered physicians to grant "mercy killings" of all individuals deemed incurable. Initially, in the *good death* program at least 5000 mentally and physically disabled children, from newborn to age 17 years, were killed by starvation or lethal overdoses. Soon extermination was extended to adults with mental or physical disabilities who lived in institutional settings, resulting in the deaths of over 70,000 adults with disabilities. After widespread public and private protest led by the German clergy, Hitler canceled the adult euthanasia program in late 1941.

Killing resumed in August 1942, however, and continued until the last days of World War II, although in a more concealed manner. Ultimately, an estimated 200,000 people were exterminated through Hitler's euthanasia program because they were regarded as "unworthy of life" (Eskay et al., 2012). Disguised as humanitarian, the basis of the decree was to eliminate genetically defective individuals from the Aryan race. Propaganda films perpetuated a utilitarian philosophy that the costs of care for mentally ill and disabled individuals did not benefit the greater good.

Particularly ironic is that the president and U.S. commander-in-chief during wartime, Franklin Delano Roosevelt (FDR), disabled by polio, administered the nation's highest office from a wheelchair. Interestingly, FDR was rarely photographed in his wheelchair. He utilized various adaptive devices to simulate his ability to stand alone or move to a speaking podium (Hamiwka et al., 2009). Contemporary disability activists often view his disguise of his disabilities as promoting an image of individuals with disabilities as weak and infirm, contradicting efforts of integration in later years.

Contemporary Conceptualizations of People With Disabilities

Soon after the conclusion of WWII, in 1950 a group of parents opposed to the concept of institutionalization for their disabled children formed the Association for Retarded Children (now called The Arc). This group began to advocate strongly for children with intellectual disabilities. Today, the Arc is the "world's largest community-based organization of and for people with intellectual and developmental disabilities" (The Arc, 2021).

The concept of independent living began with the deinstitutionalization movement in the 1960 and 1970s, when parents' groups and professionals improved institutional care and established community-based independent living centers for PWD. This corresponded with the Rehabilitation Act of 1973, which promoted disabled individuals' efforts to form community based, nonresidential programs and find resources within their geographic area. Although some PWD moved into a limited number of community settings, most remained in institutional settings.

PWD are seldom portrayed in the modern media as having a full range of personality types and unique abilities. When a television or movie role portrays people with disabilities as fully functioning, integral members of society, this is often viewed by the public as unusual or unexpected.

Global Perspective on Culture and Disability

Individuals from other parts of the globe may have varying perspectives and experiences of disability. For example, in Nigerian society, children with disability have been perceived as cursed by God for gross disobedience, having ancestral violations of societal norms, or being witches and wizards, among the range of common societal misperceptions, leading to poor treatment from others (Eskay et al., 2012). Similarly, in Chinese culture, Confucian ideology, which otherwise views all people as deserving respect and kindness, also recognizes a social hierarchy in which those with disabilities were regarded as having the lowest status (Campbell and Uren, 2011). Traditional Chinese culture focuses on the cause of disability because, culturally, there is assumed to be a link between disability and previous wrongdoing. In those areas, someone with a disability is believed to bring shame and guilt to the family (Chiang and Hadadian, 2010).

Likewise, thematic assumptions derived from qualitative research on disability in South India include the notion that increased biomedical knowledge imparted via health education programs will reduce the incidence of disability because people will learn to take preventive measures and will decrease suffering caused by disability (Staples, 2012). A common belief is that many conditions are caused or made worse by a failure to access biomedical resources or by carelessness. This implies that many disabled people, and especially those from rural, uneducated, and economically poor backgrounds, do not obtain suitable treatment for their conditions (Staples, 2012).

PREVALENCE OF DISABILITY

Worldwide, over one billion people, or 15% of the population, has some form of a disability, with between 110 and 190 million people experiencing significant functional disabilities (WHO, 2020). In the United States, prevalence estimates are that one in four or 26% of people which equates to 61 million individuals have a disability (CDC, 2018). The Disability and Health Data System (DHDS) 2018 statistics reported the largest disability by type includes those individuals with mobility issues (12.4%) followed by cognitive (11.5%), independent living (6.8%), hearing (5.9%), visual (5.0%), and self-care (3.5%) disabilities (DHDS, 2018).

The CDC (2021) noted that "Disability Impacts all of US" (Fig. 21.2). This information depicts the increased prevalence and disparities between PWD and those without disabilities in assessing heart disease, obesity, smoking, and diabetes. Of note, the most significant difference is that 14.8% more PWD smoke than their nondisabled peers. This could be attributed to not only the social factors associated with smoking but also fewer social opportunities among PWD for social interaction and employment. Other important correlates with this population are that about 36% of individuals with disabilities report not having a usual care provider, 33.5% have not had a routine checkup in 12 months, 26.6% or unemployed and 38.6% are living at or below the 100% federal poverty level (Cree et al., 2020). Most disturbing is the people with disabilities report mental distress 4.6 times more frequently than their nondisabled peers and 50% are diagnosed with depressive disorders (Cree et al., 2020).

Disability Prevalence by Age, Race, and Sex

Recent data relayed that the largest age group of PWD is comprised of those age 65 and older (43.8%), followed by those aged 45 to 64 (29.2%) and the lowest in the age group 18 to 44 (18.5%) (DHDS, 2018). More females have a disability (27.2%) than males (24.7%) and veterans comprise 28.2% of PWD (DHDS, 2018). Data for ethnicity and disability are presented in Fig. 21.3. Disparities are evident as American Indian and Alaska Natives are representative of the largest percentage of PWD (39.9%) while Asians represent the lowest percentage of PWD (16.4%) (DHDS, 2018).

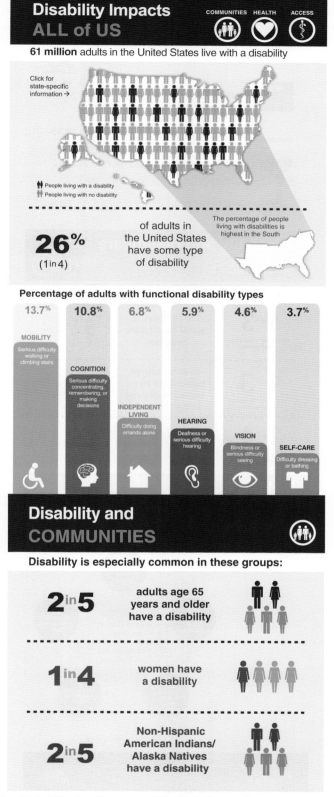

Fig. 21.2 CDC disability among US. *CDC,* Centers for disease control and prevention. (From https://www.cdc.gov/ncbddd/disabilityandhealth/disability.html.)

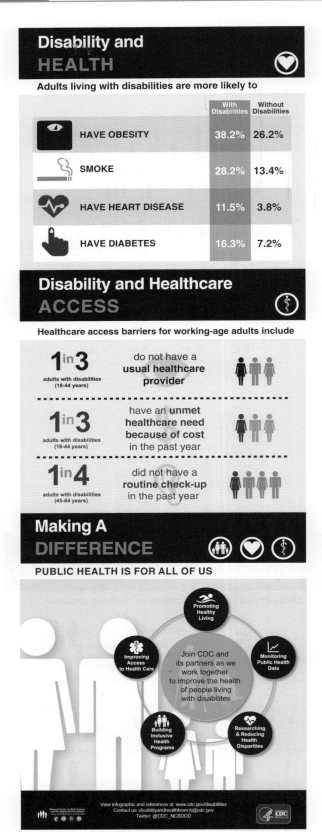

Fig. 21.2 cont'd

Prevalence of Disability in Children

Overall prevalence of children with developmental disabilities has been reported to be 17% or 1 in 6 (Zablotsky et al., 2019). Further, it is estimated that 47% of those children used Medicaid or CHIP for their health care (Musumeci and Chidambaram, 2019). Analysis of the prevalence of children with disabilities revealed a significant increase of developmental disabilities among age groups 3 to 17 years old between the years 2009 and 2017 (16.2%–17.8%) (Zablotsky et al., 2019).

Developmental disabilities among children include CP, hearing or visual loss, ID, ADHD, ASD, other developmental delays, stuttering or stammering in past 12 months and seizures (CDC, 2019).

The U.S. Department of Education provides a good source for assessment of the scope of disabilities among children who attend special education classes. Indeed, between 2011 to 2012 and 2018 to 2019 school years, the number of students receiving special education increased from 6.4 to 7.1 million (U.S. Department of Education [USDE], 2019).

According to School Year 2018 to 2019 data describing children attending special education classes, 14% of children ages 3 to 17 received special education; of those, the most prevalent disability type was reported as a "specific learning disability" (33%), followed by speech delay (19%), other health disability (15%), Autism (11%), developmental disability (7%), ID (6%), emotional disability (5%), multiple disabilities (2%), and hearing and orthopedic each comprised 1% (USDE, 2019). The race/ethnicity distribution of children receiving special education mirrors that of adults with disabilities: 18% American Indian/Alaskan Native, 16% Black, 14% White, 14% two or more races, 13% Hispanic, 11% Pacific Islander, and 7% Asian.

Intellectual and developmental disability (IDD) is defined as limitations in intellect measured by intelligence quotient (IQ) ranging from mild (IQ 50–70), moderate (IQ 35–49), severe (IQ 20–34), to profound (IQ < 20). Etiology of IDD includes genetic disorders and syndromes and TBI (APA, 2017). ID is the most common kind of developmental disability; approximately 6.5 million people in the United States have an ID, and about 1% to 3% of the global population (some 200 million people) has an ID (Special Olympics, 2021). Some of the most commonly reported developmental disabilities and IDDs are described here.

Autism Spectrum Disorder

ASD is a developmental disability that affects social, emotional, and behavioral skills. ASD is comprehensive term for a set of similar developmental disabilities, including autistic disorder, pervasive developmental disorder, and Asperger syndrome. It has been estimated that about 1 in 54 children (18.5 cases per 1000 children) have autism (CDC, 2020a). Of concern, the prevalence of autism has increased in recent years; one in 54 children had a diagnosis of ASD by age 8 in 2016, a nearly 10% increase from 2014 when the estimate was 1 in 59 (Autism

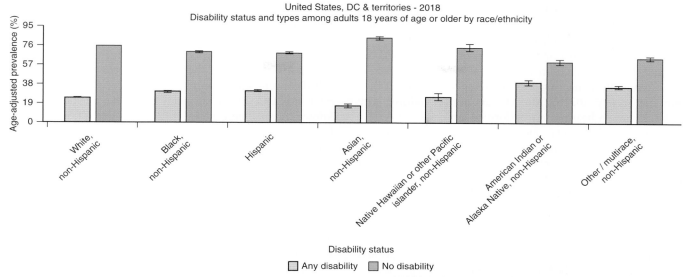

Fig. 21.3 Disability status and types by race/ethnicity. (From Centers for Disease Control and Prevention: *National Center on Birth Defects and Developmental Disabilities, Division of Human Development and Disability. Disability and Health Data System (DHDS) Data [Online].* URL: https://dhds.cdc.gov. Accessed February 27, 2021.)

Speaks, 2020). It has been observed that children diagnosed with ASD who receive intervention at an earlier age experience improvements in language and communications skills as well as higher intelligence than those who's care is delayed. As a result, *Healthy People 2030* has set a target increase of 10% (from 43.3% to 53.3%) of children receiving early, specialized services (www.healthypeople.gov).

Autism has no known etiology, but it is generally accepted that it is caused by abnormalities in brain structure or function, and more frequently occurs among children of older parents. It is about 4.5 times more common among boys than girls and cooccurs with chromosomal abnormalities such as DS and fragile X syndrome (Autism Speaks, 2020). As mentioned, early identification of autism is important for effective implementation of interventions and improvement of outcomes.

⚡ RESEARCH HIGHLIGHTS

Prevalence of Autism Spectrum Disorder

A large survey was conducted through the Early Autism and Developmental Disabilities Monitoring Network. Among the findings were a prevalence estimate for 4-year-olds at 13.4 per 1000 (20.3 male and 6.1 female). This illustrated a 30% lower prevalence than 8-year-olds, but prevalence with ASD and cognitive deficits was 20% higher among the 4-year-old age group. Additionally, female and white non-Hispanic children were more likely to be evaluated at an earlier age, 36 months, than male and non-Hispanic black children. Most

importantly, 93% of 4-year-olds and 87% of 8-year-olds had a documented record of developmental issues before age 3. Emphasis on early diagnosis is therefore imperative to improved outcomes (Christensen et al., 2016).

Down Syndrome

DS is a chromosomal disorder occurring in 1 in 700 people. Six thousand children are born with this alteration in genetic makeup each year (National Down Syndrome Society, 2021d). There are three types of DS: trisomy 21 (95%), translocation in chromosomal pairing (4%), and mosaics (1%—2%) (National Down Syndrome Society, 2021d). Children born with DS have distinctive physical characteristics as a result of changes on chromosome 21. Assessments of these children typically reveal proportionally shorter necks, small hands, almond-shaped eyes, small ears, a short stature, poor muscle tone, and "loose" joints. Of note, approximately half of children with DS present with serious cardiac anomalies, creating inadequate pulmonary and cardiovascular circulation (see the Case Study at the end of the chapter).

Individuals with DS are also prone to other comorbidities. For example, stenotic (or narrow) ear canals can occur in up to 40% to 50% of infants with DS, and consequently, children with DS and are predisposed to chronic ear infections, and adults with DS are at high risk for conductive hearing loss (National Down syndrome Society, 2021c). Therefore, audiologic testing is recommended for individuals with DS at birth and then every 6 months up to age three, or until the child can cooperate for an audiogram that includes ear-specific testing (more frequently if hearing loss is present) (National Down Syndrome Society, 2021b). After 3 years of age, children with DS should have a hearing test performed annually.

As noted, cardiovascular abnormalities are also common in DS (National Down Syndrome Society, 2021c). The most common heart defects are atrioventricular septal defect, ventricular septal defect, persistent ductus arteriosus, and tetralogy of fallot (National Down Syndrome Society, 2021b). Recommended treatment for these conditions is surgery and it must be done before age five or 6 months in order to prevent lung damage. Babies with DS also have hypotonia and ligament laxity which contributes to hip dysplasia and imposes difficulties for mothers trying to breast feed as the babies are often described as "floppy."

As they age, individuals with DS have a greatly increased risk of developing a type of dementia that is either the same as or very similar to Alzheimer's disease (Alzheimer's Association, 2021). By age 40, the brains of almost all individuals with DS have significant levels of beta-amyloid plaques and tau tangles, abnormal protein deposits considered Alzheimer's hallmarks (Alzheimer's Association, 2021). About 30% of people with DS who are in their 50s and about 50% of people with DS in their 60s have Alzheimer's dementia (National Down Syndrome Society, 2021a).

Autism is another comorbidity that can occur with DS. A growing number of children with DS are being diagnosed as also having autism (8%–9%) or ASD (16%–19%) (Down Syndrome Education International, 2021). Diagnosis of ASD is based on symptoms in three domains: social impairments, communication impairments and repetitive behaviors. Children with DS may also show behaviors associated with ASD even though they do not have ASD; therefore, experienced clinicians should use standardized assessments to make a diagnosis of ASD in children with DS. Children with DS may also show behaviors associated with ASD even though they do not have ASD (Down Syndrome Education International, 2021).

Cerebral Palsy

CP refers to a group of disorders that affect one's ability to move and maintain balance and posture. It is the most common motor disability in childhood. Cerebral means having to do with the brain, and palsy means weakness or problems with using the muscles (CDC, 2020d). CP is caused by abnormal brain development or damage to the developing brain that affects a child's ability to control his or her muscles, and recent estimates of CP range from one to nearly four per 1000 live births or per 1000 children; about 1 in 345 children (3 per 1000 8-year-old children) in the United States have been identified with CP (CDC, 2020d).

The brain damage that leads to CP can happen before birth, during birth, within a month after birth, or during the first years of a child's life, while the brain is still developing. Etiologies of CP include hypoxic ischemic injury, congenital abnormalities from brain malformation or genetic disorders, prematurity, infections, and intracranial hemorrhage. CP related to brain damage that happened before or during birth is called congenital CP, comprising the majority of CP cases (85%–90%) (CDC, 2020d). In many cases, the specific cause is not known. A small percentage of CP—acquired CP—is caused by brain damage occurring more than 28 days after birth. Acquired CP is usually associated with an infection (such as meningitis) or head injury (CDC, 2020d).

CP can be classified by type of motor disorder (spasticity, dyskinesia, ataxia, or mixed), distribution of the motor disorder (hemiplegia, diplegia, quadriplegia), or the severity of the mobility impairment. Sensory deficits such as hearing issues and strabismus or other visual acuity—related issues are frequently present with CP.

An important intervention for children with CP is use of orthotics, which refers to devices and instruments to help a child maintain his or her level of mobility, or correct physical issues that are preventing the child from being fully ambulatory (My Child at CerebralPalsy.org, 2021). Orthotics, such as externally worn braces, are complex tools or devices that are individually constructed and dictated by a child's structural and functional needs and the role expected to play in a child's development (My Child at CerebralPalsy.org, 2021). Orthotics may be utilized to help with knee or hip subluxation or dislocation; spastic movement; to correct, limit or prevent deformities; to support low-tone protonation (fallen arches, outward-turned foot due to muscle weakness) or high-tone pronation (high arch, outward-turned foot due to increased muscle tone); to correct wing-phase inconsistency (erratic movements in the foot), drop-foot (drop of the front of the foot due to weakness), eversion (outward turn), or inversion (inward turn).

Cleft Lip and Palate

Between the fourth and seventh weeks of pregnancy, the lips form (CDC, 2020c). As a baby develops during pregnancy, body tissue and special cells from each side of the head grow toward the center of the face and join together to make the face, forming the facial features, including the lips and mouth. If the tissue that makes up the lip does not join completely before birth, this results in an opening in the upper lip, called a cleft lip. The opening in the lip can be a small slit or it may be a large opening that goes through the lip into the nose (CDC, 2020c). A cleft lip can occur on one or both sides of the lip or in the middle of the lip. Children with a cleft lip can also have a cleft palate, which occurs when the tissue that makes up the roof of the mouth does not join together completely during pregnancy. Cleft lip (with or without cleft palate) affects one in 700 babies annually and is the fourth most common birth defect in the United States (WebMD, 2021). Clefts occur more often in children of Asian, Latino, or Native American descent. Surgery to repair a cleft lip usually is usually done in the first few months of life and is recommended within the first 12 months of life (CDC, 2020c).

Spina Bifida

SB occurs when there is failure of the neural tube to close during the 28th day of gestation. SB is associated with deficits in motor, sensory, and physical differences, and children born with SB also experience higher rates of epilepsy and hydrocephalus. Adequate folic acid supplementation prior to and during gestation is important for prevention of neural tube development. In the United States, mandatory fortification was instituted in 1998, to include wheat flour and maize (CDC, 2017). Birth prevalence of neural tube defects has decreased by 35% in the United States, since folic acid fortification was required in 1998 (CDC, 2017). Many developing countries experience a high prevalence of SB, cleft lip/palate, hydrocephalus, and anencephaly secondary to subpar nutritional standards—for example, cereals and flour in these areas may not be fortified with folic acid.

Science and technology have made it possible to intervene for SB in utero. Prenatal repair of myelomeningocele, the most common and severe form of SB, is a delicate surgical procedure in which fetal surgeons open the uterus and close the opening in the baby's back while they are still in the womb (Children's Hospital of Philadelphia, 2021). Because spinal cord damage is progressive during gestation, prenatal repair of myelomeningocele may prevent further damage.

Hydrocephalus

Hydrocephalus occurs in 15% to 25% of children with open myelomeningocele (one form of SB) at birth, though the proportion of patients with myelomeningocele who require shunting reaches 80% to 90% (Sgouros, 2019). Although there are a number of causes of infantile hydrocephalus, the condition is most associated with the congenital anomalies, SB, and aqueductal stenosis.

Hydrocephalus occurs when there is a buildup of fluid in the cavities (ventricles) deep within the brain. The excess fluid increases the size of the ventricles and puts pressure on the brain. The pressure of too much cerebrospinal fluid associated with hydrocephalus can damage brain tissues and cause a range of impairments in brain function (Mayo Clinic, 2021). Although hydrocephalus can happen at any age, it occurs more frequently among infants and adults 60 and over.

Signs and symptoms of hydrocephalus vary according to age of onset. Common signs and symptoms in infancy include changes in the head (an unusually large head, rapid increase in head size, or a bulging or tense fontanel on top of the head), vomiting, sleepiness; irritability, poor feeding, seizures; sunsetting of the eyes; deficits in muscle tone and strength; poor responsiveness to touch; and poor growth (Mayo Clinic, 2021). Toddlers and older children can experience headache; blurred or double vision; sunsetting of eyes; abnormal enlargement of a toddler's head; sleepiness or lethargy; nausea or vomiting;

unstable balance; poor coordination; poor appetite; seizures; urinary incontinence; behavioral and cognitive changes; irritability; change in personality; decline in school performance; and delays or problems with previously acquired skills, such as walking or talking (Mayo Clinic, 2021). Hydrocephalus manifests similarly in young and middle-aged adults, who may also experience loss of bladder control or a frequent urge to urinate, along with a decline in memory, concentration and other thinking skills that may affect job performance. In adults, 60 years of age or older more common signs and symptoms of hydrocephalus are loss of bladder control or a frequent urge to urinate; memory loss; progressive loss of other thinking or reasoning skills; difficulty walking, often described as a shuffling gait or the feeling of the feet being stuck; and poor coordination or balance (Mayo Clinic, 2021). Since some of these signs resemble those of dementia or Parkinson's disease, a thorough patient history and comprehensive diagnostic testing are important for an accurate diagnosis.

Surgical treatment for hydrocephalus can restore and maintain normal cerebrospinal fluid levels in the brain. Many different therapies are often required to manage symptoms or functional impairments resulting from hydrocephalus. Individuals with hydrocephalus will require lifelong therapy and monitoring. Options for surgical interventions for hydrocephalus include a shunt (tube) that is surgically inserted into the brain and connected to a flexible tube placed under the skin to drain the excess fluid into either the chest cavity or the abdomen so it can be absorbed by the body (National Institute of Neurological Disorders and Stroke, 2020).

Morbidity and Mortality of PWD

Epidemiological data could offer insight into disparities in care involving lack of access, income, advocacy, and into quality of care and prevention interventions. Unfortunately, standardized data are not captured comprehensively in many health visits or from national surveys, even those that aim to illuminate the extent of the data gap in both disability surveillance and morbidity and mortality reporting. In part, the variances in definitions for disability complicate the collection of measurable and generalizable data. For example, adults with any type of development disability die an average of 23.5 years earlier than those without developmental disability. Of note, individuals with CP or cooccurring developmental disabilities, die up to 34 years earlier than adults without developmental disability (Stevens, 2019). Further, persons with ID die an average of 12.7 years earlier than those without developmental disabilities, and adults with developmental disability die at extremely higher rates between ages 18 and 39 compared to those without (Stevens, 2019).

Extensive surveillance and research are warranted to determine the extent of the etiology as a consequence of the underlying disability, as opposed to the definitive disparities and inequalities that are known to occur in this vulnerable population. In the following section, fairly frequently occurring comorbidities that increase the overall risk of mortality of those with selected conditions within the disabled population will be outlined.

Epilepsy

Among those with IDD, epilepsy is prevalent as a comorbidity. Epilepsy is a significant contributor to other risk factors such as the inability to feed or care for oneself, poor communication ability, and lower IQ. Prevalence of epilepsy varies by diagnosis. A considerable body of evidence supports the understanding that psychiatric illness is overrepresented in epilepsy as compared with other chronic medical illnesses (Salpekar and Mula, 2019). People with epilepsy have a 2 to 5 times increased risk of developing any psychiatric disorder and one in three patients with epilepsy have a lifetime psychiatric diagnosis (Mula et al., 2020). Epilepsy may be present in half of children and adolescents with autism or other IDDs (Salpekar and Mula, 2019). As a whole, individuals with epilepsy have a significantly higher prevalence of psychiatric comorbid disorders involving depression, anxiety, psychotic, and attention-deficit disorders compared with the general population or patients with other chronic medical conditions (Lopez et al., 2019). A systematic and comprehensive approach to care of individuals with epilepsy has been lacking, resulting in undertreatment of these psychiatric disorders in persons with epilepsy.

Incidence of epilepsy also varies according to demographic factors, affecting both sexes and all ages with worldwide distribution (Beghi, 2020). Prevalence and the incidence of epilepsy are slightly higher in men compared to women and tend to peak among older adults, reflecting the higher frequency of stroke, neurodegenerative diseases, and tumors in this age group (Beghi, 2020).

Medical Comorbidities and IDD

Individuals with IDD are more likely to have medical comorbidities, compared to people without IDD. For example, children with intellectual disabilities have significantly higher incidence of congenital diseases, family disorders, and a higher frequency of acquired (noncongenital comorbid) disorders during early childhood compared to the children with normal psychomotor development (Markovic-Jovanovic et al., 2019). The presence of familial disorders and CNS congenital anomalies appeared to increase the risk of ID, Further, risk for congenital malformations involving other organs or organ systems is more than 7 times higher in children with intellectual deficits compared to those without developmental disorders.

Children with DS are four times more likely to develop diabetes than other children; about one child in 60 with Down's syndrome will also develop diabetes (Down Syndrome Association, 2020). Children with DS also face a high rate of congenital heart defects; as described, about 50% of infants with DS have some form of heart condition, compared with approximately 1% of typical infants (Global Down Syndrome Foundation, 2019).

Other health conditions associated with IDD include feeding and growth problems, gastroesophageal reflux disease, constipation, musculoskeletal problems including hypotonia and scoliosis, oral health problems, ear infections, sleep problems, vision and hearing problems, and dysmenorrhea (Golisano Children's Hospital, 2021). Approximately 25% of individuals with complex congenital heart disease also have IDD, which can be manifest at the outset (as in chromosomal syndromes) or appear in later childhood (Sharma, 2016).

Studies have suggested that the diagnosis of ASD is complicated by the correlation of physical activity decreasing with age and neighborhood or physical environments that are not conducive to physical activity (Jones et al., 2017). The prevalence of obesity among children ages 10 to 17 years old analyzed from a nationally representative sample with autism was significantly higher, at 23.1%, than in children without autism, at 14.1% (Must et al., 2017).

COVID-19 has very negatively affected individuals with DD. Recently, an examination was done on electronic medical record data from 42 healthcare organizations including hospitals, and primary care and specialty treatment providers designed to facilitate COVID-19 research (Turk et al., 2020). Findings revealed that across all age groups, patients with IDD and a positive diagnosis for COVID-19 demonstrated higher rates for all pre-existing conditions associated with COVID-19 disease severity and mortality (circulatory, endocrine, and pulmonary).

Lifelong monitoring and careful management of the complex healthcare needs of individuals with IDD is essential for optimal health maintenance. The leading cause of death for adults with and without IDD is heart disease (Landes et al., 2020). Further, adults with IDD, regardless of the severity of the disability, had substantially higher risk of death from pneumonitis, influenza/pneumonia and choking, while adults with mild/moderate IDD also had higher risk of death from diabetes mellitus. The importance of primary care and timely diagnoses cannot be underemphasized, as without focused and accessible health care, early mortality is likely in PWD.

Fatal Five

The "Fatal Five" refers to the top five conditions linked to preventable complications and deaths of persons with IDD and other developmental disabilities, particularly those residing in congregate care settings or in community-based residential settings (Health Risk Screening, 2020). These five conditions are: aspiration, bowel obstruction, dehydration, seizures, and infection/sepsis. The etiology of the fatal five includes polypharmacy, improper positioning, obesity, and dysphagia. Individuals with ID and/or motor disabilities are also predisposed to a variety of dental issues, including dental erosions as a consequence of GERD, dental caries, sialorrhea (drooling) due to inadequate swallowing, bruxism (grinding of teeth), malocclusion, and enamel defects (Jan and Jan, 2016).

Disability and Public Policy

Early United States public policy viewed people with disabilities as "deserving poor" who required governmental protection and provision and had little capacity for self-support or independence (Moffitt, 2015). Contemporary disability policy minimizes this disadvantaged view and maximizes opportunities for people with disabilities to live productively in their communities. Public policy on disability includes civil rights protections, skill enhancement programs, and income and in-kind assistance programs (e.g., SSDI and Medicare).

Legislation Affecting People With Disabilities

Consistent with historical and social changes and the recognition of barriers and discrimination, key federal legislation has been enacted that supports the rights of people with disabilities. This section describes a few of the most significant acts and their impact.

The Individuals With Disabilities Education Act

The Individuals with Disabilities Education Act (IDEA) (PL 94–142) ensures a free and appropriate public education to children with disabilities that is based on their needs, in the *least restrictive setting* from preschool through secondary education. Addressing special education needs requires appropriate evaluation and transition services. Parents, the student, and professionals are to join together to develop an individualized education plan (IEP) that includes measurable educational goals and related services specific for the child. The National Association of School Nurses (NASN, 2018) asserts that the registered professional school nurse is an essential member of the team participating in the identification and evaluation of students who may be eligible for services. Within the legally required process, the school nurse's responsibilities could include

- Assisting in identification of special educational or health-related service needs
- Working collaboratively with child/parent/guardian/healthcare provider assessing functional and physical health status
- Developing individualized healthcare plans and emergency care plans
- Making recommendations to the team of any health-related accommodations or services required
- Assisting the team in developing an IEP or accommodation plan that provides for required health needs and enables the student to participate in their educational program
- Assisting with identification and removal of health-related barriers to learning
- Providing in-service training for teachers and staff regarding the individual health needs of the child
- Providing and/or supervising unlicensed assistive personnel or direct service providers for provision of specialized healthcare services in the school setting
- Evaluating the effectiveness and revising as necessary the IEP health-related components (Gibbons et al., 2013; NASN, 2018).

It is the school nurse's responsibility to understand the law and to refer students who may be eligible for the services as outlined in the law. The nurse will also participate on school teams that determine eligibility for services (NASN, 2018).

The Americans With Disabilities Act of 1990 and ADA Amendments Act of 2008

The Americans with Disabilities Act (ADA) (PL 101–336) became law in July 1990. This landmark civil rights–styled legislation prohibits discrimination against people with disabilities by guaranteeing equal opportunities for people with disabilities in relation to employment, transportation, public accommodations, public services, and telecommunications (U.S. Department of Justice, 2021). It provides protection to people with disabilities similar to those provided to any person on the basis of race, color, sex, national origin, age, and religion. The U.S. Equal Employment Opportunity Commission is charged with enforcement of the employment provisions.

The ADA refers to a "qualified individual" with a disability as a person with a physical or mental impairment that substantially limits one or more major life activities or bodily functions, a person with a record of such an impairment, or a person who is regarded as having such an impairment. The ADA prohibits discrimination against people who have a known association or relationship with an individual with a disability. A qualified individual with a disability must meet legitimate skill, experience, education, or other requirements of an employment position. The person must be able to perform the essential job functions, such as those contained within a job description, with or without reasonable accommodation(s). Reasonable accommodations should make it easier to be successful in job duties and may either involve altering the duties or the tasks of the job performed. Qualifying organizations must provide reasonable accommodations unless they can demonstrate that the accommodation will cause significant difficulty or expense, producing an undue hardship.

Ticket to Work and Work Incentives Improvement Act

Historically, national public policy has defined disability as the inability to work. Typically, people with disabilities could qualify only for such benefits as health care, income assistance programs, and personal care attendant services if they chose not to work. To address employment and benefit issues for PWD, in December 1999, the Ticket to Work and Work Incentives Improvement Act (TWWIIA) (PL 106–170) was signed into law. The TWWIIA was signed into law to increase the options for PWD who wished to return to work (Social Security Administration, 2021b). The TWWIIA reduced the disincentives to work for PWD by increasing access to vocational services and provided new methods for retaining health insurance after they returned to work. In 2008, the Ticket to Work program experienced a significant overhaul when new regulations were produced that dramatically revised the payment structure available to employment networks. This provided a higher cap to accommodate earnings when beneficiaries make progress in their employment plans but before they reach the level of earnings that would terminate their benefits (Brain Injury Association of America, 2021). The Ticket to Work revision is intended to improve program effectiveness in order to maximize the economic selfsufficiency of beneficiaries.

❓ ACTIVE LEARNING

- Can a client who uses a wheelchair obtain mammography for breast cancer screening, or is the lack of adaptive equipment a barrier to participation? What can you discover online about the availability and cost of accessible transportation to the screening site? Can a woman get onto an examination table for collection of a Papanicolaou smear specimen? Office staff and equipment *should* accommodate people's limitations. Think about the office where you receive health care or the imaging laboratories in the area where you live. Can they accommodate someone in a wheelchair?
- In a primary care office, a woman presents with symptoms of a urinary tract infection. She has experienced decreased mobility due to past lower extremity amputation and is morbidly obese, so is unable to sit down on a standard toilet and hold a cup, both of which are required to collect a urine sample. How can the nurse make modifications to the environment to assist the client and collect the sample?
- The nurse working in an outpatient health clinic manages a health promotion and education program for local individuals with IDD. The time for local elections is nearing and the nurse would like to provide resources for these patients to enable them to vote. What rights do these individuals have as citizens with disabilities? What resources may they access? See https://www.eac.gov/election-officials/voting-accessibility for further information.

Public Assistance Programs

Public assistance programs include cash assistance (monetary payments, like Social Security), food stamps, and subsidized housing. Approximately 61.8% of adults aged 18 to 64 with a severe disability received some form of public assistance, while 24.0% of adults with a nonsevere disability received assistance (Taylor, 2018).

Supplemental Security Income and Social Security Disability Insurance

The Social Security Administration (2021a) defines disability as the "inability to engage in any substantial gainful activity by reason of any medically determinable physical or mental

impairment(s) which can be expected to result in death or which has lasted or can be expected to last for a continuous period of not less than 12 months." Most people who receive disability benefits qualify on the basis of their personal inability to work because of a disability; however, exceptions include people who are blind or have low vision, benefits for widows or widowers who are disabled, and benefits for children who are disabled. Table 21.2 provides a comparison of **Supplemental Security Income (SSI)** and **SSDI** programs. Information about SSI and SSDI can also be accessed online (www.ssa.gov/disability/) or be obtained at a Social Security office.

THE EXPERIENCE OF DISABILITY

PWD are commonly thought to constitute the largest minority group in the United States. Of note, most people whose lives do not end abruptly will experience disability in their later years. Regardless of the specific condition, many experiences are common in the lived experience of disability. However, the personal meaning of disability differs significantly with the time frame and the duration of the event or disease process. Those who have a temporary disability, such as a sprained ankle, have a very different experience from someone with chronic illness or permanent disability. Although the former may experience the frustrations of mobility associated with the use of a wheelchair or crutches, this condition is temporary, and the full impact of the disability is not experienced. With a temporary disability, ADLs are adjusted as needed and additional or long-term resources are generally not necessary.

In contrast, those who have a permanent disability from an accident or from a disease process, such as limb loss or stroke, must learn to incorporate the modifications required for living into their daily routines and identities. People who become disabled from the progressive decline of a chronic illness, such as multiple sclerosis, may be reluctant to use assistive devices. They might believe that accepting such a device would mean accepting the label of being disabled. Unfortunately, many falls could be prevented by the use of walkers or canes that were declined because the people did not want to appear disabled. In many progressive diseases, a benchmark event forces the person to accept their disability—for example, a driving accident caused by failing eyesight or a change in mental capacity, or a

TABLE 21.2   Comparison of SSI & SSDI

Supplemental Security Income (SSI)	Social Security Disability Insurance (SSDI)
Funded through general tax revenues	Funded through disability trust fund monies (social security taxes paid by workers, employers, and self-employed workers)
To qualify for SSI, the person with disabilities (PWD) must have limited income and resources	To qualify for SSDI, the PWD must be "insured" through Federal Insurance Contributions Act (FICA) earnings of self, parents, and/or spouse
SSI disability benefits are payable to adults and children who are disabled or blind and are eligible	SSDI disability benefits are payable to workers or widow(er)s who are disabled or adults who have been disabled since childhood and are eligible
SSI recipients receive medicaid health benefits	SSDI recipients receive medicare health benefits
Some states may elect to pay a state supplement to some PWD in SSI programs	PWD in SSDI programs are never provided with state supplements

leg amputation from diabetic complications. The person can no longer plan daily activities and expect to accomplish them independently. Because the incidence of chronic illness and disability increases with longevity, often elderly persons experience increasingly disabling changes in their daily lives.

In many cases, a disability can result in a downward spiral. For example, when people with disabling symptoms are unable to return to work, they may lose their jobs and their benefits and exhaust personal resources, which could result in the loss of their home. They may apply for state and federal disability benefits, feeling fully qualified, but are warned there is a waiting period and to expect to be initially rejected. Nurses should engage active listening to better understand a client's situation. Finally, nurses play a role in helping clients connect with comprehensive social services by maintaining knowledge of available resources.

Sexual Health, Education, and the Potential for Abuse

PWD are no different from the general population in their desire for social inclusion and intimacy. Many parents or caregivers are not comfortable addressing what is integral to the quality of life and well-being of PWD, and conservative standards may label sexual activity, marriage, or childbearing as unorthodox or difficult to condone. Most healthcare professionals receive little to no training in the intersection between disability and sexuality, may hold many misconceptions about sexuality in PWD, or think that this population is not concerned with or had no interest or perceived needs related to sexual health (Crisp-Cooper, 2018). The exclusion of PWD from a discussion about sexual health has been highlighted in recent research (Ganle et al., 2020). Studies demonstrate the lack evidence on interventions promoting access to maternal health, family planning and contraception, or safe abortion for people with disabilities (Hameed et al., 2020).

Various obstacles may interfere with the sexual health of PWD, including the societal views noted, functional or physical limitations, difficulty conceptualizing abstract concepts, and personal boundaries/privacy issues. As advocates of PWD, community health nurses should establish a rapport and initiate therapeutic conversations about healthy sexual relationships and facilitate the identification of the health-related consequences of sexual behaviors, while also assessing for potentially abusive situations.

Violence and abuse in the disabled community are more prevalent than among other populations. PWD are at a higher risk of facing interpersonal violence, as compared to individuals without disabilities (Iudici et al., 2019), and children with disabilities experience violence more than nondisabled children, and episodes of violence start at birth (Njelesani et al., 2018). Child abuse in one's family has been identified as a significant predictor of PTSD symptom severity in individuals with IDD (Catani and Sossalla, 2015). Explanations for the IDD population, in particular, being at a greater risk for sexual abuse include the potential desire for social inclusion, powerlessness, or naiveté. In one population-based study, children with IDD represented 25.9% of the maltreatment allegations, with 29% of those allegations validated (Maclean et al., 2017). Recent research shows that the COVID-19 pandemic imposed disproportionate trauma and stress on the disabled community (Lund et al., 2020).

The Family of a Child With a Disability

Challenges and stressors encountered by parents with a **CWD** are definitively different, and more numerous. Caregiver burden in terms of quality of life, employment disruption, and financial impact has been frequently documented. Uncertainty in the future of the child and worry about who will care for the child if the child outlives the parent are common themes of parents of CWD (Vasa et al., 2018).

While earlier research involving children with disabilities emphasized pathology, and impaired functioning and relationships, research has now moved away from looking at family dysfunction and increasingly recognizes the successful, resourceful ways in which families adapt and provide care (Jacques, 2019). Reasons for this include the shift away from institutional models of care; acknowledgment of the rights and value of people with disabilities within society; changes in family structure; and recognition of the importance of family care in providing support well into adulthood (Jacques, 2019).

Families quickly learn that neither governmental support nor private health plans offer adequate community-based or in-home assistance for disabled family members. Literature findings describe the associations between low income and children with special needs; associations that might go both ways. Children in poverty have experiences (lead exposure, low-birthweight, malnutrition) that tend to be more associated with disability; however, families who care for a CWD often find themselves sliding toward financial insufficiency (Goodwin, 2018). Furthermore, the extent of financial and other resources available, which can determine the possibility of compensatory strategies (such as home modifications), often is the key factor in determining whether effective adaptation can be achieved (Palmer, 2016). Being denied or delayed access to needed health services can negatively affect the health and well-being of any person.

🏠 COMMUNITY FOCUS

Bullying of Children With Disabilities

Experiences of school-age children may range from teasing to *bullying*, which is defined as unwanted, aggressive behavior among school-age children, involving a real or perceived power imbalance that is repeated or has the potential to be repeated over time (stopbullying.gov, 2020). Bullying is a very serious problem for children, regardless of disability status. Although a commonly encountered phenomenon in many situations, children with physical, developmental, intellectual, emotional, and sensory disabilities are more likely to be bullied than their peers (stopbullying.gov, 2020).

Children with special health needs may be at greater risk of being bullied or abused. Research with 89 students with ASD without ID aged 11 to 16 years validates the magnitude of the problem, finding that children with ASD are likely to have experienced bullying past 6 months. Specifically, 55 students (64%, $n = 86$) and 60 parents (70%, $n = 86$) reported face-to-face victimization, and 12 students (14%, *n* = 85) and 11 parents (13%, *n* = 85) reported cyber victimization (Ashburner et al., 2018). Children with CP had higher odds of anxiety, behavior/conduct problems, and multimorbidity, though not depression, as compared to controls in one cross-sectional study of 6 to 17-year-olds with and without CP (Whitney et al., 2019). Along with children who have medical conditions that affect their appearance (such as CP and SB), children with Asperger's, autism, ADHD, dyslexia, or any condition that sets them apart, such as food allergies or DS are also more likely to be bullied by peers (Gordon, 2020). For the child coping with a disability, the threat of bullying is an added challenge, as bullying often contributes to depression, anxiety, health complaints, and decreased academic achievement.

For individuals with disabilities, bullying may be considered "disability harassment," a behavior that is prohibited under the Rehabilitation Act of 1973 and The Americans with Disabilities Act. "Disability harassment is defined as a range of negative behaviors including, but not limited to, abusive jokes, crude name-calling, threats, and sexual and physical assault. Harassment of any kind fosters a hostile environment that severely restricts a disabled adult or child's ability to perform or function" (U.S. Department of Education, 2020). If such an event occurs, there are actions parents of children with disabilities can take to support the bullied child. This involves communicating through the proper channels within the school system. A number of resources, such as "Stopbullying.gov," provide information on how to address the problem of bullying, including strategies for bullying prevention, identification of risk factors for victimization, and resources for help.

RESEARCH HIGHLIGHTS

Body Image After Amputation

A study conducted by a team led by Freysteinson et al. (2017) described body image and self-esteem experiences that occurred when individuals viewed themselves in the mirror for the first time after the loss of a limb. Previously explored in burn patients, after mastectomy, and in the elderly, this study adds a description of the mirror trajectory of experience among amputees.

A qualitative design was employed to explore this concept with focus groups. Researchers then utilized hermeneutic phenomenology, the study of the words and meaning ascribed to them, in dwelling with the content of the discussions and shared the concepts emerging from the experience.

The mirror experience had three key moments: decision, seeing, and consent. There were four key themes: mirror shock, mirror anguish, recognizing self, and acceptance of a new normal. Participants in focus groups also shared ways that staff members could better facilitate the introduction of a mirror after an amputation, such as using it as a small tool to check skin integrity and to correct gait and balance in the larger view. As this is a little-known phenomenon, further research on educational aspects, such as preparation of patients, families, and interprofessional staff members to better support the experience, is needed. Support of a family member or friend is suggested during this experience, but as nurses develop trust and intimacy with their patients, they could be a facilitator of the discussion of what to expect.

ACTIVE LEARNING

Prepare yourself for unexpected situations in clinical practice, by remembering that the person with the disability is the expert in their care and needs. For example, if an individual with bilateral upper extremity amputations requires blood pressure screening, ask them where this measurement has been performed in the past. This demonstrates a partnering attitude and facilitates more consistent measurement than consulting another resource.

Health Promotion and Disease Prevention for PWD

Worldwide, healthcare problems frequently are unrecognized and untreated, particularly among those with IDD who may not be able to communicate their symptoms and/or are unable to share in decision making. Acquired conditions, such as TBI are also a major cause of disability, as those who survive a TBI can face effects that include impairments related to thinking or memory, movement, sensation, or emotional functioning. Falls are a leading cause of TBI, disproportionately affecting children and older adults (CDC, 2019). Falls, violence, and motor vehicle injury are also leading causes of spinal cord injury, affecting between 259,000 and 500,000 people each year, worldwide. Following spinal cord injury, there is a 2 to 5 times greater risk of premature death, lifelong (WHO, 2020).

Despite the higher prevalence of chronic conditions that can significantly compromise physical function, such as arthritis, asthma, cardiovascular disease, diabetes, high blood pressure, high cholesterol, and stroke among individuals with disabilities, improvements in primary preventative care and surveillance are slow to occur (Rotoli et al., 2020). Clients with disabilities may exhibit behavioral problems that discourage healthcare providers from caring for them, or they may resist others' attempts to care for them because of their discomfort or unfamiliarity with the healthcare setting or equipment. There may be difficulties in obtaining a client history and in determining the nature and cause of a problem. This might easily be alleviated with teaching healthcare providers about healthcare problems that accompany a specific disability (Morris et al., 2021).

For example, it is widely acknowledged that socioeconomic disadvantages account for a significant proportion of variation in health status. Specifically, women with disabilities often experience disparities in primary care services, particularly in women's health issues. Because osteoporosis develops at higher rates in women with decreased mobility, recommendations include screening at earlier and more frequent intervals, special gynecological examination techniques, and "thoughtful well-coordinated" care from primary care providers (Baylor College of Medicine, 2020). Similarly, women with cognitive limitations and functional disabilities have been noted as less likely to receive a Pap smear within the past 3 years or a mammogram within the past 2 years. Primary care assessments for this population should also include immunizations and preventive screenings, such as those for breast, colon, and testicular cancer in males (Vanderbilt Kennedy Center, n.d.). Further, health promotion questions that assess diet, exercise, alcohol, drug use, smoking, and sexual health should be routine in primary care visits for disabled individuals (Bakker-van Gijssel et al., 2017).

Strategies for the Public Health Nurse Caring for People With Disabilities

Nurses have the responsibility of caring for the needs of varying populations. Regardless of whether the nurse chooses to work in a setting that specializes in health care services for people affected by disabilities, disability is a common experience that all practicing nurses will encounter in their professional career. This will require the professional nurse to be familiar with effective strategies for communicating and caring for individuals with a variety of disabilities. The scope of responsibility in caring for individuals with disabilities includes procuring the knowledge related to health conditions that may result from or lead to the disability, as well as being aware of the resources available and legal implications that affect the PWD.

Health care professionals are taught to assess and provide interventions that promote health, and they usually assume they know what people with disabilities need. Regardless of the provider's professional experience or familiarity with disability, clients may question a provider's ability to understand their experience. Moreover, literature supports that nurses and physicians who have not had experience caring for individuals with disabilities lack confidence and exhibit attitudes that are not conducive to caring for this vulnerable population (Bu et al., 2016).

Nurses must work with the interprofessional care team to form alliances with the client and family and reduce or eliminate barriers. People affected by disabilities may have some common health care needs or utilize similar resources, but other issues will be unique to each individual situation. The

public health nurse's perspective on disability will influence the nursing role and the level of care provided to PWD and their families. Delivery of passionate, person-centered care is essential and includes concepts of care, compassion, competence, communication, courage, and commitment and ensures patients' values are a component of clinical decisions (Brown et al., 2016). The Association of Rehabilitation Nurses has proposed a competency model for nursing that can be a guide for public health nursing care of clients with disabilities in the current dynamic healthcare environment (Fig. 21.4).

Nursing care must incorporate the true essence of advocacy, where it is defined as representing the needs of the client or patient. The nurse's role should be to discern the needs and resources of the client and his or her family. Only then may the nurse act effectively as a resource themselves, working to provide information, make connections, and manage accommodations. The acronym developed that spells ADVOCATE (Table 21.3) can help remind and guide the nurse of essential principles that are integral to the care of PWD. The table provides specific strategies to ensure the nurse practices effective care, communication etiquette, and advocacy in his or her care of PWD. Basic principles for communicating with PWD are outlined in Box 21.1.

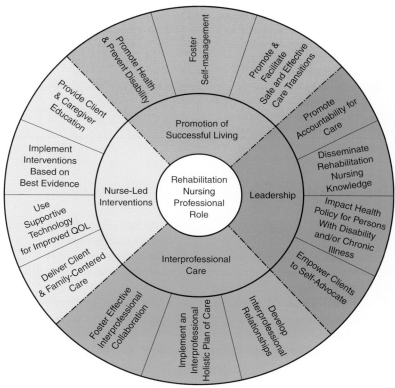

Fig. 21.4 Rehabilitation nursing professional roles. (Reprinted with permission from the Association of Rehabilitation Nursing.)

TABLE 21.3 Advocate

Advocate	Don't assume the client has a physical or cognitive deficit until you have validated it.
	Be knowledgeable and educate yourself about community resources and those pertaining to various disabilities
	Know the client's payer sources or other financial resources, as it may determine the level of assistance they obtain
	Be knowledgeable of risk for injury and abuse
	Practice forensic nursing, as clients may not be able to articulate their issues
Deficits	Determine sensory, visual, and hearing deficits
	Allocate additional time for care
	Eliminate physical environmental barriers
	Select the client's optimal time of day for education and ADLs
Vocation	Encourage vocation or "avocation," including recreational therapy that encourages social interaction (i.e., intramural teams, physical activity, hippotherapy, art classes)
	Assess employment history, interests, and employment obtainment
Outcomes	Observe for polypharmacy: Side effects/interactions
	Observe patterns of multiple hospitalizations and etiology
	Adopt the client's perspective as to what works best with no bias; cultural preferences may be a factor
	Be knowledgeable about evidence-based treatment options specific to the disability or disease
	Establish bowel and bladder routine and adequate hydration: Observe for signs and symptoms of urinary tract infection (UTI) or constipation
	Encourage weight-bearing exercises, T.E.D. hose, observe potential for postural hypotension with immobile clients
Communicate	Listen and learn from client, family, and caregiver
	Always say "Hello," "Good morning," and "Good afternoon," regardless of the client's ability to respond
	Directly speak with or to the client unless there are deficits that make it not feasible (communication, cognitive, hearing)
	At wheelchair level, by client's name, not their disability
	Reduce background noises or distractions during discussions
	Rephrase rather than repeat information if something is not understood
	Collaborate with interprofessionals for care outcomes, issues, facilitators, and barriers to care
	Professional boundaries if necessary
Assess	Determine what deficits the client deems a challenge or an issue
	Skin integrity of the immobilized and incontinent client
	Self-care ability: ADLs, feeding, bathing, and time of day where energy is optimal
	Necessary accommodations to environment (ramp, access), with communication (Braille, sign language) or adaptive devices that are used or needed; wheelchair, hearing aids, long-handled combs or shoe horns, hand braces for toothbrushes or utensils, drinking cups with weighted bases, Velcro, voice-activated technology
	Home environment, care providers, social networks
	Primary transportation preferences or use
Transition	Provide resources, information, and support when there is a change in level of care, care providers, school, or role responsibility within the family unit
Empower	Encourage learning, memory, coping skills, independence
	Reinforce abilities and success in ADLs, mobility, employment

© Allison Edwards.

Nursing Interventions

Public health nurses should partner with clients and families affected by disabilities to address barriers that negatively affect quality of life, a measure of satisfaction that reaches across physical, psychological, social, and environmental domains. Nurses cannot remedy health concerns without attending to interacting systems, such as knowledge and educational background, personal and family belief systems, religious/spiritual beliefs and supports, finances, social networks, physical resources, and cultural influences. Health promotion interventions for the community health nurse should include

• Provision of age-related health screenings

• Early surveillance of diseases based on knowledge of common comorbidities
• Maintenance of proper weight: counseling on appropriate nutrition and social inclusion through enhanced physical activity
• Identification of caregivers and support systems
• Identification of access to care issues: transportation, financial, and environmental barriers
• Safety of the physical environment: assistive technology (such as health monitoring devices and alarms, voice-activated technology, and mobility devices) and potential for abuse
• Knowledge of resources

1. Speak directly rather than through a companion or sign language interpreter who may be present.
2. Offer to shake hands when introduced. People with limited hand use or an artificial limb can usually shake hands and offering the left hand is an acceptable greeting.
3. Always identify yourself and others who may be with you when meeting someone with a visual disability. When conversing in a group, remember to identify the person to whom you are speaking. When dining with a friend who has a visual disability, ask if you can describe what is on his or her plate.
4. If you offer assistance, wait until the offer is accepted. Then listen or ask for instructions.
5. Treat adults as adults. Address people with disabilities by their first names only when extending that same familiarity to all others. Never patronize people in wheelchairs by patting them on the head or shoulder.
6. Do not lean against or hang on someone's wheelchair. Bear in mind that people with disabilities treat their chairs as extensions of their bodies. And so do people with guide dogs and help dogs. Never distract a work animal from their job without the owner's permission.
7. Listen attentively when talking with people who have difficulty speaking and wait for them to finish. If necessary, ask short questions that require short answers, or a nod of the head. Never pretend to understand; instead repeat what you have understood and allow the person to respond.
8. Place yourself at eye level when speaking with someone in a wheelchair or on crutches.
9. Tap a person who has a hearing disability on the shoulder or wave your hand to get his or her attention. Look directly at the person and speak clearly, slowly, and expressively to establish if the person can read your lips. If so, try to face the light source and keep hands, cigarettes and food away from your mouth when speaking. If a person is wearing a hearing aid, don't assume that they have the ability to discriminate your speaking voice. Never shout to a person. Just speak in a normal tone of voice.
10. Relax. Don't be embarrassed if you happen to use common expressions such as "see you later" or "Did you hear about this?" that seems to relate to a person's disability.

The ten commandments were adapted from many sources as a public service by United Cerebral Palsy Associates, Inc. (UCPA), UCPA's version of the ten commandments was updated by Irene M. Ward & Associates (Columbus, Ohio), also as a public service, and to provide the most current language possible for its video entitled, the 10 commandments of communicating with people with disabilities.

Differentiating Illness From Disability

Nurses who work in community settings must be able to differentiate between the person who has an illness and becomes disabled secondary to the illness and the person who has a disability but may not need care. Rather than assuming a need for intervention, the nurse should ask whether the client wants assistance, ask the client/family to describe the goal(s), and ask how and in what way(s) the nurse can help. PWD often confront *medicalization* issues when others view them in the *sick role* rather than as people first. Nurses should listen to understand, collaborating with the person/family to make plans and goals that meet the identified needs and that draw on strengths and improve weaknesses. Collaboration empowers and affirms the worth and knowledge of the person/family with a disability. Collaboration promotes selfdetermination and allows choices that foster personal values and preferences.

NURSING CARE GUIDELINES

Assistive Technology and Creative Solutions

A diagnosis of autism or ASD presents a myriad of issues for the provision of health care to this population. Unfamiliar individuals, places, or loud noises can overstimulate individuals with ASD. Primary care sites, including health care facilities or physicians' offices, may produce anxiety for someone with ASD. Telemedicine offers an ideal avenue for providing treatment in a convenient manner. Telemedicine involves the use of remote access to a primary care physician. Equipment necessary for accessing the primary care provider may include a video conference camera and a telephonic stethoscope, digital camera, and otoscope for a nurse-assisted visit (Langkamp et al., 2015). Telemedicine is utilized predominantly to improve access to care for individuals living in rural or underserved geographic areas; however, use in the IDD/developmental disability population could produce positive results if counseling may be more realistically delivered via conference call. Waivers issued in response to Covid-19 allowed for reimbursement by health care professionals who were previously ineligible to provide telehealth services, including physical therapists, occupational therapists, speech language pathologists, and others, and to receive payment from CMS for these services, expanding the possible uses of telehealth technology (Centers for Medicare and Medicaid Services, 2020).

"Knowledgeable Client" and "Knowledgeable Nurse"

Regardless of the cause of disability, the nurse must see beyond the disabling impairment, carefully assessing each affected person's perceptions of the disability experience. A person who lives with a disability commonly becomes an expert at knowing what works best for his or her body. This case differs significantly from the person with a new disabling illness or injury, or the parent of a child with a newly diagnosed disability, who needs information and time to adapt to their new change in circumstance. The Intersystem Model (Artinian et al., 2011) refers to the first-described person as the "Knowledgeable Client." In this case, a client has been living with disability for an extended time and has become sensitive to the needs of his or her body. The nurse should ask the client what works best for him or her and what goals the client is pursuing. The client wants the nurse to listen to his or her concerns and may benefit from a referral to health-related resources. However, if the nurse attempts to tell the Knowledgeable Client what to do without seeking input, the client may become angry and seek help elsewhere.

The clients in the second situation need the services of the "Knowledgeable Nurse" (Artinian et al., 2011). The client with a newly diagnosed condition can benefit from the nurse's information about the disability and the available community and governmental resources. It is important to note that if the nurse is unable to help a newly diagnosed client learn how to manage the disability and accept himself or herself as disabled, the nurse may compromise the client's adaptation and future client/nurse interactions.

Active collaboration between the client and nurse is required to develop a plan of care that both will find acceptable. Health care for PWD must incorporate remedies that address issues surrounding access to health care and the resolution of environmental and social barriers that prevent their full participation in society. Encouraging recreational time and physical activity provides a positive stimulus for PWD and multiple psychosocial and physiological benefits—for example, hippotherapy, a therapeutic method of horseback riding, shows evidence that it enhances motor strategies, which can improve functional task performance by enhancing reaction time among individuals with intellectual disabilities. Not only does the activity of horseback riding provide a rich social environment with the interaction between the PWD and the animal as well as other equestrians, but it also has demonstrated improvement in balance and strength in individuals with IDD, which could have a profound impact on their quality of life (Giagazoglou et al., 2012).

Ethical Issues for People Affected by Disabilities

PWD and their families are concerned about the same contemporary ethical and legal issues that concern all people. However, some of the associated issues carry particular interest for PWD and their families, including questions and problems surrounding definitions of respect for human beings, beneficence (do good), and nonmaleficence (do no harm), as well as the rights of PWD. The Patient Self-Determination Act (PSDA) of 1990 is one example. This law mandated that health decisions are communicated and protected and that patients, upon admission to a health care facility, are asked if they have a durable power of attorney or an advance directive. Families, guardians, or individuals are reluctant to address end-of-life decisions when health is good, so when conditions decline, bioethical principles must be balanced and applied, sometimes by a team or committee.

Clients' spiritual perspectives play an important role in decision making when there is a change in health status or a life-threatening illness. People who establish hope and meaning in their lives may choose to positively reframe the difficulties associated with functional limitations that others may find intolerable. Holistic caregiving requires the nurse to assess and promote spiritual health along with physical and psychological well-being.

Differences in quality of life and justice perspectives intersect with concerns about the control of healthcare costs. Advances

in neonatology are responsible for increasing numbers of very-low-birth-weight babies, who are at high risk for cognitive disorders and other serious health problems (Petrou et al., 2019). The attitudes of individuals toward impairment varies, often differentiated between congenital or stable conditions and those acquired later in life, or those with fluctuations in ability. The adoption of an identity as a disabled individual is a complex phenomenon, and it impacts views on health and function (Boardman et al., 2018).

For health care professionals to understand the end-of-life desires of the disabled population, more research is needed. Focus groups can yield beneficial information; however, feasibility is challenging. Participants may struggle to understand abstract concepts such as death; furthermore, physical environment supports and consulting for recruitment and consent among this vulnerable population are difficult (Savage et al., 2015). End-of-life decision making for children with severe developmental disabilities must involve a determination of whether the caregiver or parent will continue care necessary to sustain life, such as maintenance of a ventilator or artificial nutrition via gastrostomy tube, or cease support.

Genetic technology, such as prenatal cell-free DNA screening for chromosomal abnormalities, may lead to elective abortions but also offer hope for the prevention and cure of diseases. One study reported the elective termination rate at 67% for singleton and 60% for twins after prenatal testing resulting in aneuploidy, an abnormal number of chromosomes (Dobson et al., 2016). This prompts another question—Does selective abortion express a negative attitude that exists toward PWD? This argument might be similarly stated for end of life decisions, such as those involving physician assisted suicide or euthanasia (Reed, 2020).

ETHICAL INSIGHTS

Genome Selection and Modification by PWD Parents

The ethical principle of deontology, meaning, obligation or duty, embodies the moral principles of determining whether actions are right or wrong and not based upon their consequences.

The controversial action of preimplantation genetic diagnosis (PGD) clinics using selection or modification involves actively either selecting embryos with specific traits or modifying genetic markers to induce a diagnosis or trait. This practice was reported in 3% of PGD clinics surveyed that reported parents selecting for disabilities (Shaw, 2018). Is it ethical to impose a disability on a vulnerable population, such as a child who does not have a voice in the matter? Deontology would frame this as an active imposition of a hardship, irrespective of the child's consideration for their future choices, as opposed to passively allowing a disability to arise (Schroeder, 2018). Negative societal attitudes and perceptions of disabilities may engage the idea that disabilities somehow "reduce" well-being and therefore our moral obligation is the "reverse" those disabilities (Schroeder, 2018).

LIVING WITH A DISABILITY: CLINICAL PROFILES

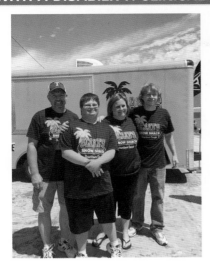

Blake is in his early 20s. His parents reported that they were told many times throughout Blake's life about what he "can't do" or "won't do." But they chose to focus on what he "can do" and even "could do" in the future. Blake was named a two-time captain of the varsity football team, Prom King, and Texas Citizen of the Year. At 20 years old, Blake became the first business owner in Texas with DS when he opened a snow cone stand, *Blake's Snow Shack*. Blake's business has achieved local, national, and international acclaim (Courtesy of Blake's Snow Shack. www.blakessnowshack.com.).

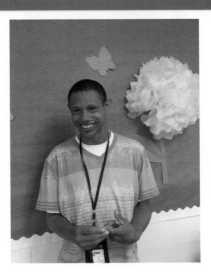

Sam is an African American in his mid-30s. Sam has autism (ASD). He is nonverbal but follows directions and performs all ADLs independently.

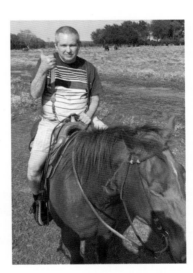

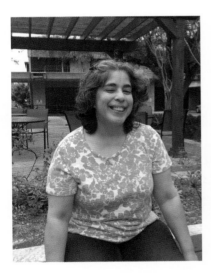

Rosa is a Hispanic female with intellectual disabilities. She is her own guardian and lives with her sister and attends a day habilitation program.

Max, age 60, is a Caucasian male, born with intellectual disabilities. He has lived in a variety of settings since the age of 12, including a specialized residential school, residential-vocation facility, long-term care, and currently a group home. He feeds and dresses himself, but personal care activities are assisted.

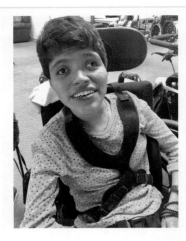

Catalina is a 32-year-old Hispanic female who was born with CP. She has some upper extremity mobility, and needs assistance eating and with ADLs. She has discernible language skills, although limited to monosyllabic words.

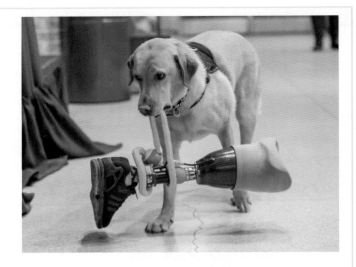

Aggie is a 4-year-old female Labrador retriever. Aggie is a Service Dog. Service Dogs are trained to help people with disabilities. Aggie helps her owner with picking up items that have fallen to the floor and retrieving personal articles as well as she assists with opening doors. Aggie came to her owner through Assistance Dogs International, a nonprofit organization that trains and provides service dogs through their worldwide coalitions. ADI sets standards and criteria for certification of dogs.

Image from: https://www.ecad1.org/index.php/resources/how-service-dogs-help.

CASE STUDY   Application of the Nursing Process

A Child With Down Syndrome

Ginger Johnson was 37 years old when she conceived her third pregnancy. Per her doctor's recommendation, Ginger underwent genetic screening tests, which revealed that the fetus was positive for DS. A very intense and emotional time followed as Ginger and her family planned to welcome the new baby they recognized would likely have physical and developmental challenges. During the pregnancy, Ginger developed gestational diabetes, and baby Jack was born 6 weeks premature by emergency caesarean section.

Assessment

Jack had feeding difficulties due to low muscle tone requiring oral motor therapy every 3 hour at birth followed by once-weekly therapy until age 2. He could not tolerate any dairy or gluten products from birth. His low muscular tone also required physical and occupational therapy one to three times per week. He had hip dysplasia that required various adaptive measures, and his feet, ankles, and lower calves required orthotic braces. Unlike over 50% of children with DS, Jack had no cardiac anomalies.

Jack had strabismus from birth, which required eye patching and glasses for far-sighted vision at approximately 18 months. He also had bilateral eustachian tubes and underwent an adenoidectomy at age 3. Jack was plagued with chronic diarrhea for his first 6 years, which resolved with elimination of intestinal bacteria and use of digestive enzymes.

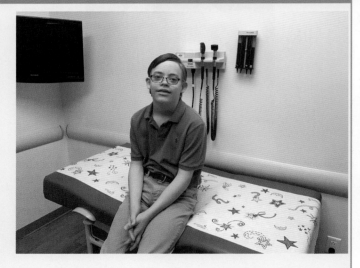

Jack, age 12, Caucasian male, was born with DS. Jack uses variety of interprofessional medical services that have yielded success in the day-to-day management of Jack's health issues.

CASE STUDY   Application of the Nursing Process—cont'd

His growth chart illustrated no growth from ages 2 to 3, and he was diagnosed with a pituitary deficiency. Human growth hormone treatment was initiated at age three and will continue through puberty. Jack was also diagnosed with ADHD but did not respond well to stimulant medications at age five; therefore a second-line medication was prescribed.

As Jack's immune system improved, he experienced fewer illnesses, with the exception of contracting pneumonia at age 7. He was hospitalized for 10 days of which 3 days were in the intensive care unit (ICU). Jack was diagnosed as borderline diabetic, and his physician recommended a Paleo diet to help normalize glucose. Jack began puberty at 10½ and was diagnosed with scoliosis at age 11. Jack attends a public high school that has a special program for children with IDDs. In elementary school he had the same teacher for the last 4 years. Jack thrived in middle school and worked in the library during his off period.

Jack's family lives in a middle-class area of a small city and consists of his mother Ginger, father Sam, and sisters Jill (15) and Jessica (17). Ginger is a stay-at-home mother, and Sam is an accountant for an insurance company. Health insurance is provided by Sam's company, but the deductible and copayments have risen dramatically in the last few years. With Jessica starting college next year, money is tight and expected to become more difficult.

Jack participates weekly in hippotherapy and maintains the horse stalls as part of his activities. His only sibling, a sister, will leave for college in a few months.

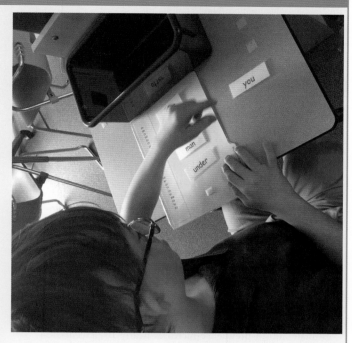

Jack has struggled with an immune-based response, alopecia.

? ACTIVE LEARNING

You are working in a urology special procedures clinic. Your patient is a 56-year-old man with a Spinal Cord Injury (SCI) resulting from a diving accident 20 years ago. His injury was at the Thoracic Spine or T5 level. He self-catheterizes and is having urodynamic procedure to assess his urethra, bladder and sphincters ability to store and release urine. You administer the blood pressure cuff to continuously monitor his blood pressure. You note he begins to complain of nausea, a slight headache and is diaphoretic. His Blood Pressure is registering 50 mm over his baseline for both systolic and diastolic. What is the cause of this? What are your first actions? What is your patient at risk for?

■ SUMMARY

Community health nurses must recognize that there are a variety of personal and societal perspectives on disability with accompanying moral or ethical issues. They should practice holistic nursing care that incorporates mind, body, and spiritual care considerations into health care practice. To this end, nurses can do the following:

- Become familiar with a variety of ethical frameworks for decision making and adopt a strategy to analyze ethical problems related to health care for people with disabilities.

- Help clients and families access information needed to make informed decisions that reflect their interests and priorities.
- Help educate the public on health care issues within the nurse's scope of practice and knowledge and skill level.
- Participate in the development of institutional policies and procedures for ethical and legal issues related to disability.
- Take a position on an ethical issue with political implications.
- Work to influence governmental policies and laws related to disability.

EVOLVE WEBSITE

http://evolve.elsevier.com/Nies/community
- NCLEX Review Questions
- Case Studies

BIBLIOGRAPHY

Alzheimer's Association: *Down Syndrome and Alzheimer's Disease*, 2021. Accessed February 12, 2021 from: https://www.alz.org/alzheimers-dementia/what-is-dementia/types-of-dementia/down-syndrome.

American Psychiatric Association: *What is intellectual disability?* 2017. January 23, 2021 Available from: https://www.psychiatry.org/patients-families/intellectual-disability/what-is-intellectual-disability.

Artinian BM, West KS, Conger M, editors: *The Artinian intersystem model: integrating theory and practice for the professional nurse*, 2011, Springer Publishing Company.

Ashburner J, Saggers B, Campbell M, Dillon-Wallace J, Hwang Y, Carrington S, Bobir N: How are students on the autism spectrum affected by bullying? Perspectives of students and parents, *J Res Spec Educ Needs* 19(1):27–44, 2018.

Autism Speaks: *CDC estimate on autism prevalence increases by nearly 10 percent, to 1 in 54 children in the U.S*, 2020. January 23, 2021 Available from: https://www.autismspeaks.org/press-release/cdc-estimate-autism-prevalence-increases-nearly-10-percent-1-54-children-us.

Bakker-van Gijssel EJ, Lucassen PLBJ, Hartman TO, Van Son L, Assendelft WJJ, van Schrojenstein Lantman-de Valk HMJ: Health assessment instruments for people with intellectual disabilities—A systematic review, *Res Dev Disabil* 64:12–24, 2017. https://doi.org/S0891-4222(17)30070-7. [pii].

Barnes C: Theories of disability and the origins of the oppression of disabled people in western society, *Disabil Soc: Emerg Issues Insights*, 1996:43–60, 1996.

Baylor College of Medicine: *Reproductive health*, 2020. Available from: https://www.bcm.edu/research/labs-and-centers/research-centers/center-for-research-on-womenwith-disabilities/a-to-z-directory/reproductive-health.

Beghi E: The epidemiology of epilepsy, *Neuroepidemiology* 54:185–191, 2020. https://doi.org/10.1159/000503831.

Boardman FK, Young PJ, Griffiths FE: Impairment experiences, identify and attitudes towards genetic screening: The views of people with spinal muscular atrophy, *J Genet Couns* 27(1):69–84, 2016.

Brain Injury Association of America: *Ticket to Work and Work Incentives Improvement Act*, 2021. January 28, 2021 Available from: https://www.biausa.org/public-affairs/public-policy/ticket-to-work-and-work-incentives-improvement-act.

Brown M, Chouliara Z, MacArthur J, et al.: The perspectives of stakeholders of intellectual disability liaison nurses: a model of compassionate, person-centered care, *J Clin Nurs* 25(7–8):972–982, 2016. https://doi.org/10.1111/jocn.13142.

Bu P, Veloski JJ, Ankam NS: Effects of a brief curricular intervention on medical students' attitudes toward people with disabilities in healthcare settings, *Am J Phys Med rehabilitation* 95(12):939–945, 2016. http://doi.org/10.1097/PHM.0000000000000535.

Campbell A, Uren M: "The invisibles"… disability in China in the 21st century, *Int J Spec Educ* 26(1):12–24, 2011.

Catani C, Sossalla IM: Child abuse predicts adult PTSD symptoms among individuals diagnosed with intellectual disabilities, *Front Psychol* 6:1600, 2015. https://doi.org/10.3389/fpsyg.2015.01600.

Centers for Disease Control (CDC) (2018). 1 in 4 US Adults live with a disability. https://www.cdc.gov/media/releases/2018/p0816-disability.html.

Centers for Disease Control and Prevention: Autism (ASD) spectrum disorders: data and statistics, 2020a. Available from: https://www.cdc.gov/ncbddd/autism/data.html.

Centers for Disease Control and Prevention: *Disability and Health Data System (DHDS)*, 2018 [Updated May 24, 2018; cited August 27, 2018]. Available from: http://dhds.cdc.gov.

Centers for Disease Control and Prevention: *Disability and health: disability overview*, 2021. Available from: https://www.cdc.gov/ncbddd/disabilityandhealth/disability.html.

Centers for Disease Control and Prevention: *Facts about Down Syndrome*, 2020b. Available from: www.cdc.gov/ncbddd/birthdefects/DownSyndrome.html.

Centers for Disease Control and Prevention: *Facts about cleft lip and palate*, 2020. February 12, 2021 Available from: https://www.cdc.gov/ncbddd/birthdefects/cleftlip.html.

Centers for Disease Control and Prevention: *What is cerebral palsy?*, 2020. January 23, 2021 Available from: https://www.cdc.gov/ncbddd/cp/facts.html#Causes.

Centers for Disease Control and Prevention: *Key findings: folic acid fortification continues to prevent neural tube defect*, 2017. January 24, 2021 Available from: www.cdc.gov/ncbddd/folicacid/features/folicacid-prevents-ntds.html#:~:text=Folic%20acid%20fortification%3A%20Folic%20acid,This%20is%20called%20fortification.

Centers for Disease Control and Prevention: *National health interview survey-about the national health interview survey*, 2019. Available from: https://www.cdc.gov/nchs/nhis/about_nhis.htm#:~:text=NHIS%20data%20are%20collected%20continuously%20throughout%20the%20year%20by%20Census%20interviewers.

Centers for Medicare & Medicaid Services (CMS). (2020). COVID-19 Emergency Declaration Blanket Waivers for Health Care providers. https://www.cms.gov/files/document/summary-covid-19-emergency-declaration-waivers.pdf.

Chiang LH, Hadadian A: Raising children with disabilities in China: the need for early interventions, *Int J Spec Educ* 25(2):113–118, 2010.

Children's Hospital of Philadelphia: *About fetal surgery for Spina Bifida (Myelomeningocele)*, 2021. February 12, 2021 Available from: https://www.chop.edu/treatments/fetal-surgery-spina-bifida/about.

Christensen DL, Bilder DA, Zahorodny W: Prevalence and characteristics of autism spectrum disorder among 4-year-old children in the autism and developmental disabilities monitoring network, *J Dev Behav Pediatr* 37(1):1–8, 2016. https://doi.org/10.1097/DBP.0000000000000235.

Cree RA, Okoro CA, Zack MM, Carbone E: Frequent mental distress among adults, by disability status, disability type, and selected characteristics—United States, 2018, *MMWR (Morb Mortal Wkly Rep)* 69(36):1238, 2020.

Crisp-Cooper M: *Our sexuality, our health: A disabled advocate's guide to relationships, romance, sexuality and sexual health*, 2018. January 28, 2021 Available from: https://odpc.ucsf.edu/advocacy/sexuality-sexual-health/our-sexuality-our-health-a-disabled-advocates-guide-to#pdf.

Desroches ML, Ailey S, Fisher K, Stych J: Impact of COVID-19: Nursing challenges to meeting the care needs of people with developmental disabilities, *Disabil Health J* 14(1):101015, 2021. https://doi.org/10.1016/j.dhjo.2020.101015.

Dirth TP, Branscombe NR: Disability models affect disability policy support through awareness of structural discrimination, *J Soc Issues* 73(2):413–442, 2017.

Dobson LJ, Reiff ES, Little SE, Wilkins-Haug L, Bromley B: Patient choice and clinical outcomes following positive noninvasive prenatal screening for aneuploidy with cell-free DNA (cfDNA), *Prenat Diagn* 36(5):456–462, 2016.

Down Syndrome Association: *Diabetes*, 2020. February 14, 2021 Available from: https://www.google.com/search?q=down+syndrome+diabetes&rlz=1C1GCEA_enUS886US886&oq=down+syndrome+diabetes&aqs=chrome..69i57j69i64.7429j0j4&sourceid=chrome&ie=UTF-8.

Down Syndrome Education International: *Autism in Down Syndrome is not typical autism*, 2021. February 12, 2021 Available from: https://www.down-syndrome.org/en-us/research/education-21/10/.

Eskay M, Onu VC, Igbo JN: *Disability within the African culture*, 2012, US-China Rev B4, pp 473–484.

Freysteinson W, Thomas L, Sebastian-Deutsch A, Douglas D, Melton D, Celia T, Reeves K, Bowyer P: A study of the amputee experience of viewing self in the mirror, *Rehabil Nurs* 42(1):22, 2017. https://doi.org/10.1002/mj.256.

Ganle JK, Baatiema L, Quansah R, Danso-Appiah A: Barriers facing persons with disability in accessing sexual and reproductive health services in sub-Saharan Africa: a systematic review, *PLoS One* 15(10):e0238585, 2020.

Giagazoglou P, Arabatzi F, Dipla K, Liga M, Kellis E: Effect of a hippotherapy intervention program on static balance and strength in adolescents with intellectual disabilities, *Res Dev Disabil* 33(6):2265–2270, 2012. https://doi.org/10.1016/j.ridd.2012.07.004.

Gibbons LJ, Lehr K, Selekman J: Federal laws protecting children and youth with disabilities in the schools. In , Philadelphia, PA, 2013, F.A. Davis & Company, pp 257–283. Selekman J, editor: *School nursing: a comprehensive text.* ed 2, Philadelphia, PA, 2013, F.A. Davis & Company, pp 257–283.

Global Down Syndrome Foundation: *Congenital Heart Defects and Down Syndrome*, 2019.

Golisano Children's Hospital: Intellectual disability, January 25, 2021 Available from: https://www.urmc.rochester.edu/childrens-hospital/developmental-disabilities/conditions/id.aspx.

Goodwin K: *Financial challenges of raising a child with disabilities*, 2018. January 30, 2021 Available from: https://www.mynoblelife.org/2018/09/financial-challenges-of-raising-a-child-with-disabilities/.

Gordon S: *10 Types of kids most likely to be bullied. Verywellfamily*, 2020. February 1, 2021 Available from: https://www.verywellfamily.com/reasons-why-kids-are-bullied-460777.

Hameed S, Maddams A, Lowe H, Davies L, Khosla R, Shakespeare T: From words to actions: systematic review of interventions to promote sexual and reproductive health of persons with disabilities in low- and middle-income countries, *BMJ Global Health* 5:1–14, 2020. e002903.

Hamiwka LD, Cara GY, Hamiwka LA, Sherman EM, Anderson B, Wirrell E: Are children with epilepsy at greater risk for bullying than their peers? *Epilepsy Behav* 15(4):500–505, 2009.

Health Risk Screening, Inc.: *The fatal five fundamentals*, 2020. January 25, 2021 Available from: https://hrstonline.com/hrsu/the-fatal-five-fundamentals/.

Iudici A, Antonello A, Turchi G: Intimate partner violence against disabled persons: Clinical and health impact, intersections, issues and intervention strategies, *Sex Cult* 23:684–704, 2019. https://doi.org/10.1007/s12119-018-9570-y.

Jacques R: *Intellectual disability and health: Family issues*, 2019. January 30, 2021 Available from: http://www.intellectualdisability.info/family/articles/family-issues.

Jan BM, Jan MM: Dental health of children with cerebral palsy, *Neurosciences* 21(4):314, 2016. https://doi.org/10.17712/nsj.2016.4.20150729.

Jones RA, Downing K, Rinehart NJ, Barnett LM, May T, McGillivray JA, Papadopoulos NV, Skouteris H, Timperio A, Hinkley T: Physical activity, sedentary behavior and their correlates in children with Autism Spectrum Disorder: A systematic review, *PLoS One* 12(2):e0172482, 2017. https://doi.org/10.1371/journal.pone.0172482.

Landes S, Stevens J, Turk M: Cause of death in adults with intellectual disability in the United States, *J Intellect Disabil Res* 65(1):47–59, 2020.

Landes SD, Turk MA, Formica MK, McDonald KE, Stevens JD: COVID-19 outcomes among people with intellectual and developmental disability living in residential group homes in New York State, *Disabil Health J* 13(4):100969, 2020. https://doi.org/10.1016/j.dhjo.2020.100969.

Langkamp DL, McManus MD, Blakemore SD: Telemedicine for children with developmental disabilities: a more effective clinical process than office-based care, *Telemed e-Health* 21(2):110–114, 2015. https://doi.org/10.1089/tmj.2013.0379.

Longmore PK: *Uncovering the hidden history of people with disabilities*, 1987.

Lopez M, Schachter S, Kanner A: Psychiatric comorbidities go unrecognized in patients with epilepsy: "You see what you know", *Epilepsy Behav* 98(B):302–305, 2019.

Lund EM, Forber-Pratt AJ, Wilson C, Mona LR: The COVID-19 pandemic, stress, and trauma in the disability community: A call to action, *Rehabil Psychol* 65(4):313–322, 2020. https://doi.org/10.1037/rep0000368.

Maclean MJ, Sims S, Bower C, et al.: Maltreatment risk among children with disabilities, *Pediatrics* 139(4):e20161817, 2017. https://doi.org/10.1542/peds.2016-1817.

Markovic-Jovanovic S, Milovanovic J, Jovanovic A, Zivkovic J, Balovic A, Nickovic V, Vasic M, Ristic M: Comorbidities in children with intellectual disabilities, *Birth Defects Res* 112(1):54–61, 2019.

Mayo Clinic: *Hydrocephalus*, 2021. February 12, 2021 Available from: www.mayoclinic.org/diseases-conditions/hydrocephalus/symptoms-causes/syc-20373604#:~:text=Hydrocephalus%20is%20the%20buildup%20of,the%20brain%20and%20spinal%20column.

Moffitt RA: The deserving poor, the family and the U.S. welfare system, *Demography* 52(3):729–749, 2015. https://doi.org/10.1007/s13524-015-0395-0.

Morris M, Wong A, Holliman B, Liesinger J, Griffin J: Perspectives of patients with diverse disabilities regarding healthcare accommodations to promote healthcare equity: A qualitative study, *J Gen Intern Med*, 2021, https://doi.org/10.1007/s11606-020-06582-8.

Mula M, Kanner A, Jette N, Sander J: Psychiatric comorbidities in people with epilepsy, *Neurol Clin Prac*, May 2020, https://doi.org/10.1212/CPJ.0000000000000874.

Must A, Eliasziw M, Phillips SM, et al.: The effect of age on the prevalence of obesity among US youth with autism spectrum disorder, *Child Obes* 13(1):25–35, 2017. https://doi.org/10.1089/chi.2016.0079.

Musumeci MB, Chidambaram P: *Issue brief medicaid's role for children with special health care needs: A look at eligibility, services, and spending*, 2019, Kaiser Family Foundation. Available from: http://files.kff.org/attachment/Medicaid%E2%80%99s-Role-for-Children-with-Special-Health-Care-Needs-A-Look-at-Eligibility,-Services-and-Spending.

My Child at Cerebral Palsy.org: Orthotic devices, February 12 Available from: https://www.cerebralpalsy.org/information/mobility/orthotics, 2021.

National Association of School Nurses. (NASN): *IDEIA and section 504 teams - the school nurse as an essential team member (position statement)*, MD, 2018, Silver Spring. Author.

National Down Syndrome Society: *Alzheimer's Disease & Down Syndrome*, 2021. February 12, 2021 Available from: https://www.ndss.org/resources/alzheimers/.

National Down Syndrome Society: *Ear, nose & throat issues & Down Syndrome*, 2021. February 12, 2021 Available from: https://www.ndss.org/resources/ear-nose-throat-issues-syndrome/.

National Down Syndrome Society: *The heart and Down Syndrome*, 2021. February 12, 2021 Available from: https://www.ndss.org/resources/the-heart-down-syndrome/.

National Down Syndrome Society: *What is Down Syndrome?*, 2021. January 24, 2021 Available from: https://www.ndss.org/about-down-syndrome/down-syndrome/.

National Institute of Neurological Disorders and Stroke: *Hydrocephalus fact sheet*, 2020. February 12, 2021 Available from: https://www.ninds.nih.gov/Disorders/Patient-Caregiver-Education/Fact-sheets/Hydrocephalus-Fact-Sheet#3125_7.

Ne'eman A: *When it comes to rationing, disability rights law prohibits more than prejudice*, 2020, Hastings Bioethics Forum. Available from: https://www.thehastingscenter.org/when-it-comes-to-rationing-disability-rights-law-prohibits-more-than-prejudice/.

Njelesani J, Hashemi G, Cameron C, Cameron D, Richard D, Parnes P: From the day they are born: a qualitative study exploring violence against children with disabilities in West Africa, *BMC Publ Health* 18:153, 2018. https://doi.org/10.1186/s12889-018-5057-x.

Norrgard K: Human subjects and diagnostic genetic testing, *Nature Education* 1(1):82, 2008.

Palmer S: Family adaptation and intervention. In Budd MA, Hough S, Wegener ST, Stiers W, editors: *Practical psychology in medical rehabilitation*, 2016, pp 415–422.

Petrou S, Yiu H, Kwon J: Economic consequences of preterm birth: A systematic review of the recent literature (2009–2017), *Arch Dis Child* 104(5):456–465, 2019.

Pfeiffer D: Overview of the disability movement: history, legislative record, and political implications, *Pol Stud J* 21(4):724–734, 1993.

Reed P: Expressivism at the beginning and end of life, *J Med Ethics* 46:538–544, 2020. https://doi.org/10.1136/medethics-2019-105875.

Rotoli J, Backster A, Sapp R, Auston Z, Francois C, Gurditta K, Mirus C, Poffenberger C: Emergency medicine resident education on caring for patients with disabilities: a call to action, *Soc Acad Emerg Med* 2020:450–460, 2020. https://doi.org/10.1002/aet2.10453.

Salpekar J, Mula M: Common psychiatric comorbidities in epilepsy: How big of a problem is it? *Epilepsy Behav* 98(B):293–297, 2019.

Sanger M: *My way to peace*, 1932. Available from: https://www.nyu.edu/projects/sanger/webedition/app/documents/show.php?sangerDoc=129037.xml.

Savage TA, Moro TT, Boyden JY, et al.: Implementation challenges in end-of-life research with adults with intellectual and developmental disabilities, *Appl Nurs Res* 28(2):202–205, 2015. https://doi.org/10.1016/j.apnr.2014.10.002.

Schroeder SA: Well-being, opportunities, and selecting for disability, *J Ethics Soc Philos* 14:1, 2018. https://doi.org/10.26556/jesp.v14i1.353.

Sharma S: Congenital heart disease. In Rubin IL, Merrick J, Greydanus DE, Patel DR, editors: *Health care for people with intellectual and developmental disabilities across the lifespan*, Cham, 2016, Springer, https://doi.org/10.1007/978-3-319-18096-0_106.

Shaw J: Selecting for disabilities: selection versus modification, *N Bioeth* 24(1):44–56, 2018. https://doi.org/10.1080/20502877.2018.1441671.

Sgouros S: *Spina Bifida Hydrocephalus and Shunts*, 2019. February 12, 2021 Available from: https://emedicine.medscape.com/article/937979-overview.

Smeltzer SC, Dolen MA, Robinson-Smith G, Zimmerman V: Integration of disability-related content in nursing curricula, *Nurs Educ Perspect* 26(4):210–216, 2005.

Social Security Administration: *Disability evaluation under social security*, 2021. January 28, 2021 Available from: www.ssa.gov/disability/professionals/bluebook/general-info.htm#:~:text=The%20law%20defines%20disability%20as,not%20less%20than%202012%20months.

Social Security Administration: *History of the ticket to work program*, 2021. January 28, 2021 Available from: https://yourtickettowork.ssa.gov/about/history.html#:~:text=The%20Ticket%20to%20Work%20and%20Work%20Incentives%20Improvement%20Act%20of,wished%20to%20return%20to%20work.&text=The%20SSI%20program%20provides%20cash,have%20limited%20income%20and%20resources.

Special Olympics: *What is intellectual disability?*, 2021. January 22, 2021 Available from: https://www.specialolympics.org/about/intellectual-disabilities/what-is-intellectual-disability.

Staples J: Culture and carelessness: constituting disability in South India (2012), *Med Anthropol Q* 26(4):557–574, 2012.

Stevens D: *People with developmental disabilities have much more life to live. Population health research brief series: lerner center for public health promotion*, 2019. January 24, 2021 Available from: https://lernercenter.syr.edu/population-health-research/.

Stopbullying.gov: *What is bullying*, 2020. January 29, 2021 Available from: https://www.stopbullying.gov/bullying/what-is-bullying.

Taylor D: *Americans with disabilities: 2014*, 2018. January 28, 2021 Available from: https://www.census.gov/content/dam/Census/library/publications/2018/demo/p70-152.pdf.

The Arc: *About us*, 2021. Available from: https://thearc.org/about-us/.

Turk M, Landes S, Formica M, Goss K: Intellectual and developmental disability and COVID-19 case-fatality trends: TriNetX analysis, *Disabil Health J* 13(3):1–4, 2020. https://doi.org/10.1016/j.dhjo.2020.100942.

U.S. Census Bureau: SIPP and estimates of disability prevalence, 2018. Available from: https://www.census.gov/programs-surveys/sipp/tech-documentation/user-notes/2018-usernotes/estimates-disability-prevalence.html.

U.S. Department of Education: *Office of Special Education Programs, Individuals with Disabilities Education Act (IDEA) database*, February 20, 2020, Available from: https://www2.ed.gov/programs/osepidea/618-data/state-level-data-files/index.html#bcc. and National Center for Education Statistics: *National elementary and secondary enrollment projection model, 1972 through 2029. See Digest of Education Statistics 2019, table 204.30.* Available from: https://nces.ed.gov/programs/coe/indicator_cgg.asp.

U.S. Department of Education: *Prohibited disability harassment*, 2020. January 30, 2021 Available from: https://www2.ed.gov/about/offices/list/ocr/docs/disabharassltr.html.

U.S. Department of Justice: *The Americans with Disabilities Act of 1990 and Revised ADA Regulations Implementing Title II and Title III*, 2021. January 26, 2021 Available from: https://www.ada.gov/2010_regs.htm.

Vanderbilt Kennedy Center: *Health care for adults with intellectual and developmental disabilities: toolkit for primary care providers-male preventive care checklist*, (n.d.). Available from: https://iddtoolkit. vkcsites.org.

Vasa R, Kreiser N, Keefer A, Singh V, Mostofsky S: Relationships between autism spectrum disorder and intolerance of uncertainty, *Autism Res* 11(4):636–644, 2018.

WebMD: *An overview of cleft lip and cleft palate*, 2021. February 12, 2021 Available from: https://www.webmd.com/oral-health/cleft-lip-cleft-palate#1.

Whitney DG, Peterson MD, Warschausky SA: Mental health disorders, participation, and bullying in children with cerebral palsy, *Dev Med Child Neurol* 61:937–942, 2019. https://doi.org/10.1111/dmcn.14175/.

World Health Organization (WHO): *Disability and health*, 2020. https://www.who.int/en/news-room/fact-sheets/detail/disability-and-health.

World Health Organization: *International Classification of Functioning, Disability and Health (ICF)*, 2002. https://cdn.who.int/media/docs/default-source/classification/icf/icfbeginnersguide.pdf?sfvrsn=eead63d3_4.

Zablotsky B, Black L, Maenner M, Schieve L, Danielson M, Bitsko R, Blumberg S, Kogan M, Boyle C: Prevalence and trends of developmental disabilities among children in the United States: 2009–2017, *Pediatrics* 144(4), 2019. https://doi.org/10.1542/peds.2019-081.

22

Veterans' Health

Bridgette Crotwell Pullis*

OBJECTIVES

Upon completion of this chapter, the reader will be able to do the following:

1. Explain basic terms and the culture associated with US military service personnel.
2. Describe elements of the Veterans Health Administration, including benefits, eligibility, costs of care, and outreach programs.
3. Explain some of the commonly occurring health issues encountered among veterans of different wars and conflicts.
4. Describe risk factors and manifestations for frequently encountered health risks among veterans.
5. Identify assessment strategies to improve the health of veterans.
6. Describe nursing interventions to improve the health of veterans.

OUTLINE

KEY TERMS

active duty
Agent Orange
burn pit
CHAMPVA
military sexual trauma (MST)
National Guard

polytrauma
posttraumatic stress disorder (PTSD)
Reserves
service-connected disability
substance use disorder (SUD)

traumatic brain injury (TBI)
TRICARE
veteran
Veterans Health Administration (VHA)

We might speak of an individual as a "World War II veteran," "a Vietnam vet," or a "veteran of the Persian Gulf War" to denote

*The author would like to acknowledge the contributions of Angelic Denise Chaison, Alison C. Sweeney, Joanna Lamkin, Robert Pullis, Sarah G. Candler, Rex Marsau, Tina Doyle-Hines, and Rola El-Serag.

service in a specific conflict or place, but a veteran is not necessarily a person who fought in war or who served in wartime. Put simply, the definition of a **veteran** is a person who has served in the military. As we'll see, this experience can impart a distinctive culture and value system, and it is also associated with certain health risks. Thus, the veteran aggregate can present in the healthcare system with unique health problems or issues associated with their experiences.

Public health nurses and others providing care in the community must be aware of the needs, histories, and experiences of this particular population. This chapter describes some of the more common health threats and issues among veterans. Also included is an overview of some of the services provided by the Veterans Health Administration (VHA), as well as an assessment of methods and strategies to help veterans manage reintegration with civilian life.

OVERVIEW OF THE AMERICAN UNIFORMED SERVICES

People join the uniformed services for many reasons: to serve their country, to learn job skills, to have the opportunity to pursue a higher education, for a sense of pride and belonging, for financial stability, for a chance to travel, or to carry on a family tradition. The US Army is the largest branch of the military, making up 39% of all military personnel. Other branches of service include the Air Force, the Navy, the Marine Corps, and the Coast Guard. Table 22.1 lists the appropriate designations for persons in each branch of the uniformed services.

Veteran Status

Legally, a veteran is an individual who has served in the active military, naval, or air service and who was discharged or released under conditions other than dishonorable. Any individual who completed service for any branch of armed forces is a veteran as long as they were not dishonorably discharged. This legal status is important to understanding a patient's eligibility for veteran benefits from the US government. Note that people who have served in the United States Public Health Service and some persons employed by the National Oceanic and Atmospheric Administration are also veterans. The number of veterans in the United States declined by about a third, from 26.4 million to 18.0 million between 2000 and 2018 with fewer than 500,000 World War II veterans living in 2018. The largest cohort of veterans alive in 2018 served during the Vietnam Era (6.4 million). The second-largest cohort of living veterans served during peacetime only (4.0 million). About 1.7 million, or 9% of veterans, were women in 2018 (Fig. 22.1). Women are the fastest growing segment of the veteran population, and it is projected that number will jump to 17% by 2040. Of note, in 2018, the median age of veterans was 65 (US Census Bureau, 2020). Table 22.2

enumerates the size of the veteran population living today from various armed conflicts.

As discussed in Chapter 13, culture is the set of shared attitudes, values, goals, and practices characterizing a group of people. Military culture is one of structure and uniformity; it is governed by rules and standards. Though each branch of the military has a different mission, common core values and norms direct the behavior of all military members. These values include leadership, teamwork, loyalty, hierarchy, obedience, and discipline. Common norms among military personnel are a strong sense of service, a hierarchal class system, solutions-focused actions, unique dialogue and expressions, and a reluctance to show weakness. These norms affect how veterans seek care and how they manage their health. For example, veterans may avoid getting needed care due to the stigma of appearing weak or out of fear of letting their colleagues down. They may not trust their information to be kept confidential, or they may fear that seeking treatment will jeopardize future promotions. They may also be concerned that seeking treatment will cause financial hardship, or they may have negative attitudes regarding providers.

ETHICAL INSIGHTS

Sexual Orientation in the Armed Forces

Prior to 1993 homosexuals were prohibited from serving in the military and were dishonorably discharged if their sexual orientation was discovered. Don't Ask Don't Tell (DADT) was an administrative regulation established by President Clinton that allowed LGB individuals to serve in the military, but required them to hide their sexual orientation. Between 1993 and 2010 more than 13,000 military members were discharged for being gay. DADT was declared unconstitutional in 2010 and repealed in 2011. Despite this change, LGB service members may face challenges to seeking health care due to concerns over:
- Threats to career advancement
- Internalized stigma and shame
- A loss of benefits after a dishonorable discharge

ACTIVE DUTY, NATIONAL GUARD AND RESERVES

The military is composed of both **active duty**, or full-time personnel, and members of the National Guard and Reserves. The service member is typically assigned to a group or unit, which is stationed either domestically or overseas. Overseas deployments generally last between 6 and 15 months; when on deployment, individuals may have periods of working nearly 24 h every day, 7 days a week. Further, military personnel may be separated from their family for long periods, even when not deployed, due to long training cycles.

Personnel serving in the **National Guard** or **Reserves** are considered part-time employees. The key difference among them is that the Reserves report to the federal government, whereas the National Guard is administered by each state (e.g., the Pennsylvania National Guard is called into action by the governor of Pennsylvania). These individuals serve no more

TABLE 22.1 Branches of the Uniformed Services	
Branch	Service member
Army	Soldier
Air Force	Airman
Navy	Sailor
Marine Corps	Marine
Coast Guard	Guardian

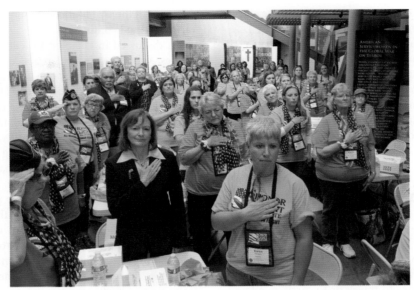

Fig. 22.1 During the All Female Honor Flight, veterans from World War II, the Korean War, the Vietnam War, and the post-9/11 era visit the Women in Military Service Memorial at Arlington National Cemetery, which honors them. (Robert Turtil/ US Department of Veterans Affairs.)

TABLE 22.2	Summary of Status of Veterans of Past Wars Involving US Service Members			
War	Number of US Service Members	Estimated Deaths	Estimated Wounded	Estimated Living Veterans (2018)
World War II (1941—45)	16,112,566	405,399 (291,557 in battle)	670,846	485,000
Korean War (1950—53)	5,720,000	54,246 (36,574 in theater)	103,284	1,306,000
Vietnam War (1964—75)	8,744,000 (estimated 3,403,000 deployed)	90,220 (58,220 in theater)	153,303 number of service members	6,384,000
Gulf War (Desert Shield/Desert Storm) (1990—2001)	2,322,000 (694,550 deployed)	1948 (383 in theater)	467	3,804,000 (2018 estimate; may include veterans who served in Iraq and Afghanistan)
The Global War on Terror (2000 to present) (e.g., actions in Afghanistan, Iraq, and Syria)	2,900,000 (2016 estimate)	6855	52,351	2,900,000 (2016 estimate)

Source: https://www.census.gov/library/visualizations/2020/comm/veteran-population-declines.html.

than 39 days a year, unless called into action. Usually, their service consists of monthly drills and 2-week annual trainings. Reservists may be called very suddenly to active duty (full-time) for deployments, requiring that they leave their family, regular job, and community for a time.

Military Rank

The military is a hierarchal organization consisting of enlisted personnel, who perform tasks according to their specific job, training and skills, and commissioned officers, who plan missions and direct the enlisted personnel. Each person in the uniformed service is assigned a rank (or *rate* in the Navy) indicating his or her position in the hierarchy:
- Enlisted Personnel (E-1 through E-9)—includes noncommissioned officers and petty officers

- Warrant Officers (W-1 through W-5)—highly specialized experts
- Commissioned Officers (0—1 through 0—10)—highest ranks, similar to managers/leaders of a company

Enlisted personnel comprise over 80% of the military workforce. Officers outrank the enlisted personnel and are referred to as "sir" or "ma'am." One can be promoted in rank based on knowledge, time in service, work performance, skills, and vacancies.

The Veterans Health Administration

Most veterans receive all or part of their health care through **the VHA** under the US Department of Veterans Affairs (VA). In order to understand the ways that veterans interact with the VHA, it is important to begin with an understanding of the VA itself. As a federal program, the overarching rules about the functions of the VA are determined at a national level. However, the implementation of those rules and guidelines is variable according to the leadership at regional and hospital levels.

Framework of the VA

The Department of Veterans Affairs has three subdivisions: the VHA, the Veterans Benefits Administration (VBA), and the National Cemetery Administration. The VHA provides all types of health care in every setting, including inpatient, outpatient, and long-term care. The VBA is an administrative arm responsible for unemployment and pension payments, home loans, vocational training, and educational benefits. The VHA is America's largest integrated healthcare system, providing care at 1293 healthcare facilities. This includes 171 medical centers and 1112 outpatient sites (VHA outpatient clinics), serving nine million enrolled veterans each year (U.S. Department of Veterans Affairs (VA), 2020c).

Eligibility and Enrollment

Veterans—and sometimes their survivors and dependents—are eligible for VA benefits when they fulfill two requirements related to service and separation. (1) Service: they must have served in active duty for 24 consecutive months or for a full period of call (Reserves and Guard). There are some exceptions to the length of service minimum, the most important being when a person is discharged for disability incurred or aggravated in the line of duty. (2) Separation: they must have been separated under any condition other than dishonorable (Scott, 2012).

Reservists and members of the National Guard can qualify for some veteran benefits depending on the length of time they were on active duty; for example, if a Guard or Reserve member is activated and serves in Afghanistan for a period of 14 months, then he or she meets eligibility requirements because the member has completed a full period of call—even though it is shorter than 24 consecutive months. However, the "active duty" requirement can prove difficult for these groups to meet. If while in the Guard or Reserves an individual is never activated for federal active duty military service, that person does not meet the active duty requirement for the definition of a veteran for VA benefits (Scott, 2012). Crucially, members of the National Guard and Reserves can face the same health issues and challenges as their active duty counterparts without being eligible for full veteran benefits. Relatedly, individuals who have been dishonorably discharged may experience the same health risks as the veteran cohort, though they are ineligible for VA benefits.

In order to receive care through the VHA, a veteran must enroll in the benefits program. It is important to understand that not all veterans who are eligible for benefits can enroll. The VA determines which veterans are able to enroll by stratifying them according to eight *priority groups* (Table 22.3), depending on urgency and need. Based on current VA funds, veterans in priority groups 1 through 7 are able to enroll in and receive care from the VHA.

TABLE 22.3 VA Enrollment Priority Groups

Priority Group	Qualifications
Priority group 1	SC $\geq$50% or unemployable as a result of SC conditions
Priority group 2	SC 30%—40%
Priority group 3	POWs, recipients of Purple Heart, Medal of Honor, disability discharge, 10%—20%, "disabling SC disability, disabled by treatment orf vocational rehabilitation"
Priority group 4	Receiving aid and attendance or housebound benefits from VA, or catastrophically disabled
Priority group 5	Non-SC or noncompensable SC rated 0% disabled with income < income limits, receiving VA pension benefits, eligible for Medicaid programs
Priority group 6	Compensable 0% SC veterans, exposed to ionizing radiation, Vietnam, Persian Gulf, Camp Lejeune, combat veterans 1998—2003 enrolled within 5 years of discharge
Priority group 7	Gross household income < income limits, who agree to pay copays
Priority group 8	Income > income limits, who agree to pay copays

POWs, Prisoners of war; *SC*, service connected; *VA*, Veterans Affairs.

One's priority group does not, however, determine which services a veteran can utilize. Instead, all veterans who enroll in care receive the same services and benefits (with the exception of dental coverage). Once a veteran is enrolled, he or she remains enrolled and maintains access to VA benefits, regardless of whether his or her priority group changes (U.S. Department of Veterans Affairs (VA), 2017a).

An individual's priority group is determined in a large part by the extent to which he or she suffers a disability related to military service. A **service-connected disability** is a disease or injury that was incurred as a result of or during the veteran's active duty, or one that was aggravated by military service. A percentage associated with service-connectedness measures the degree of disability that the veteran faces as a result of that diagnosis. For example, one veteran may be 20% service-connected for tinnitus because he gets debilitating migraines and has associated hearing loss as a result; another veteran is 0% service-connected for the same diagnosis (tinnitus) because it does not cause him any disability. These determinations are made by a third party at the regional VA offices, not by the patients' regular providers (U.S. Department of Veterans Affairs (VA), 2017b).

Notice that VA funding prohibits Priority Group 8 from enrolling in VHA services at this time. This group has no service-connected disabilities and has a higher annual income than the VA income limits.

Cost of Care

Many veterans do not realize that their care at their VA hospitals and clinics is not a type of health insurance. Instead, it is a benefit that they receive in compensation for their duty and service to the country. The difference between health insurance and VA health benefits is twofold. First, veterans do not have to "pay into" their VA benefits the way one would pay premiums for a health insurance plan. Second, the "coverage" received in the form of VA benefits is not transferable to other non-VA providers, except through formal contracts deemed appropriate by the VA and its providers.

Once veterans are enrolled, the cost of care is relatively straightforward. At the time of publication, primary care copays are $15 per visit, and outpatient specialist copays are $50 per visit (U.S. Department of Veterans Affairs (VA), 2021b). Some services are free for all veterans: care for service-connected conditions, registry exams for exposures (such as chemical exposures), compensation and pension exams, counseling/care for military sexual trauma, research, readjustment and mental health services, smoking and weight loss classes, health fairs, combat-related care post-1998, laboratory tests, electrocardiographs, and hospice (U.S. Department of Veterans Affairs (VA), 2021b).

Medications are also affordable through the VHA, and the cost is a predictable and standardized set of copays. Additionally, veterans have an annual cap (currently $700) on the amount of money they must spend on their medications (U.S. Department of Veterans Affairs (VA), 2021c).

COMMUNITY FOCUS

The Role of Private Insurance

When they enroll, veterans are required to divulge any other health coverage they have—personally or through a spouse. The VA always bills an individual's private insurance for medical care, supplies, and prescriptions provided for nonservice-connected conditions. Any monies collected from a veteran's private insurance offset his or her copayments, and furthermore, the veteran is not responsible for any balance the private insurance does not cover.

Patient-Centered Community Care and Veterans Choice Program

There are some services that the VHA may not be able to provide—either at all or in a timely manner. For these circumstances, there are programs that coordinate transfer of that care on a VA contractual basis. *Patient-Centered Community Care (PC3)* is one program for veterans needing certain primary care or inpatient-related care, particularly for female veterans after delivery and requiring limited newborn care. PC3 also covers some skilled home health care and home infusion therapy.

The *Veterans Choice Program* outsources veteran care when they cannot receive needed services at the VHA in a timely manner (within 30 days of the date clinically indicated by the veteran's VHA provider) or within reasonable distance (within 40 miles of the veteran's home). The care that is received in the community is only paid for by VA benefits if that care was approved by the veteran's VHA physician.

COMMUNITY FOCUS

Rural Outreach for the Veteran Population

Veterans are an underserved population—with more than four million veterans across the nation living in rural areas far removed from the nearest VHA or comprehensive medical center. Over 70% of rural veterans are over the age of 55 and are more likely than their urban counterparts to have at least one disabling condition. Though the VHA is seeking outreach to these veterans through community-based outpatient clinics (CBOCs), this mission is hampered by a lack of primary care providers. The Veterans Choice Act, allowing veterans unable to secure an appointment for care at a VHA within 30 days to receive care from a community provider, will increase the number of veterans seen by providers in the community. Most veterans are covered by private insurance, Medicare, Medicaid, or Tricare and do not receive care in the VHA system (U.S. Department of Veterans Affairs (VA), 2021a).

Champva and Tricare

The **Civilian Health and Medical Program of the Department of Veterans Affairs (CHAMPVA)** is a program in which the costs of *some* healthcare services for eligible civilian beneficiaries are covered by the VA. According to Benefits.gov (2017), to be eligible for CHAMPVA benefits and services, individuals must be in *one* of these categories:

- The spouse or child of a veteran who has been rated permanently and totally disabled for a service-connected disability by a VA regional office **OR**
- The surviving spouse or child of a veteran who died from a VA-rated service-connected disability **OR**
- The surviving spouse or child of a veteran who was at the time of death rated permanently and totally disabled from a service-connected disability **OR**
- The surviving spouse or child of a military member who died in the line of duty, not due to misconduct (in most of these cases, these family members are eligible for TRICARE, not CHAMPVA)

Application for CHAMPVA is made through the VHA (Benefits.gov, 2017). It is important to recognize that CHAMPVA and TRICARE are not the same. **TRICARE** is sponsored by the Department of Defense (DoD) and provides health care for active duty military personnel, their families, and their survivors. In contrast, CHAMPVA is sponsored by the VA, and eligibility for TRICARE disqualifies one for CHAMPVA.

VETERAN HEALTH RISKS

There are several health risks or threats that occur among military personnel, regardless of where or when they served. Many have experienced life-altering trauma, such as dismemberment, loss of hearing or sight, burns, or neurological conditions such as traumatic brain injuries (TBIs). In addition, mental and emotional health risks are equally important: veterans have faced many and varied stressors, such as threats to their life, loss of friends, inner conflict regarding their role in combat, survivor's guilt, and separation from family. Some may even find the quest for peace and reintegration to be harder than fighting in a war. Included in this section are common health risks for the veteran aggregate.

Traumatic Brain Injury

A **traumatic brain injury (TBI)** is a disruption of brain function caused by an external mechanical force, including blunt force trauma, penetration by a foreign object, acceleration or deceleration movements, and pressure waves from explosive blasts (Johnson et al., 2013). TBIs are categorized as mild (abbreviated mTBI), moderate, and severe (Table 22.4). The TBI is the most common, and is synonymous with the term *concussion*.

Technological advancements, such as Kevlar body armor and helmets, have greatly reduced penetrating injuries and the mortality rates from bullets and shrapnel; however, this higher survival rate has worked to increase the incidence of TBIs among veterans of combat in Iraq and Afghanistan. In addition, protective helmets do not prevent injury from pressure waves caused by blasts from improvised explosive devices (IEDs), a type of bomb favored by insurgents (Okie, 2005). Over 370,000 service members were diagnosed with TBI from 2000 to 2017 (DoD Worldwide Numbers for TBI, n.d.).

Symptoms of mTBIs can include headaches, tinnitus, sleep disorders, irritability, memory problems, mood and anxiety disorders, suicidality, chronic pain, and dizziness or balance problems (Johnson et al., 2013). Because these symptoms are often comorbid, mTBI can be difficult to identify, and beginning in 2007, all veterans who seek care at a VHA facility are screened for TBI.

Noise

Many veterans have been exposed to various levels and types of noise. This can include sound from gunfire, machinery, explosives, rockets, and heavy weapons. Others have been exposed to loud engines from tanks, large machinery, and aircraft. This exposure can lead to hearing loss and tinnitus, the top two most prevalent disabilities of all compensation recipients in 2016, affecting over 2.5 million veterans (U.S. Department of Veterans Affairs (VA), 2020a).

Radiation

Some veterans are particularly at risk from diseases caused by ionizing radiation exposure. This exposure was of particular concern among those who participated in nuclear weapons testing or who served near Hiroshima and Nagasaki after the bombings—later known as *atomic veterans*. Complications of prolonged or intense exposure to even low levels of radiation can lead to many types of cancer. It is also associated with other diseases such as thyroid and parathyroid disease, cataracts, and nervous system disorders.

Cold Injuries

The major cold injuries veterans suffer include frostbite, nonfreezing cold tissue damage, immersion foot (formerly called *trench foot*), and hypothermia (Fig. 22.2). Cold injuries may result in long-term health problems, including the following signs and symptoms (at the site of exposure):

- Changes in muscle, skin, nails, ligaments, and bones
- Skin cancer in frostbite scars
- Neurological injury with symptoms such as bouts of pain in the extremities, hot or cold tingling sensations, and numbness
- Vascular injury with Raynaud phenomenon with symptoms such as extremities becoming painful and white or discolored when cold

Amputations

Modern body armor has increased the survival rate among troops who experience an explosive ordnance in combat, and medical advances further increase the likelihood that a soldier will survive the loss of a limb (Fig. 22.3). Around 1650 men and women have lost hands, arms, legs, or feet since combat began in Afghanistan and Iraq in 2001 (DAV, 2020). The majority of the 11,879 amputation surgeries performed in 2016, however, were not combat related. Rather, the main etiology was diabetes and peripheral vascular disease, with a 78% incidence of diabetes in veterans undergoing that type of surgery in 2016. Besides the obvious physical impairment affecting activities of daily living (ADLs), body image issues from limb amputations or disfigurement may create multiple social and employment barriers (DAV, 2020).

Occupational Hazard Exposures

A veteran's particular service branch, time period of service, and activities in which the individual was engaged may have contributed to exposure to a number of other potentially harmful toxins or substances. These include exposure to asbestos, lead, industrial solvents, and other harmful chemicals. Symptoms and subsequent problems or complications might develop years later and be very hard to determine.

TABLE 22.4 Severity Rating for Traumatic Brain Injury

Severity	GCS	AOC	LOC	PTA
Mild	13–15	≤24 h	0–30 min	≤24 h
Moderate	9–12	>24 h	>30 min to <24 h	>24 h to <7 days
Severe	3–8	>24 h	≥24 h	≥7 days

AOC, Alteration of consciousness; *GCS*, Glasgow Coma Score; *LOC*, loss of consciousness; *PTA*, posttraumatic amnesia.
From U.S. Department of Veterans Affairs Office of Public Health and Environmental Hazards (13A), Force Health Protection (DoD), and the VA-DoD Deployment Health Working Group: Mild traumatic brain injury—concussion: pocket guide for clinicians, October 2010. Available at: https://www.publichealth.va.gov/docs/exposures/TBI-pocketcard.pdf.

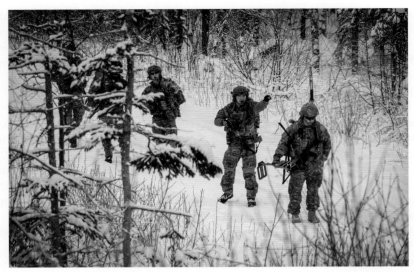

Fig. 22.2 Veterans may suffer from injuries related to their exposure to cold temperatures during their time of service. (Air Force photo by Senior Airman Curt Beach.)

Posttraumatic Stress Disorder

Although the terminology is relatively new, for centuries people have observed psychological disturbances among soldiers returning from war. Amid the devastation of the First World War (1914–18), British medical personnel noticed a series of symptoms among troops at the front lines, including anxiety attacks, hallucinations, nightmares, irritability, sleeplessness, and cardiovascular and gastrointestinal disorders. Some psychiatrists of the day theorized that these symptoms were caused by exploding artillery shells inflicting damage to the brain and dubbed the condition "*shell shock.*" Others argued it was psychological in origin, the result of witnessing killing, torture, and other horrors of war, a position confirmed by the success of psychotherapeutic treatments. Among psychiatrists and military officers, there were several different names for the condition throughout the conflicts of the twentieth century (Table 22.5) until the publication of DSM-III in 1980, which codified the diagnosis as **posttraumatic stress disorder (PTSD)**.

Put simply, PTSD is a mental illness that develops in some individuals who have experienced a shocking, frightening, or dangerous event (NIMH, 2019), and although PTSD is of special concern to the veteran cohort, it is important to recognize that the condition is not unique to the experience of warfare. For example, PTSD can develop among those involved in car accidents, natural disaster survivors, and victims of rape

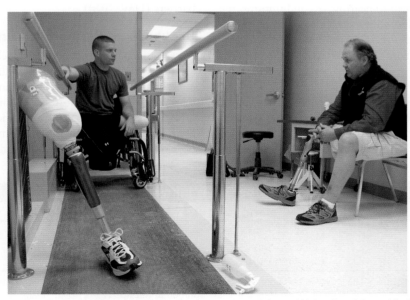

Fig. 22.3 Jack Farley, a retired federal judge and peer amputee visitor at Walter Reed Army Medical Center, talks with Marine Lance Cpl. Josh Bleill, who lost both legs in Iraq when the Humvee in which he was riding struck a bomb. (Fred W. Baker III/US Department of Defense.)

TABLE 22.5 Names for Trauma-Related Conditions in History

Time Period	Nomenclature
Seventeenth century through the American Civil War	Nostalgia
Mid-to-late 19th century	Soldier's heart
	Irritable heart
	Da costa syndrome
	Railway spine
World War I	Shell shock
World War II	Battle fatigue
Korean War	Gross stress reaction
Vietnam War	Combat stress reaction (CSR)
DSM-III (1980)	Posttraumatic stress disorder

or incest. Factors that contribute to an individual developing PTSD include getting injured or seeing another person injured, viewing a dead body, feeling helpless, having little or no social support after a traumatic event, dealing with extra stress after the event (e.g., loss of a loved one, pain, and injury), or having a history of mental illness or substance abuse (NIMH, 2019).

NURSING CARE GUIDELINES

Prevalence of PTSD

The nurse should note that not everyone exposed to dangerous events develops symptoms of PTSD; however, combat veterans are at a higher risk for the disorder. Among the general population, an estimated 8% of men and 20% of women who experience a traumatic event will develop PTSD, whereas 36% of men and 18% of women in war zones develop the disorder (Kulka, 1990; U.S. Department of Veterans Affairs (VA), 2021c).

The VA indicates that in 2011, more than 476,000 veterans received treatment at VHA facilities for primary or secondary diagnosis of PTSD (Fig. 22.4). In addition, it is estimated that PTSD will affect between 11% and 20% of veterans who served in Operations Iraqi Freedom and Enduring Freedom in a given year (U.S. Department of Veterans Affairs (VA), 2016).

Diagnosis

Typically, PTSD symptoms begin within 3 months of the traumatic incident, but they may begin years afterward. To be diagnosed with PTSD, an individual must have experienced a "stressor criterion," which means that the person has been exposed to an event that is considered traumatic (Friedman, 2016). In addition, an adult must experience all of these symptoms for at least a month:

- At least one re-experiencing symptom (e.g., flashbacks, bad dreams, frightening thoughts)
- At least one avoidance symptom (e.g., staying away from places, events, or objects that are reminders of the experience; avoiding thoughts or feelings related to the event)
- At least two arousal and reactivity symptoms (e.g., being easily startled, feeling tense or on edge, difficulty sleeping, angry outbursts)
- At least two cognition and mood symptoms (e.g., trouble remembering key features of the event, negative thoughts about oneself or the world, distorted feelings of guilt or blame, loss of interest in enjoyable activities) (NIMH, 2019)

In general, a diagnosis of PTSD has been found to be associated with chronic pain, hypertension, coronary artery disease, thyroid disorder, insomnia, back pain, swollen joints, dizziness, chronic fatigue, difficulty concentrating, high blood pressure, and heart palpitations. Women with PTSD have more than twice the number of clinic visits over a year as do women without a lifetime history of PTSD (U.S. Department of Veterans Affairs (VA), 2020b). A brief (4 min) informative video explaining PTSD is available at https://www.ptsd.va.gov/appvid/video/index.asp.

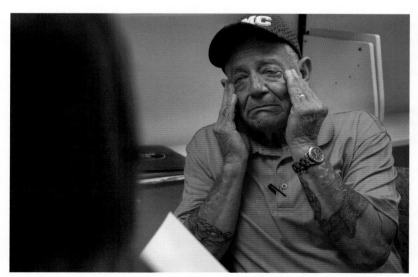

Fig. 22.4 Jim Alderman, a Vietnam veteran, receives treatment for PTSD at a VA medical center. *PTSD,* Posttraumatic stress disorder; *VA,* US Department of Veterans Affairs. (EJ Hersom/US Department of Defense.)

Military Sexual Trauma

Sexual assault and sexual harassment during military service are associated with myriad deleterious health consequences among the veteran population. The VA defines **military sexual trauma (MST)** as sexual assault or sexual harassment experienced during military service. MST includes any sexual activity that someone is involved with against their will, such as:

- Being pressured or coerced into sexual activities, such as with threats of negative treatment if you refuse to cooperate or with promises of better treatment in exchange for sex
- Sexual contact or activities without your consent, including when you were asleep or intoxicated
- Being overpowered or physically forced to have sex
- Being touched or grabbed in a sexual way that made you uncomfortable, including during "hazing" experiences
- Comments about your body or sexual activities that you found threatening
- Unwanted sexual advances that you found threatening

Anyone can experience MST, regardless of gender (U.S. Department of Veterans Affairs (VA), 2021j).

An estimated one in four female veterans and one in 100 male veterans in the VA healthcare system report experiencing MST. It is important to note that by percentage women are at greater risk of MST, but nearly 40% of veterans who disclose MST to VA are men. DAV (2020) and Box 22.1 lists common sociodemographic characteristics of MST victims. It is estimated that in one of seven women who report MST, the trauma was perpetrated by an intimate partner (Mercado et al., 2015).

A number of health conditions are more prevalent among women with a history of sexual trauma, including sexually transmitted infections, diabetes, obesity, arthritis, irritable bowel syndrome, hypertension, and eating disorders (U.S. Department of Veterans Affairs (VA), 2021j). MST is also associated with the development of significant mental health consequences and related functional impairment. In a nationally representative sample of veterans, individuals who have a history of MST are also more likely to have lifetime and current mental health conditions (Fig. 22.5). Higher rates of eating disorders—especially among male veterans—have also been documented among veterans who screen positive for MST (Blais et al., 2017). Insomnia is also a prevalent condition among veterans and is more common and more severe among

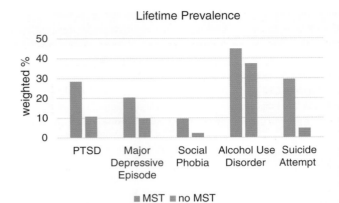

Fig. 22.5 Association between MST and mental health threats. *MST,* Military sexual trauma; *PTSD,* posttraumatic stress disorder. (Data from Klingensmith K, et al.: Military sexual trauma in US veterans, *J Clin Psychiatry* 75(10):1133–1139, 2014. https://doi.org/10.4088/jcp.14m09244.)

veterans who report a history of MST (Jenkins et al., 2015). MST is also independently associated with poorer cognitive functioning and quality of life as well as increased somatic symptoms (Klingensmith et al., 2014).

Among veterans seeking treatment for PTSD, sexual trauma has been associated with more severe PTSD than any other type of trauma, including combat trauma (Goldstein et al., 2017; U.S. Department of Veterans Affairs (VA), 2020c). Similar trends are found on the impact of MST on mental health among veterans returning from Afghanistan and Iraq. Veterans deployed to Iraq or Afghanistan who screen positive for MST when seeking services with the VHA were more likely to be diagnosed with PTSD, depressive disorders, and substance use disorders (SUD) (Gilmore et al., 2016; U.S. Department of Veterans Affairs (VA), 2020c). The VA has many resources to assist victims of MST. The MST homepage (https://www.mentalhealth.va.gov/mentalhealth/msthome/index.asp) has beneficial information regarding MST. Additionally, the VA has designed an application for victims of MST called Beyond MST (see https://mobile.va.gov/app/beyond-mst).

Polytraumatic Injuries

The term **polytrauma** refers to two or more injuries sustained in the same incident, affecting multiple body parts or organ systems, and resulting in various kinds of impairments and functional disabilities. Polytrauma is often the result of a blast-related event, and frequently includes TBI. For example, a soldier who has lost a limb, suffered a TBI, and lost his eyesight from a rocket-propelled grenade attack is said to have a polytraumatic injury. Like other types of combat health risks, incidence of polytrauma is on the rise because of IED attacks and because soldiers now survive events that would have killed them in the past (Geiling et al., 2012). Care for veterans with these injuries is especially complicated because of the presence of several overlapping physical and cognitive impairments affecting their ability to perform ADLs.

BOX 22.1   Risk Factors and Characteristics of Veterans Experiencing MST

- Female
- Younger (18–29 years of age)
- Racial ethnic minority
- Unemployed
- Single/divorced
- Enlisted
- Navy veteran

MST, Military sexual trauma.
From Klingensmith K, et al.: Military sexual trauma in US veterans, *J Clin Psychiatry,* 2014. https://doi.org/10.4088/jcp.14m09244.

Chronic Pain

Combat operations impart physical stress on the bodies of soldiers. They work long hours, carry heavy packs, and wear heavy armor, increasing the burden on the musculoskeletal system. According to a 2009 study, 29% of Operation Enduring Freedom (OEF) and Operation Iraqi Freedom (OIF) veterans report chronic widespread pain (Helmer et al., 2009). Pain is not limited to load-carrying service members in the infantry; however, one study of US Marines found that lower back pain was even more prevalent among troops in trade occupations such as construction and law enforcement than among their counterparts in the infantry (MacGregor et al., 2012). In 2015, more veterans received treatment for service-connected musculoskeletal disorders than for any other body system (Table 22.6).

Chronic pain is often comorbid with TBI and PTSD, and for some individuals, muscle tension associated with PTSD can exacerbate pain. Furthermore, constant pain can serve as a reminder of traumatic events (Johnson et al., 2013). In an effort to not only decrease chronic pain among veterans, but to decrease use of opioid medications, the VA has begun to use the Whole Health approach program. The Whole Health approach features conventional clinical care (such as medicines or counseling) and complementary and integrative care (such as acupuncture or yoga) working concurrently as part of an overall treatment plan. In a pilot study of Veterans with chronic pain engaged in Whole Health services, more than 100,000 Veterans experienced a meaningful reduction of opioid pain medications. In an important finding, opioid use among Veterans engaged in Whole Health decreased 38% compared to an 11% decrease among those not enrolled in Whole Health (U.S. Department of Veterans Affairs (VA), 2021g).

Substance Use Disorders

SUDs involve a pattern of use of alcohol, tobacco, and illegal and prescription drugs that results in marked distress and/or impairment (American Psychiatric Association [APA], 2013). Although problems with alcohol or other drugs affect veterans at about the same rates as the general population, there is a strong relationship between SUD and PTSD: more than 2 of 10 veterans with PTSD also have SUD (U.S. Department of Veterans Affairs (VA), 2017d). SUDs are also associated with other substantial negative correlates such as depression and anxiety, medical problems and disabilities, and increased rates of suicidal ideation and attempts (Teeters et al., 2017).

Binge drinking and cigarette smoking are the most prevalent types of substance use problems among male and female veterans, affecting about 11% of the veteran population, with disorders more common among males younger than 25 years of age. That this younger, male demographic associated with higher rates of SUDs in the general civilian population makes up a greater proportion of the military population could explain an increased risk of certain SUDs relative to civilians. About 4.8% of male veterans have drug use disorders, double the rate of their female counterparts (Teeters et al., 2017).

RESEARCH HIGHLIGHTS

Smoking Habits Among Veterans

Veterans are significantly more likely than nonveterans to be current smokers (28% vs. 20%). Although almost three-fourths of veterans report that they want to quit, most don't take advantage of tobacco cessation advice or counseling. A recent study at a large VHA setting by Fore et al. (2014) underscored the importance of nurses being prepared to promote smoking cessation interventions. The nurses at the facility received training on behavioral and pharmaceutical interventions that focused on evidence-based

TABLE 22.6 Number of SC Disabilities of All Compensation Recipients FY 2011 to FY 2015

Body System	2011	2012	2013	2014	2015	% Chg. FY 2014–2015
Musculoskeletal	4,721,091	5,189,302	5,780,195	6,397,255	7,117,586	11%
Auditory	1,679,146	1,883,919	2,116,528	2,352,609	2,613,285	11%
Skin	1,407,126	1,542,739	1,726,884	1,910,027	2,111,444	11%
Neurological	1,183,512	1,345,832	1,557,654	1,788,151	2,058,164	15%
Mental	878,417	986,904	1,110,050	1,230,063	1,368,427	11%
Cardiovascular	675,434	786,826	834,775	878,381	919,068	5%
Respiratory	582,933	644,675	719,770	798,353	889,002	11%
Digestive	732,523	719,598	772,021	825,345	884,368	7%
Genitourinary	464,634	515,282	570,093	627,252	684,965	9%
Endocrine	396,121	422,786	447,399	469,910	488,942	4%
The eye	187,440	200,546	216,955	233,430	252,069	8%
Gynecological	72,512	77,882	85,043	92,164	101,008	10%
Dental/Oral	58,705	64,724	72,588	80,526	89,713	11%
Hemic/Lymphatic	39,147	42,770	46,517	50,677	55,075	9%
Infection/Immune/Nutrition	47,756	48,318	48,928	49,495	50,275	2%
Total	**13,126,497**	**14,472,103**	**16,105,400**	**17,783,638**	**19,683,391**	**11%**

FY, Fiscal year; SC, service connected.
From US Department of Veteran's Affairs, Veterans Benefits Administration: Annual benefits report, fiscal year 2015. Available at: https://www.benefits.va.gov/REPORTS/abr/ABR-Compensation-FY15-05092016.pdf.

protocols to promote smoking cessation. The nurses were encouraged to provide patients with educational videos and materials as well as access to helplines and follow-up phone calls for those who wanted to stop smoking. The nurses who received the education were significantly more likely to recognize the importance of delivering smoking cessation interventions and to report confidence in their counseling efforts. The researchers concluded that nurse-delivered tobacco cessation interventions have widespread potential to increase quit rates among veterans.

From Fore AM, et al.: Nurses' delivery of the Tobacco Tactics intervention at a Veterans Affairs Medical Center, *J Clin Nurs* 23:2162–2169, 2014.

Though suicide remains a significant problem among veterans, there are some reasons to be hopeful:

- From 2017 to 2018, adjusted suicide rates fell among Veterans with recent VHA care.
- Among Veterans in VHA care, rates fell from 2005 to 2018 among those with depression, anxiety, and SUD.
- There has been a decrease in suicide risk among male Hispanic and women Veterans, engaged in VHA care.
- There is a groundswell of support for coordinated efforts at the local, regional, and national levels to implement a public health approach to end suicide (U.S. Department of Veterans Affairs (VA), 2020e).

Veteran Suicide

A November 2020 report by the VA(US Dept of VA 2020e) provided a comprehensive assessment of differences in rates of suicide among veteran and the US civilian populations. This report confirmed that veterans as a cohort are at an increased risk for suicide. Increased suicide rates were particularly evident among female veterans and veterans who did not use VHA services. The report highlighted key findings, including:

- An average of 17 veterans died by suicide each day
- In each year since 2008, the number of Veteran suicides has exceeded 6300 (6435 Veterans died by suicide in 2018, compared with 6056 in 2005 despite a decrease in the Veteran population)
- The rate for suicide was 1.2 times higher among veterans compared with US civilian adults after adjusting for differences in age and gender
- Approximately 64% of all veteran suicides resulted from firearm injuries
- Approximately 40% of all veterans who died by suicide were age 50 or older
- In both 2017 and 2018, the age-adjusted suicide rate among women Veterans was 2.1 times that of non-Veteran women. In 2018, the age-adjusted suicide rate among male Veterans was 1.3 times that of non-Veteran males.

Risk factors for suicide among veterans identified in the literature include non-Hispanic white race/ethnicity, male (Hedegaard et al., 2021), sexual minority status (Blosnich et al., 2014), preenlisted and/or current mental health conditions (history of self-directed violence (), substance use), poor physical health and functioning (McCarthy et al., 2015), intimate partner conflict (Alexander et al., 2014), lack of social support (Monteith et al., 2015), and sexual trauma (Lutwak and Dill, 2013). Veterans with any of these risk factors need to be closely screened and referred for follow-up services. Additional information on the VA's efforts to prevent suicide is described later in the chapter.

🏠 COMMUNITY FOCUS

Suicidality Following PTSD and MST

Perhaps the most crucial sequelae for both PTSD and MST is suicidality. Veterans who experienced MST are two to four times more likely to report suicidal ideation, suicide plans, and suicide attempts (Bryan et al., 2015; Monteith et al., 2016a). Suicide risk is more strongly associated with MST among male veterans compared to female veterans (Bryan et al., 2015; Monteith et al., 2016b).

Health Risks Common to Cohorts

Beyond the basic health threats, there are several health risks or problems commonly encountered for specific cohorts based on their theater, time of service, or experiences.

WWII Veterans

World War II veterans were exposed to high levels of noise. Veterans were exposed to radiation at Hiroshima and Nagasaki. WWII veterans who were in the Battle of the Bulge, fought in December 1944 through January 1945, were exposed to extreme cold and may have sustained cold injuries. Some volunteers were exposed to mustard gas experiments, in which the DoD evaluated equipment for their protection against mustard gas attacks. About 4000 soldiers were subjected to severe, full-body exposures during testing.

In addition to these, WWII veterans suffer from PTSD, at the time called *battle fatigue* or *combat stress reaction*. Despite efforts to screen soldiers for mental health as well as treatments offered on the lines, about 500,000 patients received disability pensions for neuropsychiatric disorders in 1947 (Pols and Oak, 2007).

Korean War Veterans

The Korean War, sometimes referred to as the *Korean conflict*, lasted from 1950 to 1953, with more than 5.7 million Americans serving during this time and ending in more than 54,000 American fatalities. The Korean War is often called "The Forgotten War" because it received so little attention compared with WWII.

Health concerns for Korean War veterans center around three main categories: extreme cold injuries, noise, and occupational hazards. Korean War veterans who served in the Chosin Reservoir Campaign during October through December of 1950, in particular, could have been exposed to temperatures of −50°F. Indeed, there were more casualties from cold than from battle during this campaign (NVF, 2017).

Vietnam Veterans

Approximately 8,744,000 US troops served during the Vietnam War (about 2.6 million in the theater), with 58,220 deaths, and 1611 missing in action. Actually serving "in country" is dramatically associated with increased health problems, as research indicates that veterans who were stationed in Vietnam during the war have worse health status than those who were elsewhere during the same time period. Those who served in the war theater self-report poor health status. Further, they experience significantly higher rates of other health conditions, including cancer, stroke, hypertension, and lung conditions (Brooks et al., 2008).

In addition to the common health risks of noise and occupational hazards mentioned earlier, Vietnam veterans suffer health disorders related to exposure to **Agent Orange**—an herbicide used to kill the vegetation that provided cover for the enemy. The U.S. Department of Veterans Affairs (VA) (2017e) presumes certain cancers and other conditions to be caused by Agent Orange exposure. Because of this presumptive nature, the VA awards disability compensation for the following conditions to anyone who served in the Republic of Vietnam from 1962 to 1975:

- AL amyloidosis
- Chronic B-cell leukemia
- Chloracne
- Diabetes mellitus type 2
- Hodgkin disease
- Ischemic heart disease
- Multiple myeloma
- Non-Hodgkin lymphoma
- Parkinson disease
- Peripheral neuropathy
- Porphyria cutanea tarda
- Prostate cancer
- Respiratory cancers
- Soft tissue sarcomas
- Lou Gehrig disease, or AML
- Spina bifida among children of exposed service members

Besides the physical health risks associated with serving in Vietnam, the veterans of this war contended with the effects of the political and social environment of the day. Antiwar sentiment increased in the United States from the mid-1960s to the end of the war, both among those who found the war pointless and unjust, and those who blamed the troops for the lack of a victory. When they returned home, many veterans did not speak of their experiences out of fear of criticism. Wishing to distance themselves from the war, many Vietnam veterans never received treatment for the mental impacts of their time in combat.

Gulf War and the Global War on Terror

The Gulf War, codenamed Operation Desert Shield and Operation Desert Storm, took place from 1990 to 1991 in Kuwait, Iraq, and the Saudi Arabian border. The Global War on Terror (GWOT) refers to the series of campaigns launched primarily in Iraq and Afghanistan after the September 11, 2001, attacks in the United States. Veterans of this broad series of missions include those involved in Operation Freedom's Sentinel (OFS, Afghanistan), Operation Inherent Resolve (OIR, Iraq and Syria), Operation New Dawn (OND, Iraq), Operation Iraqi Freedom (OIF, Iraq), and Operation Enduring Freedom (OEF, Afghanistan). Veterans who served in Iraq and Afghanistan have many potential health risks to consider. About 900,000 Gulf War veterans and 1 million veterans of the GWOT have received benefits from the VHA (U.S. Department of Veterans Affairs (VA), 2016). In desert conditions, they were exposed to a number of health threats, including:

- Sand, dust, and particulate matter, which can cause respiratory disorders
- **Burn pits**, open pits where waste was burned during deployment (Fig. 22.6). Toxic smoke can damage the respiratory, gastrointestinal, reproductive, peripheral nervous, and cardiovascular systems, as well as the skin and eyes (VA, OPH, WRIISC, 2013).
- Shrapnel from IEDs, bombs, mines, and shells
- TBIs from blast injuries

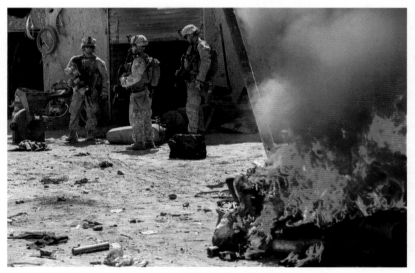

Fig. 22.6 Marines burn materials used to make IEDs in Afghanistan (2014). *IEDs,* Improvised explosive devices. (US Department of Defense.)

- Heat stroke or heat exhaustion
- Chemical exposures such as mustard agents, which can irritate the airways and cause cancer, and sarin, a nerve agent
- Chromium, which can cause cancer

In addition to these threats, veterans serving in Iraq or Afghanistan may have been exposed to a number of infectious diseases. Among them are malaria, brucellosis, *Campylobacter jejuni*, *Coxiella burnetii* (Q fever), tuberculosis, salmonella, Shigella, visceral leishmaniasis, rabies, and West Nile virus. Furthermore, many servicemen were given mefloquine (Lariam) to prevent malaria. Long-term use of this medication can cause serious neurological or psychiatric side effects (U.S. Department of Veterans Affairs [VA], 2015a).

Chronic Multisymptom Illness. Approximately 250,000 veterans of the 1991 Gulf War (about 25%—32%) returned home with multiple varied, unexplained symptoms, including fatigue, dizziness, headaches, cognitive dysfunction, musculoskeletal pain, respiratory problems, rashes, and diarrhea. Popular media of the time referred to the disorder as *Gulf War Syndrome* or *Gulf War Illness*, although today the VHA refers to this cluster of symptoms as *chronic multisymptom illness (CMI)*.

In the years immediately following the conflict, various causes for CMI were suggested, including chemical weapons exposures, depleted uranium, sarin gas, smoke from burning oil wells, vaccinations, and PTSD, many of which have been ruled out. Studies since then have narrowed in on two consistent risk factors: exposures to pesticides and pyridostigmine bromide, given to US troops as a prophylactic against nerve gas agents (White et al., 2016). The VA presumes certain illnesses to be related to service in southwestern Asia:

- Chronic fatigue syndrome
- Fibromyalgia
- Gastrointestinal illnesses (e.g., irritable bowel syndrome)
- Undiagnosed illnesses with symptoms that may include but are not limited to abnormal weight loss, fatigue, cardiovascular disease, muscle and joint pain, headache, menstrual disorders, neurological and psychological problems, skin conditions, respiratory disorders, and sleep disturbances (U.S. Department of Veterans Affairs [VA], 2017f)

Homelessness Among Veterans

Though most veterans successfully transition into civilian life, there are many who struggle, eventually becoming homeless. Though exact numbers are hard to come by, the US Department of Housing and Urban Development estimates that there are 39,471 veterans homeless on any given night. The majority of homeless veterans are single males between the ages of 31 and 50 (Fig. 22.7). The numbers of young veterans who are homeless is increasing, with approximately 12,700 veterans of OEF/OIF/OND being homeless in 2010 (Clinical Example 22.1). Only 9% of homeless veterans are females. Most homeless veterans live in urban areas and have mental health and/or substance abuse disorders. Approximately 45% of all homeless veterans are African American or Hispanic (National Coalition for Homeless Veterans, 2017).

Clinical Example 22.1

Bobby Jackson, 24, ducked into the Pontiac Health Department to get out of the January wind and settled in to one of the hard plastic chairs in the waiting room for a nap. Because everyone is required to leave the overnight shelter by 7 a.m. each morning, he has a long 14 h to fill until the shelter opens for the night. Since his discharge from the army, Bobby hasn't been able to find work, other than odd jobs shoveling walkways for strangers or washing windshields for stopped cars. Typically he spends any money he makes on a bottle or a fix—anything to calm his nerves and stop the flashbacks.

Amy Butler, RN, has worked at the Health Department for 6 months. She has noticed the young African American man asleep in the waiting room several times recently, and she knows that the army boots and flak jacket he usually wears are not warm enough for the Michigan winters. Today, she observed him twitching and trembling while he slept. Although a colleague suggested, "Ignore him, he's just a street person," Amy approached him after he awoke to offer the services of the Health Department.

When asked by Amy, Bobby explained that he had served in Operation Iraqi Freedom. Although Bobby was very polite, like many combat veterans, he seemed reluctant to seek assistance. As with every vet she cares for, Amy looked him in the eye and thanked him for his service. Then she reminded him that he is entitled to health care and other benefits through the VA. She also gave him contact information for the VHA clinic a few miles away, the local Veterans Center, so he can connect with other vets, and a flyer from the Michigan Veterans Trust Fund, which provides for temporary basic living needs of veterans. Then she pointed out the Alano Club across the street, where recovering alcoholics would be available to help Bobby with his substance abuse problem. Finally, she made an appointment for Bobby to be evaluated by the Health Department's nurse practitioner for possible elevated blood pressure and frostbite.

Before he left, Bobby promised to follow up with the VA and report back to the Health Department within 1 week.

Created by Kathleen Walsh Spencer, DNP, MA, ACNS-BC.

Nearly half of homeless veterans served during the Vietnam era, and two-thirds served our country for at least 3 years; one-third were stationed in a war zone. Approximately 89% of homeless veterans have an honorable discharge. About 1.4 million veterans are considered at risk of homelessness due to poverty, lack of support networks, and overcrowded or substandard housing (National Coalition for Homeless Veterans, 2017).

Veterans become homeless due to a number of factors. In addition to the complex set of factors influencing all homelessness—a shortage of affordable housing, lack of a livable income, and access to health care—a large number of displaced and at-risk veterans live with lingering effects of PTSD and substance abuse, which are compounded by a lack of family and social support networks. Additionally, military occupations and training are not always transferable to the civilian workforce, placing some veterans at a disadvantage when competing for employment.

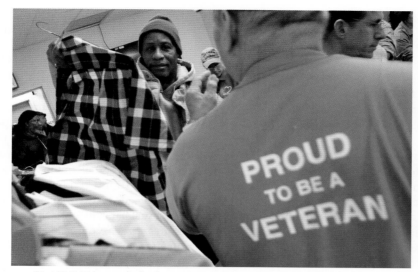

Fig. 22.7 Volunteers distribute clothing at an event for homeless veterans.

Incarceration also significantly increases the risk of a veteran becoming homeless; even a brief incarceration will increase the likelihood of homelessness. About one half of veterans participating in VA homeless assistance programs are also involved in the criminal justice system. Homelessness and criminal justice system involvement can be a vicious cycle, with the impact of one problem increasing the risk of the other. Many behaviors associated with homelessness such as trespassing, loitering, and petty theft are criminalized. Incarceration, in turn, often leads to barriers to obtaining housing and reintegrating into society. Though the incarceration rate for veterans is lower than that of civilians, 181,500 veterans were incarcerated in 2012. A greater percentage of veterans (64%) were incarcerated for violent offenses compared with nonveterans (48%).

Female Veterans and Homelessness

Men and women veterans, two groups within the homeless veteran subpopulation, have health problems similar to those of nonveteran individuals experiencing homelessness. By the end of this decade, there will be an estimated 2.5 million female veterans. Female veterans are the fastest growing demographic among the homeless population in the United States. Many women Veterans face challenges when returning to civilian life, including raising children on their own or dealing with the aftereffects of military sexual trauma. Without intervention, these and other issues can put women Veterans at greater risk of homelessness. Women veterans who experience homelessness have problems specific to their military service experience and their roles as child caregivers. A brief sketch of these problems follows. Homeless female veterans are especially likely to be undercounted. The VA has found that female veterans are at high-risk for homelessness. These veterans are more than twice as likely to be homeless as other women and more than three times as likely if they are at risk or in poverty (Rogers,

2019). The U.S. Government Accountability Office (2011) reported a study in which minor children accompanied 33% of homeless women veterans, almost two-thirds of the women were between the ages of 40 and 59 years, and more than one-third had disabilities. Additional research has demonstrated that being unemployed, disabled, or unmarried strongly predicts homelessness among women veterans (U.S. Department of Veterans Affairs [VA], 2018).

Pavao et al. (2013) found that 39.7% of the women veterans in the VHA experience MST. The U.S. Department of Veterans Affairs (VA) (2018) also documented that 60% of the housing programs serving homeless women veterans did not accommodate children and that women reported concerns about their safety in the housing facilities with regard to incidents of sexual harassment or assault. The report recommended that services for women veterans address privacy, safety, and gender-specific concerns, including accommodations for minor children.

VETERANS' HEALTH ASSESSMENT

Veterans, especially those who access care at the VHA hospitals and clinics, tend to be older, sicker, and require more complex care than nonveterans. Veterans have more diagnosed conditions such as PTSD, diabetes, hearing loss, cancer, hypertension, heart disease, and chronic conditions such as chronic obstructive pulmonary disease (COPD). Veterans are 13 times more likely to have PTSD than nonveterans. The rate of PTSD is higher among veterans who are 35 and under. These young veterans also have higher rates of TBI, amputations, blindness, and severe burns than do older veterans. Veterans of the wars in Iraq and Afghanistan are more likely to have health conditions linked to their military service than do other veterans (Watkins et al., 2011). As most veterans will access care in the community, all healthcare professionals must appropriately assess veterans, be aware of their unique needs, and develop skills to meet those needs.

It is important to ask if the person has ever served in the military, rather than asking if the person is a veteran (American Academy of Nursing, 2017). This is because many prior military service members—especially younger veterans—do not self-identify as "veterans," as they see the term as referring to "the old guys." Others may feel that if they were not deployed to a combat zone that they are not veterans. Asking if they have served in the military will allow them to tell you how they identify.

A veteran's health may be related to their theater of deployment, injuries related to combat, possible MST, and PTSD; yet over half of community providers do not ask their patients about prior military service. Training in health risks such as PTSD, CMI, MST, and TBI is an essential element of quality veteran care (Miltner et al., 2013). Box 22.2 contains assessment questions to ask the patient with prior military service.

As mentioned, PTSD is a risk factor for many veterans due to their exposure to life-threatening situations, seeing their friends killed or injured, training accidents, sexual trauma, or exposure to natural disasters. Many veterans with PTSD do not seek mental health services but present in the primary care setting, where their symptoms may go unrecognized. Traumatic stress is associated with increased health complaints, increased health services utilization, and higher morbidity and mortality (Schnurr and Jankowski, 1999). It is crucial for primary care providers to recognize signs and symptoms suggestive of a trauma history (e.g., PTSD or MST). These may include substance abuse, hostility and mistrust of the medical community, noncompliance, and frequent missed or canceled appointments. Patients who present with multiple health complaints and diagnoses, particularly those who do not respond to treatment, should alert the provider to the underlying possibility of MST or PTSD.

All veterans seeking care at the VHA are screened for MST. Models to identify women at risk for MST suggest that lower sociocultural and organizational power (young age, low education, single, lower rank, short time in service and duty unit) are predictors of administratively reported sexual assault in the military, but not self-reported MST (Street et al., 2016). Due to stigma and shame, many veterans will not volunteer information regarding sexual trauma exposure. When screening for history of MST, it is best to avoid words that are emotionally or politically loaded (e.g., "rape") or words that are poorly defined (e.g., "sexual harassment"). Nonjudgmental, descriptive general questions are recommended (National Center for Post-traumatic Stress Disorder, 2004) (see Box 22.2).

INTERVENTIONS FOR VETERAN HEALTH PROBLEMS

Nurses who encounter veterans in community-based care situations, as well as those who work with veterans on a routine basis, need to be knowledgeable about the health problems and threats common among this population. This section describes a few resources and interventions that may be helpful during these instances.

Management of PTSD

Friedman (2016) described the most effective treatment strategies for those experiencing PTSD. He noted that the most

---

BOX 22.2 Assessment Questions

General Questions
- In what branch of the military did you serve?
- Where did you serve?
- Did you serve in combat?
- What was your job in the military?
- Did you sustain any injuries related to your military service?
- What were you exposed to: chemical (pollution, solvents, etc.), biological (infectious disease), or physical (radiation, heat, vibration, etc.)?
  - What precautions were taken (avoidance, personal protective equipment [PPE], treatment, etc.)?
  - How were you exposed (inhaled, on skin, swallowed, etc.)?
  - How concerned are you about the exposure?
  - Where were you exposed?
  - When were you exposed?
  - Who else may have been affected?

Posttraumatic Stress
- Have you ever experienced a traumatic or stressful event that caused you to believe your life or the lives of those around you were in danger?
- Are you experiencing trauma-related thoughts or feelings?
- Are you having nightmares, vivid memories, or flashbacks of the event?
- Are you feeling anxious, jittery?

- Are you experiencing a sense of panic that something bad is about to happen?
- Are you having difficulty sleeping or concentrating?

Military Sexual Trauma
- During military service did you receive uninvited or unwanted sexual attention, such as touching, pressure for sexual favors, or sexual remarks?
- Did anyone ever use force or threat of force to have sexual contact with you against your will?
- Did you report the incidents to your command and/or military or civilian authorities?

Blast Concussions/Traumatic Brain Injury
- During your service, did you experience:
  - Heavy artillery fire, vehicular, or aircraft accidents
  - Explosions (improvised explosive devices [IEDs], rocket-propelled grenades, land mines, grenades) or fragment or bullet wounds above the shoulders
- Did you have any of these symptoms immediately afterward:
  - Loss of consciousness or being knocked out
  - Being dazed or seeing stars
  - Not remembering the event
  - Diagnosis of concussion or head injury

successful interventions include cognitive-behavioral therapy and medication (e.g., selective serotonin reuptake inhibitors such as sertraline [Zoloft] and paroxetine [Paxil]). Other trauma-focused psychotherapies are evidence based and highly recommended for PTSD. Here treatment focuses on the memory of the traumatic event or its meaning.

To ensure that veterans receive high-quality mental health care, the VA has increased access to evidence-based psychotherapies. Research has shown that participation in psychotherapy protocols for diagnoses such as PTSD has been shown to decrease suicidal ideation for veterans (Cox et al., 2016; U.S. Department of Veterans Affairs [VA], 2021i). There are variations of trauma-focused therapies. These include (1) prolonged exposure therapy (where the individual is repeatedly questioned by the therapist about the trauma to encourage control of the thoughts and feelings to reduce fear of the memories); (2) cognitive processing therapy, which involves talking with the therapist about the negative thoughts and beliefs and development of strategies to manage the recollection of the trauma in a way that is less upsetting; and (3) eye movement desensitization and reprocessing, which involves identification of the negative thoughts, emotions, and feelings while focusing on specific sounds or movements, helping the brain work through the traumatic memories (National Center for PTSD/VA, 2020).

The VA supports a number of programs, strategies, and experts to help veterans identify, assess, and treat PTSD. Each VHA center has PTSD specialists who provide therapy, and there are almost 200 PTSD treatment programs in the country (see the PTSD program locator at https://www.ptsd.va.gov/gethelp/find_therapist.asp). These programs offer education, evaluation, and treatment, including mental health assessment, medications, one-on-one therapy, family therapy, and group therapy. Specialized Intensive PTSD Programs provide care in inpatient or resident settings (National Center for PTSD/VA, 2020).

Home-based telemedicine is another intervention strategy that is currently being employed and investigated to increase access to PTSD treatment (U.S. Department of Veterans Affairs [VA], 2020d). This is an option that may be used in situations in which the veteran is located in a remote area or when travel is particularly difficult (e.g., when the person is bedbound or cannot leave the home). During the COVID-19 pandemic, telemedicine allowed veterans to continue their treatment and find support while maintaining social distancing. The use of telemedicine allows more veterans to access care by connecting veterans with health providers across the nation and expanding hours that care is available.

Suicide Prevention Measures

Recognizing that even one veteran suicide is one too many, the VA has worked diligently to develop and improve suicide prevention programs to help all veterans at risk for suicide, whether or not the veteran is enrolled in the VHA system. These efforts include developing better screening and assessment processes to identify veterans at risk for suicide, developing partnerships with organizations and agencies in the public and private sector to assist veterans with psychosocial concerns, and increasing access to timely and high-quality mental health services for mental health concerns such as PTSD, substance use, depression, and suicidal ideation (Pheister et al., 2014; U.S. Department of Veterans Affairs [VA], 2016).

In February 2007, the VA created a suicide prevention coordinator (SPC) position at every VHA center. The SPC's primary role is to help veterans access timely mental health care, particularly in times of crises, and to assist healthcare treatment teams with managing the care of suicidal veterans. SPCs are able to "flag" veterans' charts to prompt treatment providers to assess for suicide when appropriate. In 2018, the VA created and implemented a national suicide prevention program focused on preventing suicide through population and individual level interventions. This program calls for empowering veterans and their families through health education, access to healthcare resources, and the use of technology to expand care options (U.S. Department of Veterans Affairs [VA], 2021f).

SPCs also maintain weekly contact with the veteran and ensure that the veteran's treatment team works with him or her to develop a suicide prevention safety plan that helps the veteran cope with suicidal ideation. The safety plan is tailored to each patient and identifies crisis warning signs, internal coping resources, places the patient can go in order to maintain his or her safety, people to call with whom the veteran has close relationships, professional resources and contact information, and a plan for means restriction. Components of the safety plan can be found on the VA's website: https://www.mentalhealth.va.gov/docs/VA_Safety_Planning_manual.pdf.

A well-known suicide prevention effort is the establishment of the National Veterans Crisis Line in 2007 to provide veterans with immediate access to mental health crisis intervention and support 24 h/day, 7 days a week. Veterans may call the national suicide prevention hotline number (1-800-273-TALK), or text 838255, or use the chat service via VeteransCrisisLine.net. Hotline responders who are trained in suicide prevention and crisis intervention assist callers by initiating dispatch of emergency services to callers in imminent suicidal crisis and referring veterans to VA SPCs to ensure that veterans are connected to local mental health care.

Interventions for Mental Health Issues and Substance Abuse

The VA also expanded veteran access to timely and high-quality mental health treatment and assistance with substance use problems.

Part of increasing access has involved increased numbers of VHA CBOCs available in rural areas to provide needed mental health services, including telemental health services, available both at CBOCs and directly into the veteran's home. Free mobile phone apps have also been developed to facilitate veteran engagement in mental health treatment by providing them with tools and coaching to manage emotional and behavioral concerns.

The VA has created veteran peer support specialist positions within mental health programs. Peer support specialists are veterans who have been trained to provide recovery-oriented support and outreach that encourages other veterans to utilize VHA health services, particularly mental health, to assist with their recovery. Peer support specialists often share personal stories of recovery from mental health and SUDs using VHA resources with the purpose of helping other veterans connect to the VHA system and feel more comfortable seeking assistance.

Recognizing the mental health problems faced by female veterans and increasing numbers of female veterans accessing the VHA system, the VA has bolstered mental health services for this population. Designated women's health providers have been established at 100% of VHA centers and 90% of CBOCs to ensure that women veterans can receive a variety of healthcare services from providers who are trained specifically in women's health issues. The VA has also created a Women Veterans Call Center to contact women and inform them about available services.

In addition to seeking help at VHA facilities, veterans who served on active military duty in any combat theater or area of hostility are eligible to receive services at vet centers, which are community-based counseling centers that provide professional readjustment counseling to veterans and active duty service members. Vet center services typically include social services; psychotherapy (individual, group, and family); outreach and networking; benefits counseling; and referrals for follow-up at federal, state, and local community agencies to assist veterans with basic needs such as shelter, financial assistance, etc. There are currently 300 community-based vet centers and 80 mobile vet centers across the United States.

The VA recognizes the association between many mental health issues and substance abuse. Indeed, substance use and abuse may be the underlying problem or a way to manage the problem. Overuse or misuse of alcohol, tobacco, or drugs (both street drugs and prescription medications) can harm health, cause mood problems, destroy relationships, and result in financial problems. Effective treatment for both mental health threats, including PTSD, depression, and relationship issues, often necessitates addressing substance abuse problems. In addition to individual and group therapy focusing on treatment of substance abuse, medications are available to treat alcohol dependence or tobacco use. Medications may also be used to treat addiction to opioids; in severe cases, management may be inpatient.

In another example of programs to improve veteran's health, the VA proactively engages in education and outreach efforts that connect veterans and their families with the resources they need. Efforts often focus on increasing awareness of VA suicide prevention efforts, reducing stigma about seeking mental health treatment, and strengthening and expanding community resources available to veterans by training community providers to provide culturally competent care. The VA *Make the Connection* campaign, in particular, has been effective in highlighting veterans' true stories of mental health recovery, reducing stigma

and negative perceptions about mental health care, and connecting veterans and family members with local mental health resources (accessible at https://maketheconnection.net).

Veterans returning from combat may have sustained war-related injuries. Amputations, TBI, and hazardous exposures are some of the injuries addressed by the War-Related Illness and Injury Study Center (WRIISC). The WRIISC is a national program dedicated to Veterans' postdeployment health concerns and unique healthcare needs. The WRIISC develops and provides postdeployment health expertise to Veterans and their healthcare providers through clinical care, research, education, and risk communication. The WRIISC is part of VA's Post-Deployment Health Services (U.S. Department of Veterans Affairs [VA], 2021i).

Management of TBI

Nurses may be involved with community-based or long-term management of TBI. Even mild TBI can result in post-concussion symptoms, including headache, dizziness, nausea/vomiting, trouble concentrating, memory issues, irritability, tinnitus, and sensitivity to noise and light. If symptoms of TBI persist, referral to a specialist (e.g., neurologist or rehabilitative therapist) may be necessary (U.S. Department of Veterans Affairs [VA], 2019a).

Management of moderate to severe TBI will initially be implemented in an acute care setting. Depending on the severity and response, treatment will often be moved to a long-term care facility before the veteran goes home. With moderate to severe TBI, the individual will require treatment from a multidisciplinary team. Patient care coordination among the various providers (e.g., physical, occupational, or speech therapists) is essential, and the nurse may act as the case manager. The nurse may be called upon to assist, identify, and intervene with physical, cognitive, and emotional sequelae and help administer and evaluate the individualized treatment plan. Finally, nurses are often responsible for educating the patient and their family about available rehabilitative interventions, strategies, and options (U.S. Department of Veterans Affairs [VA], 2010). In 2008, the Department of Veterans Affairs partnered with the National Institute on Disability, Independent Living, and Rehabilitation Research (NIDILRR) to establish a VA-specific longitudinal multicenter study that examines the course of recovery and outcomes following inpatient rehabilitation for TBI. This study conducts follow-up evaluations at years 1, 2, 5, and every subsequent 5 years postinjury. The goal of this study is to define the unique needs of veterans with TBI and to design interventions to address those needs (U.S. Department of Veterans Affairs [VA], 2019a,b).

Caring for Patients With Amputations

Veterans who undergo amputations will experience a number of specific health issues and threats. The U.S. Department of Veterans Affairs (VA) (2002) described how clinicians, including nurses, should be involved in management of the physical and emotional issues related to the amputation. Specific areas that were mentioned in this report are the need for assistance during rehabilitation and long-term care, pain management, and prevention of secondary complications. Further, when the patient is physically ready for prosthetics, the nurse may be involved in prosthetic fitting and training, as well as vocational rehabilitation.

To help meet the needs, the Amputation System of Care (ASoC) was implemented by the VHA in 2007 to improve access to rehabilitation techniques and prosthetic technology for service members. The ASoC works to ensure that the veterans will have the expertise they require by incorporating the best practices in rehabilitation therapies and prosthetic technology. Using regional VHA settings, goals of the ASoC include providing state-of-the-art, holistic, interdisciplinary care; optimizing each individual's activity and participation in social roles; employing wellness and preventive strategies to minimize secondary condition, impairments, and activity limitations; and developing treatment interventions through research and outcome assessment (U.S. Department of Veterans Affairs [VA], 2015b).

Interventions for Health Problems Associated With Environmental Exposures

As explained, active duty service members are at risk for exposure to environmental toxins or agents from several sources. Interventions and resources for several of these are described here.

Chemicals

Threats to the health of veterans include exposure to a number of different chemicals, as discussed earlier. Of particular concern are Agent Orange and other herbicides. In addition is potential exposure to pesticides, industrial solvents, and polychlorinated biphenyl, which were commonly used as coolants and in insulation.

As mentioned, Agent Orange is associated with a number of significant health problems. The VA provides health care, disability compensation, and other benefits to eligible veterans and sometimes their dependents and survivors. The VA maintains a comprehensive program for health providers to educate them about health effects of exposure to Agent Orange and other pesticides. The "Agent Orange Newsletter" is a resource for health providers and exposed veterans to learn more about the health issues and the VA's programs (see https://www.publichealth.va.gov/exposures/publications/agent-orange/agent-orange-2020/index.asp). Nurses working with veterans, particularly those from the Vietnam era, should be well versed in the effects and resources related to Agent Orange exposure.

Cold Injuries

The major cold injuries suffered by veterans include frostbite, immersion foot (trench foot), and hypothermia. The risks are dependent on temperature, wind, and moisture in combination with the duration of exposure and the amount of protection. Damage from cold exposure can include changes in muscle, skin,

nails, ligaments, and bones; skin cancer in frostbite scars; or neurological or vascular injuries in the involved extremities (U.S. Department of Veterans Affairs [VA], 2017g). Those with potential health problems associated with cold injuries from military service may be eligible for disability compensation and are encouraged to contact their environmental health coordinator (https://www.publichealth.va.gov/exposures/coordinators.asp).

Radiation

Exposure to radiation among service members could have come from several situations. Some individuals from these groups might have been affected: those stationed in Japan during the Fukushima nuclear accident, the "atomic veterans" (described earlier as those involved in nuclear weapons testing and the occupation of Hiroshima and Nagasaki); nuclear weapons technicians, those exposed to pieces of depleted uranium after an explosion; Coast Guard veterans who worked at Long Range Navigation stations from 1942 to 2010; naval veterans stationed at McMurdo Station in Antarctica from 1964 to 1973; and service members (e.g., divers, submariners, and some pilots) who were given radium irradiation treatment between 1940 and the mid-1960s to prevent ear damage from pressure changes (U.S. Department of Veterans Affairs [VA], 2015c). Veterans from any of these groups are urged to discuss the potential radiation exposure to their healthcare provider or to contact their local VA environmental health coordinator (see https://www.publichealth.va.gov/exposures/coordinators.asp).

The VA reports that some diseases may be related to exposure to radiation during military service. These include many different cancers (e.g., bile duct, bone, brain, breast, colon, esophagus, gall bladder, liver, and lung, among others), as well as leukemia, lymphomas, and multiple myeloma. Other potentially related health problems include nonmalignant thyroid disease, parathyroid adenoma, subcapsular cataracts, and tumors of the brain and central nervous system (U.S. Department of Veterans Affairs [VA], 2015c). Healthcare providers, including nurses, should be aware of the resources available to address problems caused by exposure to radiation. For example, "atomic veterans" have special eligibility to enroll in VA health care (priority level 6). In addition, they are eligible to participate in the Ionizing Radiation Registry Examination Program, which coordinates care for affected veterans (U.S. Department of Veterans Affairs [VA], 2015c). Veterans should be informed of service benefits and be referred to the nearest VHA for comprehensive management and other benefits.

Air Pollutants

Exposure to a variety of air pollutants has been commonplace for veterans. Of particular concern are health threats from the burn pits that were employed to dispose of waste at military sites in Iraq and Afghanistan. Health effects associated with the smoke from burn pits include irritation of the skin and eyes as well as harm to the respiratory and cardiovascular systems and other internal organs. The health threats are dependent on the

BOX 22.3   Homeless Veteran Demographics

- 13% of the homeless adult population are veterans
- 20% of the male homeless population are veterans
- 68% reside in principal cities
- 32% reside in suburban/rural areas
- 51% of individual homeless veterans have disabilities
- 50% have serious mental illness
- 70% have substance abuse problems
- 51% are white males, compared to 38% of nonveterans
- 50% are age 51 or older, compared to 19% nonveterans

Data from National Coalition for Homeless Veterans, 2021. https://nchv.org/veteran-homelessness/.

type of waste being burned, length of exposure, and wind direction. High levels of dust and other pollutants also posed a threat to respiratory health (U.S. Department of Veterans Affairs [VA], 2017f).

Veterans of OEF/OIF, Operation Desert Shield, or Operation Desert Storm may be eligible for care and compensation. The Airborne Hazards and Open Burn Pit Registry allows veterans to document exposure and report health concerns. Findings from data analysis indicate that burn pit exposure has resulted in COPD, chronic bronchitis, or emphysema as well as asthma in a significant number of cases (U.S. Department of Veterans Affairs [VA], 2015d). Additionally, exposure to dust storms increases the likelihood of asthma, COPD, and chronic bronchitis. Hypertension was the most common cardiovascular condition associated with both burn pit and dust storm exposure. Health providers caring for veterans from these conflicts should be aware of the potential health problems and refer accordingly.

Addressing Homelessness

Addressing veteran homelessness must include initiatives to decrease incarceration, such as jail diversion programs, and efforts to help veterans obtain identification, housing, and substance abuse treatment.

Another successful initiative to divert veterans from jail is veterans' court. These courts allow veterans to avoid jail if they agree to and successfully complete a prescribed program of rehabilitation and counseling. There are over 600 of these unique courts across the country (U.S. Department of Veterans Affairs [VA], 2021d). Veterans' treatment courts have been demonstrated to be an important diversion from the cycle of incarceration and homelessness. An early sign that a veteran may have unaddressed problems may be when they break the law. The Veterans Court offers opportunities for the VA, local support organizations, and local communities to offer treatment as an alternative to time in jail. By implementing veterans treatment courts, justice system officials, the VA, and community organizations are able to attack the cycle between homelessness and incarceration, giving these veterans a much better chance for success (Military.com, 2021). The majority of these courts were established between 2011 and 2012.

Due to efforts from the VA, local and state governments, community organizations, and law enforcement, there has been dramatic progress in ending veteran homelessness. Between 2015 and 2016 veteran homelessness declined by 17%, with an overall decrease of 47% between 2010 and 2016. A housing-first orientation increases the likelihood of a veteran being successful in treatment for drug abuse, mental health disorders, and other health conditions and gaining employment. The housing-first orientation means that a veteran is housed or rehoused as quickly as possible, regardless of their state of sobriety or poor credit or financial situation or criminal history. Once housed the veteran is linked to resources to meet his or her mental and physical needs (National Coalition for Homeless Veterans, 2021). Homeless veteran demographics are broken down in Box 22.3.

Transition From Military to Civilian Life

Military service can be rewarding, positive, and life changing; however, it is sometimes difficult, demanding, and dangerous. Whether one served for a short period or retired after a long career, returning to civilian life will most often present challenges (Box 22.4). Approximately 72% of all veterans report having a smooth readjustment to civilian life, but approximately 44% of GWOT veterans report difficulty with readjustment (Morin, 2011; Romaniuk & Kidd, 2018).

Veterans' attitudes, experiences, and demographic characteristics can have a significant impact on their transition and

BOX 22.4   Voices of Veterans Upon Their Return Home

Home—the place many think is the safe haven to find relief from the stress of war—may initially be a letdown. When a loved one asks, 'What was it like?' and you look into eyes that have not seen what yours have, you suddenly realize that home is farther away than you ever imagined.

—From Down Range: From Iraq and Back, by Cantrell and Dean (2005).

I went with my wife to a new church. I sat down in the pew. All of a sudden, I was in a different church in Germany—in the middle of the war—and there were lots of bombs going off. The roof of the church was blown off and there was a woman singing.

—World War II veteran.

When in uniform, you follow orders, no matter how you feel. When given a command, you use whatever force is necessary. Then you come back to civilian life and those things land you in jail.

—Vietnam veteran.

I will only speak to another combat Marine about my experiences in the desert. No one else can understand what it means to be a Marine or what it means to be a combat Marine.

—Gulf War veteran.

After returning home, I find that I get frustrated easily with others. People here at home get upset so quickly over the little things—long lines at the grocery store, busy traffic. Don't they know that these are small things and we all need to be simply grateful that we live in a free country?

—Afghanistan veteran.

Three weeks ago I was driving Humvees and kicking down doors, and now after three weeks of demobilization, signing papers and getting medical checkups, I am suddenly back on the streets at home, but I can't yet make myself understand it or believe it.

—Iraq veteran.

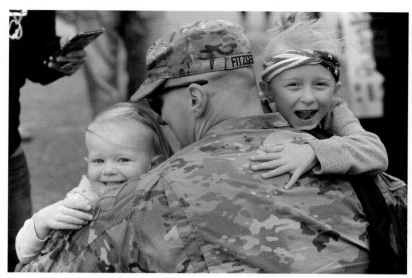

Fig. 22.8 An Army National Guardsman returns home to his family after a 10-month deployment. (South Dakota National Guard photo by Staff Sgt. Heather Trobee.)

readjustment to civilian life (Fig. 22.8). Veterans who participate in preseparation seminars, transition assistance programs, and job fairs are more likely to have easier and more successful transitions than those who do not take advantage of these resources. Military commanders require all service members to attend transition briefings to prepare these personnel for separation; however, it is imperative that veterans begin planning for civilian life 1 year, or earlier, before separation from the military.

Veterans who were commissioned officers tend to have a more positive experience transitioning, as these veterans have experienced a more focused career; they also tend to be planners and understand the importance of preparation and order. As leaders they are thorough and follow through with the "mission" of transitioning, in the same way as they would carry out their active duty job and mission.

Veterans who were noncommissioned are typically high school graduates who often held nonleadership positions. They are more likely to experience a negative transition, as they may lack the guidance, experience, and knowledge needed to prepare for separating from the military. These members tend to be younger and have not experienced a career in the military. Their separation may be based on administrative action, military downsizing, or their decision to not reenlist. Another factor that makes transitioning difficult for them may be a lack of career planning. Some veterans can transition to a civilian job similar or identical to their military job; however, this is not true for all service members. Veterans continue to have difficulty translating their job experience, qualifications, and training to the civilian job market.

🏠 COMMUNITY FOCUS

Veteran Employment

Every year thousands of veterans transition to the civilian sector to start a new life and career. With a challenging economic environment, much attention is focused helping veterans transition into civilian careers.

Unemployment rates for both male and female veterans increased in 2020, reflecting the COVID-19 pandemic. The rate for male veterans was 6.5% and 6.7% for female veterans. Additionally, unemployment rates for white, black, Asian, and Hispanic veterans were lower than for their nonveteran counterparts in 2020 (US Dept of Labor, 2021).

Enlisted service members and veterans can face unique challenges in gaining civilian credentials for military occupations because much of their education and training are attained primarily through their military service, as opposed to the traditional approaches to civilian career preparation. The military invests extensively in formal training for its enlisted personnel, complemented by extensive on-the-job training and hands-on experience. Military training is state-of-the art and, early in their careers, service members have direct experiences that are unprecedented in the civilian sector. However, the eligibility requirements for civilian credentials seldom recognize military training and experience as a means of qualification (The American Legion, 2017). It is important that future employers recognize, accept, and value the experiences, education, and training of this vital population.

An estimated 200,000 women will transition from the military during the next several years. Women veterans are younger than male veterans, with about 84% of female veterans being working age. Despite the experience and skills gained during their military service, nearly 2 in 10 female veterans aged 17 to 40 live in poverty, with about 10% of all female veterans being in poverty. A key to understanding the high poverty rate among female veterans is the perception among female veterans that their military training and experience are not relevant or helpful in transitioning to civilian jobs. Women veterans are also the fastest-growing segment of the homeless veteran population. Women veterans are two to four times more likely to be homeless than are nonveteran women. Unemployment is the biggest risk factor for homelessness among women veterans, with a lack of child care being the greatest barrier for employment. MST and PTSD are other barriers to employment for women veterans. Access to affordable housing can be a barrier for women with children; 60% of programs that serve women veterans do not house children, and the remaining programs have restrictions on the ages and numbers of children housed (Courtney, 2018).

Veterans who experienced emotional or physical trauma while serving are at a greater risk of having difficulty readjusting to civilian life (Morin, 2011). Having an emotionally distressing experience while in the military reduces the chances that a veteran will have a relatively easy transition by 26% compared with a veteran who did not have an emotionally distressing experience while on active duty. Similarly, suffering a serious injury while serving reduces the probability of an easy transition—from 77% to 58% (Morin, 2011).

It is important to understand that distress during the initial weeks of reintegration is expected and should not be medicalized. Most veterans can function well within a few weeks of returning home. If, after several months, veterans are not reintegrating well, they may be experiencing a mental health disorder and professional help should be sought.

Veterans who have families may be more likely to have a difficult time reintegrating to life after the military. Approximately 43% of service members have children. It is important that the veteran realize the changed dynamics of the family, their role within that dynamic, and how to transition into the family with as little disruption as possible. When a family member is absent due to military service, the family dynamic changes to redistribute the roles of the absent member.

Multiple deployments are common in today's military, complicating readjustment to home life. Multiple deployments are a common cause of family stress attachment problems and increase the rate for divorce among military families. The average deployment durations vary by branch of service. Military personnel often rate home life as the most stressful component of military service. Fig. 22.9 illustrates some of the sources of stress for military personnel and the impact of deployment on family life.

Predeployment is the period of training and equipping before deployment (30–90 days). Deployment is the period of a combat or humanitarian mission anywhere in the world (3–18 months). Redeployment is the return from operations to home base (30 days).

Family members need time to readjust to the veteran being home, transitioning to a new career and/or dealing with physical or mental health disorders. Veterans and their families will need time to transition into a new routine and to rebuild relationships. This could take months, as routines and responsibilities may change. The veteran and their family should seek relationship, parenting, and family counseling or classes as appropriate.

When moving to a new base or post, the military offers assistance to active duty military personnel and their families to adjust to the new environment. However, this support is not available when the veteran separates from the military. The veteran and their family will have to navigate the challenges of reintegrating and joining a new community without the assistance of the military. The VA has extensive initiatives to assist service members with the reintegration process. Counseling services and a host of resources are available (see https://www.benefits.va.gov/TAP/index.asp).

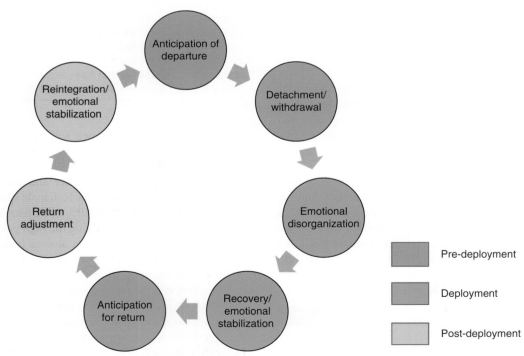

Fig. 22.9 Military deployment family life cycle.

CASE STUDY Application of the Nursing Process

A Community Intervention: Give a Vet a Smile

One of the many problems faced by homeless veterans is access to health care, and access to dental care is particularly challenging. It is difficult to obtain health care when one does not have an address or identification, and most homeless veterans have neither. The result is they go without needed health care, which leads to harmful physical and psychological consequences. Further, even if they are able to obtain health care, homeless veterans usually have no place to store medication or even personal items such as a toothbrush. Compounding the problem, many homeless veterans have mental illness, substance abuse disorders, and chronic health conditions such as diabetes and hypertension.

The US Veterans' Initiative (US Vets) is the largest nonprofit organization in the nation that serves homeless and at-risk veterans. US Vets provides transitional housing, job training, mental health services, permanent housing to disabled veterans, and crisis care to homeless veterans. The goal of US Vets is to return veterans to independent living in a home of their own.

While overseeing a community health nursing clinical group with the veterans housed at US Vets-Houston and other homeless veterans served through the drop-in center, it was observed that many veterans were reporting dental pain. The community health students and faculty saw several who had facial swelling and fever from dental infections or missing or decaying teeth. Many veterans also spoke of difficulty finding employment due to the impact of poor health and oral hygiene.

As the nursing students worked with the veterans, it become clear they had no access to dental care and therefore had neglected their oral health for years. Most sources for dental care and services are based on income and require that the patient or insurance make payment. But many of the veterans served by US Vets had very little money and no income, putting even low-cost dental care out of reach. Lack of transportation was another barrier to care faced by this population, as most homeless veterans do not have cars or transportation to clinic appointments.

Following a comprehensive assessment of the situation and validation of the needs, community-based faculty from UTHealth School of Dentistry at Houston were approached and told of the plight of these veterans. Many veterans are among the faculty, staff, and students of both the School of Dentistry and the School of Nursing, and there was considerable excitement about serving their fellow veterans. After a number of planning meetings, faculty from the nursing and dental schools developed a collaborative intervention called "Give a Vet a Smile" to provide free dental care for homeless veterans.

For the program, the faculty, students, and residents of UTHealth School of Dentistry provided dental care such as cleaning, X-rays, extractions, and other emergent care. Nursing students publicized the event at several community agencies that serve homeless veterans and completed health histories on those who chose to participate. Nursing students also solicited donations from local businesses to provide a light breakfast for the volunteers on Give a Vet a Smile Day, plus lunch for the volunteers and patients. Many veterans do not have Medicare or Medicaid and were not enrolled for care at the local VHA, so a source for medications was needed. A local pharmacist agreed to donate medications for the veterans so that they could get their prescriptions for antibiotics and pain medication filled free of charge. The veterans were given cards to remind them of the date for their appointments.

Transportation to and from the School of Dentistry was set up for the day of the event, and the veterans arrived early in the morning. Each was assessed by the dental staff for needed care, and plans of care were developed. As the process unfolded, the veterans received their requisite procedures and were scheduled for appointments for follow-up if needed.

Though the first year of Give a Vet a Smile was implemented with no donor funds—just in-kind donations such as food and dental supplies—39 veterans received dental care worth more than $18,000. The program is now in its third year, and community support is building. In year two a local private foundation

donated $2000, and in year three, a local bank donated $5000 to finance the cost of the event and to provide follow-up care such as root canals, dentures, and other complex procedures. In the third year of the event, 70 veterans received care worth more than $36,000, with several veterans receiving follow-up care.

It is gratifying for the participating professionals and volunteers to see veterans who have been helped by "Give a Vet a Smile." One veteran now has dentures and is enjoying being able to eat again. Another veteran received care that might have been lifesaving, as he had a dental infection so severe that he required several extractions and long-term antibiotics. Finally, enhanced, directed outreach to the homeless veteran community has resulted in a more trusting relationship with the veterans—encouraging and enabling them to access needed services.

Planning is under way for year four of Give a Vet a Smile.

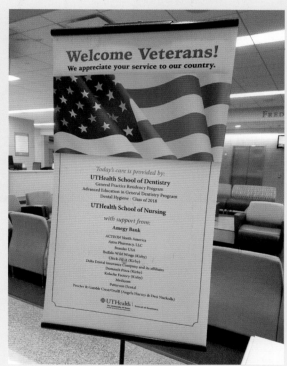

Welcome banner.

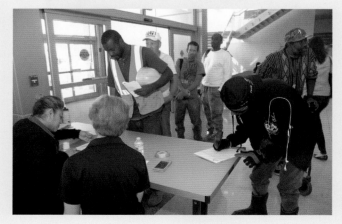

Check in for veterans.

Continued

CASE STUDY   Application of the Nursing Process—cont'd

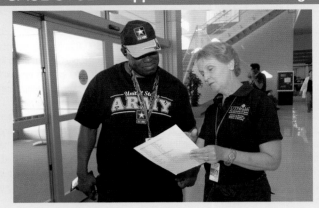

Initial intake and screening by UTHealth faculty.

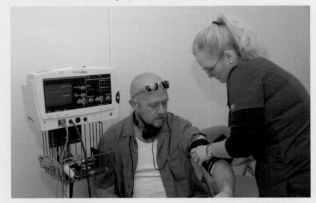

Initial health assessment by nursing students.

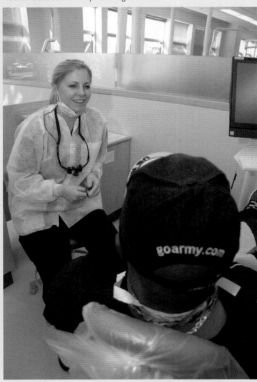

An Army Veteran and US Vets employee receives care. Initial oral assessment by a hygienist.

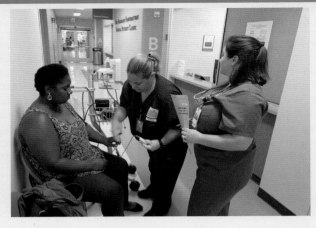

Health assessment and vital signs by nursing students.

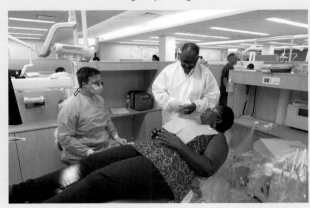

Many of the dental professionals caring for the veterans are veterans as well. They are delighted to care for other vets.

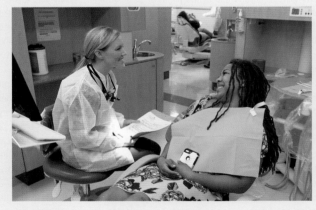

Postcare instructions.

CASE STUDY   Application of the Nursing Process—cont'd

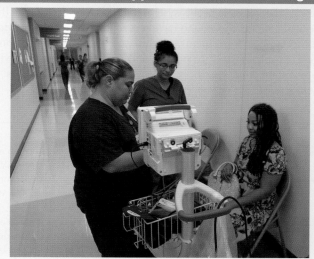

A veteran nursing student - a US Marine, welcomes fellow veterans to the event.

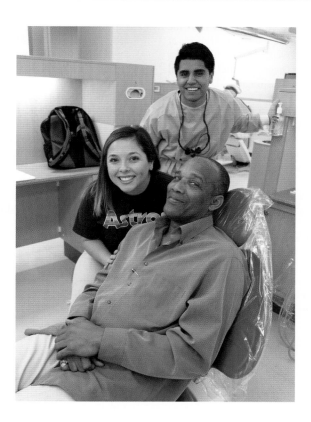

SUMMARY

The Census Bureau 2020 reports that there are almost 18 million veterans in the United States. Furthermore, there are around two million men and women currently serving in the uniformed services; they, too, will be veterans one day. This very large and very significant population requires a wide range of healthcare services. Many of these services are specific to health problems and threats directly related to the veterans' roles or activities while in the military, but many of the problems are simply those commonly found among their non-service member contemporaries. For example, WWII veterans will have problems associated with aging, and women veterans may have health concerns and issues because they are female.

Nurses working in community settings will encounter veterans in many different situations. During the assessment process, we are encouraged to include a question to elicit information on veteran status, as it may be important either with respect to underlying health problems or as a potential source for additional resources.

This chapter has presented basic information on some of the health issues and threats that commonly occur among those who have served in the military. It has also provided an overview of the veterans health system and described resources that are available for those who have served and those with service-connected health problems. All nurses should learn more about these problems and resources and be prepared to provide appropriate and specific care to meet the health needs of members of this vital population.

EVOLVE WEBSITE

http://evolve.elsevier.com/Nies/community

- NCLEX Review Questions
- Case Studies

BIBLIOGRAPHY

Alexander CL, Reger MA, Smolenski DJ, et al.: Comparing U.S. Army suicide cases to a control sample: initial data and methodological lessons, *Mil Med* 179(10):1062–1066, 2014.

American Academy of Nursing (AAN): *Have you ever served in the military? A service for America's veterans by the American Academy of Nursing*, 2017. http://www.haveyoueverserved.com/.

American Psychiatric Association (APA): *Diagnostic and statistical manual of mental disorders (DSM-5®)*, Washington, DC, 2013, American Psychiatric Publishing.

Benefits.gov: *Health care benefits for dependents (CHAMPVA)*, 2017. https://www.benefits.gov/benefits/benefit-details/318.

Blais RK, Brignone E, Maguen S, et al.: Military sexual trauma is associated with post-deployment eating disorders among Afghanistan and Iraq veterans, *Int J Eating Disord*, 2017. https://doi.org/10.1002/eat.22705.

Blosnich JR, Mays VM, Cochran SD: Suicidality among veterans: implications of sexual minority status, *Am J Public Health* 104(Suppl 4):S535–S537, 2014.

Brooks MS, Laditka SB, Laditka JN: Evidence of greater health care needs among older veterans of the Vietnam War, *Mil Med* 173(8):715–720, 2008.

Bryan CJ, Bryan AO, Clemans TA: The association of military and premilitary sexual trauma with risk for suicide ideation, plans, and attempts, *Psychiatry Res* 227(2–3):246–252, 2015. https://doi.org/10.1016/j.psychres.2015.01.030.

Counseling and Treatment for Sexual Trauma: § 38 U.S. Code Sec. 1720D violence as a form of MST: an initial investigation, *Psycholog Serv* 12(4):348–356, 2006. https://doi.org/10.1037/ser0000056.

Courtney E: *Women veterans: the challenges they face & a way forward*, 2018. Available from: https://www.nawrb.com/women-veterans/.

Cox KS, Mouilso ER, Venners MR, et al.: Reducing suicidal ideation through evidence-based treatment for posttraumatic stress disorder, *J Psychiatr Res* 80:59–63, 2016.

Defense and Veterans Brain Injury Center, (n.d.): DoD Worldwide Numbers for TBI. (n.d.). November 27, 2017. Available from: http://dvbic.dcoe.mil/dod-worldwide-numbers-tbi.

Disabled American Veterans (DAV) (2020): *Veterans with amputations/limb loss*, 2020. Available from: https://www.dav.org/veterans/resources/veterans-with-amputations-limb-loss/.

Friedman MJ: *PTSD history and overview*, 2016. Available from: https://www.ptsd.va.gov/professional/PTSD-overview/ptsd-overview.asp.

Fore AM, et al.: Nurses' delivery of the Tobacco Tactics intervention at a Veterans Affairs Medical Center, *J Clin Nurse* 23:2162–2169, 2014.

Geiling J, Rosen JM, Edwards RD: Medical costs of war in 2035: long-term care challenges for veterans of Iraq and Afghanistan, *Mil Med* 177(11):1235–1244, 2012.

Gilmore AK, Brignone E, Painter JM, et al.: Military sexual trauma and co-occurring posttraumatic stress disorder, depressive disorders, and substance use disorders among returning Afghanistan and Iraq veterans, *Wom Health Issues* 26(5):546–554, 2016. https://doi.org/10.1016/j.whi.2016.07.001.

Goldstein LA, Dinh J, Donalson R, et al.: Impact of military trauma exposures on posttraumatic stress and depression in female veterans, *Psychiatry Res* 249:281–285, 2017. https://doi.org/10.1016/j.psychres.2017.01.009.

Hedegaard H, Curtin SC, Warner M: Suicide mortality in the United States, 1999–2019, *NCHS Data Brief* 398:1–8, 2021. https://www.cdc.gov/nchs/data/databriefs/db398-H.pdf.

Helmer D, Chandler HK, Quigley KS, et al.: Chronic widespread pain, mental health, and physical role function in OEF/OIF veterans, *Pain Med* 10(7):1174–1182, 2009. Available from: https://ncbi.nlm.nih.gov/pubmed/19818029. November 28, 2017.

Jenkins MM, Colvonen PJ, Norman SB, et al.: Prevalence and mental health correlates of insomnia in first-encounter veterans with and without military sexual trauma, *Sleep* 38(10):1547–1554, 2015. https://doi.org/10.5665/sleep.5044.

Johnson BS, Boudiab LD, Freundl M, et al.: Enhancing veteran-centered care: a guide for nurses in non-VA settings, *Am J Nurs* 113(7):24–39, 2013. quiz 54, 40. https://doi.org/10.1097/01.NAJ.0000431913.50226.83.

Klingensmith K, Tsai J, Mota N, et al.: Military sexual trauma in US veterans, *J Clin Psychiat* 75(10):1133–1139, 2014. https://doi.org/10.4088/jcp.14m09244.

Kulka RA: *Trauma and the Vietnam War generation: report of findings from the National Vietnam Veterans Readjustment Study*, New York, 1990, Brunner/Mazel Publishers.

Lutwak N, Dill C: Military sexual trauma increases risk of post-traumatic stress disorder and depression thereby amplifying the possibility of suicidal ideation and cardiovascular disease, *Mil Med* 178(4):359–361, 2013.

MacGregor AJ, Dougherty AL, Mayo JA, et al.: Occupational correlates of low back pain among US Marines following combat deployment, *Mil Med* 177:845–849, 2012.

McCarthy JF, Bossarte R, Katz IR, et al.: Predictive modeling and concentration of the risk of suicide: implications for preventive interventions in the US Department of Veterans Affairs, *Am J Public Health* 105(9):1935–1942, 2015.

Mercado R, Foynes MM, Carpenter SL, et al.: Sexual intimate partner violence as a form of MST: an initial investigation, *Psychol Serv* 12(4):348–356, 2015. https://doi.org/10.1037/ser0000056.

Military.com: *Veteran treatment courts*, 2021. Available from: www.military.com/benefits/military-legal-matters/veterans-treatment-courts.html#:~:text=The%20Veterans%20Court%20offers%20opportunity%20for%20the%20VA%2C,the%20country%20are%20entitled%20to%20a%20second%20chance.

Miltner RS, Selleck CS, Moore RL, et al.: Equipping the nursing workforce to care for the unique needs of veterans and their families, *Nurse Leader* 11(5):45–48, 2013. ISSN 1541-4612. https://doi.org/10.1016/j.mnl.2013.05.013.

Monteith LL, Pease JL, Forster JE, et al.: Values as moderators of the association between interpersonal-psychological constructs and suicidal ideation among veterans, *Arch Suicide Res* 19(4):422–434, 2015.

Monteith LL, Bahraini NH, Matarazzo BB, et al.: Perceptions of institutional betrayal predict suicidal self-directed violence among veterans exposed to military sexual trauma, *J Clin Psychol* 72(7):743–755, 2016a. https://doi.org/10.1002/jclp.22292.

Monteith LL, Bahraini NH, Matarazzo BB, et al.: The influence of gender on suicidal ideation following military sexual trauma among veterans in the veterans health administration, *Psychiat Res* 244:257–265, 2016b. https://doi.org/10.1016/j.psychres.2016.07.036.

Monteith LL, Bahraini NH, Menefee DS: Perceived burdensomeness, thwarted belongingness, and fearlessness about death: associations with suicidal ideation among female veterans exposed to military sexual trauma, *J Clin Psychol*, 2017. https://doi.org/10.1002/jclp.22462.

Morin R: *The difficult transition from military to civilian life*, Washington, DC, 2011, Pew Research Center.

National Center for Posttraumatic Stress Disorder: *Iraq War clinician guide*, ed 2, 2004, Department of Veterans Affairs.

National Center for PTSD/U.S. Department of Veterans Affairs: *Understanding PTSD and PTSD Treatment*, 2017. Available from: https://www.ptsd.va.gov/public/understanding_ptsd/booklet.pdf.

National Center for PTSD/U.S. Department of Veterans Affairs: *PTSD: National Center for PTSD: PTSD treatment programs in the U.S. Department of Veterans Affairs*, 2017. Available from: https://www.ptsd.va.gov/public/treatment/therapy-med/va-ptsd-treatment-programs.asp.

National Center for PTSD/U.S. Department of Veterans Affairs: *How common is PTSD in adults? Available from: how common is PTSD in adults? - PTSD: National Center for PTSD (va.gov)*, 2020.

National Coalition for Homeless Veterans: *Background and statistics*, 2017. Available from: http://nchv.org/index.php/news/media/background_and_statistics/.

National Coalition for Homeless Veterans: *Veteran homelessness*, 2021. Available from: https://nchv.org/veteran-homelessness/.

National Institute of Mental Health (NIMH): *Post-traumatic stress disorder*, 2019. Available from: https://www.nimh.nih.gov/health/topics/post-traumatic-stress-disorder-ptsd/index.shtml.

Okie S: Traumatic brain injury in the war zone, *New Eng J Med* 352(20):2043–2047, 2005. Available from: http://nejm.org/doi/full/10.1056/nejmp058102. November 27, 2017.

Pavao J, Turchik JA, Hyun JK, et al.: Military sexual trauma among homeless veterans, *J Gen Int Med* 28(Suppl 2):536–541, 2013. https://doi.org/10.1007/s11606-013-2341-4.

Pheister M, Kangas G, Thompson C, et al.: Suicide prevention and postvention resources: what psychiatry residencies can learn from the veteran's administration experience, *Acad Psychiat* 38:600–604, 2014.

Pols H, Oak S: War & military mental health: the US psychiatric response in the 20th century, *Am J Public Health* 97(12):2132–2142, 2007. https://doi.org/10.2105/AJPH.2006.090910.

Rogers A: *Homeless female veterans: out of sight, out of mind*, 2019. Available from: https://news.psu.edu/story/598769/2019/11/18/research/homeless-female-veterans-out-sight-out-mind.

Romaniuk M, Kidd C: The psychological adjustment experience of reintegration following discharge from military service: a systematic review, *JMVH* 26(2), 2018. Available from: https://jmvh.org/article/the-psychological-adjustment-experience-of-reintegration-following-discharge-from-military-service-a-systemic-review/.

Schnurr PP, Jankowski MK: Physical health and post-traumatic stress disorder: review and synthesis, *Semin Clin Neuropsychiatry* 4:295–304, 1999.

Scott C: *Who is a veteran?—basic eligibility requirements for veterans' benefits*, 2012, Congressional Research Service. Available at: http://www.ncdsv.org/images/CRS_WhoIsAVeteran-BasicEligibilityForVeterans'Benefits_1-23-2012.pdf.

Street AE, Rosellini AJ, Ursano RJ, et al.: Developing a risk model to target high-risk preventive interventions for sexual assault victimization among female U.S. army soldiers, *Clin Psychol Sci* 4(6):939–956, 2016. https://doi.org/10.1177/2167702616639532.

Teeters JB, Lancaster CL, Brown DG, et al.: Substance use disorders in military veterans: prevalence and treatment challenges, *Subst Abuse Rehabil* 8:69–77, 2017. https://doi.org/10.2147/SAR.S116720.

The American Legion: *The state of credentialing of service members and veterans challenges, successes, and opportunities*, 2017. Available from: https://www.legion.org/sites/legion.org/files/legion/publications/25VEE0517%20The%20State%20of%20Credentialing_0.pdf.

U.S. Bureau of Labor Statistics (BLS): *Employment situation of veterans*, 2021. Available from: https://www.bls.gov/news.release/vet.toc.htm.

U.S. Census Bureau: *Census Bureau releases new report on veterans*, 2020. www.census.gov/newsroom/press-releases/2020/veterans-report.html#:~:text=Highlights%20include%3A%201%20The%20number%20of%20veterans%20in,growing%20share%20of%20veterans.%20... %20More%20items ... %20.

U.S. Department of Labor: *Veterans' employment and training service*, 2021. Available from: https://www.dol.gov/agencies/vets/latest-numbers.

U.S. Department of Veterans Affairs (VA): *Rural veterans*, 2021a. Available from: https://www.ruralhealth.va.gov/aboutus/ruralvets.asp.

U.S. Department of Veterans Affairs (VA): *About VA*, 2021b. Available from: https://www.va.gov/ABOUT_VA/index.asp.

U.S. Department of Veterans Affairs (VA): *2021 VA health care copay rates*, 2021c. Available from: https://www.va.gov/health-care/copay-rates/.

U.S. Department of Veterans Affairs (VA): *Fact Sheet: Veterans treatment courts and other veteran-focused courts served by VA veterans justice outreach specialists*, 2021d. Retrieved from: https://www.va.gov/HOMELESS/docs/VJO/Veterans-Treatment-Court-Inventory-Update-Fact-Sheet-Jan-2021.pdf.

U.S. Department of Veterans Affairs (VA): *PTSD: basics*, 2021e. Available from: www.ptsd.va.gov/understand/what/ptsd_basics.asp.

U.S. Department of Veterans Affairs (VA): *Suicide prevention*, 2021f. Available from: https://www.mentalhealth.va.gov/suicide_prevention/.

U.S. Department of Veterans Affairs (VA): *War related injury and illness study center*, 2021g. Available from: https://www.warrelatedillness.va.gov/.

U.S. Department of Veterans Affairs (VA): *Veterans' justice outreach*, 2021h. Available from: https://www.va.gov/HOMELESS/VJO.asp.

U.S. Department of Veterans Affairs (VA): *War related illness and injury study center*, 2021i. Available from: https://www.warrelatedillness.va.gov/WARRELATEDILLNESS/index.asp.

U.S. Department of Veterans Affairs (VA): *Military sexual trauma*, 2021j. Available from: https://www.mentalhealth.va.gov/msthome/index.asp.

U.S. Department of Veterans Affairs (VA): *Traumatic amputation and prosthetics: independent study course*, 2002. Available from: https://www.publichealth.va.gov/docs/vhi/traumatic_amputation.pdf.

U.S. Department of Veterans Affairs (VA): *Veterans and radiation: independent study course*, 2004. Available from: https://www.public health.va.gov/docs/vhi/radiation.pdf.

U.S. Department of Veterans Affairs (VA): *Vietnam veterans and Agent Orange: independent study course*, 2008. Available from: https://www.publichealth.va.gov/docs/vhi/VHIagentorange_text508.pdf.

U.S. Department of Veterans Affairs (VA): *Mild traumatic brain injury — concussion: pocket guide for clinicians*, 2010. Available from: https://www.publichealth.va.gov/docs/exposures/TBI-pocketcard.pdf#.

U.S. Department of Veterans Affairs (VA): *Vets in crisis get a chance, not a cell*, 2012. Available from: https://www.va.gov/health/NewsFeatures/20120216a.asp.

U.S. Department of Veterans Affairs (VA): *Iraq War exposures*, 2015a. https://www.publichealth.va.gov/exposures/wars-operations/iraq-war.asp.

U.S. Department of Veterans Affairs (VA): *Rehabilitation and prosthetic services: Amputation System of Care (ASoC)*, 2015b. Available from: https://www.prosthetics.va.gov/PROSTHETICS/asoc/index.asp.

U.S. Department of Veterans Affairs (VA): *Exposure to radiation during military service*, 2015c. Available from: https://www.publichealth.va.gov/exposures/radiation/sources/index.asp.

U.S. Department of Veterans Affairs (VA): *Report on data from the Airborne Hazards and Open Burn Pit (AH&OBP) Registry*, 2015d. Available from: https://www.publichealth.va.gov/docs/exposures/va-ahobp-registry-data-report-june2015.pdf.

U.S. Department of Veterans Affairs: *Veterans benefits administration: annual benefits report, fiscal year 2015*, 2016. Available at: https://www.benefits.va.gov/REPORTS/abr/ABR-Compensation-FY15-05092016.pdf.

U.S. Department of Veterans Affairs (VA): *Compensation: service-connected disability or death benefits*, 2020a. Available from: https://www.benefits.va.gov/REPORTS/abr/docs/2020_compensation.pdf.

U.S. Department of Veterans' Affairs (VA): *PTSD and telemental health*, 2020b. Available from: https://www.ptsd.va.gov/professional/treat/txessentials/telemental_health.asp.

U.S. Department of Veterans Affairs (VA): *Military sexual trauma*, 2020c. Available from: https://www.va.gov/health-care/health-needs-conditions/military-sexual-trauma/.

U.S. Department of Veterans Affairs (VA): *Spotlight on telehealth*, 2020d. Available from: https://www.hsrd.research.va.gov/news/feature/telehealth-0720.cfm.

U.S. Department of Veterans Affairs (VA): *VA releases 2020 National Veteran Suicide Prevention Annual Report*, 2020e. Available from: https://www.va.gov/opa/pressrel/pressrelease.cfm?id=5565.

U.S. Department of Veterans Affairs Office of Suicide Prevention: *VA suicide prevention program, facts about veteran suicide*, 2016. Retrieved on 4/19/17 from: https://www.va.gov/opa/publications/factsheets/Suicide_Prevention_FactSheet_New_VA_Stats_070616_1400.pdf.

U.S. Department of Veteran's Affairs (VA): *Health benefits: priority groups*, 2017a. Available from: https://www.va.gov/HEALTH BENEFITS/resources/priority_groups.asp.

U.S. Department of Veteran's Affairs (VA): *PTSD: National Center for PTSD*, 2017b. https://www.ptsd.va.gov/public/problems/ptsd_substance_abuse_veterans.asp.

U.S. Department of Veteran's Affairs (VA): *Veteran's diseases associated with Agent Orange*, 2017c. https://www.publichealth.va.gov/exposures/agentorange/conditions/.

U.S. Department of Veteran's Affairs (VA): *Gulf War veterans' medically unexplained illnesses*, 2017d. https://www.publichealth.va.gov/exposures/gulfwar/medically-unexplained-illness.asp.

U.S. Department of Veteran's Affairs (VA): *Cold injuries*, 2017e. Available from: https://www.publichealth.va.gov/exposures/cold-injuries/index.asp.

U.S. Department of Veteran's Affairs (VA): *Military exposures: burn pits*, 2017f. Available from: https://www.publichealth.va.gov/exposures/burnpits/index.asp.

U.S. Department of Veteran's Affairs (VA), Department of defense (DoD), the opioid therapy for chronic pain work group: *VA/DoD clinical practice guideline for opioid therapy for chronic pain*, 2017g. Available at: https://www.healthquality.va.gov/guidelines/Pain/cot/VADoDOTCPG022717.pdf.

U.S. Department of Veteran's Affairs (VA), Office of Public Health (OPH), War Related Illness & Injury Study Center (WRIISC): *Burn pits (trash and human waste exposures)*, 2013. https://www.warrelatedillness.va.gov/education/factsheets/burn-pits.pdf.

U.S. Department of Veteran's Affairs (VA): *National strategy for preventing veteran suicide, 2018—2028*, 2018. Available from: https://www.mentalhealth.va.gov/suicide_prevention/docs/Office-of-Mental-Health-and-Suicide-Prevention-National-Strategy-for-Preventing-Veterans-Suicide.pdf.

U.S. Department of Veterans Affairs/Office of Research & Development: *A new battlefront: female veterans comprise fastest-growing segment of homeless veteran population*, 2018. Available from: https://www.research.va.gov/currents/0318-Female-Veterans-comprise-fastest-growing-segment-of-homeless-Veteran-population.cfm.

U.S. Department of Veterans Affairs (VA): *Polytrauma/TBI system of care*, 2019a. Available from: https://www.polytrauma.va.gov/PolytraumaCenterDatabase/index.asp.

U.S. Department of Veterans Affairs (VA): *Polytrauma/TBI system of care/understanding traumatic brain injury*, 2019b. Available from: https://www.polytrauma.va.gov/understanding-tbi/index.asp.

U.S. Government Accountability Office: *Homeless women veterans: actions needed to ensure safe and appropriate housing*, Washington, DC, 2011, (Report to Congressional Requesters No. GAO-12—182). Also Available from: http://www.gao.gov/assets/590/587334.pdf.

VAntage Point: *Veterans with chronic pain are replacing opioid pain medications*, 2021. Available from: https://blogs.va.gov/VAntage/87384/veterans-chronic-pain-replacing-opioid-pain-medications/.

Watkins KE, Smith B, Paddock SM, et al.: *Veterans Health Administration mental health program evaluation: capstone report*, 2011. Available from: http://altarum.org/sites/default/files/uploaded-publication-files/Final%20Capstone%20Technical%20Report%20TR956_compiled.pdf. April 22, 2017.

White RF, Steele L, O'Callaghan JP, et al.: Recent research on Gulf War illness and other health problems in veterans of the 1991 Gulf War: effects of toxicant exposures during deployment, *Cortex* 74: 449—475, 2016. ISSN 0010-9452. https://doi.org/10.1016/j.cortex.2015.08.022.

23

Homeless Populations

Meredith Troutman-Jordan

OBJECTIVES

Upon completion of this chapter, the reader will be able to do the following:

1. Discuss conceptual and legal approaches used to define *homelessness*.
2. Describe strategies used to estimate the prevalence of homelessness in the United States.
3. Identify demographic characteristics of the homeless population and its subpopulations.
4. Analyze three factors that contribute to homelessness.
5. Identify major health problems among various homeless aggregates.
6. Analyze the health status of populations who are homeless using the World Health Organization (WHO) definition of health.
7. Describe the federal health centers that provide health care services to homeless populations.
8. Plan community health nursing services based on knowledge of the social determinants of health and health status in this population.

OUTLINE

KEY TERMS

annual homeless assessment report
chronically homeless
continuum of care

education for homeless children and youth
European Federation of Organisations Working with the Homeless

Federally Qualified Health Centers
FQHC look-a-likes
military sexual trauma
point-in-time (PIT) count

The purpose of this chapter is to describe the scope of the homeless problem. The chapter presents definitions, prevalence, and demographic characteristics of homelessness, and it describes the health status of selected aggregates of the homeless population. The chapter includes a discussion of the relationship between the factors that contribute to homelessness and the social determinants of health and of the implications of this relationship for community health nursing practice.

DEFINITIONS, PREVALENCE, AND DEMOGRAPHIC CHARACTERISTICS OF HOMELESSNESS

Definitions of Homelessness

Defining "homeless" and "homelessness" is not only complex but contested. Although a generally accepted agreement on the meaning of these terms is lacking, definitions are important in determining who should be counted, described, planned for, and assisted (U.S Department of Housing and Urban Development, 2021b). An exploration of the national and international homeless literature for the past decade reveals two approaches to defining homelessness, conceptual and legal. A brief overview of the conceptual approach used in Europe and Canada is presented next followed by discussion of the legal approach used in the United States.

Conceptual Approaches to Defining Homelessness

In 2005, the **European Federation of Organisations Working with the Homeless** (FEANTSA) launched the *European Typology of Homelessness and Housing Exclusion* (ETHOS) (European Federation of National Associations Working with the Homeless, 2017). In developing ETHOS, members of the *European Observatory on the Homeless*, the research arm of FEANTSA, used "home" as a basis for developing a definition of homelessness. From the ETHOS perspective, home was conceptualized as having three domains, *physical*, *social*, and *legal*. The *physical domain* meant having an adequate dwelling for which a person/family has exclusive possession; the *social domain* meant being able to maintain privacy and enjoy relations; the *legal domain* meant having exclusive possession, security of occupation, and legal title to occupation (FEANTSA, 2021a). Building on the three domains of home, the European researchers designated four broad types of living situations to classify homeless people: *rooflessness*, *houselessness*, *insecure housing*, and *inadequate housing*. Each of these four categories is subdivided into more specific living situations to provide classifications useful for different purposes, such as determining the extent of homelessness, developing policies, and evaluating interventions (FEANTSA, 2021b).

In 2012, building on ETHOS, the Canadian Homelessness Research Network provided a conceptual definition of homelessness that has four major categories: *unsheltered*, *emergency sheltered*, *provisionally accommodated*, and *at risk of homelessness*: Similar to the ETHOS, the Canadian definition is divided into more specific living situations, thereby providing more details to facilitate its use by different groups, such as governmental agents, service providers, and researchers. In contrast to ETHOS, the Canadian Research Network's definition includes a category that indicates an at-risk population (Canadian Homelessness Research Network, 2012).

For a more complete understanding of these two conceptual approaches to defining homelessness, the reader is encouraged to visit the websites of the respective organizations. Setting the browser to search for FEANTSA and then searching within the site search for ETHOS should provide access to the complete typology. To locate the Canadian definition, one should access the Research Hub website and search for "homeless definition."

Legal Approaches to Defining Homelessness

In contrast to these previously discussed European and Canadian definitions of homelessness, which were developed by researchers, the United States definition has been determined by federal governmental legislative and administrative actions. These federal actions provide the statutory and regulatory basis for local homeless service providers, including program direction, funding resources, and eligibility criteria. Responsibility for implementing and managing the many federal homeless initiatives is assigned to seven different departments within the executive branch of the federal government, the Departments of: (1) Housing and Urban Development (HUD); (2) Education (ED); (3) Health and Human Resources (HHS); (4) Veterans Affairs (VA); (5) Homeland Security (DHS); (6) Justice (DOJ); and (7) Labor (DOL) (Congressional Research Service, 2018).

Both HUD and ED administer homeless programs that hold considerable significance for community health nursing—HUD's Homeless Assistance Grants (US Department of Housing and Urban Development HUD Exchange, 2021b) and the ED's Education for Homeless Children and Youth (U.S Department of Education, 2021). A brief overview of these two programs and their definitions of homelessness follow.

HUD's Definitions of Homelessness. The *U.S. Code*, Title 42, Chapter 119 (U.S. House of Representatives, Office of the Law Revision Center, 2021) which is named "Homeless Assistance," contains two subchapters that provide homeless definitions. These are Subchapters I General Provisions and Subchapter VI Education and Training. The definitions in Subchapter I were broadened by the *McKinney-Vento Homeless Assistance (MVHA) Act as Amended by the Homeless Emergency Assistance and Rapid Transition to Housing (HEARTH) Act of 2009* (USHUD and Urban Development HUD Exchange, 2021c). Subsequent to the enactment of the HEARTH Act, the HUD issued regulations that summarized the statutory definitions in four descriptive categories, as follows (USDHHS HUD Exchange, 2021a,b,c,d)

- **Category 1**. *Literally Homeless*: Individuals and families who lack a fixed, regular, and adequate nighttime residence and includes a subset for an individual who resided in an emergency shelter or a place not meant for human habitation and who is exiting an institution where he or she temporarily resided;
- **Category 2**. *Imminent Risk of Homelessness*: Individuals and families who will imminently lose their primary nighttime residence;
- **Category 3**. *Homeless Under Other Federal Statutes*: Unaccompanied youth and families with children and youth who are defined as homeless under other federal statutes who do not otherwise qualify as homeless under this definition; and
- **Category 4**. *Fleeing/Attempting to Flee Domestic Violence (DV)*: Individuals and families who are fleeing, or are attempting to flee, DV, dating violence, sexual assault,

stalking, or other dangerous or life-threatening conditions that relate to violence against the individual or a family member.

ED's Definition of Homeless Student. The ED administers the law known as McKinney-Vento Homeless Education Assistance Improvements Act of 2001, which is located in Subchapter VI of the *U.S. Code.* One of the intents of this law is to direct state and local educational agencies to act to ensure that each child and each homeless youth has equal access to the same free, appropriate public education, including a public preschool education, as provided to other children and youths. The definitions, located in Part B, Section 11434a, are broader than the US HUD (2019) definitions listed previously. These definitions include children and youth who are (NCHE, 2019):

- Sharing the housing of other persons (frequently referred to as "doubling up")
- Abandoned in hospitals or
- Awaiting foster care placement

U.S. Department of Health and Human Services Definition of Homelessness. The U.S Department of Health and Human Services (HHS) also has definitions of who is considered homeless. The Runaway and Homeless Youth (RHY) Program is located in the Administration for Children & Families, Family and Youth Service Bureau, which are agencies within the HHS. The RHY program operates under legislation that has definitions for who is eligible for services; as defined in the statute, *runaway youth* is "a person under 18 years of age who absents himself or herself from home or place of legal residence without the permission of his or her family" and *homeless youth* is "a person under 18 years of age who is in need of services and without a place of shelter where he or she receives supervision and care" (USDHHS, Administration for Children & Families, Family and Youth Service Bureau, 2018).

In addition to these two definitions of youth, USDHHS uses a different definition in determining who is eligible for services provided through the Health Care for the Homeless (HCH) Program (see later section Health and Homeless Populations).

The next section presents information related to the number of people in the total US homeless population and also in smaller subpopulations. HUD and ED are the two primary federal agencies with responsibility for reporting US homeless prevalence estimates. The departments use their own, but differing definitions in their enumeration efforts.

Prevalence of Homelessness

Determining prevalence of homelessness requires not only definitions of who is counted but also how data are collected. Given the characteristics of the population and subpopulations of homeless people, obtaining accurate counts is difficult. Efforts to enumerate the homeless have evolved the over the past 3 decades. Earlier efforts included the U.S. Census Bureau's collections of national data on the homeless population in Census 1990 and Census 2000 (U.S. Census Bureau, 2020a,b). A brief sketch of more recent approaches to counting the homeless—those conducted by HUD and ED—follows.

HUD's Efforts to Count the Homeless

Two strategies used by HUD to strengthen the nation's efforts to reduce homelessness, including improvement in collecting prevalence data, are the **continuum of care** (CoC) concept and the Homeless Information Management System (HMIS). A brief overview of these two strategies follows.

HUD requires homeless service providers in each local community to collaborate and submit just one CoC application to HUD for funding, rather than allowing multiple providers to submit individual applications. If successful in obtaining funding, these CoC providers are then responsible for providing, to persons in the local area who are experiencing homelessness, a range of housing and related services, including emergency and preventive responses.

♥ HEALTHY PEOPLE 2030

Objectives for Social Determinants of Health
Economic Stability
SDOH-01: Reduce the proportion of people living in poverty
SDOH-02: Increase employment in working-age people
SDOH-03: Increase the proportion of children living with at least one parent who works full time

Education
SDOH-06: Increase the proportion of high school graduates in college the October after graduating.

From U.S. Department of Health and Human Services: *Healthy People 2030: Social determinants of health.* Retrieved from: https://health.gov/healthypeople/objectives-and-data/browse-objectives/economic-stability.

The CoC providers are also responsible for implementing and managing the HMIS at the local level. The HMIS is a computerized database designed to facilitate collection of client-level data used to plan for service needs of homeless populations.

As a requirement of HUD funding, all groups of CoC providers conduct a **point-in-time (PIT) count** of *sheltered* homeless people on a single night in late January of *every year* and submit these data to HUD via HMIS (USDHHS HUD Exchange, 2021d)). In addition to the annual PIT count of sheltered homeless people, HUD requires that *every 2 years*, on odd years, the PIT count include both *sheltered and unsheltered* homeless people. Although not required, some CoC providers include unsheltered homeless people in their PIT counts on both even and odd years.

Since 2007, HUD has used the data submitted by local CoC providers via the HMIS to prepare an **Annual Homeless Assessment Report** (AHAR) that is delivered to Congress. The populations and subpopulations HUD used in the AHAR reflect the legislative and administrative definitions outlined previously. In addition to total population prevalence, the AHAR includes subpopulations—individuals, families, the chronically homeless, and veterans. Homeless children and youth enrolled in public schools are not included in HUD's HMIS. Responsibility for reporting information about this important subpopulation lies with the ED. "Unaccompanied youth," children and youth who are homeless and on their own—that is, not living with their families, are often excluded from estimates of the homeless population; 4.2 million youth and young adults experience homelessness each year (School-House Connection, 2020).

ED's Efforts to Count the Homeless

One of the main differences between the HUD and ED approaches to counting homeless people is based on definitions of who is considered homeless. As previously described, the ED uses a broad definition of homelessness that includes youth and families that are living with other households, or "doubled up." Consequently, the ED provides services to homeless children and youth who are not included in HUD's programmatic services. Children and youth whom the ED defines as homeless receive services through the Education for Homeless Children and Youth (ECHY) program.

To meet ECHY requirements the ED collects data on program performance from all state education agencies (SEAs) and local education agencies (LEAs). The number of homeless students enrolled in LEAs during each school year is part of the annual performance report. In addition, the ED collects information on students' night-time residence at the time they were determined eligible for EHCY services. This information is included in the Consolidated State Performance Record, which the ED issues on an annual basis (National Center for Homeless Education, 2021a,b).

Homeless Prevalence Estimates

These two federal departments, HUD and ED, issue summary reports of the sizes of homeless populations and subpopulations. Both departments provide annual estimates. HUD provides a PIT count as well; the results of the January 2019 count are summarized in Table 23.1.

The prevalence estimates outlined in Table 23.1 provide a "snapshot" of the homeless population taken on one night in January 2019 as reported in the CoC Homeless Populations and Subpopulations Report (U.S. Department of Housing and Urban Development Exchange, 2021a,b). HUD also uses a different lens—the annual estimate—to produce another picture of the homeless population. In contrast to the one-night view, HUD's annual estimate is a count of the total number of people who used either shelters or transitional housing during the course of a year. As of this writing, the most recently available annual estimates are for fiscal year 2018 to 2019; this information follows.

Annual National Estimate of Homeless Persons Use of Shelters and Transitional Housing 2018 to 2019

HUD reported the following numbers of people in the total population and in subpopulations who used shelters or transitional housing between October 1, 2010 and September 30, 2011 (USHUD, OCPD, 2021c):

- 567, 715 people in the total homeless population an increase of nearly 3% between 2018 and 2019, or 14,885 more people;
- Adults aged 25 or older were almost nine of every 10 people experiencing unsheltered homelessness, 87% of the total number of unsheltered people.
- Children in families as well as children homeless on their own usually were sheltered. Of the 107,069 children who were experiencing homelessness, fewer than one in 10 was unsheltered (9% or 9916 children).
- Between 2018 and 2019, the number of veterans experiencing homelessness declined by 2% (793 fewer people).

The population and subpopulations HUD included in the 2019 annual estimate of shelter use are based on the legislatively and administratively derived definitions outlined previously. The ED, using a broader definition of homeless families than HUD, provides information on the population of children and youth enrolled in public schools.

ED's Annual National Estimate of Homeless Students for 2010 to 2011 School Year

According to the ED (National Center for Homeless Education, 2021a,b):

- 1, 384, 301 *homeless students* were enrolled during the 2018 to 2019 school year (SY), a decrease from 2017 to 2018 (1, 504, 544 students)

TABLE 23.1   PIT Estimates of Homeless People January 2015–16

Population	Sheltered and Unsheltered Single Night, January 2019	Change	Previous Year of Estimates
Households			
Individuals[a]	355, 212	−3%	2015
Families with children	194, 716	−6%	2015
Total	549, 928	−3%	2015
Subpopulations[b]			
Veterans	39, 471	−17%	2016
Chronically homeless	77, 486	−7%	2015

[a]Person who is not part of a family; single adults, unaccompanied youth, or in multiple-adult or multiple-child households.
[b]Categories are not mutually exclusive; it is possible for a chronically homeless person to be a veteran.
Data from U.S. Department of Housing and Urban Development: *The 2015 point-in-time estimates of homelessness*, 2019. Retrieved from: https://files.hudexchange.info/reports/published/CoC_PopSub_NatlTerrDC_2019.pdf.

- The *night-time residences* of homeless students for the 2018 to 2019 data collection period (most recent available) at the time of establishing service eligibility were:
  - 1,061,759 doubled up
  - 168,885 in shelters, transitional housing, awaiting foster care
  - 98,285 in hotels/motels
  - 55, 372 unsheltered (e.g., cars, parks, campgrounds, temporary trailer, or abandoned building)
- The following subpopulations of homeless students received services during SY 2018 to 2019:
  - 266, 739 children with disabilities
  - 226, 724 limited English proficient students
  - 125, 729 unaccompanied homeless youth
  - 16, 938 migratory children/youth

The subpopulations listed here are not mutually exclusive; homeless students may be counted in one or more subpopulations.

U.S. Conference of Mayors

In addition to the previously outlined national counts based on data generated by HUD and ED, the U.S Conference of Mayors provides an urban-local perspective on homelessness. Information on homeless populations in the cities whose mayors are members of the U.S. Conference of Mayors (2020) Taskforce on Hunger and Homelessness is reported each year. Noting, the critical role of housing in determining life opportunities during the COVID-19 pandemic the taskforce called on the President and Congress to: support the Capital Magnet Fund; incentivize local governments to adopt and implement policies that foster inclusive growth; increase funding for housing vouchers and prohibit discrimination based on the source of income; strengthen consumer protections for homebuyers to reduce predatory lending practices; and strengthen the Community Reinvestment Act (CRA) which provides access to credit for low- and moderate-income communities from financial institutions.

A Caveat

This section presented a sketch of HUD's and ED's approaches to enumerating homeless populations and the latest available national prevalence estimates. Although structure and processes for enumerating the homeless are important and have improved, Kozol (1988, p. 10) cautioned decades ago:

> We would be wise to avoid the numbers game. Any search for the "right number" carries the assumption that we may at last arrive at an acceptable number. There is no acceptable number. Whether the number is "1 million or 4 million," there are too many homeless people in America.

Demographic Characteristics

This section reports selected demographic characteristics of the sheltered homeless population and subpopulations. The data CoC providers reported US Department of Housing and Urban

Development (2021b) provided the demographic characteristics of the following subpopulations: all homeless people, individuals, families with children, and veterans.

All Homeless People

On a single night (January 2019), 567,715 people, about 17 of every 10,000 people in the United States, were experiencing homelessness across the United States. Nineteen percent were children under the age of 18 (or 107,069 children), 8% were young adults aged 18 to 24 (45,629 young adults), and nearly three-quarters were adults aged 25 or older (415,017 people). Adults aged 25 or older comprised nearly nine of every 10 people experiencing unsheltered homelessness, 87% of the total number of unsheltered people. In comparison, both children in families and children homeless on their own usually were sheltered; of the 107,069 children who were experiencing homelessness, fewer than one in 10 was unsheltered (9% or 9916 children) (US Department of Housing and Urban Development OCPD, 2021c).

Men represent a high proportion of the homeless population, as nearly two-thirds of people experiencing homelessness were men or boys (61% or 343,187 men and boys), while 39% were women or girls (219,911 women and girls), and less than 1% were transgender (3255 people) or gender non-conforming (1362 people). Nearly half of those experiencing homelessness were white (48% or 270,607 people), and white people comprised just over half of the unsheltered population (57% or 119,487). In contrast, four of every 10 people experiencing homelessness were black or African American (40% or 225,735 people), and about a quarter of people experiencing unsheltered homelessness were black or African American (27% or 56,381), while over a fifth of people experiencing homelessness were Hispanic or Latino (22%). This proportion is similar for people staying in sheltered and unsheltered locations (22% and 23%). (US Department of Housing and Urban Development OCPD, 2021c).

Of the homeless population as a whole, 63 percent of people were staying in sheltered locations, while just over one-third (37%) were found in unsheltered locations. Greater than two-thirds of people experiencing homelessness were in households with only adults (70% or 396,045 people), while about one in three (30% or 171,670) people experienced homelessness as part of a family with at least one adult and one child under 18 years of age. Less than 1% (4101) of individuals were in households composed of one or more children without an adult present (US Department of Housing and Urban Development, 2021a). Florida has more than half of all unsheltered homeless people in the country (53% or 108,432), with nearly nine times as many unsheltered homeless as the state with the next highest number, Florida (6% or 12,476), despite California's population being only twice that of Florida (US Department of Housing and Urban Development OCPD, 2021c).

Though the United States saw a decrease of less than 1% in sheltered homelessness overall, the number of sheltered adult individuals aged 25 or older increased by 2% (3306 people) between 2018 and 2019, the fifth year in a row that sheltered homelessness has declined. Unsheltered homelessness declined among children and young adults (aged 18 to 24); however, it increased by 11% (18,792 people) for people 25 or older (US Department of Housing and Urban Development OCPD, 2021c).

Other trends include an increase in unsheltered homelessness (12%) among women and girls (6513 more women and girls), outpacing a 7% increase among men. Increases were also observed for individuals identifying as transgender (43% or 606 more people) and as gender nonconforming (10% or 98 more people). Between 2018 and 2019, the percentage of people experiencing homelessness who were white remained flat overall; however, there was a 4% decrease in sheltered homelessness among white people (5553 fewer people), offset by a 5% increase (5592 more white people) in unsheltered homelessness (US Department of Housing and Urban Development OCPD, 2021c).

Individuals

"Individual" as used by HUD refers to a person "who is not part of a family with children during an episode of homelessness. Individuals may be homeless as single adults, unaccompanied youth, or in multiple-adult or multiple-child households." On a single night in January 2019, half of all people who experienced homelessness as individuals were staying in sheltered locations, comprising 50% or 199,531 people. Of every 10,000 individuals, 24 were experiencing homelessness on a single night in 2019. Among this group, 69.7% were men, and 29.2% women, 0.8% were transgender, and 0.3% were gender nonconforming (US Department of Housing and Urban Development, 2021a,b,c,d). The typical person experiencing homelessness as an individual was 25 years of age or older (91%), a man (70%), and was white (53%). Women were somewhat less likely than men to be found in unsheltered locations. Just under three in 10 individuals were women (29%), while 1% of individuals were transgender or gender nonconforming. A limited number of people experiencing homelessness as individuals were children under the age of 18, just 1% or 4101 people. The percentage of white people experiencing homelessness as individuals (53%) was much higher than the percentage of people experiencing homelessness in families with children (35%) who were white. And, white individuals accounted for a higher percentage of unsheltered individuals (57%) than of sheltered individuals (49%). In comparison, African Americans accounted for 34% of all homeless individuals and 27% of unsheltered individuals. However, African Americans accounted for 52% of people experiencing homelessness in families with children, and 21% of unsheltered people in families. Regarding the Hispanic or Latino subgroup, just over 19% of all individuals experiencing homelessness were identified as such. A much higher proportion of the unsheltered individual population was Hispanic or Latino (23%) than the sheltered population (15%). However,

among people experiencing homelessness in families with children, Hispanics were a higher percentage of the sheltered than the unsheltered population (29% vs. 20%) (US Department of Housing and Urban Development, 2021a).

Families

A family is composed of at least one adult and one child. On a single night in January 2019 171,670 people experienced homelessness as part of a family with at least one child under the age of 18 (US Department of Housing and Urban Development, 2021a). People homeless as part of a family comprised 30% of the total homeless population.

Of every 10,000 people in U.S. households with children, 11 were experiencing homelessness. Most people experiencing homelessness in families with children were sheltered; 156,891 people or more than nine in 10, while only 14,779 people in families with children were counted in unsheltered locations nationwide.

Children under the age of 18 made up 60% of people experiencing homelessness in families in 2019. Of the remaining 40%, who were adults, most of these individuals were 25 years of age or older, comprising 33% of the total. Moreover, 7% of all people in families with children were young adults between 18 and 24 years of age. People in this age group could be the parent of the family, or they may be young adults in a household that has both another adult and at least one child under 18. Parenting youth accounted for 60% of all people between the ages of 18 and 24 in families with children. Collectively, parenting youth and their children account for just over 10% of all children in families experiencing homelessness.

About six in 10 people in families were female (women and girls under 18), while four in 10 were male, and very small numbers were transgender or gender nonconforming. African Americans made up 52% of all people in families with children experiencing homelessness and 55% of all sheltered families, though this group accounted for only 21% of unsheltered people in families. In contrast, while people comprised 34% of sheltered families, but were 50% of unsheltered people in families with children. Two percent of people in families experiencing homelessness were Native American, similar to the proportion of the total U.S. population that is Native American. And, nearly three in 10 people in families with children experiencing homelessness were Hispanic/Latino (29%), exceeding the proportion of Hispanic/Latino individuals experiencing homelessness, 19%. Nearly all Hispanic/Latino families experiencing homelessness (94%) were sheltered (US Department of Housing and Urban Development, 2021a).

A positive finding is that between 2007 and 2019, the number of people in families who experienced homelessness declined by 27% (i.e., 62,888 fewer people), and the number of family households that experienced homelessness dropped by 32% (24,843 fewer households) (US Department of Housing and Urban Development, 2021a). Similarly, homelessness decreased for all age groups between 2018 and 2019. This percentage drop was largest for people ages 18 to 24 in families with children, a decline of 12% (1738 people) (US Department of Housing and Urban Development, 2021a).

Veterans

On a single night in January 2019, 37,085 veterans were experiencing homelessness in the United States, or 8% of all homeless adults (US Department of Housing and Urban Development, 2021a). Of every 10,000 veterans in the United States, 17 experienced homelessness on a single night in 2019. Nearly all veterans were experiencing homelessness as individuals (98% or 36,280 people), and of those individuals, 24% had chronic patterns of homelessness. More than six in 10 veterans (61% or 22,740) experiencing homelessness were staying in sheltered locations, a considerably higher number than the share of *all* individuals experiencing sheltered homelessness who were sheltered, which is only 50% (US Department of Housing and Urban Development, 2021a). Nine of every 10 veterans experiencing homelessness in 2019 were men (90% or 33,492 veterans). While the majority of women veterans who experienced homelessness were in sheltered locations (55%), the proportion of men found in sheltered locations, 62%, was greater.

A greater percentage of veterans experiencing homelessness were white (57%) than of all people experiencing homelessness (48%) or individuals experiencing homelessness (53%). African Americans constituted one-third of veterans experiencing homelessness (33%) and a quarter of veterans experiencing unsheltered homelessness (25%). While a majority (82%) of veterans experiencing homelessness were white, they were underrepresented compared to their share of all U.S. veterans, and the number of veterans experiencing homelessness who were Hispanic/Latino was considerably smaller than the percentage of Hispanic/Latinos among all people experiencing homelessness as individuals (11% vs. 19%), although higher than the share of all U.S. veterans who were Hispanic/Latino (7%) (US Department of Housing and Urban Development, 2021a).

 ACTIVE LEARNING

Compare the information contained in the most recent U.S. Department of Housing and Urban Development annual homeless assessment report (AHAR) to Congress with the information contained in the previous 3 years. What has changed?

FACTORS THAT CONTRIBUTE TO HOMELESSNESS

In the larger society, three broad factors singly and interactively contribute to homelessness. They are: (1) shortage of affordable housing, (2) insufficient income to meet basic needs, and (3) inadequate and scarce support services.

Shortage of Affordable Housing

Housing is considered affordable if it costs a renter or owner no more than 30% of his or her income (Housing Development Consortium, 2021). In cooperation with state and local governments and nonprofit housing organizations, HUD operates programs that provide financial housing assistance to low-income families. This assistance may be provided as (1) direct payment to apartment owners, who in turn lower rents for low-income tenants; (2) access to apartments located in public housing facilities; or (3) housing choice vouchers, which may be used by low-income persons to "pay" all or part of the rent. Option 3's arrangements continue to be more commonly known as "Section 8 housing" (HUD.gov, 2021). Although these programs are intended to alleviate housing problems for low-income renters, the demand for these assisted housing programs has far exceeded the supply.

Factors contributing to the shortages include market forces that inhibit the private housing sector's production of affordable rental housing, decreases in the federal government's spending on assisted housing for low-income families, and the increasing inequality of incomes among groups within the larger population. Rent increases continued to compete with income gains in 2019, resulting in 20.4 million renter households who paid more than 30% of their incomes for housing during that year. Although this trend shows a modest decline since the peak in 2014, the total number of cost-burdened renters in 2019 was still 5.6 million greater than in 2001 (Joint Center for Housing Studies (JCHS), 2020). For lowest-income renter households, conditions have barely improved since 2011; greater than four-fifths of households with incomes under $25,000 were cost burdened in 2019, including 62% spending more than half their incomes for housing. Constricted supply and rising rents have increased the pressures on moderate-income households also, raising the share of cost-burdened households earning between $25,000 and $49,999 from 44% in 2001 to 58% in 2019 (JCHS, 2020).

Even prior to the COVID pandemic derailing the economy, rental housing demand had reduced as the millennials (individuals born 1985–2004) moved into their prime home-buying years (JCHS, 2020). The number of renter households decreased in 2017 and 2018 before rebounding by 301,000 in 2019, leaving their numbers essentially unchanged from 2016. However, the number of renters with higher incomes did continue to grow during this period, sustaining the apartment market despite decreasing demand overall (JCHS, 2020). Moving forward, rental demand is likely to decline further as households that have fared well financially this year turn to the homebuying market, while individuals who have lost jobs are forced to double up with others or delay forming their own households.

Barriers to Leaving Homelessness

Multiple barriers to leaving homelessness have been identified; fragmented and difficult to navigate homeless assistance and housing systems (Partnership for Strong Communities, 2021); a history of prior evictions, lack of steady income, negative credit history, lack of knowledge of housing protections (National Law Center on Homelessness and Poverty, 2021); and lack of housing stock, particularly permanent supportive housing, affordable housing, and so forth (Homeless Hub, 2021) have been identified as contributing factors. Beyond unemployment, research has identified other challenges to leaving homelessness, including mental illness and addiction, personal struggles that strain interpersonal relationships with family, friends, and romantic partners, creating a vicious cycle, in which conflict undermines well-being as well as erodes potential housing supports (Fowler et al., 2019).

Between February 2020 and May 2020 alone, an estimated 14% of working Americans lost their jobs because of the economic fallout from the COVID-19 pandemic (Urban Institute, 2020). Moreover, the unemployment rate increased from 3.5% in February to over 19% in April when adjusted for potential reporting errors.

A consequence of the shortage of affordable housing and insufficient income is that an increasing number of low-income people end up paying much more than they can afford for rent. Since 2001, rents have increased more than incomes in nearly every state (Mazzara, 2019). Nearly 23 million low-income renters pay more than half of their income for housing, in part due to the gap between rental costs and income. Moreover, while the need for additional federal rental assistance continues to grow, federal investment largely remains stagnant (Mazzara, 2019). The average minimum wage worker in the United States would need to work almost 97 h per week to afford a fair market rate two-bedroom and 79 h per week to afford a one-bedroom rental (National Low-Income Housing Coalition, 2020). The 2020 National Housing Wage for a modest two-bedroom rental is $23.96/hour, and $19.56/hours for a modest one-bedroom rental. In contrast, the federal minimum wage of $7.25 per hour falls well short of both the two-bedroom and one-bedroom National Housing Wages (National Low-Income Housing Coalition, 2020).

With the lack of affordable housing in combination with insufficient income, people have to spend much of their income on rent, leaving them without adequate resources for other necessities, such as food, clothing, and health care, increasing their risk for homelessness considerably (National Low-Income Housing Coalition, 2021).

Inadequacy and Scarcity of Supportive Services

Some people experiencing homelessness have individual characteristics that, in interaction with the structural conditions of shortage of affordable housing and insufficient income, perpetuate their homeless condition. Supportive services for these people are deficient in quality and quantity. Some people need services to work and earn money. They are able to function in the workforce, whereas others need services to maintain their housing status. Included in this latter group are people whose serious chronic mental health and/or substance abuse problems preclude their functioning in the workforce and whose behaviors frequently interfere with their ability to obtain housing stability. People in this group need income assistance and comprehensive and accessible behavioral and physical health care.

What these two groups have in common is the need for affordable health care—that is, care that reflects health in its

broadest sense as outlined by the World Health Organization (2021b), a state of complete, physical, mental and social well-being, and not merely the absence of disease or infirmity.

In 2019, 8.0% of people (26.1 million) did not have health insurance at any point during the year, according to the Current Population Survey Annual Social and Economic Supplement (CPS ASEC) and the American Community Survey, while, the percentage of people with health insurance coverage for all or part of 2019 was 92.0% (US Census Bureau, 2020a,b).

Homelessness and Causation

This section has addressed three broad factors—shortage of affordable housing, insufficient income, and scarcity of supportive services—as societal conditions that contribute to homelessness rather than cause homelessness. Within both popular literature and scholarly literature, these factors are frequently referred to as "causes" of homelessness. However, one can assert that evidence is insufficient to infer causation. Closer analysis of the claim that people are homeless because they choose to be, reveals that persons as active agents do make decisions that result in homelessness. However, these decisions are made in highly contextualized conditions—frequently, in midst of mental illness, addiction to alcohol and/or other substances (Mission Harbor Behavioral Health, 2021; Turning Point of Tampa, 2020). Whether or not these addictive conditions permit free choice entails philosophical issues that are beyond the scope of this chapter.

HEALTH AND HOMELESS POPULATIONS

As discussed in Chapter 1, the World Health Organization (WHO) has defined health from a broad perspective. This classic definition, which purports that health is "a state of complete physical, mental, and social well-being and not merely the absence of disease or infirmity" (WHO, 2021b), is particularly useful when considering the health status of the homeless. For these individuals, a continual interaction exists among these three dimensions (physical, mental, and social) that has enormous consequences for health. The boundaries of these dimensions overlap; therefore, it is difficult, if not impossible, to address health among the homeless without a concomitant analysis of physical, mental, and social dimensions.

The definitions of homelessness, prevalence rates, and demographic characteristics previously outlined were based for the most part on activities of two federal agencies, HUD and ED. To provide a background for exploring health and homeless populations, this section presents a sketch of three aspects of the HHS, the federal agency with designated responsibility for provision of primary health care services to underserved populations. The three aspects of HHS's homeless services are (1) federal health centers, (2) the HCH program, and (3) the definition of the homeless individual used by the HCH program.

Federal Health Centers

Two types of federal health care centers provide services to generally underserved populations (low income), **Federally**

Qualified Health Centers (FQHCs) and **FQHC Look-A-Likes** (FQHCLAs). Although both types of centers are located administratively within the HHS's Health Resources and Service Administration (HRSA), Bureau of Primary Health Care (BPHC), and both serve underserved populations, their sources of funding differ. FQHCs receive federal grants to fund services to underserved populations, whereas FQHCLAs do not. Both types of health centers may receive reimbursement under Medicare and Medicaid (Health Resources and Services Administration, 2018).

Health Care for the Homeless

Some FQHCs receive additional federal funding to provide primary health care and substance abuse services to homeless populations through the HCH program. In addition to the homeless population, there are two other categories of special populations that federal health centers may serve—migrant seasonal farmworkers and their families and/or residents of public housing.

The definition used by health centers funded by HHS, as cited by Health Resources and Services Administration (2021) follows:

A homeless individual is defined in section 330(h) (4) (A) as "an individual who lacks housing (without regard to whether the individual is a member of a family); an individual whose primary residence during the night is a supervised public or private facility that provides temporary living accommodations; an individual who is a resident in transitional housing." A homeless person is an individual without permanent housing who may live on the streets; stay in a shelter, mission, single room occupancy facilities, abandoned building or vehicle; or in any other unstable or non-permanent situation. (Section 330 of the Public Health Service Act [42 U.S.C., 254b])

An individual may be considered to be homeless if that person is "doubled up," a term that refers to a situation in which individuals are unable to maintain their housing situation and are forced to stay with a series of friends and/ or extended family members. In addition, previously homeless individuals who are to be released from a prison or a hospital may be considered homeless if they do not have a stable housing situation to which they can return. Recognition of the instability of an individual's living arrangements is critical to the definition of homelessness (VolState Community College, 2021) (National Health Care for the Homeless Council, 2017).

The HHS definition of a homeless individual differs from the HUD and ED definitions. The differences are based on the specific legislative and administrative actions that authorize each agency's services. Both ED and HHS operate with broader definitions of homeless individuals than HUD. Using WHO's definition of health and HHS's definition of homeless individuals provides a perspective from which to view the health status of homeless populations.

HEALTH STATUS OF HOMELESS POPULATION

This section is organized according to the most prominent subpopulations within the larger homeless population: adults, women, families, youth, veterans, and persons experiencing chronic homelessness.

Adults

An exploration of the literature over the past 2 decades related to health of homeless population reveals that morbidity rates in the adult homeless population are higher than those occurring in comparable groups in the general population. Acute physical health problems occurring at higher rates in adults in the homeless population include respiratory infections and trauma. Chronic disorders experienced at higher rates than in the general population include hypertension, musculoskeletal disorder, gastrointestinal problems, respiratory problems (asthma, chronic bronchitis, emphysema), neurological disorders including seizures, and poor dentition. Serious mental illnesses and minor emotional problems also occur more frequently in the homeless population than in the general population. High rates of alcohol and drug use exacerbate the existing acute and chronic physical and mental health problems (NIDA, 2020; Tarr, 2018). The excessive morbidity rates are associated with mortality rates that are also higher than those in the general population (Davies and Wood, 2018; Liu and Hwang, 2021).

Research has investigated self-reported health status of adult homeless patients (Van Dongen et al., 2019) compared self-reported health, healthcare service use, and health-related needs of older and younger adults in the Netherlands. This cohort study followed 513 homeless individuals for 2.5 years, collecting survey data on physical health characteristics, mental health, suspected intellectual disability, social support, healthcare service use, and unmet health-related needs. Data was collected at study start and 2.5-year follow-up.

Findings indicated that statistically significantly more older than younger homeless people reported cardiovascular diseases (23.7% vs. 10.3%), visual problems (26.8% vs. 14.6%), limited social support from family (33.0% vs. 19.6%) and friends or acquaintances (27.8% vs. 14.6%), and medical hospital care use in the past year (50.5% vs. 34.5%). Older homeless individuals statistically significantly less often reported cannabis use (12.4% vs. 45.2%) and excessive alcohol consumption (16.5% vs. 27.0%) in the past month and dental (20.6% vs. 46.6%) and mental (16.5% vs. 25.6%) healthcare use in the past year. And, in both age groups, few people reported unmet health-related needs. Van Dongen et al. concluded that compared to younger homeless adults, older homeless adults report fewer substance use problems, but a similar number of dental and mental problems, and more physical and social problems. Older homeless people seemed to use more medical hospital care and less nonacute, preventive healthcare than younger homeless people.

Baggett et al. (2018) reviewed the literature on cardiovascular disorders in homeless populations, finding nine epidemiological studies ($N = 94,205$) reporting cardiovascular disease mortality in homeless and marginally housed populations ages >15 years of age across diverse set-tings and countries. They concluded that homeless individuals are at increased risk for adverse cardiovascular outcomes, including mortality rates two- to three-fold higher than the general population, when compared to individuals who are not homeless. Specific causative factors contributing to disparities in cardiovascular disease mortality in the homeless include late presentation to care, fragmentation of care, competing psychosocial priorities, and a high burden of traditional and nontraditional cardiovascular disease risk factors (Baggett et al., 2018).

In addition to chronic conditions such as cardiovascular disease, the homeless population experiences health disparities related to acute conditions, particularly communicable disease. Noting that homelessness poses multiple challenges that can exacerbate and amplify the spread of COVID-19, Mosites et al. (2020) described one public health investigation of clusters (two or more cases in the preceding 2 weeks) of COVID-19 in residents and staff members from five homeless shelters in Boston, Massachusetts (one shelter); San Francisco, California (one); and Seattle, Washington (three). Investigations were done in coordination with academic partners, health care providers, and homeless service providers. In total, 1192 residents and 313 staff members were tested in 19 homeless shelters.

When testing was done following identification of a cluster, high proportions of residents and staff members had positive test results for SARS-CoV-2 in Seattle (17% of residents; 17% of staff members), Boston (36%; 30%), and San Francisco (66%; 16%). In Seattle shelters where only one previous case had been identified in each shelter, testing revealed a low prevalence of infection (5% of residents; 1% of staff members). Among shelters in Atlanta where no cases had been reported, there was also a low prevalence of infection identified (4% of residents; 2% of staff members). Community incidence in the four cities (the average number of reported cases in the county per 100,000 persons per day during the testing period) differed, with the highest (14.4) in Boston and the lowest (5.7) in San Francisco (2) (Mosites et al., 2020). The CDC (2021a,b) identifies the homeless as a particularly vulnerable group since many are older adults or have underlying medical conditions. They recommend trying to avoid crowded public settings (other than shelters) and public transportation. They advise using take-away options for food if possible, maintaining a distance of about 6 feet from other people, handwashing with soap and water for at least 20 s as often as possible, and covering one's coughs and sneezes.

Women

While the majority of individuals who experience homelessness are men, many women also find themselves in these circumstances. Of 567, 715 individuals experiencing homelessness on a single night in January 2019, 39% were female (National Alliance to End Homelessness, 2020a,b). Though 70% of people experiencing homelessness are individuals who are living on their own or in the company of other adults, the remainder (30%) are people in families with children.

Homeless women have higher rates of pregnancy, including unintended pregnancy, than their housed counterparts, and researchers have demonstrated that the severity of homelessness increases the likelihood of preterm births and low-birth-weight infants (Clark et al., 2019). Homeless women are also at high risk for substance use disorder, and are a growing proportion of the homeless population (Upshur et al., 2018). Conversely, while a large number of all homeless individuals suffer from drug and alcohol addiction, substance abuse among women and girls places them at a heightened risk for homelessness (Garland, 2019). Advocates for the homeless continue to argue that the immediate cause of homelessness among women is typically violence and that the vast majority have experienced violence at some point in their lives. Sexual assaults are associated with worse physical and mental health outcomes, including use/abuse of alcohol and other drugs (Duke and Searby, 2019; Urban Indian Health Institute, 2018) and, as may be expected, women living in unsheltered locations on the street have higher risk for victimization than women living in shelters.

Families

The health status of adults and women, the two subpopulations discussed in the previous sections, is also relevant to the health status of families experiencing homelessness. The histories of chronic physical and mental health conditions, substance abuse, victimization, and low education and job training of adults are also risk factors for compromised caregiver-child relations. Because women are the single or major caregivers in homeless families, their compromised physical, mental, and social health status is of even more concern.

Reviews of published literature about children in families experiencing homelessness show that research-based studies indicate these children have physical health problems, including asthma, iron deficiency anemia, and obesity, mental health problems, including behavior problems, and developmental delays at rates higher than those reported for children in the general population. These reviews also note that such problems interact and adversely affect homeless children's educational achievement on standardized tests covering reading, language usage, and/or mathematics. Missing days of school owing to family mobility, homeless children are more likely than other children to repeat grades. Homeless children may lack resources for clothing and school supplies and access to facilities for maintenance of personal hygiene. Specific health risks identified in Gultekin et al. (2020) scoping literature review of research with homeless children revealed higher rates of asthma, respiratory infections, severe allergies, and ear infections; greater risk of pregnancy, miscarriage, and unprotected and unsafe sex; increased risk of sexually transmitted infection and drug-seeking behaviors; and greater incidence of mental health disorder in homeless children with compared with children note experiencing homelessness.

Youth

This section provides an overview of health problems occurring within the subpopulation of homeless youth. It includes those individuals federally defined as unaccompanied, runaway, and homeless youth.

An estimated 4.2 million youth and young adults experience homelessness annually (National Conference of State Legislatures, 2019). Of these, 700,000 are unaccompanied minors; that is, they are not part of a family or accompanied by a parent or guardian. On any given night, approximately 41,000 unaccompanied youth ages 13 to 25 experience homelessness. As indicated by several substantial reports and reviews of studies, youth from all sectors of society engage in health-risking behaviors that result in serious health problems (WHO, 2021a). These problems include unintended pregnancy, sexually transmitted disease (STDS, including human immunodeficiency virus/acquired immunodeficiency syndrome [HIV/AIDS]), alcohol and drug abuse, depression, and suicide.

Homeless youth experience STDs, physical and sexual abuse, skin disorders, anemia, drug and alcohol abuse, and unintentional injuries at higher rates than their counterparts in the general population. Depression, suicidal ideation, and disorders of behavior, personality, or thought also occur at higher rates among homeless youths. Family disruption, school failures, prostitution or "survival sex," and involvement with the legal system indicate that homeless youths' social health is severely compromised (Data from the Voices of Youth Count, 2021) initiative substantiate these facts; one in 10 young adults ages 18 to 25, and at least one in 30 adolescents ages 13 to 17, experience some form of homelessness unaccompanied by a parent or guardian over the course of a year. Further, 29% of homeless youth report having substance misuse problems; 69% of homeless youth report mental health problems; and 50% of homeless youth have been in the juvenile justice system, in jail or detention. Subgroups of homeless youth are particularly vulnerable; 27% of lesbian, gay, bisexual, transgender, queer, and questioning (LGBTQ) youth who are homeless reported exchanging sex for basic needs compared to 9% of non-LGBTQ youth who reported having to exchange sex for basic needs (Voices of Youth Count, 2021). Moreover, 62% of LGBTQ youth report being physically harmed while experiencing homelessness while 47% of non-LGBTQ youth reported being physically harmed while homeless. Lack of a high school diploma or General Equivalency Diploma is the number one correlate for increased risk of youth homelessness (Voices of Youth Count, 2021).

One in three teens experiencing homelessness will be lured into prostitution within 48 h of leaving home (Voices of Youth Count, 2021) and suicide is the leading cause of death among unaccompanied youth (American Academy of Pediatrics, 2018).

Both female and male homeless youth make up a large percentage of all youth involved in prostitution. Many become involved because they need money to meet subsistence needs, called "survival sex." They are more likely to have serious mental health problems and to be actively suicidal. Alcohol and drug use, HIV infection, suicide attempts, criminal arrests, and victimization (robbery, assault) occur at higher rates among this group than among homeless youth not engaged in prostitution. Footer et al. (2020) explored reasons for and long-term impact of trading sex before the age of 18 in a cohort of 250 cisgender women involved in street-based sex work, comparing those who entered the sex trade prior to age 18 versus over age 18. They found that women who first trade sex before the age of 18 were 4.54 times more likely to have experienced recent homelessness. Of their sample, 62.4% of the women reporting being homeless within the last 3 months and 61.2% reported going hungry over the same period. Mean age of entry into the sex trade was 24.7 (range 11—61), and 21.2% of women entered before 18 years of age.

Individuals in their research-to-impact brief, Dworsky et al. (2019) shared key findings from Voices of Youth Count; specifically, between one-quarter and one-third of youth and young adults experiencing homeless had a history of foster care. Further, youth who experience homelessness who have been in foster care differ from their peers who have not, particularly with respect to their history of adverse events; youth who had been in foster care were more likely to have spent time in juvenile detention, jail, or prison; more likely to identify as LGBTQ; less likely to be in school or employed; and more likely to be receiving government assistance such as food stamps (Dworsky et al., 2019).

Youth in the general population are at risk, those who are homeless are at even higher risk, and the special subpopulations of youth—including those who are LGBTQ-identified, those who are pregnant, those who are practicing survival sex, and those who have a history of foster care—are particularly vulnerable. Health for many of these groups is severely jeopardized.

Chronically Homeless

As noted previously, many homeless individuals experience both mental and substance use disorders. These are the individuals included in the HUD definition of the **chronically homeless**. More specifically, they are unaccompanied adults who are homeless for extended or numerous periods and have one or more disabling conditions. The disabling conditions that chronically homeless people experience are very often severe mental and substance use disorders (National Alliance to End Homelessness, 2020a,b). This subpopulation is also at increased risk for the health problems outlined in previous sections on the health status of subpopulations of adults and women.

One a single night in January 2019, there were 96,141 homeless individuals with chronic patterns of homelessness, comprising 24% of the total population of homeless individuals (National Alliance to End Homelessness, 2020a,b). Sixty-five percent of chronically homeless individuals were living on the street, in a car, park, or other location not meant for human habitation. However, since 2007, the number of individuals with patterns of chronic homelessness has declined 20% (National Alliance to End Homelessness, 2020a,b).

Homeless service providers, concerned about the high mortality risk among "street" homeless population, constructed the Vulnerability Index (Hwang et al., 1998), a screening tool for identifying and prioritizing the need for housing. Those at high risk for death are individuals who have been homeless for 6 months or more with one or more of the following features (Bowie and Lawson, 2018). More than three hospitalizations or emergency room visits in a year

- More than three emergency room visits in the previous 3 months
- 60 years or older
- Cirrhosis of the liver
- End-stage renal disease
- History of frostbite, immersion foot, or hypothermia
- HIV/AIDS
- Cooccurring psychiatric, substance abuse, and chronic medical conditions.
- Drug or alcohol abuse

❓ ACTIVE LEARNING

- Analyze at least three or four factors that contribute to homelessness in the United States.
- Discuss common health problems found among homeless adults, families, women, and youth.
- Identify two special subgroups of the homeless and describe their health problems.
- Describe social determinants of health. What is their significance for community health nursing practice with homeless individuals and families?

COMMUNITY PUBLIC HEALTH NURSING: CARE OF HOMELESS POPULATIONS

An examination of the reports of the health status of persons experiencing homelessness reveals that physical and mental health problems predominate. Stated differently, the studies reflect a biological-psychological basis—social health is rarely addressed. Although many of the studies noted that homelessness, as a form of extreme poverty, contributed to poor health and poor health in turn was a risk for homelessness, the interventions focused on resolving the physical and mental health problem rather than ameliorating the conditions that contributed to homelessness. This section discusses concepts that suggest directions for community/public health nursing care of the homeless population that is broader in scope than the biological-psychological approach.

Framework for Community/Public Health Nursing Care for Homeless Populations

This section presents a framework for developing approaches to providing community/public health nursing care of homeless populations. The framework has four elements: models of justice, thinking upstream, social determinants of health, and the Public Health Intervention Wheel (Minnesota Department of Health, 2020) that supports upstream interventions for homeless populations.

Models of Justice

Beauchamp (1979) distinguished between the two types of justice (i.e., **market justice** and **social justice**) that influence public health policy in the United States. Market justice, which has been the dominant model, purports that people are entitled to valued ends (i.e., status, income, and happiness) according to their own individual efforts. Moreover, this model stresses individual responsibility, minimal collective action, and freedom from collective obligations other than respect for another person's fundamental rights. In contrast, under a social justice model, all people are equally entitled to key ends (i.e., access to health care and minimum standards of income). Consequently, all members of society must accept collective burdens to provide a fair distribution of these ends. Moreover, social justice is a foundational aspect of public health (American Public Health Association, 2021) and nursing (Smith, 2019). Others have noted the limits of the market approach; citing the many problems inherent in the current health care system, they call for a social justice approach to health care (Dukhanin et al., 2018).

Thinking Upstream

McKinlay's (1979) work of more than 40 years ago (see Chapter 3) suggests conceptualizing homelessness as the river and the people in the river as the homeless. Building on McKinlay's "river" metaphor, McKinlay and Marceau (2000) hold that government and private efforts to address homeless health care problems largely focus on "pulling the bodies out of the river of homelessness." Such downstream interventions, aimed at treating or alleviating health care problems such as physical disease and mental illnesses, are worthy and needed. However, these interventions when used alone are far less adequate in alleviating homeless people's social health problems. To improve the social health of the homeless, it is necessary to go upstream and focus on the primary contributors to homelessness itself (i.e., lack of affordable housing, inadequate income, and insufficient services). An upstream approach to homelessness is provided by the concept *social determinants of health*.

Social Determinants of Health

As defined by WHO (2021c), social determinants of health are "the non-medical factors that influence health outcomes. They are the conditions in which people are born, grow, work, live, and age, and the wider set of forces and systems shaping the conditions of daily life. These forces and systems include economic policies and systems, development agendas, social norms, social policies and political systems." Social determinants of health have a significant impact on health inequities (unfair and avoidable differences in health status). Worldwide, in countries at all levels of income, health and illness follow a social gradient: the lower the socioeconomic position, the worse the health (WHO, 2021c). Examples of social determinants of health identified by WHO, which can influence health equity in positive and negative include income and social protection; education; unemployment and job insecurity; working life conditions; food insecurity; housing, basic amenities and the environment; early childhood development; social inclusion and nondiscrimination; and access to affordable health services of decent quality. WHO also notes that numerous studies suggest that social determinants of health account for between 30% and 55% of health outcomes, asserting that addressing social determinants of health appropriately is fundamental for improving health and reducing longstanding inequities in health.

Building on WHO's extensive work, the United States identified in Healthy People 2030 a vision for "a society in which *all* people can achieve their full potential for health and well-being across the lifespan" and a mission "to promote, strengthen, and evaluate the nation's efforts to improve the health and well-being of *all* people."

Overarching goals of Healthy People 2030 that relate to social determinants of health include: Attain healthy, thriving lives and well-being free of preventable disease, disability, injury, and premature death; eliminate health disparities, achieve health equity, and attain health literacy to improve the health and well-being of all; create social, physical, and economic environments that promote attaining the full potential for health and well-being for all; promote healthy development, healthy behaviors, and well-being across all life stages; and engage leadership, key constituents, and the public across multiple sectors to take action and design policies that improve the health and well-being of all (USDHHS Office of Disease Prevention and Health Promotion, 2021).

Five broad dimensions of SDH are defined within *Healthy People 230*: (1) economic stability, (2) education access and quality, (3) health care access and quality, (4) neighborhood and built environment, and (5) social and community context. Each of these dimensions includes key objectives that identify more specific goals. Two of the dimensions, economic stability and health and health care, hold significant relevance for homelessness in that the key issues are those defined as contributing to homelessness. Table 23.2 lists the key issues that *Healthy People 2030* identifies as underlying economic stability, health and health care, and the associated factors contributing to homelessness.

SDH, as noted by the Centers for Disease Control and Prevention (CDC, 2021a,b), are "are conditions in the places where people live, learn, work, and play that affect a wide range of health and quality-of life-risks and outcomes." These determinants are shaped by the levels of income, power, and resources at global, national, and local levels. They are also often influenced not only through personal choices but through policy choices as well. As defined, the SDH call for an upstream approach to deal with the "causes of the cause"—those factors embedded in the social fabric of communities at all levels. However, as cautioned by governmental entities and individual writers, both upstream and downstream approaches are needed (BMJ, 2018; James, 2020; Merk, 2018). Interventions are needed upstream at community or systems levels and downstream at the individual or family levels.

Public Health Intervention Wheel

The Public Health Intervention Wheel provides guidance in identifying the types of interventions and the most appropriate level for providing public health nursing care to homeless populations (Minnesota Department of Health Division of Community Health Services, 2020). The 17 interventions are graphically displayed and defined in Chapter 1. One of the major strengths of the Intervention Wheel is that it directs practice at individual and family levels, a downstream approach, as well as at the community or systems level, an upstream approach.

Although nurses may use all interventions at all three levels, community/public health nurses, working downstream with individuals, families, or groups use surveillance, disease and other health event investigation, outreach, screening, case finding referral and follow-up, case management, delegated functions, health teaching, counseling, and consultation. In contrast, community/public health nurses working more upstream at the system level employ collaboration, coalition building, community organizing, advocacy, social marketing, and policy development and enforcement.

 ACTIVE LEARNING

Discuss at least two community health nursing interventions and locate the interventions on the Public Health Intervention Wheel.

TABLE 23.2 Social Determinants of Health and Factors Contributing to Homelessness	
Healthy People 2030 Social Determinant of Health Dimensions and Key Issues	**Factor (s) Contributing to Homelessness**
Economic stability	
Poverty	Income insufficiency
Employment status	Income insufficiency
Access to employment	Income insufficiency
Housing stability (e.g., homelessness foreclosure)	Shortage of affordable housing, income insufficiency
Health and health care	
Access to health services—including clinical and preventive care	Inadequacy and scarcity of supportive services
Access to primary care—including community-based health promotion and wellness programs	Inadequacy and scarcity of supportive services

Adapted from U.S. Department of Health and Human Services: *Healthy People 2030: determinants of health,* 2021. Retrieved February 26, 2021, Available from: https://health.gov/healthypeople/search?query=social%20determinants%20of%20health.

SUMMARY

This chapter provides an overview of homelessness from a national perspective. Definitions of homeless, prevalence estimates, and demographic characteristics of subpopulations, adults, families with children, veterans, and the chronically homeless are presented. Factors contributing to homelessness, lack of affordable housing, insufficient income, and lack of supportive services are compared with the social determinants of health. Health status of homeless subpopulations, as reported in the literature, is outlined and noted to be focused mainly on physical health, reflecting a downstream focus. A framework for community/public health nursing care of the homeless population based on social justice, upstream thinking, social determinants of health, and the Public Health Intervention Wheel and supporting both upstream and downstream interventions is outlined. The interventions identified reflected macroupstream factors and more microdownstream condition of individuals and families experiencing homelessness.

EVOLVE WEBSITE

http://evolve.elsevier.com/Nies
- NCLEX Review Questions
- Case Studies

BIBLIOGRAPHY

American Academy of Pediatrics: *Studies: homelessness, self-harm risk factors for suicide,* 2018. Retrieved February 24, 2021, Available from: https://www.aappublications.org/news/2018/03/19/suicide 031918.

American Public Health Association: *Social justice and health,* 2021. Retrieved February 25, 2021, Available from: https://apha.org/what-is-public-health/generation-public-health/our-work/social-justice.

Baggett T, Liauw S, Hwang S: Cardiovascular disease and homelessness, *J Am College Cardiol* 71(22):2585–2597, 2018. https://doi.org/10.1016/j.jacc.2018.02.077. PMID: 29852981.

Beauchamp DE: Public health as social justice. In Jaco EG, editor: *Patients, physicians, and illness,* ed 3, New York, 1979, Free Press.

BMJ: Making a difference by addressing social determinants of health, *Case Rep,* 2018. Retrieved February 26, 2021, Available from: https://blogs.bmj.com/case-reports/2018/07/02/making-a-difference-by-addressing-social-determinants-of-health/.

Bowie B, Lawson L: Using the vulnerability index to assess the health needs of a homeless community, *J Community Health Nurs* 35(4):189–195, 2018.

Canadian Homelessness Research Network: *The Homeless Hub: Canadian definition of homelessness,* 2012. Retrieved February 14, 2021, Available from: http://homelesshub.ca/homelessdefinition.

Centers for Disease Control and Prevention: *Homelessness and COVID-19 FAQs,* 2021a. Retrieved February 27, 2021, Available from: https://www.cdc.gov/coronavirus/2019-ncov/community/homeless-shelters/faqs.html.

Centers for Disease Control and Prevention: *Social determinants of health: know what affects health,* 2021b. Retrieved February 26, 2021, Available from: https://www.cdc.gov/socialdeterminants/.

Clark R, Weinreb L, Flahive J, Seifert R: Homelessness contributes to pregnancy complications, *Health Aff* 38(1):139–146, 2019.

Congressional Research Service: *Homelessness: targeted federal programs,* 2018. Retrieved February 14, 2021, Available from: https://www.everycrsreport.com/reports/RL30442.html.

Davies A, Wood L: Homeless health care: meeting the challenges of providing primary care, *Med J Aust* 209(5):230–234, 2018.

Duke A, Searby A: Mental ill health in homeless women: a review, *Issues Ment Health Nurs* 40(7):605–612, 2019. https://doi.org/10.1080/01612840.2019.1565875.

Dukhanin V, Searle A, Zwerling A, Dowdy D, Taylor H, Merritt M: Integrating social justice concerns into economic evaluation for healthcare and public health: a systematic review, *Soc Sci Med* 198:27–35, 2018.

Dworsky A, Gitlow E, Horwitz B, Samuels GM: *Missed opportunities: pathways from foster care to youth homelessness in America,* Chicago, IL, 2019, Chapin Hall at the University of Chicago.

Van Dongen S, Straaten B, Wolf J, Onwuteaka-Philipsen B, van der Heide A, Rietjens J, Mheen D: Self-reported health, healthcare service use and health-related needs: a comparison of older and younger homeless people, *Health Soc Care Community* 27(4):E379–E388, 2019.

European Federation of National Associations Working with the Homeless: *ETHOS typology on homelessness and housing exclusion,* 2017. Retrieved February 14, 2021, Available from: https://www.feantsa.org/download/en-16822651433655843804.pdf.

Fédération Européenne d'Associations Nationales Travaillant avec les Sans-Abri AISBL. (FEANTSA): *ETHOS—European typology of homelessness and housing exclusion,* 2021a. Retrieved February 14, 2021, Available from: https://www.feantsa.org/download/en-16822651433655843804.pdf.

Fédération Européenne d'Associations Nationales Travaillant avec les Sans-Abri AISBL. (FEANTSA): *FEANTSA,* 2021b. Retrieved February 14, 2021, Available from: https://www.feantsa.org/en.

Footer K, White R, Park J, Decker M, Lutnick A, Sherman S: Entry to sex trade and long-term vulnerabilities of female sex workers who enter the sex trade before the age of eighteen, *J Urban Health* 97(3):406–417, 2020. https://doi.org/10.1007/s11524-019-00410-z. PMID: 32034655; PMCID: PMC7305278.

Fowler P, Hovmand P, Marcal K, Das S: Solving homelessness from a complex systems perspective: insights for prevention responses, *Annu Rev Publ Health* 40(1):465–486, 2019.

Garland T: *Homelessness and female drug and alcohol addiction,* 2019, Wiley Online Library. Retrieved February 27, 2021, Available from: https://onlinelibrary.wiley.com/doi/abs/10.1002/9781118929803.ewac0274.

Gultekin L, Brush B, Ginier E, Cordom A, Dowdell E: Health risks and outcomes of homelessness in school-age children and youth: a scoping review of the literature, *J Sch Nurs* 36(1):10–18, 2020.

Health Resources and Services Administration: *Glossary,* 2021. Retrieved February 20, 2021, Available from: https://bphc.hrsa.gov/program requirements/compliancemanual/glossary.html.

Health Resources and Services Administration: *Service area overlap: policy and process,* 2018. Retrieved February 20, 2021, Available from: https://bphc.hrsa.gov/programrequirements/policies/pin200709.html.

Homeless Hub: *Potential barriers and challenges to integration of homelessness services,* 2021. Retrieved February 18, 2021, Available from: https://www.homelesshub.ca/solutions/why-do/potential-barriers-and-challenges-integration-homelessness-services.

Housing Development Consortium: *Glossary*, 2021. Retrieved February 27, 2021, Available from: https://www.housingconsortium.org/glossary/#affordable-housing.

HUD.gov: *Housing choice vouchers fact sheet*, 2021. Retrieved February 27, 2021, Available from: www.hud.gov/topics/housing_choice_voucher_program_section_8#:~:text=The%20housing%20choice%20voucher%20program,housing%20in%20the%20private%20market.&text=A%20housing%20subsidy%20is%20paid,behalf%20of%20the%20participating%20family.

Hwang S, Lebow J, Bierer M, O'Connell J, Orav E, Brennan T: Risk factors for death in homeless adults in Boston, *Arch Intern Med* 158:1454—1460, 1998.

James T: *What is upstream healthcare? Boston Medical Center Healthcity Newsletter*, 2020. Retrieved February 26, 2021, Available from: https://www.bmc.org/healthcity/population-health/upstream-healthcare-sdoh-root-causes.

Joint Center for Housing Studies (JCHS) of Harvard University: *State of nation's housing 2020*, 2020. Retrieved February 18, 2021, Available from: https://www.jchs.harvard.edu/sites/default/files/reports/files/Harvard_JCHS_The_State_of_the_Nations_Housing_2020_Report_Revised_120720.pdf.

Kozol J: *Rachel and her children: homeless families in America*, New York, 1988, Crown.

Liu M, Hwang S: Health care for homeless people, *Nat Rev Dis Prim* 7, 2021. https://doi.org/10.1038/s41572-020-00241-2.

Mazzara A: *Rents have risen more than incomes in nearly every state since 2001. Center on Budget and Policy Priorities*, 2019. Retrieved February 19, 2021, Available from: https://www.cbpp.org/blog/rents-have-risen-more-than-incomes-in-nearly-every-state-since-2001.

McKinlay JB: A case for refocusing upstream; the political economy of illness. In Jaco EG, editor: *Patients, physicians, and illness*, ed 3, New York, 1979, Free Press.

McKinlay JB, Marceau LD: To boldly go, *Am J Publ Health* 90(1):25—33, 2000.

Merk A: *The upstream-downstream parable for health equity*, 2018. Salude America! Retrieved February 26, 2021, Available from: https://salud-america.org/the-upstream-downstream-parable-for-health-equity/#:~:text=Public%20health%20advocates%20talk%20about,and%20other%20people%20of%20color.

Minnesota Department of Health Division of Community Health Services: Public health interventions: Applications for nursing practice. In *The Wheel manual*, ed 2. Retrieved February 19, 2021, Available from: https://www.health.state.mn.us/communities/practice/research/phncouncil/wheel.html.

Mission Harbor Behavioral Health: *What's the connection between homelessness and addiction?*, 2021. Retrieved February 19, 2021, Available from: https://sbtreatment.com/homelessness-addiction/.

Mosites E, Parker E, Clarke K, Gaeta J, Baggett T, Imbert E, Sankaran M, Scarborough A, Huster K, Hanson M, Gonzales E, Rauch C, Page L, McMichael T, Keating R, Marx G, Andrews T, Schmit K, Morris S, Dowling N, Peacock G: Assessment of SARS-CoV-2 infection prevalence in homeless shelters—four U.S. cities, March 27—April 15, 2020, *MMWR (Morb Mortal Wkly Rep)* 69:521—522, 2020. https://doi.org/10.15585/mmwr.mm6917e1external icon.

National Alliance to End Homelessness: *Chronically homeless*, 2020. Retrieved February 25, 2021, Available from: https://endhomelessness.org/homelessness-in-america/who-experiences-homelessness/chronically-homeless/.

National Alliance to End Homelessness: *State of homelessness: 2020 edition*, 2020. Retrieved February 22, 2021, Available from: https://endhomelessness.org/homelessness-in-america/homelessness-statistics/state-of-homelessness-2020/.

National Center for Homeless Education at SERVE: *"10 in 10" Orientation Tutorial for New State Coordinators*, 2019. Retrieved July 1, 2022, Available from: https://nche.ed.gov/wp-content/uploads/2019/01/2.pdf.

National Center for Homeless Education: *Education for homeless children and youth program: guide to developing an annual plan for state-level activities*, 2021. Retrieved February 15, 2021, Available from: https://nche.ed.gov/education-for-homeless-children-and-youth-program/.

National Conference of State Legislatures: *Youth homelessness overview*, 2019. Retrieved February 24, 2021, Available from: https://www.ncsl.org/research/human-services/homeless-and-runaway-youth.aspx.

National Institute on Drug Abuse: *Common comorbidities with substance use disorders research report*, 2020. Retrieved February 20, 2021, Available from: https://www.drugabuse.gov/publications/research-reports/common-comorbidities-substance-use-disorders/why-there-comorbidity-between-substance-use-disorders-mental-illnesses.

National Law Center on Homelessness and Poverty: *Breaking the cycle of homelessness: ensuring housing & educational stability for survivors of domestic violence and their children*, 2021. Retrieved February 18, 2021, Available from: https://safehousingpartnerships.org/sites/default/files/2017-01/Breaking%20the%20Cycle%20of%20Homelessness%20-%20Hsg%20and%20Educ%2C%20Stability%20for%20Survivors_0.pdf.

National Low-Income Housing Coalition: *Out of reach 2020*, 2020. Retrieved February 19, 2021, Available from: https://reports.nlihc.org/sites/default/files/oor/OOR_BOOK_2020.pdf.

National Low-Income Housing Coalition: *The problem*, 2021. Retrieved February 19, 2021, Available from: https://nlihc.org/explore-issues/why-we-care/problem.

National Center for Homeless Education: *National overview*, 2021. Retrieved February 15, 2021, Available from: http://profiles.nche.seiservices.com/ConsolidatedStateProfile.aspx.

Partnership for Strong Communities: *Barriers to ending homelessness: from those who experience it*, 2021. Retrieved February 18, 2021, Available from: https://www.pschousing.org/files/RH_ConsumerFeedback_final.pdf.

SchoolHouse Connection: *Unaccompanied youth*, 2020. Retrieved February 15, 2021, Available from: https://schoolhouseconnection.org/learn/unaccompanied-youth/.

Smith MA: The promotion of social justice in healthcare, *Nurs Made Incred Easy* 17(2):26—32, 2019. https://doi.org/10.1097/01.NME.0000553091.78584.a9.

Tarr P: *Homelessness and mental illness: a challenge to our society*, 2018. Retrieved February 20, 2021, Available from: https://www.bbrfoundation.org/blog/homelessness-and-mental-illness-challenge-our-society.

Turning Point of Tampa: *Homelessness and substance use disorder*, 2020. Retrieved February 19, 2021, Available from: https://www.tpoftampa.com/homelessness-and-substance-use-disorder/.

Upshur V, Jenkins D, Weinreb L, Gelberg L, Orvek E: Homeless women's service use, barriers, and motivation for participating in substance use treatment, *Am J Drug Alcohol Abuse* 44(2):252—262, 2018. https://doi.org/10.1080/00952990.2017.1357183.

Urban Indian Health Institute: *Our bodies, our stories*, 2018. Retrieved February 23, 2021, Available from: https://www.uihi.org/resources/our-bodies-our-stories/.

Urban Institute: 2020 poverty projections, Retrieved February 18, 2021, Available from: https://www.urban.org/sites/default/files/publication/102521/2020-poverty-projections.pdf, 2020.

U.S. Census Bureau: *1990 Overview*, 2020. Retrieved February 15, 2021, Available from: https://www.census.gov/history/www/through_the_decades/overview/1990.html.

U.S. Census Bureau: *Health insurance coverage in the United States: 2019*, 2020. Retrieved February 19, 2021, Available from: https://www.census.gov/library/publications/2020/demo/p60-271.html.

U. S. Conference of Mayors: *Make housing more affordable and address homelessness*, 2020. Retrieved February 16, 2021, Available from: https://www.usmayors.org/2020-vision/make-housing-more-affordable-and-address-homelessness/.

U.S. Department of Education: *Education for homeless children and youths grants for state and local activities*, 2021. Retrieved February 14, 2021, Available from: https://www2.ed.gov/programs/homeless/index.html.

U.S. Department of Health and Human Services: *Administration for children & families; family and youth service bureau. Runaway and homeless youth program authorizing legislation*, 2018. Retrieved February 14, 2021, Available from: http://www.acf.hhs.gov/programs/fysb/resource/rhy-act.

U.S. Department of Health and Human Services: *Office of disease prevention and health promotion, Search Healthy People for "social determinants of health"*, 2021. Retrieved February 26, 2021, Available from: https://health.gov/healthypeople/search?query=social%20determinants%20of%20health&f%5B0%5D=content_type%3Ahealthy_people_objective.

U.S. Department of Housing and Urban Development: *Criteria and recordkeeping requirements for definition of homelessness*, 2021. Retrieved February 14, 2021, Available from: https://www.hudexchange.info/resource/1974/criteria-and-recordkeeping-requirements-for-definition-of-homeless/.

U.S. Department of Housing and Urban Development: *Housing CHOICE VOUCHERS FACT Sheet*, 2021. Retrieved February 18, 2021, Available from: https://www.hud.gov/topics/housing_choice_voucher_program_section_8.

U.S. Department of Housing and Urban Development Exchange: *ESG eligible participants*, 2021. Retrieved February 14, 2021, Available from: https://www.hudexchange.info/sites/onecpd/assets/File/ESG-Eligible-Participants-Slides.pdf.

U.S. Department of Housing and Urban Development Exchange. *Continuum of care (CoC) program*, 2021b. Retrieved February 15, 2021, Available from: https://www.hudexchange.info/programs/coc/.

U.S. Department of Housing and Urban Development: office of community planning and development. In *2019 AHAR: part 1—PIT Estimates of Homelessness in the U.S.* Retrieved February 15, 2021, Available from: https://www.hudexchange.info/resource/5948/2019-ahar-part-1-pit-estimates-of-homelessness-in-the-us/.

US Department of Housing, and Urban Development: *AHAR reports*, 2021. Retrieved February 16, 2021, Available from: https://www.hudexchange.info/homelessness-assistance/ahar/#2019-reports.

US Department of Housing and Urban Development HUD Exchange: *CoC homeless populations and subpopulations reports*, 2021. Retrieved February 15, 2021, Available from: https://www.hudexchange.info/programs/coc/coc-homeless-populations-and-subpopulations-reports/?filter_Year=2019&filter_Scope=NatlTerrDC&filter_State=&filter_CoC=&program=CoC&group=PopSub.

US Department of Housing and Urban Development HUD Exchange: *Homelessness assistance*, 2021. Retrieved February 14, 2021, Available from: https://www.hudexchange.info/homelessness-assistance/.

US Department of Housing and Urban Development HUD Exchange: *Homeless emergency assistance and rapid transition to housing act*, 2021. Retrieved February 14, 2021, Available from: https://www.hudexchange.info/homelessness-assistance/hearth-act/.

US Department of Housing and Urban Development HUD Exchange: *Point-in-time count and housing inventory count*, 2021. Retrieved February 15, 2021, Available from: https://www.hudexchange.info/programs/hdx/pit-hic/.

USHUD: *HUD's Definition of Homelessness: resources and Guidance*, 2019. Retrieved July 1, 2022, Available from: https://www.hudexchange.info/news/huds-definition-of-homelessness-resources-and-guidance/.

U.S: *house of representatives; Office of the Law Revision Center: U.S. Code*, 2021. Retrieved February 14, 2021, Available from: https://uscode.house.gov/browse/prelim@title42/chapter119&edition-prelim.

Voices of Youth Count: *Understanding and ending youth homelessness*, 2021. Retrieved February 24, 2021, Available from: https://www.chapinhall.org/project/voices-of-youth-count/.

VolState Community College: *What is the official definition of homelessness?*, 2021. Retrieved February 20, 2021, Available from: https://www.volstate.edu/homelessness.

World Health Organization: *Adolescent and young adult health*, 2021. Retrieved February 24, 2021, Available from: https://www.who.int/news-room/fact-sheets/detail/adolescents-health-risks-and-solutions.

World Health Organization: *Constitution: WHO remains firmly committed to the principles set out in the preamble to the constitution*, 2021. Retrieved February 19, 2021, Available from: www.who.int/about/who-we-are/constitution#:~:text=Health%20is%20a%20state%20of,belief%2C%20economic%20or%20social%20condition.

World Health Organization: *Social determinants of health*, 2021. Retrieved February 25, 2021, Available from: https://www.who.int/health-topics/social-determinants-of-health#tab=tab_1.

FURTHER READING

Centers for Disease Control and Prevention (CDC): *Homelessness and COVID-19 FAQs*, 2020. Retrieved February 22, 2021, Available from: https://www.cdc.gov/coronavirus/2019-ncov/community/homeless-shelters/faqs.html.

Rural and Migrant Health

Patricia L. Thomas and Carol G. Enderle

OBJECTIVES

Upon completion of this chapter, the reader will be able to do the following:

1. Compare and contrast characteristics of rural and urban communities.
2. Describe features of the healthcare system and population characteristics common to rural aggregates.
3. Discuss the impact of structural and personal barriers on the health of rural aggregates.
4. Identify factors that place farmers and migrant workers at risk for illness and accidents.
5. Discuss the importance of the informal care network to rural health and social services.
6. Describe the characteristics of rural community health nursing practice.
7. Apply an upstream perspective to health promotion and illness prevention for rural and migrant populations.
8. Discuss rural health policy and relevant resources

OUTLINE

KEY TERMS

collaborative leadership
community health
disparities

frontier
healthy people 2030
metropolitan

migrant
pesticide
post-acute

rural   seasonal   urban
rural nursing   upstream

RURAL UNITED STATES

There are many different versions of rural America, in that each rural area is somewhat unique but shares certain features with other rural regions. Geographic, demographic, environmental, economic, and social factors all influence health, access to health care, and quality of health care. When aggregated, these characteristics may be contrasted with those of **urban** populations. In this section, we present a "snapshot" of rural populations and health characteristics that contribute to challenging health **disparities** for many of the people living in the most rural areas of America.

Although the urban growth rate has been steadily climbing since 1890, with numbers of urban dwellers surpassing those in rural areas around 1920, the number of rural residents is the highest in the country's history. Until 2016, nonmetro populations had seen steady declines but slight growth (33,000 people) was experienced between July 2016 and June 2017. Metro areas grew by 0.82% where nonmetro areas grew by 0.07%. This was the first period of growth in 6 years after steady decline between 2010 and 2016 in the United States as a whole (USDA, 2020a).

Populations stabilized after 2014 in nonmetro populations after years of decline likely related to improved rural employment growth. The postrecession recovery for rural populations has been slower and more gradual compared to previous recessions (USDA, 2019a). Current census estimates are that 17.5% of the nation's elderly and more than 16% of the nation's poor live in rural areas. Rural residents have long been thought to be family farmers and ranchers, but today, rural America is a diverse and important marketplace to marketers of consumer products, and demographers and economists consider trends in farm and farm-related employment much more broadly. They characterize agriculture as a "food and fiber system" that encompasses all aspects of agriculture, from core materials sectors (farm, food processing, textiles, and other manufacturing) to wholesale and retail trade and the food service sector (USDA, National Institute of Food and Agriculture, 2020b). Despite the shrinking number of family farms and full-time farmers, agriculture continues to be an important part of the rural and U.S. economy, with agriculture-related employment representing 5.2% of the gross domestic product (GDP) and farms representing 0.5% of the GDP.

Poverty, a key health determinant, continues to be greater in rural America than in urban areas. Whereas the nonmetropolitan population had a poverty rate of 16%, the metropolitan poverty rate was 13% in 2018, and child poverty rates were 23% nonmetropolitan and 19% metropolitan (U.S. Department of Agriculture, ERS, Poverty Overview, 2020). This overall gap may not seem large, but when the degree of rurality or the poverty rate for particular subpopulations (e.g., minorities, children under 18 years of age, or the elderly) are examined, the

gap increases. In 2019, poverty rates declined to the lowest point overall at 10.5% since the inception of its measurement in 1959. That said, the gains were not even for all groups. While non-Hispanic whites and Asians had a 7.3% poverty rate, non-Hispanic black populations were at 18.8% and Hispanic populations were at 15.7% (U.S. Census Bureau, 2020a,b,c,d,e). See Box 24.1 for the 2020 U.S. Department of Health and Human Services' (DHHS) Poverty Guidelines.

Not only is the economic base shifting but the age composition is as well. For the first time in decades, 2010 to 2014 showed a decline in nonmetropolitan populations, stabilizing in 2015. Younger people are leaving rural areas for jobs in urban centers, so that those who remain behind are increasingly older and isolated and have diminished access to health care. Recent demographic changes in rural areas identify the 18% of rural areas are 65 and older and 2% are 85 and older (Rural Health Information Hub, Rural Aging, 2018). Three trends—aging in place, outmigration of young adults, and immigration of older

BOX 24.1   The 2020 U.S. Department of Health and Human Services Poverty Guidelines

In concept, the U.S. Department of Health and Human Services (DHHS) determines the poverty guidelines by estimating the minimum income level needed by a family or individual to just meet the basic needs of food, shelter, clothing, and other essential goods and services. Official poverty guidelines adjusted for family size and composition are set by DHHS for use by all federal agencies to determine financial eligibility for certain federal programs (e.g., Medicaid). Some programs (e.g., State Children's Health Insurance Program) also use multiples of the guidelines to determine eligibility of participants. For example, participants may be eligible for programs if they are classified as being at or near poverty, with poverty being defined as 100%, and near poverty as 125% or 150% of the poverty level. Poverty guidelines are adjusted periodically by DHHS to reflect price changes and are published in the *Federal Register*. As required by law, this update is accomplished by increasing the latest published Census Bureau poverty thresholds by the relevant percentage change in the Consumer Price Index for All Urban Consumers (CPI–U). The guidelines in this 2020 notice reflect the 1.8% price increase between calendar years 2018 and 2019. After this inflation adjustment, the guidelines are rounded and adjusted to standardize the differences between family sizes. The 2020 guidelines reflect just the size of the "persons in family/household" rather than the family unit or composition. The poverty level for persons in a family/household of one in the contiguous 48 states, for example, was $12,760; it was $26,200 for a family unit of four and $44,120 for a family of eight. Each household's cash income (including pretax income and cash welfare assistance, but excluding in-kind welfare assistance, such as food stamps and Medicare) is compared with the poverty line for the household.

Modified from U.S. Department of Health and Human Services; Federal Register: *Annual Update of the HHS Poverty Guidelines*, 2020d. Available from: https://www.federalregister.gov/documents/2020/01/17/2020-00858/annual-update-of-the-hhs-poverty-guidelines.

persons from metro areas—present challenges to already stressed communities that must provide adequate health care, housing, transportation, and other human services (Rural Health Information Hub, Rural Aging, 2018).

The rural population is also becoming more ethnically diverse. Generations ago, many families began farming when they came to the United States as European immigrants. In the 1990s, new immigrants began buying and operating their own small family farms, and others found employment in rural agriculture and manufacturing. Today, more than one half of rural Hispanics live outside the Southwest, and "high-growth Hispanic counties" are mostly in the South and Midwest (U.S. Census Bureau, 2019a,b,c).

Policies and programs developed to close the health disparities gap must take a population health view of the special circumstances of rural life. Although 75% of U.S. counties are classified as rural, they contain only 15% of the U.S. population (CDC, 2017a,b,c).

Members of rural populations also are more likely to be older, to be less educated, to live in poverty, to lack health insurance, and to experience a lack of available health care providers and access to health care (Farrigan and Parker, 2012; RHIHub, 2019d). Access Only 10% of U.S. physicians practice in rural counties, and the ratio of physicians in rural population size is 40 per 100,000 people, compared to 53 per 100,000 people in urban settings (National Rural Health Association [NRHA], 2021).

Rural residents more often assess their health as fair or poor and have more disability days associated with acute conditions than their urban counterparts. Rural people also tend to have more problems related to negative health behaviors (e.g., untreated mental illness; obesity; and alcohol, tobacco, and drug use) that contribute to excess deaths and chronic disease and disability rates. The literature suggests, for example, that the highest death rates for children and young adults are in the most rural counties. Residents of rural areas are nearly twice as likely to die from unintentional injuries, including motor vehicle accidents, then urban residents (NRHA, 2021).

Noting a prominent and persistent pattern of risky health behaviors in rural dwellers, McClelland et al. (2010) suggested "rural culture" may itself be a key determinant of health in rural communities and that these behaviors vary along the rural–urban continuum and within rural populations by geographical areas. A decade later, this persists (NRHA, 2021; Probst et al., 2016). These behaviors, including unintentional injury, smoking, and suicide, are discussed in more detail in the section titled "Composition: Health Disparities Related to Persons."

Defining Rural Populations

Multiple definitions of rural populations have been formulated to describe the characteristics of areas with low population density. Previous definitions have simply included either those towns with a population of less than 2500 or towns located in open country as **rural**. This definition has often been further differentiated into the subcategories farm and rural nonfarm. A second classification of interest used the term *rural* for

populations with fewer than 45 persons per square mile and the term **frontier** for geographical areas with fewer than six persons per square mile (Rural Assistance Center, n.d.). Many counties of the Great Plains, Intermountain West, and Alaska are designated as frontier.

The rural–urban continuum distinguishes counties by population and adjacency to metropolitan areas. Residences can range from small towns to large metropolitan areas. Statistical reporting has been in use since 1990 with the term *metropolitan statistical areas (MSAs)* used to differentiate nonmetropolitan and **metropolitan** areas. In June 2003, the Office of Management and Budget (OMB) released a new classification scheme to better reflect trends in population distribution across the nation (OMB, 2021). The MSA designation has been replaced by county-level *Core Based Statistical Areas (CBSAs)* to simplify the multilevel designations. Within CBSAs, *metropolitan areas* are those counties that contain at least one urbanized area (UA) of 50,000 or more people. A micropolitan area contains a cluster of 10,000 to 50,000 persons. Counties that are neither metropolitan nor micropolitan are called "outside CBSAs," also known as *noncore areas* (U.S. Census, 2013, 2017, 2019, 2021).

Describing Rural Health and Populations

Rural populations differ in complex geographical, social, and economic ways. Although older, poorer, and less educated people are usually overrepresented in rural areas, this finding may not apply to all rural areas or to everyone in a particular rural area.

The health profiles discussed here are shared by rural areas in general and may be contrasted with overall patterns of health, health habits, and health care in urban settings. However, the reader should note that it is difficult to interpret differences between urban health and rural health. First, statistically significant differences between urban and rural health indicators may seem small when data are aggregated to "rural areas" in general. The differences tend to become larger when data are available for particular rural areas (e.g., certain counties), particular rural subgroups (e.g., minorities), or specific characteristics (e.g., percentage of uninsured children). Second, heterogeneity of race, age, economic status, regional distribution, and cultural groupings makes health data for rural populations useful only as estimates of individual health. For example, in 2018, about 16.1% of people in nonmetro areas compared to 13.1% of people in metro areas had income below the poverty level in the United States. This is contrasted with 2010 when the metro and nonmetro populations represented 15% and 16%, respectively. In 2018, nonmetro children in poverty were 22% for compared to 17% metro children. https://www.ers.usda.gov/topics/rural-economy-population/rural-poverty-well-being/#historic.

The family poverty rate in 2019 was 10.5% (representing the fifth consecutive year of decline) and a 1.5% decrease from 2018 estimates (U.S. Census Bureau, 2020a,b,c,d,e).

Infant mortality, a major health status indicator, varies greatly by geographical area, even within rural areas, and dramatizes the importance of both contextual and compositional data. The infant mortality rate 2017 to 2018 was six infants per 1000 live births. In rural and micropolitan locations the infant mortality rate was 6.8 and 6.4 per 1000 births contrasted with 5.6 per 1000 in metropolitan areas. The infant mortality rate also differs with race. In 2017 to 2018 the non-Hispanic-Black infant mortality was 11 per 1000 births, nine per 1000 for American Indian/Alaska Native non-Hispanic, and five per 1000 Hispanic (Forum on Child and Family Statistics, 2020).

Examination of the infant mortality rate comparisons between rural and urban areas noted stark differences. The overall infant mortality rate was 2.1 per 1000 births across the U.S in 2018. Infant mortality in high poverty locations was twice that of low poverty locations. Neonatal mortality was 38% higher and postnatal mortality was 37% higher in high poverty locations. In addition to poverty, mortality increased with mothers who had less than high school education, unmarried, non-Hispanic Black or Hispanic families with low access to prenatal care (Mohamoud et al., 2019). Mohamoud et al. (2019) also identified that infant deaths also increase with rurality.

The 2018 infant mortality in the United States was 5.7 per 1000 births. The rate of infant deaths for non-Hispanic Black Americans was 10.8, more than twice that of Whites, Asians, and Hispanics (4.6, 3.6, and 4.9 respectively) per 1000 births (CDC, 2020a,b,c,d; infant mortality, Mohamed et al., 2019) identified that infant deaths increase with rurality.

One needs to also consider the health disparities that exist among rural racial and ethnic minorities. Although limited because the phenomenon has only recently been studied, research findings support the conclusion that rural racial and ethnic minorities—Native Americans, Alaska Natives, Hispanics/Latinos, and African Americans—concentrated in the South and West are more disadvantaged relative not only to rural majority members but also to urban racial and ethnic minorities. The disparities include employment, income, education, health insurance, mortality, morbidity, and access to health care (Healthy People 2020 Disparities, 2010, Healthy People 2020, n.d. -a, Healthy People, 2030, n.d. -b).

Because population numbers are small, national rural data, limited as they are, can only suggest the health needs of a particular area, racial or ethnic mix, or age distribution, for example. Program planners still need to determine whether certain health or health care delivery problems apply to their specific service area. Useful data sources include state-, county-, and census tract—level data on health and demographics available from state and federal government agencies, such as those cited in the References at the end of this chapter. In planning for health-related programs, nurses can also gather community-level data from healthcare providers, local records, focus groups, and older residents who know the area's history.

RURAL HEALTH

Minority Health and Healthy People 2030

Healthy People 2030 represents the health promotion and disease prevention agenda for the nation (U.S. Department of Health and Human Services [USDHHS], Office of Disease Prevention and Health Promotion, n.d.-b) Additionally, Healthy People 2030 is the United States' contribution to the World Health Organization "Health for All" program. The framework for Healthy People 2030 *is based on the* Healthy People 2020 *priorities and represents a streamlining and consolidation of objectives for clarity and less redundancy. The Healthy People plans were* developed through public consensus, builds on the national health program established since the 1980s (U.S. Department of Health and Human Services, n.d.). It has the broad goals of increasing quality of life and years of life, eliminating disparities in health among different population groups, and improving access to preventive health services.

Healthy People 2030 is an evidence-based, 10-year plan with the goal to "attain high-quality, longer lives free of preventable disease, disability, injury, and premature death." Every 10 years, the plan and goals are updated and revised. Achieving the goals will accomplish health equity, elimination of disparities, and improvement of the health of all groups through social and physical environments to promote quality of life, healthy development, and healthy behaviors across all life stages (Bolin and Bellamy, n.d., Healthy People, 2030, n.d.). The challenges are great, but public health professionals and planners in every state have a plan patterned on *Healthy People* goals to direct their efforts.

RURAL HEALTH DISPARITIES: CONTEXT AND COMPOSITION

To improve understanding of the health of populations and health disparities, there is a growing emphasis on the distinction between context, which is defined by the characteristics of places of residence, and composition, which is the collective health effects that result from a concentration of persons with certain characteristics. Most public health problems include elements of both context and composition, though they may be predominantly one or the other. The Centers for Disease Control is the primary public health organization in the United States and, working with its partners, focuses on factors leading to health disparities among racial, ethnic, geographic, and socioeconomic barriers (CDC Health Disparities, 2020a, CDC Social Determinants of Health, 2020c). The CDC recognizes health disparities and inequalities exist and highlight disparities are demonstrated across diseases, behavioral risk factors, exposures, social determinants of care, and healthcare access by sex, race and ethnicity, income, education, disability status, and other social characteristics (CDC Health Disparities, CDC Social Determinants of Health, 2020c). It is noteworthy that rural health, particularly for children, identified mental, behavioral, and developmental disorders begin early in childhood affecting lifelong health and well-being. People in rural areas report more health-related disparities, including less access to health resources, poorer health, and more health risk behaviors, than counterparts in urban areas (Robinson et al., 2017).

Health issues in rural areas are contextual when they derive from characteristics of place. Characteristics of place include not only natural features of geography and environment but also the political, social, and economic institutions that build and support communities within a given geographical area. For example, limited economic opportunities, low wages, or agricultural accidents might be considered to have contextual effects on the health of populations. Problems in rural areas are compositional when they derive from individual characteristics of groups of people residing in rural settings. Examples of compositional sources of health disparities include such characteristics as age, education, income, ethnicity, and health behaviors.

Consideration of both context and composition enables us to take a more deliberate and refined approach to study, plan programs for, and deliver health care services to rural populations. Although the overall health of rural Americans is worse than that of urban Americans, the relationship between rurality and health is not necessarily linear. Many differences exist among rural areas in both the nature and extent of health problems. Furthermore, some rural populations share more in common with people in urban core areas than with people in other rural areas. Effective planning depends on understanding and documenting needs that take into account context, composition, and their interaction. The next section presents data for problems of both contextual and compositional sources of health disparities in rural America.

Context: Health Disparities Related to Place

Regardless of their diverse demographic and geographical attributes, rural groups share certain health patterns, difficulties, and delays in obtaining health care (see Ethical Insights box). Many of the contextual issues that contribute to rural health disparities are described in the introduction to the chapter ("Rural United States"). Many rural regions that are already sparsely populated are losing residents, a process that often triggers a downward spiral. People leave and services are lost; the local drugstore closes; the tax base will not support an ambulance service, so most seriously ill persons must be transported long distances to get health care; jobs become scarce and younger people leave the area. Retirees may be attracted to the lower costs, but they need public health and other services that must be provided by counties without the tax base to support them. Racial and ethnic minorities are migrating to rural areas to find employment opportunities. Structural, financial, and personal barriers to accessing health care services exist in all environments, but rural residents are unique in how they experience structural barriers.

Access to Care

Rural health leaders have identified 10 priorities for health care in rural America, with access to and affordability of care topping the list. Because most people in rural America are selfemployed or part of small businesses, insurance tied to employment will not serve them (Bailey, 2009; U.S. Census Bureau, 2019a). In 2019, rural populations were less likely to have insurance than their urban counterparts. Those in mostly

rural and completely rural lacked insurance 11.3% and 12.3% of the time and those without insurance in urban settings was 11.3% (Cheeseman-Day, 2019).

Agency for Healthcare Research and Quality (AHRQ) published the *National Healthcare Quality and Disparities Report: Chartbook on Rural Health Care* (2017b), *a comprehensive overview of healthcare in the U.S. population and disparities experienced by different* racial, ethnic, and socioeconomic groups. The report assesses and evaluates health delivery using over 250 indicators centered on three focus areas: access to health care, quality of health care, and priorities of the National Quality Strategy (NQS). For rural populations, the quality of healthcare services improved from 2000 to 2015 but the pace of improvement varied by priority area:

- Person-Centered Care: About 80% of measures improved overall.
- Patient Safety: Almost two-thirds of measures improved overall.
- Healthy Living: About 60% of measures improved overall.
- Effective Treatment: More than half of measures improved overall.
- Care Coordination: About half of measures improved overall.
- Care Affordability: About 70% of measures did not change.

Overall, disparities were smaller but persist particularly for poor and uninsured populations in all priority areas. Twenty percent of the measures showed improvements for Blacks and Hispanics, but more than half of measures showed poor and low-income households (about 40%) had worse care than other income groups. Nearly two-thirds of the measures show that uninsured people had worse care than privately insured people (AHRQ, 2017b).

Primary Care. Rural areas have fewer primary care physicians than urban areas, fueling concerns about inadequate access and gaps in U.S. healthcare equity in many rural areas. Several improvements have been made since the inception of the Affordable Care Act (ACA) in 2010 through training grants, reimbursement modifications, expanded scope of practice for nurse practitioners (NPs) in select states, and Medicaid expansion. Despite these efforts, the disparities for access to and availability of primary care providers still exist.

About 20% of the U.S. population lives in rural areas, yet only 10% of the nation's physicians practice in a rural area. This is a contributing factor for the higher death rates, disabilities, and chronic conditions rural populations experience compared with urban populations. "Of the 2050 rural U.S. counties, 77% are designated as health professional shortage areas (HPSAs). Notably, nearly 30% of rural primary care practitioners are at or nearing retirement age, and those under 40 account for 20% of the current rural workforce. Existing shortages coupled with replacement requirements for retirees escalate concerns regarding equitable care for rural populations. As a result of the ACA, an additional five million rural Americans (16%) will have health insurance coverage by 2019, so when combined with demands of an aging population, an already burdened rural healthcare delivery system will be stretched further.

ETHICAL INSIGHTS

Racial and Ethnic Disparities in Health Care

Because public health is a societal approach to protecting and promoting health that usually acts through social rather than individual means (Sorrell, 2012; Fields, 2015), many of the most pressing ethical dilemmas are considered in public domains. Perhaps no more important ethical challenge facing our public today revolves around the just distribution of healthcare resources. With the enactment of the Patient Protection and Affordability Act, ethical concerns persist related to access to care, the underserved, and coverage. Recently, this discussion has encompassed private-public insurance programs and the ethical questions remain (Sorrell, 2012; Fields, 2015).

For example, in 2019 there were 27.5 million people or 8.5% of the U.S. population was uninsured (U.S. Census Bureau, 2019a,b,c). People living in rural areas represented about 12% of the uninsured (Cheeseman-Day, 2019). Of the uninsured living in rural areas, poverty was a confounding variable. Keith (2018) identified statistically significant drops in insurance coverage based on family status, geography (urban vs. rural), race, and immigration status. Notably, there were also statistically significant decreases in coverage rates irrespective of full or part time employment, marital status, educational level, and disability status. The uninsured distribution by race in 2019 was 13.6% of Blacks, 7.4% of Asians, and 9.8% of non-Hispanic whites. Hispanics had the highest uninsured rate at 27% up from a historic low of 16.9% in Statista and Elflein (2019). These individuals were also often poor with 18.8% of Blacks, Hispanics 15.7%, 7.3% for Asians and non-Hispanic whites living in poverty level (U.S. Census Bureau, 2020b). While there were improvements compared to previous decades, the rates remained high. These data may help explain why minorities are more likely to not seek care, use less prenatal care, and make fewer visits to physicians.

Differences in care resulting from patient or care process-level variables (e.g., patient attitudes, preferences or expectations, provider bias, stereotyping, or uncertainty) are problems of professional ethics. Disparities in care resulting from system-level variables, such as financing, accessibility, and geographical location, are problems of justice (Institute of Medicine [IOM], 2001; Rural Health Information Hub, Rural Health Disparities, 2019f). Subsequently, solutions for justice issues in disparities in care require public discourse aimed at solving system-level problems.

From an ethical perspective, the theory of justice as fairness was formulated to specify terms of social cooperation that are "fair" and ensure that people of equal basic liberties have equal opportunity (Daniels et al., 1999). The Civil Rights Act of 1964 specifically bars discrimination in health care for all entities that receive federal funds, and both the American Nurses Association (ANA) and American Medical Association codes of ethics endorse the principle of justice. However, despite overall agreement that justice is an important practice concept, difficulty arises in implementing changes in the health system to address disparities in care. Recently, growing interest in health inequities in vulnerable populations and recognition of social determinants of health have highlighted how justice and social justice in nursing could be a lever to address long-standing disparities (Garrigues, 2021; Healthy People 2030).

Solutions to disparities in care were suggested by the IOM (2003) and include the following policy, health system, and patient education and empowerment interventions:

Policy Interventions

1. Medical care financing should discourage fragmentation of health care into separate tiers of providers who adhere to different standards of care and serve separate racial and ethnic minority segments of society. Government programs that require enrollment in managed care should be prepared to pay plans at rates comparable to those paid to plans for privately insured patients.
2. Strengthen the stability of patient–provider relationships in publicly funded health plans and create policy to create consistency, limit patient loads for providers, and provide reasonable time allowances for initial and follow-up visits.
3. Increase the proportion of underrepresented U.S. racial and ethnic minorities among health professionals.
4. Apply the same managed care protections to publicly funded health maintenance organization (HMO) enrollees that apply to private HMO enrollees.
5. Provide greater resources to the USDHHS Office for Civil Rights to enforce civil rights laws.

Health Systems Interventions

1. Promote the consistency and equity of care through evidence-based guidelines. These guidelines should be published to allow public and professional scrutiny.
2. Construct payment systems to enhance available services to minority patients, and limit provider incentives that may promote disparities.
3. Enhance patient–provider communication and trust by providing financial incentives for practices that reduce barriers.
4. Support the use of interpretation services where community need exists.
5. Institute programs that use community health workers among medically underserved and racial and ethnic minority populations.
6. Support greater use of multidisciplinary treatment and preventive care teams to improve and streamline care for racial and ethnic minority patients.

Patient Education and Empowerment Interventions

1. Implement patient education programs to increase patients' knowledge of how to access care and participate in treatment decisions.

With the enactment of the Patient Protection and Affordability Act, improvements have been made related to care access and Medicaid expansion; however, issues persist related to equity.

Recommendations for scholarships, loan repayment, focused recruitment for rural practitioners, and medical residencies in rural health are being considered. Today, nonphysician primary care practitioners (NPs and physician assistants) make up nearly half (46%) the providers in rural federally qualified health centers (National Conference of State Legislatures, n.d.). In a joint statement, the NRHA and the American Academy of Family Physicians said medicine has become specialized, centralized, and urban and challenged educators to be responsive to the needs of rural underserved communities (AAFP, 2013).

Availability of providers and healthcare facilities in rural areas is an important determinant of the quality of the health care delivery system and the likelihood of positive health outcomes for rural residents. McQueen et al. (2017) identified fewer than 12% of providers practice in rural locations. Further, the National Rural Health Association (2021) identified the shortage of primary care providers in rural versus urban locations is highlighted in the patient to provider ratios. In rural areas there 40 physicians for every 100,000 people were in urban areas there are 53. Compounded by less density in population, the access to care concerns becomes amplified. A good example of the lack of specialists is the lack of mental health services available for rural dwellers of any age. The incidence of mental illness in rural areas is the same as that of urban areas, but there is far less access to mental health services in rural areas. Additionally, primary care doctors, nurses, and physician assistants, rather than mental health specialists, provide most of the mental health care in rural regions (RHIHub, 2019a—h). Medicare beneficiaries saw a physician assistant or NP for all (17%) or some (24%) of their primary care in 2012 (National Conference of State Legislatures, n.d.).

General Health Services. A study by the National Academy of Medicine (NAM), formerly called the Institute of Medicine (IOM), reported rural medical access problems in these areas, with some hospital and pharmacy closures, greater distances to travel for physician services, and limited (if any) choice of providers (IOM, 2005). Lack of local access to primary care and health care facilities forces rural residents to either go without or travel long distances—often over rural roads in dangerous weather conditions—to access needed care. Access to health care may become a particularly challenging and expensive proposition for the elderly who do not drive and depend on limited public transportation. Geography, health care costs, and lack of available services also are contextual problems that keep many rural adults and children from obtaining needed primary, secondary, and tertiary preventive services.

Health Insurance. With economic decline and rising costs of health care, health insurance—or, more importantly, the lack of health insurance—for Americans has become a major issue for the health of the nation. An estimated 25.7 million people were without health insurance in 2018 compared to 45.7 million in 2010 (U.S. Census Bureau, 2011, 2018). While gains have been made, significant work remains.

As with poverty and unemployment data, insurance coverage varied with race and ethnicity coverage in 2007, as did age and residence (rural or urban). For example, 10.4% of non-Hispanic whites, 19.5% of Blacks, and 16.8% of Asians were uninsured for all or part of 2007; young adults were more likely to lack health insurance than older persons; and 18% of poor or near-poor children lacked coverage (U.S. Census Bureau, 2012). Lack of insurance coverage was greatest in the South (14.2%) and West regions (12%), and in general, rural residents were more likely than urban residents to lack insurance (20% vs. 17%) (IOM, 2005). In 2018 there were notable gains across race and ethnicity. Rates of uninsured Hispanics was 19%, followed by Blacks 11.5%, Asians 6.8% and non-Hispanic whites at 7.5% (Artiga et al., 2020). About 18% of the persons living in rural counties were at the poverty level, with 14% of rural children living in poverty (USDA, 2016).

The impact of health insurance and decision making related to healthcare practices since the Patient Protection and Affordability Act of 2010 demonstrate improvements for states with Medicaid expansion and dire outcomes for rural hospitals. What is known is that the number of uninsured patients nationwide has decreased. However, 2019 represented the worst year for rural hospitals. It brought the highest number of rural hospital closures with 19 rural hospitals closing. In the last

decade more than 120 rural hospitals have closed. Medicaid expansion has been beneficial, but 14 states chose not to expand Medicaid and the impact was immense on those living in rural areas. Nearly two-thirds of uninsured people in rural areas live in states that did not expand Medicaid coverage (Scott, 2020). Additionally, the linkage of provider influence on health promotion and health literacy cannot be assumed. Although early research points to a strong relationship among health insurance status, chronic illnesses, and poverty, Benitez and Seiber (2018) noted gains for rural Americans in Medicaid expansion states after the Patient Protection and Affordability Act was implemented. While rural areas improved at rates higher than urban counterparts, there is room for improvement with the most rural areas. Rural people are often employed in industries characterized by seasonal work, economic uncertainty and decline, high unemployment risk, and occupational accidents and death (e.g., agriculture, mining, forestry, and fisheries). Rural industries are often small and offer low wages, thereby contributing to the growing number of uninsured rural families. Farm families also tend to be two-parent households, so they are less likely to qualify for Medicaid, even with incomes below the federal poverty level. Unlike the uninsured population nationally, individuals in rural areas face challenges in accessing care related to transportation and workforce shortages in providers (Rural Health Information Hub, 2019a—h).

Health insurance has been identified as one of the 10 leading health indicators because it is generally a reliable predictor of overall health status (Bailey, 2009; Center on Budget and Policy Priorities, 2012; Sommer et al., 2017). Public health professionals and health planners are most concerned with the impact of increasing numbers of uninsured children. In 2019, the overall percentage of children who were uninsured was 5.7% per million which works out to 726,000 children in the United States. While the lowest rate of uninsured children in a 3-year period 2016 to 2019, was 3.6% per million in 2016, this rate has steadily increased over the last 3 years. 2017 saw 4.1% per million and 2018 had 4.1% per million. The uninsured rate of children in 2008 was 7.6% per million and declined annually until 2015 in large part because of state programs.

However, rural children are still uninsured at a higher rate than the national average and urban counterparts. Disproportionate high rates of uninsured children occur in the south with the Midwest and West also seeing increases (Alker and Corcoran, 2020). In the absence of health insurance, poverty becomes an even more powerful predictor of poor health for all age groups and particularly for children.

In 1997, the State Children's Health Insurance Program was enacted to improve health insurance coverage of children less than 19 years of age in poor and near-poor families (see the "Legislation and Programs Affecting Rural Public Health" section in this chapter). In the years following passage of this program, the overall percentage of children who were uninsured declined. Health insurance coverage of children as well as adults varies from state to state and is influenced by employment patterns, the percentage of children in the population, state Medicaid policies, poverty levels, and racial and ethnic composition.

Composition: Health Disparities Related to Persons

To review, health problems in rural areas are compositional when they result from a concentration of persons with certain characteristics. Examples of compositional sources of health disparities include such characteristics as income, health behaviors, education, occupation, gender, and ethnicity. In the *Rural Healthy People 2020* survey, 80% of respondents listed access to health care as the top rural health priority (Bolin and Bellamy, n.d., Healthy People 2020). Additional priorities listed by respondents as leading health problems are largely compositional but may also have a contextual dimension. For example, problems such as obesity, chronic pulmonary disease, and higher levels of infant mortality have a strong compositional component because their variation is related to the health behaviors and the educational, socioeconomic, racial, and ethnic characteristics of the rural groups. The variation may also be contextual, because the groups have fewer educational opportunities, have low-wage jobs, lack insurance, or have genetic propensities for certain health problems. The Healthy People 2030 disparities and defines these attributes as social determinants of health and health literacy (Healthy People 2030, n.d.).

Income and Poverty

Income, education, and type of employment help determine socioeconomic status, and in the aggregate, rural dwellers have lower educational levels, higher unemployment rates, higher poverty rates, and lower income levels than urban aggregates (Healthy People 2020, Social Determinants). The poverty rate is one of the most important indicators of the health and well-being of all Americans, regardless of where they live (see Ethical Insights box).

The U.S. Department of Agriculture's ERS tracks economic trends and demographic characteristics of rural dwellers to help develop policies and services. In the most recent report, the ERS reported the number of people living in nonmetro counties had increased slightly in 2016 to 2017 ending a six-year trend of declining populations. The growth rate gap between rural and urban narrowed slightly but remain with 0.07% growth in nonmetro areas and 0.82% growth in metro areas. Employment and populations in rural areas have also stabilized. The population of rural counties was 46.1 million representing 14% of the U.S. population (USDA, ERS, 2020).

In 2018, the nonmetro poverty rate was 16.1% compared to 12.6% in metro areas. The nonmetro poverty rate has decreased 2.3% since the peak of 18.4% in 2013. This decline represents one million fewer rural residents in poverty in just 5 years. Metro poverty rates declined at a higher rate between 2013 and 2018, resulting in increase of the metro-nonmetro poverty rate gap of 3.5 percentage points in 2018 (ERDS, Rural Poverty and Wellbeing) (Fig. 24.1 and Table 24.1). As noted earlier in this section, however, data averaged across all rural counties in the United States do not give planners and providers much information about their own counties, or even regions. The following discussion gives examples of available data that can be used to make an analysis of local and regional conditions and characteristics.

Regional Differences. Consistent with the idea that there are many rural Americas in rural America, rural poverty varies by

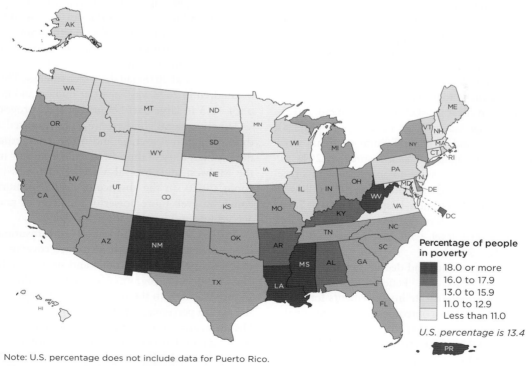

Note: U.S. percentage does not include data for Puerto Rico.

Fig. 24.1 Individuals Below the Poverty Level by State. (From U.S. Census Bureau. (2017). Available at: https://www.census.gov.)

TABLE 24.1 Percentage of Population in Poverty by State (2019)

| | ALL PEOPLE IN POVERTY (2019) | | | CHILDREN AGES 0–17 IN POVERTY (2019) | | |
| | 90% CONFIDENCE INTERVAL OF ESTIMATE | | | 90% CONFIDENCE INTERVAL OF ESTIMATE | | |
Name	Percent	Lower Bound	Upper Bound	Percent	Lower Bound	Upper Bound
Alabama	15.6	15.2	16.0	21.9	21.1	22.7
Alaska	10.2	9.6	10.8	13.2	12.2	14.2
Arizona	13.5	13.2	13.8	19.2	18.4	20.0
Arkansas	16.0	15.6	16.4	21.7	20.8	22.6
California	11.8	11.7	11.9	15.6	15.3	15.9
Colorado	9.4	9.1	9.7	11.2	10.5	11.9
Connecticut	9.9	9.6	10.2	13.5	12.7	14.3
Delaware	11.2	10.6	11.8	16.3	15.2	17.4
District of Columbia	14.1	13.2	15.0	20.8	17.6	24.0
Florida	12.7	12.5	12.9	18.2	17.6	18.8
Georgia	13.5	13.2	13.8	19.5	18.8	20.2
Hawaii	9.0	8.5	9.5	11.2	10.1	12.3
Idaho	11.0	10.5	11.5	12.7	11.8	13.6
Illinois	11.4	11.2	11.6	15.6	15.1	16.1
Indiana	11.9	11.6	12.2	15.1	14.4	15.8
Iowa	11.0	10.6	11.4	12.8	12.1	13.5
Kansas	11.3	11.0	11.6	14.3	13.6	15.0
Kentucky	16.0	15.6	16.4	20.9	20.1	21.7
Louisiana	18.8	18.4	19.2	26.4	25.5	27.3
Maine	10.9	10.4	11.4	13.8	12.9	14.7
Maryland	9.1	8.9	9.3	12.3	11.6	13.0
Massachusetts	9.5	9.3	9.7	12.0	11.3	12.7
Michigan	12.9	12.7	13.1	17.5	16.9	18.1
Minnesota	8.9	8.7	9.1	11.0	10.4	11.6
Mississippi	19.5	19.0	20.0	27.6	26.5	28.7
Missouri	12.9	12.6	13.2	17.0	16.4	17.6
Montana	12.6	12.1	13.1	15.4	14.4	16.4
National	12.3	12.2	12.4	16.8	16.6	17.0
Nebraska	9.9	9.5	10.3	11.5	10.7	12.3
Nevada	12.7	12.3	13.1	17.6	16.7	18.5
New Hampshire	7.5	7.0	8.0	8.1	7.2	9.0
New Jersey	9.1	8.9	9.3	12.2	11.6	12.8
New Mexico	17.5	17.0	18.0	23.5	22.4	24.6
New York	13.1	12.9	13.3	18.2	17.7	18.7
North Carolina	13.6	13.4	13.8	19.3	18.7	19.9
North Dakota	10.5	9.9	11.1	10.9	9.9	11.9
Ohio	13.0	12.8	13.2	18.1	17.5	18.7
Oklahoma	15.1	14.8	15.4	19.7	19.1	20.3
Oregon	11.5	11.2	11.8	13.6	12.8	14.4
Pennsylvania	12.0	11.8	12.2	16.5	15.9	17.1
Rhode Island	11.6	11.0	12.2	16.5	15.3	17.7
South Carolina	13.9	13.5	14.3	19.9	19.1	20.7
South Dakota	11.9	11.4	12.4	14.9	13.9	15.9
Tennessee	13.8	13.5	14.1	19.4	18.7	20.1
Texas	13.6	13.4	13.8	19.2	18.8	19.6
Utah	8.8	8.5	9.1	9.6	8.9	10.3
Vermont	10.1	9.5	10.7	10.8	9.8	11.8
Virginia	9.9	9.7	10.1	13.3	12.7	13.9
Washington	9.8	9.5	10.1	12.0	11.4	12.6
West Virginia	16.2	15.7	16.7	20.8	19.8	21.8
Wisconsin	10.4	10.2	10.6	13.5	12.9	14.1
Wyoming	9.9	9.2	10.6	11.7	10.6	12.8

U.S. Census Bureau: *Small area income and poverty estimates. Table modified. U.S. Department of Agriculture, Economic Research Service: County-level data sets: Poverty,* 2019d. Available from: https://data.ers.usda.gov/reports.aspx?ID=17826#P6b9ac9c741c747f8824c66382472c7bb_3_225iT3.

rural region. For example, there are 353 counties with persistent poverty rates in the United States (persistent poverty is defined as being in poverty over the last 30 years), comprising 11% of all U.S. counties. Of these, 301 are in nonmetropolitan areas. Persistent poverty is highest in the South (22%), followed by the West (16.2%), and then the Northeast and Midwest (13%). The higher persistent poverty rate in the South is particularly important, because an estimated 43% of the nonmetro population lived in this region in 2010 (USDA, ERS, 2019c) descriptions and maps persistent poverty. Poverty is also highest in the most rural areas and in completely rural counties (i.e., not adjacent to any metropolitan counties), the poverty rate is 35% with 26% residing in persistent poverty counties (USDA, ERS, 2014, 2019c).

Racial and Ethnic Minorities. When poverty rates among rural dwellers are analyzed by race, ethnicity, age, and family structure, the statistics on poverty are even more dramatic than residence or region. Racial and ethnic minorities (mainly nonwhite Hispanics, Blacks, and Native Americans) constitute 20% of the rural population. Non-Hispanic Blacks comprise 8% of the rural population (compared to 13% in urban areas), Hispanics comprise 9% (compared to 20% in urban areas) and American Indians comprised 2% and were the only group with a higher rural concentration compared to 0.5% in urban areas (Cromaratie and Vilorio, 2019). According to the ERS, poverty rates among rural and racial minorities were two to three times higher (67%) than poverty rates for rural Whites (13%). A high incidence of poverty often reflects the low income of their racial/ethnic minorities. Nonmetro Blacks/African Americans had the highest incidence of poverty in 2018 (31.6%) followed by American Indians/Alaska Natives (30.9%), Hispanics (23.8%), and Whites (14%) (USDA, 2020c).

Family Composition. Families with two or more adults are less likely to be poor, whether in rural or urban areas, because they are more likely to have multiple sources of income. Families with more than one adult have lower out-of-pocket childcare costs and are less likely to have to limit their working hours. More than 63% of rural families are headed by a married couple, and these constitute only 6% of families living in poverty. On the other hand, people living in female-headed families have higher poverty rates (44%) than single male–headed families (17.3%) in rural areas. The ERS attributes the high rate of poverty for female-headed families to "lower labor force participation rates, shorter average work weeks, and lower earnings" (USDA, ERS, 2020c).

Children. Children are particularly vulnerable to outcomes of poverty, and they are among the poorest citizens in rural America, constituting 25%, of the overall population of rural poor (CDC, 2017a,b,c; USDA, 2017, 2019 child poverty chart gallery). The heaviest concentrations of child poverty are in the South and West. Understanding how poverty is distributed in rural populations is important for planning and delivering programs that ameliorate the impact of poverty, such as food stamps, school lunch programs, school health nursing interventions, and health insurance coverage (CDC, 2017a,b,c;

RHIHub, 2019a—h). https://www.ruralhealthinfo.org/topics/healthcare-access.

When race and ethnicity are taken into account, the poverty profile of children worsens dramatically. Racial and ethnic minorities fare far worse than the general rural population of children from birth to 18 years of age. When family composition is also taken into account, we find that almost half of children (44.3%) of children who lived in a female-headed household were poor compared to children in coupled homes (5.8%) (USDA, 2020c).

Health Risk, Injury, and Death

Health behaviors vary along the rural—urban continuum and within rural populations by geographical area. For example, researchers have noted that adults in nonmetropolitan areas use seat belts less often and are less likely to use preventive screening (although the latter trend is confounded by access problems). Marshal and Ferenchak (2017) compared the prevalence of unlicensed teenaged drivers and that of licensed drivers and found that the former was more likely to be Black or Hispanic and to live in rural areas. Rural teens are equally likely as or more likely than both suburban and urban teens to report being victims of violent behavior, to engage in suicide behaviors, and to use drugs. Rural residents in the Southern states are more likely to be obese, to smoke more heavily if they do smoke, to use smokeless tobacco, and to engage in sedentary lifestyles. In the rural West, rates of smoking, seat belt use, and obesity are lower and those of alcohol and smokeless tobacco use are higher. For example, 19% of adolescents living in the most rural counties are smokers, compared with 11% in large metropolitan counties (National Rural Health Association, n.d.).

Other risk factors include alcohol use (higher in rural areas and highest among persons living in the most rural areas and more commonly among men than women), obesity (higher in rural areas, most particularly rural areas of the South), and physical inactivity during leisure time, which varies by level of urbanization (National Rural Health Association, 2021).

Intentional injuries, against the self or another, are most often the result of firearms usage. In rural counties, nonfatal firearm injuries occur most often at home, whereas in urban counties such injuries occur most often in the streets. Furthermore, numerous studies have noted that firearm suicide in rural counties is an important public health concern. Nationally, suicide is the 10th leading cause of death, but in rural America, it is the second leading cause of death. The rate of suicide in some rural areas is 800% higher than the national average. Nationally, 14.5 people in 100,000 died by suicide in 2020 (CDC, Suicide & Self Injury, 2021a; Pettrone and Curtin, 2020). There was also variation by race and ethnicity. Notable increases have been experienced in rural versus urban locations and with rural women. Decreased access to mental health services for treatment of depression may contribute to these higher rates. Among suicide victims, racial and ethnic disparities exist. During a 20-year period (1998—2018), the total suicide rate in the United States increased 35% from 10.5 per 100,000 in 1999 to 14.2 per 100,000 in 2018. While rates for male suicide are 3.7 times higher (22.8 per 100,000) than females (6.2 per 100,000), this trend is shifting noting more female suicides at younger ages. The age of suicide also differs by gender with the highest female rate (10.2 per 100,000) between 45 and 64 where for men, the highest suicide rate (39.9 per 100,000) were aged 75 and older (National Institute of Mental Health, 2021).

Suicide rates were highest for American Indian, non-Hispanic males (34.8 per 100,000) and females (10.5 per 100,000), followed by White, non-Hispanic males (30.4 per 100,000) and females (8.3 per 100,000) in 2018 (National Institute of Mental Health, 2021).

Unintentional injuries are the leading cause of death in the United States for both sexes, for all races and ethnicities, and for all age groups from ages 1 to 44 years. Overall, unintentional injuries occur most often as the result of driving a vehicle (automobile, all-terrain vehicle, bicycle). In the latest available reports, unintentional injuries continue to be higher in rural areas of the United States. The mortality rate for unintentional injuries reported in the *Urban and* Rural Health Chartbook 2020 was 50% higher for rural residents than metropolitan residents at 54.1 per 100,000 (AHRQ, 2017a,b).

According to the CDC's National Center for Health Statistics, unintentional injury was ranked third the leading causes of death in 2019 (CDC, 2019). This category of death includes "transport accidents," including motor vehicle accidents, and "nontransport accidents," which include falls, firearm accidents, drowning, fire-related deaths, and accidental poisoning. Overall, deaths from unintentional injuries were approximately higher for males than females in the most rural counties than for those in suburban areas of metropolitan counties in 2018. Driving at high speeds, driving long distances, driving in winter conditions, not using seat belts, and consuming alcohol have been cited as contributing factors to higher levels of injury deaths and disability for rural residents (CDC, 2019; CDC, National Center for Injury Prevention and Control, 2020). Lack of ready access to counseling, emergency medical services (EMS), and rehabilitation are also thought to be contributing factors to these high levels.

Vulnerable Groups

Demographic and personal characteristics, such as age, education, gender, race, ethnicity, language, and culture, round out the examples of factors that affect health and that may block access to existing services. Age is an important consideration in the planning of health care services for rural communities. As noted in previous sections, many retirees are moving into rural areas, and many younger people are moving out. Because the incomes of many elderly may be lower, the tax base of counties and municipalities may be inadequate to cover the disproportionate share of the healthcare services used by the elderly (age 65 years and over) (Saint Onge and Smith, 2020).

The population of the elderly is expected to double by 2050. Elderly women tend to live at or near the poverty level and to achieve poverty status twice as often as men. Along with educational attainment, this is a critical indicator of well-being for the elderly and the young. The elderly poor tend to be isolated and to lack access to support services, health care, prescription drugs, adequate nutrition, and transportation (Saint Onge and Smith, 2020).

There are about 13.4 million children under the age of 18 who live in the rural areas of the nation. While poverty rates were lower in rural (18.9%) versus urban (22.3%) areas, more were uninsured (7.3% compared to 6.3%). The number of children 0 to 18 has declined in rural areas (U.S Census, 2016a).

In rural America, racial and ethnic diversity has increased. Today, the proportion of Hispanic children is the fastest-growing component of the rural population, regardless of region representing 8% of the population. The population of Black children has remained steady, and the majority of rural Black children are still concentrated in the South. Native American children constitute only 3% of the total nonmetropolitan population, although in areas of the country (mainly West and Central) with high concentrations of Native Americans, this percentage is higher. Evidence suggests that fetal, infant, and maternal mortality rates are slightly higher in nonmetropolitan than metropolitan areas and that prenatal care in the later pregnancy stages is problematic. Nonmetropolitan children, like nonmetropolitan adults, are more likely to live in poverty, and proportionately fewer rural children were covered by health insurance (Johnson, 2017, ; USDA, 2018). Review of adverse childhood events in the United States highlighted increased risk for rural children in rural communities centered on single parent homes, lower parental education levels, higher poverty, and economic hardship (Crouch et al., 2019).

Education and Employment

Research on the socioeconomic determinants of health has revealed a strong positive correlation between health and length of schooling. Demographics of a minority group often influence and result from social and economic factors. Age and education are indicators for employment. For the aged and for ethnic and racial minorities, a pattern of lower educational attainment and unfavorable economic circumstances emerges with increasing rurality (Fig. 24.2). Although the education picture is changing, many women now in their 70 and 80s grew up before public education was mandatory. Families could not afford to send them to school, or they were simply expected to learn to read and write, seek employment, and marry. Education, with its links to economic and health variables, is still a serious problem for rural America (Fig. 24.3). Low education and employment levels characterize all rural minority groups except Asians. Children living in precarious economic conditions have additional challenges to doing well in school and remaining in school through high school graduation. Generally, rural students perform better than students in cities and town, but not as well as suburban students, on the National Assessment of Educational Progress (NAEP). Students in rural

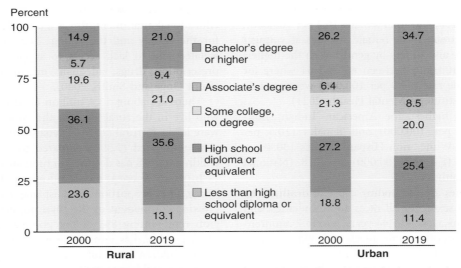

Note: Educational attainment for adults 25 and older; Urban and rural status is determined by Office of Management and Budget's 2018 metropolitan area definitions.

Fig. 24.2 Educational Attainment Rates for Rural Adults. (From U.S. Department of Agriculture, Economic Research Service: *Employment & education: high school completion rates (adults 25 and older)*, 2020. Available from: https://www.ers.usda.gov/topics/rural-economy-population/employment-education/rural-education.aspx.)

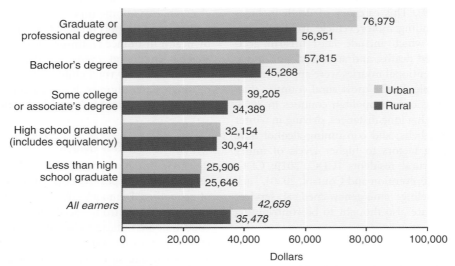

Note: Median earnings in 2019 dollars for all earners 25 and older; Urban and rural status is determined by Office of Management and Budget's 2018 metropolitan area definitions.

Fig. 24.3 Rural and Urban Earnings by Educational Level. (From USDA Rural Education; Farrigan, T: *Rural education*, 2020. Available from: https://www.ers.usda.gov/topics/rural-economy-population/employment-education/rural-education/.)

districts had higher graduation rates than in cities and towns. Educational attainment is a challenge in rural America, and skill requirements for rural employment continue to rise. Lack of education is correlated with persistent poverty, and poverty is a predictor of poor health.

Furthermore, counties that have a low-wage economy have difficulty providing the infrastructure needed to provide education, public health, and health care services for low-wage families. They also have difficulty attracting new employers who might contribute to the economic development of a rural area but need a more highly educated workforce.

Occupational Health Risks

In the United States, approximately 5333 workers died from work-related illnesses and injuries in 2019, up 2% from 2018. The overall fatal work injury rate for the United States in 2019 was 3.5 fatal injuries per 100,000 full-time equivalent workers, the same in 2018. This rate has been consistent for the last decade (Bureau of Labor Statistics, 2019).

Tractors contributed to 416 farm and farmworker deaths representing a fatality rate of 20.4 deaths per 100,000 workers. Transportation incidents that include tractors were the leading cause of death (NIOSH, 2020d; Agricultural Safety). Occupational injuries, fatalities, and illnesses play a significant role in rural health, because rates of disabling injuries and injury-related mortality are dramatically higher in the rural population. Industries with the highest death rate were construction and transportation, followed by agriculture, forestry, and fishing (NIOSH, 2020; U.S. Department of Labor, 2019).

Occupational death and disability can also be attributed to nonfatal injuries and occupational diseases, such as cancer, asbestosis, silicosis, and anthracosis, associated with both organic and inorganic exposures (CDC, NIOSH Program Portfolio, 2012). Work-related injuries, deaths, and illness data must be interpreted with caution. Although surveillance of occupational injuries, illnesses, and fatalities has improved through the collaboration of the states and NIOSH, data still come from many sources, and underreporting continues to be problematic (NIOSH, 2021a,b).

Perceptions of Health
Gender, Race, and Ethnicity

Both rural men and rural women are less likely than metropolitan residents to report their health as good or excellent. Rural areas, particularly in the rural South, have higher incidents of heart disease and cancer. Higher prevalence of chronic disease is consistent with the composition of rural populations, which tend to be older, poorer, and less educated (Artnak et al., 2011; James et al., 2017). Rural men and women also smoke or use smokeless tobacco more. In the aggregate, they exercise fewer preventive behaviors, have less contact with physicians, and often have less access to care than people with similar problems in urban areas (NRHA, 2021). Rural men and youths are also more likely to die or become disabled from unintentional injuries due to risky behavior or work-related causes and are more likely to commit suicide than women or urban men and youths (James et al., 2017).

Although rural populations overall are at lower risk for most cancers, certain rural subpopulations are at greater risk. For example, Appalachia has a much higher rate than the national figure. The CDC (2017) reported rural Americans are more likely to die from preventable disease, including heart disease (25,000), cancer (19,000), unintentional injury (12,000), chronic lower respiratory disease (11,000), and stroke (4000). The percentages of deaths that were potentially preventable were higher in rural areas than in urban areas. Residents in low-income areas and the uninsured, particularly African Americans, tend to have more late-stage cancer diagnoses; and rural residents in general may have less access to quality health care, including both medical care and screening and prevention programs. A particularly serious problem for minorities and the elderly is the lack of cancer screening, including screening for breast and cervical cancer for women and prostate cancer for men. Preventive care is especially important for African American men, for whom the prostate cancer rate is higher than for any other racial or ethnic group.

Seigel (2018) highlighted woman aged 40 and older who had screening mammograms improved for urban and rural women, but rural women lagged behind. Nationally, the rate for mammogram improved overall with 75.8% of urban and 70.8% rural populations. In rural populations, age, race, ethnicity and income influenced screening mammography. The population was predominantly 65 years or older, non-Hispanic white, married, making more than $25,000 annually with at least a high school education. The percentages for ever having a screening mammogram were lower for all racial and ethnic minorities. Use of mammography was the lowest among the poor, most particularly in the 40- to 49-year age bracket and among the least educated (Seigel, 2018; Tran and Tran, 2019). Health objectives for 2030 called for at least 71% American women aged 40 years and older to have received a mammogram and clinical breast examination in the previous 2 years (Healthy People, 2030; National Advisory Committee on Rural Health and Human Services, 2013).

Similarly, women who are poor, elderly, and less educated are less likely to receive Papanicolaou (Pap) smear tests. In racial and ethnic groups, the percentages of women who get Pap tests are lower for Hispanics, American Indians, and Alaska Natives. The lowest percentage is found in Asian women.

The percentage of Hispanics and Latinos in the U.S. population in 2019 was 19% and African Americans were 13%. In 2011, Hispanic and African Americans as part of the whole were (13% 16%) It was noted a decade ago that the Hispanic population would become the largest minority group in the United States, and this is now true (U.S. Census Bureau, 2010a,b, 2019a,b,c). They are the predominant minority in the West. Hispanics have diverse cultures, histories, and socioeconomic and health status. The largest Hispanic subgroups are of Mexican, Cuban, and Puerto Rican descent, although Mexican is the largest by far (accounting for 58% of the Hispanic population living in the United States). In nonmetropolitan areas, the population of Hispanics has doubled, and almost half of all Hispanics in rural areas are living outside the traditional areas of settlement in the Southwestern states. As emphasized previously, this growing segment of the population continues to be overrepresented among the rural poor. In 2019, the U.S. Census Bureau reported the lowest ever observed poverty rates for Hispanics (15.7%), compared to the prior low of 17.6% in 2018. The Asian poverty rate of 7.3% was also the lowest on record. The 2019 poverty rate of 7.3% for non-Hispanic Whites was not statistically different than the previous low (historically adjusted) of 7.2%. U.S. Census Bureau (2019) Poverty rates for Blacks and Hispanics.

Elderly Hispanics were also 2.5 times more likely to live below the poverty line than white non-Hispanics. Hispanics are most likely to report barriers to obtaining needed health care and are least likely to have a usual source of care; for those Blacks and Hispanics reporting a usual source of care, the source is most likely to be hospital based (U.S. Census Bureau, 2019a,b,c).

In 2019, Blacks represented 13.2% of the population but their share in poverty was 23.8% or 1.8 times their share in the population. Likewise, Hispanics comprised 18.7% of the population but 28.1% of the population in poverty, 1.5 times more than their share in the general population. In contrast, non-Hispanic Whites and Asians were underrepresented in the poverty population with Whites comprising 59.9% of the population and only 41.6% of the poverty population. Asians made up 6.1% of the population and 4.3% of the population in poverty (U.S. Census Bureau, 2020b, Inequalities Persist Despite Decline in Poverty For All Major Race and Hispanic Origin Groups).

SPECIFIC RURAL AGGREGATES

Agricultural Workers

Health Disparities

An example of health disparities among agricultural workers is the group of farm workers that support fruit and vegetable production. In general, migrant and seasonal farmworkers (MSFWs) may have the poorest health of any aggregate in the United States and the least access to affordable health care. Seventy-eight percent of MSFWs are Hispanic, Latino, or African American. The rest are largely white seasonal workers who follow the harvests to drive combines or haul crops from the fields to storage, market, or seaports. These populations, estimated as between three and five million people each year, are vulnerable to a host of health problems and diseases that center on occupational and environmental hazards and other health correlates (USDA, 2020d, Farm Labor).

Accidents and Injuries

Working in highly variable environmental conditions (e.g., temperature extremes, a wide variety of work tasks, and unpredictable circumstances) is associated with an increased frequency of accidents and fatalities. Farm-related activities are extremely heterogeneous and vary significantly with the season, types of crops produced, and types of machinery used. Farmers are located in geographically isolated areas and often work alone. This constellation of factors puts farmers and their families at increased risk for accidental injury and delayed access to emergency or trauma care.

In 2019, the rate of fatal injuries per 100,000 full-time equivalents employed in the agricultural sector was 22.8, equal to those in fishing and forestry for the highest rates followed by transportation and moving materials (15.0) and construction and extraction (12.2) (Americas Health Rankings, 2018).

According to the CDC's NIOSH Program (2020), agricultural machinery is the most common cause of fatalities and nonfatal injuries of U.S. agricultural workers, including on-farm fatalities among youth (<20 years). Tractor-related accidents, especially rollovers, are the most frequent causes of farm accidents, accounting for more than one fourth of farm fatalities.

The actual causes of death and serious injury are associated with rollovers of equipment that lacks rollover protective structures and seat belts (CDC, NIOSH Program, 2020).

With such statistics, it is easy to see why accident prevention programs for farm children and families have focused heavily on tractor safety awareness.

Acute and Chronic Illnesses

Several types of farming activities are associated with more occurrences than expected of acute and chronic respiratory conditions. Individuals with long-term exposure to grain dusts, such as grain elevator workers and dairy workers, have diminished respiratory function and increased frequency of respiratory symptoms (National Center for Farmworker Health [NCFH], 2018).

Occupational asthma and more exotic fungal or toxic gas—related conditions also occur in higher frequency in agricultural than nonagricultural populations. Community health nurses, who are familiar with local farming practices in rural areas, often make links between farm work and respiratory symptoms. In such situations, the role of the nurse is to refer patients to appropriate health care providers and to provide support and education for affected people and their families.

Exposure to pesticides, herbicides, and other chemicals is also a major concern for farmers and their families. From an occupational perspective, farming is unusual because the home and the worksite are the same. Exposure risks to children and spouses may be heightened when farmers wear contaminated clothing and boots into the home. Homes are often located in close proximity to fields and animal containment facilities, which are treated with a variety of chemicals.

Nurses in rural emergency rooms or other ambulatory care settings may be the first providers to encounter farmers and others with acute **pesticide** poisoning. During discussions with farmers, ranchers, or other high-risk groups (e.g., nursery workers and tree planters), community health nurses may note a pattern of headaches and nausea that occurs during planting or spraying seasons. In such an instance, the nurse can serve as an important resource by obtaining a careful history of signs and symptoms, the temporal nature of symptom occurrence, and the types of pesticides and personal protection used (e.g., respirators and protective clothing). When evidence suggests pesticide-related illness, appropriate referral and follow-up are imperative to ensure the safety of the affected person and the family.

Signs and symptoms of acute pesticide poisoning are fairly clear, and most health providers in rural communities would recognize them. Common symptoms include headache, dizziness, diaphoresis, nausea, and vomiting. If left untreated, those affected may experience a progression of symptoms, including dyspnea, bronchospasm, and muscle twitching. Deaths are relatively uncommon, but they do occur.

Several demographic, environmental, economic, and social factors might put rural residents at higher risk of death from these public health conditions. Residents of rural areas in the United States tend to be older and sicker than their urban counterparts. They have higher rates of cigarette smoking, high blood pressure, and obesity. Rural residents report less leisure-time physical activity and lower seat belt use than their urban counterparts. They also have higher rates of poverty, have less access to health care, and are less likely to have health insurance (CDC, 2017a,b,c).

Migrant and Seasonal Farmworkers

Although the discussion of agricultural issues has focused primarily on farmers and farm families, it is important to understand the role of **migrant** (i.e., migrate to find work) and **seasonal** (i.e., reside permanently in one place and work locally when farm labor is needed) farmworkers in U.S. agricultural production and the health risks to this population. Older references to farmworkers often referred to three "migrant streams," in which workers entered the country through Mexico and migrated north. The current reality is that migrant workers enter the country through a variety of access points and follow any route necessary to obtain work. Seasonal workers reside in agricultural areas permanently and take various farm jobs during harvesting times. For example, a seasonal worker may be employed in restaurant work during the winter and may spend the summer months picking apples or working in a local apple shed or cannery (Migrant Clinicians Network, 2017, USDA, ERS, 2013). Definitions and Overview.

MSFWs comprise a vulnerable population in regard to health risks because they have a low-income and migratory status. In many rural areas, community health nurses form the central link between farmworkers and health services. Through standing or mobile clinic sites, nurses have established a leadership role in the provision of episodic and preventive services for workers and their families. Lacking access to many types of preventive services, farmworkers often visit a migrant clinic with any number of health problems, including severe dental problems, unresolved communicable diseases, and untreated injuries. In addition to the direct provision of care, nurses in many communities have served as important advocates on behalf of farmworkers and have worked to ensure health care access for those traveling through their areas (Migrant Clinicians Network, 2017).

Cultural, linguistic, economic, and mobility barriers all contribute to the nature and magnitude of health problems observed in farmworkers. Cultural and linguistic barriers are the most overt because many of the communities where farmworkers work consider them outsiders. In many settings, migrant workers live isolated from the agricultural communities they serve. Although some workers travel in extended family groups and have the support that comes with being together, other workers leave their families at home. Often the latter are male workers who work and live together. A common misconception among U.S. health care providers is that these farmworkers are from Mexico and that Spanish is their primary language. Farmworkers originate from many communities in Mexico, the Caribbean, and Central and South America, and they may speak the language of their home country, English, or several languages (Migrant Clinicians Network, 2017).

Enumeration of Migrant and Seasonal Farmworkers

To increase access to primary and preventative care for MSFW populations, information is needed on the numbers and distribution of farmworkers at the national, state, and local levels. Because MSFWs move frequently for work, census estimates generally provide a poor assessment of this population's needs for health care services. Additionally, the legislation that created the Migrant Health Program (MHP) (Section 330g of the Public Health Service Act), under the direction of the Bureau of Primary Health Care (BPHC) (2000) and the Health Resources and Services Administration (HRSA), requires that priorities be established according to where the greatest need exists. Hence the MHP has supported the ongoing and comprehensive assessment of the numbers of MSFWs and published the Migrant and Seasonal Farmworker Enumeration Profile Study (National Advisory Council on Migrant Health, 2018).

Health Needs and Opportunities for Preventive Care

Similarities in exposure and work practices make some of the farmworkers' health needs similar to those of farmers and their families. Generally, these health needs reflect the increased rates of accidents and injuries, dermatological conditions, and pulmonary problems observed in the two populations. However, there are additional challenges in both the identification and the treatment of farmworkers with health problems. One of the biggest problems that nurses face in designing health programs is understanding the full magnitude of these health problems. Many farmworkers who become ill eventually return to their countries of origin to obtain treatment and to be with family. This phenomenon makes it difficult to get complete, reliable numbers about disease rates. A variety of public health indicators are likely to undercount farmworkers as a group, ranging from tumor registries to workers' compensation injuries (NCFH, 2018). In addition, farmworkers may be less likely to seek treatment for health problems that do not require emergency treatment or surgery.

Studies of farmworkers' health status have provided data indicating that they are less likely to receive preventive care from any health source. Preventive needs include dental care, vision screening and treatment, and gynecological and breast examinations. Many farmworkers, because they move from community to community, are often unaware of clinical and social services they could receive and that are available at reduced or no cost to low-income families (NCFH, 2018).

❓ ACTIVE LEARNING

1. University libraries commonly subscribe to newspapers published within the state. Visit the library and select three to four small town or rural county newspapers. Read them for information about healthcare activities and concerns related to the health of the individuals, families, and community.

- Report findings to the class about rural health concerns and activities.
- Identify one priority problem that could be researched in the community and has relevance to rural community health nursing practice.

2. Choose one of the major causes of morbidity and mortality in migrant populations.
   - On the basis of risk factor and natural history, specify interventions for primary, secondary, and tertiary prevention of this problem.
   - Identify which of these interventions are examples of upstream thinking.

3. Locate a telephone book, a community resource directory, or a resource website from a rural community.
   - List and evaluate the resources that are available for prevention, assessment, intervention, and follow-up care for the major cause of mortality and morbidity identified in Learning Activity 2.
   - Would it be necessary to go outside the rural town or county for any of the needed resources? Which ones? Where might they be located?

RURAL HEALTHCARE DELIVERY SYSTEM

Healthcare Provider Shortages

In a National Advisory Committee on Rural Health and Human Services brief (2013), the authors indicate that the quality and functionality of a health care delivery system depend on the availability of medical personnel and infrastructure to provide needed services. Rural communities generally have fewer physicians, nurses, specialists, and other healthcare workforce. The small population size and scale make the loss or shortage of a single health provider likely to have far-reaching impacts.

The health care labor shortage in the United States has been widely documented and is expected to last for the foreseeable future. The increase in population—aging and growing racial and ethnic diversity—is partially responsible for the health care labor shortage. As the health care workforce ages, the demographics of the U.S. population over the age of 65 will dramatically shift, with projections to increase to 21% by 2030 and an aging population that is expected to outnumber that of children (Vespa et al., 2020). In addition to the shortage of health professionals, maldistribution is another prevalent obstacle rural Americans face in accessing timely and appropriate primary healthcare services (National Rural Health Association, 2012). Workforce shortages are especially serious in remote frontier communities, many of which are located in the Western region of the United States.

Nursing is by far the largest healthcare profession in the United States, with more than 3.8 million RNs practicing in hospitals and other settings nationwide. Despite their large numbers, many more qualified nurses must be prepared in programs offered by community colleges and 4-year institutions to meet the nation's growing demand for health care and to replace a large wave of nurses nearing retirement (American Association of Colleges of Nursing, 2019). The Bureau of Labor Statistics projects demand for RN's will continue as the fastest-growing occupation with a 7% increase or 221,900 positions in addition to 175,900 RN job openings each year by 2029 (American Association of Colleges of Nursing, 2020). More than 1.2 million RNs will be needed to work in acute care hospitals, long-term care facilities, community health centers (CHC), nursing schools, and other areas by 2029 (American Association of Colleges of Nursing, 2021). Although approximately 20% of the U.S. population, equating to one in five Americans or 60 million people, live in nonmetropolitan counties, with only 18% of RNs practicing in nonmetropolitan countries an inequitable distribution of the nursing workforce exists across rural areas (U.S. Census Bureau, 2016a; U.S. Bureau of Labor Statistics, 2020).

Clearly, the growing nursing shortage continues to affect all of America. This is both a supply shortage and a demand shortage (U.S. Department of Health and Human Services, 2017). The inability for nursing schools to expand capacity to meet the increased need for nurses, the retirement of current nurses and the increased need for care of an aging population make the situation especially critical (American Association of Colleges of Nursing, 2020). A survey by the American Organization of Nurse Executives found that it takes significantly longer to fill vacancies in small hospitals, usually located in rural areas, than in larger urban facilities (Thrall, 2007; Zhang et al., 2018). Rural nurses earn less than their urban counterparts, compounding recruitment difficulties. Nurses with baccalaureate and master's degrees, other than master's degree-prepared NPs, are compensated less for this additional education (Thrall, 2007; Probst et al., 2019).

A solution proposed for the shortage of health care providers is for rural communities to "grow their own." A rural community, a group of small communities, or a county could support local students attending college and recruit students currently attending professional schools. The students would make a commitment to work in the community in return for monetary support for their educations (Thrall, 2007; Rural Health Information Hub, 2019b). Tuition reimbursement and access to distance learning programs can assist practicing nurses. Continuing education and baccalaureate and master's degrees are available through e-mail, Internet-based courses, interactive video classes, and by-mail videos. Some programs are provided exclusively via the internet. Nebraska's rural communities are enthusiastic about the University of Nebraska College of Nursing Internet courses. The program is helping them grow their own nurses. Research shows that nurses educated in rural communities are more apt to stay and work there than those who move away to attend school (Thrall, 2007; Rural Health Information Hub, 2019b).

Once new graduates are hired into healthcare positions in rural communities, it is imperative that they are assisted in their transition to practice. An opportunity exists to transform nurses' professional development and improve healthcare quality and affordability through nurse residency programs. These programs need to go beyond basic orientation and provide a clinical preceptorship focused not just on delivering competent care but also on developing and growing in the nursing profession. A survey of new nurses found many challenges: a lack of confidence, difficulty with work relationships, frustrations relating to the work environment, lack of time, and guidance for developing organizational and priority-setting abilities, and overall high levels of stress. These factors likely contribute to the high turnover rate among new nurses, estimated at between 35% and 60% within the first year (Kosman, 2011; Van Camp and Chappy, 2017).

Telemedicine

In light of provider storages and recruitment difficulties with the physician, nurse, and other healthcare worker shortages, coupled with the difficulty in recruiting them to rural areas, alternatives to improve access must be identified. Telemedicine is expanding across the country as an alternative way to address the health care disparities that have long existed in rural communities. Telemedicine is viewed as a cost-effective alternative to the more traditional face-to-face way of providing medical care (Medicaid.gov, n.d.).

The American Telemedicine Association (2021) largely views telemedicine and telehealth as interchangeable terms, encompassing a broad definition of remote health care, although telehealth may not always involve clinical care. Yet, regardless of how you refer to it, what is now indisputable is how telemedicine greatly improves the quality, equity, and affordability of health care throughout the world.

Distinctions can be made between telehealth and telemedicine. *Telehealth* includes technologies such as telephones, facsimile machines, electronic mail systems, and remote patient monitoring devices for the collection and transmission of patient data for monitoring and interpretation. Conversely, telemedicine seeks to improve a patient's health by permitting two-way, real-time, interactive communication between the patient and the physician or practitioner at the distant site and is centered on efficiency, effectiveness, and safety. This electronic communication means the use of interactive telecommunications equipment that includes, at a minimum, audio and video equipment. This definition is modeled on Medicare's definition of telehealth services (Medicaid.gov, n.d.).

Recent projects geared toward extending telemedicine services to rural areas include the Frontier Health Projects support of new models of health care and the Medicare expansion of telehealth services that have been implemented during ongoing public health emergencies (American Hospital Association, 2019). Although several states in the Midwest and West have taken advantage of telemedicine in rural areas, the patchwork approach in legislation has contributed to varying degrees of implementation and financial support (Alexander, 2013).

Managed Care in the Rural Environment

Managed care has recently changed healthcare delivery in the United States. In rural areas, healthcare delivery networks with managed care elements are being developed as the expanded insurance coverage in Medicaid expansion and insurance marketplaces accounts for a projected demand of an additional 19,300 nurses by 2030 (U.S. Department of Health and Human Services, 2017). Potential benefits and risks of managed care for rural areas have been identified, with recognition of the difficulty rural providers in solo or small group practices face in delivering cost-effective, complex health care. Possible benefits to managed

care include lowering primary care costs, improving the quality of care, and stabilizing the local rural health care system. Risks are also apparent, including probable high startup and administrative costs and the volatile effect of large, urban-based, for-profit, managed care companies (Allender et al., 2014).

Outside of Medicaid, managed care has yet to become a significant presence in much of rural America because small disperse populations, few visits per individual, and large numbers of elderly on Medicare with low-level reimbursements do not make the aggregate financially attractive to a managed care organization (MCO). In fact, despite the existence of federally qualified health centers that provide care to underserved populations through Medicare or Medicaid or on sliding fee scales, few rural people were enrolled in sponsored health plans (Allender et al., 2014). Providers in rural markets face severe financial constraints and greater financial vulnerability to policy changes in the payment of services as HMOs. Rural providers increasingly cope with smaller numbers of enrollees and reduced provider reimbursement, reflected in less reimbursement than the cost of providing care to the patient (American Hospital Association, 2019).

Team-based care models, such as Patient-Centered Medical Homes (PCMHs) and Patient-Centered Medical Neighborhoods play a vital role in delivering care to rural communities. The medical home model holds promise to improve health care in America by transforming how primary care is organized and delivered. Building on the work of a large and growing community, the Agency for Healthcare Research and Quality (2014) defines a medical home not simply as a place but as a model of the organization of primary care that delivers the core functions of primary health care. The medical home encompasses five functions and attributes: comprehensive care, patient-centered, coordinated care, accessible services, and quality and safety.

We conceptualize the medical neighborhood as a PCMH and the constellation of other clinicians providing health care services to patients within it, along with community and social service organizations and state and local public health agencies. Defined in this way, the PCMH and the surrounding medical neighborhood can focus on meeting the individual patient's needs and incorporate aspects of population health and overall community health needs in its objectives.

Postacute Care

The complexity of health care takes on many transitions throughout the patient's hospital stay. As a differentiator from larger hospitals, many rural hospitals can accommodate and offer services as patients transition from acute care to **postacute** care. One such service that accommodates such a transition is that of providing Swing Bed services. The Centers for Medicare and Medicaid Services (2019) defines Swing Bed services as a hospital room that can switch from acute care status to skilled care. This allows the rural health hospital with fewer than 100 beds to provide post-skilled care for patients in the community.

Approximately 15% of total Medicare spending is comprised of postacute care offered in the settings of long-term care, inpatient rehabilitation, skilled nursing facilities, and home health (American Hospital Association, 2021). Patients and families in the community benefit from Swing Bed services that provide daily therapy, care, and activities to return to independence before going home, providing patients that qualify for these services with an additional level of individualized care and access to provider and hospital services. Rural hospitals that are certified to provide Swing Bed services can also receive patients who require postacute care from larger facilities, reducing acute care length of stays, readmissions and increasing access to health care for a rural population. By offering postacute care services, rural hospitals facilitate the improvement of community health by keeping the care of the patient close to home in further caring for their community.

Community-Based Care

In the mid-1990s, the phrase *community-based care* became a popular term for the myriad of services provided outside the walls of an institution. Health care services are no longer provided exclusively in the hospital setting. Community-based care includes services that are provided where individuals live, work, or go to school. Examples of community-based services are home health and hospice care, occupational health programs, community mental health programs, ambulatory care services, school health programs, faith-based care, and elder services such as adult day care. The concept also includes community participation in decisions about health care services, a focus on all three levels of prevention, and an understanding that the hospital is no longer the exclusive health care provider.

Home Health, Hospice, and Palliative Care

Rural populations are disproportionately older than their urban counterparts, and this disparity will only increase as baby boomers continue to age. The elderly growth rates in nonmetropolitan areas have tripled since 1990, with the fastest growth rate of those that are 85 years of age or older. The elderly growth rate is expected to grow from four million in 2000 to 21 million by 2050, with much of the growth expected in rural areas (National Conference of State Legislatures, 2011). Aside from being older, rural residents have higher rates of age-adjusted mortality, disability, and chronic illness than their urban counterparts. As the elderly comprise a larger percentage of the rural population, access to high-quality end-of-life care in rural areas will become increasingly important.

Home health, hospice, and palliative care programs vary in structure. A national study on Medicare hospice use found that only one-third of rural counties have a hospice based within the county, but nearly two-thirds of urban counties do (Virnig et al., 2004; Medicare Payment Advisory Commission, 2020). Urban hospices are more likely to be freestanding, whereas rural hospices tend to be hospital-based. Larger communities may support a hospital-based home care agency with hospice service, a freestanding full-service agency, or both. In sparsely populated rural locations, home health, hospice, and palliative care services may be contracted from a larger regional agency, with a local nurse hired to provide services.

While home health, hospice, and palliative care can improve the quality of life for patients in both rural and urban communities, Virnig and associates (2004) and the Medicare Payment Advisory Commission (2020) found that the more remote the rural environment, the less likely hospice services were used. Nurse case management and development of local resources, using the county extension services as a bridge for outreach services, can improve home care for patients needing hospice and palliative care while also providing support for their families. A partnership between the public health nurse and county extension service could provide support and information groups and caregiving classes for the important informal provider network.

Given the more fragile financial margins and lower patient volumes in rural areas, rural hospice and palliative care providers face different challenges from their urban counterparts. A one-size-fits-all policy reform may have negative consequences for rural hospice and palliative care providers, despite data indicating that hospice and palliative care provider density in rural areas is comparable to and even higher than in urban areas. Rural and frontier Medicare decedents continue to utilize hospice and palliative care at lower rates than their urban peers (National Advisory Committee on Rural Health and Human Services, 2013). Chapter 34 discusses home health, hospice, and palliative care in greater detail.

Faith Communities and Parish Nursing

Rural residents are perceived as having strong traditional values. At the heart of these values are a strong sense of community, family life, and religious faith. Since the conceptualization of parish nursing in the early 1980s, RNs have developed and expanded the role. The Canadian Association for Parish Nursing Ministry (2020) defines the parish nurse's role as to promote the integration of faith and health in a variety of ways that reflect the context of the faith community. Specific examples include health advocacy, health counseling, health education, and resource referral. The Westberg Institute (2021) develops and supports faith community or parish nurses. They define the role as licensed, registered nurses who practice holistic health for self, individuals, and the community using nursing knowledge combined with spiritual care. They function in paid and unpaid positions as members of the pastoral team in a variety of religious faiths, cultures, and countries. The focus of their work is on the intentional care of the spirit, assisting the members of the faith community to maintain and/or regain wholeness in body, mind, and spirit.

In a comparison of experiences of rural and urban faith-based programs, rural nurses are more likely to be involved in case management and coordination of services than their urban counterparts (Molanari et al., 2011; National Rural Health Association, 2017). In urban settings, contact with parishioners is primarily at the church, whereas contacts in rural settings are most often in the home, on the phone, or in other community-based settings. Collaboration between faith communities and other organizations can help extend limited rural community health resources. Such partnerships have been promoted by federal and state governments to enhance public health efforts (Zahner and Corrado, 2004; U.S. Department of Health and Human Services, 2020a).

In 1997, the ANA designated parish nursing a specialty practice and was recognized in 2005 by the ANA as Faith Community Nursing to acknowledge the full range of faiths in the United States (Anaebere and DeLilly, 2012). At the same time, the Health Ministries Association (n.d.), a membership organization for parish nurses and others in health ministry, developed the "Scope and Standards of Parish Nursing Practice," revised in 2017, these standards are now called "Faith Community Nursing: Scope and Standards of Practice." According to the Parliament of the World's Religions, over 50 religions are recognized by the fundamental core values of nursing, which include the respect for life and the promotion of service to others (Anaebere and DeLilly, 2012). Chapter 33 Faith Community Nursing provides an in-depth discussion of faith communities and parish nursing.

As described in an article by the American Nurses Association (2010), the International Parish Nurse Resource Center preparation curriculum describes the philosophy of parish nursing as follows:

The spiritual dimension is central to parish nursing practice. Personal spiritual formation is an intentional process of intimacy with god to foster spiritual growth. It is an ongoing, essential component of practice for the parish nurse and includes both self-care and hospitality through opening the heart to self and others. the parish nurse role reclaims the historic roots of professional nursing … each parish nurse practices under the scope and standards of practice and the ethical code of nursing as set forth in their country … shalom, God's intent for harmony and wholeness, serves as a foundation for understanding health.

Informal Care Systems

Limited availability of and accessibility to formal healthcare resources in rural areas, combined with the self-reliance and self-help traits of rural residents, have resulted in the development of strong informal care and social support networks in rural communities. Rural residents are more apt to entrust care to established informal networks than to new formal care systems. Examining perceptions of rural health and social systems, Thorngren (2003) and the Harvard T.H. Chan School of Public Health (2018) found that rural residents agreed that experiences inherent in rural life both contribute to and ameliorate health-related concerns, attributed to higher levels of family and community involvement, problem-solving abilities, and connections to the land, all factors which may be present in the formation and use of informal systems.

Informal care systems or networks include people who have assumed the role of the caregiver based on their individual qualities, life situations, or social roles. These informal care providers are often referred to as *lay caregivers*. Family caregivers play an important role in patient-centered health care. Lay caregivers are individuals who are not licensed health professionals but often care for patients after a hospital stay.

Those designated caregivers are usually friends or members of a patient's family (Miller, 2015). People who participate in these networks may provide direct help, advice, or information.

Informal caregivers often find themselves in stressful circumstances (Sanford and Townsend-Rocchiccioli, 2004; Roth, Fredman, & Haley, 2015). Rural residents who find themselves in need of assistance are usually elderly, have chronic illness, have fewer resources, and must travel long distances for health care. In a U.S. Census Bureau Report (2015) that analyzes U.S. population projections, it is projected that by 2060, the U.S. minority population as a whole is expected to rise to 56% of the total population as compared to 38% in 2014, with 45% of the U.S. population over the age of 65 belonging to a minority group (Scommenga et al., 2018).

Disparities already exist in the physical and mental health status, service availability, service access, and socioeconomic status for minorities. Americans in rural communities and in the black community rely heavily on community-based informal care systems. Currin et al. (2019) studied gaps in communication between primary family caregivers of older adults and respite caregivers and found that those who could potentially benefit from respite care were reluctant to seek it for various reasons. This finding has enormous implications for nursing practice. Since informal health care is an important, cost-effective component of healthcare systems, different forms of respite care have been implemented to support caregivers. Not only do many patients prefer receiving care from someone familiar in their home environment, in many cases, such care will help them avoid placement in a long-term care facility. Nurses are uniquely positioned to build impactful relationships with informal caregivers and have a role in looking for alternatives to improve the delivery of care. Community relationships with informal caregivers, provides nurses with the knowledge, skills, and resources to discuss the potential benefits of support that is available for both the family and the care recipient.

RURAL PUBLIC HEALTH DEPARTMENTS

There are more than 2800 local and state health departments in the United States and 61% of the majority are small, located in populations of fewer than 50,000 people, serving less than 10% of the U.S. population (National Association of County & City Health Officials, 2019). Since 1980 the *Healthy People* initiative has been launched to set measurable objectives to increase community health and wellbeing (Healthy People.gov, n.d.). The purpose of Healthy People (2010) objective 24-11 was to increase the proportion of state and local public health departments (LHDs) that meet national performance standards for public health services. Both in 2010 and 2020, substantial progress has been made in achieving the *Healthy People* objectives. The 2020 results show that 25% of the *Healthy People* objectives outlined for public health have been improved upon, with 50% exceeding or meeting the target. Leaving 25% in further decline or with no change to the public health infrastructure (U.S. Department of Health and Human Services, n.d. -g). The transition to Healthy People (2030) will consist of a more streamlined approach.

Consisting of wide-range initiatives and targets that are focused on core, developmental, and research objectives relative to monitoring community health, reporting health disparities, and utilizing evidence-based research to impact the health and well-being of rural communities (U.S. Department of Health and Human Services, n.d.-a.).

State and local public health departments are uniquely positioned within rural communities as a potential catalyst for addressing the long-standing challenges associated with urban-rural health disparities. While focused on improving the health of populations, LHDs provide a wide array of services focused on assessing health status, mobilizing action to address health-related issues, and ensuring the delivery of important health services in the community. The ability of rural health departments to develop and cultivate partnerships is essential for the integration of public health within the larger healthcare delivery system.

Nonetheless, rural LHDs remain subject to the same persistent challenges facing the larger health care delivery system in rural communities. Limited by budget, staffing, and capacity constraints, both the number and type of public health services provided in rural health departments often differ markedly from what is observed among urban LHD counterparts. These differences ultimately limit the ability of rural health departments to respond to national public health and health care policy initiatives. Even so, some examples, as illustrated in the outcomes of the *2010* and *2020 Healthy People* objectives, point to important advances in meeting the health needs of rural communities (Hale, 2015).

Rural Mental Health Care

Much like the economic crisis in the 1980s, the Covid-19 Pandemic in 2000 has affected a considerable number of the rural population and contributed to mental health problems. Public health pandemics, such as Covid-19 and natural disasters, such as drought and flood, in addition to the economic downturns in the late 1990s, are all contributing factors to continuing chronic stress. Those affected are most apt to work in the traditional ranching, farming, mining, forestry, and fishing industries. Although mental health disorders widely affect rural and urban residents throughout the lifespan, nearly one in five rural residents face some form of mental illness (Bailey, 2016). Factors such as poverty, race, age, social isolation, and rural dwelling lower the prospect of accessing mental health services. Clearly, large sections of at-risk rural populations are without mental health care (Bailey, 2009; Rural Health Information Hub, 2019c).

Three key factors have been identified as contributing to mental illness in rural areas. First, there is a lack of specialized mental health providers in rural areas. The most recent figures show that 75% of rural counties with populations between 2500 and 20,000 do not have a psychiatrist and that 95% do not have a child psychiatrist. Next, because of the lack of qualified mental healthcare providers, rural residents often receive services from primary care providers. Many rural primary care providers are ill-equipped to provide mental health services,

and there are limited NP and physician assistant resources to support the mental health care that is needed. Both specialized mental health care and primary health care providers are confronted with barriers related to rural practice. These include a more diverse practice, fewer opportunities for ongoing education, and fewer professionals to consult with than their colleagues in urban practice. Lastly, rural residents often do not seek mental health services because of perceived stigma and because they do not always recognize a need for mental health services (Bailey, 2009; Rural Health Information Hub, 2019g).

Rural America is dominated by factors of self-employment and small businesses, leading to lower rates of employer-sponsored health insurance, and residents who are less insured or are underinsured with greater rates of mental health difficulties than their urban counterparts. Possessing unique attitudes and beliefs that are characterized by much less mental health literacy than their urban peers, knowing the symptoms and the issues that surround behavioral health disorders, and the available choices and options for care is a constant challenge for rural residents who find themselves navigating a complex healthcare system for mental health (National Institute of Mental Health, 2018). Nurses and rural care providers have the unique opportunity to join forces in their community to develop the use of mental health resources, such as partnering with schools and public health centers, promoting telehealth and telepsychiatry, and developing advocacy programs to create further awareness and community outreach to provide resources and reduce the stigma surrounding mental health for those who may be in need of mental health care.

EMERGENCY SERVICES

Access to EMS has become a safety net for underserved rural communities, often becoming the only guaranteed access to health services, EMS been identified as one of the most significant health care issues for rural residents and (Bailey, 2009; Bryant, 2009; National Rural Health Association, 2018a). As an integrated service operating at the crossroads between health care, public health, and public safety, EMS is an essential public service intended to enhance the health and safety of a community (DC.gov, n.d.). As a widely regarded system, EMS provides transport to definitive care for patients with emergency illnesses and injuries and includes the provision of pre-hospital care, hospital or health center-based emergency care, and trauma systems.

Rural residents depend on EMS because of the propensity to high risk for unintentional injury. Low population density, such as that in rural areas, has been shown to be a strong predictor of higher injury-related morbidity and mortality rates (Peek-Asa et al., 2004; Jarman et al., 2016). In medically underserved areas, EMS systems play an increasingly important role in decreasing the morbidity and mortality of individuals needing emergency care. Getting patients from the place of injury to the trauma center within the "golden hour" is imperative and frequently not possible in rural areas because of barriers imposed by distance, terrain, climatic conditions, and communication methods. Some rural facilities are more than 1 hour away by air from the nearest trauma center or tertiary care hospital (Hsia and Shen, 2011; National Rural Health Association, 2018a). For those rural residents, the death rate remains twice that of urban residents.

There is an enormous variability in EMS systems across the rural landscape; with declining federal and state funding, some EMS systems are organized through the local fire department while other systems are operated through local municipal or county governments. EMS may also be delivered by volunteers or may be provided by hospital-based systems or private companies (Institute of Medicine, 2006; Homeland Security, 2017). Challenges faced by rural EMS systems include a shortage of volunteers, obtaining and maintenance of equipment necessary for patient transport, a lower level of training than among urban providers, reduced funding for training and education, training curricula that often do not reflect rural hazards (e.g., farm equipment trauma), lack of guidance from physicians, and a lack of physician training about and orientation to the EMS system (Bryant, 2009; National Rural Health Association, 2018a). Low population density; large, isolated, or inaccessible areas; severe weather; poor roads; and lower density of telephones or other communication methods also contribute to difficult public access for emergency care. These problems make the challenges of developing EMS in rural areas substantial (National Rural Health Association, 2018a).

Emergency Preparedness in Rural Communities

Emergency preparedness refers to actions that should be performed before an emergency, such as planning and coordination meetings, procedure writing, team training, emergency drills and exercises, and positioning of emergency equipment. Emergency response is generally described as the tactical planning and practical activities designed to protect life and property immediately after some type of event. Emergency response plans prioritize protecting people first and property second. Some of the key elements of an emergency response program include evacuation planning and assembly; escalation protocols; damage assessment and reporting; hazmat response and spill control; medical response; salvage and reclamation; and specialty issues such as fire brigades, first aid, high angle or confined space rescue, and so forth. (Ready.gov, 2021; Rural Health Information Hub, 2019e). Rural areas are not exempt from disasters. Challenges of emergency preparation and management are different for rural communities from those for urban ones. As written in the *Rural Emergency Preparedness and Response* guide, The Rural Health Information Hub (2019e) categorized these challenges into five major themes: resource limitations, access to healthcare, remoteness and geography, low population density, and communication.

Resources needed in a disaster include human capital, financial capital, and social capital. Due to the increase in urbanization, the decline in the overall rural population, and the rise in the rural population age, the human and financial resources available to prepare and respond to disasters are limited. Social capital becomes the focus to meet the challenges

of rural communities. Building relationships among emergency agencies, community organizations, and local businesses is essential to secure human and financial resources. Rural areas also depend on networks of volunteers (e.g., first responders).

The remoteness of rural areas results in longer response times. Population density may affect the funding of rural communities' emergency preparedness. As state and federal programs often consider population size and density in many funding decisions, so densely populated areas receive the most attention for mitigation and recovery activities (Bryant, 2009; Rural Health Information Hub, 2019e). Finally, communication education about emergency preparation is more expensive in rural areas. This higher cost leads to reduced outreach before disasters and throughout the event. Warning systems are often absent or neglected in remote areas, placing the burden on the individual to access emergency information.

Nurses can help assist in responding to community health problems and health-endangering situations by reviewing disaster plans and policies, determining when, where and how evacuations should occur, and studying operation protocols for protective equipment, immunization, security, and safety measures. Nurses can assume a variety of roles by actively participating in emergency drills to obtain the necessary skills for planning and preparation in response to any type of community health problem or situation. The variety of roles for nurses who acquire this knowledge includes that of providing consumer and community education, administering aid and medications, assessing victims and vulnerable populations, or monitoring the mental health needs of responders and victims (Mississippi College, 2018).

Emergency Preparedness During the COVID-19 Pandemic

When emergencies happen in rural communities, especially those that are severe and prolonged, the demand can quickly consume available resources. The 2020 nationwide response to the COVID-19 pandemic demonstrates the importance of emergency preparedness.

During the height of the COVID-19 pandemic, rural residents accounted for 27% of all the COVID-19 deaths and accounted for more case infections per 100,000 adults than their urban counterparts, averaging two weekly rural deaths per 100 cases. Contributing factors that accounted for these deaths include an older population that lives farther away from access to hospitals and a population more likely to have underlying healthcare issues and comorbidities who are less likely to have health insurance (U.S. Department of Agriculture Economic Research Service, 2020a).

During the COVID-19 pandemic, rural healthcare systems experienced episodes of fluctuating volumes. Patients who visited hospitals and clinics were of higher acuity, the result of patients waiting to seek treatment due to the fear associated with contracting the Coronavirus. Residents of rural nursing homes were considered a high-risk and vulnerable population to contracting the Coronavirus, resulting in fear, deaths, and further social isolation away from family members. Government restrictions on activity, social distancing requirements, and other measures in response to the pandemic adversely affected the U.S. economy. The Centers for Disease Control and Prevention (CDC) identified two personal characteristics of a highly vulnerable population to the Coronavirus, an older aging population—especially those over the age of 75, and the presence of underlying health problems. In addition to the difficulty in accessing health care and the geography of residing far away from hospitals and healthcare centers, the implications for the rural population is devastating, as the COVID-19 pandemic continued to affect a higher magnitude of the rural population living in a highly vulnerable area (U.S. Department of Agriculture Economic Research Service, 2020a).

Throughout the COVID-19 pandemic, rural healthcare systems have been faced with additional financial vulnerabilities. As care providers have become ill, healthcare systems have been tasked with the increased demands of hiring and paying for additional and contract staffing, obtaining additional equipment and supplies for intensive services, and canceling or postponing services that are financially beneficial to keeping the hospital viable within the community.

Learning from these burdens can strengthen the opportunity for change and advocacy in health care. Specifically, for rural health care, further opportunities exist in the expansion of coverage of telemedicine and telehealth services, legislative policies that support increased bed capacity in rural hospitals and expanding legislative advocacy for health care in rural communities (Nickels, 2020).

As a result of the COVID-19 pandemic from a social standpoint, the increased stress on healthcare resources has created an opportunity for increased collaboration from healthcare facilities and service organizations. Such collaborative forces are necessary to ensure adequate manpower exists to complete and fulfill community testing requirements, administer personal protective equipment (PPE) and administer vaccines throughout the rural community. Every community must prepare and respond to hazardous events as they will continue to occur, posing devastating economical, health, and social consequences. Whether a natural disaster or disease outbreak, social vulnerability factors such as poverty, housing, lack of access to transportation, geographical access, and healthcare services continue to threaten rural populations and weaken a community's ability to prevent human suffering and financial loss in a disaster (Pfankuch, 2020).

? ACTIVE LEARNING

Select a rural community health nurse (i.e., public health or home care) and conduct an interview in person or by telephone if distance prohibits a face-to-face meeting.
- Identify what the nurse sees as the pros and cons of rural nursing.
- If negative aspects of rural nursing are identified, discuss how the nurse deals with them.
- Ask the nurse to discuss the three highest-priority efforts related to his or her rural practice.

UPSTREAM INTERVENTIONS

Upstream and prevention-oriented approaches have several implications for nurses in rural practice. Descriptions of three strategies for upstream interventions follow: attack community-based problems at their roots, emphasize the "doing" aspects of health, and maximize the use of informal networks.

Attacking Community-Based Problems at Their Roots

Upstream approaches to community health problems can be multifaceted and complex, directing the nurse toward an understanding of the precursors of poor health within populations of interest. Individual nurses can be effective forces in uncovering and enhancing community awareness of health-endangering situations. Environmental health issues in rural communities, such as pesticide exposure and health hazards from point-source factory emissions, are more effectively assessed and remedied on a community level than on a case-by-case basis. Nurses' involvement in helping people understands health problems in a larger context can be the genesis of change. Nurses and other community members can take social action on behalf of those affected. For example, by heightening awareness of sulfur dioxide levels from a local refinery and the relationship of those emission levels to respiratory problems in vulnerable populations, nurses can help citizens gain an understanding of the collective rather than individual burden of the refinery on their community's health.

Additional avenues that nurses can use to become involved in upstream interventions include advocating at public council meetings when issues affecting community health are discussed. Working with community members and employers to promote health opportunities and healthy work environments, utilize community data to identify and discuss threats to health and responding to disease outbreaks, advocating for the promotion of healthy behaviors, and promoting connectedness within communities for healthy behaviors. Rural nurses have a powerful voice in community-based disease prevention efforts, advocating for patient health initiatives, and in decreasing emerging risk factors to promote healthy behaviors in the prevention of illness for their community.

? ACTIVE LEARNING

Meet with an elected community official or community hospital board member or participate in a community group organized around a community health problem. Speak about the risk factors that may be presently threatening the health of your community. Discuss how you can actively take part in promoting connectedness and healthy behaviors in your community by completing the following:
- Identify three precursors of poor health in your population.
- What initiatives can you support from the precursors that you have identified to improve the health in your community?
- Develop a strategy to promote connectedness within your community in promoting healthy behaviors to eliminate community health issues.

Emphasizing the "Doing" Aspects of Health

There are consistent differences between the ways rural and nonrural residents perceive health. The primary difference is the relative importance of "work" and "being able to work" in selfreported definitions of health (Weinert and Long, 1987; Gessert et al., 2015). Rural attitudes generally emphasize the "doing" aspects of health in functioning and performing the activities that are fundamentally important in their daily lives. The high value placed on "being able to do" can give astute nurses intervention opportunities for both families and communities. Examples of nursing interventions and strategies that capitalize on this attitude include accident prevention programs for children, exercise and nutrition programs for seniors, and participation of local industries in risk reduction programs for workers. Active involvement of the target population in all phases of program planning and implementation is key to the success of these programs.

Emphasizing the "doing" aspects of health is a cultural attribute for rural residents, independence and self-reliance are survival values that are ingrained in rural residents who live long distances away from services and other people - identifying a sense of pride in being part of a community where neighbors look out for and care for one another. Rural families possess more traditional and conservative values built upon family traditions and customs, and their position or status in the community is almost always tied to the family.

Rural residents are also often slow to adopt new advances in modern technology and demonstrate a sense of security in keeping the status quo in "the way things have always been done." Modifications to their health behavior patterns are adopted more slowly and gradually, and minor health issues can turn into severe problems. This creates additional challenges to community prevention initiatives and the ability to achieve sustainable, positive, and transformational outcomes when addressing community determinants of health in a rural community.

Maximizing the Use of Informal Networks

Recognizing and using informal networks in the community is essential to the "doing" concept of prevention programs. As most people who have been involved in community empowerment programs will attest, accomplishing the involvement of these important entities is not an easy or straightforward task. Territorial issues and collateral agendas can obstruct rather than facilitate change. However, failure to elicit community involvement in population-based health interventions will have unfavorable consequences. Frequently, superimposed change tends to fit poorly with the community it is intended to serve. Rural change strategies will be short-lived unless community members understand them and invest in their own well-being.

Working with informal networks for collaborative problem solving and decision making requires **collaborative leadership**. A process that involves all stakeholders who take responsibility to solve a problem to work collaboratively together (Rabinowitz, 2020). Collaborative leadership consists of the process of utilizing informal networks to consider a problem and working together

with key stakeholders to develop and collectively decide upon possible interventions to deploy. By utilizing collaborative leadership, partnerships with informal networks can be developed to obtain ownership and "buy-in" to a common purpose. Responsibility and involvement in initiatives also deepen as action plans are developed, and trust grows within the group as individuals find common ground in working together (Rabinowitz, 2020).

The process of collaborative leadership also offers additional advantages, such as access to new information and ideas, empowerment, and increased opportunities to obtain sustainable outcomes. Collaborative leadership can also lead to a fundamental change in the way that organizations, networks, and communities' function and operate together. Collaboration breeds more collaboration that ultimately leads to a different way of looking at and solving community problems (Rabinowitz, 2020). Prevention-oriented approaches will require collaborative leadership to successfully identify community problems in working within a diverse culture to collectively initiate fundamental change within a rural community.

LEGISLATION AND PROGRAMS AFFECTING RURAL PUBLIC HEALTH

Programs That Augment Health Care Facilities and Services

On September 23, 2020, the Federal Office of Rural Health Policy (FORHP) designated areas to be eligible for rural health grant programs published in the Federal Register, adding MSA counties that contain no UA population to the areas eligible for rural health grant programs. The FORHP collected stakeholder comments describing a change to the definition of rural for the determination of geographic areas eligible to apply for or receive services funded by rural health grants. Issuing a rural change and new grant opportunities for rural communities in 2022 (Health Resources and Services Administration, 2021).

Several programs exist that are particularly important for meeting the public health needs of rural communities. Rural health programs continue to evolve with changes in healthcare reform, so why this is not a comprehensive list of all the programs that are available for rural health facilities and providers, it provides a good understanding of the programs that are available to meet the public health needs of rural populations.

The Community Health Centers (CHC) program authorized by the United States Public Health Service Act. The CHC program benefits underserved areas and populations by providing primary health care and, in some cases, supplemental secondary and tertiary health care, such as hospital care, long-term home health care, and rehabilitation. Rural health clinics (RHCs) are designed to improve access to primary care. As an incentive to rural communities to apply as an RHC, Medicare, and Medicaid are reimbursed at a higher rate than usual at such centers (Health Resources Services Administration, n.d.-a; Electronic Code of Federal Regulations, 2021).

The MHP comes under the Bureau of Primary Health Care and the HRSA, Department of Health and Human Services

(DHHS). Through the MHP, Community and Migrant health centers (MHCs) provide comprehensive nursing and medical care and support services to Migrant and Seasonal Farm Workers and their families. MHCs provide culturally sensitive care to a racially and culturally diverse farm labor force from many countries in Latin America and the Caribbean. Bilingual, bicultural health personnel, including lay outreach workers, use culturally appropriate protocols to provide primary care, preventive health care, transportation, dental care, pharmaceuticals, and environmental health services. The MHC must provide the same services as the CHC and may also offer supplemental services, such as environmental health services, infectious disease and parasite control, and accident prevention programs (Health Resources and Services Administration, n.d.-a).

Medicare's Rural Hospital Flexibility grant program (the Flex Program) replaces earlier demonstration programs. Funded by the FORHP, the Flex Program allows small hospitals the flexibility to reconfigure operations and be licensed as Critical Access Hospitals (CAHs) (Flex Monitoring Team, n.d.; Health Resources and Services Administration, n.d.-b). The program also provides cost-based reimbursement for inpatient Medicare and outpatient services. Grants are also awarded for planning, implementing, and establishing networks of care and improving EMS. The Flex Monitoring Team (FMT) examines data from the Flex Program. It operates and maintains The Critical Access Hospital Measurement and Performance Assessment System (CAHMPAS) to conduct research and benchmarking on CAHs and address the performance of quality, financial, and community measures at the national, state, and hospital level. The FMT publishes its findings each year to assist in optimizing the performance of state Flex Programs and CAHs (Flex Monitoring Team, n.d.).

Primary Care Association Cooperative Agreements (PCAs) facilitate the development of primary care services and attract primary care providers to rural HPSA (Health Resources and Services Administration, n.d.-d). Special legislation for HPSAs has also created programs to attract primary and mental health providers to acute care facilities to provide inpatient and outpatient services for primary care and mental health services (U.S. Department of Health and Human Services, 2020b).

The Rural Healthcare Provider Transition Project, authorized by the HRSA and the U.S. DHHS as a cooperative agreement, helps provide technical assistance to small rural communities with nonprofit hospitals, tribal organizations, and RHCs. To adjust to changes in clinical practice patterns and in-hospital use, shifts from hospital to community-based care, and changes in emergency care delivery patterns to strengthen their foundation in the elements of value-based care, including quality, efficiency, patient experience, and safety of care (Health Resources and Services Administration, n.d.-c).

On September 3, 2020, the US DHHS released the Rural Action Plan, an assessment of rural healthcare efforts as administered by the DHHS Rural Task Force. This assessment provides an action plan to strengthen health care coordination efforts for Americans who live in rural communities. The Rural Action Plan examines the key challenges facing rural communities related to issues such as emerging health disparities, chronic disease, maternal mortality, and access to mental health services. These key challenges are the focus of existing strategies that have been implemented by the DHHS Rural Task Force to build a sustainable health and human services model for rural communities, leveraging technology and innovation, preventing disease and mortality, and increasing rural access to care (U.S Department of Health and Human Services, 2020c). The Rural Action Plan builds upon funding opportunities as those previously mentioned in addition to other opportunities for rural communities.

Health centers have become part of the nation's primary health care foundation, distinguished by their quality of care, affordability, and accessibility to all community residents, and their mission to the community.
RCHN, Community Health Foundation (2021)

RURAL COMMUNITY HEALTH NURSING

One of the most important messages for nurses practicing in a rural environment is that perhaps a more accurate title than rural community health nursing would be "community health nursing along the rural continuum." Nonmetropolitan areas would be at one end of the continuum, with metropolitan areas at the other end.

Practice in a rural area may require working as the only nurse at a health department in a remote Western Great Plains frontier county with a population of 6000, at a full-service health department in a town of 50,000 people, or at a large health department in a rural area next to an urban population. A practice in a rural area adjacent to a large metropolitan area often appears to have more in common with the urban end of the continuum in terms of agency size, distances, and resources. For the purposes of this discussion, the practice setting is at the more "rural" end of the continuum.

The following definition illustrates the broad-based, generalist focus of the modern rural community health nurse. It includes the important geographical and cultural environment in which community health practice is implemented and helps define appropriate nursing interventions.

Rural nursing is the practice of professional nursing within the physical and sociocultural context of sparsely populated communities. It involves the continual interaction of the rural environment, the nurse, and his or her practice. Rural nursing includes the diagnosis and treatment of a diversified population of people of all ages and a variety of human responses to actual (or potential) occupational hazards or to actual (or potential) health problems existent in maternity, pediatric, medical/surgical, and emergency nursing in a given rural area (Bigbee, 1993; Lee and Winters, 2004; Rosenthal, 2005; Williams et al., 2012).

Characteristics of Rural Nursing

The uniqueness of rural nursing practice has been in question. Some believe that nursing care for rural clients is the same as for other individuals and that health problems and patient care needs are similar, regardless of the setting. Others argue that rural practice should be designated as a specialty or subspecialty because of factors such as isolation, scarce resources, and the need for a wide range of practice skills that must be adapted to emerging social and economic structures. Whether generalist or specialist, nurses being prepared for rural practice must be equipped with additional community health assessment skills (Kulbok et al., 2012).

The study of Rural Nurses: Lifestyle Preferences and Education Preferences (Molanari et al., 2011), and the article, Importance of Nursing in Rural Communities (University of North Carolina Wilmington, 2019). Identifies several positive attributes of rural nursing in the ability to provide holistic care, to know everyone well, and to develop close relationships with the community and coworkers where nurses enjoyed a rural lifestyle as reasons to practice rural nursing. Autonomy, professional status, and being valued by the organization and community to deliver quality care to the whole patient have been reported as favorable and positive components of job satisfaction. Of those components identified as negative, both healthcare and professional organizations are most actively addressing professional isolation. The use of distance education technologies is one way to address the isolation many rural nurses experience. University degree programs and continuing education courses are readily available online or through full-motion interactive or simulation multimedia. Using these technologies, rural nurses can update their skills and network with other nurses without having to leave their home communities to develop multiple proficiencies that are required of a rural nurse.

The conceptual framework so eloquently described in the book *Conceptual basis for rural nursing* (Scharff, 1998) still applies to the rural nurse of the present (Molinari and Bushy, 2012). Considering the distinctive nature of the rural nurse's practice, Scharff found that the rural nurse is a generalist and remarked that "generalist" is not synonymous with "boring." Interviews with rural nurses show that they feel an "intensity of purpose" that makes rural nursing distinctive. Nurses living and practicing in the same place have a strong sense of integration and continuity between practice and community. The conceptual framework of rural nursing applies to the rural nurse of today, as Scharff goes on to eloquently describe the transition of a rural nurse:

The newcomer practices nursing in a rural setting, unlike the more experienced nurse, who practices rural nursing. Somewhere between these extremes lies the transitional period of events and conditions through which each nurse passes at her or his own pace. It is within this time zone that nurses experience rural reality and move toward becoming professionals who understand that having gone rural, they are not less than they were, but rather, they are more than they expected to be. Some may be conscious of the transition, and others may not, but in the end, a few will say, "I am a rural nurse."

Scharff (1998, p.38)

Rural community health nursing services can include maternal and child health, adult and geriatric health, school health, mental health, and occupational health. Rural nurses also work in surgery, intensive care units, and emergency departments in caring for acutely ill patients.

The uniqueness of rural nursing, unlike nurses who practice in urban areas, is the ability to have a higher level of autonomy. Simultaneously, rural nurses must anticipate patient needs and be acutely aware of their own boundaries and scope of practice limitations to demonstrate a level of self-awareness in autonomous nursing practice. The nurse practicing with the autonomy common in rural practice brings knowledge and competence in other clinical specialties. This level of autonomy is directly related to the need for rural nurses to acquire the necessary skills to float or work in multiple clinical areas, adding additional skills and opportunities to the nurse's repertoire by training in multiple clinical areas. For example, rural nurses who are trained to work in the emergency department and in the intensive care units will cross-train to each of these areas as part of a critical care specialty. Rural nurses acquire diverse clinical experiences that evolve from advanced knowledge and increased autonomy over their ability to expand upon their area of practice and their ability to make autonomous decisions based on their training and professional knowledge in caring for their patients.

Autonomy is also exhibited in working as part of a team, collaborating with other nurses in supporting one another, and involving other nurses by sharing their knowledge and skills when making clinical decisions. Rural nurses also exhibit increased autonomy by being more involved in taking part in informal shared governance and decision-making committees, often asked to serve on multiple committees and unit councils to make decisions that affect their areas of nursing practice. While autonomy also exists for urban nurses, it is rural nurses who are more often involved in extensive practice areas, providers gain increased interdependence and trust in the nurse's clinical judgment, and team cohesiveness is developed within the rural healthcare team, maximizing the full potential of the healthcare team in designing and implementing improvements in rural health.

Rural nursing requires a discriminating, solid practitioner who can perform general nursing at a skill level beyond that of the outdated "mile wide and inch deep" general nursing. To be able to move seamlessly and confidently across patient populations with scare resources, requires an independent spirit, flexibility, creativity, constant adaptability, strong networking and communication skills, and a commitment to the ongoing pursuit of professional development (Molinari and Bushy, 2012). The rural nurse must be an "expert generalist," developing multiple proficiencies in technical and clinical competency, self-confidence, leadership, adaptability, flexibility, sound decision making, and interest in continuing education, together with skills in handling emergencies, teaching, and public relations to provide any care that is needed (Molinari and Bushy, 2012).

Community Health Needs Assessments

Rural communities have limited services to address many of the health-related needs of their community. Research and needs assessments can help determine where and how resources and program evaluations should be targeted as an area of focus when determining interventions or approaches that work well in a rural environment. **Community health** needs assessments (CHNA) are tools utilized to identify the current state of affairs in a community, organization, or program and is used as a decision-making aid for stakeholders in determining what is needed to strengthen health resources in a rural community (Rural Health Information Hub, 2019a).

Key audiences for completing a CHNA are local public health departments, which include community health assessments (CHA) and the development of community health improvement plans (CHIP) as an element to obtain federal funding and maintain accreditation standards. Likewise, to maintain their tax-exempt status, charitable and nonprofit hospitals have a federal requirement to complete a CHNA once every 3 years and, on an annual basis, must provide a description of the actions taken and the implementation strategy to address the needs that have been identified in the CHNA for the rural community (Rural Health Information Hub, 2019a).

CHNAs can fulfill a variety of functions, such as identifying community strengths and weaknesses, determining a particular healthcare service or strategy to address a need in the community, identifying the healthcare status of a specific population or demographic, defining the need for rural healthcare workers, and identifying particular health conditions in a rural community. CHNAs also provide a better understanding of how to utilize resources by distinguishing the underlying culture and social structure that is present in a rural community (Center for Community Health and Development, 1994–2020).

Community stakeholders, government officials, community-based organizations, schools, colleges, and businesses are a key resource involved in the assessment process to provide information and perspectives on the necessary services that are important in the community. Methods for gathering information include the use of data collection, surveys, interviews, focus groups, and community forums. Data obtained to form the CHNA is analyzed and implemented into action plans that become part of the assessment and evaluation process to direct community funding and resources to the highest identified priority needs. The completion of the CHNA involves sharing findings with the community to gain valuable input and feedback on the progress of implementation. Additionally, continuous engagement with rural stakeholders on the outcomes of the CHNA improvement plan is essential to collaborate and join efforts and to make positive and sustainable health changes in the community (Center for Community Health and Development, 1994–2020).

RURAL HEALTH RESEARCH

There are multiple policy-relevant resources that exist for decision making and tracking progress on efforts to improve the health and lives of rural residents and families. The following resources provide a good understanding of some of the research

programs currently available to meet the needs of rural communities.

The HRSA provides access to and support for research through the Research Centers Program. The Research Centers Program is the only federal research program entirely dedicated to producing policy-relevant research on health care and population health in rural areas. Each research center has its own identity (although it may be part of a larger organization), Website, and core staff that includes a disciplinary mix of health services research, epidemiology, public health, geography, medicine, and mental health. Over the 4-year award cycle, each research center develops a portfolio of several research projects per year in conjunction with input from the FORHP and other experts (Health Resources and Services Administration, 2019).

To strengthen the dissemination of research results, the HRSA launched the Rural Health Research Gateway in early 2006. The gateway is a "one-stop-shop" for the research centers, providing easy access to projects funded by the FORHP and summaries of research in progress. The gateway's research alerts provide e-mail updates when new publications become available (Health Resources and Services Administration, 2019).

The HRSA has also developed the Community-Based Division (CBD) grant programs. These programs provide funding to increase access to care in rural communities and to address the unique health care challenges of rural communities. Most of the CBD's programs require community organizations to share resources and expertise using evidence-based models of care in networks of two or more healthcare services providers (Health Resources and Services Administration, 2020).

The Robert Wood Johnson Foundation (RWJF) emerged as the nation's second-largest wealthiest philanthropic foundation more than 45 years ago and is driven by a continuous cycle of research with the aim of identifying the root cause of health disparities in America and potential solutions to improve health, equity, and well-being. Grant programs are preference to provide funding to higher education, public entities, and nonprofit organizations, with research funded to help address some of America's most pressing health challenges in the key areas of targeted research, policy and systems research, and research-driven demonstrations. Through four broad areas of health systems, healthy children and families, healthy communities, and leadership for better health, research is conducted with a specific focus that addresses health outcomes and key determinates of health and improving population health and health equity. The RWJF has a specific collection dedicated to rural health and well-being in America to understand strengths, challenges, and opportunities for achieving health and well-being in rural communities (Robert Wood Johnson Foundation, 2001–2020).

Universities across the country have created centers for rural health research. North Dakota State University has The Center for Rural Health (2021), which undertakes research initiatives to support rural and tribal communities by identifying and describing health disparities; examining issues related to health care service delivery and systems, health workforce, and population health; and supporting the development of research expertise. The University of Minnesota has the Rural Health Research Center (2021). The research center has been producing focused, top-quality research for 2 decades now. The Rural Health Research Center was first established with funding from the FORHP in 1992. Their projects address key forces that are shaping quality of care and quality improvement in rural areas.

For example:

- Employing quality measurement and public reporting as tools to upgrade quality of care.
- Using technology and health professional staffing in innovative ways to improve quality of care and patient safety.
- Devising financial incentives that can help improve care in rural hospitals and clinics.

Capacity to Manage Improvements in Rural Health

Healthy People (2020) outlines health-related objectives for Americans and forms the rationale for efforts to intervene in disease trends to improve health where disparities have been identified. The health disparities in rural health have been highlighted, and specific areas of focus for rural health have been established, with over 300 objectives outlined for this area of improvement (HealthyPeople.Gov, 2020).

Determining the status of health indicators, such as rates of morbidity, mortality from common diseases or injury, and, perhaps most important, access to health care services, allows for priorities to be determined for which improvements in health are needed. Importantly, Healthy People 2020 objectives and intervention strategies have been analyzed for rural-urban disparities that may exist along geographic, demographic, and cultural dimensions to provide a more specific picture of potential research priorities concerning improvements in health. The Healthy People 2020 box presents data from a survey of 1214 national and state rural health experts that identify percentages of respondents who indicated giving priority status for various health issues.

Interestingly, in their position statement, The National Organization of State Offices of Rural Health (NOSORH, 2019) indicates that for *Healthy People 2030*, foundation documents do not include any rural specific objectives. Noting the multiple demonstrable health disparities between populations in rural, nonmetropolitan areas and populations in urban, metropolitan areas. Given the size of the rural population and the continuing health disparities between rural and urban populations, NOSORH recommends creating a separate Rural Health category for *Healthy People 2030*. While the transition from *Healthy People 2020* to *Healthy People 2030* consists of a more streamlined approach to include a new focus on social determinants of health (SDOH), the overall objectives for this goal are to improve the health for all demographics and populations "in

attaining the full potential for health and well-being for all" (U.S. Department of Health and Human Services, n.d.).

The NOSORH proposed rule-specific objectives for *Healthy People 2030* box presents the creation of a separate Rural Health category for *Healthy People 2030* with key objectives and rationale for their inclusion.

Research questions directed toward improving health may be suggested for any of the *Healthy People 2020* and *2030* objectives but may have the greatest potential to address salient rural trends if they relate to issues of access to care, mental health, oral health, educational and community-based programs, diabetes, or injury and violence prevention. Additionally, investigators may want to consider how these established rural priorities may be consistent or different within specific populations of concern. Because the availability of surveillance data is often limited as researchers concern themselves with increasingly smaller populations (e.g., from state to county), efforts to gather additional primary data may be needed to set research priorities for improvements to health.

❤ HEALTHY PEOPLE 2020
Rural Health Priorities

Rural Priorities (Identified by Rural Health Survey Priority Votes)	Percentage (%) of Respondents (*N* = 1214)
Access to health care	76.3
Nutrition and weight status	54.5
Diabetes	54.4
Mental health and mental disorders	53.6
Substance abuse	45.4
Heart disease and stroke	45.3
Physical activity and health	44.7
Older adults	39.7
Maternal, infant and child health	37.0
Tobacco use	35.3
Cancer	35.2
Education and community-based programs	33.2
Oral health	31.4
Quality of life and well-being	26.9
Immunizations and infectious diseases	26.7
Public health infrastructure	26.0
Family planning and sexual health	22.9
Injury and violence prevention	21.8
Social determinants of health	21.3
Health communication and IT	21.2

Data from Bolin JN, Bellamy G, Ferdinand AO, Kash B, Helduser JW, editors: *Rural Healthy People 2020: A companion document to Healthy People (2020). Table modified* (Vol. 1). College Station, TX, 2015, The Texas A&M Health Science Center, School of Public Health, Southwest Rural Health Research Center. Available from: https://srhrc.tamhsc.edu/docs/rhp2020-volume-1.pdf.

HEALTHY PEOPLE 2030

The National Organization of State Offices of Rural Health (NOSORH) Proposed Rural-Specific Objectives and Rationale for Healthy People 2030

Category of Key Objectives for Rural Health—Healthy People 2030

Fair or poor health status
Functional limitation
Adult obesity
Serious psychological distress
Heart disease mortality
Suicide mortality
Unintentional injury mortality

Infant mortality
Child vaccination
Access to healthcare
Access to dental care
Health insurance
Financial barriers to prescription drugs

Rationale for key objectives for rural health—Healthy People 2030

Proposed objective	Rationale	Proposed baseline unit of measure
Fair or poor health status Decrease the percent of persons in rural areas reporting fair or poor health status, decreasing the disparity between rural and urban percentages for this measure. Proposed data source: National health interview survey data made available by NCHS is proposed as the source of data for this objective. Anticipated number of data points: Annual updates of these files should provide 10 additional data points for the decade.	Summary tables made available by the National Center For Health Statistics (NCHS) show that in 2016, 11.4% of persons in rural non-metro areas reported being in fair or poor health, as compared to 8.6% of persons in metro areas. Similar rural-urban disparities exist in previous years.	The percent of persons in rural (nonmetro) and urban (metro) areas reporting fair or poor health status is recommended as the unit of measure for this objective. Nonmetro and metro areas are as defined in the latest urbanization categories used by CDC. The 2016 data for this measure is suggested as a proposed baseline.
Functional limitation Decrease the percent of persons age 18 and older in rural areas reporting a complete inability or a lot of difficulty in performing routine functions, decreasing the disparity between rural and urban percentages for this measure. Proposed data source: National health interview survey data made available by NCHS is proposed as the source of data for this objective. Anticipated number of data points: Annual updates of these files should provide 10 additional data points for the decade.	Summary tables made available by the National Center For Health Statistics (NCHS) show that in 2016, 11.3% of persons age 18 and older in rural non-metro areas reported a complete inability or a lot of difficulty in performing routine functions, as compared to 8.1% of persons age 18 and older in metro areas. Similar rural-urban disparities exist in previous years.	The percent of persons in rural (nonmetro) and urban (metro) areas reporting a complete inability or a lot of difficulty in performing routine functions is recommended as the unit of measure for this objective. Nonmetro and metro areas are as defined in the latest urbanization categories used by CDC. The 2016 data for this measure is suggested as a proposed baseline.
Adult obesity Decrease the percent of obese persons age 18 and older in rural areas, decreasing the disparity between rural and urban percentages for this measure. Proposed data source: Behavioral risk factor surveillance system (BRFSS) data made available by CDC is proposed as the source of data for this objective. Anticipated number of data points: Annual updates of these files should provide 10 additional data points for the decade.	Summary tables made available by the Centers for Disease Control and Prevention (CDC) show that in 2016, 34.2% of persons age 18 and older in rural non-metro areas self-reported obesity, as compared to 28.7% of persons age 18 and older in metro areas. Similar rural-urban disparities exist in previous years.	The percent of persons age 18 and over in rural (non-metro) and urban (metro) areas selfreporting obesity is recommended as the unit of measure for this objective. Nonmetro and metro areas are as defined in the latest urbanization categories used by CDC. The 2016 data for this measure are suggested as a proposed baseline.
Serious psychological distress Decrease the percent of persons age 18 or over in rural areas reporting serious psychological distress, decreasing the disparity between rural and urban percentages for this measure. Proposed data source: National Health Interview Survey data made available by NCHS is proposed as the source of data for this objective. Anticipated number of data points: Annual updates of these files should provide 10 additional data points for the decade.	Summary tables made available by the National Center For Health Statistics (NCHS) show that in 2015—16, 5.1% of persons age 18 and older in rural non-metro areas reported having serious psychological distress in the last 30 days, as compared to 3.3% of persons in metro areas. Similar rural-urban disparities exist in previous years.	The percent of persons age 18 and older in rural (non-metro) and urban (metro) areas reporting serious psychological distress in the last 30 days is recommended as the unit of measure for this objective. Nonmetro and metro areas are as defined in the latest urbanization categories used by CDC. The 2015—16 data for this measure is suggested as a proposed baseline.

Heart disease mortality

Reduce the death rate from heart disease in rural areas, decreasing the disparity between rural and urban heart disease mortality rates.

Proposed data source: The multiple cause of death files maintained in the CDC wonder online database are proposed as the source of data for this objective.

Anticipated number of data points: Annual updates of these files should provide 10 additional data points for the decade.

Detailed mortality tables made available by the Centers For Disease Control And Prevention (CDC) show that for each of the years 2015—17, the age-adjusted death rates from heart disease in rural (non-metro) areas was substantially higher than the corresponding rates in metro areas. For the entire 3-year period in non-core (non-metro) areas, the age-adjusted rate was 196.9 per 100,000 population as compared to 157.6 per 100,000 population in large central metro areas. Similar rural-urban disparities exist in all categories of urbanization.

The age-adjusted death rate from heart disease per 100,000 population in rural (non-metro) and urban (metro) areas is recommended as the unit of measure for this objective. Nonmetro and metro areas are as defined in the latest urbanization categories used by CDC. The 3-year combined rate for 2015—17 is suggested as a proposed baseline.

Suicide mortality

Reduce the suicide death rate in rural areas, decreasing the disparity between rural and urban suicide mortality rates.

Proposed data source: The multiple cause of death files maintained in the CDC wonder online database are proposed as the source of data for this objective.

Anticipated number of data points: Annual updates of these files should provide 10 additional data points for the decade.

Detailed mortality tables made available by the Centers For Disease Control And Prevention (CDC) show that for each of the years 2015—17, the age-adjusted death rates from suicide in rural (non-metro) areas was substantially higher than the corresponding rates in metro areas. For the entire 3-year period in noncore (nonmetro) areas the age-adjusted rate was 19.0 per 100,000 population as compared to 10.7 per 100,000 population in large central metro areas. Similar rural-urban disparities exist in all categories of urbanization.

The age-adjusted death rate from suicide per 100,000 population in rural (non-metro) and urban (metro) areas is recommended as the unit of measure for this objective. Nonmetro and metro areas are as defined in the latest urbanization categories used by CDC. The 3-year combined rate for 2015—17 is suggested as a proposed baseline.

Unintentional injury mortality

Reduce the unintentional injury death rate in rural areas, decreasing the disparity between rural and urban mortality rates from this cause.

Proposed data source: The multiple cause of death files maintained in the CDC wonder online database are proposed as the source of data for this objective.

Anticipated number of data points: Annual updates of these files should provide 10 additional data points for the decade.

Detailed mortality tables made available by the Centers For Disease Control And Prevention (CDC) show that for each of the years 2015—17, the age-adjusted death rates from unintentional injury in rural (non-metro) areas was substantially higher than the corresponding rates in metro areas. For the entire 3-year period in non-core (non-metro) areas the age-adjusted rate was 62.6 per 100,000 population as compared to 39.2 per 100,000 population in large central metro areas. Similar rural-urban disparities exist in all categories of urbanization.

The age-adjusted death rate from unintentional injury per 100,000 population in rural (nonmetro) and urban (metro) areas is recommended as the unit of measure for this objective. Nonmetro and metro areas are as defined in the latest urbanization categories used by CDC. The 3-year combined rate for 2015—17 is suggested as a proposed baseline.

Infant mortality

Reduce the infant mortality rate in rural areas, decreasing the disparity between rural and urban mortality rates from these causes.

Proposed data source: The infant death files maintained in the CDC wonder online database are proposed as the source of data for this objective.

Anticipated number of data points: Annual updates of these files should provide 10 additional data points for the decade.

Detailed mortality tables made available by the Centers For Disease Control And Prevention (CDC) show that the infant mortality rate in rural (non-metro) areas was 6.69 per 1000 live births for the 3-year period 2013—15 in rural (non-metro) counties as compared to 5.49 per 1000 live births in large urban counties. Similar rural/urban disparities exist for neonatal and postneonatal mortality rates.

The infant mortality rate per 1000 live births in rural (non-metro) and urban (metro) counties is recommended as the unit of measure for this objective. Nonmetro and metro areas are as defined in the latest urbanization categories used by CDC. The 3-year combined rate for 2015—17 is suggested as a proposed baseline.

Child vaccination

Increase the percent of children aged 19—35 months in rural areas with the recommended 7-vaccine series, decreasing the disparity between rural and urban vaccination percentages.

Proposed data source: The national immunization survey data made available by NCHS is proposed as the source of data for this objective.

Anticipated number of data points: Annual updates of these files should provide 10 additional data points for the decade.

Summary tables made available by The National Center For Health Statistics (NCHS) show that in 2016 67.0% of children aged 19—35 months in non-metro areas received the recommended 7-vaccine series on a timely basis as compared to 71.3% of the same group in central city metro areas. Similar rural-urban disparities exist in other categories of urbanization.

The percent of children aged 19—35 months with the appropriate 7-vaccine series in rural (non-metro) and urban (metro) areas is recommended as the unit of measure for this objective. Nonmetro and metro areas are as defined in the latest urbanization categories used by CDC. The 2016 data for this measure is suggested as a proposed baseline.

Continued

♥ HEALTHY PEOPLE 2030—cont'd

Category of Key Objectives for Rural Health—Healthy People 2030

Access to healthcare

Increase the percent of persons in rural areas who had a health care visit in the last 12 months, decreasing the disparity between rural and urban percentages for this measure.

Proposed data source: National health interview survey data made available by NCHS is proposed as the source of data for this objective.

Anticipated number of data points: Annual updates of these files should provide 10 additional data points for the decade.

Summary tables made available by the National Center For Health Statistics (NCHS) show that in 2016, 16.4% of persons in rural nonmetro areas had no healthcare visit (in doctor's office, emergency department or home visit) in the last 12 months as compared to 14.2% of persons in metro areas. Similar rural-urban disparities exist in previous years.

The percent of persons in rural (nonmetro) and urban (metro) areas who had a health care visit (in doctor's office, emergency department or home visit) in the last 12 months is recommended as the unit of measure for this objective. Nonmetro and metro areas are as defined in the latest urbanization categories used by CDC. The 2016 data for this measure is suggested as a proposed baseline.

Access to dental care

Increase the percent of persons age 2 and over in rural areas who had a dental care visit in the last 12 months, decreasing the disparity between rural and urban percentages for this measure.

Proposed data source: National health interview survey data made available by NCHS is proposed as the source of data for this objective.

Anticipated number of data points: Annual updates of these files should provide 10 additional data points for the decade.

Summary tables made available by the National Center For Health Statistics (NCHS) show that in 2016, only 61.3% of persons age 2 and over in rural non-metro areas had a dental care visit in the last 12 months as compared to 69.9% of persons age 2 and over in metro areas. Similar rural-urban disparities exist in previous years.

The percent of persons age 2 and over in rural (non-metro) and urban (metro) areas who had a dental care visit in the last 12 months is recommended as the unit of measure for this objective. Nonmetro and metro areas are as defined in the latest urbanization categories used by CDC. The 2016 data for this measure is suggested as a proposed baseline.

Health insurance

Increase the percent of persons under age 65 in rural areas with health insurance coverage, decreasing the disparity between rural and urban health insurance coverage percentages.

Proposed data source: National health interview survey data made available by NCHS is proposed as the source of data for this objective.

Anticipated number of data points: Annual updates of these files should provide 10 additional data points for the decade.

Summary tables made available by the National Center For Health Statistics (NCHS) show that in 2016 13.3% of persons under age 65 in rural nonmetro areas had no health insurance coverage as compared to 9.9% of persons under age 65 in metro areas. Similar rural-urban disparities exist in previous years.

The percent of persons under age 65 with no health insurance in rural (nonmetro) and urban (metro) areas is recommended as the unit of measure for this objective. Nonmetro and metro areas are as defined in the latest urbanization categories used by CDC. The 2016 data for this measure is suggested as a proposed baseline. Proposed data source: National health interview survey data made available by NCHS is proposed as the source of data for this objective.

Financial barriers to prescription drugs

Decrease the percent of persons in rural areas who did not receive prescription drugs in the last 12 months due to cost, decreasing the disparity between rural and urban percentages for this measure.

Proposed data source: National health interview survey data made available by NCHS is proposed as the source of data for this objective.

Anticipated number of data points: Annual updates of these files should provide 10 additional data points for the decade.

Summary tables made available by the National Center For Health Statistics (NCHS) show that in 2016, 9.5% of persons in rural nonmetro areas did not receive prescription drugs in the last 12 months due to cost, as compared to 6.2% of persons in metro areas. Similar rural-urban disparities exist in previous years.

The percent of persons in rural (non-metro) and urban (metro) areas who did not receive prescription drugs in the last 12 months due to cost, is recommended as the unit of measure for this objective. Nonmetro and metro areas are as defined in the latest urbanization categories used by CDC. The 2016 data for this measure is suggested as a proposed baseline.

National Organization of State Offices of Rural Health. (2019): *Proposed rural-specific objectives for Healthy People 2030. Table modified. (NOSORH) Position statement. Sterling Heights, MI.* Available from: https://nosorh.org/wp-content/uploads/2019/02/HP-2030.pdf.

Information Technology in Rural Communities

As the distribution of technology expands across rural populations, more research is needed to examine the impacts of readily accessible information for both rural citizens and the health care delivery system. Rural patients are able to access specialty services such as radiological or dermatological examinations through telemedicine, and people in rural communities are increasingly taking advantage of the World Wide Web to access information to make health decisions, with 71% of rural residents owning a smartphone (Pew Research Center, 2019). The federal government has tied healthcare reimbursement to compliance with requirements of hospitals and physician practices to implement an electronic health record. Federal efforts directed toward disaster and terrorism preparedness have strengthened rural technological infrastructure so that communication pathways remain open during times of need. Just as patients access healthcare services from isolation, rural citizens are accessing health education through distance programs both for continuing education for entry-level and advanced degree programs in various health sciences. Employers are utilizing technology in the hiring process to recruit, hire, and onboard new employees, filling rural recruitment needs and vital workforce roles of medical professionals and healthcare personnel.

Telehealth (or telemonitoring) is the use of telecommunications and information technology (IT) to provide access to health assessments, diagnosis, intervention, consultation, supervision, and information across distance. Telehealth includes technologies such as interactive video (e.g., teleconsultation, teleradiology), patient monitoring (e.g., home monitoring, electronic intensive care unit [E-ICU], telehospitalist), and medication order review. Advancements in telehealth continue in the disciplines of mental health, diabetes prevention, and community-based health, wound care, oncology, acute care patient monitoring, and primary care services (Frontier Community Health Integration Project, Telehealth, 2014).

Advances in healthcare and innovative thinking create new models of healthcare delivery, including telehealth and virtual exam opportunities to increase access to care for rural patients across the care continuum. For example, a patient can go into a radiology department in a local community hospital to have a radiology exam completed by a technician, and a doctor 200 miles away can read the exam and meet with the patient virtually to immediately provide test results and follow-up with the patient regarding their care. This is a wonderful service for patients in a rural community. It provides access to care, removes geographic barriers, and eliminates the need for patients to travel long distances for specialized care, keeping the care of the patient close to home. Fig. 24.4 shows the telehealth opportunities for rural communities.

The use of telehealth services has expanded over the past decades, along with the use of technology in improving and coordinating care. The benefits in the expansion of IT and telehealth adoption continue to evolve for rural communities, as

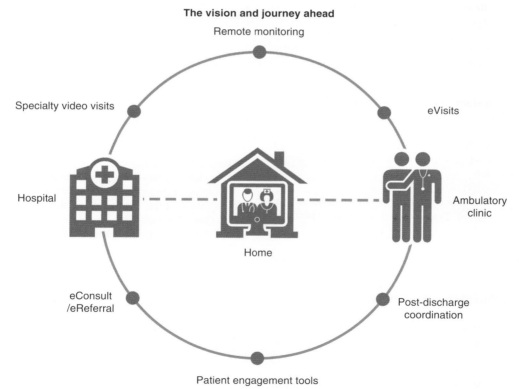

Fig. 24.4 Telehealth Opportunities for Rural Communities. (From Kung, P: *Telehealth from the Business Perspective. Telehealth alliance of oregon*, 2017. Available at https://slidetodoc.com/telehealth-from-the-business-perspective-peter-kung-mba/.)

federal and state opportunities exist in expanding coverage and reimbursement for telehealth services, lifting federal and state telehealth restrictions, and allowing a broader number of providers to engage in offering telehealth services to their patients.

Rural and public health resources are available to provide grant funding for the expansion of IT and telehealth technologies in addition to rural health research opportunities for incorporating telehealth into standard of care practices. The need to address new research questions has grown alongside the rapid expansion of IT, and questions abound relating to the application and evaluation of technology for improving systems of care and care outcomes.

Questions related to IT for public health in rural areas include

- What is the role of telehealth in public health?
- What impact is distance learning having on the skills of rural public health professionals?
- What are the costs and infrastructure implications of ensuring access to IT in rural areas?
- How can IT be used to fill the gaps in epidemiology and surveillance capacity in rural health departments?

PERFORMANCE STANDARDS IN RURAL PUBLIC HEALTH

The National Public Health Performance Standards Program (NPHPSP) was a collaborative effort, organized through the CDC, whose mission is to improve the quality of public health practice and the performance of local public health systems by providing and evaluating standards of performance.

The NPHPSP utilized the "*10 Essential Public Health Services*" to establish three assessment instruments that can be used by local and state public health systems for evaluation and improvement. Standards describe an optimal level of performance by public health systems, including all public, private, and voluntary entities that contribute to activities directed toward public health in an assessment area. The assessment can be used to improve collaborations among key public health partners, educate participants about public health, strengthen the network of public health partners, identify strengths and weaknesses, and provide benchmarks for public health practice improvements (Centers for Disease Control and Prevention, 2018).

🔍 RESEARCH HIGHLIGHTS

Defining Rural Areas: Old and New Classifications

The Census Bureau delineates urban areas after each decennial census by applying specified criteria to decennial census and other data (U.S. Census Bureau, 2020d).

Old Classification System (Before Census 2000)

Metropolitan (Metro) or Urbanized Areas (UAs):
- Cities of 50,000 or more residents *or*
- UAs of 50,000 or more residents and a total area population of 100,000 or more.

Nonmetropolitan (Non-Metro) or Non-UAs:
- All counties not classified as metropolitan or Urban.

New Classification System—Core-Based Statistical Area (Census 2000–2010)

Metropolitan (Metro) or UAs:
- Central counties with 50,000 or more residents, regardless of total area population; includes outlying counties with 25% or more of the employed population commuting daily.

Micropolitan (Micro) or Non-UAs:
- Central counties with one or more urban clusters of 10,000–50,000 persons; includes outlying counties with 25% or more of the employed population commuting daily.

  Noncore areas:
- All counties not meeting the new "metro" or "micro" classification are classified as "Outside Core Based Statistical Areas."

Newest and Most Recent Classification System (Census 2010)

Metropolitan (Metro) or Urbanized (UA) Core Based Statistical Areas (CBSAs):
- A CBA associated with at least one UA that has a population of at least 50,000.
- Each CBSA must contain at least one UA of 10,000 or more population.
- The MSA comprises the central county or counties containing the core, plus adjacent outlying counties having a high degree of social and economic

integration with the central county or counties as measured through commuting.

Micropolitan (Micro) or Non-Urbanized Core Based Statistical Areas (CBAs):
- A CBA associated with at least one urbanized cluster (UC) that has a population of at least 10,000 but less than 50,000.
- Each CBSA must contain at least one UA of 10,000 or more population.
- The Micropolitan Statistical Area comprises the central county or counties containing the core, plus adjacent outlying counties having a high degree of social and economic integration with the central county or counties as measured through commuting.

Noncore Areas or Non-Metro (not synonymous of rural areas)
- Counties that do not qualify for inclusion in a CBSA.

Rural Areas
- "Rural" encompasses all population, housing, and territory not included within an urban area (Figs. 24.5 and 24.6).

Notes for 2010 U.S. Census Classification

The Census Bureau's urban-rural classification is a delineation of geographical areas, identifying both individual urban areas and the nation's rural areas. The Census Bureau's urban areas represent densely developed territory and encompass residential, commercial, and other nonresidential urban land uses (U.S. Census Bureau. 2016b).

Metropolitan and micropolitan statistical areas are collectively referred to as "Core Based Statistical Areas" (CBSAs).

UA—A statistical geographic entity delineated by the Census Bureau, consisting of densely settled census tracts and blocks and adjacent densely populated territory that together contain at least 50,000 people.

Urban cluster—A statistical geographic entity delineated by the Census Bureau, consisting of densely settled census tracts and blocks and adjacent densely populated territory that together contain at least 2500 people. For purposes of delineating Core Based Statistical Areas, only those urban clusters of 10,000 more population are considered.

The Census Bureau provides the official, statistical definition of rural, based strictly on measures of population size and density. According to the current delineation, released in 2012 and based on the 2010 decennial census, rural areas comprise open country and settlements with fewer than 2500 residents.

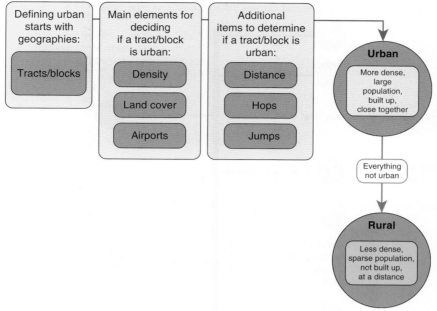

Fig. 24.5 Graphic Depiction of Urban/Rural Classification. (Data from U.S. Census Bureau: Ratcliffe, M, Burd, C, Holder, K, Fields, A: *Defining Rural at the U.S. Census Bureau. American community survey and geography brief*, 2016b.)

The Public Health Act and Prevention and Public Health Fund were created in 2012 as part of the Patient Protection and Affordable Care Act (Public Law 111−148). With this law and allocation of resources, the National Public Health Improvement Initiative—part of the CDC's larger effort to increase the performance management capacity of public health departments to ensure that public health goals are effectively and efficiently met—was born. The focal point of this work is to strengthen the public health infrastructure in the improvement of health outcomes.

Research questions that need to be addressed in rural areas may focus on the extent to which state and local performance assessments outlined by NPHPSP have been carried out, as well as on the ability of rural public health systems to respond to needed changes to comprehensively address essential services. Additionally, rural areas may benefit from research examining resource constraints and the need to expand partnerships to address essential services that may be difficult to provide in isolated rural populations.

RURAL PUBLIC HEALTH QUALITY PATIENT CARE AND OUTCOMES

In 2007, The National Rural Health Association (NRHA) adopted the 2001 IOM's quality of care definition as: "the degree to which health services for individuals and populations increase the likelihood of desired health outcomes and are consistent with current professional knowledge" (Agency for Healthcare Research and Quality, 2020). The NQS identifies the aims of better care: healthy people/healthy communities and affordable care (Agency for Healthcare Research and Quality,

2017a). These aims were adopted by the NRHA to emphasize patient and family engagement, care coordination, and population health in rural communities (National Rural Health Association, 2015). In alignment with the six aims of quality improvement (safe, effective, patient-centered, timely, efficient, equitable) as defined in the *Institute of Medicine's Crossing the Quality Chasm report*, as stated by Driesen et al. (2015) in an NRHA policy brief, initiatives to improve rural healthcare quality should include the following:

- Relevant to rural community conditions and health service realities.
- Equitably distributed and appropriate in scale to achieve improvement
- Comprehensive, involving multiple stakeholders and health service sectors.

Quality improvement is not a spectator sport but a team event that is continuously evolving across the continuum of care, involving both the health care team and the patient at the center of the care team. Many rural hospitals and public health facilities have demonstrated the capacity to improve health services and, in some areas, now perform better than, or equivalent to their urban counterparts. Rural community residents often report being more satisfied with care and rural hospitals and public health facilities have comparable performance with urban hospitals in quality, patient satisfaction, and operational efficiency for the type of care provided (National Rural Health Association, 2015).

Even so, many rural and public health facilities, especially the smaller, independent facilities that operate in remote geographic regions with lower case volumes, face significant financial and operational barriers, have limited time, and have fewer providers,

Decennial census urban definitions over time

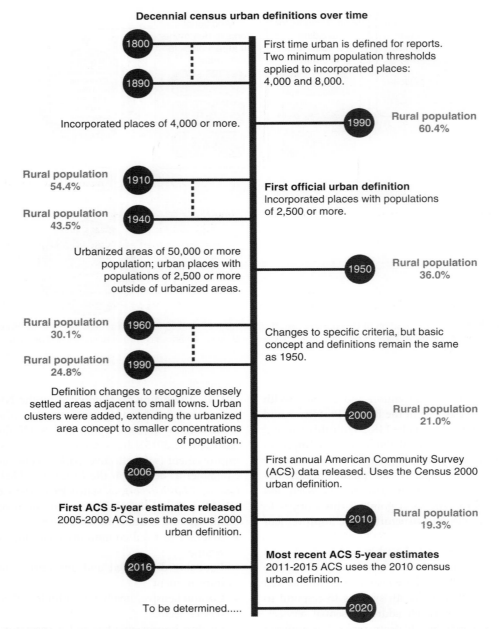

Fig. 24.6 Decennial Census Urban Definitions Over Time. (Data from U.S. Census Bureau: *Rural America— How does the U.S census bureau define "Rural?" interactive maps,* 2010b.)

staff, and resources available, making it difficult to demonstrate quality improvement. These limitations affect how healthcare is provided between rural and urban settings, as well as socioeconomic and cultural differences of the populations served, making it challenging to compare healthcare quality.

Resources, initiatives, funding, and grant programs help assist in the development of rural quality improvement programs. However, research to support rural quality measures with an understanding of these differences is one of the greatest challenges in comparing quality outcomes. Additional research is necessary for the implementation of relevant federal and state rural quality indicators and outcomes to decrease the gaps in

quality measurements and showcase the value that is present in rural facilities and the impact upon improving the quality of care in rural communities. Many questions will have to be answered by additional research, such as:

- What quality measures are relevant in rural and public health facilities that positively impact patient experience, care outcomes, and population health?
- How can relevant rural quality indicators be measured and benchmarked to improve the quality of care provided in rural and public health facilities?
- How do rural public health providers and facilities measure with relevant quality performance initiatives, and what is the

impact of these quality initiatives on patient outcomes and population health?

- How can federal and state programs implement relevant rural quality measures?

LEADERSHIP AND WORKFORCE CAPACITY FOR RURAL PUBLIC HEALTH

Consequences can be costly when health and environmental impacts are not placed at the center of decisions affecting the health of a nation. Nothing has reminded us of this more than the COVID-19 pandemic. Showing us the impact of how imperative and essential a strong public health workforce and infrastructure is for a community to address the fundamental drivers of health and establishing readiness and resilience to crisis.

In 2003, the IOM published the results of a report intended to improve our understanding of what is needed to prepare the public health workforce for the 21st century (Gebbie et al., 2003; U.S. Department of Health and Human Services, 2013). Workforce capacity challenges cited by the IOM report include globalization, which increases travel and allows for distribution of emerging and reemerging diseases (e.g., HIV and AIDS, tuberculosis, hepatitis B, malaria, cholera, diphtheria, Ebola virus, and the Coronavirus); advances in scientific and medical technologies that challenge the public health workforce in areas of ethics, data security, and communication; and demographic transformations that require new skills and services as our population ages and become more diverse.

The *Centers for Disease Control and Prevention—Public Health Improvement Initiative* (2017b), aims to accelerate public health accreditation readiness activities; to provide additional support for performance management and improvement practices; and to develop, identify, and disseminate innovative and evidence-based policies and practices. This program supports the *Healthy People 2020* and *2030* focus area of addressing public health infrastructure. Cross-jurisdictional (state, local, tribal, territorial, regional, community, and border) collaboration is encouraged to increase the impact of limited resources, to improve efficiency, and to leverage other related health reform efforts and projects. This initiative suggests that an initial strategy should be to monitor workforce composition and conduct research to validate a methodology to enumerate the public health workforce.

Building on the extraordinary circumstances of the past, the U.S. Department of Health and Human Services (2016) *Public Health 3.0* initiative has transformed public health from a behind-the-scenes discipline to a widely recognized leader of community and global initiatives. Leaders serve as new health strategists partnering across multiple sectors and leveraging data and resources to address social, environmental, and economic conditions that affect health and health equity. A strong public health accredited infrastructure, effective leadership, useable data, and adequate funding are the necessary components to prepare the public health workforce from an essential government function to an enhanced and broadened public health practice. Developing and implementing performance

standards and becoming increasingly professionalized as they engage community collaboration to drive initiatives to address upstream social determinants of health in both urban and rural communities.

COMMUNITY HEALTH SYSTEMS, MANAGED CARE, AND PUBLIC HEALTH

The evolution of managed care into rural environments has limited the safety-net role of some local health departments to provide primary care by preventing fee-for-service reimbursement and contracting care to networks of providers or organizations. This statement is especially true for Medicaid managed care, which serves the same population of people who traditionally receive primary care services through local public health departments. Medicaid's importance for rural areas is likely to grow as broader healthcare developments, such as declining inpatient use of rural hospitals and reductions in Medicare reimbursement, and the expansion in Medicaid eligibility provoke more interest in using the Medicaid system to support threatened rural infrastructure (American Hospital Association, 2019).

Consequently, the administration of the Medicaid program will increasingly seek the cost savings promised by managed care, and the role of rural public health departments may increasingly narrow into areas that are currently without any type of reimbursement. Finding ways to integrate public health into rural primary care at the community level will become more and more important (American Academy of Family Physicians, 2020).

These combined efforts work as a dyad within the health care system. Primary care activities, such as clinical preventive services, early diagnosis and intervention, quality-driven and evidence-based care, health promotion, and health advocacy, reinforce public health activities. Such as population surveillance, disease control, health promotion, and interventions based on determinants of health, injury prevention, and policy formation facilitate primary care's ability to function within the healthcare system (American Academy of Family Physicians, 2020). This integration between public health and rural primary care, with a common goal of both individual and population health, results in a substantial interdisciplinary relationship in the care continuum in improving the health outcomes of a community or population (Fig. 24.7).

According to the American Academy of Family Physicians (2020) position paper on the *Integration of Primary Care and Public Health*, the health of a population is not simply a product of functionality or funding of health care services. Rather, it includes the conditions in which people are born, grow, live, work, and age and encompasses inequities in power, money, and resources. The emphasis on population health supports a greater focus on health equity, disaster preparedness, and the upstream and downstream causations to reshape the community environments that affect health and behaviors. Leveraging available technologies, including telehealth, patient portals, and even social media, provides multiple access points for patients

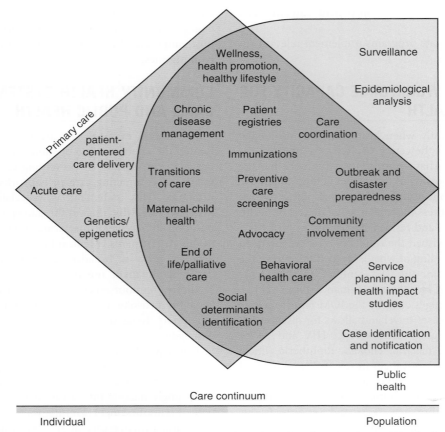

Fig. 24.7 Primary Care and Public Health Continuum. (Data from American Academy of Family Physicians: *Integration of Primary Care and Public Health. (Position Paper)*, 2020.)

to meet a variety of needs in the community. This approach must also define the value of health care, addressing managed care payment and reimbursement models and systems that align with Medicare funding. Amid this changing and challenging landscape, there are many opportunities for implementing changes that will impact the structure of the health care system and support further integration efforts.

Many questions will have to be answered by additional research to include

- What factors are associated with the successful integration of public health and managed care in rural environments?
- What capacity do rural health departments have for contracting arrangements with MCAs?
- What are the effects of local public health and managed care contracts on the direct provision of services?

NEW MODELS OF HEALTHCARE DELIVERY FOR RURAL AREAS

The healthcare delivery system is undergoing dramatic change, with an emphasis on finding new approaches and organizational frameworks to improve health outcomes, control costs, and improve population health (Rural Health Information Hub, 2021). Several innovative pilot projects have been implemented to address care delivery in rural areas. The

Frontier Community Health Integration Project, authorized by the Public Health Service Act and guided by the Medicare Improvements to Patients and Provider Act of 2008, is testing new models of care delivery to frontier areas in critical access hospitals and through the use of telemedicine. Four frontier states have been identified: Alaska, Montana, North Dakota, and Wyoming. A frontier area is defined as a county with six or fewer people in a square mile and a daily hospital census of five or less (Frontier Community Health Integration Project, 2014). The telehealth application can include home monitoring and electronic ICU and telehospitalist services; other applications include remote medication review by a pharmacist and consultation by a specialist at a distance. Payment for these services varies by a third-party payer, and distinct challenges in credentialing providers and leveraging technology exist.

The Centers for Medicare and Medicaid Services (CMS) Innovation Center (2020) develops payment and service delivery models in accordance with the requirements of the Social Security Act (Section 115A). Additionally, Congress has defined, both through the Affordable Care Act and previous legislation, a number of specific demonstrations to be conducted by CMS. To continue their collaboration to transform rural health and address inequities in rural health care, CMS has announced a Community Health Access Rural Transformation

Track (CHART) to begin in 2021 as a pilot program to provide funding, regulatory and operational flexibilities, and technical assistance for rural communities to transform their systems of care. Further, in 2021, through an additional Innovation Center pilot program, CMS enables providers to participate in value-based payment models where they are paid for quality and outcomes, instead of volume, through an Accountable Care Organizations (ACO) Transformation Track. Fifteen lead organizations will be selected for the community transformation track, and 20 lead organizations will be chosen for the ACO transformation track, which will be responsible for working closely with key entities such as participant hospitals and the state Medicaid agency—driving healthcare delivery system redesign by leading the development and implementation of transformation plans with their community partners (Centers for Medicare and Medicaid Services, 2020). These transformation plans are a detailed description of the strategy that outlines the community's plan to implement the redesign of

rural healthcare delivery. Throughout these programs, CMS is initiating waivers for many of the operational and regulatory stipulations that have been placed on providers and rural facilities and providing incentives to transform the delivery of care in rural communities.

Rural transformation models exist to ensure the delivery of health care in rural communities is sustainable for both the health system and the communities that are served. The formation of such models indicates an understanding that there are differences in access, needs, and resources to obtain healthcare in rural communities. Rural healthcare providers are often paid outside of the traditional prospective payment systems and fee schedules; there is less known about how new and emerging models of care might function in rural communities and the relevancy of quality improvement initiatives. As a result, policymakers and rural providers need to continue to understand the implications of new and emerging models of care for the delivery of care in rural communities.

SUMMARY

Clearly, the growing nursing shortage will affect all of America. Rural nurses are uniquely positioned to build impactful relationships and have a role in looking for alternatives to improve the delivery of rural healthcare. There are nearly 60 million residents in rural America spread across 80% of the country's landmass. The places where we live, learn, work, and play, the choices we make, and the opportunities we have all matter to our physical, mental, and social well-being and are influences in health. Rural individuals and organizations pull together for a common goal and make the most of limited

resources. Rural health care is not a small-scale version of urban health care, and successful rural improvement models exist and should be replicated in other rural service areas. Significant progress has been made during the past decade in improving access to care and the quality of rural health services. However, improvements in rural health care must be a continuous process in addressing the health, public health, infrastructure, emergency, and economic needs of rural areas. Rural nursing is distinctive. It is different from working in any other nursing context.

BIBLIOGRAPHY

Agency for Healthcare Research and Quality: Updates on primary care research: the AHRQ patient-centered medical home resource center, *Ann Fam Med* 12(6):586, 2014. Available from: https://www.ncbi.nlm.nih.gov/pmc/articles/PMC4226788/.

Agency for Healthcare Research and Quality: *About the national quality strategy*, 2017a. Available from: https://www.ahrq.gov/workingforquality/about/index.html.

Agency for Healthcare Research and Quality: *National healthcare quality and disparities report, chartbook on rural health care*, 2017b. Available from: https://www.ahrq.gov/sites/default/files/wysiwyg/research/findings/nhqrdr/chartbooks/qdr-ruralhealthchartbook-update.pdf.

Agency for Healthcare Research and Quality: *Understanding quality measurement*, 2020. Available from: https://www.ahrq.gov/patient-safety/quality-resources/tools/chtoolbx/understand/index.html.

Alexander L: *Where do states stand on private coverage of telemedicine? Check out this map*, 2013. Available from: https://medcitynews.com/2013/05/where-do-states-stand-on-private-coverage-of-telemedicine-check-out-this-map/.

Allender JA, Rector C, Warner KD: *Community health nursing: promoting and protecting the public's health*, ed 8, 2014, Philadelphia, PA: Lippincott Williams & Wilkins.

American Academy of Family Physicians: *Integration of primary care and public health (Position Paper)*, 2020. Available from: https://www.aafp.org/about/policies/all/integration-primary-care.html.

American Association of Colleges of Nursing: *Joint statement on academic progression for nursing students and graduates, Downloaded January 28*, 2021. Available from: https://www.aacnnursing.org/News-Information/Position-Statements-White-Papers/Academic-Progression.

American Association of Colleges of Nursing: *Nursing fact sheet*, 2019. Available from: https://www.aacnnursing.org/News-Information/Fact-Sheets/Nursing-Fact-Sheet#:~:text=Nursing%20is%20the%20nation%27s%20largest%20healthcare%20profession%2C%20with,will%20be%20created%20each%20year%20from%202016—202026.%202.

American Association of Colleges of Nursing: *Nursing shortage*, 2020. Available from: https://www.aacnnursing.org/News-Information/Fact-Sheets/Nursing-Shortage.

American Hospital Association: *Rural Report—Challenges facing rural communities and the roadmap to ensure local access to high-quality, affordable care*, 2019. Available from: https://www.aha.org/system/files/2019-02/rural-report-2019.pdf.

American Hospital Association: *Post-acute care*, 2021. Available from: https://www.aha.org/advocacy/long-term-care-and-rehabilitation.

American Nurses Association: Parish nursing: reclaiming the spiritual dimensions of care, *Am Nurse Today*, 2010. Available from: https://

www.myamericannurse.com/parish-nursing-reclaiming-the-spiritual-dimensions-of-care-2/.

American Telemedicine Association: *Telehealth is health*, 2021. Available from: https://www.americantelemed.org/.

Anaebere AK, DeLilly CR: Faith community nursing: supporting mental health during life transitions, *Issues Ment Health Nurs* 33(5):337–339, 2012. Available from: https://www.ncbi.nlm.nih.gov/pmc/articles/PMC3710745/.

Artiga S, Orgera K, Damico A: *Changes in health coverage by race and ethnicity since the ACA, 2010–2018*, 2020. Available from: https://www.kff.org/racial-equity-and-health-policy/issue-brief/changes-in-health-coverage-by-race-and-ethnicity-since-the-aca-2010-2018/.

Artnak K, McGraw R, Stanley V: Health care accessibility for chronic illness management and end-of-life care: a view from rural America, *J Law Med Ethics* 39(2):140–155, 2011.

Bailey J: *Rural behavioral and mental health is still overlooked. Center for rural affairs*, 2016. Available from: https://www.cfra.org/blog/rural-behavioral-and-mental-health-still-overlooked.

Bailey J: *The top 10 rural issues for health care reform: a series examining health care in rural America. Center for rural affairs*, 2009. Available from: https://citeseerx.ist.psu.edu/viewdoc/download?doi=10.1.1.493.7252&rep=rep1&type=pdf.

Benitez JA, Seiber EE: US health care reform and rural America: results from the ACA's medicaid expansions, *J Rural Health* 34(2):213–222, 2018. https://doi.org/10.1111/jrh.12284. Epub 2017 Nov 6. PMID: 29105809.

Bigbee JL: The uniqueness of rural nursing, *Nurs Clin* 28(1):31–144, 1993.

Bolin JN, Bellamy G, Ferdinand AO, Kash B, Helduser JW, editors: *Rural Healthy People 2020: a companion document to healthy people 2020* (vol. 1), College Station, TX, 2015, The Texas A&M Health Science Center, School of Public Health, Southwest Rural Health Research Center. Available from: https://srhrc.tamhsc.edu/docs/rhp2020-volume-1.pdf.

Bryant D: *Challenges of rural emergency management*, 2009. Homeland1 News.

Canadian Association for Parish Nursing Ministry: *Definition of parish nurses*, 2020. Available from: https://www.capnm.ca/resources/parish-nurse-fact-sheet/.

ChildStats.gov Forum on Child and Family Statistics: *America's children in brief: key national indicators of well-being, 2020, Infant Mortality*, 2020. Available from: https://www.childstats.gov/americaschildren/infant_mortality.asp.

Center for Community Health and Development. Developing a plan for assessing local needs and resources. The community tool box 3(1) 1994–2020. The University of Kansas. Available from: https://ctb.ku.edu/en/table-of-contents/assessment/assessing-community-needs-and-resources/develop-a-plan/main

Centers for Disease Control and Prevention: *About rural health*. Rural health, 2017a. Available from: https://www.cdc.gov/ruralhealth/about.html.

Centers for Disease Control and Prevention: *Advancing public health: the story of the national public health improvement initiative*, Atlanta, GA, 2017b, U.S. Department of Health and Human Services. Available from: https://www.cdc.gov/publichealthgateway/docs/nphii/compendium.pdf.

Centers for Disease Control and Prevention: *Defining health disparities. Health disparities in HIV/AIDS, Viral Hepatitis, STD, and TB*, 2020. Available from: https://www.cdc.gov/nchhstp/healthdisparities/default.htm.

Centers for Disease Control and Prevention: *Infant mortality*, 2020. Available from: https://www.cdc.gov/reproductivehealth/maternalinfanthealth/infantmortality.htm.

Centers for Disease Control and Prevention: *National public health performance standards program*, 2018. Available from: https://www.cdc.gov/publichealthgateway/nphps/index.html?CDC_AA_refVal=https%3A%2F%2Fwww.cdc.gov%2Fnphpsp%2Findex.html.

Centers for Disease Control and Prevention: *Rural Americans at higher risk of death from five leading causes*, 2017. Available from: https://www.cdc.gov/media/releases/2017/p0112-rural-death-risk.html.

Centers for Disease Control and Prevention: *Suicide and self-harm injury. National Center for Health Statistics*, 2021. Available from: https://www.cdc.gov/nchs/fastats/suicide.htm.

Centers for Disease Control and Prevention: *What are social determinates of health?* About social determinants of health (SDOH), 2020. Available from: https://www.cdc.gov/socialdeterminants/about.html.

Centers for Disease Control and Prevention; National Institute for Occupational Safety and Health (NIOSH): *Agricultural Safety*, 2020. Available from: https://www.cdc.gov/niosh/topics/aginjury/.

Centers for Disease Control and Prevention; National Institute for Occupational Safety and Health (NIOSH): *State Surveillance Program*, 2021. Available from: https://www.cdc.gov/niosh/oep/statesurv.html.

Centers for Medicare and Medicaid Services: Community health access and rural transformation (CHART) model fact sheet, *Newsroom*, 2020. Available from: https://www.cms.gov/newsroom/fact-sheets/community-health-access-and-rural-transformation-chart-model-fact-sheet.

Centers for Medicare and Medicaid Services: *Swing bed services. MLN fact sheet*, 2019. Available from: https://www.cms.gov/Outreach-and-Education/Medicare-Learning-Network-MLN/MLNProducts/Downloads/SwingBedFactsheet.pdf.

Crouch E, Probst JC, Radcliff E, Bennett KJ, McKinney SH: Prevalence of adverse childhood experiences (ACEs) among US children, *Child Abuse & Neglect* 92:209–218, 2019. Available from: https://doi.org/10.1016/j.chiabu.2019.04.010.

Currin F, Razo G, Min A: Give me a break: design for communication among family caregivers and respite caregivers, *CHI'19 Extended Abstracts*, May 4–9, 2019. Glasgow, Scotland, UK. Available from: https://dl.acm.org/doi/pdf/10.1145/3290607.3309687.

Daniels N, Kennedy BP, Kawachi I: Why justice is good for our health: the social determinants of health inequalities, *Daedalus* 128:215–251, 1999.

DC.gov. (n.d.): *What is EMS? DC health*, Available from: https://dchealth.dc.gov/service/what-ems.

Electronic Code of Federal Regulations: *Grants for community health services*, 2021. Available from: https://www.ecfr.gov/cgi-bin/text-idx?SID=4655ec57ce96e5c9d9a016de226b0bb7c&node=42:1.0.1.4.27&rgn=div5.

Fields R: The ethics of expanding health coverage through the private market, *AMA J Ethics* (7):665–671, 2015. Available from: https://journalofethics.ama-assn.org/article/ethics-expanding-health-coverage-through-private-market/2015-07.

Flex Monitoring Team: *The flex program*, n.d. Available from: https://www.flexmonitoring.org/the-flex-program.

Frontier community health integration project: *White paper #2 case study on frontier telehealth*, 2014. Available from: https://www.ruralhealthinfo.org/new-approaches/pdf/case-study-on-frontier-telehealth.pdf.

Garrigues LJ: Addressing health inequities in vulnerable populations through social justice. In Vermeesch A, editor: *Integrative health* nursing interventions for vulnerable populations, 2021, Springer, pp 11−25. Available from: https://doi.org/10.1007/978-3-030-60043-3_2.

Gebbie K, Rosenstock L, Hernandez L: *Who will keep the public healthy? Educating public health professionals for the 21st century*, Washington, DC, 2003, The National Academies Press. Available from: https://www.nap.edu/catalog/10542/who-will-keep-the-public-healthy-educating-public-health-professionals.

Georgetown University Health Policy Institute Center for Children and Families, Alker J, Corcoran A: *Children's uninsured rate rises by largest annual jump in more than a decade*, 2020. Available from: https://ccf.georgetown.edu/wp-content/uploads/2020/10/ACS-Uninsured-Kids-2020_10-06-edit-3.pdf.

Gessert C, Waring S, Bailey-Davis L, Roberts M, VanWormer J: Rural definition of health: a systematic literature review, *BMC Publ Health* 15:378, 2015. Available from: https://www.ncbi.nlm.nih.gov/pmc/articles/PMC4406172/.

Hale NL: "*Rural public health systems: challenges and opportunities for improving population health*," Academy Health, 2015. Available from: https://academyhealth.org/sites/default/files/AH_Rural%20Health%20brief%20final2.pdf.

Harvard TH: Chan school of public health. In *NPR, RWJF, Harvard School of Public Health. (Eds.). Life in rural America: experiences and views from rural America on health issues and life in rural communities.* NPR, RWJF, Harvard School of Public Health, 2018, Public Opinion Poll Series. Available from: https://www.rwjf.org/en/library/research/2018/10/life-in-rural-america.html#:~:text=%E2%80%9CLife%20in%20Rural%20America%E2%80%9D%20illustrates%20that%20rural%20Americans,in%20particular,%20drug%20addiction/abuse%20and%20troubled%20local%20economies.

Health Ministries Association, Inc. (n.d.).: *Nursing practice support*, Available from: https://hmassoc.org/practice-support/#FCNS&S3rd Edition.

Health Resources and Services Administration: *Defining rural population. Federal Office of Rural Health Policy—about FORHP*, 2021. Available from: https://www.hrsa.gov/rural-health/about-us/definition/index.html.

Health Resources and Services Administration: *Medicare rural hospital flexibility program*, (n.d.-b). Available from: https://www.hrsa.gov/grants/find-funding/hrsa-19-024.

Health Resources and Services Administration: *Rural community programs*, 2020. Available from: https://www.hrsa.gov/rural-health/community/index.html.

Health Resources and Services Administration: *Rural healthcare provider transition project*, (n.d.-c). Available from: https://www.hrsa.gov/grants/find-funding/hrsa-20-099.

Health Resources and Services Administration: *Rural health research and policy programs*, 2019. Available from: https://www.hrsa.gov/rural-health/research/index.html.

Health Resources and Services Administration: *State and regional primary care association (PCA) cooperative agreements.* Health Center Program, (n.d.-d). Available from: State and Regional Primary Care Associations | Official web site of the U.S. Health Resources & Services Administration (hrsa.gov).

HealthyPeople.gov; Healthy People. (n.d.).: *Home*, 2020. Available from: https://www.healthypeople.gov/2020.

Healthy People.gov; Healthy People 2020. 2010. *Disparities*, 2010. Available from: https://www.healthypeople.gov/2020/about/foundation-health-measures/Disparities.

Homeland Security: *Emergency services sector profile*, 2017. Available from: https://www.cisa.gov/sites/default/files/publications/NPPD_emergency-services-sector-profile-v3.pdf.

Hsia R, Shen Y: Possible geographical barriers to trauma center access for vulnerable patients in the United States: an analysis of urban and rural communities, *Arch Surg* 146(1):46−52, 2011. Available from: https://jamanetwork.com/journals/jamasurgery/fullarticle/406563.

Institute of Medicine: *Crossing the quality chasm: a new health system for the 21st century*, Washington, DC, 2001, National Academy Press. Available from: https://www.med.unc.edu/pediatrics/files/2018/01/crossing-the-quality-chasm.pdf.

Institute of Medicine: *Emergency medical services at the crossroads*, Washington, DC, 2006, National Academy Press. Available from: https://nasemso.org/wp-content/uploads/EMS-at-Crossroads.pdf.

Institute of Medicine: *Quality through collaboration: the future of rural health care*, Washington, DC, 2005, National Academy Press.

James CV, Moonesinghe R, Wilson-Frederick SM, Hall JE, Penman-Aguilar A, Bouye K: Racial/ethnic health disparities among rural adults—United States, 2012−2015, *MMWR Surveill Summ* 66(23):1−9, 2017. Available from: https://www.ncbi.nlm.nih.gov/pmc/articles/PMC5829953/.

Jarman MP, Castillo RC, Carlini AR, Kodadek LM, Haider AH: Rural risk: geographic disparities in trauma mortality, *Surgery* 160(6):1551−1559, 2016. Available from: https://www.ncbi.nlm.nih.gov/pmc/articles/PMC5118091/.

Johnson K: Where is rural America and who lives there? In Tickamyer A, Sherman J, Warlick J, editors: *Rural poverty in the United States*, New York, 2017, Columbia University Press.

Keith K: *Uninsured rate rose in 2018, Says census bureau report*, September 2019. Available from: https://www.healthaffairs.org/do/10.1377/hblog20190911.805983/full/.

Kosman S: *Nurse residencies: building a better future for patients and nurses*, 2011. Available from: https://www.rwjf.org/en/blog/2011/10/nurse-residencies-building-a-better-future-for-patients-and-nurses.html.

Kulbok PA, Thatcher E, Park E, Meszaros PS: Evolving public health nursing roles: focus on community participatory health promotion and prevention, *Online J Issues Nurs* 17(2), 2012. Available from: http://ojin.nursingworld.org/MainMenuCategories/ANAMarketplace/ANAPeriodicals/OJIN/TableofContents/Vol-17-2012/No2-May-2012/Evolving-Public-Health-Nursing-Roles.html.

Kung P: *Telehealth from the business perspective.* Telehealth alliance of Oregon, 2017. Available from: https://www.ortelehealth.org/content/telehealth-business-perspective.

Lee H, Winters C: Testing rural nursing theory: perceptions and needs of service providers, *Online J Rural Nurs Health Care* 4(1):51−63, 2004. Available from: https://rnojournal.binghamton.edu/index.php/RNO/article/view/212/185.

Marshall WE, Ferenchak NN: Assessing equity and urban/rural road safety disparities in the US. *J Urbanism, Int Res Placemaking Urban Sustain* 4(10):422−441, 2017. Available from: https://doi.org/10.1080/17549175.2017.1310748.

McClelland SL, Steel S, Marsh L, et al.: *Dimensions in health: a sample of rural and global health issues*, 2010. Available from: https://digitalrepository.unm.edu/cgi/viewcontent.cgi?article=1001&context=rural-cultural-health.

Medicaid.gov: Keeping America healthy (n.d.) *Telemedicine*, Available from: https://www.medicaid.gov/medicaid/benefits/telemedicine/index.html.

Medicare Payment Advisory Commission: *Hospice services: assessing payment adequacy and updating payments.* Report to the congress, *Med Payment Pol* 12:325−362, 2020. Washington, DC: MedPAC. Available from: http://www.medpac.gov/docs/default-source/reports/mar20_medpac_ch12_sec.pdf.

Migrant Clinicians Network: *The migrant/seasonal farmworker*, 2017. Available from: https://www.migrantclinician.org/issues/migrant-info/migrant.html.

Miller, Geneva: *Lay caregivers, HB 3378. The Bandon western world*, 2015, Mary. Available from: https://theworldlink.com/lifestyles/thrive/lay-caregivers-hb/article_bd2d484e-8f27-5783-93d3-5d8752186159.html.

Mississippi College: *How nurses can help during disasters*, 2018. Available from: https://online.mc.edu/degrees/nursing/rn-to-bsn/how-nurses-can-help-during-disasters/.

Molinari D, Bushy A. In *The rural nurse: transition to practice*, New York, 2012, Springer Publishing Company. Available from: https://www.ncsbn.org/9780826157560_chapter.pdf.

Molanari D, Jaiswal A, Hollinger-Forrest T: Rural nurses: lifestyle preferences and education perceptions, *Online J Rural Nurs Health Care* 11(2):16—26, 2011. Available from: https://rnojournal.binghamton.edu/index.php/RNO/article/view/27/19.

Mohamoud YA, Kirby RS, Ehrenthal DB: Poverty, urban-rural classification and term infant mortality: a population-based multilevel analysis, *BMC Pregnancy Childbirth* (19):40, 2019. Available from: https://doi.org/10.1186/s12884-019-2190-1.

National Advisory Committee on Rural Health and Human Services: *Rural implications of changes to the medicare hospice benefit. Policy brief*, 2013. Available from: https://www.hrsa.gov/sites/default/files/hrsa/advisory-committees/rural/publications/2013-medicare-hospice.pdf.

National Association of County & City Health Officials: *2019 National Profile of Local Health Departments*, 2019. Available from: https://www.naccho.org/uploads/downloadable-resources/Programs/Public-Health-Infrastructure/NACCHO_2019_Profile_final.pdf.

National Center for Farmworker Health, Inc: *Farmworker occupational health and safety fact sheet*, 2018. Available from, http://www.ncfh.org/occupational-health-and-safety.html.

National Conference of State Legislatures. 2017: Closing the gaps in the rural primary care workforce, 2017. Available from: https://www.ncsl.org/research/health/closing-the-gaps-in-the-rural-primary-care-workfor.aspx.

National Conference of State Legislatures: *Home and community based services: meeting the long-term care needs of rural seniors. The rural health connection*, 2011. Available from: https://www.ncsl.org/Portals/1/documents/health/RHHCBS.pdf.

National Institute of Mental Health: *Mental health in rural America: challenges and opportunities*, 2018. Available from: https://www.nimh.nih.gov/news/media/2018/mental-health-and-rural-america-challenges-and-opportunities.shtml.

National Institute of Mental Health, 2021: *Suicide*, January 2021. Available from: https://www.nimh.nih.gov/health/statistics/suicide.shtml.

National Organization of State Offices of Rural Health: *Proposed rural-specific objectives for Healthy People 2030*, Sterling Heights, MI, 2019, NOSORH position statement. Available from: https://nosorh.org/wp-content/uploads/2019/02/HP-2030.pdf.

National Rural Health Association: *About rural health care*, 2021. Available from: https://www.ruralhealthweb.org/about-nrha/about-rural-health-care.

National Rural Health Association, Burrows E, Suh R, Hamann D: *Health care workforce distribution and shortage issues in rural America. National rural health association policy brief*, 2012. Available from: https://www.ruralhealthweb.org/getattachment/Advocate/Policy-Documents/HealthCareWorkforceDistributionandShortageJanuary2012.pdf.aspx?lang=en-US.

National Rural Health Association, Driesen K, Holms H, Smith M: *Comprehensive quality improvement in rural health care. Policy brief*, 2015. Available from: https://www.ruralhealthweb.org/getattachment/Advocate/Policy-Documents/ComprehensiveQualityImprovementinRuralHealthCareFeb2015.pdf.aspx?lang=en-US.

National Rural Health Association, King N, Pigman M, Huling S, Hanson B: *EMS services in rural America: challenges and opportunities. National rural health association policy brief*, 2018a. Available from: https://www.ruralhealthweb.org/NRHA/media/Emerge_NRHA/Advocacy/Policy%20documents/05-11-18-NRHA-Policy-EMS.pdf.

National Rural Health Association, Martin D, Williams J, Crawford P, King N: *Health disparities: closing the gaps using faith-based institutions. National rural health association policy brief*, 2017. Available from: https://www.ruralhealthweb.org/NRHA/media/Emerge_NRHA/Advocacy/Policy%20documents/2017-NRHA-policy-paper-Health-Disparities-Closing-the-Gaps-Using-Faith-Based-Institutions.pdf.

National Rural Health Association, Seigel J: *Breast cancer in rural America*, 2018b. https://www.ruralhealthweb.org/blogs/ruralhealthvoices/october-2018/breast-cancer-in-rural-america.

Nickels T: *What's next for rural hospitals? Additional COVID-19 relief and beyond*. American Hospital Association, 2020. Available from: https://www.aha.org/news/blog/2020-11-18-whats-next-rural-hospitals-additional-covid-19-relief-and-beyond https://ruralhealth.und.edu/what-we-do/research-and-evaluation.

North Dakota State University: *Center for rural health*, 2021. Available from: https://ruralhealth.und.edu/what-we-do/research-and-evaluation.

Peek-Asa C, Zwerling C, Stallones L: Acute traumatic injuries in rural populations, *Am J Publ Health* 94(10):1689—1693, 2004. Available from: https://ajph.aphapublications.org/doi/full/10.2105/AJPH.94.10.1689.

Healthy People.gov: *Healthy People*, 2020. Available from: https://www.healthypeople.gov/2020/about/foundation-health-measures/Disparities.

Pew Research Center, Internet & Technology: *Mobile phone ownership over time. Mobile fact sheet*, 2019. Available from: https://www.pewresearch.org/internet/fact-sheet/mobile/.

Pfankuch P: *Special report: Pandemic threatens fragile rural health-care system in South Dakota. South Dakota News Watch*, 2020. Available from: https://www.sdnewswatch.org/stories/small-towns-big-challenges-pandemic-burdens-fragile-rural-healthcare-system-in-sd/.

Probst JC, Barker JC, Enders A, Gardiner P: Current state of child health in rural America: how context shapes children's health, *J Rural Health*, 2016. Available from: https://doi.org/10.1111/jrh.12222.

Probst JC, Mckinney SH, Odahowski C: *Rural registered nurses: Educational preparation, workplace, and salary. Rural & Minority Health Research Center*, 2019. Findings Brief, October 2019. Available from: https://www.sc.edu/study/colleges_schools/public_health/research/research_centers/sc_rural_health_research_center/documents/ruralregisterednurses.pdf.

Rabinowitz P: *Section 11. Collaborative leadership. Community tool box. Center for Community Health and Development at the University of Kansas*, 2020. Available from: https://ctb.ku.edu/en/table-of-contents/leadership/leadership-ideas/collaborative-leadership/main.

RCHN Community Health Foundation: *Community Health Centers: Chronicling their history and broader meaning. chronicles: the community health centers story*, 2021. Available from: https://www.chcchronicles.org/stories/community-health-centers-chronicling-their-history-and-broader-meaning.

Ready.gov: *Emergency response plan*, 2021. Available from: https://www.ready.gov/business/implementation/emergency.

Robert Wood Johnson Foundation: *Research, evaluation and learning*, 2001—2020. Available from: https://www.rwjf.org/en/how-we-work/rel.html.

Rosenthal K: What rural nursing stories are you living? *Online J Rural Nurs Health Care* 5(1), 2005. Available from: https://rnojournal.binghamton.edu/index.php/RNO/article/view/189/164.

Roth D, Fredman L, Haley W: Informal caregiving and its impact on health: a reappraisal from population-based studies, *Gerontol* 55(2):309–319, 2015. Available from: Informal Caregiving and Its Impact on Health: a Reappraisal From Population-Based Studies | The Gerontologist | Oxford Academic (oup.com).

Rural Health Information Hub: *Conducting rural health research, needs assessment, and program evaluation,* 2019a. Available from: https://www.ruralhealthinfo.org/topics/rural-health-research-assessment-evaluation.

Rural Health Information Hub: *Education and training of the rural healthcare workforce,* 2019b. Available from:https://www.ruralhealthinfo.org/topics/workforce-education-and-training#grow-your-own.

Rural Health Information Hub: *Factors that impact mental health in rural areas. Mental health in rural communities toolkit,* 2019c. Available from: https://www.ruralhealthinfo.org/toolkits/mental-health/1/outside-factors.

Rural Health Information Hub: *Healthcare access in rural communities,* 2019d. Available from: https://www.ruralhealthinfo.org/topics/healthcare-access.

Rural Health Information Hub: *Rural aging,* 2018. Available from: https://www.ruralhealthinfo.org/topics/aging.

Rural Health Information Hub: *Rural emergency preparedness and response,* 2019e. Available from: https://www.ruralhealthinfo.org/topics/emergency-preparedness-and-response/about-this-guide.

Rural Health Information Hub: *Rural health disparities,* 2019. Available from: https://www.ruralhealthinfo.org/topics/rural-health-disparities.

Rural Health Information Hub: *Testing new approaches—Why rural-specific demonstration projects are needed,* 2021. Available from: https://www.ruralhealthinfo.org/new-approaches.

Rural Health Information Hub, *University of Minnesota rural health research center and NORC Walsh center for rural health analysis. Mental health in rural communities toolkit,* 2019. Available from: https://www.ruralhealthinfo.org/toolkits/mental-health.

Rural Health Information Hub: *What is rural?,* 2019. Available from: https://www.ruralhealthinfo.org/topics/what-is-rural.

Saint Onge JM, Smith S: Demographics in rural populations, *Surg Clin North Am* 100(5):823–833, 2020. Available from: https://doi.org/10.1016/j.suc.2020.06.005.

Sanford JT, Townsend-Rocchiccioli J: The perceived health of rural caregivers, *Geriatr Nurs* 25(3):145–148, 2004. Available from: https://doi.org/10.1016/j.gerinurse.2004.04.007.

Scharff KE: The distinctive nature and scope of rural nursing practice: philosophical bases. In *Lee HJ, editor: Conceptual basis for rural nursing,* New York, 1998, Springer Publishing Company.

Scommenga P, Mather M, Kilduff L: *Eight demographic trends transforming America's older population. Population reference bureau,* 2018. Available from: https://www.prb.org/eight-demographic-trends-transforming-americas-older-population/.

Sommers B, Gawande A, Baicker K: Health insurance coverage and health—what the recent evidence tells us, *N Engl J Med* 377(6):589–593, 2017. Available from: https://www.nejm.org/doi/full/10.1056/NEJMsb1706645.

Sorrell J: Ethics: the patient protection and affordable care act: ethical perspectives in 21st century health care, *Online J Issues Nurs* 18(1), 2012. Available from: http://ojin.nursingworld.org/MainMenuCategories/ANAMarketplace/ANAPeriodicals/OJIN/Columns/Ethics/Patient-Protection-and-Affordable-Care-Act-Ethical-Perspectives.html.

Statista, Elflein J: *Percentage of U.S. Americans without health insurance by ethnicity from 2010 to June 2019, by ethnicity,* 2019. Available from: https://www.statista.com/statistics/200970/percentage-of-americans-without-health-insurance-by-race-ethnicity/.

Thorngren JM: Rural mental health: a qualitative inquiry, *J Rural Community Psychol* E6(2):1–6, 2003.

Thrall T: Rural recruitment, *Hosp Health Network* 81(12):45–48, 2007.

Tran L, Tran P: US urban-rural disparities in breast cancer-screening practices at the national, regional, and state level, 2012–2016, *Cancer Causes Control* 30:1045–1055, 2019. Available from: https://doi.org/10.1007/s10552-019-01217-8.

University of Minnesota: *Rural health research center,* 2021. Available from: https://rhrc.umn.edu/.

University of North Carolina Wilmington: *Importance of nursing in rural communities,* 2019. Available from: https://onlinedegree.uncw.edu/articles/nursing/importance-nursing-rural-communities.aspx.

U.S. Bureau of Labor Statistics: *Census of fatal occupational injuries in 2019,* 2020. Available from: https://www.bls.gov/opub/hom/cfoi/pdf/cfoi.pdf.

U. S. Bureau of Labor Statistics: *Number and rate of fatal work injuries, by industry. Census of fatal occupational injuries summary sector,* 2019. Available from: https://www.bls.gov/charts/census-of-fatal-occupational-injuries/number-and-rate-of-fatal-work-injuries-by-industry.htm.

U.S. Census Bureau, Cheeseman-Day J: *Rates of uninsured fall in rural counties, remain higher than urban counties,* 2019a. Available from: https://www.census.gov/library/stories/2019/04/health-insurance-rural-america.html.

U.S. Census Bureau: *Health Insurance coverage in the United States: 2018,* 2019b. Available from: https://www.census.gov/library/publications/2019/demo/p60-267.html.

U.S. Census Bureau: *In some states, more than half of older residents live in rural areas,* 2020a. Available from: https://www.census.gov/library/stories/2019/10/older-population-in-rural-america.html#:~:text=More%20than%201%20in%205,to%2013.8%25%20in%20urban%20areas.

U.S. Census Bureau: *Inequalities persist despite decline in poverty for all major race and hispanic origin groups,* 2020c. Available from: https://www.census.gov/library/stories/2020/09/poverty-rates-for-blacks-and-hispanics-reached-historic-lows-in-2019.html.

U.S. Census Bureau: *Income and poverty in the United States: 2019,* 2020d. https://www.census.gov/library/publications/2020/demo/p60-270.html.

U.S. Census Bureau: *2017 metropolitan and micropolitan Statistical Areas (CBSAs) of the United States and Puerto Rico,* 2019c. Available from: https://www.census.gov/geographies/reference-maps/2017/geo/cbsa.html.

U.S Census Bureau: *New census data show differences between urban and rural populations,* 2016a. Available from: https://www.census.gov/newsroom/press-releases/2016/cb16-210.html#:~:text=About%2013.4%20million%20children%20under,percent%20compared%20with%206.3%20percent.

U.S. Census Bureau: *Office of management and budget: metropolitan and micropolitan statistical areas main,* 2020e. Available from: https://www.census.gov/programs-surveys/metro-micro/about.html.

U.S. Census Bureau: *Overview of race and hispanic origin: 2010; Census briefs,* 2010a. Available from: https://www.census.gov/prod/cen2010/briefs/c2010br-02.pdf.

U.S. Census Bureau, Ratcliffe M, Burd C, Holder K, Fields A: *Defining rural at the U.S. census bureau. American community survey and geography brief,* 2016b. Available from: https://www.census.gov/content/dam/Census/library/publications/2016/acs/acsgeo-1.pdf.

U.S. Census Bureau: *Rural America—How does the U.S census bureau define "rural?", interactive maps*, 2010b.

U.S. Census Bureau: *Urban and rural*, 2020f. Available from: https://www.census.gov/programs-surveys/geography/guidance/geo-areas/urban-rural.html.

U.S. Census Bureau: *Quick facts United States*, 2019e. Available from: https://www.census.gov/quickfacts/fact/table/US/PST045219.

U.S. Department of Agriculture Economic Research Service, Cromartie J, Dobis EA, Krumel TP, McGranahan D, Pender J: *Rural America at a Glance 2020 Edition*, 2020a. Available from: https://www.ers.usda.gov/webdocs/publications/100089/eib-221.pdf?v=8019.8.

U.S. Department of Agriculture Economic Research Service, Cromaratie J, Vilorio D: *Rural population trends. Statistic: rural economy & population*, 2019a. Available from: https://www.ers.usda.gov/amber-waves/2019/february/rural-population-trends/.

U.S. Department of Agriculture Economic Research Service: *Description and maps*, 2019b.

U.S. Department of Agriculture Economic Research Service: *Employment & education: rural education*, 2020. Available from: https://www.ers.usda.gov/topics/rural-economy-population/employment-education/rural-education.aspx.

U.S. Department of Agriculture Economic Research Service: *Farm labor*, 2020. Available from: https://www.ers.usda.gov/topics/farm-economy/farm-labor#employment.

U.S. Department of Agriculture Economic Research Service, Farrigan T, Parker T: *The concentration of poverty is a growing rural problem*, 2012. Available from: https://www.ers.usda.gov/amber-waves/2012/december/concentration-of-poverty.

U.S. Department of Agriculture Economic Research Service: *Rural child poverty chart gallery*, 2019. Available from: https://www.ers.usda.gov/data-products/rural-child-poverty-chart-gallery/.

U.S. Department of Agriculture; National Institute of Food and Agriculture: *Ag and food sectors and the economy*, 2020b. Available from: https://www.ers.usda.gov/data-products/ag-and-food-statistics-charting-the-essentials/ag-and-food-sectors-and-the-economy.aspx.

U.S. Department of Health and Human Services: *Health professional shortage area physician bonus program. Mln fact sheet*, 2020. Available from: https://www.cms.gov/Outreach-and-Education/Medicare-Learning-Network-MLN/MLNProducts/Downloads/HPSAfctsht.pdf.

U.S. Department of Health and Human Services: *Rural action plan*, 2020. Available from: https://www.hhs.gov/sites/default/files/hhs-rural-action-plan.pdf.

U.S. Department of Health and Human Services; Health Resources and Services Administration: *Supply and demand projections of the nursing workforce: 2014–2030*, 2017. Available from: https://bhw.hrsa.gov/sites/default/files/bureau-health-workforce/data-research/nchwa-hrsa-nursing-report.pdf.

U.S. Department of Health and Human Services National Advisory Council on Migrant Health (NACMH), 2018. Available from: https://bphc.hrsa.gov/sites/default/files/bphc/qualityimprovement/strategicpartnerships/nacmh/may2018minutes.pdf.

U.S. Department of Health and Human Services National Center for Health Statistics, Pettrone K, Curtin S: *Urban—rural differences in suicide rates, by sex and three leading methods: United States, 2000–2018. NCHS Data Brief*, 2020. Available from: https://www.cdc.gov/nchs/data/databriefs/db373-h.pdf.

U.S. Department of Health and Human Services Office of Disease Prevention and Health Promotion: *Who will keep the public healthy? Educating public health professionals for the 21st century*, 2013. Available from: https://health.gov/healthypeople/tools-action/browse-evidence-based-resources/who-will-keep-public-healthy-educating-public-health-professionals-21st-century.

U.S. Department of Health and Human Services Office of the Assistant Secretary for Health: *Healthy People 2020: an end of a decade snapshot*, (n.d.-g). Available from: https://health.gov/sites/default/files/2020-12/HP2020EndofDecadeSnapshot.pdf.

U.S. Department of Labor; Bureau of Labor Statistics: *National census of fatal occupational injuries in 2019. News Release*, 2019. Available from: https://www.bls.gov/news.release/pdf/cfoi.pdf.

Van Camp J, Chappy S: The effectiveness of nurse residency programs on retention: a systematic review, *AORN J* 106(2):128–144, 2017.

Vespa J, Medina L, Armstrong D: Demographic turning points for the United States: population projections for 2020 to 2060, *Curr Popul Rep* P25–P1114, 2020. U.S. Census Bureau, Washington, DC. Available from: https://www.census.gov/content/dam/Census/library/publications/2020/demo/p25-1144.pdf.

Virnig BA, Moscovice IS, Durham SB, Casey MM: Do rural elders have limited access to medicare hospice services, *J Am Geriatr Soc* 52(5):731–735, 2004. Available from: https://doi.org/10.1111/j.1532-5415.2004.52213.x.

Weinert C, Long KA: Understanding the health care needs of rural families, *Fam Relat* 36(4):450–455, 1987.

Westberg Institute: *Philosophy of faith community nursing*, 2021. Available from: https://westberginstitute.org/faith-community-nursing/.

Williams MA, Andrews JA, Zanni KL, Fahs P, Stewart S: Rural nursing: searching for the state of the science, *Online J Rural Nurs Health Care* 2(12):102–117, 2012.

Zahner SJ, Corrado SM: Local health department partnerships with faith-based organizations, *J Publ Health Manag Pract* 10(3):258–265, 2004.

Zhang X, Tai D, Pforsicch H, Lin VW: United States registered nurse workforce report card and shortage forecast: a revisit, *Am J Med Qual* 33(3):229–236, 2018. Available from: https://edsource.org/wp-content/uploads/2019/02/Zhang-Daniel-Pforsich-Lin-2017-United-States-Registered-Nurse-Workforce-Report-Card-and-Shortage-Forecast_-A-Revisit.pdf.

FURTHER READING

Agency for Healthcare Research and Quality: *Coordinating care in the medical neighborhood: critical components and available mechanisms*, 2011. Available from: https://pcmh.ahrq.gov/sites/default/files/attachments/coordinating-care-in-the-medical-neighborhood-white-paper.pdf.

Aldwin C, Gilmer D: *Health, illness, and optimal aging: biological and psychosocial perspectives.* (3), New York, 2018, Springer Publishing.

Bureau of Primary Health Professions, 2016. Available from: https://bphc.hrsa.gov/.

County Economic Types: *Edition*, 2015. Available from: https://www.ers.usda.gov/data-products/county-typology-codes/descriptions-and-maps.aspx#ppov.

Health Resources and Services Administration: *Bureau of primary health care. Health Center Program*, n.d. Available from: https://bphc.hrsa.gov/.

U.S. Bureau of Labor Statistics Occupational Employment Statistics: *Occupational employment and wages*, 2020. May 2019. Available from: https://www.bls.gov/oes/current/oes291141.htm#st.

U.S. Census Bureau: *New census bureau report analyzes U.S. population projections. Release number CB15-TBS*, 2015. Available from: https://www.census.gov/newsroom/press-releases/2015/cb15-tps16.html.

U.S. Census Bureau, Creamer J: *Inequalities persist despite decline in poverty for all major race and hispanic origin groups*, 2020. Available from: https://www.census.gov/library/stories/2020/09/poverty-rates-for-blacks-and-hispanics-reached-historic-lows-in-2019. html#:~:text=Poverty%20rates%20declined%20between% 202018,Hispanics%2C%20it%20was%2015.7%25.

U.S. Department of Agriculture Economic Research Service: *Rural America at a glance, 2018 edition*, 2018. Available from: https:// www.ers.usda.gov/webdocs/publications/90556/eib-200.pdf.

U.S. Department of Agriculture Economic Research Service: *Rural economy & well-being*, 2020g. Available from: https://www.ers.usda. gov/topics/rural-economy-population/rural-poverty-well-being/ #demographics.

U.S. Department of Health and Human Services: *About HHS center of faith and opportunity initiatives*, 2020a. Available from: https:// www.hhs.gov/about/agencies/iea/partnerships/about-the- partnership-center/index.html.

U.S. Department of Health and Human Services: *Office of disease pre- vention and health promotion. Health People 2030 building a healthier future for all*, (n.d. -e). Available from: https://health.gov/healthypeople.

U.S. Department of Health and Human Services; Federal Register: *Annual update of the HHS poverty guidelines*, 2020d. Available from: https://www.federalregister.gov/documents/2020/01/17/2020- 00858/annual-update-of-the-hhs-poverty-guidelines.

U.S. Department of Health and Human Services; Healthy People 2030: *Healthy People 2030: Building a healthier future for all*, (n.d.-a). Available from: https://health.gov/healthypeople.

U.S. Department of Health and Human Services Office of the Assistant Secretary for Planning and Evaluation: *Public Health 3.0: A call to action to create a 21st century public health infrastructure*, 2016. Available from: https://www.healthypeople.gov/sites/default/files/ Public-Health-3.0-White-Paper.pdf.

U.S. Department of Health and Human Services Office of the Assistant Secretary for Planning and Evaluation (ASPE): *U.S. Federal Poverty Guidelines used to determine financial eligibility for certain federal programs. 2020 Poverty guidelines*, 2020f. Available from: https:// aspe.hhs.gov/2020-poverty-guidelines.

U.S. Department of Health and Human Services Office of Disease Prevention and Health Promotion: *Social determinants of health.*

Healthy People 2030, (n.d.-d). Available from: https://health.gov/ healthypeople/objectives-and-data/social-determinants-health.

U.S. Department of Health and Human Services Office of Minority Health: *Infant mortality and African Americans*, 2019. Available from: https://minorityhealth.hhs.gov/omh/browse.aspx?lvl=4&lvlid=23.

U.S. Bureau of Labor Statistics Occupational Employment Statistics: *Occupational employment and wages*, 2020. May 2019. Available from:https://www.bls.gov/oes/current/oes291141.htm#st.

U.S. Department of Health and Human Services Office of Disease Prevention and Health Promotion: *Healthy People 2030*, (n.d.-c). Available from: https://health.gov/healthypeople.

U.S. Department of Agriculture Economic Research Service: *Rural economy and population: population overview*, 2020i. Available from: https://www.ers.usda.gov/topics/rural-economy-population/ population-migration/.

U.S. Department of Health and Human Services Office of Disease Prevention and Health Promotion: *Healthy People 2020, social de- terminants of health, interventions, poverty*, (n.d.-b). Available from: https://www.healthypeople.gov/2020/topics-objectives/topic/social- determinants-health/interventions-resources/poverty.

U.S. Department of Health and Human Services Office of Disease Prevention and Health Promotion: *Healthy People 2030: How has healthy people changed?*, (n.d. -f). Available from: https://health.gov/ healthypeople/about/how-has-healthy-people-changed.

U.S. Department of Agriculture Economic Research Service: *Rural economy & population*, 2020e. Available from: https://www.ers.usda. gov/topics/rural-economy-population/.

U.S. Department of Agriculture Economic Research Service: *Rural economy & population and migration overview*, 2020f. Available from: https://www.ers.usda.gov/topics/rural-economy-population/ population-migration/.

U.S. Department of Agriculture Economic Research Service: *Rural poverty & wellbeing*, 2020. Available from: https://www.ers.usda.gov/ topics/rural-economy-population/rural-poverty-well-being/#historic.

25

Populations Affected by Mental Illness

Meredith Troutman-Jordan

OBJECTIVES

Upon completion of this chapter, the reader will be able to do the following:

1. Explain the concepts of community mental health, and discuss the importance of community mental health promotion in special populations.
2. Discuss the historical context for contemporary community mental healthcare.
3. Describe biological, social, and political factors associated with mental illness.
4. Illustrate the impact of natural and human-made disasters on the mental health of communities.
5. Describe some of the most common types of mental illnesses encountered in community settings.
6. Discuss the problem of suicide and recognize suicide warning signs.
7. Describe different types of evidence-based treatment for mental disorders, including use of psychotropic medication management, community case management, and crisis intervention.
8. Describe the role of mental health nurses in the community.

OUTLINE

KEY TERMS

agoraphobia
anorexia nervosa
anxiety disorders
anosignosia
Assertive Community Treatment
attention deficit disorder
attention deficit/hyperactivity disorder
bipolar disorder
bulimia nervosa
case management

Community Mental Health Centers Act
cooccurring
comorbidity
Crisis Intervention Team
deinstitutionalization
depression
generalized anxiety disorder
major depression
mental health, mental health consumer

mental illness
obsessive-compulsive disorder
panic disorder
phobia, posttraumatic stress disorder
psychotropic/psychotherapeutic medications
schizophrenia
severe emotional disorder
severe mental illness
stigma

Mental health refers to the absence of mental disorders and includes emotional, psychological, and social well-being, and importantly, it affects how we think, feel, and act (USDHHS, 2020). **Mental illness** consists of a major disturbance in an individual's thinking, feelings, or behavior that reflects a problem in mental function, and causes distress or disability in social, work, or family activities (American Psychiatric Association, 2020). Other effects of mental illnesses including disruptions of daily function and lifestyle, such as incapacitating personal, social, and occupational impairment as well as premature death.

Mental health can be affected by numerous factors, such as biological and genetic vulnerabilities, acute or chronic physical dysfunction, environmental conditions, and stressors. Twenty-first century community mental health necessitates comprehensive mental health services, including inpatient, outpatient, home-based, school, and community-based programs for individuals, families, and populations in need. Threats such as vulnerability, poverty, homelessness, cost, and limited accessibility to mental healthcare can be pervasive. Whether populations live in rural, suburban or urban settings, people need mental health services. Community mental healthcare exists throughout all levels of prevention and can be designed to supplement and decrease the need for more costly inpatient mental healthcare delivered in hospitals. A community's mental health is a reflection of community as a whole. Community-based mental health professionals work with populations at risk such as homeless veterans, families, children, and the elderly.

Nearly 21% (1 in 5) of U.S. adults experienced mental illness in 2019 (51.5 million people) (SAMHSA, 2019) and 5.2% (1 in 20) of U.S. adults experienced serious mental illness in 2019 (13.1 million people). Further, mental illness is a significant public health problem affecting not only the person with mental illness but their family, friends, schoolmates, work mates, and others. Mental illness is associated with lower use of healthcare, reduced adherence to treatment therapies for chronic diseases, and higher risks of adverse health outcomes.

The costs of mental healthcare can be estimated much the way that other healthcare costs are determined. There are significant studies that look at **co-occurring** mental illness and chronic diseases such as cardiovascular disease, diabetes, obesity, asthma, epilepsy, and cancer. Similarly, there is increased cooccurring use of tobacco products and abuse of alcohol in mental illness populations (SAMHSA, 2020a,b,c). Rates for intentional and unintentional injuries are higher among people with a mental illness as compared to the general population. For example, one recent study (Shadloo et al., 2016) almost half of those who had a history of psychiatric disorder in the past 12 months, also reported a history of injury during the same period. Furthermore, major risk factors for intentional injuries from interpersonal or selfinflicted violence includes mental illness, as well as other factors including access to firearms, history of interpersonal violence, and alcohol abuse (Maine Center for Disease Control and Prevention, 2021). The recognition that most mental illnesses can be managed successfully offers hope, and increasing access to and use of mental health treatment services can substantially reduce the associated morbidity. There are evidence-based practice (EBP) models consisting of community-based programs of intervention, education, and collaboration. Continual monitoring of mental illness is critical in providing appropriate organizations the data they require to assess the need for mental and behavioral health services and to inform the provision of those services.

The **Affordable Care Act** (ACA) built on the **2008 Mental Health Parity and Addiction Equity Act** (Dahukey et al., 2020)

to extend federal parity protections to more American the ACA addressed problems of denial of coverage, exclusion and capping mental health services, increases in premiums and cost-sharing, and restriction of access to drugs by pairing coverage expansions with access to mental healthcare (Baumgartner et al., 2020). Subsequently efforts to expand coverage, including allowing young people to stay on parents' plans until age 26 and expanding the Medicaid program, led to a significant drop in the number of uninsured by 2018. The ACA builds on the parity law by requiring coverage of mental health and substance use disorder benefits for millions of Americans who currently lack these benefits. This parity law helps ensure that when coverage for mental health and substance use conditions is provided, it is generally comparable to coverage for medical and surgical care. More recently, the COVID-19 relief stimulus legislation included a section titled "Strengthening Parity in Mental Health and Substance Use Disorder Benefits" that introduced additional "Mental Health Parity" compliance requirements (Ballard Spahr, 2021).

More than ever, community-based mental health nurses and interdisciplinary community teams face multiple challenges such as complex patient **comorbidity**, lack of resources, competent mental health professional workforce and law enforcement, physical facility inadequacies, and the stigma of mental illness. The purpose of this chapter is to describe critical issues that affect the mental health of individuals, families, groups, and special populations and to explore the potential influences and advocacy issues that nurses can be involved with. The chapter depicts issues that affect individuals, families, groups, and populations and explores promising EBP programs and educational models utilized in community mental health.

Severe mental illness (SMI) is a diagnosis applied to any adult who currently or at any time during the past year has had a diagnosable mental, behavioral, or emotional disorder with moderate, severe, or extreme functional behavior effects in specific lifestyle areas. These mental health disorders of persons 18 years of age or older present emotional or behavioral functioning that is so impaired as to interfere substantially with their capacity to remain in the community without supportive treatment or services of a long-term or indefinite duration. SMI mental disability is severe and persistent, associated with overrepresentation in the justice system (Bonfine et al., 2019), homelessness, arrest, incarceration, victimization, suicidality, family violence, and danger to others (Advocacy Treatment Center, 2018). Integrated models of care and nonintegrated models of care, contingency management, cognitive behavioral therapy, motivational interviewing, skills training, and cognitive behavioral therapy plus motivational interviewing have all been compared to standard care for individuals with SMI. On review, no high-quality evidence has been found to support any one psychosocial treatment over standard care for important outcomes such as remaining in treatment, reduction in substance use or improving mental or global state in people with serious mental illnesses and substance misuse (Hunt et al., 2019). The World Health Organization (WHO, 2018) notes that individuals with SMI generally have a life-expectancy 10 to

20 years shorter than the general population, and the majority of these premature deaths are due to physical health conditions. WHO encourages access to comprehensive health services which offer health promotion, screening and treatment for physical as well as mental health conditions, noting, however, that such services remain out of reach for the majority of people with severe mental disorders.

OVERVIEW AND HISTORY OF COMMUNITY MENTAL HEALTH: 1960 TO THE PRESENT DAY

The National Institute of Mental Health (NIMH) initially developed a Community Mental Health Center (CMHC) program in the 1960s. CMHCs were designed to provide comprehensive services for people with mental illness, locate these services closer to home, and provide an umbrella of integrated services for catchment areas of 125,000 to 250,000 people. These centers were intended to provide prevention, early treatment, and continuity of care in communities, promoting social integration of people with mental health needs. In 1963 President John F. Kennedy signed the **Community Mental Health Centers Act** (CMHCA) which resulted in deinstitutionalization and the closing of many mental institutions (NIMH, 2017). As a result, patients were released into communities, too often without supporting community services. Further cuts in housing and other services throughout the 1980s and beyond has resulted in growing numbers of homeless individuals in the United States.

The 1999 *Surgeon General's Report on Mental Health* defined mental health as a state of successful performance of mental function that results in productive activities, fulfilling relationships with others, and an ability to adapt to change and cope with adversity.

Table 25.1 provides a snapshot of the development of community mental health from the 1960s to present day.

Deinstitutionalization Cause and Effects

Deinstitutionalization is the release of institutionalized people, especially mental health patients, from an institution for placement and care in the community. In 2016, the U.S. had 37,679 state psychiatric beds, down about 13% since 2010 (Treatment Advocacy Center, 2018). Deinstitutionalization moved patients with psychiatric illnesses out of state-run "insane asylums" into federally funded CMHCs beginning in the 1960s as a way to improve the treatment of the mentally ill while also cutting government budgets (Amadeo, 2020). This national movement was also concerned with civil rights issues and the conditions of the state institutions. These questions and concerns led courts throughout the country to limit involuntary institutionalization and to set minimum standards for care in institutions. At that time there were not sufficient community resources, such as adequate housing, supported employment, community mental health professional workforce, and other community mental healthcare services, available throughout the country to meet the needs of patients coming back to communities. There was a beginning evolution in the structure, practice, experiences, and purposes of community mental healthcare in the United States. The CMHCA of 1964 provided federal support for mental health services (National Council for Behavioral Health, 2021). The Act supported measures to implement facilities to care for those who were mentally retarded and to construct CMHC.

Following passage of the Act, individuals with serious mental illness were returned to families and communities who were ill prepared to care for them, and funding did not follow the change in policy. Too many individuals with mental illness found themselves homeless, in shelters, or in prisons or jails. There was a critical need for more effective mental health treatment, improvements in the social welfare system, and provision of community support for this population, and shortly thereafter, the federal government recommended

TABLE 25.1	Community Mental Health Movement From the 1960 to the Present Day	
1960	Blue Ribbon Panel Report *Action for Mental Health*	Recommendations for intensive care of acutely ill mental patients and Community Mental health clinics
1963	Community Mental Health Clinics Legislation	Community mental health centers in some urban communities
1960s	Deinstitutionalization	Discharged mentally ill from state hospitals, patients returned to communities with inadequate resources (i.e., finances, housing, healthcare, supportive employment)
1981	Mental Health Block Grant, as part of the Omnibus Reconciliation Act	States develop comprehensive mental health plans for persons with serious mental illness
1986	State Mental Health Planning Act	
1999	U.S. Surgeon General's Report on Mental Health	Acknowledging mental illness as a disease
2008	Mental Health Parity and Addiction Equity Act of 2008	Insurance coverage for mental health and substance use conditions
2010	Affordable Care Act	Builds on the Mental Health Parity and Addiction Equity Act of 2008 to extend federal parity protections to 62 million Americans
2016	Helping Families in Mental Health Crisis Act (21st Century CURES)	Clarified Medicare reimbursement for mental health services and enhances crisis services, provides grants and promotes early intervention and support for mental health substance abuse and primary care
2018	Substance Use Disorder Prevention That Promotes Opioid Recovery and Treatment (SUPPORT) for Patients and Communities Act	Works to prepare providers to standardize delivery of addiction medicine and expand access to care for opioid addiction

linking community mental health services with informal community support services to improve treatment options.

Present-Day Community Mental Health Reform

It is estimated that one in seven patients presenting to U.S. Emergency Departments are the result of behavioral emergencies, thus the need for emergency psychiatric services cannot be understated (Zeller, 2021). In addition, resources and support for long term management of chronic psychiatric illness are also insufficient. As of 2018, 11.4 million people experienced serious mental illness; of those, only 64% received treatment for their disease (Amadeo, 2020). One reason for this is that 13.4% don't have insurance coverage. Mental health reform works toward monitoring federal legislation, administration activity, and public education initiatives. Such reform policies make community mental health a national priority and establish early access, recovery, and quality in mental health services as quality standards in our nation's mental healthcare delivery systems. There remains great need for mental health reform.

Several bills introduced in the 116th Congress are pertinent to mental health; H.R.3180, RISE from Trauma Act, which aims to improve the identification and support of children and families who experience trauma (Congress.gov, 2021b), and H.R.1109—Mental Health Services for Students Act of 2020 (Congress.gov, 2021a), which seeks to revise and extend projects relating to children and to provide access to school-based comprehensive mental health programs. Outcomes for these and subsequent legislation should prove to be beneficial.

Medicalization of Mental Illness

The American Psychiatric Association's (APA) *Diagnostic and Statistical Manual of Mental Disorders, Fifth Edition* (DSM V) (APA, 2017); has supported the medicalization of mental illness and has helped put mental disorders on parity with other diseases. The DSM V is an evidence-based manual that is useful to clinicians in helping them accurately diagnose mental disorders (APA, 2017). For example, with mental health parity, schizophrenia and depression may be treated as vigorously with treatment as diabetes. Medicalization can be described as the process in which conditions and behaviors are labeled and treated as medical issues (NYU Grossman School of Medicine, 2020). Medicalization may reduce social discrimination and stigma for those with mental illness. This, along with Federal laws barring health insurers from imposing lower coverage limits on mental health services than they do on other medical treatments have improved access and care for those with mental illness.

Brain Neuroimaging, Genetics, and Hope for New Treatments

Brain imaging scans, also called neuroimaging scans, are being used more and more to help detect and diagnose a number of medical disorders and illnesses. Currently, the main use of brain scans for mental disorders is in research studies to learn more about the disorders.

Researchers use neuroimaging to study healthy brain development and the effects of mental illnesses or the effects of mental health treatments on the brain. Brain scans alone, however, cannot be used to diagnose mental illness when used by themselves or predict risk of getting a mental illness (NIMH, 2021a,b,c,d).

 ACTIVE LEARNING

1. Locate the National Alliance for Mental Illness (NAMI) and Suicide Prevention Action Network (SPAN) chapters in your community. What services do these agencies offer? How might those services be helpful in the community mental health nursing role?

HEALTHY PEOPLE 2030: MENTAL HEALTH AND MENTAL DISORDERS

Healthy People 2030 is a collaboration among federal, state, and territorial governments and private, public, and nonprofit organizations to set national disease prevention and health promotion objectives (Healthypeople.gov, 2021a,b). The *Healthy People 2030* box lists several objectives that cover issues related to mental health. Major mental health objectives target prevention and access to psychiatric and substance abuse treatment. There are objectives for treatment expansion, and providing adequate community resources for adults, children, and families struggling with mental illnesses.

 HEALTHY PEOPLE 2030

Objectives Related to Mental Illness and Health
Mental Health Status Improvement
  MHMD–1: Increase the number of children and adolescents with serious emotional disturbance who get treatment.
  MHMD–2: Reduce suicide attempts by adolescents.
  MHMD–3: Increase the proportion of children with mental health problems who get treatment.
  MHMD–4: Increase the proportion of adults with serious mental illness who get treatment.

Treatment Expansion
  MHMD–5: Increase the proportion of adults with depression who get treatment.
  MHMD–6: Increase the proportion of adolescents with depression who get treatment.
  MHMD–7: Increase the proportion of people with substance use and mental health disorders who get treatment for both.
  MHMD–8: Increase the proportion of primary care visits where adolescents and adults are screened for depression.
  MHMD-R01 Increase the proportion of homeless adults with mental health problems who get mental health services.

From HealthyPeople.gov: *Healthy People 2030: Mental health and mental disorders,* 2021. Available from: https://health.gov/healthypeople/objectives-and-data/browse-objectives/mental-health-and-mental-disorders.

FACTORS INFLUENCING MENTAL HEALTH

Although treatment of mental disorders has dramatically improved, the cause of most mental illnesses is not well understood. Research has identified a number of biological and sociological factors that contribute to mental health and mental illness. Some of these factors are discussed here.

Biological Factors

For centuries, mental illnesses were viewed as conditions that needed to be contained in institutions. Neuroscience research has provided a better understanding of the biology of mental illnesses; however, many questions remain unanswered. Biological factors associated with mental illness include genetic factors, neurotransmission, and abnormalities of brain structure and functioning.

Genetic Factors

Genetic expressions, combined with neurochemical and metabolic changes and environmental insults, may result in the display of mental disorder indicators. There is evidence of predisposition to mental illnesses in families, suggesting that people who have a family member with a mental illness are more likely to experience one themselves. Experts believe that some mental illnesses are linked to abnormalities in several genes, not just one. People may inherit a susceptibility to a mental illness and do not necessarily go on to have a mental illness. Mental illnesses more likely occur from the interaction of multiple genetic factors and some other factors, such as stress, abuse, and traumatic events. These factors can influence, trigger, or exacerbate an illness in a person who has an inherited susceptibility to it. Psychiatric genetics has generated very promising results in terms of risk variants associated with major psychiatric disorders and treatment outcomes; however, psychiatry still lags behind other areas of medicine in terms of translation of existing knowledge into diagnostic genetic tests that could facilitate early diagnosis and accurate classification of disorders (Hoehe & Morris-Rosendahl, 2018).

Abnormalities of Brain Structure and Functioning

Evidence indicates that structural brain abnormalities can be related to some mental illnesses, such as schizophrenia, depression, and Alzheimer's disease. As the science of neuroimaging evolves, a more refined view of the role of brain structure and functioning is unfolding. For example, molecular, biological, and psychological links between stress exposure and the pathogenesis of anxiety and mood disorders have been extensively studied, leading to and ensuing in the quest for novel psychopharmacological strategies aimed at targets of the hypothalamic-pituitary-adrenal (HPA) axis (Tafet & Nemeroff, 2020). Scientists are also recognizing how other systems of the body can impact brain functioning. For example, research demonstrates that sleep plays a housekeeping role that removes toxins in the brain that build up while one is awake (NIH, 2019).

Although a number of theories on the etiology of mental disorders have been developed, information is insufficient to establish a definitive biological cause for mental illness. Scholars have concluded that mental disorders are multifactorial, complex phenomena. The important point for community health nurses to understand is that mental illnesses have a very strong biological basis, much like other chronic conditions such as diabetes and heart disease, but that other factors are highly influential.

Social Factors

Some community occurrences and phenomena, such as school shootings, public bombings, bullying, domestic violence, and other tragic events, have identified critical gaps in the need for public education, advocacy, and treatment of mental illness (National Council for Behavioral Health, 2019). Throughout history, the symptoms of mental illness have been perceived as permanent, dangerous, frightening, and shameful. People with a diagnosis of mental illness have been described as lazy, idle, weak, immoral, irrational, and too often criminal. On the basis of these characterizations and assumptions, many people with a diagnosis of mental illness have experienced widespread social rejection that may lead to isolation, discrimination, unwarranted legal restrictions, and social control (National Council for Behavioral Health, 2019).

Clinical Example 25.1

Photographer Michael Nye has spent hundreds of hours photographing and taping illness narratives of individuals living with serious mental illness. Viewing his photographs and listening to the accounts of those living with these conditions are valuable experiences for nurses who care for this population (http://michaelnye.org/fineline/index.html). Han and Oliffe (2016) reviewed the use of photovoice in mental illness, in nine qualitative studies. They reported how participants described feelings of loneliness, being marginalized, and their support care needs to build selfconfidence.

Another social concern is the tendency of communities to make use of prisons rather than psychiatric hospitals as a solution to the "mental health problem." About 0.7% of United States residents are currently in a federal or state prison or local jail (Wagner & Bertram, 2020). It has been observed that while less than 5% of the world's population live in the United States, but 20% of the world's incarcerated people are located here.

U.S. prisons and jails incarcerate a disproportionate amount of people who have a current or past mental illness. Indeed, 37% of the people in state and federal prisons have been diagnosed with a mental illness, but 66% of those with mental illness in federal prisons reported not receiving any mental healthcare while incarcerated (Prison Policy Initiative, 2020). Prisons are sadly unprepared to provide adequate care to the mentally ill. To help address this problem, in 2008, Senate Bill S.2304, the Mentally Ill Offender Treatment and Crime Reduction Reauthorization and Improvement Act, was signed into law. This bill provided grants aimed at improving the mental health treatment provided to criminal offenders with a mental illness. Other related initiatives have focused on establishing specialty courts or problem-solving courts. There may be mental health courts in communities to address the needs of the community and those who are charged with a criminal offense and also experience a mental illness (Mental Health America, 2017).

Gender, Racial, and Sexual Orientation Disparities

Racial and ethnic minorities are the fastest-growing population groups in the United States. The NIMH's Office for Research on Disparities and Global Mental Health (ORDGMH) (NIMH, 2021a,b,c,d) is active in working to reduce mental health disparities. The ORDGMH collects local and global mental health disparities data, including movements of populations, global economic relationships, and communication technologies. Culturally diverse groups often bear a disproportionately high burden of disability due to mental disorders. For example, African Americans with severe depression are more likely to be misdiagnosed as having schizophrenia than white patients (Gara et al., 2019).

Because of the lack of access in their communities, Hispanic Americans use mental health services far less than other ethnic and racial groups. Yet, 18.3% of the U.S. population identifies as Hispanic or Latino, and of these, over 16% (over 10 million people) reported having a mental illness within the past year (Mental Health America, 2021b). This population also constitutes the largest group of uninsured in the United States. In addition, American Indian and Alaska Natives experience the higher rates of mental disorders compared to the overall population. These groups experience far greater psychological distress are at greater risk for mental disorders such as depression, substance abuse, anxiety, and posttraumatic stress disorder (PTSD). In some American Indian groups, the rates of alcoholism and illicit drug use disorder are much higher than the U.S. average.

COMMUNITY FOCUS

Percentages of depression and anxiety reveal ethnic differences. In the Mental Health America (2021a) over 2.6 million people completed a mental health online screening program that took place from January to December 2020 (largely through COVID-19). Among the findings was that the proportion of people with moderate to severe symptoms of anxiety was highest (84%) among Native American or American Indians. The largest increase in the proportion of people scoring for moderate to severe anxiety was among individuals who identified their race as "Other" (4.67% increase) and Asian or Pacific Islander screeners (4.53% increase). The proportion of people with moderate to severe symptoms of depression was highest among people who identified with more than one race in 2020 (90%). Interestingly, rates of moderate to severe depression were lower in 2020 than in 2019 for individuals of nearly every race/ethnicity, except for Native American or American Indians, although the percentage of people with moderate to severe symptoms of depression in December 2020 was higher than December 2019 average for every racial/ethnic group.

Those from the lesbian, gay, bisexual, and transgendered (LGBT) community are at increased risk for a number of mental health problems. LGBT individuals face health disparities associated with societal stigma, discrimination, and denial of their civil rights (Healthypeople.gov, 2021a,b). Moreover, discrimination against LGBT persons has been linked with high rates of psychiatric disorders, substance abuse, and suicide.

Natural and Human-Made Disasters and Mental Illness

Natural and human-made disasters, such as hurricanes, floods, violence, terrorism, war, and the global economic crisis, are profound stress-inducing events that can lead to mental illness. Community mental health nurses must be prepared not only to respond to the mental health needs of a community during a disaster but also to maintain vigilance in caring for survivors many years thereafter.

PTSD is highly prevalent among combat veterans returning from war. PTSD is associated with extreme anxiety that can result in suicide. Veterans are twice as likely as civilians to die by suicide (U.S. Department of Veterans Affairs, 2018). Veterans, who comprise more than 14% of all suicides, account for only 8% of the total population. Lack of access to mental healthcare, a growing sense of disconnection in society, economic, and relationship difficulties are proposed contributing factors for this trend (U.S. Department of Veterans Affairs, 2019). Early intervention is key to prevention and treatment. The U.S. Department of Defense (DOD, 2021) recognizes the urgency of intervention and resource availability for service members and veterans. Based on their 2019 Annual Suicide Report, the DOD identified the need to target: young and enlisted members, specifically addressing perceived barriers to seeking help and encouraging use of support resources, addressing common risk factors with an integrated violence prevention approach and supporting the rollout of a new "988" crisis line number. The DOD also acknowledges military families, identifying the need to teach influencers such as spouses, chaplains, and students in DOD schools of risk factors for suicide, the importance of encouraging help-seeking and promoting safe storage of lethal means. Further, they intend to focus on measuring program effectiveness, via the DOD-wide program evaluation framework and enhancing research, data and evaluation capabilities.

The onset of the global COVID-19 pandemic in early 2020 had devastating social, economic, mental, and physical health consequences. While initial concerns were on transmission of the virus, and physical health of communities, families, and individuals, as months progressed, the pandemic began to exert its toll on mental health of these groups. For instance, individuals with personal experiences related to COVID-19 diagnosis or death were more likely to have psychological symptoms (Gallagher et al., 2020). Unusual public health emergencies such as this affect health, safety, and well-being of individuals (causing, for example, insecurity, confusion, emotional isolation, and stigma) and communities (due economic loss, work and school closures, inadequate resources for medical response, and deficient distribution of necessities) (Pfefferbaum & North, 2020). These effects may translate into a range of emotional reactions (such as distress or diagnosable psychiatric conditions), unhealthy behaviors (such as excessive substance use) in those who contract the disease as well as in the general population. Therefore, it is critical for community health nurses to be sensitive to mental health needs of all patients in times of such public health crises, even those with no prior history of psychiatric illness.

Political Factors

Political factors can dramatically influence how mental disorders are managed. One significant factor in the politics of mental illness is parity in healthcare coverage—that is, the equal access to healthcare for physical and mental illnesses, as mentioned previously. Historically, health insurance companies have provided less access to treatment for a mental disorder than for a physical disorder. Since 2008, when the Paul Wellstone and Pete Domenici Mental Health Parity and Addiction Equity Act was enacted, there are laws requiring health insurance to cover treatment for mental illness on the same terms and conditions as physical illness. Although this legislation was a victory for mental health, there has been inconsistency in how the legislation has moved forward.

Healthcare disparities have become a key issue in public health policy discussions. As discussed, members of ethnic minority groups have less access to mental health services than do their white counterparts. For example, Black adults in the U.S. are more likely than white adults to report persistent symptoms of emotional distress, such as sadness and hopelessness (U.S. Department of Health and Human Services Office of Minority Health, 2019); and in 2017, suicide was the second leading cause of death for African Americans, ages 15 to 24 (CDC, 2019). Similarly, Hispanic/Latinx communities experience disparities in access to and quality of mental health treatment. It has been observed that over half of Hispanic young adults ages 18 to 25 with serious mental illness may not receive treatment, and approximately 34% of Hispanic/Latinx adults with mental illness receive treatment each year compared to the U.S. average of 45% (NAMI, 2021a,b,c,d). This inequality puts these members of these aggregates at a greater risk for more severe and persistent forms of mental health conditions.

The disparities in minority mental health diagnosis and treatment is a pressing issue, heightened by increasing population diversity in the U.S. Recommended responses to close this gap include nurses' consideration of their own awareness of values and how perceptions may influence interactions with patients from other cultures. Additionally, community health nurses and policymakers should strongly support legislation and policies that address health disparities, and provide access to necessary resources and additional assistance such as education, awareness, advocacy, and integration of behavioral health with primary care for all patients (USC Department of Nursing, 2021).

MENTAL DISORDERS ENCOUNTERED IN COMMUNITY SETTINGS

The influence of untreated mental illness on communities and their social structure has been vastly understated. SAMHSA (2020a,b,c) reports an estimated 51,495,000 (20.6%) Americans 18 years and older experienced some form of mental illness in the past year. In addition, more than 8 million adults age 12 or older (3%) adults had a substance use disorder, and among persons age 18 or older, more than 9 million had cooccurring SUD and some form of mental illness in the past year. The sheer number of those with mental illness is highly concerning as it is one of the leading causes of disability in the United States (NIMH, 2020a,b). The problem is worldwide as mental illness and substance use disorders affected more than 1 billion people globally in 2016, causing 7% of all global burden of disease (Rehm & Shield, 2019). In the United States, spending mental healthcare increased by more than 50% from 2009 to 2019, and in 2019 mental health spending reached $225 billion, accounting for nearly 5.5% of all health spending (Open Minds, 2020).

Because most mental illnesses are identified and managed in community settings, it is essential that community health nurses be familiar with frequently occurring mental disorders. There is a need for screening, referring, and follow-up for people with mental health problems in order to meet their needs (NAMI, 2021a,b,c,d).

Overview of Selected Mental Disorders

The *DSM* V (American Psychiatric Association [APA], 2017) classifies mental illnesses and outlines diagnostic criteria for more than 300 disorders. Children with mental disorders are often referred to as children with **severe emotional disorder** (SED). SED disturbance suggests broad ranges of behaviors that might result in classification of a student with SED as eligible for special education. A child with SED may demonstrate emotional disturbance with hallucinations, may have a very short attention span, may hurt others physically, may destroy property, or may have severe presentations of depression, anger, or fear. Among students with SED, externalizing behaviors such as acting out are significantly more prevalent than internalizing behaviors such as withdrawal or depression.

Schizophrenia

Schizophrenia is the most severe of all mental illnesses. The prevalence of schizophrenia (i.e., the number of cases in a population at any one time point) approximates 1% both nationally and globally (Fisher & Buchanan, 2021). The effect of this condition on the community is enormous in terms of social and economic burden. To the individual and families affected by schizophrenia, the impact is incalculable. The affected person may present with positive symptoms, including hallucinations, delusions, disorganized thinking and speech, and bizarre behavior, or negative symptoms, such as flat affect, poor attention, lack of motivation, apathy, lack of pleasure, and lack of energy. Onset typically occurs during late adolescence and early adulthood in males and somewhat later in females. There is an increased risk for alcohol use, depression, suicide, and diabetes among persons with schizophrenia. These factors compound the problems associated with living with a psychotic disorder.

About 30% of people with schizophrenia experienced "severe" lack of awareness of their diagnosis, known as anosignosia (NAMI, 2021a,b,c,d). Anosignosia contributes to noncompliance with medications and treatment. Research indicates that a lifetime rate of suicide in individuals with schizophrenia is between 4% and 13%, while rates of suicide attempts in patients with schizophrenia vary between from 18% to 55% (Sher & Khan, 2019).

Treatment for schizophrenia must be intensive and generally involves hospitalization (initially), antipsychotic medications, and psychotherapy/counseling. Long-term follow-up by mental health professionals is necessary to monitor medication compliance and to watch for side effects and complications, which may be severe and life-threatening, and to evaluate the patient's ability to integrate into the community.

Depression

Depression is the most frequently diagnosed and one of the most disabling mental illnesses in the United States. Approximately 17.3 million (7.1%) adults in the United States reportedly had at least one major depressive episode during the past year (NIMH, 2019a,b,c). Of these individuals, 63.8% had severe impairment. Depressive disorders include major depressive disorder, dysthymic disorder, and bipolar disorders. Depression often cooccurs with serious physical disorders, such as heart attack, stroke, diabetes, and cancer. Although effective treatments exist, many people with depressive illness do not get help. Of note, approximately 65% received combined care by a health professional and medication treatment, while 6% received treatment with medication alone; and about 35% of adults with major depressive episode did not receive treatment (NIMH, 2019a,b,c). Having a family or personal history of depression, childhood trauma, serious or chronic illness, traumatic or stressful events, such as physical or sexual abuse, the death or loss of a loved one, a difficult relationship, or financial problems are among the risk factors for depression (Mayo Clinic, 2017). Health education for patients with depression should include risk factor identification as well as when and how to obtain treatment. Symptoms of depression are listed in Box 25.1.

RESEARCH HIGHLIGHTS

Measuring Mental Illness—Related Stigma Imposed by Healthcare Providers

Knowing that mental illness-related stigma can lead to low rates of seeking help, lack of access to care, undertreatment, and social marginalization, Kassam et al. (2012) developed and tested the *Opening Minds Scale for HealthCare Providers* (OMS-HC) with 787 healthcare providers/trainees across Canada. The OMS-HC provides hope in demonstrating that it that can be

utilized in evaluation of programs with goals to reduce mental illness—related stigma imposed by healthcare providers.

Data from Kassam A, Papish A, Modgill G, Patten S: The development and psychometric properties of a new scale to measure mental illness related stigma by healthcare providers: the Opening Minds Scale for Healthcare Providers (OMS-HC). *BMC Psychiatry* 12:62, 3—12, 2012.

Depression in Children and Adolescents. About 7% of children ages 3 to 17 have anxiety, and around 3% deal with depression (Cleveland Clinic, 2021). Further, both depression and anxiety tend to be higher in older children and teenagers between the ages of 12 and 17. Approximately 3.2 million adolescents aged 12 to 17 (13.3% of population aged 12—17) in the United States have had at least one major depressive episode, and an estimated 31.9% of adolescents have had an anxiety disorder (Cleveland Clinic, 2021). A family history of depression is a major risk factor for childhood depression. Other associated factors that may increase the risk of depression in children and adolescents are a history of verbal, physical, or sexual abuse; frequent separation from, or loss of, a loved one; poverty; mental retardation; attention deficit/hyperactivity disorder; hyperactivity; chronic illness; alcohol or drug use; physical illness; and stressful life events (Cleveland Clinic, 2021).

Treatment for depression includes pharmacological therapy, psychotherapy, behavior therapy, electroconvulsive therapy, or a combination of these (NIMH, 2019a,b,c). In general, the most effective, first-line treatment is a combination of antidepressant medication and psychotherapy.

Bipolar Disorder

Bipolar disorder refers to a group of mood disorders that manifest as changes in mood from depression to mania. The depressed phase manifests as symptoms seen in major depressive disorder. The manic phase is characterized by a persistent abnormally elevated or irritable mood, impaired judgment, flight of ideas, pressured speech, grandiosity, distractibility, excessive involvement in goal-directed activities,

BOX 25.1 Symptoms of Depression

- Persistent sad, anxious, or "empty" feelings
- Feelings of hopelessness or pessimism
- Feelings of guilt, worthlessness, or helplessness
- Irritability, restlessness
- Loss of interest in activities or hobbies once pleasurable, including sex
- Fatigue and decreased energy
- Difficulty concentrating, remembering details, and making decisions
- Insomnia, early-morning wakefulness, or excessive sleeping
- Overeating or appetite loss
- Thoughts of suicide, suicide attempts
- Aches or pains, headaches, cramps, or digestive problems that do not ease even with treatment

From National Institute of Mental Health: *Depression* (NIH publication No. 11—3561), Rockville, MD, 2000, Revised 2011, Author.

spending few hours sleeping, and impulsivity. These symptoms may cooccur with psychotic features such as hallucinations and delusions. Persons with bipolar disorder are at increased risk for alcohol and substance abuse as well as suicide. The presence of bipolar disorder results in poor occupational and social functioning.

Management of bipolar disorder must be ongoing and must involve close monitoring. Treatment generally involves use of mood-stabilizing medication, often in combination with a second-generation ("atypical") antipsychotic (NIMH, 2020a,b). Often, providers prescribe antidepressant medication to treat depressive episodes in bipolar disorder, combining this with a mood stabilizer to prevent triggering a manic episode (NIMH, 2020a,b). When working with persons with bipolar disorder, nurses need to monitor symptoms and response to psycho-pharmacological treatment.

Anxiety Disorder

Anxiety disorders are a group of conditions characterized by feelings of anxiety. Anxiety disorders affect 40 million U.S. adults age 18 and older, or 18.1% of the population, every year (Anxiety and Depression Association of America, 2020). Though highly treatable, only 36.9% of individuals experiencing anxiety disorders receive treatment. Anxiety disorders may be attributed to the genetic makeup and life experiences of the individual. Some of the more commonly encountered anxiety disorders are generalized anxiety disorder (GAD), panic disorder (sometimes accompanied by agoraphobia), social anxiety disorder, phobias, obsessive-compulsive disorder (OCD), and PTSD (NIMH, 2018). They are discussed briefly here.

Generalized Anxiety Disorder.
GAD is characterized by chronic, unrealistic, and exaggerated worry and tension about one or more life circumstances lasting 6 months or longer (NIMH, 2018). Approximately half of cases of GAD begin in childhood or adolescence, and the disorder is more common in women than in men. Symptoms of GAD include trembling, twitching, muscle tension, headaches, irritability, sweating or hot flashes, dyspnea, and nausea (Anxiety and Depression Association of America, 2020). Periods of increasing symptoms are usually associated with life stressors or impending difficulties. GAD is probably the most underdiagnosed mental disorder.

Panic Disorder.
Approximately 6 million adults (2.7% of the U.S. population) have panic disorder, with women twice as likely to be affected as men (Anxiety and Depression Association of America, 2020). **Panic disorder** can strike at any age, and while symptoms often begin before age 25, they may also occur in the mid-30s (Medline Plus, 2021). Children can also have panic disorder, but it is often not diagnosed until they are older. Approximately 2% to 3% of Americans experience panic disorder in a given year and it is twice as common in women than in men (Anxiety and Depression Association of America, 2020). A panic attack consists of a period of intense fear that develops abruptly and unexpectedly. The initial attack may occur while the client is performing everyday tasks. Typically, he or she experiences tachycardia; dyspnea; dizziness; chest pain; nausea; numbness or tingling of the hands and feet; trembling or shaking; sweating; choking; or a feeling that he or she is going to die, go crazy, or do something uncontrolled. It can be extremely frightening. A diagnosis of panic disorder is made when attacks occur with some degree of frequency or regularity.

As the disorder evolves, the anxiety attacks become increasingly frequent and severe, and anticipatory anxiety (fear of having a panic attack) develops. During this phase, events and circumstances associated with the attack may be selectively avoided, leading to phobic behaviors. Thus, the client's life may become progressively constricted.

As the avoidance behavior intensifies, the client begins to withdraw further to avoid being in places or situations from which escape may be difficult or embarrassing or in which help may be unavailable in the event of a panic attack (e.g., church, elevators, movie theaters). The fear of being in these situations or places can lead to **agoraphobia** (literally, fear of the marketplace or open places). Individuals with agoraphobia frequently progress to the point that they cannot leave their homes without experiencing anxiety. Cognitive behavioral treatment and short-course benzodiazepines therapy are used to treat panic disorder.

Phobias.
A **phobia** is an irrational fear of something (an object or situation), and an estimated 19 million Americans have a phobia that results in difficulty in some area of their lives (Healthline.com, 2021). Adults with phobias realize that their fears are irrational, but facing the feared object or situation might bring on severe anxiety or a panic attack. Although phobias may begin in childhood, they usually first appear in adolescence or adulthood.

Social phobia, or social anxiety disorder, is a persistent and intense fear of, and compelling desire to avoid, something that would expose the individual to a situation that might be humiliating and embarrassing (NIMH, 2017). It has a familial tendency and may be accompanied by depression or alcoholism. The most common social phobia is a fear of public speaking. Other examples include being unable to urinate in a public bathroom and not being able to answer questions in social situations. Most people with social phobias can be treated with cognitive-behavioral therapy and medication.

Simple phobias involve a persistent fear of, and compelling desire to avoid, certain objects or situations. Common objects of phobias are spiders, snakes, dogs, cats, and situations such as flying, heights, and closed-in spaces. The person often recognizes that the fear is unreasonable but avoids the situation or endures it with intense anxiety. Systematic desensitization and normal exposure are the most effective treatments for simple phobias.

Obsessive-Compulsive Disorder. OCD is characterized by anxious thoughts and rituals that the individual has difficulty controlling. The person with OCD feels compelled to engage in some ritual to avoid a persistent frightening thought, idea, image, or event. *Obsessions* are recurrent thoughts, emotions, or impulses that cannot be dismissed. *Compulsions* are the rituals or behaviors that are repeatedly performed to prevent, neutralize, or dispel the dreaded obsession. When the individual tries to resist the compulsion, anxiety increases. Common compulsions include hand washing, counting, checking, and touching (NIMH, 2019a,b,c). Most individuals recognize that what they are doing is senseless but are unable to control the compulsion. Lifetime prevalence rates of OCD worldwide have been estimated at 1.5% for women and 1.0% for men (Fawcett et al., 2020). Depression and other anxiety disorders often accompany OCD. Behavioral therapy and medication aimed at reducing accompanying symptoms have been found to be helpful.

Posttraumatic Stress Disorder. **Posttraumatic stress disorder** is a debilitating condition that follows a shocking, scary or dangerous event. About 7% to 8% of the population will have PTSD at some point in their lives, and approximately 8 million adults have PTSD during a given year (U.S. Department of Veterans Affairs, 2019). Around 10% women develop PTSD sometime in their lives compared with about 4% of men. Individuals with PTSD have recurring, persistent, frightening thoughts, and memories of their ordeal. The event may involve "shell shock" or "battle fatigue" common to war veterans, a violent attack, serious accident, or natural disaster, or having witnessed a mass destruction or injury, such as an airplane crash. Sometimes the individual is unable to recall an important aspect of the traumatic event. The highest incidence of PTSD occurs among combat-experienced military personnel.

People with PTSD repeatedly relive the trauma in the form of nightmares or disturbing recollections or flashbacks during the day, resulting in sleep disturbances, depression, feelings of detachment or emotional numbness, or being easily startled. They may avoid places or situations that bring back memories (e.g., a woman raped in an elevator may refuse to ride in elevators), and anniversaries of the event are often very difficult. PTSD occurs at all ages and may be accompanied by depression, substance abuse, and/or anxiety. It usually begins within 3 months of the trauma, and the course of the disorder varies. Some individuals recover within 6 months; the condition becomes chronic in others. Infrequently, the illness does not manifest until years after the traumatic event. Treatment includes antidepressants and antianxiety medications and psychotherapy. Support from family and friends can be very beneficial.

Eating Disorders

Eating disorders—anorexia nervosa and bulimia nervosa—are increasingly prevalent in the United States. An estimated 20 million women and 10 million men in America will have an eating disorder at some point in their lives (National Eating Disorders Association, 2018). The definition of anorexia nervosa was revised for the Fifth Edition of the Diagnostic and Statistical Manual (DSM-5) (Mustelin et al., 2016). One of the leading reasons for the revision was to reduce the number of patients who were diagnosed with eating disorder not otherwise specified, who constituted over half of patients in specialized eating disorder units.

DSM-5 introduced three changes to the criteria defining anorexia nervosa: the weight loss criterion was revised, fear of weight gain does not need to be verbalized if behaviors interfering with weight gain can be observed, and amenorrhea was no longer required. Another revision in the DSM-5 is the introduction of a body mass index (BMI) based severity rating (Mustelin et al., 2016).

Eating disorders primarily affect females, and most clients with a diagnosis of eating disorders are white; however, the reason may be socioeconomic factors rather than race. Anorexia and bulimia are often triggered by developmental milestones (e.g., puberty, first sexual contact) or another crisis (e.g., death of a loved one, ridicule over weight, starting college).

Bulimia nervosa refers to binge eating; recurrent and frequent episodes of eating unusually large amounts of food, and feeling a lack of control over the eating. For example, a person with bulimia might eat an entire pie, half a cake, or a half gallon of ice cream at one sitting. This binge-eating is followed by a type of behavior that compensates for the binge, such as purging (e.g., vomiting, excessive use of laxatives or diuretics), fasting, and/or excessive exercise (NIMH, 2017).

Bulimia nervosa typically begins in adolescence or during the early 20s, usually in conjunction with a diet. High school and college students, as well as members of certain professions that emphasize weight and/or appearance (e.g., dancers, flight attendants, cheerleaders, athletes, actors, models), are at risk. The condition may lead to electrolyte imbalance, resulting in fatigue, seizures, muscle cramps, arrhythmias, and decreased bone density. Vomiting can damage the esophagus, stomach, teeth, and gums.

The person with **anorexia nervosa** becomes obsessed with a fear of fat and with losing weight. Anorexia nervosa often develops as a fairly gradual decrease in caloric intake. However, the decrease continues until the person is consuming almost nothing. Anorexia usually begins in early adolescence (12–14 years is the most common age-group) and may be limited to a single episode of dramatic weight loss within a few months, followed by recovery, or may last for many years.

Risk factors for eating disorders are perfectionism, low selfesteem, stress, poor coping skills, sexual/physical abuse, poor self-image, dependency on others' opinions and deference to others' wishes, and being emotionally reserved. In response to the severely decreased caloric intake, the body tries to compensate by slowing down body processes. Menstruation ceases; blood pressure, pulse, and respiration rates slow; and thyroid activity diminishes. Electrolyte imbalance can become very severe. Other symptoms are mild anemia, joint swelling, and reduced muscle mass. Anorexia nervosa can be life threatening and has a mortality rate of 5% to 21%.

Treatment for eating disorders involves long-term nutrition counseling, psychotherapy, and behavior modification. Hospitalization may be required for clients with serious complications. Self-help groups and support groups can be very beneficial for both the client and the family.

Nurses need to be aware of the resources available from the American Academy of Child and Adolescent Psychiatry (AACAP), which has a section for families and youth. Such knowledge is important, as community health nurses assess the social influences that contribute to the condition.

Attention Deficit/Hyperactivity Disorder

Two of the most common conditions encountered by nurses who work with children in community settings are **attention-deficit/hyperactivity disorder** (ADHD) and **attention deficit disorder** (ADD). In children ages 5 to 17, 10.8% have ever been diagnosed with ADHD; 14.8% of boys and 6.7% of girls (CDC, 2020). Behaviors that might indicate ADHD/ADD usually appear before age 7 years and are often accompanied by related problems, such as learning disability, anxiety, and depression. The three major characteristics of ADHD/ADD are inattention, hyperactivity, and impulsivity.

The cause of ADHD/ADD is not known, but it is important to note that the disorder is not caused by minor head injuries, birth complications, food allergies, too much sugar, poor home life, poor schools, or too much television watching. Maternal substance use and abuse (e.g., alcohol, cigarettes, cocaine) may affect the brain of the developing baby and produce symptoms of ADHD/ADD later in life. This possibility, however, accounts for only a small percentage of those affected. Attention disorders run in families.

Most children with ADHD/ADD receive a diagnosis during the elementary school years (NIMH, 2019a,b,c). Experts caution that diagnosis of attention disorders should be made following a comprehensive physical, psychological, social, and behavioral evaluation and should not be based solely on anecdotal reports from parents or teachers. The evaluation should rule out other possible reasons for the behavior (e.g., emotional problems, poor vision or hearing, physical problems) and should include input from teachers, parents, and others who know the child well. Intelligence and achievement testing may also be performed to rule out or identify a learning disability.

Symptoms of ADHD/ADD are typically managed through a combination of behavior therapy, emotional counseling, and practical support. Use of medication is now becoming increasingly commonplace in the management of ADHD/

ADD. It is very important, however, that children with attention disorders and their families understand that medication does not cure the disorder; it just temporarily controls symptoms.

Stimulants have been shown to be successful in treating attention disorders. The most commonly used medications are methylphenidate (Ritalin), dextroamphetamine and amphetamine (Adderall), and dextroamphetamine (Dexedrine). Appetite suppression and poor sleep are common side effects.

Suicide

There are approximately 1 million deaths by suicide per year throughout the world. The American Foundation for Suicide Prevention (2021) reported that nearly 50,000 (48,344, to be exact) Americans died by suicide in 2020 (average of 132 each day), In addition, about 1.4 million Americans attempted suicide that year. Moreover, suicide was the second leading cause of death in the U.S. for ages 10 to 34 and the fourth leading cause of death for ages 35 to 54. American Indian and Alaska Native youth and middle-aged persons have the highest rate of suicide, followed by non-Hispanic White middle-aged and older adult males (NIMH, 2021a,b,c,d). Although younger preteens and teens have a lower rate of suicide than older adolescents, there has been a significant rise in the suicide rate among youth ages 10 to 14 (NIMH, 2021a,b,c,d).

Historically, risk and protective factors have been used to identify those at highest risk for suicide. The American Association of Suicidology (AAS, 2020) has recommended recognition of warning signs as more relevant than risk and protective factors in preventing death by suicide. The AAS has organized the warning signs according to the easily remembered mnemonic, IS PATH WARM (Table 25.2). Warning signs that indicate acute risk for suicidality may be observed in individuals who are threatening to hurt or kill themselves, attempting to identify access to lethal weapons or other means that could result in death, or communicating about dying when these thoughts or actions are out of the ordinary for them.

Risk factors include previous suicide attempts, mental illness, substance abuse, and barriers to accessing mental health treatment. Protective factors may decrease the risk of suicide include appropriate mental healthcare, easy access to treatment, community support, and continuing support from medical and mental healthcare providers. Box 25.2 lists protective factors and risk factors that all community health nurses should recognize, and Box 25.3 provides warning signs of suicide.

Thus, it is important that all community health nurses become familiar with assessing for suicide warning signs and accessing appropriate resources. Nurses should refer the person exhibiting suicide warning signs to a mental health clinic or provider as soon as possible. This may involve taking emergency action by calling the local emergency services number in the community and staying with the person until help arrives. Table 25.3 provides a list of suicide information resources.

TABLE 25.2 Suicide Warning Signs: "Is Path Warm"

Ideation	Does the person state that he or she is having thoughts of suicide?
Substance abuse	Is the person demonstrating increased use of alcohol or drugs?
Purposelessness	Does the person state that he or she feels as if there is no purpose in his or her life?
Anxiety	Is the person demonstrating anxiety-related behaviors such as: talking about being overly worried about things, ruminating, difficulty concentrating, or exhibiting increased psychomotor agitation?
Trapped	Does the person state that he or she feels trapped, that there is no way out of the current situation except to die?
Hopelessness	Does the person state that he or she feels hopeless? Is the person able to describe something to look forward to?
Withdrawal	Is the person withdrawing from others such as family and friends? Is the person isolating?
Anger	Is the person demonstrating uncontrolled anger? Is the person acting with rage or seeking revenge?
Recklessness	Is the person engaged in risk-taking behaviors? Is the person acting as if he or she "doesn't care" or isn't thinking about the consequences of the risk-taking behavior?
Mood changes	Is the person experiencing dramatic mood changes?

From American Association of Suicidology: *Know the warning signs of suicide*, 2017. Available from: http://www.suicidology.org/resources/warning-signs. Contact information: American Association of Suicidology 5221 Wisconsin Ave. NW Second Floor Washington, DC 20015–2032 Phone (202) 237–2280, Fax (202) 237–2282. www.suicidology.org, info@suicidology.org.

BOX 25.2 Suicide: Protective Factors and Risk Factors

Protective Factors
- Effective clinical care for mental, physical, and substance abuse disorders
- Easy access to a variety of clinical interventions and support for help seeking
- Family and community support (connectedness)
- Support from ongoing medical and mental healthcare relationships
- Skills in problem solving, conflict resolution, and nonviolent ways of handling disputes
- Cultural and religious beliefs that discourage suicide and support instincts for selfpreservation

Risk Factors
- Family history of suicide
- Family history of child maltreatment
- Previous suicide attempt(s)
- History of mental disorders, particularly clinical depression
- History of alcohol and substance abuse
- Feelings of hopelessness
- Impulsive or aggressive tendencies
- Cultural and religious beliefs (e.g., belief that suicide is noble resolution of a personal dilemma)
- Local epidemics of suicide
- Isolation, a feeling of being cut off from other people
- Barriers to accessing mental health treatment
- Loss (relational, social, work, or financial)
- Physical illness
- Easy access to lethal methods
- Unwillingness to seek help because of the stigma attached to mental health and substance abuse disorders or to suicidal thoughts

Adapted from Substance Abuse and Mental Health Services Administration, National Suicide Prevention Lifeline: *Risk factors for suicide*, n.d. Available at: http://www.suicidepreventionlifeline.org/learn/riskfactors.aspx.

BOX 25.3 Warning Signs of Suicide

Seek help as soon as possible by contacting a mental health professional or by calling the National Suicide Prevention Lifeline at 1-800-273-TALK if you or someone you know exhibits any of the following signs:
- Threatening to hurt or kill oneself or talking about wanting to hurt or kill oneself
- Looking for ways to kill oneself by seeking access to firearms, available pills, or other means
- Talking or writing about death, dying, or suicide when these actions are out of the ordinary for the person
- Feeling hopeless
- Feeling rage or uncontrolled anger or seeking revenge
- Acting reckless or engaging in risky activities—seemingly without thinking
- Feeling trapped—like there's no way out
- Increasing alcohol or drug use
- Withdrawing from friends, family, and society
- Feeling anxious, agitated, or unable to sleep or sleeping all the time
- Experiencing dramatic mood changes
- Seeing no reason for living or having no sense of purpose in life

From Suicidepreventionlifeline.org: *Talk to someone now*. Available at: https://suicidepreventionlifeline.org/talk-to-someone-now/.

IDENTIFICATION AND MANAGEMENT OF MENTAL DISORDERS

Early identification, appropriate treatment, and rehabilitation can significantly reduce the duration and level of disability associated with mental disorders and decrease the possibility of relapse. Interventions to promote mental health and decrease mental disorders include focusing on decreasing stressors and/or increasing the capacity of the individual to cope with stress. Other interventions include the use of pharmacological agents and psychosocial interventions such as strengthening interpersonal, psychological, and physical resources through counseling, support groups, and psychoeducation.

The accessibility of mental health service is pivotal in promoting and maintaining the health. Decreased funding for services, managed care limitations on mental health coverage, and the inequality of coverage by the insurance industry has caused downsizing or forced closure in the traditional places of treatment, such as CMHC and community hospitals. Consequently, the accessibility to community mental health services has become an issue of significant concern. In addition, the

TABLE 25.3   Suicide Prevention and Referral Resources

National Suicide Prevention Lifeline	1-800-273-TALK (8255) www.suicidepreventionlifeline.org/
American Association of Suicidology	https://suicidology.org/
Suicide Prevention Resource Center	www.sprc.org/
Suicide Awareness Voices of Education	www.save.org/
Suicide Prevention: A Resource Manual for the Army	http://www.armyg1.army.mil/dcs/docs/Suicide%20Prevention%20Manual.pdf
Veterans Crisis Line	1-800- 273—8255 Text to 838255 www.veteranscrisisline.net/ChatTermsOfService.aspx?account=Veterans%20Chat
American Foundation for Suicide Prevention	www.afsp.org/
Local emergency resource	Dial 911

symptoms of mental illness often interfere with an individual's ability to access services. Alterations in thoughts and perceptions, anxiety, and decreased energy are common symptoms of mental illness, all of which interfere with negotiating the complex systems that currently surround the provision of mental health services. This section describes actions that may be taken by community health nurses to identify mental illness and outlines potential treatment options.

Identification of Mental Disorders

Whether the nurse is working in a physician's office, a community clinic, a school, or home health and hospice, occupational health, or other setting, recognition of signs and symptoms that might indicate a mental disorder is an important component of practice. More than ever, public health nurses work in collaboration with crisis housing agencies and school district managers for homeless families. In these situations, the nurse should continue to assess for other signs and symptoms that might indicate a mental disorder and should be prepared to intervene if they appear.

Often, the assessment process includes direct questioning or observation. At other times, a standardized assessment tool or questionnaire might be employed. Figs. 25.1 and 25.2 contain examples of instruments that are available to elicit information about symptoms of anxiety or depression. Whenever using these or other screening tools, the nurse should be prepared in advance to intervene on the basis of assessment data. Often, this intervention incorporates referral to other health professionals for further assessment, testing, counseling, treatment, and follow-up by all health professionals involved.

Evidence-Based Practice Management of Mental Disorders

The website of the Substance Abuse and Mental Health Services Agency's (SAMHSA) National Registry of Evidence-Based Programs and Practices lists EBP programs and interventions that demonstrate positive outcomes in community mental health. The goals of treatment for mental illness are to reduce symptoms, improve occupational and social functioning, develop and strengthen coping skills, and promote behaviors to improve the individual's life. Crisis housing programs, supportive employments programs, Assertive Community Treatment (ACT) team models, **Crisis Intervention Team** (CIT) models, psychotropic medication management programs, community **case management** programs, mobile crisis units, Cognitive Behavioral Intervention for Trauma in Schools programs, and many more are listed. Basic approaches to the treatment of mental disorders are detailed; see the website (https://www.samhsa.gov/nrepp).

Psychotropic or Psychotherapeutic Medications

Psychotropic/psychotherapeutic medications treat symptoms of mental illness. The appropriateness of psychopharmacological agents and their prescribed regimen depends on the diagnosis, side effects, and client response. Some of the psychotropic medications prescribed are classified as antipsychotics, antidepressants, mood stabilizers, anticonvulsants, antianxiety agents, and hypnotics. Information about medication profiles and treatment regimens often changes as new information becomes available, so nurses should be aware of up-to-date medication information from Internet resources such as www.nlm.nih.gov/medlineplus/druginformation.html or www.rxlist.com.

Psychotherapy

Psychotherapy, also referred to as talk therapy, is a way to help people with a broad variety of mental illnesses and emotional difficulties, by helping eliminate or control troubling symptoms so one can function better and can increase well-being and healing (American Psychiatric Association, 2019). In nursing, psychotherapy is an intervention used predominantly by psychiatric/mental health advanced practice nurses. Psychotherapy involves the use of a professional, therapeutic relationship and the application of psychotherapy theories and best practices to change a client's attitudes, feelings, beliefs, defenses, personality, and behaviors. Therapy approaches vary among schools of psychotherapy and with the nature of the client's problem. Psychotherapy is often used in conjunction with medication to treat many mental disorders. Various types of psychotherapy include the following (NIMH, 2016):

Individual therapy focuses on the client's current life and relationships within the family, social, and work environments.

Family therapy involves problem-solving sessions with members of a family.

Couple therapy is used to develop the relationship and minimize problems through understanding how individual conflicts are expressed in the couple's interactions.

Group therapy involves a small group of people with similar problems who, with the guidance of a therapist, discuss individual issues and help one another with problems.

During the Past Week	Rarely or None of the Time (Less Than 1 Day)	Some or a Little of the Time (1–2 Days)	Occasionally or a Moderate Amount of the Time (3–4 Days)	Most or All of the Time (5–7 Days)
1. I was bothered by things that don't usually bother me.	0	1	2	3
2. I did not feel like eating; my appetite was poor.	0	1	2	3
3. I felt that I could not shake off the blues even with the help of my family or friends.	0	1	2	3
4. I felt that I was just as good as other people.	3	2	1	0
5. I had trouble keeping my mind on what I was doing.	0	1	2	3
6. I felt depressed.	0	1	2	3
7. I felt everything I did was an effort.	0	1	2	3
8. I felt hopeful about the future.	3	2	1	0
9. I thought my life had been a failure.	0	1	2	3
10. I felt fearful.	0	1	2	3
11. My sleep was restless.	0	1	2	3
12. I was happy.	3	2	1	0
13. I talked less than usual.	0	1	2	3
14. I felt lonely.	0	1	2	3
15. People were unfriendly.	0	1	2	3
16. I enjoyed life.	3	2	1	0
17. I had crying spells.	0	1	2	3
18. I felt sad.	0	1	2	3
19. I felt that people disliked me.	0	1	2	3
20. I could not get "going."	0	1	2	3

Fig. 25.1 Center for Epidemiologic Studies depression scale. Interpretation: A total score of 22 or higher is indicative of depression when the scale is used in primary care. (From Radloff LS: The CES-D scale: a self-report depression scale for research in the general population, *Appl Psychol Meas* 1:385–401, 1977. Copyright 1977, West Publishing Company/Applied Psychological Measurement, Inc.)

Play therapy is a technique used for establishing communication and resolving problems with young children.

Cognitive-behavioral therapy may be used in individual, family, couples, or group therapy. The goal is to identify and change thinking and behavior patterns that are harmful or ineffective, replacing them with more accurate thoughts and functional behaviors (American Psychiatric Association, 2019).

Behavioral therapy uses learning principles to change thought patterns and behaviors systematically; it is used to encourage the individual to learn specific skills to obtain rewards and satisfaction.

Psychotherapy may be short term or long term, depending on the nature of the problem and the availability of resources.

Rank	Life Event	Mean Value	Rank	Life Event	Mean Value
1	Death of spouse	100	23	Son or daughter leaving home	29
2	Divorce	73	24	Trouble with in-laws	29
3	Marital separation	65	25	Outstanding personal achievement	28
4	Jail term	63			
5	Death of close family member	63	26	Wife begins or stops work	26
6	Personal injury or illness	53	27	Begin or end school	26
7	Marriage	50	28	Change in living conditions	25
8	Fired at work	47	29	Change in personal habits	24
9	Marital reconciliation	45	30	Trouble with boss	23
10	Retirement	45	31	Change in work hours or conditions	20
11	Change in health of family member	44			
12	Pregnancy	40	32	Change in residence	20
13	Sex difficulties	39	33	Change in schools	20
14	Gain of new family member	39	34	Change in recreation	19
15	Business readjustment	39	35	Change in church activities	19
16	Change in financial state	38	36	Change in social activities	18
17	Death of close friend	37	37	Mortgage or loan less than $10,000	17
18	Change to different line of work	36			
19	Change in number of arguments with spouse	35	38	Change in sleeping habits	16
			39	Change in number of family get-togethers	15
20	Mortgage over $10,000	31			
21	Foreclosure on mortgage or loan	30	40	Change in eating habits	15
22	Change in responsibilities at work	29	41	Vacation	13
			42	Christmas	12
			43	Minor violations of the law	11

Life Crisis Categories and LCU Scores*

No life crisis	0–149
Mild life crisis	150–199
Moderate life crisis	200–299
Major life crisis	300 or more

*The LCU score includes those life event items experienced during a 1-year period.

Fig. 25.2 Social readjustment rating scale. *LCU*, Life change unit(s). (From Holmes TH, Rahe RH: The social readjustment rating scale, *J Psychosom Res* 11:213–217, 1967, Elsevier Science Inc.)

COMMUNITY-BASED MENTAL HEALTHCARE

Over the past several decades, there have been a number of initiatives directed toward improving and promoting community-based care of those with mental illness. One of those initiatives is the ACA. The ACA, one of the largest expansions of mental health and substance use disorder coverage in a generation, requires that most individual and small employer health insurance plans, cover mental health and substance use disorder services (MentalHealth.gov, 2017). Mental and behavioral health services are recognized as essential health benefits. Consequently, the ACA stipulated that all plans must cover: behavioral health treatment, such as psychotherapy and counseling; mental and behavioral health inpatient services; and substance abuse treatment (HealthCare.gov, 2021). Similarly, preexisting mental and behavioral health conditions are covered, and spending limits aren't allowed. And, Marketplace plans can't deny one coverage or charge more on the basis of any preexisting condition, including mental health and substance use disorder conditions. Parity protections now exist for mental health services.

Marketplace plans must provide certain "parity" protections between mental health and substance abuse benefits on the one hand, and medical and surgical benefits on the other. As a rule, this means limits applied to mental health and substance abuse services can't be more restrictive than limits applied to medical and surgical services. The ACA has been a tremendous step forward for mental healthcare in the U.S.

The Center for Mental Health Services (CMHS) was formed in the early 1990s to improve prevention and mental health treatment services for all Americans. The CMHS helps states improve and increase the quality and range of treatment, rehabilitation, and support services for people with mental health problems, their families, and their communities. Objectives of the CMHS are to strengthen the nation's mental health system by helping states improve and increase the quality and range of their treatment, rehabilitation, and support; to make it easier for people to access mental health programs; to encourage a range of programs such as systems of care to respond to the increasing number of mental, emotional, and behavioral problems among America's children; to support outreach and case management programs for Americans who are homeless and the improvement of these services; and to ensure that scientifically-established findings and practice-based knowledge are applied in preventing and treating mental disorders (SAMHSA, 2020a,b,c).

One of the programs promoted by the CMHS is the Community Support System. The Community Support System uses case management strategies to comprehensively provide care for those with serious mental illness. Components of the Community Support System include client identification and outreach, mental health treatment, crisis response service, health and dental care, housing, income support and entitlement, peer support, family and community support, rehabilitation services, and protection and advocacy. The case management approach serves to link the service system to the client and to coordinate their service received (NCBI, 2017).

The **ACT** model is another example of a community-based initiative to help meet the needs of those with mental illness. ACT, which has been in existence since the late 1960s, has become the exemplar of community mental health treatment models. The ACT program moves the traditional 24-hour treatment model of acute care settings into the community and serves people with mental illness in a highly individualized fashion (National Alliance on Mental Illness [NAMI], 2021a,b,c,d). The ACT model is based around the idea that people receive better care when their mental healthcare providers work together. ACT team members help the individual address every aspect of their life, whether it be medication, therapy, social support, employment, or housing. ACT is primarily used for people who have transferred out of an inpatient setting but would benefit from a similar level of care and having the comfort of living a more independent life than would be possible with inpatient care (NAMI, 2021). The ACT model provides supportive therapy, mobile crisis intervention, psychiatric medications, hospitalization, education, and skill teaching for consumers and their families. ACT programs have been implemented in countries such as the United States, Canada, Australia, and the United Kingdom. Specifically, in the United States, ACT was implemented across the country by the Department of Veterans Affairs (Cuncic, 2020). Box 25.4 gives additional details about ACT programs.

The CIT program originates from the Memphis Model, an educational and advocacy training program (International Crisis Intervention Team, 2021). The Memphis Police Department joined with the Memphis Chapter of the NAMI, mental health providers, the University of Memphis, and the University of Tennessee in organizing, training, and implementing a specialized unit. CIT programs partner with **mental health consumers** and family members, mental health professionals, and advocacy organizations. Law enforcement personnel are trained in developing a more intelligent, understandable, and safe approach to mental crisis events (See Box 25.5 for the core elements of the CIT).

Specialty courts—also called treatment courts, accountability courts, and problem-solving courts—deal with a number of problem areas within the criminal justice system. These specialty courts can deal with adult, juvenile, users, and family drug problems, mental health disorders, military veterans, and

---

BOX 25.4 Key Features of the Assertive Community Treatment (ACT) Program

- Psychopharmacological treatment
- Individual supportive therapy
- Mobile crisis intervention
- Hospitalization
- Substance abuse treatment
- Behaviorally oriented skill teaching
- Supported employment
- Support for resuming education
- Collaboration with families and assistance to clients with children
- Direct support to help clients obtain legal and advocacy services

---

people found to be driving under the influence of alcohol or drugs. These programs incorporate assessment and screening to examine problematic behavior due to mental health problems and substance abuse. Specialty courts provide education regarding mental and substance use disorders and medication monitoring and drug testing.

ROLE OF THE COMMUNITY MENTAL HEALTH NURSE

More than ever, there are opportunities for the community mental health nurse to make a difference. For the psychiatric–mental health nurse there are EBP models of care providing promising outcome in communities. Applications of the nursing process are and always can be facilitated to help special populations affected by mental illness in the community. There certainly are challenges to the effective provision of mental health services in the community, such as accessibility, disparity, and cost. Community health nursing is challenging and filled with professional and personal satisfaction (Gerber, 2017). When nurses are providing care to individuals, families, groups, and communities, there is a hope for change, progress, and improved health promotion for everyone. In spite of multiple challenges, the role of a community mental health nurse can be extremely rewarding (ExploreHealthCareers.org, 2017).

Community mental health nursing roles are multidimensional (e.g., participant in mental health courts, veterans' courts, other specialty or problem-solving courts; educator, researcher, collaborator, consultant, case managers, content expert, administrator, activist, politician, advocate, initiator, evaluator, grant writer, practitioner, and coordinator). Mental health nurses serve on ACT, Crisis Intervention, community case management, mobile crisis, and crisis housing coordination teams. Community mental health nurses as educators and activists dispel myths, provide accurate information about mental illness, and influence policy and legislation advocating for those with mental illness.

As practitioner and coordinator, the nurse works directly with individuals, groups, and families. Besides intervening to assist consumers in controlling or alleviating the symptoms of mental

BOX 25.5 Core Elements of Crisis Intervention Teams (CITs)

Ongoing Elements
1. Partnerships: law enforcement, advocacy, mental health
2. Community ownership: planning, implementation, and networking
3. Policies and procedures

Operational Elements
1. CIT: officer, dispatcher, coordinator
2. Curriculum: CIT training
3. Mental health receiving facility: emergency services

Sustaining Elements
1. Evaluation and research
2. In-service training
3. Recognition and honors
4. Outreach: developing CIT in other communities

From the University of Memphis, School of Urban Affairs and Public Policy, Department of Criminology and Criminal Justice, CIT Center CIT International, Randolph Dupont, PhD, Major Sam Cochran MS, and Sarah Pillsbury, MA: Crisis intervention team core elements, 2007. Available from: http://www.citinternational.org/resources/Documents/CoreElements.pdf. Accessed February 12, 2021.

illness, the practitioner and coordinator also helps the consumer "navigate" the segmented web of agencies and other service providers. A list of organizations that advocate for mental health is shown in Table 25.4. Community mental health nurses not only act to solve an immediate problem, but also plan and intervene to ensure safety, continuity, and quality of care for consumers. Therefore, the practitioner and coordinator roles require skills in anticipating and evaluating the actions of other providers and communicating with consumers, families, rehabilitation services, and government or social agencies.

Within this aspect of community mental health nursing, individual-, family-, and community-level crises are anticipated and prevented or, failing these, contained. For example, as practitioners and coordinators, nurses might organize people taking psychotropic medications to share experiences about interacting with a psychiatrist, managing side effects of medications, and enhancing their coping strategies. Such a proactive stance may help prevent problems that lead clients to discontinue medications and the consequences of such actions. In the practitioner and coordinator roles, community mental health nurses work toward matching consumers and families with culturally appropriate and sensitive providers to achieve the "best fit."

TABLE 25.4 Organizations That Promote Education and Advocate for Mental Health

Resource	Services	Contact Information
Substance Abuse and Mental Health Services Administration (SAMHSA)	Programs, policies, information and data, contracts, and grants Vision: Behavioral health is essential for health, prevention works, treatment is effective, people can recover from mental illness diagnosis and substance abuse	http://www.samhsa.gov/
National Alliance on Mental Illness (NAMI)	Consumer education regarding various mental health disorders, medication and treatment, research, public policy issues; links to find support at state and local level including support groups and online discussion groups; tips for becoming politically involved in mental health public policy issues	http://www.nami.org/
Mental Health America (MHA)	Inform, advocate, and enable access to quality behavioral health services for all Americans	http://www.mentalhealthamerica.net/
National Institute of Mental Health (NIMH)	Education on mental health topics and research Vision: Understanding and treatment of mental illnesses through basic and clinical research, paving the way for prevention, recovery, and cure	http://www.nimh.nih.gov/index.shtml
Depression and Bipolar Support Alliance	Education on depression and bipolar disorder; online discussion and support groups; assistance in finding treatment resources	http://www.dbsalliance.org
National Education Alliance for Borderline Personality Disorder	Education about borderline personality disorder and treatment	www.borderlinepersonalitydisorder.com/
Obsessive-Compulsive Foundation	Education about obsessive compulsive and anxiety disorders and treatment	www.ocfoundation.org/
Postpartum Support International	Education and resource information for individuals experiencing symptoms of prenatal or postpartum mood or anxiety disorders	http://postpartum.net/
U.S. Department of Veteran Affairs National Center for PTSD	Public and professional sections for education, training materials as well as information and tools to help you with assessment and treatment	http://www.ptsd.va.gov/
Brain and Behavior Research Foundation, formerly called National Association for Research on Schizophrenia And Depression (NARSAD)	Alleviating the suffering caused by mental illness by awarding grants that will lead to advances and breakthroughs in scientific research	http://bbrfoundation.org/
National Council for Community Behavioral Healthcare	Behavioral healthcare, holistic approach to meet needs of the individuals and families	www.thenationalcouncil.org/cs/home

CASE STUDY Application of the Nursing Process

Joseph Green, a divorced 52-year-old veteran of Operation Iraqi Freedom, was discharged from the hospital with a referral to cardiac rehabilitation. Joseph has a ventricular pacemaker that was inserted 2 years ago. Last week he was brought into the emergency department for failure of the pacemaker. He was experiencing syncope and hypotension. His pacemaker was corrected and he was discharged back into the community, where he is currently living at a men's shelter.

Joseph has a history of a congestive heart failure, depression, alcoholism, chronic obstructive pulmonary disease, traumatic brain injury, and PTSD. He has prescriptions for citalopram, carvedilol, and an Advair inhaler. He admits to being noncompliant at times with taking his prescriptions. He has access to healthcare services from the nearest VA medical center, which is 350 miles away. He takes a Disabled American Veterans (DAV) van to the medical center once or twice a month where he fills his prescriptions and sees mental health counselors. There is cardiac rehabilitation at the center, but Joseph does not want to go as often as the VA doctors have recommended. Joseph has no income and cooks meals at the men's shelter for his room and board. Because he cannot drink alcohol at the shelter, he has been abstinent for 9 months. He smokes a pack of cigarettes daily when he has cigarettes.

Joseph has difficulty sleeping most nights and awakens from nightmares. He was diagnosed with major depression and PTSD 5 years ago and reports having suicidal thoughts occasionally. He has been estranged from his grown children for several years. He has a sister living in the same city and his relationship with her strained. The ACT team makes visits to the shelter to assist other men, and Joseph has inquired how to become a consumer of ACT services. There is a local veterans' support group at the Veterans of Foreign Wars (VFW) building that Joseph and others from the shelter go to several nights a week.

Assessment
On his first trip to the VA medical center after his recent discharge, the outpatient clinic nurse notes that Joseph was noncompliant with his medications only 2 days the previous week. He reports that he is not depressed, and he denies having suicidal thoughts. He has had no syncope or chest palpations.

Diagnosis
Individual
- History of mental illness (depression, PTSD, and alcoholism)
- Difficulty following treatment regimen
- Less than adequate social skills
- Poor selfworth
- History of suicidal ideation

Family and Social Relationships
- Inability to communicate with family members effectively
- Jeopardy of reoccurring homelessness

Planning
Planning for Joseph is primarily through collaboration in the community where he resides at the men's shelter. His relationships with others at the shelter and the VFW are important. The staff at the men's shelter are familiar with the VA's homeless program information: 1-877-4AID-VET (1-877-425-3838) and http://www.va.gov/HOMELESS/for_homeless_veterans.asp.

The men's shelter also supports Joseph by helping him get to the DAV van when he has appointment at the VA medical center. The shelter offers chaplain services and also utilizes the community CIT law enforcement officers at times to help talk with residents when they are experiencing stress or need deescalation of their behavior. A CIT officer who is a veteran stops in once in a while to see the men as a proactive visit.

Individual
Long-Term Goal
- Joseph will progress with community supportive services and relationships with people

Short-Term Goals
- Joseph will remain medication compliant
- Joseph will remain abstinent from alcohol

Family and Social Relationships
Long-Term Goals
- Safe housing
- Compliance with medications
- Sobriety
- Case management with ACT Team and VA

Short-Term Goals
- Working with shelter staff and ACT Team
- Sobriety
- Compliance with medications

Intervention
The staff at the men's shelter meet with Joseph regularly to evaluate compliance with medications. The staff also will know when his appointments are at the VA in order to plan transportation on the DAV van. The relationships that Joseph has with other veterans are helpful in a support milieu.

Individual
- Joseph has agreed to work with the staff at the shelter in a team effort to keep him in safe housing. He has agreed to work with the ACT Team, VA case management, and his Alcoholics Anonymous (AA) community.

Family and Social Relationships
- Joseph will continue to work with VA case management, the ACT Team, and the staff at the shelter.
- He will call his sister weekly.

Evaluation
Joseph verbalized understanding of the importance of safe housing, the ACT Team intervention, and social relationships with VA peers and AA peers. He also agreed to call his AA or VA contact when needed if he is beginning to feel agitated or wanting to isolate himself. The ACT Team will consistently contact Joseph and be available on weekends. Joseph has agreed to give permission for the ACT Team to report his status to the VA case managers.

Levels of Prevention
Primary
- Maintaining housing at shelter
- Assisting Joseph with compliance with medications

Secondary
- Encouraging maintenance of social relationships (shelter staff, other veterans, AA peers) and relationship with sister

Tertiary
- Monitoring of medical health status and psychological health status
- Group therapy at AA meetings and the VA medical center

▮ SUMMARY

Like all other aspects of nursing, community mental health nursing is developing, applying, and utilizing EBP models of community treatment, such as ACT, community case management, or CITs. The 21st century community mental health multidisciplinary team approaches can promote improvement in the identification of and care for those with mental illness. Improved information and EBP may result in greater understanding of the factors that contribute to mental disorders and lead to more effective treatment.

As discussed in this chapter, the vast majority of individuals with diagnosable mental disorders are found in the community, and many, if not most, never seek professional help. The framework for community mental health nursing presented in this chapter should prove useful in improving the lives of individuals, families, and groups of people with mental illness. Further, it is hoped that all nurses will become advocates for the mentally ill and will support social and political change to improve the mental health of all.

EVOLVE WEBSITE

http://evolve.elsevier.com/Nies
- NCLEX Review Questions
- Case Studies

BIBLIOGRAPHY

Advocacy Treatment Center: *Consequences of non–treatment*, 2018. Available from: https://www.treatmentadvocacycenter.org/key-issues/consequences-of-non-treatment. Accessed February 3, 2021.

Amadeo K: *Deinstitutionalization, its causes, effects, pros and cons*, 2020. Available from: https://www.thebalance.com/deinstitutionalization-3306067#citation-18. Accessed February 4, 2021.

American Association of Suicidology: *Know the warning signs of suicide*, 2020. Available from: http://www.suicidology.org/resources/warning-signs. Accessed February 9, 2021.

American Foundation for Suicide Prevention: *Suicide statistics*, 2021. Retrieved February 9, 2021 from: https://afsp.org/about-suicide/suicide-statistics/.

American Psychiatric Association: *Diagnostic and statistical manual of mental disorders*, ed 3, Arlington, VA, 2017, American Psychiatric Publishing.

American Psychiatric Association: *What is psychotherapy?*, 2019. Retrieved February 9, 2021 from: https://www.psychiatry.org/patients-families/psychotherapy.

American Psychiatric Association: *Understanding mental disorders: your guide to DSM-5*, 2020. Retrieved February 1, 2021 from: https://www.psychiatry.org/patients-families/understanding-mental-disorders.

Anxiety and Depression Association of America: *Facts and statistics*, 2020. Retrieved February 8, 2021 from: https://adaa.org/about-adaa/press-room/facts-statistics.

Ballard Spahr, LLC: *New stimulus law seeks to strengthen mental health parity compliance*, 2021. Retrieved February 2, 2021 from: https://www.jdsupra.com/legalnews/new-stimulus-law-seeks-to-strengthen-5190964/.

Baumgartner J, Aboulafia G, McIntosh A: *The ACA at 10: how has it impacted mental healthcare?*, 2020. Retrieved February 2, 2021 from: https://www.commonwealthfund.org/blog/2020/aca-10-how-has-it-impacted-mental-health-care.

Bonfine N, Wilson A, Munetz M: Meeting the needs of justice-involved people with serious mental illness within Community Behavioral Health Systems, *Psychiatr Serv* 71(4):355–363, 2019.

Centers for Disease Control and Prevention (CDC): *Attention deficit hyperactivity disorder (ADHD)*, 2018. Retrieved February 9, 2021 from: https://www.cdc.gov/nchs/fastats/adhd.htm.

Centers for Disease Control and Prevention: *National center for injury prevention and control. Web-based Injury Statistics Query and Reporting System (WISQARS)*, 2019. Retrieved February 5, 2021 from: http://www.cdc.gov/injury/wisqars/index.html.

Centers for Disease Control and Prevention: *Attention-deficit hyperactivity disorder*, 2020. Retrieved February 2021 from: https://www.cdc.gov/nchs/fastats/adhd.htm.

Cleveland Clinic: *Depression in children*, 2021. Retrieved February 8, 2021 from: https://my.clevelandclinic.org/health/diseases/14938-depression-in-children.

Congress.gov: *H.R.1109—mental health services for students act of 2020*, 2021a. Retrieved February 4, 2021 from: https://www.congress.gov/bill/116th-congress/house-bill/1109/text.

Congress.gov: *H.R.3180—rise from trauma act*, 2021b. Retrieved February 4, 2021 from: https://www.congress.gov/bill/116th-congress/house-bill/3180/text.

Cuncic A: *The basics of assertive community treatment*, 2020. Retrieved February 10, 2021 from: https://www.verywellmind.com/assertive-community-treatment-4587610.

Dahukey A, Yood K, Cohen S: *Venture capital and private equity investors take note: primary care may be the next behavioral health*, 2020. Retrieved February 2, 2021 from: https://www.natlawreview.com/article/venture-capital-and-private-equity-investors-take-note-primary-care-may-be-next.

ExploreHealthCareers.org: *Public health nurse*, 2017. Available at: https://explorehealthcareers.org/career/nursing/public-health-nurse/.

Fawcett E, Power H, Fawcett J: Women are at greater risk of OCD than men: a meta-analytic review of OCD prevalence worldwide, *J Clin Psychiatr* 81(4), 2020. Epub 2020 Jun 23.

Fisher B, Buchanan R: *Schizophrenia in adults: epidemiology and pathogenesis*, 2021. Retrieved February 6, 2021 from: https://www.

uptodate.com/contents/schizophrenia-in-adults-epidemiology-and-pathogenesis.

Gallagher M, Zvolensky M, Long L, Rogers L, Garey L: The impact of Covid-19 experiences and associated stress on anxiety, depression, and functional impairment in American Adults, *Cognit Ther Res* 44:1043–1051, 2020. https://doi.org/10.1007/s10608-020-10143-y.

Gara M, Minsky S, Silverstein S, Miskimen T, Strakowski S: A naturalistic study of racial disparities in diagnoses at an outpatient behavioral health clinic, *Psychiatr Serv* 70(2):130–134, 2019.

Gerber L: Community health nursing: a partnership of care, *Nursing* 42(1), 2017. Available at: http://www.nursingcenter.com/journal article?Article_ID=1287272.

Han B, Oliffe J: Photovoice in mental illness research: a review and recommendations, *Health Interdisc J Soc Study Health Illness & Med* 20(2):110–126, 2016.

Healthcare.gov: *Read the Affordable Care Act*, 2021. Retrieved February 10, 2021 from: https://www.healthcare.gov/where-can-i-read-the-affordable-care-act/.

Healthline.com: *Phobias*, 2021. Retrieved February 9, 2021 from: https://www.healthline.com/health/phobia-simple-specific.

HealthyPeople.gov: *Healthy people 2030*, 2021a. Retrieved February 4, 2021 from: https://health.gov/healthypeople.

HealthyPeople.gov: *Lesbian, gay, bisexual, and transgender health*, 2021b. Retrieved February 5, 2021 from: https://www.healthy people.gov/2020/topics-objectives/topic/lesbian-gay-bisexual-and-transgender-health.

Hoehe M, Morris-Rosendahl D: The role of genetics and genomics in clinical psychiatry, *Dialogues Clin Neurosci* 20(3):169–177, 2018. https://doi.org/10.31887/DCNS.2018.20.3/mhoehe.

Hunt G, Siegfried N, Morley K, Sitharthan T, Cleary M: Psychosocial interventions for people with both severe mental illness and substance misuse, *Cochrane Syst Rev*, 2019. Retrieved February 3, 2021 from: https://www.cochranelibrary.com/cdsr/doi/10.1002/14651858.CD001088.pub4/abstract.

International Crisis Intervention Team: *Welcome to CIT international*, 2021. Retrieved February 10, 2021 from: https://www.citinter national.org/Learn-About-CIT.

Kassam A, Papish A, Modgill G, et al.: The development and psychometric properties of a new scale to measure mental illness related stigma by health care providers: the opening minds scale for health care providers (OMS-HC), *BMC Psychiatr* 12(62):3–12, 2012.

Maine Center for Disease Control and Prevention: *Intentional injury*, 2021. Retrieved February 2, 2021 from: https://www.maine.gov/dhhs/mecdc/population-health/inj/intentional.html.

Mayo Clinic: *Depression: risk factors*, 2017. Retrieved February 12, 2021 from: http://www.mayoclinic.org/diseases-conditions/depression/basics/risk-factors/con-20032977.

Medline Plus: *Panic disorder*, 2021. Retrieved February 8, 2021 from: https://medlineplus.gov/ency/article/000924.htm#:~:text=But%20panic%20disorder%20often%20occurs,diagnosed%20until%20they%20are%20older.

Mental Health America: *How race matters: what we can learn from Mental Health America's Screening in 2020*, 2021a. Retrieved February 5, 2021 from: https://www.mhanational.org/mental-health-data-2020.

Mental Health America: *Latinx/hispanic communities and mental health*, 2021b. Retrieved February 5, 2021 from: https://www.mhanational.org/issues/latinxhispanic-communities-and-mental-health.

Mental Health America: *Position statement 53: mental health courts*, 2017. Available at: http://www.mentalhealthamerica.net/positions/mental-health-courts.

MentalHealth.gov: *Health insurance and mental health services*, 2017. Available at: https://www.mentalhealth.gov/get-help/health-insurance/.

Mustelin L, Silén Y, Raevuori A, Hoek H, Kaprio J, Keski-Rahkonen A: The DSM-5 diagnostic criteria for anorexia nervosa may change its population prevalence and prognostic value, *J Psychiatr Res* 77:85–91, 2016.

National Alliance on Mental Illness: *Anosignosia*, 2021a. Retrieved February 6, 2021 from: https://www.nami.org/About-Mental-Illness/Common-with-Mental-Illness/Anosognosia.

National Alliance on Mental Illness: *Hispanic/latinx*, 2021b. Retrieved February 5, 2021 from: https://www.nami.org/Your-Journey/Identity-and-Cultural-Dimensions/Hispanic-Latinx.

National Alliance on Mental Illness: *Mental health screening*, 2021c. Retrieved February 6, 2021 from: https://www.nami.org/Advocacy/Policy-Priorities/Intervene-Early/Mental-health-screening#:~:text=Mental%20health%20screenings%20allow%20for,and%20prevent%20years%20of%20suffering.

National Alliance on Mental Illness: *Psychosocial treatments*, 2021d. Retrieved February 10, 2021 from: https://nami.org/About-Mental-Illness/Treatments/Psychosocial-Treatments.

National Council for Behavioral Health: *Mass violence in America*, 2019. Retrieved February 4, 2021 from: https://www.thenational council.org/wp-content/uploads/2019/08/Mass-Violence-in-America_8-6-19.pdf?daf=375ateTbd56.

National Council for Behavioral Health: *Community mental health act*, 2021. Retrieved February 4, 2021 from: https://www.thenationalcouncil.org/about/national-mental-health-association/overview/community-mental-health-act/.

National Eating Disorders Association: *What are eating disorders?*, 2018. Retrieved February 9, 2021 from: https://www.national eatingdisorders.org/what-are-eating-disorders.

National Institute of Mental Health: *Eating disorders among adults—bulimia nervosa*, 2017. Retrieved February 11, 2021 from: https://www.nimh.nih.gov/health/statistics/prevalence/eating-disorders-among-adults-bulimia-nervosa.shtml.

National Institute of Mental Health: *Anxiety disorders*, 2018. Retrieved February 8, 2021 from: https://www.nimh.nih.gov/health/topics/anxiety-disorders/index.shtml.

National Institute of Mental Health: *Obsessive-compulsive disorder*, 2019a. Retrieved February 9, 2021 from: https://www.nimh.nih.gov/health/topics/obsessive-compulsive-disorder-ocd/index.shtml.

National Institute of Mental Health: *Attention-deficit/hyperactivity disorder*, 2019b. Retrieved February 9, 2021 from: https://www.nimh.nih.gov/health/topics/attention-deficit-hyperactivity-disorder-adhd/index.shtml.

National Institute of Mental Health: *Major depression*, 2019c. Retrieved February 8, 2021 from: https://www.nimh.nih.gov/health/statistics/prevalence/major-depression-among-adults.shtml.

National Institution of Mental Health: *Bipolar disorder*, 2020a. Retrieved February 8, 2021 from: https://www.nimh.nih.gov/health/topics/bipolar-disorder/index.shtml#part_145404.

National Institute of Mental Health: *Mental illness*, 2020b. Retrieved February 6, 2021 from: https://www.nimh.nih.gov/health/statistics/mental-illness.shtml.

National Institute of Mental Health: *Neuroimaging and mental illness: a window into the brain NIH publication No. 09-7460*, 2021a. Retrieved February 4, 2021 from: https://www.naminys.org/images/uploads/pdfs/Neuroimaging%20(FAQ).pdf.

National Institute of Mental Health: *Neuroimaging and mental illness: a window into the brain: frequently asked questions about brain scans*, 2021b. Retrieved February 11, 2021 from: https://www.naminys.org/images/uploads/pdfs/Neuroimaging%20(FAQ).pdf.

National Institute of Mental Health: *Office for research on disparities and global mental health (ORDGMH)*, 2021c. Retrieved February

5, 2021 from: https://www.nimh.nih.gov/about/organization/gmh/index.shtml.

National Institute of Mental Health: *Suicide in America: frequently asked questions*, 2021d. Retrieved February 9, 2021 from: https://www.nimh.nih.gov/health/publications/suicide-faq/index.shtml.

National Institutes of Health: *Brain basics: understanding sleep*, 2019. Retrieved February 4, 2021 from: https://www.ninds.nih.gov/Disorders/Patient-Caregiver-Education/Understanding-sleep#:~:text=Sleep%20is%20important%20to%20a,up%20while%20you%20are%20awake.

NYU Grossman School of Medicine: *Medicalization: scientific progress or disease mongering?*, 2020. Retrieved February 4, 2021 from: https://med.nyu.edu/departments-institutes/population-health/divisions-sections-centers/medical-ethics/education/high-school-bioethics-project/learning-scenarios/medicalization-ethics.

Open Minds: *The U.S. mental health market: $225.1 billion in spending in 2019: an open minds market intelligence report*, 2020. Retrieved February 6, 2021 from: https://openminds.com/intelligence-report/the-u-s-mental-health-market-225-1-billion-in-spending-in-2019-an-open-minds-market-intelligence-report/.

Pfefferbaum B, North C: Mental health and the Covid-19 pandemic, *N Engl J Med* 383(6):510–512, 2020.

Prison Policy Initiative: *Mental health: policies and practices surrounding mental health*, 2020. Retrieved February 4, 2021 from: https://www.prisonpolicy.org/research/mental_health/.

Rehm J, Shield K: *Global burden of disease and the impact of mental and addictive disorders*, 2019. Retrieved February 6, 2021 from: https://pubmed.ncbi.nlm.nih.gov/30729322/.

Shadloo B, Motevalian A, Rahimi-Movaghar V, et al.: Psychiatric disorders are associated with an increased risk of injuries: data from the Iranian Mental Health Survey (IranMHS), *Iran J Public Health* 45(5):623–635, 2016.

Shen G, Snowden L: Institutionalization of deinstitutionalization: a cross-national analysis of mental health system reform, *Int J Ment Health Syst* 8(47), 2014. https://doi.org/10.1186/1752-4458-8-47.

Sher L, Kahn R: Suicide in schizophrenia: an educational overview, *Medicina* 55(7):361, 2019. https://doi.org/10.3390/medicina55070361.

Substance Abuse and Mental Health Services Administration (SAMHSA): *Key substance use and mental health indicators in the United States: results from the 2019 National Survey on Drug Use and Health*, 2019. Retrieved February 1, 2021 from: https://www.samhsa.gov/data/sites/default/files/reports/rpt29393/2019NSDUHFFRPDFWHTML/2019NSDUHFFR1PDFW090120.pdf.

Substance Abuse and Mental Health Services Administration (SAMHSA): *Center for mental health services*, 2020a. Retrieved February 10, 2021 from: https://www.samhsa.gov/about-us/who-we-are/offices-centers/cmhs.

Substance Abuse and Mental Health Services Administration (SAMHSA): *Mental and substance use disorders*, 2020b. Retrieved February 1, 2021 from: https://www.samhsa.gov/disorders.

Substance Abuse and Mental Health Services Administration (SAMHSA): *Table of contents for the 2019 NSDUH detailed tables*, 2020c. Retrieved February 6, 2021 from: https://www.samhsa.gov/data/report/2019-nsduh-detailed-tables.

Tafet G, Nemeroff C: Pharmacological treatment of anxiety disorders: the role of the HPA axis, *Front Psychiatr*, 2020, https://doi.org/10.3389/fpsyt.2020.00443.

Treatment Advocacy Center: *Going, going, gone; trends and consequences of eliminating state psychiatric beds, 2016*, 2018. Retrieved February 11, 2021 from: http://www.treatmentadvocacycenter.org/evidence-and-research/studies.

USC Department of Nursing: *Understanding barriers to minority mental health care*, 2021. Retrieved February 6, 2021 from: https://nursing.usc.edu/blog/discrimination-bad-health-minority-mental-healthcare/.

U.S. Department of Defense: *Defense suicide prevention office*, 2021. Retrieved February 11, 2021 from: https://www.dspo.mil/.

United States Department of Health and Human Services: *What is mental health?*, 2020. Retrieved February 1, 2021 from: https://www.mentalhealth.gov/basics/what-is-mental-health/.

United States Department of Health and Human Services Office of Minority Health: *Mental and behavioral health—African Americans*, 2019. Retrieved February 5, 2021 from: https://www.minorityhealth.hhs.gov/omh/browse.aspx?lvl=4&lvlid=24/.

U.S. Department of Veteran Affairs: *Veteran suicide data and reporting*, 2018. Retrieved February 5, 2021 from: https://www.mentalhealth.va.gov/mentalhealth/suicide_prevention/data.asp.

U.S. Department of Veterans Affairs: *How common is PTSD in adults?*, 2019. Retrieved February 9, 2021 from: https://www.ptsd.va.gov/understand/common/common_adults.asp.

Wagner P, Bertram W: "What percent of the U.S. is incarcerated?" (And other ways to measure mass incarceration). *Prison Policy Initiative*, 2020. Retrieved February 4, 2021 from: https://www.prisonpolicy.org/blog/2020/01/16/percent-incarcerated/

World Health Organization: *WHO guidelines: management of physical health conditions in adults with severe mental disorders*, 2018. Retrieved February 4, 2021 from: https://www.who.int/mental_health/evidence/guidelines_severe_mental_disorders_web_note_2018/en/.

Zeller S: The promise and potential of emergency psychiatry, *Psychiatr Times* 38(1), 2021. Retrieved February 3, 2021 from: https://www.psychiatrictimes.com/view/promise-potential-emergency-psychiatry.

26

Communicable Disease

Deanna E. Grimes and Barbara E. Hekel

OBJECTIVES

Upon completion of this chapter, the reader will be able to do the following:

1. Review principles related to the occurrence and transmission of infection and infectious diseases.
2. Describe the focus areas in *Healthy People 2030* objectives that apply to infectious diseases.
3. Describe the chain of transmission of infectious diseases.
4. Apply the chain of transmission to describing approaches to control infectious disease.
5. Review types of immunity, including herd immunity.

6. Review principles of immunization, and specify the immunization recommended for all age groups in the United States.
7. Describe the legal responsibility for control of communicable diseases in the United States.
8. Describe the chain of transmission and control for priority infectious disease.
9. Identify nursing activities for control of infectious diseases at primary, secondary, and tertiary levels of prevention.

OUTLINE

KEY TERMS

acquired immunity   active immunity   agent

antigenicity
carriers
case
cold chain
communicable disease
communicable period
control
direct transmission
elimination
endemic
environment
epidemic
eradication
fomites
herd immunity
host
immunity
immunization

incidence
incubation period
indirect transmission
infection
infectious disease
infectivity
isolation
latency
multicausation
natural immunity
notifiable infectious diseases
outbreak
pandemic
passive immunity
pathogenicity
portal of entry
portal of exit
primary vaccine failure

quarantine
reservoir
resistance
secondary vaccine failure
subclinical infection
susceptible
toxigenicity
universal precautions
vaccination
Vaccine Adverse Event Reporting
  System (VAERS)
vaccine hesitancy
Vaccine Information Statements
  (VISs)
vectors
virulence

Throughout history, epidemics have been responsible for the destruction of entire groups of people. Despite amazing advances in public health and health care, control of communicable diseases continues to be a major concern of health care providers. The emergence of new pathogens, the reemergence of old pathogens, and the appearance of drug-resistant pathogens are creating formidable challenges in the United States and worldwide. The COVID-19 pandemic is an example of an emergence of a new pathogen, which began quietly in 2019 but quickly spread throughout the world causing major suffering and death.

Despite global eradication campaigns, malaria, ebola, and other vector-borne diseases and life-threatening gastrointestinal infections continue to cause significant morbidity and mortality in the developing world. Although the incidence rate of tuberculosis (TB) has been declining, in 2019 there were an estimated 10 million new cases of TB worldwide, with 1.4 million people dying from the disease (World Health Organization [WHO], 2020c, TB). To add to the world's growing infectious disease burden, human immunodeficiency virus (HIV) and acquired immunodeficiency syndrome (AIDS) continue to spread worldwide, as evidenced by the estimate that 38.0 million adults and children were living with HIV/AIDS globally at the end of 2019. Although new HIV infections have been declining slowly since 2001, there were approximately 1.7 million new infections worldwide in 2019 (UNAIDS, 2020).

Great strides have been made in the United States with respect to vaccine-preventable diseases, yet segments of the population remain unimmunized or underimmunized. Both measles and pertussis can be prevented with a vaccine, and indigenous measles had been virtually eliminated in the United States, with only 55 cases reported in 2012, This number has varied yearly since then, to reach another high of 1282 cases in 2019 (CDC, 2021c, Measles Cases and Outbreaks). Unvaccinated US residents traveling internationally are at risk for acquiring measles. These cases mainly have occurred in outbreaks among close-knit communities and populations unimmunized because of philosophical or religious preferences. It is interesting to note that new cases of measles in the US dropped to 13 reported cases during 2020, a time when pandemic precautions were in place (CDC, 2021c, Measles Cases and Outbreaks). Pertussis incidence in the US has varied from a low of 1010 cases in 1976 when the vaccine was new, to a high of 48,277 cases in 2012. Fortunately, the number of new cases of pertussis declined in 2019 to 18,617 (CDC, 2019d, Pertussis Cases by Year). Cases of hepatitis A, B, and C have been significantly reduced since the 1990s through administration of vaccines for hepatitis A and B and testing of the blood supply for hepatitis C. Yet these diseases persist. Treatable sexually transmitted diseases (STDs), such as gonorrhea, Chlamydia, and syphilis, are still occurring at significant rates. Gonorrhea cases increased 56% since 2015 in the US to 616,392 cases in 2019. Chlamydia, the most commonly reported bacterial disease in the United States, reached 1.8 million cases in 2019 (CDC, 2021d, STD surveillance). Rates of primary and secondary syphilis also have increased to an all-time high in 2019 to 129,813 cases (CDC, 2021d, STD surveillance).

In the United States, there have been significant accomplishments in preventing foodborne and waterborne infections through environmental sanitation. The incidence, however, of vector-borne infections, such as Lyme disease, Rocky Mountain spotted fever, St. Louis encephalitis, West Nile encephalitis, and Zika, appears to be increasing. Slight progress has been achieved in recent years to reduce new HIV infections in the U.S. In 2016 there were approximately 40,000 new HIV infections diagnosed in the United States, whereas in 2019 there were just over 36,000 new cases diagnosed (CDC, 2021b, HIV surveillance). On another note, there were just over 1,000,000 diagnosed adults and teenagers living with HIV in the United States in 2019 (CDC, 2021a, HIV prevalence). There may be many more who do not know that they are HIV positive.

Probably one of the most profound failures in infectious disease control in the United States and elsewhere is that the successes are not equally distributed in the general population. Infectious diseases continue to be differentially distributed by

BOX 26.1 Antimicrobial-Resistant Pathogens by Priority

Urgent Threats (Potential to Become Widespread)
- Carbapenem-resistant *Acinetobacter*
- *Candida auris*
- *Clostridioides difficile* (CDIFF)
- Carbapenem-resistant Enterobacteriaceae (CRE)
- Drug-resistant *Neisseria gonorrhoeae*

Serious Threats (May Become Urgent if Incidence Increases)
- Drug-resistant Campylobacter
- Drug-resistant Candida
- Extended-spectrum Enterobacteriaceae (ESBL)-producing Enterobacterales
- Vancomycin-resistant Enterococcus (VRE)
- Multidrug-resistant *Pseudomonas aeruginosa*
- Drug-resistant nontyphoidal *Salmonella*
- Drug-resistant *Salmonella* serotype *typhi*
- Drug-resistant Shigella
- Methicillin-resistant *Staphylococcus aureus* (MRSA)
- Drug-resistant *Streptococcus pneumoniae*
- Drug-resistant tuberculosis

Concerning (Serious Conditions With Multiple Therapeutic Options Currently)
- Erythromycin-resistant Group A *Streptococcus*
- Clindamycin-resistant Group B *Streptococcus*

Watch List (Resistance Not Spread Widely in US but Could Become Common)
- Azole-resistant *Aspergillus fumigatus*
- Drug-resistant *Mycoplasma genitalium*
- Drug-resistant *Bordetella pertussis*

Centers for Disease Control and Prevention: *Antibiotic resistance threats in the United States*, 2019. U.S. Department of Health and Human Services. https://doi.org/10.15620/cdc:82532. Available from: www.cdc.gov/DrugResistance/Biggest-Threats.html. Accessed June 25, 2021.

BOX 26.2 Centers for Disease Control and Prevention List of Potential Bioterrorism Agents and Diseases by Priority Category

Category A
Highest priority; easily transmitted with high mortality and social disruption:
- Anthrax (*Bacillus anthracis*)
- Botulism (botulinum toxin)
- Plague (*Yersinia pestis*)
- Smallpox (variola virus)
- Tularemia (*Francisella tularensis*)
- Viral hemorrhagic fevers
  - Filoviruses (Ebola, Marburg)
  - Adenaviruses (Lassa, Machupo)

Category B
Moderately easy to disseminate; high morbidity with low mortality:
- Brucellosis (*Brucella* spp.)
- Epsilon toxin of *Clostridium perfringens*
- Food safety threats:
  - Salmonellosis (*Salmonella* spp.)
  - *Escherichia coli* O157:H7
  - Shigellosis (*Shigella* spp.)
- Glanders (*Burkholderia mallei*)
- Melioidosis (*Burkholderia mallei*)
- Psittacosis (*Chlamydia psittaci*)
- Q fever (*Coxiella burnetii*)
- Ricin toxin
- Staphylococcal enterotoxin B
- Typhus fever (*Rickettsia prowazekii*)
- Viral encephalitis (alphaviruses)
- Water safety threats:
  - Cholera (*Vibrio cholerae*)
  - *Cryptosporidium parvum*

Category C
Emerging pathogens that could be engineered for mass dissemination because of availability, ease of production and dissemination, and potential for major impact on health with high morbidity and mortality rates.
- Such as Nipah virus and hantavirus

Centers for Disease Control and Prevention: *Emergency preparedness and response: bioterrorism agents/diseases.* Page last reviewed April 4, 2018. Available from: https://emergency.cdc.gov/agent/agentlist-category.asp. Accessed June 25, 2021.

income and ethnic groups, and the poor and minorities continue to experience the greater burden.

Although there has been marked improvement, infectious and communicable diseases persist. Scientific discoveries about the infectious etiology of stomach ulcers, coronary artery disease, and cervical cancer, for example, suggest that infectious agents may be responsible for more morbidity and mortality than previously recognized. New concerns include the rapid proliferation of drug-resistant organisms (Box 26.1) and the threat that deadly pathogens may be weaponized by terrorists (Box 26.2). Other threats are emerging infectious diseases, those diseases for which the incidence in humans has increased within the past 2 decades or threatens to increase in the near future. For more information, see the Centers for Disease Control (CDC), National Center for Emerging Zoonotic Infectious Diseases website at https://www.cdc.gov/ncezid/.

This chapter provides nurses with the knowledge necessary to help control infectious diseases. The terms *communicable disease* and *infectious disease* are synonymous and will be used interchangeably.

COMMUNICABLE DISEASE AND *HEALTHY PEOPLE 2030*

The U.S. Department of Health and Human Services program *Healthy People* was established to "promote, strengthen, and evaluate the nation's efforts to improve the health and well-being of all people" (Office of Disease Prevention and Health Promotion, n.d.). Health People *2030* contains 355 measurable objectives as well as additional developmental and research objectives to improve health. These objectives are used to evaluate national prevention and control efforts and can guide local prevention and control efforts. The objectives are organized into 38 topic areas that are organized as health conditions, health behaviors, specific populations, settings and systems, and social determinants of health. Two of the topic areas (Infectious Diseases and STDs) are categorized under Health Conditions. It must be noted that objectives referent to infectious diseases are sometimes located within categories other than the specific one for health conditions. Objectives for vaccination are covered within the category of Health Behaviors as well as in the Infectious Disease category. The *Healthy People 2030* box lists examples of objectives related to infectious diseases, including STDs and immunizations, with headings that refer to where the objective appears in the Healthy People 2030 classifications. Additional information, including baseline and target data for all objectives, can be found on the *Healthy People 2030* website: https://health.gov/healthypeople/objectives-and-data/browse-objectives.

PRINCIPLES OF INFECTION AND INFECTIOUS DISEASE OCCURRENCE

Nurses in all settings must be aware of potential threats related to communicable diseases and be prepared to intervene (see Ethical Insights box). To help prepare nurses for this

responsibility, biological and epidemiological principles inherent in infection and infectious disease occurrence are reviewed and major terms are defined in this section.

ETHICAL INSIGHTS

Nurse's Responsibility Regarding Communicable Diseases

Rapid proliferation of drug-resistant organisms, bioterrorism, and emerging infectious diseases are all concerns that have great implications for nursing practice. Every nurse should be knowledgeable about recognizing, reporting, preventing, and controlling infectious diseases. Infectious disease control can no longer be limited to the jurisdiction of the public health department or the hospital infection control nurse; it is every nurse's responsibility.

Equitable distribution of resources is an ethical issue. During the COVID-19 pandemic the lack of personal protective equipment (PPE) was not anticipated and rationing of PPE occurred, putting healthcare providers at risk. Fair distribution of scarce resources such as PPE and immunizations are advocacy opportunities for nurses. The equitable distribution of immunizations is also a priority to ensure access for vulnerable populations. Policies must be ethical and transparent.

❤ HEALTHY PEOPLE 2030

Communicable/Infectious Disease Objectives

Topic Area—Infectious Disease. Accessed in March 2021 from: https://health.gov/healthypeople/objectives-and-data/browse-objectives/infectious-disease
Infectious Disease—General:
  Reduce cases of pertussis among infants—IID-05
  Reduce TB cases—IID-17
  Reduce the rate of hospital admissions for urinary tract infections among older adults—OA-07
Health Care-Associated Infections:
  Reduce C. diff infections that people get in the hospital—HAI-01
  Reduce MRSA blood stream infections that people get in the hospital—HAI-02
  Reduce inappropriate antibiotic use in outpatient settings—HAI-D01
Sexually Transmitted Infections (STI):
  Reduce infections of human papilloma virus (HPV) types prevented by the vaccine in young adults—IID-07
  Reduce the rate of hepatitis A—IID-10
  Reduce the rate of acute hepatitis B—IID-11
  Reduce the rate of acute hepatitis C—IID-12
  Increase the proportion of people who know they have chronic hepatitis B—IID-13
  Increase the proportion of people who know they have chronic hepatitis C—IID-14
  Reduce the rate of deaths with hepatitis B as a cause—IID-15
  Reduce the rate of deaths with hepatitis C as a cause—IID-16
Vaccination:
  Maintain the elimination of measles, rubella, congenital rubella syndrome and polio—IID-01
  Increase the proportion of people with vaccination records in an information system—IID-D02
  Increase the proportion of adults age 19 or older who get recommended vaccines—IID-D03
Topic Area—STIs. Accessed from: https://health.gov/healthypeople/objectives-and-data/browse-objectives/sexually-transmitted-infections
  Reduce the syphilis rate in females—STI-03

Reduce the rate of new HIV infections—HIV-01
Reduce gonorrhea rates in male adolescents and young men—STI-02
Reduce the proportion of adolescents and young adults with genital herpes—STI-06
Reduce rates of pelvic inflammatory disease in young women—STI-07
Increase knowledge of HIV status—HIV-02
Reduce the number of new HIV diagnoses—HIV-03
Increase linkage to HIV medical care—HIV-04
Increase viral suppression—HIV-05
Reduce the rate of mother-to-child transmission—HIV-06
Reduce congenital syphilis—STI-04
Increase the proportion of sexually active female adolescents and young women who get screened for chlamydia—STI-01
Reduce the syphilis rate in men who have sex with men—STI-05
Increase the proportion of adolescents who get recommended doses of the HPV vaccine—IID-08
Topic Area: Vaccination. Accessed from https://health.gov/healthypeople/objectives-and-data/browse-objectives/vaccination (The only objectives included here are those not included in the sections on Infectious Disease or STIs).
Increase the proportion of people who get the flu vaccine every year—IID-09
Increase the proportion of women who get the Tdap vaccine during pregnancy—IID-D01
Reduce the proportion of children who get no recommended vaccines by age 2 years—IID-02
Maintain the vaccination coverage level of one dose of the measles-mumps-rubella (MMR) vaccine in children by 2 years—IID-03
Maintain the vaccination coverage of two doses of the MMR vaccine for children in kindergarten—IID-04
Increase the coverage level of four doses of the DTaP vaccine in children by age 2 years—IID-06
Increase the proportion of adults aged 19 years or older who get recommended vaccines—IID-D03

Multicausation

During the early years of medical and nursing history, science promulgated cause-and-effect theories of disease that relied on specifying one cause for each disease. Today, we understand that disease etiology is complex and multicausal. Infectious diseases are the result of interactions among the human **host**, an infectious **agent**, and the **environment** that surrounds the human host where transmission can occur. This interaction is pictured in the epidemiological triangle of agent, host, and environment. The principle of **multicausation** emphasizes that an infectious agent alone is not sufficient to cause disease; the agent must be transmitted within a conducive environment to a susceptible host. Of special note, nurses are part of the environment and, consequently, must maintain their own up-to-date immunization status and must practice optimum infection control.

Spectrum of Infection

Not all contact with an infectious agent leads to infection, and not all infection leads to an infectious disease. The processes, however, begin in the same way. An infectious agent may contaminate the skin or mucous membranes of a host but not invade the host. Or it may invade, multiply, and produce a **subclinical infection** (unapparent or asymptomatic) without producing overt symptomatic disease. Or the host may respond with overt symptomatic infectious disease. **Infection**, then, is the entry and multiplication of an infectious agent in a host. **Infectious disease** and **communicable disease** refer to the pathophysiological responses of the host to the infectious agent manifesting as an illness. When the disease is diagnosed in a person, the occurrence would be considered a **case**. A case is determined by a set of standard criteria for classifying the disease or health condition. Once infectious agents replicate in a host, they can be transmitted from the host irrespective of the presence of disease symptoms. Some persons become **carriers** and continue to shed the infectious agent without any symptoms of the disease.

Stages of Infection

An infectious agent that has invaded a host and found conditions hospitable will replicate until it can be shed from the host. This period of replication before shedding is called the *latent period*, or **latency**. The **communicable period**, or communicability, follows latency and begins with shedding of the agent. The **incubation period** is the time from invasion to the time when disease symptoms first appear. Frequently the communicable period begins before symptoms are present. Understanding the distinctions among these terms is important in controlling transmission. These stages of infection are depicted in Fig. 26.1. The stages of infection vary with different infectious agents.

Spectrum of Disease Occurrence

The principles covered to this point apply to individuals and their acquisition of infections and infectious diseases. Control of infectious diseases in a population requires identifying and

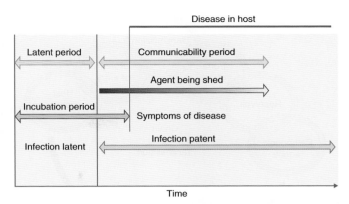

Fig. 26.1 Stages of infection. (From Grimes DE: *Infectious diseases*, St Louis, 1991, Mosby.)

monitoring the occurrence of new cases (**incidence**) in a population. Some infectious diseases are **endemic** and occur at a consistent, expected level in a geographic area. Such is the case with some STDs and with TB. An **outbreak** is an unexpected occurrence of an infectious disease in a limited geographic area during a limited period. Outbreaks of pertussis and salmonellosis, for example, are not uncommon. An **epidemic** is an unexpected increase in occurrence of an infectious disease in a geographic area over an extended period. Epidemics are defined relative to the infectious agent and the history of the disease in the area. One case of smallpox anywhere would constitute an epidemic, whereas 1000 new cases of gonorrhea would not be considered an epidemic in an area where gonorrhea is common. A **pandemic** is a steady occurrence of a disease, or an epidemic, that covers a large geographic area or is evident worldwide. For example, on March 11, 2020 the WHO Director-General characterized COVID-19 as a pandemic (WHO, 2020a).

CHAIN OF TRANSMISSION

Transmission is frequently conceptualized as a chain with six links, all connected, as in Fig. 26.2. Each of the links (infectious agent, reservoir, portal of exit, mode of transmission, portal of entry, and host susceptibility) represents a different component that contributes to transmission. The chain of transmission and its elements are summarized in Table 26.1.

Infectious Agents

Because the process of transmission is different for every infectious agent, one might envision a different configuration of the chain and its links for each infectious agent and infectious disease that exist. Infectious agents act differently, depending on their intrinsic properties and interactions with their human host. For example, an agent's size, shape, chemical composition, growth requirements, and viability (ability to survive for extended periods) have an impact on transmission and the type of parasitic relationship it establishes with its host. These characteristics determine the classifications of different agents (e.g., prions, viruses, bacteria, fungi, and protozoa), and

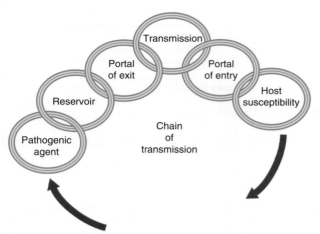

Fig. 26.2 Chain of transmission. (From Grimes DE: *Infectious diseases*, St Louis, 1991, Mosby.)

Reservoirs

The environment in which a pathogen lives and multiplies is the **reservoir**. Reservoirs can be humans, animals, arthropods, plants, soil, water, or any other organic substance. Some agents have more than one reservoir. Knowing the reservoirs for infectious agents is important, because in some cases, transmission can be controlled by eliminating the reservoir, such as eliminating the standing water where mosquitoes breed.

Portals of Exit and Entry

Agents leave the human host through a **portal of exit** and invade through a **portal of entry**. Portals of exit include respiratory secretions, vaginal secretions, semen, saliva, lesion exudates, blood, and feces. Portals of entry are associated with the portal of exit and include the respiratory passages, mucous membranes, skin and blood vessels, oral cavity, and the placenta.

Modes of Transmission

Direct transmission is the immediate transfer of an infectious agent from an infected host or reservoir to an appropriate portal of entry in the human host through physical contact, such as a touch, bite, kiss, or sexual contact. Direct projections of mucous secretions by droplet spray to the conjunctiva or mucous membranes of the eye, nose, or mouth during coughing, sneezing, or laughing are also considered direct transmission. Direct person-to-person contact is responsible for the transmission of many communicable diseases (e.g., STDs, influenza).

Indirect transmission is the spread of infection through a vehicle of transmission outside the host. These may be contaminated fomites or vectors. **Fomites** can be any inanimate objects, materials, or substances that act as transport agents for a microbe (e.g., water, a telephone shared by many, or a contaminated tissue). The infectious agent may or may not reproduce on or in the fomite. Substances such as food, water, and blood products can provide indirect transmission through ingestion and intravenous transfusions. Botulism is an example of an indirectly transmitted foodborne enterotoxin disease.

knowing the classification is helpful in understanding how specific agents are transmitted and produce disease. Also important are how the agent interacts with its host and its mode of action in the body. For example, it may kill cells, like *Mycobacterium tuberculosis* (*MTB*), or interfere with circulation, like the spirochete that causes syphilis. Or maybe it produces a toxin (**toxigenicity**), as does *Clostridium botulinum,* or stimulates an immune response in the host (**antigenicity**), as does rubella virus. Other considerations for understanding the action of agents are their power to invade and infect large numbers of people (**infectivity**), their ability to produce disease in those infected with the agent (**pathogenicity**), and their ability to produce serious disease in their hosts (**virulence**). If we apply the preceding concepts to the chickenpox virus, we see that it has high infectivity, high pathogenicity, and very low virulence. On the other hand, *MTB* has low infectivity and low pathogenicity but high virulence if untreated. Smallpox virus is high on all three concepts. Last, one must consider how adaptable an agent is to its human host and whether the agent changes, or mutates, over time, as do HIV and COVID-19.

TABLE 26.1	Chain of Transmission	
Link of the Chain	**Definition**	**Factor(s)**
Infectious agent	An organism (virus, rickettsia, bacteria, fungus, protozoan, helminth, or prion) capable of producing infection or infectious disease	Properties of the agent: Morphology, chemical composition, growth requirements, and viability; interaction with the host: mode of action, infectivity, pathogenicity, virulence, toxigenicity, antigenicity, and ability to adapt to the host
Reservoir(s)	The environment in which a pathogen lives and multiplies	Humans, animals, arthropods (bugs), plants, soil, or any other organic substance
Portal(s) of exit	Means by which an infectious agent is transported from the host	Respiratory secretions, vaginal secretions, semen, saliva, lesion exudates, blood, and feces
Mode(s) of transmission	Method whereby the infectious agent is transmitted from one host (or reservoir) to another host	*Direct:* Person to person
Indirect: Implies a vehicle of transmission (biological or mechanical vector, common vehicles or fomites, airborne droplets)
Portal(s) of entry	Means by which an infectious agent enters a new host	Respiratory passages, mucous membranes, skin, percutaneous new host space, mouth, and through the placenta
Host susceptibility	The presence or absence of resistance to an infectious agent	Biological and personal characteristics (e.g., gender, age, genetics), general health status, personal behaviors, anatomical and physiological lines of defense, immunity

Vectors can be animals or arthropods, and they can transmit through biological and mechanical routes. The mechanical route involves no multiplication or growth of the parasite or microbe within the animal or vector. Such is the case when a housefly carries gastrointestinal agents from raw sewage to uncovered food. Biological transmission occurs when the parasite grows or multiplies inside the animal, vector, or arthropod. Examples of diseases spread by this method of transmission include arthropod-borne diseases such as malaria, hemorrhagic fevers, and viral encephalitis. Transmission from a vector to the human host usually occurs through a bite or sting. Such is the case with the mosquito vector that transmits St. Louis encephalitis, West Nile, and Zika viruses.

Fecal-oral transmission can be direct or indirect. It can occur indirectly through the ingestion of water that has been fecally polluted or through consumption of contaminated food. Direct transmission occurs through engagement in oral sexual activity. Poliovirus and hepatitis A are spread through fecal-oral routes.

Airborne transmission occurs mainly through dissemination of microbial aerosols and droplet nuclei (small residues that result from evaporation of droplets of fluid from an infected host). The time frame in which an airborne particle can remain suspended greatly influences the virility and infectivity of the organism. The size of the particle can also determine how long it remains airborne and how successful it will be at penetrating the human lung. Aerosols are extremely small solid or liquid particles that may include fungal spores, viruses, and bacteria. Droplet nuclei, such as the spray from sneezing or coughing, may make direct contact with an open wound or with a mucous membrane, or they may be inhaled into the lung. TB is spread through inhalation of contaminated droplets.

Host Susceptibility

Not all humans are equally **susceptible** to, or at risk for, contracting an infection or development of an infectious disease. Biological and personal characteristics play an important role. Just as the young are at greater risk for diphtheria, older adults are at greater risk for bacterial pneumonia. Further, a fetus is at greater risk for harm from the Zika virus than is the pregnant woman. General health status is important, as evidenced by the increased risk for gastrointestinal parasites in children living in poverty. Personal behaviors certainly influence susceptibility, as does the presence of healthy lines of defense. The immune system and immunization status play important roles in the increased number of infections in unimmunized and immunocompromised persons.

BREAKING THE CHAIN OF TRANSMISSION

Picture a situation in which one of the links in the chain of transmission is broken (see Fig. 26.2). Breaking just one link of the chain at its most vulnerable point is, in fact, what is done to control transmission of an infectious agent. Of course, where the chain is broken depends on all of the factors that have just been discussed—characteristics of the agent, its reservoir,

portals of exit and entry, how the agent is transmitted, and susceptibility of the host.

Controlling the Agent

Controlling the agent is an area in which technology and medical science have been extremely effective. Inactivating an agent is the principle behind disinfection, sterilization, and radiation of fomites that may harbor pathogens. Antiinfective drugs, such as antibiotics, antivirals, antiretrovirals, and antimalarials, play important roles in controlling infectious diseases. Not only do they permit recovery of the infected person, but they also play a major role in preventing transmission of the pathogens to another. The first step in preventing transmission of TB and syphilis is to treat the infected person with antibiotics. Early screening and treatment of an HIV infection is also key to decreasing transmission of HIV: at the end of 2019%, 67% of people living with HIV were receiving antiretroviral therapy (ART) and 59% achieved viral suppression with no risk of infecting others (WHO, 2020b, HIV/AIDS).

Eradicating the Nonhuman Reservoir

Common nonhuman reservoirs for pathogens in the environment include water, food, milk, animals, insects, and sewage. Treating or eliminating them is an effective method of preventing replication of pathogens and thus preventing transmission.

Controlling the Human Reservoir

Treating infected persons, whether they are symptomatic or not, is effective in preventing transmission of pathogens directly to others. **Quarantine** is an enforced isolation or restriction of movement of those who have been exposed to an infectious agent during the incubation period; this is another method of controlling the reservoir. Quarantine was used effectively during the outbreak of severe acute respiratory syndrome (SARS) in 2003, when some hospitals required that their staff exposed to patients with SARS remain at the hospital until proven to be symptom-free at the end of the incubation period. Quarantine of unvaccinated persons exposed to COVID-19 has been routinely used during the recent pandemic.

Controlling the Portals of Exit and Entry

The transmission chain may be broken at the portal of exit by properly disposing of secretions, excretions, and exudates from infected persons. Additionally, **isolation** of sick persons from others and requiring that persons with an infection such as Covid-19 wear a mask in public can be effective.

The portal of entry of pathogens also can be controlled by using barrier precautions (masks, gloves, condoms); avoiding unnecessary invasive procedures, such as indwelling catheters; and protecting oneself from vectors, such as mosquitoes. In response to the risk of exposure to bloodborne pathogens (e.g., HIV, hepatitis B, and hepatitis C) the CDC developed a set of guidelines, called **universal precautions**, to prevent transmission of diseases found in blood and other body fluids. These guidelines were developed because infected people may be asymptomatic and have no knowledge of their conditions;

therefore, health care workers must assume that every patient is infectious and must protect themselves, other health care workers, and other patients.

Improving Host Resistance and Immunity

Many factors, such as age, general health status, nutrition, and health behaviors, contribute to a host's **resistance**, or ability to ward off infections. Immunity, however, is an incredible defense against infection. There are several kinds of **immunity**, each providing resistance in different ways to different pathogens. **Natural immunity** is an innate resistance to a specific antigen or toxin. **Acquired immunity** is derived from actual exposure to the specific infectious agent, toxin, or appropriate vaccine. There are two types of acquired immunity: active and passive. **Active immunity** occurs when the body produces its own antibodies against an antigen, from either infection with the pathogen or introduction of the pathogen, or some element of the pathogen, in a vaccine. **Passive immunity** is the temporary resistance that has been donated to the host either through transfusions of plasma proteins, immunoglobulins, or antitoxins or transplacentally (from mother to fetus). Passive immunity lasts only as long as these substances remain in the bloodstream. Types of acquired immunity with examples are summarized in Table 26.2.

When administered, according to established guidelines and protocols, vaccines provide acquired immunity in most cases. However, there are exceptions. **Primary vaccine failure** is the failure of a vaccine to stimulate any immune response. It can be caused by improper storage that may render the vaccine ineffective, improper administration route, or exposure of a light-sensitive vaccine to light. Additionally, seroconversion never occurs in some immunized persons, either because of failure of their own immune system or for some other unknown reason. **Secondary vaccine failure** is the waning of immunity after an initial immune response. It often occurs in patients with immunosuppression and in those who have undergone organ transplantation in whom the immune memory is essentially destroyed.

Herd immunity is a state in which those not immune to an infectious agent are protected if a certain proportion (generally considered to be 80%) of the population has been vaccinated or is otherwise immune (Fig. 26.3). The percent necessary varies with the infectious agent. This effect applies only if those who are immune are distributed evenly in the population. This is especially true for the transmission of diseases, such as diphtheria, that are found only in the human host and that have no invertebrate host or other mode of transmission. Without the presence of a susceptible population to infect, the organism will be unable to live because the vast majority of the population is immune. Unfortunately, herd immunity for COVID-19 has shown to be elusive with gaps among those fully vaccinated and an unknown number and location of those who have contracted the virus and therefore have antibodies.

PUBLIC HEALTH CONTROL OF INFECTIOUS DISEASES

Most human diseases (e.g., cancer or diabetes) can be classified as personal health problems. Individuals with personal health problems can be treated by the health care system one person at a time. By contrast, infectious diseases are categorized as public or community health problems. Because of their potential to spread and cause community-wide or worldwide emergencies, infectious diseases require organized, public efforts for their prevention and control.

Such organized public efforts are under the jurisdiction of official public health agencies at local, state, national, and international levels. Each government unit obtains its powers through a complex array of laws. It is important to remember that in areas of health within a state, state laws usually prevail over federal law. The reason for this hierarchy is that the US Constitution did not address health and the 10th Amendment reserved power to the states over all issues not addressed in the Constitution (Schneider, 2006). Historically, states have accepted this responsibility. For example, all states have laws addressing infectious disease control, such as what diseases must be reported and who has authority to implement quarantines. Every state has a board of health and a department of health to implement state laws.

The CDC is the national public health entity responsible for infectious disease control across the states. It has responsibility

TABLE 26.2 Types of Acquired Immunity

Type of Immunity	How Acquired	Example	Duration of Resistance
Natural			
Active	Natural contact and infection with the antigen	Acquiring measles	May be temporary or permanent
Passive	Natural contact with antibody transplacentally	Infant born with temporary antibodies to measles	Temporary or through colostrum and breast milk
Artificial			
Active	Inoculation of antigen	Tetanus vaccine to stimulate production of antibodies to tetanus	May be temporary or permanent
Passive	Inoculation of antibody or antitoxin	Injection of tetanus antitoxin to an unimmunized person	Temporary

Modified from Grimes DE: Infectious diseases. In Thompson JM, et al., editors: *Mosby's clinical nursing*, St Louis, 1991, Mosby.

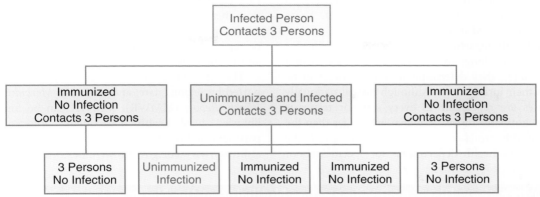

Fig. 26.3 Example of herd immunity.

for monitoring infectious diseases and for supporting local and state governments to control outbreaks and epidemics if such assistance is needed. Although there are many aspects of public health control of infectious diseases, only four are presented here: common control terminology, reporting diseases, responding and controlling, and preventing diseases by vaccination.

Terminology: Control, Elimination, and Eradication

Control of a communicable disease is, by definition, the reduction of incidence (new cases) or prevalence (existing cases) of a given disease to a locally acceptable level as a result of deliberate efforts (Dowdle, 1999). The WHO Expanded Program on Immunizations is a global attempt to control morbidity and mortality for many vaccine-preventable diseases, with each country adapting these guidelines as necessary. Countries have incorporated increasingly broad immunization agendas and are routinely reaching over 80% of children under 1 year of age (WHO, 2021, Immunizations).

Elimination of a communicable disease occurs when it is controlled within a specified geographic area, such as a single country, an island, or a continent, and the prevalence and incidence of the disease is reduced to near zero. Elimination is the result of deliberate efforts, but continued intervention measures are required (Dowdle, 1999). Such would be the case if no new cases of polio were reported in the United States during the year after an aggressive immunization campaign. Localized elimination of a vaccine-preventable condition, however, does not suggest eradication of the condition. Continued vaccination is still necessary.

The International Task Force for Disease Eradication defines **eradication** as reducing the worldwide incidence of a disease to zero as a function of deliberate efforts, without a need for further control measures (Dowdle, 1999). Eradication is possible under certain conditions. Criteria for assessing eradicability are listed in Box 26.3.

Smallpox was eradicated in 1977, and the virus now exists only in storage in laboratories. Many factors contributed to the

BOX 26.3   Criteria for Assessment of Disease Eradicability

Criteria for assessment of the possibility of disease eradication include the following:
- Human host only; no host in nature
- Easy diagnosis; obvious clinical manifestations
- Limited duration and intensity of infection
- Natural lifelong immunity after infection
- Highly seasonal transmission
- Availability of vaccine, curative treatment, or both
- Substantial global morbidity and mortality rates
- Cost-effectiveness of campaign and eradication
- Integration of eradication with additional public health variables
- Eradication is preferred over use of control measures only

From Centers for Disease Control and Prevention: Recommendations of the international task force for disease eradication, *MMWR Morb Mortal Wkly Rep* 42:1–38, 1993; and Dowdle WR: The principles of disease elimination and eradication, *MMWR Morb Mortal Wkly Rep* 48(suppl 1):23–27, 1999.

successful eradication of the disease, including the mode of transmission, the isolated geographic distribution of the infection, the ease of administration of the freeze-dried vaccine, the establishment of an effective surveillance system, the increase in national and international political will, and tremendous community participation.

Defining and Reporting Communicable Diseases

Standardized definitions of diseases are necessary for public health monitoring and surveillance throughout all levels of government. Diseases are defined and classified according to confirmed cases, probable cases, laboratory-confirmed cases, clinically compatible cases, epidemiologically linked cases, genetic typing, and clinical case definition. Once defined, disease occurrences can be compared across time, populations, and geographic areas, and appropriate control efforts can be implemented.

The CDC is responsible for monitoring communicable disease in the United States. Along with the Council of State and Territorial Epidemiologists, the CDC has designated notifiable infectious diseases, meaning that healthcare providers who encounter cases of these diseases must report them to, or notify, the local or regional health department. These notifiable diseases are listed in Box 26.4.

Because state health departments have the responsibility for monitoring and controlling communicable diseases within their respective states, they determine which diseases will be reported within their jurisdictions. Although not all nationally notifiable diseases are reportable in every state or territory, some states have notifiable disease lists that are longer than the CDC's list. All health professionals are advised to check the websites of their state health departments for specifics about

reporting laws in their states. The processes for reporting also vary by state, and this information usually is available on the state health department's website. Generally, providers are encouraged to report cases of infectious diseases to their local or regional health departments, who then report to the state and to the CDC.

The CDC publishes a weekly list of notifiable diseases reported by region, state, and nation in *Morbidity and Mortality Weekly Report* (MMWR). MMWR can be found in medical libraries, local health departments, infection control departments in hospitals and medical centers, and on the Internet at https://www.cdc.gov/mmwr/index.html.

BOX 26.4 Infectious Diseases Designated as Notifiable at the National Level, 2021

- Anthrax
- Arboviral neuroinvasive and nonneuroinvasive diseases: California serogroup virus disease, Chikungunya virus disease, Eastern equine encephalitis, Powassan virus disease, St. Louis encephalitis, West Nile virus disease, and Western equine encephalitis
- Babesiosis
- Botulism (foodborne, infant, wound, and other)
- Brucellosis
- Campylobacteriosis
- *Candida auris*, clinical
- Carbapenemase producing carbapenem-resistant Enterobacteriaceae (CP-CRE): CP-CRE *Enterobacter* spp., CP-CRE *Escherichia coli*, CP-CRE *Klebsiella* spp.
- Chancroid
- *Chlamydia trachomatis*, genital infections
- Cholera
- Coccidioidomycosis
- Congenital syphilis: syphilitic stillbirth
- Coronavirus disease 2019 (COVID-19)
- Cryptosporidiosis
- Cyclosporiasis
- Dengue virus infections (dengue, dengue-like illness, severe dengue)
- Diphtheria
- Ehrlichiosis/anaplasmosis (*Anaplasma phagocytophilum, Ehrlichia chaffeensis, Ehrlichia ewingii,* undetermined human ehrlichiosis/anaplasmosis)
- Giardiasis
- Gonorrhea
- *Haemophilus influenzae*, invasive disease
- Hansen disease (leprosy)
- Hantavirus infection
- Hantavirus pulmonary syndrome
- Hemolytic uremic syndrome, postdiarrheal
- Hepatitis A, acute
- Hepatitis B, acute, and chronic
- Hepatitis B, perinatal virus infection
- Hepatitis C, acute and chronic, perinatal
- HIV infection
- Influenza-associated pediatric mortality
- Invasive pneumococcal disease
- Legionellosis
- Leptospirosis

- Listeriosis
- Lyme disease
- Malaria
- Measles
- Meningococcal disease
- Mumps
- Novel influenza A virus infections
- Pertussis
- Plague
- Poliomyelitis, paralytic
- Poliovirus infection, nonparalytic
- Psittacosis
- Q fever (acute and chronic)
- Rabies (animal and human)
- Rubella
- Rubella, congenital syndrome
- *Salmonella* Paratyphi Infection
- *Salmonella* Typhi Infection
- Salmonellosis
- SARS—associated coronavirus disease
- Shiga toxin—producing *E. coli*
- Shigellosis
- Smallpox
- Spotted fever rickettsiosis (formerly Rocky Mountain spotted fever)
- Streptococcal toxic-shock syndrome
- Syphilis (all stages)
- Tetanus
- Toxic shock syndrome (other than streptococcal)
- Trichinellosis (trichinosis)
- Tuberculosis
- Tularemia
- Vancomycin-intermediate *Staphylococcus aureus* (VISA)
- Vancomycin-resistant *Staphylococcus aureus* (VRSA)
- Varicella (morbidity and death)
- Vibriosis
- Viral hemorrhagic fevers (Crimean—Congo hemorrhagic fever virus, Ebola virus, Lassa virus, Lujo virus, Marburg virus, New World Arenaviruses [Guanarito, Machupo, Junin, and Sabia viruses])
- Yellow fever
- Zika virus disease and infection (all stages)

From Centers for Disease Control and Prevention: *Infectious diseases designated as notifiable at the national level during 2021.* Available from: https://www.cdc.gov/nndss/index.html and https://wwwn.cdc.gov/nndss/conditions/notifiable/2021/infectious-diseases; Centers for Disease Control and Prevention: *National Notifiable Disease Surveillance System (NNDSS). 2021 National Notifiable Infectious Diseases Tables.* Page reviewed May 17, 2021. Available from: https://www.cdc.gov/nndss/data-statistics/infectious-tables/index.html. Accessed June 25, 2021.

RESPONDING AND CONTROLLING EPIDEMIC AND PANDEMICS

Public health control of epidemics and pandemics requires strong collaboration with the community including healthcare providers. Nurses are part of a community's first line of defense in the response and control and of epidemics and pandemics (Edmonds et al., 2020). A public health crisis occurs with an unexpected increase in an infectious disease, an epidemic, or when the epidemic has spread to other regions and countries causing a pandemic. Nurses take on additional roles in many settings including: health departments, schools, outpatient clinics, community health centers, and hospitals, for example (Corless et al., 2018). The nurses' normal roles often have to adjust to take on additional responsibilities during the duration of the pandemic, for example, an ICU nurse may be called to assist with mass-vaccination clinics.

Early identification of cases is key to decrease spread of the infectious disease (Corless et al., 2018). Nurses are on response teams investigating cases, exploring case-contacts and conducting contact tracing to identify cases of the infectious disease. Nurses provide education to cases and case-contacts to decrease the spread of the disease including; self-isolation and quarantine, available supportive care or treatments, and provide most recent guidelines from the CDC. Nurses also assist with providing education to the population on prevention measures, assist with screening, and provide interventions and treatments such as vaccinations. Nurses also advocate for vulnerable populations such as socioeconomically and under-resources communities who are at higher risk during a public health crisis (Edmonds et al., 2020). The CDC provides detailed step by step information on case investigation at https://www.cdc.gov/coronavirus/2019-ncov/php/contact-tracing/contact-tracing-plan/investigating-covid-19-case.html.

ACTIVE LEARNING

1. Subscribe to the e-mail Listserv to receive *Morbidity and Mortality Weekly Report (MMWR)* (www.cdc.gov/mmwr).
2. Attend an immunization clinic at your local health department to observe a nurse in the process of screening children for immunizations; and participate in screening, if appropriate.
3. Obtain and evaluate health education materials regarding childhood immunizations from your local health department; help distribute in your community, if appropriate.
4. Log on to your state health department website to learn about the process of reporting notifiable diseases in your state. Who is responsible for the reporting process? To whom do they report, what information is reported, and how often are diseases reported?

VACCINES AND INFECTIOUS DISEASE PREVENTION

This section contains comprehensive information on vaccines and vaccine-preventable diseases. Diseases for which there are

BOX 26.5 Vaccine-Preventable Diseases

- Adenovirus
- Anthrax
- Chickenpox (varicella)
- Cholera
- Diphtheria
- Flu (Influenza)
- *Haemophilus influenzae* type b (Hib)
- Hepatitis A
- Hepatitis B
- Human papilloma virus (HPV)
- Japanese encephalitis (JE)
- Measles
- Meningococcal disease
- Mumps
- Pertussis
- Pneumococcal disease
- Poliomyelitis
- Rabies
- Rotavirus
- Rubella
- Shingles (herpes zoster)
- Smallpox
- Tetanus
- Tuberculosis
- Typhoid fever
- Yellow fever

From Centers for Disease Control and Prevention: *Recommended vaccines by disease and vaccines recommended for travel and some specific groups,* Page reviewed: November 22, 2016. https://www.cdc.gov/vaccines/vpd/vaccines-diseases.html. Accessed June 25, 2021.

vaccines are listed in Box 26.5. Recommended vaccination schedules for selected groups are available on the CDC website, which is listed in Table 26.3 along with other resources.

Vaccines: A Word of Caution

As with other areas of health care, information and recommendations on immunizations and vaccine usage change regularly. Therefore, health care providers should seek the most current information on the CDC website. Recommendations, policies, and procedures concerning international immunization practices are determined by the WHO. In the United States, national governance is provided by the American Academy of Pediatrics Committee on Infectious Diseases and the U.S. Public Health Service Advisory Committee on Immunization Practices (ACIP). Occasionally these agencies differ in their recommendations.

Precautions must be taken when giving any immunization. The most recent recommendations—which immunizations to give; to whom they should be given; how they should be given; and how they are to be transported, stored, and administered—can be obtained from the CDC (Table 26.3).

The CDC produces **Vaccine Information Statements (VISs)** that explain vaccine benefits and risks to vaccine recipients, their parents, or their legal representatives. Federal law requires that VISs be handed out before each dose whenever certain

TABLE 26.3   Resources for Recommended Vaccine Schedules for Selected Population Groups

Advisory Committee on Immunization Practices	https://www.cdc.gov/vaccines/hcp/acip-recs/index.html
General immunization schedules	https://cdc.gov/vaccines/schedules/
Children/adolescents aged 18 years or younger	https://www.cdc.gov/vaccines/schedules/hcp/imz/child-adolescent.html
Adults	https://www.cdc.gov/vaccines/schedules/hcp/imz/adult.html
Travelers	https://wwwnc.cdc.gov/travel/destinations/list
Pregnant and breast-feeding women	https://www.cdc.gov/vaccines/pregnancy/index.html
Health care workers	https://www.cdc.gov/vaccines/adults/rec-vac/hcw.html
Adults with chronic health conditions	https://www.cdc.gov/vaccines/adults/rec-vac/health-conditions/
Adults with weakened immune systems	https://www.cdc.gov/vaccines/adults/rec-vac/health-conditions/weakened-immune.html

TABLE 26.4   Examples of Available Vaccines by Type

Type/Description	Name of Vaccine and/or Name of Disease
Live Attenuated/Modified Disease Producing Virus or Bacterium	
Viral	MMR: Measles, mumps, rubella
	Vaccinia, yellow fever, varicella zoster, rotavirus, influenza (intranasal), adenovirus
Bacterial	Typhoid vaccine (Ty21a) used to prevent typhoid fever.
	BCG (bacillus Calmette-Guérin: Used for preventing mycobacterium tuberculosis and leprosy in some countries; not used as vaccine in the United States).
Recombinant (genetically engineered vaccine antigens)	Oral typhoid vaccine
Inactivated (virus or bacterium grown in media and inactivated by chemical or heat, cannot replicate or cause disease from infection)	
Viral	Influenza, polio, rabies, hepatitis A
Bacterial	Typhoid, cholera, plague
Subunit (fractional)	Influenza, acellular pertussis, anthrax, Japanese encephalitis, typhoid VI
Toxoid (inactivated bacterial toxin)	Diphtheria and tetanus
Recombinant (genetically engineered vaccine antigens)	Hepatitis B, human papilloma virus (HPV), serogroup B meningococcal and influenza
Conjugate polysaccharide (polysaccharide, long chains of sugar molecules, chemically linked to a protein)	*Haemophilus influenzae* type b and pneumococcal 13-valent
Pure polysaccharide (pure cell wall polysaccharide from bacteria)	Pneumococcal disease, meningococcal disease, and *Salmonella typhi* (VI)
Genetic Vaccines (contain a segment of genetic material that codes for a specific protein, may be DNA or RNA)	
mRNA vaccine (messenger RNA)	SARS-CoV-2 for COVID-19

From Centers for Disease Control and Prevention: *Epidemiology and prevention of vaccine-preventable diseases.* Hamborsky J, Kroger A, Wolfe S, editors, ed 3. Washington, DC, 2015, Public Health Foundation. https://www.cdc.gov/vaccines/pubs/pinkbook/index.html 18 out of 22 chapters updated in 2020–21. U.S. Department of Health and Human Services: *Vaccine Types.* Last reviewed April 29, 2021. Available from: https://www.hhs.gov/immunization/basics/types/index.html. Accessed June 25, 2021.

vaccinations are given. VISs can be downloaded from the Internet at http://www.cdc.gov/vaccines/hcp/vis/index.html.

Types of Immunizations

Immunization is a broad term used to describe a process by which active or passive immunity to an infectious disease is induced or amplified. Immunizing agents can include vaccines, immune globulins, or antitoxins. **Vaccination** is a narrower term referring to the administration of a vaccine or toxoid to confer active immunity by stimulating the body to produce its own antibodies. Vaccination does not subject the recipient to the disease and possible complications.

Vaccines can be prepared in several ways. They may be suspensions in a variety of solutions; protected with preservatives, stabilizers, or antibiotics; or mixed with adjuvants, which are used to increase immunogenicity. Vaccines can be live and attenuated (with the virulence reduced), or they may be killed or inactivated (with the virulence removed), leaving only the antigenic property necessary to stimulate the human immune system to produce antibodies. Types of inactivated vaccines include toxoids and polysaccharide vaccines. Inactivated conjugate vaccines, containing chemically linked polysaccharides and proteins, and genetically engineered "recombinant" vaccines are also now being administered. Inactivated vaccines can be fractions or subunits or whole "killed" bacteria or viruses. Immune globulins and antitoxins are solutions that contain antibodies from human or animal blood and are introduced into a patient to provide passive protection without initiating the immune system to produce an immunogenic response. An example of a genetic vaccine is the messenger RNA (mRNA) vaccine approved for COVID-19. The mRNA vaccine contains a segment of the genetic material for a specific protein, which stimulates an immune response to the antigen produced (U.S. Department of Health and Human Services, 2021). Table 26.4 presents information on types of available vaccines.

Vaccine Storage, Transport, and Handling

Vaccines should be safely stored, transported, and handled at all times to ensure their efficacy. A **cold chain** is a system used to ensure that vaccines are kept at a designated temperature from the time they are manufactured until they are used for vaccination. Failing to maintain the cold chain and exposing the vaccines to higher or lower temperatures than recommended may result in loss of potency and vaccine failure. Several methods are available for ensuring that the appropriate temperature has been maintained throughout vaccine transport and storage. These include liquid crystal thermometers, dial thermometers, recording thermometers, digital thermometers, ice pack indicators, shipping indicators that change color if the temperature exceeds or falls below the recommended level, freeze-watch indicators, and cold chain monitors. Vaccine storage and handling information can be obtained at https://www.cdc.gov/vaccines/hcp/admin/storage-handling-toolkit.pdf.

Vaccine Administration

The efficacy of a vaccine can be adversely affected if it is not administered appropriately. Information on the correct dosage can be found on the package insert. If more than one vaccine is being administered simultaneously, different anatomical sites should be used. Additionally, it is important to follow the same safety procedures one would use to administer any intramuscular or subcutaneous injection (i.e., use sterile technique, use the correct size needle, avoid injecting in a blood vessel, and dispose of the needle and syringe properly).

Vaccine Spacing

Wherever possible, all children should be age-appropriately immunized and their immunization status kept up to date according to current recommendations. The same applies to adolescents, adults, persons with chronic illness, pregnant women, healthcare workers, and international travelers.

The number of injections for any one immunobiological substance should be administered according to recommendations of the ACIP. An interruption in the schedule does not require that the entire series begin again. However, if vaccines are administered at less than the recommended intervals, they should not be counted as part of the primary series of immunization. Completion of the primary vaccine series and receiving periodic booster doses as recommended, are necessary to ensure protective levels of immunity. Additional information is available at www.cdc.gov/vaccines.

Vaccine Hypersensitivity and Contraindications

Minor and common side effects may include redness and/or pain at the injection site and mild fever. Although adverse reactions are not common after immunization, they can occur in some individuals. These reactions can be to vaccine components such as eggs, egg proteins, antibiotics, preservatives, and adjuvants. Patient allergies should be considered before administration of specific vaccines. For additional precautions and contraindications, refer to the vaccine package insert and the latest instructions from the CDC at https://www.cdc.gov/vaccines/hcp/acip-recs/contraindications.html.

Mild illness with or without low-grade fever is not a contraindication to vaccination. However, vaccination should be postponed in cases of moderate or severe febrile illness to avoid any confusion between a vaccine side effect and an unknown underlying cause.

Pregnancy is not a contraindication to immunization using inactivated vaccines, antitoxins, or immune globulins. However, pregnant women should avoid live vaccines, including those for MMR, varicella, and yellow fever, unless the risk of infection is very high (see the link to guidelines for vaccinating pregnant women in Table 26.3).

In general, immunocompromised patients should not receive live vaccines. There are, however, situations in which an immunocompromised patient may receive vaccines as determined by the patient's physician. Updated information on this issue is provided by the CDC on a regular basis. Killed or inactivated vaccines can be given, but they may not produce an optimal antibody response (see the link to guidelines for vaccinating specific groups of people in Table 26.3).

Vaccine Documentation

Legal documentation of vaccinations is important for both the individual and the provider for future administration and follow-up of hypersensitivity reactions. Both individual and provider immunization records should be maintained. The healthcare provider is responsible for maintaining accurate records, including patient name; dates immunized; vaccine type; vaccine manufacturer; vaccine lot number; date of the VIS; and the name, title, and address of the person administering the vaccine. VISs can be downloaded from http://www,cdc.gov/vaccines/hcp/vis/index.html.

Vaccine Safety and Reporting Adverse Events and Vaccine-Related Injuries

No drug is perfectly safe or effective, and vaccines are no exception. They are biological rather than chemical, and when introduced into the human biological system, they can and do produce a variety of responses, both positive and negative. Furthermore, vaccines are administered to healthy people; they are given to prevent illness and not treat it; and vaccines are given to far greater numbers of people than other pharmaceuticals.

Public concern regarding the health risks associated with vaccines has increased as the risk of contracting the diseases has declined. For example, wild polio virus has been eliminated in the United States, yet between 1979 and 1997 cases of poliomyelitis were reported in the United States in association with use of the oral, live virus vaccine. The health risk of the oral vaccine exceeded that of the risk of the disease. This led to a change in vaccine policy from the use of the live oral vaccine to the inactivated polio vaccine (IPV) (CDC, 1999). Likewise, whole cell pertussis vaccine has been changed to an acellular pertussis vaccine because of the adverse side effects, most notably convulsions, associated with the whole cell vaccine.

To enable monitoring of actual and potential vaccine-related problems, health care providers must report specific post-vaccination "adverse events" to the **Vaccine Adverse Event**

Reporting System (VAERS). Information and reporting forms are available at https://www.cdc.gov/vaccinesafety/ensuringsafety/monitoring/vaers/index.html. The National Vaccine Injury Compensation Program reviews all VAERS reports and provides assistance for individuals and families who experience a vaccine-related injury, including disability and death.

VACCINE HESITANCY

Vaccine hesitancy may be found in many communities and nurses may need to address vaccine hesitancy when caring for specific population groups. Vaccine hesitancy was defined by SAGE Working Group on Vaccine Hesitancy as a "delay in acceptance or refusal of vaccination despite availability of vaccination services. Vaccine hesitancy is complex and context specific, varying across time, place and vaccine" (MacDonald, 2015, p. 4161). Vaccine hesitancy includes lack of trust: in vaccine safety, in the healthcare providers delivering the vaccine, or in the decision makers who approve the vaccine. Personal factors may include fear of needles, lack of concern about the preventable disease, availability of vaccine, and cost of services. There also is a continuum found from full acceptance of all vaccines to outright refusal of all vaccines. Vaccine hesitancy may be found in a population and the reasons for population level vaccine hesitancy may be very different from the personal reasons.

Vaccine hesitancy undermines demand, it is important to determine the reasons a population or a person has vaccine hesitancy. A rapid community assessment can elicit a community's needs and gaps (Association of State and Territorial Health Officials [ASTHO], 2021). Active listening and good communication are important when assessing a person's vaccine hesitancy. Strategies to reinforce confidence in vaccines includes actions to build trust and relationships, empower the healthcare provider and families, stop myths, increase vaccine availability, and engage communities and individuals (ASTHO, 2021; CDC, 2019a, vaccine confidence; CDC, 2021e, vaccine confidence).

> ### ⍰ ACTIVE LEARNING
> Log on to the website of an advocacy group against immunizations to understand the messages that they are communicating to the public. Then explore the CDC strategies to reinforce confidence when you talk with families about vaccines. https://www.cdc.gov/vaccines/partners/vaccinate-with-confidence.html.

VACCINE NEEDS FOR SPECIAL GROUPS

Recommendations on immunizations and schedules for vaccination are routinely updated and published by the CDC on its website. Practitioners are encouraged to check regularly for updates. Travelers can obtain the most current recommendations from the CDC through its telephone hotline, 1-800-CDC-info (1-800-232-4636), or at its website: http://wwwnc.cdc.gov/travel.

HEALTHY PEOPLE 2030 FOCUS ON IMMUNIZATION AND INFECTIOUS DISEASES

Healthy People 2030 objectives, discussed earlier in this chapter, detailed three topic areas for infectious diseases. Immunization and Infectious Diseases (IID), as listed in the *Healthy People 2030* table, highlights vaccine-preventable and other priority infectious diseases, excluding STI and HIV. This section provides tables summarizing the chain of transmission and control of such conditions. Table 26.5 covers childhood vaccine–preventable diseases, excluding hepatitis, which is summarized in Table 26.6. Table 26.7 summarizes TB. For more information see the *Healthy People 2030* Website: https://health.gov/healthypeople.

HEALTHY PEOPLE 2030 FOCUS ON SEXUALLY TRANSMITTED INFECTIONS

STIs include the more than 25 infectious organisms that are transmitted primarily through sexual activity. STIs, even those for which treatment exists, continue to be a major public health problem. The rates of STIs in the United States are among the highest in the industrialized world, approaching those in some developing countries. More than 26 million new cases of STIs occur each year in the United States and rates are increasing with half of them in persons aged 15 to 24 years (CDC, 2021d, STDs Adolescents and young adults).

Concern over the persistence and increases in STIs led those formulating the *Healthy People 2030* objectives to create a topic area specific to STIs (Healthy People 2030, 2021c Objectives). For easy reference, the chain of transmission and control of STIs addressed in the *Healthy People 2030* objectives is presented in Table 26.8. The CDC regularly updates STD treatment guidelines, which are available on the website.

HEALTHY PEOPLE 2030 FOCUS ON HIV/AIDS

No other infection or infectious disease in recent history has inflicted as much destruction and pain on individuals, families, and communities and created as many challenges for healthcare professionals as HIV/AIDS. Indeed, HIV stands out as the one condition that touches nurses everywhere. HIV affects persons of every age, ethnicity, socioeconomic status, gender, and occupation. Eventually, HIV/AIDS has an impact on every organ and function of the human body. Every nurse, regardless of area of practice, will eventually care for someone with HIV infection. Currently, there is no cure or vaccine, although early treatment with ART has shown signs of effectively reducing transmission of the HIV virus (The INSIGHT START Study Group, 2015). Due to the worldwide spread of HIV, it is not surprising that *Healthy People 2030* has a Workgroup, https://health.gov/healthypeople/about/workgroups/hiv-workgroup, with HIV expertise who developed six objectives specific to HIV/AIDS (Healthy People 2030, 2021c, STIs).

Continued

TABLE 26.5 Chain of Transmission and Control: Childhood Vaccine—Preventable Diseases

	Chickenpox	Diphtheria	Pertussis	Tetanus	Polio
Occurrence	Worldwide in all populations; primarily a childhood disease in temperate climates; acquired by older children in tropical areas, resulting in an increase in cases in adults.	Rare where immunization rates are high; affects unimmunized children under 15 years and adults whose immunity has waned, increased cases in winter and spring in temperate climates.	Worldwide and common in children; declined with immunization; some outbreaks in recent years in US adults whose immunity has waned	Worldwide; occurs sporadically and affects all ages; more common in agricultural areas and among parenteral drug users; rare in areas with high immunization rates	Worldwide before immunization; is now rare in countries with adequate immunization rates
Etiological agent(s)	Human (alpha) herpesvirus 3 (varicella zoster virus)	Corynebacterium diphtheriae, of gravis, mitis, intermedius, and belfanti biotypes	Bordetella pertussis	Clostridium tetani (an anaerobic pathogen)	Poliovirus types 1, 2, and 3; all are paralytogenic
Reservoir	Humans	Humans	Humans	Soil and intestines and feces of some animals	Humans, particularly children with subclinical infections
Transmission	Direct and indirect contact with droplets from respiratory passage or vesicle fluid; enters through respiratory tract and conjunctiva; extremely contagious	Direct through respiratory droplets. Direct or indirect contact with exudates from mucous membrane lesions of infected person or carrier; raw milk has served as a vehicle	Direct contact with droplets from respiratory passages; exposure to fomites	Tetanus spores enter body through a wound (usually a puncture wound) contaminated with soil and feces; spores germinate in anaerobic conditions; necrotic tissue favors the growth of the anaerobic bacillus	Highly infectious; direct and indirect contact with respiratory discharges and feces; oral-oral and fecal-oral routes
Incubation period	14–16 days; range 2–3 weeks; prolonged in immunocompromised persons and in those who have received postexposure prophylaxis with varicella specific immune globulin	2–5 days; range of 1–10 days, occasionally longer in untreated people	7–10 days; range 4–21 days	8 days; range 1–21 days; rarely, several months	3–6 days nonparalytic poliomyelitis, 7–21 days for onset of paralytic poliomyelitis; range 3–35 days. Postpolio syndrome, 15–40 years; 25%–40% paralytic poliomyelitis
Communicability period	1–2 days before onset of rash till all lesions have crusted	Until bacilli have disappeared from discharges and lesions (usually 2 week); effective antibiotic therapy interferes with shedding; a carrier may transmit for 6 mo.	Highly communicable during early catarrhal and coughing stages; gradually decreasing until week 3; communicability is negligible after 5 days with effective antibiotic therapy	Not transmitted directly person to person	Highly communicable during first days immediately before and after onset of symptoms; virus is in throat secretions within 36 h and in feces 72 h after infection; remains 1 week in throat and 6 weeks in feces

TABLE 26.5 Chain of Transmission and Control: Childhood Vaccine–Preventable Diseases—cont'd

	Chickenpox	Diphtheria	Pertussis	Tetanus	Polio
Susceptibility and resistance	General population not previously infected or vaccinated are at risk; can be severe or fatal in adults and immuno-compromised persons	General unimmunized population are at risk; infants born of immune mothers have passive immunity for 6 mo; recovery from disease or asymptomatic infection usually confers lifetime immunity; immunization confers prolonged, but not lifetime, immunity	General unimmunized population are at risk; unimmunized children under 5 years are most susceptible; no passive immunity from mother; disease confers prolonged, but not lifetime, immunity	General unimmunized population are at risk; active immunity from tetanus toxoid persists for 10 years; tetanus immune globulin confers temporary immunity; infants born to immune mothers are protected at birth; active disease does not confer lifetime immunity	General unimmunized population is at risk; active immunization confers lifetime immunity; disease or subclinical infection confers type-specific lifetime immunity
Prevention and control	Two-dose vaccination of children: first dose between 12 and 15 mo of age; second dose between 4 and 6 year (see Table 26.3)	After initial immunization with diphtheria-pertussis-tetanus vaccine (DPT), immunization with diphtheria toxoid boosters every 10 years (see Table 26.3)	Childhood immunization with DPT (see Table 26.3) Immunization with DTaP or Tdap as indicated, an antibiotic effective against pertussis should be administered to all exposed persons, including health care workers, regardless of vaccination status	Active immunization with tetanus toxoid boosters every 10 year, and as prophylaxis after penetrating injuries for those whose last booster was more than 10 year ago	Active immunization with inactivated polio vaccine (IPV) in childhood as recommended (see Table 26.3) Adults at risk without record of polio vaccination should receive immunization (see Table 26.3)
Disease manifestations	Sudden mild fever and malaise, rash, or both; rash is progressive, changing from maculopapular to vesicular and then forming a crust or scab; lesions tend to be more numerous on covered parts of the body; can be on all mucous membranes and are highly pruritic; complications are more common in persons over 15 year old, infants under 1 year old, persons with HIV, and immunocompromised persons; virus can persist in a dormant state in sensory nerve endings and can reactivate, causing herpes zoster, or shingles	Acute onset; usually affecting the upper respiratory tract. Malaise, sore throat, anorexia, and low-grade fever. Lesions are caused by the release of a cytotoxin and manifest as a patch or patches of inflammation surrounding a grayish membrane; complications may result in severe swelling of the neck, thrombocytopenia, nephritis, polyneuropathies, and myocarditis	Pertussis (whooping cough) begins with upper respiratory cough and proceeds to a paroxysmal stage of coughing, often ending in vomiting; paroxysmal stage may last 1–2 mo or longer; complications include seizures, pneumonia, encephalopathy, and death	Tetanus (lockjaw) is an acute neurological illness caused by an anaerobic bacterium that produces an exotoxin in the portal of entry in the human host; tetanus causes gradually worsening neurological symptoms, including painful muscle contractions and spasms frequently resulting in death	Symptoms may range from inapparent illness, minor nonspecific illness (low fever and sore throat) to severe paralysis or death

Diagnosis	By symptoms	By symptoms with confirmatory bacteriological culture of nasal and throat secretions and from lesions	Paroxysmal stage diagnosis suspected; bacteriological culture of nasal or throat secretions	History of injury plus clinical symptoms; bacterium is rarely found in wound cultures	Isolation of the virus from fecal or oropharyngeal specimens
Treatment	Antiviral drugs within 1 week of exposure may modify severity; varicella-zoster immune globulin administered within 96 h of exposure can modify or prevent the disease	Single dose of equine antitoxin followed by a full course of antibiotic therapy	Treatment with antibiotics reduces the period of infectivity and may lessen the severity of the disease if given before the paroxysmal stage	Tetanus antitoxin and/or tetanus immune globulin (TIG), wound care with removal of necrotic tissue, supportive care	Supportive care
Report to local health authority?	Yes	Yes	Yes	Yes	Yes

	Measles	Mumps	Rubella	H. Influenza B	Pneumonia	Influenza
Occurrence	Worldwide; endemic and epidemic occurrences where immunization rates are low; still a major killer of children worldwide	Worldwide; recently increase in cases and outbreaks in close-contact settings among vaccinated persons; one-third of infected persons have subclinical infections	Worldwide and endemic where immunization rates are low; epidemics occur every 5–9 year; primarily a disease of children	Worldwide; most common in children 2 mo to 5 year of age; rare with widespread immunization	Worldwide; most common in children 2 mo to 3 year of age, the elderly, and immunocompromised adults	Worldwide; in pandemics, epidemics, localized outbreaks, and sporadic cases
Etiological agent(s)	Measles virus, a paramyxovirus	Mumps virus, a paramyxovirus	Rubella virus	H. influenzae serotype B (Hib)	Streptococcus pneumoniae	Orthomyxovirus family, three types affect humans: A, B, and C, each with many subtypes;
Reservoir	Humans	Humans	Humans	Humans	Humans (often found in respiratory passages of healthy persons)	Humans; some mammals (e.g., pigs, horses, mink, and ferrets) and birds
Transmission	Direct or indirect contact with nasal or throat secretions of infected person via respiratory droplets; highly communicable; transmission may occur for up to 2 h after a person with measles occupied an area	Direct contact with saliva (airborne or droplets) from infected person	Direct or indirect contact with nasopharyngeal secretions of infected person; transplacental transmission leads to congenital rubella syndrome (CRS)	Direct or indirect contact with droplets of nasopharyngeal secretions of infected person, close contact with a case-patient can lead to outbreaks	Direct or indirect contact with droplets of nasopharyngeal secretions of infected person, or by autoinoculation in persons carrying the bacteria in their upper respiratory tract	Direct or indirect via large droplets or aerosol small droplets, exposure to fomites
Incubation period	11–12 days until fever that lasts 2–4 days; 14 days until rash, range 7–21 days	16–18 days; range 12–25 days	14 days; range 12–23 days	Unknown; probably 2–4 days	Unknown; probably 1–3 days	2 days, range, 1–4 days

Continued

TABLE 26.5 Chain of Transmission and Control: Childhood Vaccine–Preventable Diseases—cont'd

	Measles	Mumps	Rubella	H. Influenza B	Pneumonia	Influenza
Communicability period	4 days before to 4 days after appearance of the rash	2 days before to 5 days after onset of parotitis; but the range can be 7 days before to 15 days after onset; can be transmitted by persons with subclinical infections	7 days before to 7 days after onset of rash; highly communicable; infants with CRS may shed virus for months after birth	Variable as long as organisms are in nasopharynx; noncommunicable within 24–48 h after onset of effective antibiotic therapy	Unknown, presumably as long as organism is found in nasopharynx; may be prolonged in immunocompromised persons	Day before symptom onset to 5–7 days after clinical onset in adults; up to 10 days after clinical onset in children
Susceptibility and resistance	General population who has not had disease or immunization is at risk; lifetime immunity after illness; infants of mothers who have had the disease are protected for 6–9 mo; infants of immunized mothers have variable level of passive antibody; length of immunity following immunization is unknown; revaccination is recommended for some groups	Lifetime immunity develops after subclinical or clinical illness; however, increase in mumps cases since 2006 with most cases in persons fully vaccinated	General unimmunized or previously uninfected population is at risk; lifetime immunity after illness; infants born to immune mothers are protected for 6–9 mo; long-term immunity following immunization	General unimmunized or previously uninfected population is at risk; immunity acquired transplacentally, by infection, and by immunization	General population is probably at risk; immunity is acquired transplacentally, from prior infection, or from immunization	General population is at risk; persons over 65 years, pregnant women, and children younger than 5 years are at risk for complications, infection and immunization produce immunity to only one subtype of the virus
Prevention and control	Active immunization with live, attenuated measles vaccine (see Table 26.3)	Active immunization with live, attenuated mumps virus vaccine (see Table 26.3)	Active immunization with live, attenuated rubella virus vaccine in childhood (see Table 26.3); immunity in adolescent girls should be ensured	Active immunization with Hib conjugate vaccine (see Table 26.3)	Pneumococcal conjugate vaccine (PCV) for infants and children; pneumococcal polysaccharide vaccine (PPV) for high-risk groups (see Table 26.3)	Active immunization yearly prior to influenza season
Disease manifestations	Acute-onset fever of 101°F or higher, cough, coryza, conjunctivitis, Koplik spots on the buccal mucosa, and a red rash usually lasting 5–6 days that begins on the face and becomes generalized down and outward to hands and feet; measles can progress into severe complications, including pneumonia, encephalitis, and death	Acute-onset fever and painful swelling of the salivary and parotid glands; nonspecific myalgia, malaise, headache, low-grade fever; may be asymptomatic; complications range from pancreatitis, meningoencephalitis to permanent hearing impairment and orchitis in postpubescent males, but rarely sterility	Maculopapular rash and postauricular, occipital, and posterior cervical lymphadenopathy; children are usually relatively asymptomatic, but adults may experience fever, headache, and malaise; rare complications include encephalitis and thrombocytopenia; congenital defects in fetuses of pregnant women who are infected: Congenital rubella syndrome	Hib can affect multiple organ systems, resulting in meningitis, epiglottitis, otitis media, pneumonia, arthritis, and cellulitis, with symptoms associated with those conditions; complications are serious and include septic arthritis, life-threatening airway obstruction, fulminating infection, and death	Acute-onset symptoms of fever and chills, meningitis, bacteremia, or pneumonia	Acute-onset dry cough, fever, headache, myalgia, sore throat, and other generalized symptoms; symptom severity depends on the subtype of the virus; complications include pneumonia, otitis media, meningitis, Reye syndrome, and death

Diagnosis	Throat swab specimen for reverse transcriptase polymerase chain reaction (RT-PCR) and a serum specimen for IgM, viral genotyping can help track transmission	Clinical presentation; RT-PCR or viral culture of virus from oral and throat spray, and urine	Serological testing, clinical diagnosis is unreliable as many rash illnesses mimic rubella	Identification of organisms in blood or cerebrospinal fluid	Isolation of the organism from the blood or other sterile body site	Clinical findings, isolation of virus from nasal or pharyngeal secretions, serological testing, antigen detection, gene amplification, and rapid diagnostic test
Treatment	Supportive care	Supportive care	Supportive care	10–14 days of antibiotics	Antibiotics	Antiviral drugs may be indicated for prevention or treatment
Report to local health authority?	Yes	Yes	Yes	Yes	Varies by state, epidemics only	Varies by state; influenza-associated deaths among children younger than age 18 years and a human infection with a novel influenza a virus are nationally notifiable

Modified from Grimes DE, Grimes KA, Zack CM: Infectious diseases. In Thompson JM, et al., editors: *Mosby's clinical nursing*, ed 5, St. Louis, 2002, Mosby; with data from Heymann DL, editor: *Control of communicable diseases manual*, ed 20, Washington, DC, 2015, American Public Health Association; Centers for Disease Control and Prevention: *Immunization schedules: for health care providers*. Last reviewed February 11, 2021. Available from: https://www.cdc.gov/vaccines/schedules/index.html. Accessed June 25, 2021; Centers for Disease Control and Prevention: *Epidemiology and prevention of vaccine-preventable diseases*. Hamborsky J, Kroger A, Wolfe S, editors, ed 13, Washington DC, 2015, Public Health Foundation. Updated. Available from: https://www.cdc.gov/vaccines/pubs/pinkbook/chapters.html. 18 out of 22 chapters updated in 2020–21.

RESEARCH HIGHLIGHTS

Human Papilloma Virus Immunization

Humans are subject to infection from more than 100 human papilloma viruses (HPVs). HPV is the most common STI in the United States with an estimated 43 million infections in 2018. HPV infects skin and mucous membrane cells and is transmitted by direct contact. Pathogenic HPV has been recovered from fingertips, nails, breast tissue, sinonasal areas, nipples, and hair follicles. In addition, it has been found in 6.5% of the oral cavities of a random sample of Americans and can readily be transmitted from infected mothers to their children during childbirth and by touch after birth. The vast majority of HPVs are not pathogenic—low-risk HPVs, but a small number are known to be oncogenic—high-risk HPBs. High-risk HPVs can cause several types of cancer. There are about 14 high-risk HPVs including HPV 16, 18, 31, 33, 35, 39, 45, 51, 52, 56, 58, 59, 66, and 68. Two of these, HPV16 and HPV18, are responsible for most HPV-related cancers and to be causative agents for cancers of the cervix, vulva, vagina, anus, penis, and oropharynx; they may also contribute to prostate and breast cancer. In addition, HPV six and HPV 11 are known to cause genital warts.

Three vaccines that protect against oncogenic HPVs have been approved for use in the United States; however, only Gardasil 9 is distributed in the United States. Gardasil 9 protects against HPV types 6, 11, 16, d 18, 31, 33, 45, 52, and 58. Currently, the CDC recommends that both boys and girls between 11 and 12 years of age (minimum age 9 years) be immunized against HPV. For those who did not receive the vaccine at these ages, it can be administered up to age 26 (CDC, 2020c, Epidemiology). HPV vaccination is not recommended for adults over the age of 26 years. A two-dose series is recommended when first dose is before their 15th birthday (with exceptions such as immunocompromising conditions). A three-dose series is recommended for those who receive the first dose on or after their 15th birthday.

Widespread HPV vaccine use in other countries has proved to be extremely effective, in 2019 54.2% of US adolescents were up to date with the recommended vaccination schedule. Uptake of the vaccine in the United States has been poor for several reasons, including cost, parental concerns that children will become sexually active, concerns about the safety of the vaccine, lack of understanding of the nature of transmission of HPV, and failure of health professionals to promote and adhere to the recommendations (Wilson et al., 2016). CDC provides strategies for healthcare providers to improve vaccination rates: bundle recommendation with other adolescent vaccines; consistent message from all office staff; take every patient encounter to check, recommend and administer vaccines; share personal examples; and answer all questions (CDC, 2019b, HPV).

Research has shown that girls and boys who were vaccinated did not have sexual debut earlier and did not have an increase in sexual partners (Brouwer et al., 2019). Unfortunately, many health professionals are not aware of the widespread nature of HPV, its association with certain cancers, or of the vaccine and its safety. Some health professionals have viewed the transmission of HPV as occurring only during sex and have not allayed parental concerns about potential increases in sexual behavior or the safety of the vaccine. Education is critical, because research shows that young women are three times more likely to undergo immunization if it is strongly recommended by their healthcare providers. Furthermore, even partial immunization, both at the individual level and within a community, has been very effective in reducing overall prevalence of HPV through the effects of herd immunity.

Implications for Nurses

1. Nurses need to educate patients and others that HPV is not only sexually transmitted, but can be transmitted by other means.
2. Nurses can be central to reduction of a number of cancers by encouraging widespread use of the HPV vaccine for both males and females as recommended by the CDC.

Further Reading

Centers for Disease Control and Prevention: *HPV vaccination coverage data*, n.d.a. https://www.cdc.gov/hcp/vacc-coverage.html.

Centers for Disease Control and Prevention: *Human papilloma virus (HPV) for healthcare professionals*, n.d.b. https://www.cdc.gov/hpv/hcp/index.html.

Centers for Disease Control and Prevention: *Confidentiality issues and use of sexually transmitted disease services among sexually experienced persons aged 15–25 years—United States, 2013–2015*, 2017, 2017. https://www.cdc.gov/mmwr/volumes/66/wr/mm6609a1.htm.

Centers for Disease Control and Prevention: *Vaccine safety: human papilloma virus (HPV) vaccine*, 2020, 2020. http://www.gov/vaccinesafety/Vaccines/HPV/indx.html.

Grimes RM, Benjamins LJ, Williams KL: Counseling about the HPV vaccine: desexualize, educate, and advocate, *J Pediatr Adolesc Gynecol* 26(4):243, 2013.

HIV, a retrovirus, is the organism that causes the syndrome known as AIDS. In 2019, an estimated 1.2 million persons 13 years and older were living with HIV infection, and 13% had not yet been diagnosed (CDC, 2021b, HIV surveillance). After initial infection and a possible flulike illness during the first few weeks, the disease is typically asymptomatic for months to years. In most cases, the infected person does not know that he or she is infected and continues to transmit the virus to others. HIV usually manifests gradually as conditions that result from inadequate immune system function as the virus slowly attacks the body's immune system. Over time, the body loses its ability to fight illnesses, and opportunistic infections occur and become recurrent. A standardized case definition for AIDS was specified by CDC in 1993. An updated case definition for AIDS as well as revised classifications for HIV infection can be found at http://www.cdc.gov/hiv/statistics/recommendations/. The critical elements for both HIV and AIDS are summarized for easy reference in Table 26.9.

Screening is recommended as routine health care, once for everyone between 13 and 64, and yearly for those at higher risk. For people who are at high risk for HIV infection and do not have HIV, may prevent or decrease risk of HIV with pre-exposure prophylaxis (PrEP) when taken daily and consistently (CDC, 2020b, HIV PrEP).

HIV infection is defined by laboratory criteria using three types of diagnostic tests: nucleic acid tests (NAT), antigen/antibody tests, and antibody tests. NAT, not routinely used for screening, can detect HIV infection 10 to 33 days after exposure. Antigen/antibody tests, common in the United States, are based on detection of HIV antibodies and/or p24 antigen and can detect HIV infection 18 to 45 days after an exposure. Antibody tests look for antibodies in oral fluid or blood, and can detect within 23 to 90 days after exposure. Further information on testing for HIV can be found at http://www.cdc.gov/hiv/testing/index.html.

Treatment for HIV and AIDS is complex and changes frequently. Of note, early treatment with ART is preferred as a

TABLE 26.6 Chain of Transmission and Control: Hepatitis

	Hepatitis A	Hepatitis B	Hepatitis C	Hepatitis D	Hepatitis E
Occurrence	Worldwide; endemic in some areas, sporadic and epidemic with cyclic recurrence; outbreaks in institutions where sanitation is poor	Worldwide; endemic; highest in young adults, homosexually active men, persons engaging in unprotected sex, injection drug users, health care and public safety workers	Worldwide; directly related to prevalence of injection drug use in the population, HCV in the donated blood supply, and lack of use of parenteral precautions in health care	Worldwide; occurs epidemically and endemically in population at risk for HBV infection; declining in areas where chronic carriers of HBsAg have declined	Epidemic and sporadic cases, particularly in developing countries; highest in young adults; rare in children or the elderly
Etiological agent(s)	Hepatitis a virus (HAV)	Hepatitis B virus (HBV); made up of a core antigen, HBcAg, and a surface antigen, HBsAg; HBV has at least 10 different genotypes	Hepatitis C virus (HCV), which has 7 genotypes and 67 subtypes	Hepatitis delta virus (HDV), which consists of a coat of HBsAg and an internal antigen, the delta antigen	Hepatitis E virus (HEV)
Reservoir(s)	Humans are only natural hosts	Humans and some primates in Africa and Southeast Asia are infected with HBV	Humans; virus has been transmitted experimentally to chimpanzees	Humans; virus can be transmitted experimentally to chimpanzees and to woodchucks	Humans and nonhuman primates, pigs, chickens, and cattle
Transmission	Person-to-person by fecal-oral route; ingestion of contaminated food, water, shellfish, etc.	Direct and indirect contact with blood and serum-derived fluids; sexual contact; perinatal	Parenteral; sexual and perinatal transmission are less likely to occur	Similar to that of HBV; must coinfect with HBV	Person-to-person by fecal-oral route; contaminated food or water. Consumption of uncooked/undercooked pork or deer meat
Incubation period	28–30 days; range 15–50 days	60–90 days; range 45–180 days	6–9 week; range 2 week –6 mo	3–7 week	26–42 days; range 15 –60 days
Communicability period	Latter half of incubation period to 1 week after onset of jaundice	During incubation period and throughout clinical course of disease; infectious any time that HBsAg present, carrier state may persist for years	Virus persists indefinitely	Throughout acute and chronic disease	Unknown; virus has been detected in stools 1 week prior to onset to 30 days after onset of symptoms and 4 week after ingestion of contaminated food or water
Susceptibility and resistance	General population is at risk; usually affects children and young adults; probable lifetime immunity after infection	General population is at risk; disease is mild in children; lifetime immunity follows infection if antibody to HBV develops and test for HBV is negative	General population is at risk; degree of immunity after infection is not known	All persons susceptible to HBV or who have an HBV infection and are coinfected with HDV	Pregnant women in third trimester have mortality reaching 10%–30%, may be serious threat to people with preexisting chronic liver disease and organ-transplant recipients
Prevention and control	Active immunization with inactivated whole-virus vaccines (see Table 26.3); eliminate common sources of infection with sanitation; improve hygienic practices and hand washing; cook shellfish; immunize high-risk groups or persons in high-risk situations with HAV vaccine; for postexposure: Administer vaccine and immune globulin (IG) within 2 week; use universal precautions	Routinely immunize infants, children, and high-risk groups (see Table 26.3); at birth give HBIG and Hep B vaccine to infants born to HBsAg-positive mothers, followed by additional vaccine doses at 1 and 6 months of age; immunize persons exposed to HBV; test all donated blood for HBV antigen; practice safe sex; use universal precautions	Apply HBV control measures except immunization; no vaccine exists at this time, and IG does not prevent HCV infection	Apply HBV prevention and control measures; however, HBIG, IG, and hepatitis B vaccine do not prevent HDV infection in those already infected with HBV	No vaccine; IG not effective; sanitation appears to be the only effective measure of prevention; access to clean drinking water, avoid raw pork and venison

Continued

TABLE 26.6 Chain of Transmission and Control: Hepatitis—cont'd

	Hepatitis A	Hepatitis B	Hepatitis C	Hepatitis D	Hepatitis E
Disease manifestations	Acute-onset fever, anorexia, malaise, dark urine, and jaundice, usually lasting 2 mo; has a very low fatality rate and, although rare, can last up to 6 mo	Insidious onset that ranges from asymptomatic illness to generalized nonspecific symptoms, such as anorexia, nausea, vomiting, and dark urine before jaundice, occasionally resulting in fulminant fatal hepatitis	Like HBV, has an insidious onset; symptoms vary from completely asymptomatic (80%) to the rare fulminating, fatal disease; mild symptoms are same as those for HBV; chronic hepatitis develops in half of those infected with HCV	Abrupt onset with range of symptoms similar to those of HBV; always associated with HBV infection, either coinfection or as a suprainfection in persons with chronic hepatitis B,	Clinical course similar to that of HAV: Fatigue, fever, poor appetite, stomach pain, nausea, jaundice, dark urine, clay-colored stool, joint pain; no chronic form
Diagnosis	Serologic testing; serum antibodies (anti-HAV) detectable 5—10 days postexposure	Presence in sera of HBsAg, anti-HBsAg (antibodies), HBcAg and anti-HBcAG, HBeAG and anti-HBeAG	Presence of serum antibodies to HCV (anti-HCV) and HCV RNA. Tests to detect antibodies do not distinguish between acute, chronic, and resolved infection	Presence of serum antibodies to HDV (anti-HDV) and/or HDV RNA	Exclusion of other causes of hepatitis, particularly HAV; presence of serum antibodies, anti-HEV; presence of HEV RNA in feces and serum
Treatment	Supportive care	Supportive care	Treatment no longer depends on genotype. Regimen may include interferon, peginterferon, ribavirin, or any HCV direct-acting antiviral (DAA) agent	Pegylated-interferon has some efficacy and new therapies are being evaluated	Supportive care; no specific antiviral therapy for acute hepatitis E
Report case to local health authority?	Yes	Yes	Yes	Yes	Yes

Modified from Grimes DE, Grimes KA, Zack CM: Infectious diseases. In Thompson JM, et al., editors: *Mosby's clinical nursing*, ed 5, St. Louis, 2002, Mosby; with data from Heymann DL, editor: *Control of communicable diseases manual*, ed 20, Washington, DC, 2015, American Public Health Association; Centers for Disease Control and Prevention: *Vaccines and preventable diseases: diseases and the vaccines that prevent them*. Last reviewed November 22, 2016. Available from: https://www.cdc.gov/vaccines/vpd/index.html. Accessed June 10, 2021. Centers for Disease Control and Prevention: *Epidemiology and prevention of vaccine-preventable diseases*. Hamborsky J, Kroger A, Wolfe S, editors, ed 13, Washington, DC, 2015, Public Health Foundation. Updated. Available from: https://www.cdc.gov/vaccines/pubs/pinkbook/chapters.html. 18 out of 22 chapters updated in 2020–21.

TABLE 26.7 Chain of Transmission and Control: Tuberculosis

TUBERCULOSIS

Occurrence	Worldwide; tuberculosis (TB) cases have declined in the United States since 1993; multidrug-resistant cases continue to be reported but in the US the percentage has remained stable; the US 2019 case count was the lowest number of TB cases on record; most newly reported cases in the United States occur in non-US born persons and persons having diabetes, excessive alcohol use, coinfected with HIV, using both noninjectable and injectable drugs, homeless, or living in correctional settings. Some reported cases are a reactivation of a latent infection in older age groups and those with chronic diseases.
Etiological agent	*Mycobacterium tuberculosis*; less often *Mycobacterium bovis* or *Mycobacterium africanum*
Reservoir	Humans; diseased cattle for *M. bovis*
Transmission	Inhalation of airborne droplets from the sputum of persons with active disease; children rarely transmit TB because they do not cough forcefully; infrequently by ingestion or skin penetration

	Infection (New or Latent)	Active Disease (Case)
Incubation period	2–10 week	Anytime during one's lifetime
Communicability period	Not communicable unless there are viable bacilli in the sputum	As long as bacilli are in sputum; may be communicable for years in inadequately treated persons
Susceptibility and resistance	Anyone, such as healthcare workers, family members, or the institutionalized, working or living in close contact with a person who has active disease can become infected	Vulnerable persons such as children and persons who are older than 65 years, have chronic diseases or compromised immune systems, are malnourished, etc.
Prevention and control	Perform skin testing in high-risk groups (e.g., healthcare workers), and treat those with new infections to prevent progression to active disease; routine skin testing, particularly of children, is no longer recommended in United States; bacille Calmette-Guérin (BCG) vaccine is still used in some parts of the world	Promptly identify, diagnose, and treat those with active disease; ensure compliance with treatment; initiate respiratory isolation until sputum is clear of bacilli; have patient wear a mask; examine close contacts of TB cases and treat, if infected
Disease manifestations	Initial infection goes unnoticed; 5%–10% of infected persons eventually have active disease, 50% of those within the first 2 years	Onset of active disease can occur immediately after an initial infection or after a variable latency period for untreated persons; disease onset is usually insidious, with fever, night sweats, and weight loss; cough with pulmonary disease; extrapulmonary symptoms correspond with the location of disseminated bacilli and lesions
Diagnosis	TB skin test reaction and/or blood tests (interferon-gamma release assays); immunosuppressed persons may have a negative skin test reaction due to anergy. Skin test results: 5-mm induration = positive for the immunosuppressed and close contacts with active cases; 10 mm induration = positive for infections in persons <2 year and persons with high-risk conditions; 15 mm induration = positive for all low-risk persons	10%–20% of those with active disease have a negative skin test reaction; demonstration of acid-fast bacilli in stained smears of sputum or other body fluids; isolation of organism from cultured specimen; radiological evidence of TB in lungs or elsewhere
Treatment	Treat with isoniazid (INH) for 6–9 mo for all new/latent infections to prevent progression to active disease; treat HIV-infected persons with INH in combination with antiretrovirals	Treat with combination of antimicrobial drugs to which the strain of *Mycobacterium* is susceptible, such as isoniazid (INH), rifampin (RIF), pyrazinamide (PZA), and ethambutol (EMB), for 6–12 mo or until sputum cultures are negative; monitor adherence to therapy carefully because nonadherence is increasing drug resistance
Report to local health authority?	No	Yes

Data from Heymann DL, editor: *Control of communicable diseases manual*, ed 20, Washington, DC, 2015, American Public Health Association; Centers for Disease Control and Prevention: *Tuberculosis (TB): data and statistics*. Last reviewed October 29, 2020. Available from: https://www.cdc.gov/tb/statistics/default.htm. Accessed June 25, 2021; Duetch-Feldman M, Pratt RH, Price SF, Tsang CA., Self JL: Tuberculosis-United States, 2020. *Morb Mortal Wkly Rep* 70(12):409–414, 2021. https://doi.org/10.15585/mmwr.mm7012a1. Available from: https://www.cdc.gov/mmwr/volumes/70/wr/pdfs/mm7012a1-H.pdf.

TABLE 26.8 Chain of Transmission and Control: Sexually Transmitted Infections (STIs)

	Gonorrhea	Chlamydia Trachomatis	Syphilis	Genital Herpes	Warts, Human Papilloma Virus (HPV) Infection
Occurrence	Worldwide; highest in males and females 15–30 year old	Worldwide; most prevalent STD; continues to increase	Worldwide and increasing; highest in males and females 20–30 year old	Worldwide and increasing; highest in males and females 15–30 year old	Worldwide; most common STD (see research highlights box)
Etiological agent	Neisseria gonorrhoeae, the gonococcus	Chlamydia trachomatis	Treponema pallidum	Herpes simplex virus (HSV) types 1 and 2	HPV, which has 100 types
Reservoir	Humans	Humans	Humans	Humans	Humans
Transmission	Contact with exudates from mucous membranes of infected persons; usually by direct sexual contact, although the pathogens can be transmitted during childbirth	Contact with exudates from mucous membranes of infected persons; usually by direct sexual contact, although the pathogens can be transmitted during childbirth	Direct sexual contact with infectious exudates from lesions; transplacental; blood transfusion early in infection of donor	Direct contact with secretions from mucous membranes and lesions; transplacental	Direct contact with infected skin and mucous membranes; autoinoculation; during childbirth
Incubation period	2–7 days	7–10 days	3 week; range 10 days to 3 mo	2–12 days	2–3 mo; range 1–20 mo
Communicability period	Months if untreated	Unknown	When moist lesions are present during the primary and secondary stages, generally 1 year	During and up to 7 week after primary lesions; transient shedding of virus occurs in the absence of lesions for years	Unknown, presumed to be high, probably as long as lesions persist
Susceptibility and resistance	General population is at risk; antibodies are not protective against reinfection	General population is at risk; no acquired immunity	General population is at risk; however, only 30% of exposures lead to infection; some immunity develops over time	General population is at risk; immune response does not prevent recurrence	General population is at risk; immunosuppressed persons are more susceptible
Prevention and control	Safer sexual practices; detect and treat cases and contacts; test pregnant women for infection and treat		Safer sexual practices; cesarean delivery if lesions are present during late pregnancy		Routinely immunize females and males aged 11–12 year against HPV, can start at age 9, with "catch-up" vaccination for everyone through age 26; HPV vaccination may be recommended for some adults 27–45 years who were not vaccinated; safer sexual practices

Disease manifestations	*Males:* Urethritis with purulent discharge from anterior urethra. *Females:* Mucopurulent cervicitis, often asymptomatic; 20% progress to endometritis, salpingitis, and pelvic peritonitis. Both genders may have pharyngeal or anorectal infections, depending on their sexual practices; individuals are frequently coinfected with N. gonorrhoeae and C. trachomatis	*Males:* Urethritis with purulent discharge from anterior urethra. *Females:* Mucopurulent cervicitis; 20% progress to endometritis, salpingitis, and pelvic peritonitis. Both genders may have pharyngeal or anorectal infections depending on their sexual practices; individuals are frequently coinfected with N. gonorrhoeae and C. trachomatis	*Primary:* Moist lesion appearing within 3 week at area of contact. *Secondary:* Symmetrical maculopapular rash in 4–6 week. *Latency:* Indefinite time, no symptoms. *Tertiary:* Late lesions of bone, viscera, central nervous system (CNS), and cardiovascular system	Local, primary, vesicular lesions, period of latency and recurring, localized lesions; lesions start at area of contact but may spread to surrounding tissues or be disseminated in body, even to the CNS; other disease symptoms depend on extent of dissemination	Skin and mucous membrane lesions that are circumscribed, hyperkeratotic, and of varying sizes and shapes; certain types of HPV, specifically 16 and 18, have been found to be associated with cancer of the cervix, vulva, anus, penis, vagina, and oropharynx; HPV 16 and 18 account for more than 70% of these cancers
Diagnosis	Gram staining of discharges, bacteriological cultures, or tests that detect gonococcal nucleic acid	Failure to detect N. gonorrhoeae in discharges from symptomatic persons; mononuclear antibody tests of discharges	Serological testing of blood and cerebrospinal fluid, if indicated	Detection of cell changes in tissue scrapings or biopsy specimens; isolation of virus from lesions or other affected tissue; serological tests	Visualization of the lesion; excision and histological examination of the lesion
Treatment	Treat with antibiotics, preferably with single dose, intramuscular antibiotics, such as ceftriaxone; treatment depends on extent of infection; follow-up testing is recommended	Treat with antibiotics such as single-dose azithromycin or 7 days of doxycycline; advisable to treat for gonorrhea and chlamydia concurrently	Treat with antibiotics; treatment differs with stage of the disease	Treatment with antivirals; treatment varies depending on area of lesions and whether they are disseminated	Removal of the warts by freezing with liquid nitrogen or other chemical; treatment of cancers
Report to local health authority?	Yes	Yes	Yes, including congenital syphilis	No	No

Modified from Grimes DE, Grimes KA, Zack CM: Infectious diseases. In Thompson JM, et al., editors: *Mosby's clinical nursing*, ed 5, St. Louis, 2008, Mosby; with data from Heymann DL, editor: *Control of communicable diseases manual*, ed 20, Washington, DC, 2015, American Public Health Association; Centers for Disease Control and Prevention: *HPV vaccine*, 2009. Last reviewed March 17, 2020. Available from: www.cdc.gov/vaccines/vpd-vac/hpv/default.htm#vacc. Accessed June 25, 2021; Centers for Disease Control and Prevention: *Sexually transmitted diseases (STD): human papilloma virus (HPV)*. Last reviewed 2021. Available from: http://www.cdc.gov/std/hpv/. Accessed June 20, 2021; Centers for Disease Control and Prevention: *Sexually transmitted diseases (STDs): treatment and screening*, 2015. Available from: https://www.cdc.gov/mmwr/pdf/rr/rr6403.pdf; Centers for Disease Control and Prevention: *Epidemiology and prevention of vaccine-preventable diseases*. Hamborsky J, Kroger A, Wolfe S, editors, ed 13, Washington, DC, 2015, Public Health Foundation. Updated. Available from: https://www.cdc.gov/vaccines/pubs/pinkbook/chapters.html. 18 out of 22 chapters updated in 2020–21.

TABLE 26.9 Chain of Transmission and Control: Human Immunodeficiency Virus/Acquired Immunodeficiency Syndrome (HIV/AIDS)

	HIV/AIDS	
Occurrences	Worldwide estimates in 2020: About 37.6 million persons were living with HIV; 1.5 million new infections in 2020 and 690,000 deaths. Since the start of the epidemic, approximately 78 million people have become infected with HIV	
Etiological agent	HIV is a retrovirus with two serologically and geographically distinct types (HIV-1 and HIV-2); HIV-1 makes up 90%–95% of the world's cases; it may be more pathogenic, lead to more rapid disease progression, and have higher mother-to-infant transmission than does HIV-2; multiple subtypes (sometimes called *clades*) have been identified for both HIV-1 and HIV-2	
Reservoir	Humans; HIV may have evolved from a chimpanzee virus	
Transmission	Direct person-to-person through unprotected sexual contact or from mother to fetus or mother to infant (during birth or by breastfeeding) Indirect through contact of abraded skin or mucous membranes with infected blood or body fluids, injection of contaminated blood or fluids, use of contaminated needles, or transplantation of organs from infected persons	

	HIV Infection	**AIDS**
Incubation period	9 days–6 mo before antibodies are detectable	<1–15 year; may be longer with effective antiretroviral therapy
Communicability period	Presumed to be <10 days after infection and lasting throughout life; may be highest in early infection when viral load is highest, and again later when clinical status worsens	
Susceptibility and resistance	General population is at risk; increased risk for infection with untreated ulcerative STDs and in uncircumcised males; evidence that some persons are less susceptible because of chemokine-receptor polymorphisms; very small percentage of infected persons do not progress to AIDS, for an unknown reason	
Prevention and control	Preexposure prophylaxis (PrEP) with tenofovir-emtricitabine is highly effective in preventing HIV infection; postexposure prophylaxis (PEP) is recommended as a prevention option after a single high-risk exposure to HIV during sex, through sharing needles or syringes, or from a sexual assault; practice universal precautions and safer sex; treat pregnant women with antiretrovirals to prevent transmission to fetus; teach infected women to avoid breastfeeding; treat drug users and provide needle exchange programs for injection drug users; treat STDs to decrease chance of acquisition of HIV through sores on mucous membranes; maintain a safe blood supply; encourage autologous blood transfusions, when possible, early treatment of HIV-infected persons suppresses the virus enough to decrease risk of transmission to others	Adherence to effective antiretroviral therapy delays progression to AIDS; prophylactic treatment for opportunistic infections delays onset of conditions associated with AIDS diagnosis
Disease manifestations	Within 10 days to several weeks an infected person experiences an acute, self-limiting illness lasting for 1–2 weeks with symptoms that mimic other conditions (fever, rash, pharyngitis, myalgia, lymphadenopathy, and malaise); although immune deficiency may progress, the person may be without further symptoms for years	Progressive immune deficiency and increasing susceptibility to life-threatening infections and cancers in untreated populations
Diagnosis	*Early after infection:* The HIV p24, or HIV-1 RNA tests; recommended laboratory-based screening test for HIV is a combination antigen/antibody assay that detects antibodies against HIV, as well as p24 antigen. *99% within 6 week after infection, may take 6 weeks to 6 months.* Earliest diagnosis is 9 days with HIV-1 RNA	A standardized case definition for AIDS was specified by the CDC in 1993 An updated case definition for AIDS and revised classifications for HIV infection can be found in the CDC document cited in the "resources" portion
Treatment	Treatment with antiretroviral drugs to suppress the virus, not eradicate it Currently seven classes of drugs are available: Nucleoside reverse transcriptase inhibitors, nonnucleoside reverse transcriptase inhibitors, protease inhibitors, integrase inhibitors, fusion inhibitors, postattachment inhibitors, and CCR5 antagonists; each attacks a different target in the reproduction process of the virus. Treatment requires almost perfect adherence to regimen because development of drug-resistant HIV is common. Current guidelines recommend early treatment to suppress the virus to prevent transmission and treatment as preexposure prophylaxis (PrEP) for high-risk persons	

Continued

TABLE 26.9 Chain of Transmission and Control: Human Immunodeficiency Virus/Acquired Immunodeficiency Syndrome (HIV/AIDS)—cont'd

Report to local health authority?	Yes, in all states	Yes, in all states

Resources for Information on HIV/AIDS
Case Definition:
CDC definition (http://www.cdc.gov/hiv/pdf/statistics_HIV_Case_Def_Consult_Summary.pdf) **OR** *2016 UNAIDS Report on the Global AIDS Epidemic* (https://www.unaids.org/en/resources/fact-sheet and https://www.unaids.org/en)
Statistics: https://www.hiv.gov/hiv-basics/overview/data-and-trends/statistics
Testing: www.cdc.gov/hiv/testing
Treatment: https://clinicalinfo.hiv.gov/en or https://hivinfo.nih.gov/
Treatment as prevention and pre-exposure prophylaxis: https://www.cdc.gov/hiv/guidelines/index.html or https://www.cdc.gov/hiv/guidelines/preventing.html

Data from Heymann DL, editor: *Control of communicable diseases manual,* ed 20, Washington, DC, 2015; UNAIDS: *Global HIV and AIDS statistics—fact sheet,* Preliminary UNAIDS 2021 epidemiological estimates. Available from: https://www.unaids.org/en/resources/fact-sheet; HIV.gov: *Global Statistics,* 2020. Accessed June 10, 2021 from: https://www.hiv.gov/hiv-basics/overview/data-and-trends/global-statistics; Centers for Disease Control and Prevention: *CDC yellow book, traveler health: chapter 4 travel-related infectious diseases HIV infection* by Philip J. Peters and John T. Brooks, 2019. Available from: https://wwwnc.cdc.gov/travel/yellowbook/2020/travel-related-infectious-diseases/hiv-infection. Accessed June 10, 2021.

way of controlling transmission of the virus, extending health, reduction of viral load, and reducing HIV-related illness (CDC, 2020a, HIV testing). The benefit of treatment is HIV medication can lower the viral load to an undetectable level. An undetectable viral load ensures no risk of transmitting HIV to an HIV-negative partner through sex (CDC, 2020b, PrEP).

The U.S. Food and Drug Administration has approved many drugs for HIV infection and AIDS-related conditions. At present, there are nine classes of antiretroviral drugs, each corresponding to different mechanisms whereby HIV invades the cells of the immune system. Current information on treatment is available at https://www.cdc.gov/hiv/basics/livingwithhiv/treatment.html and the National Institutes of Health (NIH) Office of Aids Research at https://hivinfo.nih.gov/understanding-hiv-fact-sheets/fda-approved-hiv-medicines.

Exposure of health care personnel to HIV, although rare, remains a concern for the CDC and health care workers. The CDC continues to update recommendations for postexposure prophylaxis for occupational exposures. These guidelines are among the many that can be downloaded from the CDC's website. Additional resources include a postexposure hotline for clinicians, the PEPline, at 1-888-448-4911, which is available 9 to 2 a.m. eastern time. Current information from the CDC is the postexposure prophylaxis with resources and guidelines at https://www.cdc.gov/hiv/risk/pep/.

Eradication of HIV/AIDS depends on safe and effective HIV prevention options, access to ART, and development of a vaccine and the infrastructure necessary to vaccinate populations at risk worldwide. In 2021, the NIH research includes two late-stage vaccine trials taking place in multiple nations (National Institute for Health, 2020, HIV vaccine development). Until a vaccine is available control of HIV/AIDS currently depends on preventing transmission of the virus and ART. Problems with

adherence to the therapy are interfering with the "treatment as prevention" approach.

 ACTIVE LEARNING

Log on to the CDC website to obtain the most recent guidelines for treating persons with HIV/AIDS, STIs, or TB.

PREVENTION OF COMMUNICABLE DISEASES

All practicing nurses have a role in primary, secondary, and tertiary prevention of communicable diseases. Examples of appropriate interventions for individuals are reviewed here and in Table 26.10, which also provides applications of levels of prevention to the individual and population levels.

Primary Prevention

Primary prevention of communicable diseases involves measures to prevent transmission of an infectious agent and to prevent pathology in the person exposed to an infection. All of the activities described in the section on breaking the chain of transmission are primary prevention activities. Immunization is primary prevention. Changing the behaviors that lead to exposure to a pathogen is primary prevention. See Tables 26.5–26.9 for primary preventions specific to the conditions listed in those tables.

Secondary Prevention

Secondary prevention consists of activities to detect infections early and effectively treat persons who are infected. These actions prevent not only progression of the infectious disease but also transmission of the pathogen to others. Reporting infectious diseases, investigating contacts, notifying partners, finding

TABLE 26.10   Examples of Primary, Secondary, and Tertiary Prevention Activities for Control of Infectious Diseases at the Individual and Population Levels

Infectious Disease	Individual	Population
Primary Prevention		
Sexually transmitted infections	Teach safe sex practices. Provide education and access to HPV vaccine.	Place condom machines in accessible areas in places where young adults congregate. Marketing campaign for PrEP (preexposure prophylaxis) to prevent HIV from sex or injection drug use.
Diseases caused by blood-borne pathogens	Teach barrier precautions to all healthcare workers. Teach injecting drug users about dangers of sharing needles.	Provide an adequate supply of gloves and sharps containers in patient care areas. Initiate citywide needle exchange programs and methadone programs.
Vaccine-preventable diseases	Ensure that all children who come to the clinic have age-appropriate immunizations.	Work with community groups to cosponsor immunization clinics in areas where immunization rates are low. Work to counteract parental fears of vaccines. Educate on the value and safety of HPV vaccine.
Hepatitis A, gastrointestinal infections	Teach safe food-handling practices in the home.	Require as part of the licensing of restaurants that food handlers take a course in safe food handling.
Hepatitis A and B	Provide immune globulin after exposure to hepatitis A or B.	Mandate immunization of health care workers for hepatitis A and B.
HIV/AIDS	Teach safe sex practices in all clinics. Provide preexposure prophylaxis (PrEP) for high-risk patients.	Provide education on safe sex practices to community groups. Educate public about the concept of treatment as prevention. Make PrEP widely available in the community.
Secondary Prevention		
STIs	Screen and treat for all STIs.	Institute an STI partner notification program in a population.
Tuberculosis	Screen close contacts of persons with TB. Treat persons with a recent skin test "conversion" (from negative to positive).	Initiate a program of yearly testing of health care workers for TB. Provide treatment to all with recent skin test conversions free of charge at their workplace.
HIV/AIDS	Provide testing and treatment for HIV in local clinics. Encourage and monitor patient adherence to antiretroviral therapy.	Ensure all hospitals and health care clinics have PEP (postexposure prophylaxis) available to anyone in the community to prevent HIV after a recent (72 h) possible exposure to HIV from sex or injection drug use.
Meningitis	Provide immunization and chemoprophylaxis to persons exposed to meningitis.	Provide immunization and chemoprophylaxis to all students in a school following an exposure.
Tertiary Prevention		
Tuberculosis	Provide therapy for persons with active TB. Teach patients to take all doses of prescribed antibiotics, and monitor adherence.	Initiate a directly observed therapy (DOT) program in the community shelters, jails, and to other high-risk groups. Initiate community education campaigns about the problem of drug resistance associated with incomplete antibiotic use.

HPV, Human papilloma virus; *TB,* tuberculosis.

new cases, and isolating infected people also are examples of secondary prevention.

Tertiary Prevention

Tertiary prevention includes activities involved in caring for persons with an infectious disease to ensure that they are cured, or that their quality of life is maintained, or management of disability related to the disease sequela. Perhaps the most important part of the treatment process is to ensure that people take their antimicrobial agents completely and effectively. In a time of increased resistance to pathogens, helping patients adhere to a drug regimen is critical. Additionally, caregivers should be taught to protect themselves and their environment by using appropriate precautions when caring for an infected family member.

The case study is based on current guidelines, and follow-up including the number of days and time may change according to CDC guidelines.

CASE STUDY Application of the Nursing Process

Employee With a Communicable Disease

Adrienne Zack is the employee health nurse for a large city hospital. On a recent workday, she saw Beverly Yancy, a staff nurse in the newborn nursery of the hospital, who presented to the employee health clinic with a productive cough, wheezing, low-grade fever, chills, and fatigue lasting more than 1 month. Beverly stated that she had been treating her symptoms with over-the-counter antihistamines, cough suppressants, and antipyretics. When weighed in the clinic, Beverly was surprised that she had lost 10 lb since she was weighed last. She told Adrienne that she has no history of asthma or lung disease.

Beverly's employee health record revealed that she had had a positive tuberculin skin test (TST also called Mantoux tuberculin skin test) reaction of 15-mm induration when she was screened 11 years earlier for employment at the hospital. A chest radiograph at that time showed no evidence of TB. Because Beverly was without TB symptoms at the time of employment and declined to take isoniazid (INH) for treatment of the latent TB infection, she believed that the positive TST reaction was the result of having received bacille Calmette-Guérin (BCG) vaccination at birth in the Philippines. Furthermore, she has had no symptoms during her annual symptom screen by the employee health clinic.

A chest X-ray showed suspicious areas indicating that Beverly most likely had active, infectious pulmonary TB. The diagnosis was confirmed when testing of three sputum smear examinations were positive for acid-fast bacilli (AFB). False-positive and false-negative are common and testing of three specimens is recommended by the CDC (CDC, 2017c, TB testing and dx). On the basis of the timing of Beverly's symptoms, Adrienne determined that Beverly's disease probably has been communicable for 3 months.

Diagnosis

Individual
- Active TB
- Potential for spread of TB to close contacts

Family
- Potential for undiagnosed TB

Community
- At risk for exposure to TB

Planning

MTB is transmitted by airborne droplets of sputum from persons with active disease who cough or otherwise discharge respiratory droplets into the air. Health care workers are at risk for TB infection because of frequent exposure to patients with active disease. Beverly could not have been infected by the newborns in the nursery where she worked. Most likely she was exposed to TB before her screening 11 years previously. For Beverly, the skin test reaction of 15-mm induration suggested a latent TB infection (LTBI) rather than a BCG vaccination at birth. There are three cut points to determine if skin test is positive depending on two factors: measurement in mm of the induration, and the person's risk and history. Current information on TB can be obtained at https://www.cdc.gov/tb/. LTBI can become active TB disease at any time. In this case, latency lasted more than 11 years. Current guidelines encourage all health care workers be treated for LTBI unless medically contraindicated (Sosa et al., 2019).

Healthcare workers, like anyone with active TB, can transmit the infection to close contacts such as coworkers, high-risk patients, and personal contacts. Newborns and children younger than 2 years are at high risk for acquiring TB infection and for progressing to TB disease. Such contacts must be found, screened, and treated as soon as possible. The incubation period for a detectable infection is generally 2–10 weeks after exposure. Recent contacts whose skin test results are negative now should be retested in 2–3 months.

Goals

Individual

Short-Term Goals
- Beverly will begin her course of medications immediately using directly observed therapy (DOT). DOT is recommended for treatment of all persons with TB disease and all persons with LTBI.
- Beverly will take short-term disability and will not return to work until her sputum culture results are negative and she is cleared by the employee health clinic.
- Beverly will monitor and report: her improvement in TB symptoms (e.g., cough, fever, fatigue, night sweats) and any medication adverse effects (e.g., jaundice, dark urine, nausea, vomiting, abdominal pain, fever, rash, anorexia, malaise, neuropathy, arthralgias)

Long-Term Goals
- Beverly will complete her course of medications as directed.

Beverly will provide sputum cultures at baseline, then monthly until two consecutive specimens are negative. She will undergo chest X-ray examination at baseline, at month two if baseline cultures are negative and as necessary for employee health clinic.

Family

Short-Term Goals
- All of Beverly's family members will be tested for TB within 3 days.
- Any family member testing positive will be started on a course of medication as recommended by the health department and his or her healthcare provider.

Long-Term Goal
- All family members will be retested in 6 months.

Community (Hospital)

Short-Term Goals
- Beverly's coworkers will be tested for TB within 3 days.
- The parents of all of Beverly's patients from the past 3 months will be contacted to encourage that they be tested and have their babies tested.
- Any contact or patient testing positive will be started on a course of medications as recommended by the local health department and his or her healthcare provider.

Long-Term Goal
- All contacts will be retested in 6 months.

Intervention

TB must be reported to local public health authorities, who are responsible for control of TB in the community. Control relies on identifying and adequately treating all active TB cases and those with latent infections. The public health department will investigate Beverly's contacts inside and outside the hospital during the previous 3 months. This process will identify and treat persons, including the discharged newborns, to whom Beverly might have transmitted MTB. Adrienne and the other health clinic employees may be asked to assist with screening hospital workers exposed to Beverly and providing education about treatment.

TST reactions are determined to be positive under the following conditions (CDC, 2017c, TB testing and dx):

1. Induration of 5 mm in persons with HIV infection, those in close personal contact with someone with active TB, persons who have fibrotic chest radiographs, or patients with organ transplants and other immunosuppressed patients (receiving 15 mg/d of prednisone for 1 month).
2. Induration of 10 mm in other high-risk persons, such as children less than 5 years of age; infants, children, and adolescents exposed to adults at high risk for developing active TB; injecting drug users, persons with chronic disease that places them at high risk; residents and employees of high-risk congregate settings; and those from countries or communities where TB prevalence is high.

Continued

CASE STUDY   Application of the Nursing Process—cont'd

3. Induration of 15 mm for persons with no known risk factors for TB, for anyone who does not meet the preceding criteria.

All persons with a positive skin test reaction should be tested for active disease. Those for whom AFB are identified in a stained smear of sputum, mycobacteria are isolated from a cultured specimen, or there is radiological evidence of TB must be treated for active disease with a combination of drugs according to protocols established by the CDC.

Multidrug-resistant TB (MDR TB) is a major health threat globally and is caused by MTB resistant to at least isoniazid and rifampin, used to treat TB disease. Globally of all new TB cases, it is estimated 3.5% are MDR TB and 20.5% of previously treated cases are MDR TB (CDC, 2015a, TB fact sheet). A rare type of MDR TB, extensively drug resistant TB (XDR TB), is resistant to most potent TB drugs and patients have less effective treatment available. People with weakened immune systems, such as people living with HIV, XDR TB is a special concern and outcomes are often worse. Patients must be helped to meticulously adhere to the prescribed regimen. Studies have demonstrated that healthcare workers are as poor as the general public at adhering to long-term drug therapy.

Persons with a recent "conversion" to a positive TST result should undergo treatment for latent TB according to CDC protocols. Such treatment reduces lifetime risk that a latent infection will progress to active disease. Persons taking INH should be taught the symptoms of side effects to the drug, including hepatotoxicity, peripheral neuropathy, and central nervous system (CNS) changes.

Teaching should include the following information:

- The importance of isolating oneself from contact with others and wearing a mask in public until sputum is clear of bacilli—around 4–8 weeks with effective treatment.
- Will have a 2-month intensive phase of TB treatment, followed by 4 or 7 additional months (total of 6–9 months treatment).
- Proper discharge of sputum and materials contaminated with sputum.
- Drug therapy must be continued uninterrupted for the designated period even after sputum tests are negative for bacilli and even if no longer feel sick.

Drug toxicity and side effects must be reported to the physician immediately. These include, but are not limited to the following (Payam et al., 2016): First-line drugs

- *INH:* Hepatotoxicity, peripheral neuropathy, CNS changes
- *Rifampin:* Red-orange urine, hepatotoxicity, CNS symptoms
- *Ethambutol:* Reduced visual acuity with inability to see the color green
- *Pyrazinamide:* Hypersensitivity, hepatotoxicity, gastrointestinal disturbances, renal failure
- *Rifabutin:* Red-orange urine, gastrointestinal disturbances

- *Rifapentine:* Red-orange urine, hepatotoxicity, gastrointestinal disturbances
- Second-line drugs
  - *Cycloserine:* CNS effects
  - *Ethionamide:* Gastrointestinal disturbance and symptoms of hepatotoxicity
  - *Streptomycin:* Rash, fever, malaise, vertigo, deafness, gastrointestinal disturbance, CNS changes
  - *Fluoroquinolone:* CNS effects tendon, joint and muscle pain

Sputum must be reexamined until recommended specimens test negative for bacilli following local health department guidelines.

Evaluation

Beverly and anyone else with active TB can return to work when the results of AFB testing of three sputum smear specimens collected 8–24 h apart, at least one of which is an early morning specimen, are negative. Adrienne will refer to the CDC's latest guidelines for preventing transmission of TB in health care settings, available at www.cdc.gov/tb/topic/infectioncontrol/default.htm and will update the hospital's infection control plan in accordance with the guidelines.

Levels of Prevention
Primary
- Educate healthcare workers and others about TB infection and disease.
- Educate staff on airborne precautions and the proper use of respiratory protection.
- Design and implement signage throughout the hospital to remind staff and patients about respiratory hygiene, cough etiquette, and hand hygiene.

Secondary
- Establish regular screening of health care workers for positive skin test conversions.
- Establish mechanisms for detection, referral, and treatment of staff with LTBIs and with active TB.
- Implement procedures for rapid detection and treatment of patients with active TB.
- Coordinate efforts with the local health department.

Tertiary
- Monitor medication compliance and follow-up testing.
- Support policies and organizations that provide TB education and care with goal to reduce global TB stigma.
- Create opportunities to minimize disability.

SUMMARY

This chapter presents the challenges of infectious diseases that all nurses face. It reviews principles that are the foundation for the occurrence, transmission, and control of infectious diseases and applies those principles to infectious diseases that are emphasized in the *Healthy People 2030* objectives. Most important, because nurses will be affected by infectious diseases wherever they practice, resources from which any nurse can obtain up-to-date information on any infectious disease at any time are included.

EVOLVE WEBSITE

http://evolve.elsevier.com/Nies/community

- NCLEX Review Questions
- Case Studies

BIBLIOGRAPHY

Association of State and Territorial Health Officials: *State strategies to increase access, administrative capacity, and confidence for COVID-19 vaccines*, 2021. Available from: https://www.astho.org/COVID-19/State-Strategies-to-Increase-Access-Administrative-Capacity-and-Confidence-for-COVID-19-Vaccines/. Accessed May 26, 2021.

Brouwer AF, Delinger RL, Eisenberg MC, et al.: HPV vaccination has not increased sexual activity or accelerated sexual debut in a college-aged cohort of men and women, *BMC Pub Health* 19(1):821, 2019. https://doi.org/10.1186/s12889-019-7134-1.

Centers for Disease Control and Prevention: *Advisory Committee on Immunization Practices (ACIP) recommended immunization schedules for persons aged 0 through 18 years and adults aged 19 years and older—United States*, 2016a. https://www.cdc.gov/vaccines/vpd/index.html.

Centers for Disease Control and Prevention: *CDC fact sheet: TB drug resistance in the U.S*, 2015. Last Reviewed May 4, 2016. Available from: https://www.cdc.gov/tb/publications/factsheets/drtb/mdrtb.htm.

Centers for Disease Control and Prevention: *Estimated HIV incidence and prevalence in the United States, 2015—2019, HIV Surveill Suppl Rep* 26(1), 2021a. Available from: http://www.cdc.gov/hiv/library/reports/hiv-surveillance.html. Accessed May 28, 2021.

Centers for Disease Control and Prevention: *For immunization partners: vaccinate with confidence*, 2019. Available from: https://www.cdc.gov/vaccines/partners/vaccinate-with-confidence.html. Accessed May 28, 2021.

Centers for Disease Control and Prevention: *HIV: HIV testing*, 2020a. https://www.cdc.gov/hiv/testing/index.html.

Centers for Disease Control and Prevention: *HIV: pre-exposure prophylaxis (PrEP)*, 2020. Available from: https://www.cdc.gov/hiv/risk/prep/index.html. Accessed May 28, 2021.

Centers for Disease Control and Prevention: *HIV surveillance report, 2019: diagnoses of HIV infection in the United States and dependent areas* vol. 32, 2021. Available from: http://www.cdc.gov/hiv/library/reports/hiv-surveillance/vol-32/index.html. Accessed June 2021.

Centers for Disease Control and Prevention: *HPV: Boosting vaccination rates*, 2019b. https://www.cdc.gov/hpv/hcp/boosting-vacc-rates.html.

Centers for Disease Control and Prevention. In Hamborsky J, Kroger A, Wolfe S, editors: *Epidemiology and prevention of vaccine-preventable diseases*, ed 13, Washington, DC, 2015b, Public Health Foundation, pp 2020—2021. https://www.cdc.gov/vaccines/pubs/pinkbook/index.html 18 out of 22 chapters updated in.

Centers for Disease Control and Prevention: *Infectious diseases designated as notifiable at the national level during*, 2017. Available from: https://wwwn.cdc.gov/nndss/conditions/notifiable/2017/infectious-diseases.

Centers for Disease Control and Prevention: *Informatics and surveillance*, 2020. Available from: https://www.cdc.gov/pertussis/downloads/pertuss-surv-report-2019-508.pdf.

Centers for Disease Control and Prevention: *Measles cases and outbreaks*, 2021. Available from: https://www.cdc.gov/measles/cases-outbreaks.html. Accessed June 2021.

Centers for Disease Control and Prevention: Measles—United States, January 1—April 26, 2019, *MMWR Morb Mortal Wkly Rep* 68(17):402—404, 2019c.

Centers for Disease Control and Prevention: *National center for emerging zoonotic infectious diseases*, 2017. Available from: https://www.cdc.gov/ncezid/.

Centers for Disease Control and Prevention: National, regional, state, and selected local area vaccination coverage among adolescents aged 13—17 years—United States, 2015, *MMWR Morb Mortal Wkly Rep* 65:850—858, 2016b.

Centers for Disease Control and Prevention: *Pertussis surveillance and reporting, pertussis cases by year (1922—2019)*, 2019. Available from: www.cdc.gov/pertussis/surv-reporting/cases-by-year.html. Accessed June 2021.

Centers for Disease Control and Prevention: Recommendations of the advisory committee on immunization practices: revised recommendations for routine poliomyelitis vaccination, *MMWR Morb Mortal Wkly Rep* 48(27):590, 1999.

Centers for Disease Control and Prevention: *Sexually transmitted diseases: adolescents and young adults*, Last reviewed April 8, 2021. Available from: https://www.cdc.gov/std/life-stages-populations/adolescents-youngadults.htm. Accessed June 2021.

Centers for Disease Control and Prevention: *Sexually transmitted disease surveillance, 2019*, 2021. Available from: www.cdc.gov/std/statistics/2019/default.htm. Accessed June 2021.

Centers for Disease Control and Prevention: Sexually transmitted diseases treatment guidelines, *MMWR Morb Mortal Wkly Rep* 64(3):1—137, 2015c. Available from: https://www.cdc.gov/mmwr/pdf/rr/rr6403.pdf.

Centers for Disease Control and Prevention: *Tuberculosis (TB): testing & diagnosis*, 2020. Available from: https://www.cdc.gov/tb/publications/guidelines/testing.htm.

Centers for Disease Control and Prevention: Tuberculosis—United States, 2016, *MMWR Morb Mortal Wkly Rep* 66(11):289—309, 2017c. Available from: https://www.cdc.gov/mmwr/volumes/66/wr/pdfs/mm6611a2.pdf.

Centers for Disease Control and Prevention: *Vaccines*, 2017. Available from: https://www.cdc.gov/vaccines/vpd/index.html.

Centers for Disease Control and Prevention: *Vaccines & Immunizations: vaccinate with confidence*, 2021. Available from: https://www.cdc.gov/vaccines/covid-19/vaccinate-with-confidence.html. Accessed May 28, 2021.

Corless IB, Nardi D, Milstead JA, et al.: Expanding nursing's role in responding to global pandemics, *Nurs Outlook* 66(4):412—415, 2018. https://doi.org/10.1016/j.outlook.2018.06.003.

Dowdle WR: The principles of disease elimination and eradication, *MMWR Morb Mortal Wkly Rep* 48(suppl 1):23—27, 1999.

Edmonds JK, Kneipp SM, Campbell L: A call to action for public health nurses during the COVID-19 pandemic, *Public Health Nurs* 37(3):323—324, 2020. https://doi.org/10.1111/phn.12733.

Healthy People 2030, HealthyPeople.gov: *Browse objectives: health conditions*, 2021. Available from: https://health.gov/healthypeople/objectives-and-data/browse-objectives.

Healthy People 2030, HealthyPeople.gov: *Infectious disease: vaccination*, 2021. Available from: https://health.gov/healthypeople/objectives-and-data/browse-objectives/infectious-disease https://health.gov/healthypeople/objectives-and-data/browse-objectives/vaccination.

Healthy People 2030, HealthyPeople.gov: *Objectives: sexually transmitted infections: HIV*, 2021. Available from: https://health.gov/healthypeople/objectives-and-data/browse-objectives/sexually-transmitted-infections.

Heymann DL. In *Control of communicable diseases manual*, ed 20, Washington, DC, 2015, American Public Health Association.

MacDonald NE: SAGE working group on vaccine hesitancy: vaccine hesitancy: definition, scope and determinants, *Vaccine* 33(34):4161—4164, 2015. https://doi.org/10.1016/j.vaccine.2015.04.036.

National Institute for Health: *An empirical approach to HIV vaccine development*, 2020. Last reviewed February 5, 2020. Available from: https://www.niaid.nih.gov/diseases-conditions/empirical-approach. Accessed June 2021.

National Notifiable Disease Surveillance System: *Week 52, 2019 final pertussis surveillance report*, Atlanta, GA, 2021, CDC Division of Health. Available from: https://www.cdc.gov/pertussis/surv-reporting.html.

Office of Disease Prevention and Health Promotion. *Healthy People 2030 framework. Healthy People 2030, n.d.* U.S. Department of Health and Human Services. Available from: https://health.gov/healthypeople/about/healthy-people-2030-framework. Accessed April 7, 2021.

Payam N, Dorman SE, Alipanah N, et al.: Executive summary: Official American Thoracic Society/Centers for Disease Control and Prevention/Infectious Diseases Society of America Clinical Practice Guidelines: treatment of drug-susceptible tuberculosis, *Clin Infect Dis* 63(7):853—867, 2016. https://doi.org/10.1093/cid/ciw566.

Schneider MJ: *Introduction to public health*, ed 2, Boston, 2006, Jones and Bartlett.

Sosa LE, Njie GJ, Lobato MN, et al.: Tuberculosis screening, testing, and treatment of U.S. Health Care Personnel: recommendations from the National Tuberculosis Controllers Association and CDC, 2019, *MMWR Morb Mortal Wkly Rep* 68(19):439—443, 2019. https://doi.org/10.15585/mmwr.mm6819a3.

The INSIGHT START Study Group: Initiation of antiretroviral therapy in early asymptomatic HIV infection, *N Engl J Med* 373:795—807, 2015.

UNAIDS: *Global HIV & AIDS statistics-2020 fact sheet*, 2020. Available from: http://www.unaids.org/en/resources/fact-sheet. Accessed March 24, 2021.

U.S. Department of Health and Human Services: *Vaccine types*, 2021. Available from: https://www.hhs.gov/immunization/basics/types/index.html. Accessed June 2021.

Wilson KL, White A, Rosen BL, et al.: Factors associated with college students' intentions to vaccinate their daughters against HPV: protecting the next generation, *J Commun Health* 41(5):1078—1089, 2016. https://doi.org/10.1007/s10900-016-0192-8.

World Health Organization: *Global Health fact sheets: tuberculosis*, 2020c. Available from: https://www.who.int/news-room/fact-sheets/details/tuberculosis. Accessed June 21, 2021.

World Health Organization: *HIV/AIDS*, 2020b. Available from: https://www.who.int/news-room/fact-sheets/detail/hiv-aids. Accessed April 7, 2021.

World Health Organization: *Immunizations, vaccines and biologicals: National programmes and systems*, 2021. Available from: https://www.who.int/immunization/programmes_systems/en/. Accessed April 7, 2021.

World Health Organization: *WHO Director-General's opening remarks at the media briefing on COVID-19-11 March 2020*, 2020a. Available from: https://www.who.int/director-general/speeches/detail/who-director-general-s-opening-remarks-at-the-media-briefing-on-covid-19—-11-march-2020. Accessed April 7, 2021.

27

Substance Abuse

Meredith Troutman-Jordan

OBJECTIVES

Upon completion of this chapter, the reader will be able to do the following:

1. Discuss the historical trends and current conceptualizations of the cause and treatment of substance abuse.
2. Describe the current social, political, and economic aspects of substance abuse.
3. Describe the ethical and legal implications of substance abuse.
4. Detail the typical symptoms and consequences of substance abuse.
5. Identify issues related to substance abuse in various populations encountered in community health nursing practice.
6. Apply nursing care standards related to the patients with substance abuse problems.

OUTLINE

KEY TERMS

abstinence
Addiction
Alcoholics Anonymous
case management
cooccurring disorders
delirium tremens
detoxification
dual diagnosis

harm reduction
initiation
intensive outpatient treatment
intervention
mutual help groups
National Institute on Drug Abuse
opioid use disorder (OUD)
professional enablers

social consequences
Substance Abuse and Mental Health Services
substance abuse
substance abuse treatment
substance use disorder (SUD)
War on Drugs

Perhaps no other health-related condition has as many far-reaching consequences in contemporary Western society as substance abuse. These consequences include a wide range of social, psychological, physical, economic, and political problems. Drug abuse and addiction have negative consequences for individuals, families, and communities. Estimates of the total overall costs of substance abuse in the United States, including productivity and health- and crime-related costs, exceed $740 billion annually (NIDA, 2020a–r). This figure includes approximately $193 billion for illicit drugs, $300 billion for tobacco, and $249 billion for alcohol. These numbers in dollars do not describe the extent of public health and safety implications (SAHMSA, 2016; Wilkinson et al., 2016). Some of these critical implications are family disintegration, loss of employment, failure in school, domestic violence, and child abuse.

Excessive alcohol use led to approximately 95,000 deaths and 2.8 million years of potential life lost annually in the United States from 2011 to 15, shortening the lives of those who died by an average of 29 years (Esser et al., 2020). Moreover, excessive drinking was responsible for one in 10 deaths among working-age adults aged 20 to 64 years (CDC, 2021). In 2010, the financial costs of excessive alcohol consumption were estimated at $249 billion, or $2.05 a drink (Sacks et al., 2015). According to the SAMHSA (2019a,b) National Survey on Drug Use and Health, 14.1 million adults ages 18 and older had alcohol use disorder (AUD). This includes 8.9 million men and 5.2 million women. An estimated 414,000 adolescents ages 12 to 17 had AUD. This number includes 163,000 males and 251,000 females. Unfortunately, only about 5% of you with AUD in the past year received treatment (SAMHSA, 2019a,b). The **social consequences** of substance abuse include its role in crime, need for money to buy substances, specific theft of drugs, and irreversible health consequences/disabilities that can result from use. These outcomes present a nationwide burden; an estimated 95,0005 people (approximately 68,000 men and 27,000 women) die from alcohol-related causes annually, making alcohol the third leading preventable cause of death in the United States (CDC, 2019a,b). In 2018, there were 67,367 drug overdose deaths in the United States. Opioids—primarily synthetic opioids (other than methadone)—are currently the main driver of drug overdose deaths. Opioids were involved in 46,802 overdose deaths in 2018 (69.5% of all drug overdose deaths) (Hedegaard et al., 2020). Two out of three (67.0%) opioid-involved overdose deaths involve synthetic opioids (Wilson et al., 2020).

Research indicates that an estimated 65% percent of the United States prison population has an active substance use disorder (SUD) (NIDA, 2020a–r). In 2019 there were 1,558,862 total drug-related arrests in the United States; 545,602 of these involved marijuana, 495,871 involved violent crime, and 1,074,367 involved property crime (McVay, 2020). However, a recent National Academy of Sciences report on Medications for Opioid Use Disorder revealed that only 5% of people with opioid use disorder in jail and prison settings receive medication treatment.

All aggregates in society are potentially affected by substance abuse problems. Infants exposed in utero to alcohol, amphetamines, or opiates are at risk for withdrawal syndromes and later developmental problems. Indirect social effects of substance abuse include relationship conflicts, divorce, job loss/lack of employment, spousal and child abuse, and child neglect.

In the past, alcoholism and drug addiction were considered problems of the urban poor; society and most health professionals virtually ignored them. Substance abuse problems now pervade all levels of U.S. society, and awareness has increased. Community health nurses must be knowledgeable about substance abuse because it is a problem that frequently intertwines with other medical and social conditions.

This chapter focuses on helping community health nurses recognize substance abuse in their clients and in the larger community. It reviews historical trends, the causes of substance abuse, the most common symptoms of these disorders, and treatment options. The chapter also suggests nursing interventions appropriate for assisting those with substance-related problems in a community context.

ETIOLOGY OF SUBSTANCE ABUSE

Substance abuse has an impact on virtually every aspect of individual and communal life, and many institutions and academic fields have addressed it. Several theories attempt to explain the cause and scope of the problem and offer solutions. Some theories address individual, physiological, spiritual, and psychological factors. Others deal with social influences involving family, ethnicity, race, access to drugs, environmental stressors, economics, political status, culture, and sex roles. Most theories suggest that a combination of factors is the underlying impetus for substance abuse.

Although previous research studies have suggested a link between genetics and alcoholism, there is growing evidence that genetic variations may contribute to the nature of alcoholism within families. Individual and environmental factors also contribute to an increased risk for alcohol abuse. On the individual level, a person's inherited sensitivity to alcohol is a predictor for the development of alcohol abuse. Personality traits can influence risk for drug experimentation, addictive behaviors and uncontrolled overeating (Ramirez et al., 2020). Many of studies have revealed that personality factors of extraversion, neuroticism, openness to experience, agreeableness, and conscientiousness were influential for alcohol use (Chen et al., 2019). For example, it has been consistently found that high neuroticism, low agreeableness, and low conscientiousness were significantly associated with alcohol use problems. Alcohol expectancies (i.e., beliefs about anticipated consequences of drinking) are also a predictor of alcohol abuse. If one expects a certain effect, such as relief, one is more likely to feel it after use of a drug. The satisfied expectancies may set up neural pathways that are interpreted as pleasurable.

Medical models of alcoholism and other substance abuse conditions may not provide an understanding of commonalities among addictive behaviors (e.g., excessive drinking, gambling, eating, drug use, and sexual behavior). Cross-addiction, or multidrug use, is more prevalent now than in the past, and more studies point to the presence of both automatic and nonautomatic factors in physiological and psychological dependence. Specific biological medical models are giving way to multicausal models.

In the biopsychosocial model, risk factors interact with protective factors to develop a predisposition toward drug or alcohol use (SAHMSA, 2021). This predisposition is then influenced by exposure to the substance, availability, and the experiential interpretation of the drug experience (e.g., pleasant or unpleasant). Continued availability of the substances and a social support system that enables or supports their use is also necessary. These factors combine to determine whether addiction develops and is maintained.

HISTORICAL OVERVIEW OF ALCOHOL AND ILLICIT DRUG USE

During the 20th century, fluctuations in the use of alcohol and illicit drugs were influenced by shifts in public tolerance and political and economic trends. In general, alcohol use gained more social acceptance than other drug use. Alcohol consumption in the United States was higher during World Wars I and II and decreased during Prohibition and the Great Depression. In 1971, when the voting age was lowered from 21 to 18, 30 states concurrently lowered the drinking age (Devenyns, 2019). However, the decrease in the minimum legal drinking age was shown to drastically increase the number of alcohol-related car accidents. In fact, by the mid-1970s, 60% of traffic accident fatalities involved alcohol. In 1984, Congress passed legislation that would withhold federal highway construction funds from any state that had not adopted a minimum legal drinking age of 21 (CDC, 2020a). After all states adopted an age 21 minimum legal drinking age, drinking during the previous month among persons aged 18 to 20 years declined from 59% in 1985 to 40% in 1991.7, while drinking among people aged 21 to 25 also declined significantly when states adopted the age 21 MLDA, from 70% in 1985 to 56% in 1991 (CDC, 2020a).

The decline in alcohol consumption through the 1990s and into the 21st century is attributed to less tolerant national attitudes toward drinking, increased societal and legal pressures and actions against drinking and driving, and increased health concerns among Americans. The identification of, and response to, driving under the influence of alcohol or another drugs is an example of a shift in thinking from addiction as the primary concern to other problems linked with, for example, alcohol use. These problems are thus termed *substance-related problems* and have become a significant community concern.

Public attitudes and governmental policies also have influenced the history of illicit drug use. Although 19th-century physicians prescribed morphine for a large variety of ailments, the discovery of the addictive properties of cocaine and opiates led to increased governmental regulation at the beginning of the 20th century. The Harrison Narcotic Act of 1914, and subsequent laws, lessened the medical profession's control over the use of addictive drugs Kmiec (2017); the legislation specified that the physician could prescribe these drugs only in the course of general practice and not to maintain an addiction. This limitation on the physician's power to prescribe and dispense addictive drugs, and made it illegal to sell or give away these drugs without a written order on a form issued by the commissioner of Revenue (Kmiec) (see https://www.naabt.org/documents/Harrison_Narcotics_Tax_Act_1914.pdf). At that time, an increase in illegal drug trafficking caused heroin use to proliferate, particularly in inner cities.

By the 1970s, drugs were increasingly available. During this period, a counterculture population, composed largely of young people, focused their efforts on enhancing social justice, ending the Vietnam War, and lessening "repressive" sexual mores; many conceptualized drug use as a way to liberate the mind. Marijuana use occurred in communal, social settings; alcohol use was less favored because it was associated with the "establishment" the young people were critiquing (PBS, 2014). Consequently, the use of hallucinogens, cannabis, and heroin spread beyond urban drug subcultures to the general population. Alarmed by the social and personal problems inherent in this change, the public grew less tolerant of drug use, and prevention and treatment programs were given more attention and resources. After peaking in 1979, illicit drug use decreased among most segments of the population throughout the 1980s, reaching a low in the early 1990s. The Anti-Drug Abuse Acts of 1986 and 1988 increased funding for treatment and rehabilitation, and also stiffened penalties for drug offenses (Sterling, 2021); the 1988 act created the Office of National Drug Control Policy. The director, referred to as the "drug czar," is responsible for coordinating national drug control policy.

To combat concerns about the physical, social, and psychological impacts of drug abuse and dependence, federal drug policy has emphasized law enforcement and interdiction—the **War on Drugs**—to reduce the supply. Trends have shown renewed interest in prevention and treatment efforts to decrease the amount of illicit drug use in society and to lessen its impact (SAMHSA, 2016). Federal government resources targeting illicit drug use have increased during the last decade; over $34.6 billion were requested in the Fiscal Year 2020 Drug Control Budget to help communities, states, and law enforcement respond to the drug crisis and curb drug trafficking (Office of National Drug Control Policy, 2020). Goals of the 2020 National Drug Control Policy include reducing the number of Americans dying from drug overdose significantly within 5 years; educating the public about drug used, specifically opioids; increasing nationwide accessibility of evidence-based addiction treatment, including medication assisted therapy; increasing mandatory prescriber education and continuing training on best practices and current guidelines; reducing nationwide opioid prescription refills; increasing Prescription Drug Monitoring Program interoperability and usage across the nation; significantly reducing availability of illicit drugs in the United States by preventing their production outside of the United States; significantly reducing the availability of illicit drugs in the United States by disrupting their sale on the internet, and stopping their flow into the country through the mail and express courier environments, and across our borders; and decreasing availability of illicit drugs in the United States.

There are numerous federal resources that nurses and other health care professionals need to be familiar with. For instance, there is the **National Institute on Drug Abuse** (NIDA) (http://www.drugabuse.gov/). NIDA's mission is to lead the United States in research on drug abuse and addiction. NIDA's strategic goals address substance abuse as a complex disease and underlying causes. The institute works with research programs in basic, clinical, and translational science, including genetics, functional neuroimaging, social neuroscience, medication and behavioral therapies, prevention, and health services. There are four strategic goals: Identify the biological, environmental, behavioral, and social causes and consequences of drug use and addiction across the lifespan; Develop new and improved strategies to prevent drug use and its consequences; Develop new and improved treatments to help people with substance use disorders achieve and maintain a meaningful and sustained recovery; and, Increase the public health impact of NIDA research and programs (NIDA, 2017a,b). NIDA gathers data on health disparities related to drug addiction and its many effects. The institute has many education programs encompassing criminal justice, medical, and educational systems. NIDA continues to promote research addressing nicotine addiction, HIV/AIDS, and emerging trends as well as training and dissemination of science-based information on drug abuse.

The **Substance Abuse and Mental Health Services Administration** (SAMHSA), at https://www.samhsa.gov/, leads public health efforts to advance the behavioral health of the nation. SAMHSA's mission is to reduce the impact of substance abuse and mental illness on America's communities (SAMHSA, 2020a—f). https://www.samhsa.gov/data/report/2019-nsduh-detailed-tables.

PREVALENCE, INCIDENCE, AND TRENDS

The growing recognition of the widespread effects of substance abuse has initiated extensive collection of data by multiple agencies. This section describes selected statistics and current trends. The U.S. National Survey on Drug Use and Health is an annual survey conducted by SAMHSA that estimates the prevalence of illicit drug and alcohol use in the United States. Findings from a 2019 report include the following (SAMHSA, 2019a,b):

Alcohol

In the 2018 survey, 139.8 million Americans age 12 or older were current drinkers of alcohol, an increase from the 138.3 million reported in the 2015 survey. In 2018, 67.1 million (48%) American alcohol users age 12 or older were binge drinkers, while 16.6 million (11.8% of alcohol users and 24.7% binge users) were heavy drinkers (SAMHSA, 2019a,b). Of these 66.7, approximately 9% of teens age 12 to 17 in 2018 were current alcohol users; 2.2 million adolescents consumed alcohol in the past month. Rates of alcohol consumption in this age range in 2018 decreased from percentages in most years from 2002 through 2017, with approximately one in 11 adolescents being current alcohol users in 2018 (SAMHSA, 2019a,b).

Approximately 1.2 million adolescents ages 12 to 17 (4.7% adolescents) were past month binge drinkers in 2018. This equates to about one in 21 adolescents who were current binge drinkers, similar to rates reported in 2016 and 2017, yet less than the percentage in 2015, 5.8% (SAMHSA, 2019a,b). Roughly 34.9% of young adults ages 18 to 25 in 2018 were

binge drinkers in the past month, which equals about 11.9 million young adults; greater than a third of young adults in 2018 were current binge drinkers (SAMHSA, 2019a,b). However, the proportion of young adults who were current binge drinkers in 2018 was lower than rates in 2015 to 2017 (which range from 39.0% in 2015 to 36.9% in 2017).

Excessive drinking is responsible for more than 3500 deaths and 210,000 years of potential life lost among people under age 21 each year (CDC, 2020a—e). Underage drinking cost the U.S. $24 billion in 2010 (most recent date available) (Sacks et al., 2015). The CDC (2019a,b) Youth Risk Behavior Survey found that among high school students, 29% drank alcohol; 14% binge drank; 5% of drivers drove after drinking alcohol; and 17% rode with a driver who had been drinking alcohol, during the past 30 days. These alarming trends have grave consequences for communities; youth who consume alcohol are more likely to have school problems, such as higher rates of absences or lower grades; social problems, such as fighting or lack of participation in youth activities; legal problems, such as arrest for driving or physically hurting someone while drunk; physical problems, such as hangovers or illnesses.; unwanted, unplanned, and unprotected sexual activity; disruption of normal growth or sexual development; physical and sexual violence; increased risk of suicide and homicide; alcohol-related motor vehicle crashes and other unintentional injuries, such as burns, falls, or drowning; memory problems; misuse of other substances; changes in brain development that may have lifelong effects; and alcohol poisoning (Esser et al., 2019; Jones et al., 2020; USDHHS, 2016).

Illicit Drug Use

An estimated 53.2 million (19.4% of the population) people aged 12 or older in 2018 had used an illicit drug in the past year (SAMHSA, 2019a,b). This means that nearly one in five people age 12 and older in the United States used illicit drugs in the past year. Illicit drugs included marijuana, cocaine (including crack), heroin, hallucinogens, inhalants, methamphetamine (MA), as well as misuse of prescription stimulants, misuse of tranquilizers or sedatives, and misuse of pain relievers. The proportion of the population in 2018 who used illicit drugs in the past year was higher than the percentages in 2015 and 2016, yet similar to the percentage in 2017, 19.0% (SAMHSA, 2019a,b). Further findings are as follows:

- Marijuana continues to be the most commonly used illicit drug as of 2019 (SAMHSA, 2019a,b), with 43.5 million Americans, 15.9% of the population, reporting use during the past year. This is an increase from the rate of 22.2 million current users, or 8.3% of the population age 12 and older, from 2015.
- There have long been advocates for legalization of marijuana, citing therapeutic benefits. A total of 36 states, District of Columbia, Guam, Puerto Rico and U.S. Virgin Islands have approved comprehensive, publicly available medical marijuana/cannabis programs (National Conference of State Legislatures, 2021), while 11 states and the District of Columbia have made recreational marijuana use legal;

Alaska, California, Colorado, Illinois, Maine, Massachusetts, Michigan, Nevada, Oregon, and Vermont (Mohanty, 2020).

- An estimated 808,000 people aged 12 or older (about 0.3% of the population) in 2018 reported heroin use in the past year. This estimate exceeds reported rates of use from most years between 2002 and 2008, though it is comparable to estimates from years between 2009 and 2017 (SAMHSA, 2019a,b).

- Hallucinogens include LSD, PCP, peyote, mescaline, psilocybin mushrooms, "Ecstasy" (MDMA or "Molly"), ketamine, DMT/AMT/"Foxy," and *Salvia divinorum* (SAMHSA, 2019a,b). In 2018, nearly 5.6 million people age 12 or older (2% of the population) were users of hallucinogens during the past year, similar to percentage reported in 2017.

- Due to the changes that were made to the prescription drug questions in 2015, a new baseline started in 2015 for all prescription drug measures. The four categories of prescription drugs (pain relievers, tranquilizers, stimulants, and sedatives) cover numerous medications that currently are or have been available by prescription.

- Prescription psychotherapeutic drugs comprise prescription stimulants, tranquilizers or sedatives (including benzodiazepines), and pain relievers (SAMHSA, 2019a,b). In 2018, an estimated 16.9 million Americans aged 12 or older (6.2% of the population) misused prescription psychotherapeutic drugs at least once during the past year.

- Stimulants include amphetamine products, methylphenidate products, weight-loss stimulants, and Provigil (for narcolepsy). In 2018, an estimated 5.1 million people age 12 or older (1.9% of the population) misused prescription stimulants in the past year. In 2018, about 369,000 teens aged 12 to 17 (1.5% adolescents) were past year misusers of prescription stimulants, a number similar to percentages in 2016 and 2017 (SAMHSA, 2019a,b).

- Approximately 4.2 million adolescents aged 12 to 17 (16.7%, or one in six teens) in 2018 were past year illicit drug users, an increased percentage from the illicit drug use rates of 2.2 million (8.8% adolescents) in this age group reported in 2015.

- In 2018, 3.1 million adolescents (about one in 8, or 12.5%) aged 12 to 17 were past year marijuana users (SAMHSA, 2019a,b). The rate of illicit drug use during the past year among young adults aged 18 to 25 in 2018 was 38.7% (approximately two in 5, or about 13.2 million young adults [SAMHSA, 2019a,b]). This rate of use is in contrast to 7.8 million (22.3%) young adults in 2015 who were current users of illicit drugs.

- In 2018, an estimated 16.9 million Americans aged 12 or older misused prescription psychotherapeutic drugs at least once in the past year. This number of past year prescription, corresponding to 6.2% of the population (SAMHSA, 2019a,b).

- Prescription pain relievers were the most commonly misused in individuals aged 12 or older, with 9.9 million who misused prescription pain relievers in that period, 5.1 million who misused prescription stimulants, and approximately 6.4 million who misused prescription tranquilizers or sedatives (SAMHSA, 2019a,b).

Illicit drug use among adults aged 50 or older was projected to increase from 2.2% to 3.1% between 2001 and 2020, with the number of older Americans with SUD expected to rise from 2.8 million in 2002 to 2006 to 5.7 million by 2020 (Matteson et al., 2017).

- While illicit drug use typically declines after young adulthood, nearly one million adults aged 65 and older live with a substance use disorder, according to 2018 data from SAMHSA (2019a,b).

- In 2018, 20.5 million people aged 16 or older drove under the influence of alcohol in the past year and 12.6 million drove under the influence of illicit drugs (SAMHSA Center for Behavioral Health Statistics and Quality, 2019).

- Among persons aged 12 or older who misused prescription pain relievers in the past 12 months, 38.6obtained the drug from a friend or relative for free; 9.5% bought the drug from a friend or relative, 3.2% took the drug from a friend or relative without asking, and 37.6% reported they either got it through prescriptions (36.7%) or stole from a health care provider (0.9%) (SAMHSA, 2019a,b). An annual average of 6.5% people got pain relievers from a drug dealer or other stranger, and 4.6% obtained them some other way (SAMHSA, 2019a,b).

Nonmedical Use of Prescription-Type Psychotherapeutics

Nonmedical use and abuse of prescription drugs constitute a serious public health problem in this country. An estimated 18 million people (more than 6% of those aged 12 and older) have misused such medications at least once in the past year (NIDA, 2020a–r). The NIDA Monitoring the Future (MTF) annual survey (2020) of 11,800 8th, 10th, and 12th grade students across the U.S. found that nonmedical use of prescription drugs continued to decline from previous years; Vicodin use in the past year was down to 1.1% in 2019, and OxyContin use was at 1.7% as for 2019. Marijuana use has in this age group has remained steady, with 11.4%, 28%, and 35.2% of 8th, 10th, and 12th graders reporting past year use, respectively (NIDA, 2020a–r). Regarding daily use, these percentages were 1.1%, 4.4%, and 6.9%, respectively. Trends in vaping remain concerning; 22.1% of 12th graders, 19.1% of 10th graders, and 8.1% of eight graders reported past year marijuana vaping in 2020. However, rates of vaping any substance in the past year were 39%, 34.6%, and 19.2%, respectively.

Hallucinogen, Inhalant, and Heroin Use

Hallucinogen drugs cause hallucinations by disrupting the interactions of nerve cells and the neurotransmitter serotonin. There are profound distortions of perceptions of reality. People may see things, hears sounds, and feel sensations that seem real but do not exist. Some hallucinations may also produce emotional changes in behavior. There may be changes in mood, hunger sensations, body temperature, sexual behavior, and muscle coordination.

LSD (D-lysergic acid diethylamide), which was discovered in 1938 and is manufactured from lysergic acid, has unpredictable psychological effects, "trips" that may last 12 h. Some doses of LSD may cause delusions and hallucinations. LSD may be sold in tablets, capsules, or, occasionally, liquid form; thus, it is usually taken orally. LSD is often added to absorbent paper, which is then divided into decorated pieces, each equivalent to one dose. Behavior of someone using LSD may manifest as psychosis. There may be other symptoms, such as increases in body temperature, heart rate, and blood pressure; sleeplessness; and loss of appetite (NIDA, 2016a,b). LSD use has increased in the U.S. by 56.4% from 2015 to 2018 (Yockey et al., 2020). Past-year LSD use in individuals 18 and older increased from 2015 to 2018.

Peyote is a small, spineless cactus, *Lophophora williamsii*, in which the principal active ingredient is the hallucinogen mescaline. The peyote cactus has been used by natives in northern Mexico and the southwestern United States as a part of religious ceremonies. Tops (buttons) of the peyote cactus are cut from the roots and dried, then are chewed or soaked in water to produce an intoxicating liquid. Extracts are bitter and may be prepared into a tea by boiling the cacti for several hours. A hallucinogenic dose of mescaline is about 0.3 to 0.5 g, and its effects last about 12 h (NIDA, 2015a–f).

Psilocybin (4-phosphoryloxy-*N,N*-dimethyltryptamine), also known as magic mushrooms, is obtained from certain types of mushrooms that are indigenous to tropical and subtropical regions of South America, Mexico, and the United States. Mushrooms containing psilocybin are available fresh or dried and are typically taken orally. They may be brewed as a tea or added to other foods to mask their bitter flavor. Hallucinatory effects may appear within 20 min of ingestion and may last up to 6 h (NIDA, 2015a–f).

PCP (phencyclidine) was developed in the 1950s as an intravenous anesthetic for surgery but was never approved for human use because of problems during clinical studies, including intensely negative psychological effects. PCP is a white crystalline powder that is readily soluble in water or alcohol. PCP can also be mixed easily with dyes and is often sold on the illicit drug market in a variety of tablet, capsule, and colored powder forms that are normally snorted, smoked, or orally ingested. PCP has a distinctive bitter chemical taste. When smoked, it is often applied to a leafy material such as mint, parsley, oregano, or marijuana. Depending on concentration and route of ingestion, its effects can last approximately 4 to 6 h (Drugs.com, 2021; NIDA, 2015a–f).

During their lifetime, 9.1% individuals age 12 and older reported inhalant use, with a corresponding 0.7% during the past year (NIDA, 2020a–r). Inhalants can be found in many products readily available in the home or workplace. Spray paints, markers, glues, and cleaning fluids contain volatile substances that have psychoactive properties when inhaled. They can be used especially, but not exclusively, by young children and adolescents. Most often these substances produce a rapid high that resembles alcohol intoxication, resulting in a loss of sensation and even unconsciousness. Serious and irreversible effects include hearing loss, limb spasms, central nervous system or brain damage, and bone marrow damage. Inhaling high concentrations of these substances may result in death from heart failure or suffocation.

According to the United Nations Office on Drug and Crime (UNODC, 2020), the global prevalence of opiate use in 2018 was estimated at 1.2% of the population, or 57.8 million people. Levels of opiate use were much higher than the global average in North America (3.6%), Australia and New Zealand (3.3%), the Near and Middle East and South-West Asia (2.6%) and South Asia (2.0%). As prescription opioids have become pricier and harder to get on the street, heroin has gotten cheaper and easier to obtain (SAMHSA, 2020a–f). It is estimated that about 23% of individuals who use heroin become dependent on it. An opioid drug, heroin is synthesized from morphine. Heroin initiation has decreased significantly with a 57% decline from 2018 (SAMHSA, 2020a–f). Heroin usually is a white or brown powder or as a black sticky substance, known as black tar heroin. Injection of drugs like heroin brings about the highest risk of contracting HIV and hepatitis C. These diseases are transmitted through contact with blood or other bodily fluids, which can occur with sharing of needles or other injection drug use equipment. Hepatitis C is the most common blood-borne infection in the Unites States. HIV can also be contracted during unprotected sex, which drug use makes more likely. There is close association between drug abuse and the increased of infectious diseases.

Gender Differences

In general, higher proportions of males than females are involved in illicit drug use, especially heavy use, and overall, more males than females abuse prescription drugs in all age-groups except those 12 to 17 years old. Females in this age group exceed males in the nonmedical use of all psychotherapeutics, including pain Women experience unique issues related to substance use, due to differences based in biology and on culturally defined roles for men and women (NIDA, 2020a–r). Women frequently use substances differently than men, such as using smaller amounts of certain drugs for less time before they become addicted. They can also respond to substances differently; they may have more drug cravings and may be more likely to relapse after treatment. Women may be more sensitive than men to the effects of some drugs, due to sex hormones. There may also be more physical effects on the heart and blood vessels in women who use drugs, and brain changes can be different from those in men. Lastly, women may be more likely to go to the emergency room or die from overdose or other effects of certain substances, compared to men (NIDA, 2020a–r).

Demographics

Comprehensive data sources the U.S. Census Bureau, Bureau of Labor Statistics, Centers for Disease Control and Prevention, Federal Bureau of Investigation, Substance Abuse and Mental Health Services Administration, U.S. Drug Enforcement Administration, Child and Adolescent Health Measurement Initiative, Project Know, the Pew Charitable Trusts, Guttmacher Institute, OHS Health & Safety Services, IMS Institute for

Healthcare Informatics, Recovery.org and WalletHub research (Kiernan, 2020) make it possible to compare 50 states and the District of Columbia across 22 key metrics, ranging from arrest and overdose rates to opioid prescriptions and employee drug testing laws.

According to their analysis, the five top-ranking states with drug use as their "biggest problem" were Missouri, West Virginia, Michigan, District of Columbia, and New Hampshire. Drug use and addiction were determined by a panel of physician and doctorally prepared drug-addiction experts who compared all 50 states according to 22 metrics, with each metric graded on a 100-point scale. A score of 100 represents the biggest drug problem. Next, they determined each state and the District's weighted average across all metrics to calculate its overall score. This total score was the basis for the final ranking. So the state ranked first in this study has the biggest drug problem, based on the data, while the state ranked 51st has the smallest drug problem.

Constructs representing *drug use and addiction* were the portion of teens who used illicit drugs in the past month; share of teens who tried marijuana before age 13; the number of teens offered, sold, or given an illegal drug on school property during the past year; portion of adults who used illicit drugs in the past month; number of children who lived with anyone who had a problem with alcohol or drugs; number of opioid pain reliever prescriptions per 10 people; number of clandestine drug laboratories or dumpsites; overdose deaths per capita; and over dose deaths growth. Top-ranking states for drug abuse and addiction were Vermont, Delaware, District of Columbia, West Virginia, and New Mexico.

Law enforcement constructs were comprised of drug arrests per capita; drug arrests on college campuses; prescription drug monitoring laws; maternity drug policies (i.e., whether substance abuse during pregnancy is considered a crime); and whether the state has employee drug testing laws. Top ranking states for law enforcement were Missouri, Wyoming, West Virginia, Indiana, and North Dakota.

Drug health issues and rehab constructs were states offering coronavirus support scores; share of adults who could not get treatment for illicit drug use in the past year; number of substance abuse facilities per 100,000 people using illicit drugs; admissions to substance abuse treatment services per 1000 people; drug treatment program availability to pregnant women; share of addiction treatment medication paid by Medicaid; Narcotics Anonymous and Alcoholics Anonymous (AA) meetings accessibility; and substance abuse and behavioral disorder counselors per capita. Top-raking states for drug health issues and rehab were Nevada, District of Columbia, Alabama, Oregon, and Montana.

Additionally, rates of current illicit drug use vary significantly among major racial/ethnic groups. As of 2019, demographic breakdown of the U.S. population by race was: White: 60.1%; Hispanic or Latino: 18.5%; Black or African American: 13.1%; Asian American: 5.9%; American Indian or Alaskan Native: 1.3%; and Native Hawaiian and Other Pacific Islander: 0.3% (U.S. Census Bureau, 2019). In contrast, alcohol

and drug abuse was reported in the following percentages for each racial group: White: 7.7%; Hispanic or Latino 7.1%; Black or African American 6.9%; Asian American: 4.8%; American Indian or Alaskan Native: 10.1%; and Native Hawaiian and Other Pacific Islander: 9.3% (SAMHSA, 2019a,b). Discrepancies in the percentages of American Indian or Alaskan Native and Native Hawaiian and Other Pacific Islander affected by alcohol and drug abuse relative to the proportion of the U.S. population they comprise highlight this health disparity.

Among White Americans alcohol use is the most frequently used substance in individuals age 12 or older in the past year, occurring in 67% of this group, followed by tobacco (in 29.4%) and illicit drugs (in 20.2%) (SAMHSA, 2019a,b). The most commonly used illicit drug in the White Americans, marijuana, was used by 16.5% White Americans. These proportions are slightly different in Hispanic/Latino Americans, of whom 67.9% reported alcohol use, 19.6% tobacco, and 17.1% illicit drugs. Similar to White Americans, in this group marijuana was the most frequently reported illicit drug, used by 13.6% Hispanic/Latino individuals. Black Americans also had these three substances as the most frequently used ones, in 57.3%, 27.2%, and 17.8% of this group, respectively. In Asian Americans, use of these three substances was similarly ranked, though tobacco and illicit drug use frequencies were much closer, used by 12.8% and 8.9% of the Asian American group (Alcohol use was reported in 53.6% Asian Americans). Like each of these groups, Native Hawaiians and other Pacific Islanders' most common substance used was also alcohol, in 54.3% of this group, with tobacco use in 33.6% and marijuana in 17.7%. American Indians had parallel rates of use, with alcohol use in 55%, tobacco in 41%, and marijuana in 23% of this group.

Within each population subgroup are varying trends. For example, in White Americans, particularly White men, are the highest rates of opioid misuse and deaths due to over dose, with over 35,000 White Americans dying from opioid overdose in 2018 (Kaiser Family Foundation, 2018). Hispanic Americans, particularly those ages 26 and over, have experienced a significant increase in marijuana use, and substance abuse occurs more often among Latino Americans with cooccurring mental health disorders. Latino Americans generally have worse outcome in addiction treatment program, though the reason for this is not clear (Close, 2020).

Black Americans in middle and high school have experienced a decline in alcohol use since 2015, about a 25% decrease, and prescription opioid misuse has also decline in all age groups of Black Americans (SAMHSA, 2019a,b). There has been a significant increase in marijuana use in Black Americans, especially those aged 26 and older (Close, 2020). Though Asian Americans have low rates of reported substance abuse, statistics may not be representative; substance abuse may be perceived as atypical or unusual to the culture, thus stigmatizing substance-abusing individuals and possibly making it less likely that Asian Americans will seek treatment for addiction (SAMHSA, 2006). Culture constraints may order that substance abuse is been handled within the family; family dysfunction may be considered a private affair, not up for discussion publicly or even within the family, creating a potential social stigma that may act as a barrier to treatment (Close et al., 2020). Visit the SAMHSA Office of Applied Studies website, at https://www.samhsa.gov/data/ for more information about substance abuse trends and statistics.

Native Hawaiian and Other Pacific Islanders tend to abuse substances at rates much higher than the national average and higher than other minority groups, perhaps due to the fact that many live on islands that may have limited care available and depressed economies (Wong and Barnett, 2010). Easy and regular access to drugs and alcohol at a young age may be common, and Native Hawaiian and Other Pacific Islanders may be less likely to seek health care than other population groups. Individuals of this ethnic group may abuse stimulant drugs more often than other ethnic groups, as these drugs are common in their cultures, may be affordable and easy to obtain (Wong and Barnett, 2010). Compared to White Americans, Native Hawaiian, and Other Pacific Islanders are less likely to complete substance abuse treatment (Godinet et al., 2020).

American Indian and Alaskan Native individuals have experienced significant increases in MA use in those aged 26 and up (SAMHSA, 2019a,b). However, there has been a significant decline in cocaine use in the 18 to 25 subset of American Indians and Alaskan Natives (SAMHSA, 2019a,b). A general mistrust of outside healthcare providers and cultural differences may prevent members of this ethnic group from seeking mental health and/or substance abuse treatment, and these individuals tend to be less likely to enter into treatment programs and may instead focus on traditional healing methods (SAMHSA, 2018).

Access to care, availability of culturally and ethnically congruent care, environmental, social, and financial concerns may be barriers to treatment for people of color or minority groups. It is important for the community health nurse to recognize one's extent of acculturation, spiritual and religious beliefs, primary language and socioeconomic status all must be considered when planning substance use treatment and related nursing care. Respect and sensitivity are essential.

Trends in Substance Use

Research has revealed that problems associated with substance abuse may or may not relate to classically or clinically defined dependence or addiction. Many people are turning to recovery before they have developed physiological dependence. Thus, many in the field have begun to differentiate between use and misuse (*misuse* being interchangeable with *abuse*), and these terms now appear in the literature. This section describes significant trends in substances that are being abused and discusses substance abuse among special populations.

Healthy People 2030 and Substance Abuse

The U.S. Department of Health and Human Services (USDHHS) set goals and objectives related to substance abuse

in *Healthy People 2030* (USDHHS Office of Disease Prevention and Health Promotion, 2021). Healthy People provides measurable public health objectives and tools to help track progress toward achieving them (USDHHS Office of Disease Prevention and Health Promotion, 2021). These objectives are evaluated and reestablished every 10 years. Healthy People identifies public health priorities to help individuals, organizations, and communities across the U.S. to improve health and well-being. The initiative's fifth iteration, Healthy People 2030 builds on knowledge gained over the first 4 decades. The Healthy People 2030 vision is for a society in which all people can achieve their full potential for health and well-being across the lifespan, with a mission to promote, strengthen, and evaluate the nation's efforts to improve the health and well-being of all people (USDHHS Office of Disease Prevention and Health Promotion, 2021). The *Healthy People 2030* box presents selected objectives and targets from *Healthy People 2030* related to substance abuse.

 HEALTHY PEOPLE 2030

Selected Proposed Objectives for Substance Abuse

Goal: Reduce Misuse of Drugs and Alcohol
Drug and Alcohol Use-General
- Reduce drug overdose deaths
- Reduce the proportion of adults who used drugs in the past month
- Reduce the proportion of adults who use marijuana daily or almost daily
- Reduce the proportion of people aged 21 years and over who engaged in binge drinking in the past month
- Reduce the proportion of motor vehicle crash deaths that involve a drunk driver
- Reduce the proportion of people who misused prescription drugs in the past year
- Reduce the proportion of people who used heroin in the past year
- Reduce the proportion of people who started using heroin in the past year

Addiction
- Increase the proportion of people with a substance use disorder who got treatment in the past year
- Reduce the proportion of people who had alcohol use disorder (AUD) in the past year
- Reduce the proportion of people who had drug use disorder in the past year
- Reduce the proportion of people who had opioid use disorder in the past year
- Increase the number of admissions to substance use treatment for injection drug use
- Increase the rate of people with an opioid use disorder getting medications for addiction treatment

Adolescents
- Reduce the proportion of adolescents who drank alcohol in the past month
- Reduce the proportion of adolescents who used drugs in the past month
- Reduce the proportion of adolescents who used marijuana in the past month
- Reduce the proportion of people under 21 years who engaged in binge drinking in the past month
- Increase the proportion of adolescents who think substance abuse is risky

Methamphetamine

MA has evolved as the most widely produced controlled substance in the United States. It is appearing in mass quantities, in part because of the ease with which the fertilizer anhydrous ammonia can be converted into MA, which has attracted more individuals to this clandestine business. MA is a powerful, highly addictive stimulant that affects the central nervous system. Crystal MA is a form of the drug with the appearance of glass fragments or shiny, bluish-white rocks. It is chemically comparable to amphetamine, a drug used to treat attention-deficit hyperactivity disorder (ADHD) and narcolepsy, a sleep disorder (NIDA, 2019a,b). Illegal street forms of MA, often called crank, crystal, or meth, are available as a powder that can be injected, inhaled, or taken orally. In addition, a smokable form, known as ice or glass, is widely available.

The pleasurable effects of MA are due to the release of high levels of dopamine in the brain, leading to increased energy, a sense of euphoria, and greater productivity. Short-term effects are increased heart rate, insomnia, excessive talking, excitation, and aggressive behavior. Prolonged use results in tolerance and physiological dependence. MA has multiple negative effects for users, their families, and communities. It appears to damage the brain in ways that are different from, and more severe than, damage from using other drugs. Negative consequences range from anxiety, convulsions, and paranoia to brain damage.

MA user profiles represent the most common categories reported by officials and treatment professionals: high school and college students and college athletes; and White, blue-collar workers and men and women in their 20s and 30s who are jobless (Rehab International, 2021). Meth abuse occurs across rural and urban boundaries. Usage is divided equally among both women and men. Approximately 964,000 people aged 12 or older (about 0.4% of the population) had a MA use disorder in 2017, as number significantly higher than the 684,000 people who reported having MA use disorder in 2016 (NIDA, 2019a,b). The 2018 reported that about 0.5% of eighth, 10th, and 12th graders had used MA within the past year. Use of MA by adolescents has declined significantly since 1999, when this drug was first added to the MTF survey of adolescent drug use and attitudes (NIDA, 2019a,b). The impact of MA abuse on communities, families, and social networks is considerable. Highest estimated rates of MA use (from 2015 to 2018) were among adults aged 26 to 34 (11.0%), 18 to 25 (9.3%), and 35 to 49 (8.3%) years and among non-Hispanic whites (7.5%), Hispanics (6.7%), and non-Hispanic other races (5.6%) (Jones et al., 2020). MA manufacturing and distribution has been shown to cause significant damage to the environment; is hazardous to innocent children and others in close proximity to where it is being manufactured; can have a negative impact on the economy, crime rates and infrastructure of communities; and has proven to be a drain on vital resources (National Neighborhood Watch, 2021). Furthermore, exposure to combustible secondhand fumes puts children at risk for not only complications related to primary ingestion but also fatalities and injuries related to the highly combustible nature of the chemicals used in manufacture of the drug.

Steroids

Anabolic steroids are synthetic variants of the male sex hormone testosterone. The proper term for these compounds is anabolic-androgenic steroids. They can build muscle and are said to be androgenic, referring to increased male sexual characteristics. These steroids are taken orally, injected into the muscles, or applied topically. Doses taken may be 10 to 100 times higher than the doses prescribed to treat medical conditions (NIDA, 2018b). Steroids taken continuously can decrease the body's responsiveness to the drugs, increasing tolerance as well as causing the body to stop producing its own testosterone. Though prior evidence suggested that steroid use among adolescents was decreasing, more recent dat shows steroid use in this group trending upward. In 8th, 10th, and 12th graders, rates of lifetime and past year steroid use increased from 2017 to 2020, while past month use increased for 10th and 12th graders and stayed the same for eight graders in the MTF Study (NIDA, 2020a—r). Steroid use is more common in athletes and other individuals willing to risk potential and irreversible health consequences to build muscle. There are other more potentially fatal risks, including blood clots, liver damage, premature cardiovascular changes, and increased cholesterol (NIDA, 2018b). Evidence also points at behavioral changes leading to an increased potential for suicide and aggressive and risky behaviors among steroid users. Collaborative treatment programs that monitor both psychological and physical issues, including options of the drug use route as injection, are necessary to combat steroid abuse.

Although anabolic steroids do not cause the same high as other drugs, use of this type of steroid can lead to substance use disorder. Steroid use may persist despite physical problems and negative effects on social relationships that it causes. Steroid abusers typically spend large amounts of time and money obtaining the drug. Individuals who abuse steroids often experience withdrawal symptoms when they stop using them, including mood swings, fatigue, restlessness, loss of appetite, insomnia, reduced sex drive, and steroid cravings. One of the most dangerous withdrawal symptoms is depression. Persistent depressive symptoms can sometimes lead to suicide attempts. Research has found that some steroid abusers turn to other drugs, such as opioids, to counteract the negative effects of steroids (NIDA, 2018a—h).

ADOLESCENT SUBSTANCE ABUSE

Youth are a particularly susceptible aggregate for substance abuse. Recent use of illicit substances is most common among people in their mid-teens to mid-20s; similarly, rates of substance abuse and dependence were highest among people aged 18 to 25 (Shaffer, 2020). Roughly 23% of people in that age group had problems with abuse and dependence, compared with just under 9% of the general population (Shaffer).

In 2019, the majority (45.9 million) of the 58.1 million current tobacco users were current cigarette smokers, and among past month tobacco product users, the percentage who used only cigarettes increased with age (35.4% of adolescents aged 12—17,

49.6% of young adults ages 18 to 25, and 68.% of adults aged 26 or older). However, the percentage who used only noncigarette tobacco products decreased with age (39.6% of adolescents, 27.9% of young adults, and 19.5% of adults aged 26 or older) (SAHMSA, 2020a). Cigarettes are still highly available to the young, and concerned groups continue to monitor advertising that targets new potential smokers, such as youth and women.

The 2019 National Survey on Drug Use and Health (NSDUH) measured perceived risk as the percentage of youth reporting that there is great risk in the substance use behavior (SAMHSA, 2019a,b).

With legalization of marijuana in 11 states and District of Columbia, there is definitely skepticism about the drug's danger. There is research that marijuana use during adolescence has the potential to set young people up for a cascade of life-altering events, impeding their success and hindering them from fulfilling their potential. Teens too often do not believe this to be true. The MTF survey of drug use has for years demonstrated a steady drop in the number of middle- and high-school students who think occasional or even regular marijuana users risk harming themselves physically or in other ways (SAMHSA, 2020a–f).

In order to effectively plan for the present and future needs of the community, the community health nurse needs the most current overall perspective. Information on the prevalence, incidence, and trends in the amount and types of substance abuse at the general, state, and local levels is readily available on the Internet. As harmful, illicit substances come in and out of vogue, particularly among young people, the community health nurse must develop a good understanding of drug culture, terminology, and differing signs and symptoms.

CONCEPTUALIZATIONS OF SUBSTANCE ABUSE

Conceptualizations of substance abuse and dependence have changed over the years, often for political and social reasons rather than for scientific reasons. Some conceptualizations focus on the phenomenon of **addiction**, which is manifested by compulsive use patterns and the onset of withdrawal symptoms when substance use is abruptly stopped. Other views focus on the problems resulting from the substance use itself, regardless of whether an addictive pattern is present. Problematic consequences of substance use include intoxication, psychological dependence, relational conflicts, employment or economic difficulties, legal difficulties, and health problems. For example, addiction need not be present for individuals to experience legal consequences of illicit drug use, such as driving while intoxicated or alcohol- or drug-related domestic violence.

Drawing fine distinctions among ideas of dependence, addiction, and abuse concerning substance use may seem irrelevant if there is evidence that the substance use has become problematic. Indeed, the DSM-5 revisions included combining abuse and dependence criteria into a single substance use disorder. The DSM-5 has 11 criteria for substance use disorders

based on decades of research and has helped change how we think about addictions by not overly focusing on withdrawal (Addiction Policy Forum, 2020).

In the DSM-5, symptoms of substance abuse disorders fall into four categories: (1) impaired control, (2) social problems, (3) risky use, and (4) physical dependence (Box 27.1).

The DSM-5 provides guidelines for clinicians to determine how severe a substance use disorder is, based on the number of symptoms one has. Two or three symptoms indicate a mild substance use disorder; four or five symptoms indicate a moderate substance use disorder, and six or more symptoms indicate a severe substance use disorder. A severe SUD is also known as having an addiction. It is also becoming increasingly evident that specific interventions may be needed for each separate addictive problem (e.g., overeating and gambling). Moreover, in each specific group, there is wide individual diversity.

Definitions

The DSM-5 acknowledges substance-related disorders resulting from the use of 10 separate classes of drugs: alcohol; caffeine; cannabis; hallucinogens (phencyclidine or similarly acting aryl-cyclohexylamines, and other hallucinogens, such as LSD); inhalants; opioids; sedatives, hypnotics, or anxiolytics; stimulants (including amphetamine-type substances, cocaine, and other stimulants); tobacco; and other or unknown substances (Verywellmind, 2020). There are two groups of substance-related disorders: substance-use disorders and substance-induced disorders. Substance-use disorders are patterns of symptoms resulting from the use of a substance that one continues to take, despite experiencing problems as a result, while substance-induced disorders, including intoxication, withdrawal, and other substance/medication-induced mental disorders, are detailed alongside substance use disorders (APA, 2013). Traditional conceptualizations of substance use focus solely on alcohol and illicit street drugs. Other conceptualizations include prescription medications such as tranquilizers and analgesics. In eating disorders such as bulimia and compulsive overeating, food is viewed as the abused substance. Table 27.1 shows a classification scheme for commonly used substances.

BOX 27.1 DSM-5 Categories of SUD Symptoms

Impaired Control	Social Problems	Risky Use	Physical Dependence
Using more of a substance or more often than intended	Neglecting responsibilities and relationships	Using in risky settings	Needing more of the substance to get the same effect (tolerance)
Wanting to cut down or stop using but not being able to	Giving up activities they used to care about because of their substance use	Continued use despite problems	Having withdrawal symptoms when a substance isn't used
	Inability to complete tasks at home, school, or work		

SUD, Substance use disorder.

TABLE 27.1   Classification of Commonly Used and Abused Substances

Substance	Desired Effect(s)	Possible Withdrawal Symptoms
Central Nervous System Depressants		
Alcohol	Euphoria, disinhibition, and sedation	Anxiety, irritability, seizures, delusions, hallucinations, and paranoia
Barbiturates	Euphoria and sedation	Restlessness, tremors, and anxiety
Sedative-hypnotics (e.g., benzodiazepines [Rohypnol])	Sedation and amnesia	Insomnia, anxiety restlessness, and tremors
Tranquilizers (e.g., GHB [gamma-hydroxybutyrate], the "date rape" drug)	Depress consciousness	Confusion, psychosis, agitation
Central Nervous System Stimulants		
Amphetamines (e.g., methamphetamine)	Euphoria, hyperactivity, omnipotence, insomnia, and anorexia	Depression, apathy, lethargy, and sleepiness
Cocaine	Increased sense of energy and alertness	Depression and anxiety
Nicotine	Calmness concentration	Restlessness and agitation
Caffeine	Concentration, energy	Restlessness and agitation
Narcotics-opioids	Euphoria and sedation	Restlessness, pain, and agitation
Codeine	Euphoria and sedation	Anxiety, irritability, agitation, runny nose, watery eyes, chills, sweating, nausea and vomiting, diarrhea, tremors, and yawning
Meperidine and acetaminophen (e.g., Demerol)	Euphoria and sedation	Restlessness, pain, and agitation
Hydromorphone (e.g., Dilaudid)	Euphoria and sedation	Restlessness, pain, and agitation
Fentanyl	Euphoria and sedation	Restlessness, pain, and agitation
Heroin	Euphoria and sedation	Restlessness, pain, and agitation
Methadone	Euphoria and sedation	Restlessness, pain, and agitation
Morphine	Euphoria and sedation	Restlessness, pain, and agitation
Opium	Euphoria and sedation	Restlessness, pain, and agitation
Oxycodone (e.g., Percodan)	Euphoria and sedation	Restlessness, pain, and agitation
Hallucinogens		
Mescaline	Hallucinations, illusions, and heightened awareness	Depression
LSD	Hallucinations, illusions, and heightened awareness	Depression
PCP (phencyclidine) (e.g., ketamine)	PCP: Violent dissociative and anesthetic effect Ketamine: Agitation, confusion, psychosis, (including delusions and hallucinations), loss of motor skills, rage, nausea, decrease in respiratory and cardiac functions, insomnia, tremors, Hearing loss, fatigue	
STP (2,5-dimethoxy-4-methylamphetamine) and MDMA (methylenedioxymethamphetamine (i.e., Ecstasy)	Hallucinations, illusions, and heightened awareness	Depression
Psilocybin (e.g., mushrooms)	Hallucinations, illusions, and heightened awareness	Depression
Cannabis		
Marijuana	Hallucinations, illusions, and heightened awareness	Depression
Hashish and THC (tetrahydrocannabinol)	Hallucinations, illusions, and heightened awareness	Depression
Inhalants		
Gasoline	Euphoria	Restlessness, anxiety, and irritability
Toluene acetate	Euphoria	Restlessness, anxiety, and irritability
Cleaning fluids	Euphoria	Restlessness, anxiety, and irritability
Airplane cement	Euphoria	Restlessness, anxiety, and irritability
Amyl nitrate	Euphoria	Restlessness, anxiety, and irritability

Modified from Faltz B, Rinaldi J: *AIDS and substance abuse: a training manual for health care professionals*, San Francisco, 1987, Regents of the University of California.

In addition to varying in their abuse potential, substances vary in their degree of potential harm to those who use them and to others in the immediate environment. Tobacco is an example of a substance that is unsafe to the smoker and to those who inhale secondhand smoke. Those who abuse alcohol may also harm others by driving under its influence, and its lowering of inhibitions may foster violent activities in some users (e.g., child or partner abuse).

The APA (2021) focused on the following psychoactive substances that affect the nervous system: alcohol, amphetamines, caffeine, cannabis, cocaine, hallucinogens, inhalants, tobacco, opioids, phencyclidine, sedatives, and hypnotics or anxiolytics. Substance use disorders can also be categorized as being in early remission ($\geq$3 to <12 months without meeting substance use disorders criteria, except craving) and sustained remission ($\geq$12 months without meeting substance use disorders criteria, except craving) (APA, 2013). A diagnosis of substance use disorder indicates a maladaptive pattern of substance use that is manifested as recurrent and significant adverse consequences related to repeated use of a substance. These adverse consequences include failure to fulfill major role obligations, repeated use in physically hazardous situations, multiple legal problems, and recurrent social and interpersonal problems.

The criteria for the diagnosis of dependence include a cluster of cognitive, behavioral, and physiological symptoms that indicate continued use of the substance despite significant substance-related problems, use a criteria count (from 2 to 11) as an overall severity indicator, and use number of criteria met to indicate mild (2–3 criteria), moderate (4–5), and severe (6 or more) disorders. A pattern of repeated, self-administered use results in tolerance, withdrawal, and compulsive drug-taking behaviors, which are frequently accompanied by a craving or strong desire for the substance. This craving then motivates the user to be preoccupied with supply, money to purchase drugs, and getting through time between periods of use, all of which take up mental energy, effort that is diverted from work or school and from connectedness to significant others. This process is how the use becomes problematic and how others around the user become confused and eventually often feel rejected, hurt, ignored, angry, or even responsible for the user's behavior.

SOCIOCULTURAL AND POLITICAL ASPECTS OF SUBSTANCE ABUSE

Within community settings, substance-related problems are not always easy to identify. For example, the consequences of the sale and use of crack cocaine in an inner-city, African American neighborhood may be apparent through media attention. The traffic of these drugs into the middle classes, on the other hand, is less easily recognized. The increasing tendencies of elderly persons to rely on alcohol and other, even illicit, drugs may be shocking to some nurses. It can be understood contextually, however, and may be the result of multiple factors, such as isolation, fears, uncontrolled chronic pain, anxiety, and sleep

disturbances. Nurses must incorporate sociocultural and political dimensions into caring for clients in the community. Nurses must also possess knowledge that is useful in countering media stereotypes and allows them to model a more holistic, multifaceted approach to prevention and management of substance abuse.

Although there are subcultural and regional variations, drinking norms of the dominant culture in the United States are relatively permissive. Traditional ethnic ceremonial and symbolic substance use patterns vary significantly. As acculturation occurs, however, cultural definitions of "appropriate" use of alcohol and drugs have been dulled, leaving a void regarding social expectations. Subcultural groups such as gay, lesbian, bisexual, and transgender persons have often had a social center that was a bar, and alcohol use was historically a way of demonstrating and celebrating differentiation from a more repressive majority. These cultural conditions create ambiguity in clearly determining when a substance abuse problem exists. Furthermore, each subculture may define *abuse* differently. It can be theorized that stigmatized minorities might be under more stress, and perhaps more likely to use substances, but this cannot be assumed in any individual case.

Substances are also given economic value and are bought and sold as commodities in a variety of social arenas, both legal and illegal. The ways in which drugs, including nicotine, medications, and alcohol, are produced and distributed among the various segments of the population are determined largely by economic, cultural, and political conditions.

COURSE OF SUBSTANCE-RELATED PROBLEMS

There is no predictable course of addictive illness and no "addictive personality type." When habitual use is well established, behaviors may be clinically visible and similar; this observation has led to assumption of a singular, addiction-prone personality. However, not everyone who initiates drug or alcohol use progresses to dependence or displays associated behaviors. Because the path from **initiation** to dependency is multidimensional, the context of client and community experiences is key to understanding and responding to problems encountered. Nurses need to take a comprehensive health and substance use history and place it in a context of cultural, historical, family, and social factors. Neither addiction nor dependency is a unitary phenomenon with a single isolated cause; rather, it is the result of interactions among a host of variables.

A variety of screening and assessment tools are available (NIDA, 2018a–h). It is important to consider the person, substance, and the context (Patrick et al., 2016). The person assessment involves demographic information, medical history, comorbidities, and known perceptions and meanings the individual displays. The drug assessment consists of the qualities of the substance itself, physiopharmacological effects, pattern of use, availability, and toxicity. Context assessment should cover family, social, employment, legal, cultural, and economic contingencies.

The progression from initiation to continuation, transition to abuse, and, finally, addiction and dependency varies. Individuals often describe a progression that began with initiation through social interactions. For some, the substance and setting are reinforcing and prime the individual for a pattern of use. For others, the experience is unpleasant enough to prevent further use. It cannot be assumed, however, that an unpleasant initiation will always be preventive. In the case of stimulants, such as MA, the drug produces such strong feelings of euphoria, alertness, control, and increased energy that future use is enticing, especially when the drug is easily accessible.

The continuation stage of substance abuse is a subsequent period in which substance use persists but does not appear to be detrimental to the individual. In stimulant abuse, continued use often occurs in a binge pattern. Individuals are able to exercise some control over use, but use becomes more frequent. Neither the individual nor the social network views use during this stage as problematic.

A critical point is the transition stage from substance use to substance abuse. It may be evident to both the user and his or her social network that the use of the substance is having adverse effects. During this stage, users begin to use more often and in more varied settings. Rationalizations that deny the seriousness and consequences of the substance use are commonly constructed during this stage.

The research on correlates and antecedents of substance abuse points to a variety of personal and social motivations. For many young people, motivators are the attraction of a rebellious subculture, peer pressure, and nationwide fads. Considerable research exists on the self-medication aspects of individuals with comorbid mental illnesses. Once the addiction is established, unpleasant physical and emotional withdrawal symptoms are strong motivators to continue use. Abstinence in the stimulant abuser can result in symptoms such as depression, lethargy, and anhedonia (i.e., inability to feel pleasure). The depression experienced by the user when not using stimulants is contrasted with the recalled euphoria produced by the use of the drug. These factors, coupled with associated cues, help initiate the cycle of binge use, with increased craving and continued self-administration to relieve symptoms. Brain imaging techniques have demonstrated that abuse of drugs such as cocaine and amphetamine produce immediate and long-lasting physical changes that are likely to contribute to the maintenance of dependency. Nurses can learn more about this research from the NIDA's web page on addiction science, at http://www.drugabuse.gov/related-topics/addiction-science.

The development of addiction or dependency is marked by changes in both behavior and cognition. There is a growing focus on the substance and a narrowing of interests, social activities, and relationships. The process of becoming dependent or addicted requires the individual to deny or ignore evidence or information that may challenge the behavior or the rationalization of the behavior. There is a preoccupation with the substance and its procurement during this stage, even in the face of negative consequences. Table 27.2 outlines the stages in the process of stimulant addiction.

TABLE 27.2 Typical Course of Addictive Illness: Stages in Continuum From Initiation to Dependency

Stage	Characteristics
Initiation	First use of the substance
	Exposure frequently occurs through family or friends
Continuation	Continued, more frequent use of substance
	Usually social use only, with no detrimental effects
Transition	Beginning of change in total consumption, frequency, and occasions of use
	More than just social use, with beginning of loss of control
Abuse	Adverse effects and consequences of substance use
	Rationalizations for continued use and denial of adverse effects present in user and significant others
	Unsuccessful attempts at control of use
Dependency and addiction	Physical or psychological dependency, or both, on the substance; marked by behavioral and cognitive changes
	Preoccupation with the substance and its procurement, despite negative consequences
	Narrowing of interests, social activities, and relationships to only those related to the substance use

LEGAL AND ETHICAL CONCERNS RELATED TO SUBSTANCE ABUSE

For the past 30 years, the United States has pursued a drug policy based on prohibition and the active application of criminal sanctions against the use and sale of illicit drugs. During this time, the number of criminal penalties for drug offenses has climbed to 1.5 million offenses. This increase in drug-related imprisonment is a result of harsher enforcement policies and longer mandatory sentences for possession of smaller quantities of drugs. Although some individuals are in prison for violent crimes (Drugwarfacts.org, 2016) or major drug trafficking, many drug offenders are arrested for small-scale drug deals made to support their personal use (Drugwarfacts). Of the approximately 1,558,862 arrests for drug law violations in the United States in 2019, 86.7% (1,351,533) were for possession of a controlled substance, and 13.3% (207,328) were for sale or manufacture of a drug (Common Sense for Drug Policy, 2021). Of the arrests for possession, 500, 395 of these were for marijuana, 305,537 for heroin, cocaine and derivatives, and 62,354 were for synthetic or manufactured drugs. Arrests for sale/manufacturing were heroin, cocaine, and derivatives (65,472), marijuana (45,207), and synthetic or manufactured drugs (26,501).There were 68,590 arrests for other dangerous nonnarcotic drugs.

Alcohol use and abuse are different issues because the possession and sale of alcoholic beverages is illegal only if the individual involved is a minor. Concerns arise when individuals are intoxicated during work, while driving, or in situations that may affect the welfare of others. Legal penalties have increased for driving under the influence of alcohol because groups such as Mothers Against Drunk Driving have influenced legislation (Box 27.2).

BOX 27.2 Drunk Driving

In 2018, 10,511 people were killed in alcohol-impaired crashes, a decrease of 3.6% from the 10,908 deaths in 2017. Alcohol-impaired driving accidents involve at least one driver or motorcycle operator with a blood alcohol concentration (BAC) of 0.08 g per deciliter (g/dL) or higher. There has been progress in reducing alcohol-impaired crashes; in 1982, 48% of all traffic deaths involved alcohol-impaired crashes. This proportion has decreased to 29% of deaths in 2018. The percentage of lower BAC alcohol-involved crashes (from 0.01 to 0.07 g/dL) has been very stable over the decades, fluctuating between 5% and 7%.

From National Safety Council: *Motor vehicle safety issues*, 2020. https://injuryfacts.nsc.org/motor-vehicle/motor-vehicle-safety-issues/alcohol-impaired-driving/

BOX 27.3 Substance Abuse and Pregnancy

Use of a drug, alcohol, or tobacco by a pregnant woman, thereby exposing her developing fetus to the substance, can have potentially deleterious and even long-term effects on the exposed child. Smoking during pregnancy can increase risks of stillbirth, infant mortality, sudden infant death syndrome, preterm birth, respiratory problems, slowed fetal growth, and low birth weight. Alcohol use during pregnancy can lead to the development of fetal alcohol spectrum disorders, characterized by low birth weight and enduring cognitive and behavioral problems. Prenatal use of opioids and other drugs may cause a withdrawal syndrome in newborns called neonatal abstinence syndrome (NAS). These infants are at greater risk of seizures, respiratory problems, feeding difficulties, low birth weight, and even death. There are evidence-based treatments for pregnant women (and their babies), including medications. Methadone maintenance combined with prenatal care and a comprehensive drug treatment program can improve many of the detrimental outcomes associated with untreated maternal heroin abuse. However, newborns exposed to methadone during pregnancy still require treatment for withdrawal symptoms. A medication option for opioid dependence, buprenorphine, has been shown to produce fewer NAS symptoms in babies than methadone, resulting in shorter infant hospital stays. In general, it is important to closely monitor women who are trying to quit drug use during pregnancy and to provide treatment as needed.

Data from National Institute on Drug Abuse: *Principles of drug addiction treatment: a research*-based guide, ed 3, 2012b. NIH Publication No. 12–4180.

One area that has also received the attention of the legal system is the use by pregnant women of substances known to increase risks to their fetuses in terms of future long-term developmental and behavioral problems (Box 27.3). Pregnant addicts have been imprisoned and forced into treatment, and their children have been removed from their custody after birth. Many treatment providers and patient advocates view this approach as punitive and counterproductive to assisting these women and their children. There is concern that such sanctions may prevent addicted women from seeking treatment, for fear of legal consequences.

Military veterans are an aggregate in great need of quality **substance abuse treatment** (American Addiction Centers, 2021). The U.S. Department of Veterans Affairs (VA) can address the following areas in substance abuse: screenings for alcohol or tobacco use, outpatient counseling, intensive outpatient treatment (IOT), marriage and family counseling, self-help groups, and drug substitution therapies.

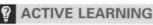 **ACTIVE LEARNING**

Locate resources in your community that help veterans with substance abuse.

MODES OF INTERVENTION

Correlating with the numerous theories about substance abuse is the wide variety of **intervention** strategies incorporating all levels of prevention. National, state, and local legislative measures have attempted to limit access to potentially addictive pharmaceuticals and illicit street drugs. The growing social demand for smoke-free environments in public buildings, restaurants, airplanes, and similar areas exemplifies how perceptions of tobacco and its risks have changed over the past 50 years. Alcohol taxes, zoning schemes for liquor outlets, a legal drinking age, and legal sanctions on driving while intoxicated are other examples of community efforts to prevent or contain substance abuse.

Media campaigns provide public service communications about the risks of substance abuse and the availability of treatment for these problems. However, these efforts must have culturally relevant and realistic goals. Some have proved to be quite successful. The Partnership for a Drug-Free America conducted an antiinhalant media campaign. Several goals of *Healthy People 2030* are reduction of the proportion of adolescents who drank alcohol in the past month; who used drugs in the past month; who used marijuana in the past month; reduction in the proportion of people under age 21 who engaged in binge drinking in the past month; and increasing the proportion of adolescents who think substance abuse is risky (U. S. Department of Health and Human Services Office of Disease Prevention and Health Promotion, 2021). Educational programs administered through schools and penal institutions have been developed, but evaluation and evidence of success or failure of the interventions have been sporadic. National organizations such as the Partnership for a Drug-Free America and the National Alliance on Mental Illness (NAMI) have national, state, and local chapters and affiliates that support community education, research, and support.

Prevention

The principles of prevention are paramount in community nursing practice. Primary prevention in the community includes working with other providers to perform a needs assessment. This process identifies high-risk situations and potential problems that threaten the integrity of the community and its inhabitants—in particular, what factors in the community are encouraging initiation of substance abuse, how effective school- and community-based programs are, and what political issues in the community may be influencing resource allocation.

On the federal level, primary prevention efforts have been overshadowed by the ongoing "War on Drugs." A significant amount of fiscal resources has been allocated to law enforcement, interdiction, crop eradication, and harsh, punitive laws to prosecute drug users and manufacturers. Debate continues at both the state and federal levels regarding the cost-benefit ratio of drug legalization or decriminalization. Supporters argue that legalization and decriminalization would lead to a reduction in crime and would move the drug problem out of the realm in which it is regarded as the moral failure of individuals toward more humane treatment approaches. Thus, public support for the war on drugs has waned in recent decades, with some Americans and policymakers asserting that the campaign has been ineffective or has led to racial divide (History.com, 2019). Between 2009 and 2013, some 40 states took steps to soften their drug laws, lowering penalties and shortening mandatory minimum sentences, according to the Pew Research Center (2014). Though the War on Drugs is still being fought, it with less intensity and publicity than in its early years.

There is no question that substance abuse is a costly medical, social, and legal problem. Until society can effectively deal with the serious effects of two lethal but legal drugs, alcohol and nicotine, there will be an argument for adding further sanctions that is difficult to accept and justify. Other preventive efforts at government and private levels include community-based programs, training of health professionals, faith-based initiatives, volunteer consumer groups, organized sports programs, and employer programs.

The secondary prevention role of the community health nurse involves screening and finding resources and solutions specific to the particular community. It is important for the community health nurse to be aware of the evidence base for certain programs and to modify or discard those programs that have not proved successful over time.

Screening tools such as the CAGE (Ewing, 1984) test are brief and simple and allow health providers to talk about substance abuse by incorporating relevant questions into the interview and history of any client. A positive response to any of the CAGE questions does not constitute a diagnosis of alcohol or drug dependence, but it should raise suspicion and mandate further investigation.

Prevention efforts should be specific to aggregates rather than directed at the general public. The Clinical Institute Withdrawal Assessment (CIWA) is a continual assessment protocol commonly utilized in the medical setting that helps patients transition through alcohol withdrawal with less risk of **delirium tremens** (DTs) and other medical problems (Jesse et al., 2017; Sen et al., 2017). The CIWA focuses on common withdrawal symptoms, such as nausea and vomiting, anxiety, paroxysmal sweats, tactile disturbances, tremors, agitation, orientation, auditory disturbances, and headaches.

Prevention efforts and interventions focusing on minority groups such as African Americans have been limited (De Kock, 2020). A possible reason is that such treatment programs fail to incorporate culturally sensitive and appropriate interventions and strategies. The demand for a culturally specific approach is

evidence that previous approaches, and the assumptions that underlie them, are insufficient for understanding and explaining the etiology of substance abuse among members of minority groups. Successful prevention efforts are usually not focused solely on alcohol and drug abuse but are appropriately matched with cultural traditions, respect the values of clients, and are grounded in partnership with communities (Blume, 2016).

Treatment

Substance abuse problems are socially defined and frequently attributed to sufferers who do not recognize their substance use as a problem. Furthermore, the substance abuse treatment system has increasingly taken on social welfare and criminal justice tasks. In this sense, substance abuse differs from many other health-related problems. Most states have laws pertaining to involuntary treatment of substance abusers. Employers and families are often enlisted to assist or coerce the identified client into accepting treatment. This aspect of substance abuse as a health concern raises some crucial questions for health care providers in terms of the encroachment of therapeutic interventions on individual rights to privacy, informed consent, and self-determination.

On the individual level, those providing substance abuse treatment should take into consideration the cultural and educational background and resources of the person, the attitudes of significant others, the degree of invasiveness of the effects of the substance use, and the existence of alternatives. Interventions have been developed to assist some individuals in achieving moderation. Additionally, some research has shown that a small percentage of individuals who recognize a harmful pattern of substance use are able to stop using the substance or to achieve a controlled, nonpathological pattern of use. There are those who, because they experience an important life change, such as graduating from college or getting married, appear to change from excessive alcohol use to social alcohol use.

Nevertheless, people exhibit serious problems related to their use of substances and are usually not able to stop or control their use without outside intervention. Research on identified problem drinkers' ability to return to social alcohol use is still inconclusive. Consequently, most scientists and health care providers advocate **abstinence** as a cornerstone of recovery.

Abstinence is difficult to maintain on a long-term basis. Therefore, an important area of continuing research is relapse prevention (i.e., a behavioral approach that aims to prepare the client for the relapse situation in the hope of preventing it or minimizing its impact on recovery). Relapse prevention models can be applied to alcohol, drug, and behavioral addictive problems (e.g., overeating and compulsive gambling) and can have either controlled use or abstinence as their goal. In relapse prevention, relapses are reframed as learning opportunities, and the client makes plans for coping with negative mood states, meeting the challenge of craving, and stopping a relapse quickly if it should occur.

Inpatient and outpatient are the two main types of treatment programs for substance abuse. Each of these programs may or may not include a detoxification component. Treatment programs also differ in the following ways: they may be voluntary or compulsory and pharmacologically based or drug free. In general, although treatment is intricately tied to the concept of recovery, disciplinary philosophy guides specific treatment approaches. There are a variety of treatment approaches and models, which are sometimes contradictory. The treatment models vary by such factors as the composition of staff and the philosophical approach (i.e., social vs. psychological vs. medical models) to substance abuse problems.

Inpatient treatment isolates individuals from the external world and provides an opportunity to focus only on substance abuse issues. Outpatient treatment is appropriate for those who do not require such structure and protection, those with strong supportive social networks and high levels of motivation, and those who need to continue working while in recovery.

The severity of the individual's alcohol or drug problems and pertinent cultural factors determine the necessity and type of treatment. Therefore, the assessment process is of primary importance and begins with an accurate social and medical history. The history taking begins with more general questions about lifestyle, employment, relationships, and self-perception. This general line of questioning permits the development of a therapeutic relationship with the client.

A therapeutic relationship based on trust is essential to collecting information about sensitive issues such as drug and alcohol use. The assessment should then proceed to determining risky behavior patterns and stressors. The interviewer assesses dietary practices; prior health problems; allergies; hospitalizations, including psychiatric disorders; and family history of similar problems, including drug- and alcohol-related problems. This general line of questioning can be followed by more specific questions about harmful behaviors, such as smoking, drinking, and illicit drug use. This ordering of questions progresses from the more socially sanctioned behaviors to more "socially disapproved" behaviors and from the general to the more specific. Positive responses to questions about drug and alcohol use should be probed in a nonjudgmental, direct way and treated as "routine" in healthcare encounters.

A physical examination is another valuable tool in evaluating the client for potential or actual alcohol and drug problems. Although at-risk clients may not have physical signs of alcohol and drug problems and may even deny obvious consequences of such, certain physical findings warrant further investigation. Complaints such as vague, nonspecific abdominal pain, insomnia, depression, chronic fatigue, back pain, chronic anxiety, refractory hypertension, and night sweats require more intensive investigation. Consistent and heavy users of MA commonly experience extensive and rampant tooth decay, known as "Meth Mouth," owing to the acidic nature of the drug. Although laboratory tests may not yield clues to drug or alcohol use, certain laboratory findings (e.g., abnormal liver function), in the absence of other etiological agents, may raise the index of suspicion.

Intervention strategies frequently begin with information about the effects of alcohol and drugs and a discussion of the solutions to substance abuse–related problems. This initial educational approach can defuse frequently encountered barriers to intervention, such as shame, guilt, fear, and the client's erroneous perceptions regarding risks. Presenting information and solutions in a nonjudgmental and clear manner may help minimize defensiveness. Reframing interventions within the context of health maintenance or health promotion and education minimizes the sense of stigma.

Ambivalent clients may respond to education and decide to abstain from substances or seek treatment. Other clients, however, even when confronted with legal, financial, physical, and psychological consequences of substance abuse, may resist treatment offers. Therefore, the clinician must continue to work with clients and involve important members of their social network to remove internal and environmental barriers and move clients toward readiness for change and treatment. Potential discrimination in group settings and logistical problems, such as lack of child care, may be barriers to treatment.

Much of the effort for substance abuse treatment has been invested in detoxification, residential, and outpatient treatment programs. Secondary problems related to drug and alcohol abuse are intoxication, overdose, and withdrawal. Overdose may be accidental or intentional and requires acute interventions to stabilize the client. As a client advocate, the community health nurse can be an important ally in ensuring that adequate follow-up is conducted for those admitted to emergency departments for overdose. **Detoxification** is best described as a short-term treatment intervention designed to manage acute withdrawal from the substance. It involves medical management to reduce the adverse side effects of the substance and help stabilize the client. It may be performed on an inpatient or outpatient basis, depending on the substance and severity of dependence.

Addressing acute withdrawal symptoms is of utmost importance in detoxification. The cocaine abuser may experience extreme depression with suicidal ideation. Withdrawal from central nervous system depressants, including alcohol, produces the most life-threatening medical consequences, including anxiety, tremors, delirium, convulsions, and possible death, unless medically managed. Symptoms of withdrawal from narcotics, although less life threatening, are temporarily disabling and painful; they include chills, sweating, cramps, and nausea. Such feelings may cause the individual who is withdrawing from treatment to begin the cycle of abuse again. Detoxification is one of the most crucial periods in the recovery process. Clinicians should be aware of the level of services offered in any detoxification program in order to make appropriate referrals.

Outpatient and inpatient treatment programs vary, but they usually include group and individual therapy and counseling, motivational interviewing, family counseling, education, and socialization into 12-step mutual self-help groups. Many programs are integrating psychotherapy, such as cognitive-behavioral therapy, with pharmacotherapy. The medications used are discussed more fully in the next section. Other strategies are hypnosis, occupational therapy, confrontation, assertiveness training, blood alcohol—level discrimination training, and other behavior modification approaches. Relapses are common; therefore, the most effective treatment programs incorporate some form of relapse prevention as a part of the healing process.

Therapy that involves the family has proved to be most effective in aiding recovery. Family and social contacts can be helped to initiate change in the abuser, to aid in recovery, and to assist in maintenance of treatment gains. A well-known family involvement motivational technique is the Johnson Institute Intervention, which involves a confrontation of the abuser with guidance from therapists (American Psychological Association, 2021). A less coercive version is called A Relational Sequence for Engagement (ARISE) (Association of Intervention Specialists, 2017), whereby significant others are educated and coached over time. Another effective strategy is Community Reinforcement and Family Training (CRAFT) (Center for Motivation and Change, 2014). With this approach, a concerned significant other is trained in techniques such as positive reinforcement, identification of dangerous situations, and stress reduction. NIDA (2014) published a research-based guide to drug addiction treatment. Important points from this publication are listed in Box 27.4.

Treatment programs have been unprepared for the influx of users of MA and the unique problems associated with its use. Prolonged MA use may lead to serious acute psychotic

disorders with intensive physical and psychological withdrawal, characterized by protracted anhedonia and dysphoria and accompanied by severe craving. Currently, there are no medications to reverse overdoses of and no reliable drugs to treat the paranoia and psychosis associated with MA. However, combination of injectable naltrexone and oral bupropion, appears safe and effective in treating adults with moderate or severe MA use disorder, and thus shows promise (Trivedi et al., 2021). Complications of treatment include high dropout rates, severe behavioral and psychotic states, and severe craving. Various treatments for MA abuse and addiction are being tried, with mixed results. The effect of MA on brain functioning suggests a need for longer treatment plans. The most promising is a long-term comprehensive case study approach, using home visits and assisting with transportation and emergency fund provision. While there are evidence-based psychosocial treatments (including cognitive-behavioral therapy) available for the treatment of MA, there are no FDA-approved medications for this SUD (National Institutes of Health, 2021).

Studies show that clients respond favorably to treatment for MA use, but because of the multiple dimensions, it is a very challenging problem. Women with MA problems who have young children require a higher level of care. Specifics may include an environment of security and safety with social and emotional support (New Beginnings, 2021). Because many abusers lack a supportive environment, the potential for relapse is high. Also, because of MA addicts' typical inability to recognize the problematic nature of their use, combined drug court and outpatient treatment strategies are being developed.

Having a substance abuse problem does not mean that all problems are attributable to the addiction. Many substance-abusing clients also have other psychiatric problems (e.g., schizophrenia, depression, bipolar affective disorder, dissociative disorder, posttraumatic stress disorder). The coexistence of both a mental health and a substance use disorder is referred to as cooccurring disorders, formerly known as dual diagnoses (National Alliance on Mentally Illness, 2022) Likewise, many of these clients have chronic medical problems (Sunrise House, 2017). In cases with compounding problems, specialized attention involving a **case management** approach is warranted.

Research demonstrates that treatment for substance abuse can be more effective than no treatment, but evaluation of treatment alternatives requires establishment of appropriate criteria to measure effectiveness (SAMHSA, 2016). Examples of criteria that have been used are shown in Box 27.5. It is clear that treatment programs vary and that certain programs will be more culturally appropriate and therefore more effective than others for particular aggregates of individuals.

Pharmacotherapies

In the search for successful treatment of those susceptible to drug and alcohol problems, several pharmacotherapeutic adjuncts to formalized treatment have been developed. Medications include drugs used to assist in the initiation and maintenance of abstinence, drugs used as substitutes for illegal

---

BOX 27.4 Guidelines for Drug Abuse Treatment

- Drug addiction is a brain disease that affects behavior.
- Recovery from drug addiction requires effective treatment, followed by management of the problem over time.
- Treatment must last long enough to produce stable behavioral changes.
- Assessment is the first step in treatment.
- Tailoring services to fit the needs of the individual is an important part of effective drug abuse treatment for criminal justice populations.
- Drug use during treatment should be carefully monitored.
- Treatment should target factors that are associated with criminal behavior.
- Criminal justice supervision should incorporate treatment planning for drug abusing offenders, and treatment providers should be aware of correctional supervision requirements.
- Continuity of care is essential for drug abusers reentering the community.
- A balance of rewards and sanctions encourages prosocial behavior and treatment participation.
- Offenders with cooccurring drug abuse and mental health problems often require an integrated treatment approach.
- Medications are an important part of treatment for many drug abusing offenders.
- Treatment planning for drug abusing offenders who are living in or reentering the community should include strategies to prevent and treat serious, chronic medical conditions, such as HIV/acquired immunodeficiency syndrome (HIV/AIDS), hepatitis B and C, and tuberculosis.

From National Institute on Drug Abuse: *Principles of drug abuse treatment for criminal justice populations: a research-based guide*, 2014. Retrieved from: http://www.drugabuse.gov/sites/default/files/podat_cj_2012.pdf.

drug use, and drugs used to treat comorbidities. This section discusses pharmacotherapies that providers currently use. Good clinical judgment and patient motivation should guide the use of any pharmacotherapy, and therapy should be combined with psychosocial support.

Pharmacotherapeutics are used in detoxification, stabilization, and maintenance; as antagonists; and as treatment for coexisting disorders. Clinically, it is considered better to prevent withdrawal symptoms with medication than to wait for symptoms to appear. Methadone is the treatment of choice in withdrawal from heroin and other opiates. As a detoxification agent, methadone is dispensed over an 8-day period in a tapering dose. Dosage depends on the severity of opiate withdrawal symptoms present. A widely used example of the use of medication for long-term stabilization is methadone maintenance. The client is prescribed daily administration of a long-acting opioid (methadone) as a substitute for the illicit use of opiates (typically heroin). A large body of research confirms its effectiveness in treatment retention and in reduction of risks such as human immunodeficiency virus (HIV) (http://www.drugabuse.gov/publications/drugfacts/heroin).

However, there are continuing varying philosophical opinions about abstinence versus sanctioned use in the debate over the use of methadone. Methadone maintenance is more controversial because the individual remains dependent on the drug. It is dispensed under medical supervision as part of a treatment program. Maintenance may minimize or abate illegal activity, eliminate the infection hazards of injection drug use, reduce the social disruption typically seen with opiate use, and facilitate increased levels of functioning. A myth about maintenance programs is that methadone produces a euphoric "high" and is therefore merely a legal substitute for heroin.

Naltrexone is a long-acting narcotic antagonist traditionally used as an adjunct in the treatment of opiate dependence. It blocks the effects of opiates via competitive binding, but it does not block the effects of other substances, such as benzodiazepines, cocaine, and alcohol (SAMHSA, 2016). Studies indicate that naltrexone is also effective in reducing craving, rates of relapse to alcohol, and severity of alcohol-related problems.

Buprenorphine is an opioid agonist-antagonist that has been used in the treatment of opiate-dependent clients and those with concurrent cocaine dependence (SAHMSA, 2020a–f). Buprenorphine does not produce severe withdrawal on abrupt cessation of its use, giving it an advantage over methadone. Its antagonist component helps reduce the possibility of lethal overdose. Clinical studies support the use of buprenorphine in reducing the frequency of heroin and cocaine self-administration.

Use of disulfiram (Antabuse) to promote cessation of alcohol abuse (NIH, 2016) is rare today because of serious safety issues. A select group (i.e., those who are relapse prone, those who have supportive networks, and those who have histories of abstinence) may benefit from its short-term use. Requests for disulfiram should not be granted in the absence of treatment and supportive relationships. Disulfiram, when combined with alcohol, produces the classic disulfiram ethanol reaction (DER) (i.e., flushing, tachycardia, nausea, headache, chest tightness, and chest pain). The DER is thought to be the result of a disturbance in alcohol metabolism. The response, which typically begins within minutes after alcohol consumption, is dose dependent and highly variable. Significant risks of the DER are cardiovascular symptoms of tachycardia, hypotension, dysrhythmia, and shock. Preexisting cardiac disease is an absolute contraindication to disulfiram. Emergency treatment of the DER is symptomatic.

Benzodiazepines are considered effective tools for alcohol withdrawal because they decrease the likelihood of seizures and delirium (Buell et al., 2019; Wolf et al., 2020). Acamprosate (calcium acetyl homotaurinate; Campral) has been used successfully in Europe over the past decade and was approved for use in the United States in 2004. The main efficacy is in reducing frequency of drinking and maintenance of abstinence. Acamprosate reduces glutaminatergic transmission and neuronal hyperexcitability during withdrawal from alcohol. This drug has a low incidence of side effects but should be used under the care of a physician and prescribed cautiously in patients with liver or kidney problems.

Mutual Help Groups

Mutual help groups are associations that are voluntarily formed, are not professionally dominated, and operate through face-to-face supportive interaction focusing on a mutual goal. Many mutual help groups exist, and they are usually organized by recovering substance abusers or those recovering from compulsive behavior patterns. The first mutual help group was AA (2017), founded in 1935. Initially, a small group of male alcoholics found a way to stay sober "1 day at a time" through meeting regularly with others like themselves. The early AA members developed 12 steps to guide the recovery process, which are summarized in Box 27.6.

As a nonprofessional ongoing source of assistance, AA is viewed as an invaluable resource to the community. However, not all of those with alcohol problems find AA comfortable, culturally relevant, and socially supportive. Because of the realities of social discrimination and regional variation in

BOX 27.6 Basic Tenets of 12-Step Programs

- Admission of defeat and surrender to a higher power
- Inventory of past shortcomings and strengths
- Spiritual practices (e.g., prayer and meditation)
- Willingness to change
- Making amends
- Extension of this process into daily life

TABLE 27.3 Modes of Intervention for Substance Abuse

Level	Intervention
Individual and family levels	Education
	Treatment: detoxification, inpatient, outpatient, and residential
	Mutual help groups (e.g., Alcoholics Anonymous, Narcotics Anonymous, Cocaine Anonymous, Al-Anon)
Community level	Law enforcement measures to limit access to and distribution of addictive substances (e.g., street drugs)
	Alcohol taxes and zoning schemes for liquor outlets
	Legal drinking age and legal sanctions on driving while intoxicated
	Educational programs at schools and penal institutions
	Television and radio public service communications concerning the risks of substance abuse and the availability of treatment
State and federal levels	Formation of national associations such as the National council on Alcoholism and Drug Dependence
	Establishment of federal research entities such as the National Institute on Drug Abuse and the National Institute on alcohol abuse and alcoholism to centralize research, education, and treatment efforts
	Specialty courts/problem-solving courts (drug courts, veteran courts)

customs, AA should not be considered a universal form of assistance for alcohol problems. Predominantly in large cities, women and members of racial, ethnic, religious, or sexual preference minority groups with alcohol problems have formed their own AA groups and other mutual help organizations for support in recovery.

Other 12-step programs have developed through the adaptation of AA's approach to similar addictive problems. Narcotics Anonymous, Gamblers Anonymous, Debtors Anonymous, Cocaine Anonymous, Overeaters Anonymous, and Sex and Love Addicts Anonymous are examples. Because they became organized more recently than AA, these groups may not be as well-known or as widely available, and they may not exhibit as much diversity among their membership as AA. Children, partners, and close associates of substance abusers have also founded self-help groups, such as Al-Anon, Codependents Anonymous, and Adult Children of Alcoholics. Although these groups initially had a predominance of female members, the trend is moving toward participation by equal numbers of men and women.

AA meetings are not standardized. Customs shaping the actual format and sequence of the meeting vary according to region, group size, ethnic and sex composition, and other cultural variations of the members. In general, 12-step meetings follow one of the following formats:

- Uninterrupted talks by one or more speakers about "what it was like, what happened, and what it is like now."
- Each person at the meeting being given the opportunity to speak briefly during discussion.
- A combination of the first two options.
- Meetings either closed or open to the general public.

At least two mutual help groups have developed in response to their founders' negative experiences in AA or their failure to succeed in AA. Women for Sobriety were organized in 1976 to replace or augment AA for women; it addresses women's needs to overcome depression, guilt, and low self-esteem (Women for Sobriety, 2021). Secular Sobriety Groups were organized to meet the needs of individuals who are unable to accept the concept of, or to depend on, a "higher power" in their recovery from alcohol problems. Other mutual help groups that do not follow the 12 steps are available for a variety of addictive problems. AA does not require dues or fees, but some groups, such as Weight Watchers, require monetary commitment. Other groups, such as Recovery Incorporated, have more

professional involvement. Any of these groups could be a resource for selected people with substance abuse problems.

To be effective, interventions for substance abuse must take place at multiple levels and must involve a number of individuals, activities, policies, and substances. Table 27.3 summarizes some of the many interventions available for substance abuse at various levels.

Harm Reduction

New approaches reflecting a changing view of drug and alcohol addiction have been proposed for substance use problems that are not amenable to traditional approaches. Some of these have been grouped under the general term **harm reduction**. Harm reduction consists of individual and collective approaches to the treatment of substance use that are not primarily aimed at complete abstinence from all substances. Instead, incremental change is sought, which involves elimination of the more harmful effects of substance use through behavior and policy modifications. Harm reduction is a process rather than a static approach or an end in itself. It is used in various ways, depending on the context and the needs of individual clients (Harm Reduction Coalition, 2020).

Harm reduction strategies remain controversial, although some see them as evidence of a paradigm shift with the potential to significantly improve treatment results. They are often the only options that will preserve a therapeutic relationship when people continue to use or drink problematically. An early example of harm reduction is the substitution of methadone for heroin. Although they are still using an opiate, individuals taking methadone can be functional without getting high and without the need to engage in criminal activity for drugs. Harm reduction psychotherapy aims to support the process of self-transformation through empathetic resonance, raising awareness of harm, setting goals, and understanding the multiple meanings of the substance. Harm reduction has been used in response to alcohol, illicit drugs, and tobacco use. In the case of alcohol, harm reduction might involve decreasing the number of drinks, decreasing the number of days in which drinking occurs, or avoiding drinking when driving.

On a community level, harm reduction may include attempts to legislate for decreased access to alcohol or raising the legal age for drinking. More controversial public health projects aimed at harm reduction are legalization of some illicit drugs and needle exchange programs. Needle exchange programs have had some success, and although they may not lead the intravenous drug user to abstinence, they do, in fact, serve to break the link in the deadly chain of exposure to and transmission of AIDS.

Viewed from a community health perspective, harm reduction involves planned social and policy changes. "Harm reduction is a movement for social justice built on a belief in, and respect for, the rights of people who use drugs (Harm Reduction Coalition, 2020)." Although harm reduction strategies are not usually sanctioned by lay support systems (e.g., 12-step groups), they can have an important impact. Community health nurses using harm reduction strategies can help reduce drug- and alcohol-related social problems by advocating for programs that "bridge the gap" for those who cannot immediately reach the goal of abstinence.

? ACTIVE LEARNING

1. Attend a local AA, Narcotics Anonymous, or Cocaine Anonymous meeting, and share impressions with classmates.
2. Visit a local treatment center that provides detoxification, inpatient, or outpatient treatment, and determine the center's treatment philosophy and the types of services it provides to patients and their families.

SOCIAL NETWORK INVOLVEMENT

Family and Friends

The social network of the substance abuser either can be highly influential in helping the individual alter behavior or can aid and abet the substance abuser in self-destruction. There is evidence for both positive and negative effects of social support in either mitigating or supporting the behaviors of substance abusers (Alcoholrehab.com, 2022). Evidence suggests that particularly among adolescents and young adults, substance use and abuse often occur in the context of social interactions. Adolescents may use alcohol and other substances as social lubricants during an often-troubled developmental period. Family treatment is considered essential because of the potential for enabling behavior. In addition, the family has suffered the effects of substance abuse emotionally, socially, economically, physically, and spiritually. The family's wounds must be

acknowledged and treated in order for the substance abuser to return to an environment supportive of recovery.

A user's social network may play a role in allowing the substance abuse to continue. Spouses may call to work to report that their partner is "sick" or may remain silent after discovering evidence of abuse. Complex community and family interactions that serve to promote certain behaviors are commonly known as *codependency* and *enabling*. The boundaries between the nonaddicted family members and addict waver, with the result that the excessive substance-abusing behavior is covered up or excused. Social network members may compensate for the fact that the student is absent from school, the car payment is late, or an important appointment is canceled or forgotten. These distress signals are common but often go unrecognized because periods of use are often interspersed with periods of abstinence. This behavior reinforces the individual's, and often the significant other's, perceived sense of control over the substance use. There are mutual help groups for addressing codependency that are founded on the principles of AA and provide opportunities to discuss the issues germane to the alcoholic or addicted family system or network. Families participating in treatment should also be encouraged to participate in these mutual help groups.

Codependency cannot be concretely defined the same way in each culture. Cultural groups vary in the degree to which individuals are expected to anticipate the needs of others and care for them. The danger in applying a rigid definition of codependency in all cases is that it might unfairly and inappropriately label it as a disease in some cultures that value interdependency over individualism.

Through development of a therapeutic relationship and comprehensive assessment, the community nurse should identify the important members of the social network for each client and the ways in which these individuals provide support for the client. The nurse must also recognize that the concept of family refers not only to nuclear families but also to alternative family systems. Whatever the constellation of family, significant others should be included in the treatment and intervention. Substance abuse, addiction, and recovery do not occur in a vacuum, and many relapses are precipitated by interpersonal conflicts.

Effects on the Family

Substance abuse has been called a family disease because it affects the entire family system and holds potential adverse psychological and physical consequences for the family members in addition to the abuser. Family theorists view families, whether the traditional nuclear form or an alternative, as social systems that try to stay in balance (Wright and Leahy, 2019). Professionals may see families as either functional or dysfunctional, depending on how well they fulfill the social tasks expected of them by society. Substance-abusing families are frequently observed to be dysfunctional in clinical terms. However, cultural and political factors should also be considered, because families may have developed these patterns for historical reasons rather than as the effects of substance abuse.

A functional family system is open and flexible and allows its members to be themselves. In the nuclear family model, the parents model intimacy for the children, differences are negotiated, boundaries are defined and maintained, and communication is consistent and clear. In functional family systems, whether the traditional nuclear family or other nontraditional forms, there is trust, individuality, and accountability among family members. All family members are able to have their needs met in a reasonable way.

On the other hand, dysfunctional families are closed systems with fixed, rigid roles. In the case of substance abuse, a major purpose of the system is to deny the substance abuse of the affected family member and keep it a "shameful" family secret. Generally, ego boundaries between the family members are weakened or nonexistent, with enmeshment of the members and an intolerance of individual differences. Rules are rigid and communication is unbalanced; the dynamics are either always conflicting or always superficially pleasant. Children may become involved in a "role reversal" in which they act as caretakers of their parents.

When one or more family members are substance abusers, family functions revolve around the substance abuser and accommodate or compensate the abuser's behavior (Palombi, 2017). The individual needs of other family members are often unmet. Denial is central to a "dysfunctional" family system. The spouse of the substance abuser may gradually take over latter's role, functions, and control of the family. The children are cast into various roles in their struggle for survival in this environment and to maintain the family.

Adult children from dysfunctional families often carry these roles and coping mechanisms into adult life, with many becoming substance abusers or partners of substance abusers. Children of alcoholics also have a higher risk for many other behavioral and emotional problems (Pierce, 2019). Frequently, they have difficulties with intimacy and parenting. Many have lifelong emotional problems, such as depression and anxiety, and physical illnesses often associated with these conditions (e.g., ulcers, colitis, migraine headaches, and eating disorders). The risk for developing alcoholism is greater for children raised in alcoholic homes, whether children are biological children of alcoholic parents or adopted children who grow up with the daily influence of alcohol in the home (Alcoholism-Statistics.com, 2013). Thus, alcoholism is influenced by environment and genetics, or by a combination of both. One in five adult Americans has lived with an alcoholic relative while growing up. Generally, these children are at greater risk for having emotional problems than children whose parents are not alcoholics. Children of alcoholics are four times more likely than other children to become alcoholics themselves (American Academy of Child and Adolescent Psychiatry, 2019).

In addition to psychological burdens that substance abuse places on families, there are the financial burdens related to medical costs, loss of income from job difficulties or unemployment, and the financial losses attributable to divorce. Furthermore, spousal violence and child abuse and neglect are strongly associated with substance abuse.

Professional Enablers

Health care professionals can also contribute to the initiation and continuation of substance abuse and dependency in various ways, becoming **professional enablers**. One obvious way is the physician's role in prescribing psychoactive medications. The medical model advocates the treatment of symptoms with medication. The relief of pain, anxiety, and insomnia is not an exception. The addictive potential of narcotic analgesics and antianxiety agents is often ignored if quick symptom relief is the main goal. Long-term goals for the treatment of medical problems and nonmedication management of pain and anxiety are more thoughtful approaches. However, undermedication or refusal to use "addictive" medicines can lead susceptible clients to self-medicate with illegal drugs or alcohol.

Physicians and nurses are often the first to see the physical effects of substance abuse and are in an excellent position to intervene. By focusing on the health consequences of substance abuse, they can form trusting relationships, provide information, and refer patients to the appropriate treatment. Too often, this opportunity is missed because the health care professional is reluctant to bring up this taboo subject. This reluctance may be based on professionals' inability to examine their own drinking or drug-taking behaviors, or those of significant others, or on concerns about negative responses from clients.

In the past, many psychiatrists and psychotherapists have focused on the reasons the client uses substances rather than on the dependency itself. The assumption was that insight would lead to a change in behavior. This approach has usually not proved to be effective, especially if the psychiatrist is concurrently prescribing other potentially addictive antianxiety medications or hypnotics. Complete abstinence from all mood-altering medication is a model for preventing the cross-addiction common in substance abusers (i.e., substituting one substance for another, such as a benzodiazepine for alcohol). Exceptions to this approach are patients with serious medical conditions requiring pain medication and those who also have a second psychiatric disorder that requires medication (i.e., schizophrenia, depression, bipolar affective disorder). The recovering substance abuser often needs support when he or she must take medication for these psychiatric conditions because others may criticize the use of any medication and place the patient in a difficult situation.

Caregivers have become more aware of signs of client substance abuse. Some providers are willing to begin therapy with a nonabstinent client under the stipulation that, if therapeutic gains are not made, the client will be referred for treatment or the caregiver will withdraw services. Clients who lack social support may succeed using this strategy, which allows the formation of a trusting relationship before taking the leap to abstinence. Clinical wisdom and research continue to point toward more tailored, individualized approaches to substance abuse.

VULNERABLE AGGREGATES

When viewed from a community perspective, substance abuse problems clearly affect some populations more severely than others. Some groups are more susceptible to experiencing substance abuse problems, may tend to deteriorate more quickly in the process, or may have fewer sources of support for recovery. These groups, termed *vulnerable aggregates*, require special attention in terms of prevention, intervention, and rehabilitation strategies.

Current resources for prevention, treatment, and mutual support may not be flexible enough to meet the needs of various vulnerable aggregates who are at risk of experiencing substance abuse problems and are often excluded or alienated from services by policies, provider attitudes, economic constraints, and social isolation. This section describes the issues of substance abuse with several vulnerable aggregates, including adolescents, the elderly, women, and racial and ethnic minorities.

Preadolescents and Adolescents

Why do young people use drugs? It is clear that drug and alcohol use among adolescents is a pervasive problem with many devastating consequences. The trend data in some aspects are undoubtedly worse for adolescents than for adults. The teenage years may be a turbulent time for some because of the necessary developmental tasks of discovering their own unique identity, learning how to form intimate relationships, and developing autonomy. Currently, this maturing is accomplished in a confusing era in which the cultural status of adolescents is undefined. Today's teenagers are an increasingly independent subculture with more money available than any time before, yet they have not attained full adult status.

The teenage years may be a time of experimentation, searching, confusion, rebellion, poor self-image, alienation, and insecurity. There is no such thing as the typical adolescent substance abuser, and there are multiple theories of causation for the abuse. Researchers have concluded that adolescent drug use is a symptom and not the cause of maladjustment. Those with significant difficulty are usually using substances as coping mechanisms.

Studies have identified various predictors of adolescent substance abuse. For example, use of legal substances (e.g., tobacco, alcohol) almost always precedes use of illegal drugs. Risk factors for adolescent substance abuse can be separated into two categories; broad societal and cultural (i.e., contextual) factors, and factors that lie within individuals and their interpersonal environments (GenPsych, 2020). Contextual risk factors include laws and norms, drug availability, extreme economic deprivation, and neighborhood disorganization. Examples of individual risk factors are experiencing problem behaviors from an early age (such as aggressiveness, negative moods and withdrawal, impulsivity), having a coexisting mental health diagnosis (e.g., conduct disorder, ADHD, depression) or a learning disorder, problems in the family (e.g., low bonding to parent, parent abuse of substances, poor parenting practices), problems in school (e.g., low academic achievement, low commitment to school), and association with drug-using peers, and early initial use of drugs (GenPsych, 2020). In adolescents, two particular individual risk factors are

having a family member who abuses substances and associating with drug-using peers (GenPsych, 2020).

The younger the initiation, the greater the probability of prolonged and accelerated substance use. Other contributing factors are the feeling of powerlessness and selling drugs as a viable economic solution to poverty. Subculture theory describes the status and power that charismatic leaders have to influence members of peer groups. In drug-using peer groups, such leaders have influence over inexperienced drug users and acculturate them into the drug scene. Thus it is crucial that communities work to maintain strong family and social bonds.

The community health nurse can play an important part in advocating for these vulnerable children and educating teachers on the vital importance of maintaining a validating, nonjudgmental attitude toward these students.

It is especially important that families are supported in the community. Substance abuse is less likely in families who give clear messages and have open communication and more likely in families in which parents are alcoholic, condemning, overly demanding, or overly protective. Committed family involvement helps retain the adolescent in treatment. However, it must be remembered that many well-functioning families have children who succumb to substance abuse.

There are positive outcomes with wraparound recovery programs (Rutman et al., 2020). Wraparound programs take a team approach, with children, parents, counselors, and other invested team members involved in the adolescent's successful recovery through abstinence, education, and life skills. Families whose teenagers are substances abusers also may experience significant community rejection and judgmental attitudes.

The preadolescent years are a particularly vulnerable time for initiation into and subsequent problematic substance use. When drug use escalates in adolescents, it can have devastating long-lasting consequences. There is a strong relationship between adolescent behavior problems, such as aggressiveness, delinquency, and criminal activity, and heavy alcohol use between the ages of 12 and 17 years.

Escalating use of substances enhances the risk of school and social failure, criminal activities, violent behavior, sexual risk taking, sexual violence, depression, suicide, and unintended injuries. Primary prevention for adolescents is typically focused on education aimed toward complete abstinence, which some say is unrealistic. Education plays an important role. A striking feature is the strong inverse relationship between perceived risk and drug use. Historically for all drugs, with no change in drug availability, when students perceive a drug as harmful, fewer students actually use it.

Responsible media efforts can bring about change but only with accompanying parental and community efforts. Early detection of predisposing factors, such as underlying psychiatric illness, is important. Other strategies are providing structured clubs and organizations and facilitating school success, career skills, family communication skills, and conflict resolution. Secondary prevention is targeted at inpatient and outpatient treatment and harm reduction.

However, almost as important as intervention and treatment is recognizing when treatment is unnecessary. Not all drug use requires therapy, nor is it even desirable. Not all young drug users are antisocial or mentally unstable, nor should they be labeled as such. Most will develop a responsible philosophy concerning substance use if given support and opportunity.

Huhn et al. (2018) analyzed data from state-certified addiction treatment centers collected via the Treatment Episode Data Set—Admissions between 2004 and 15, looking at trends in first time treatment admissions for opioid use disorder (OUD) in adults 55 and older ($n = 400, 421$). They determined that the percentage of older adults seeking treatment for OUD rose steadily between 2004 and 13 (41.2% increase of statistical significance, with $P < .046$), then rapidly between 2013 and 15 (53.5%, $P < .009$). Further, they found that the proportion of older adults with primary heroin use more than doubled between 2012 and 15 ($P < .001$); these individuals were increasingly male ($P < .001$), African American ($P < .001$), and using via the intranasal route of administration ($P < .001$). Huhn et al. note that previous comparisons of older and younger adults in OMT reported that older adults initiated their substance use later in life, speculating that some older adults have a long history of OUD, while others may have a form of "late-onset" OUD brought on by prescription opioid exposure later in life.

Older Adults

Older adults are considered vulnerable to substance abuse problems because of diminished physiological tolerance, increased use of medically prescribed drugs, and cultural and social isolation life. Misuse of prescription drugs may be the most common form of drug abuse among older adults. Chronic health conditions which tend to develop as part of aging, the fact that older adults are often prescribed more medicines than other age groups, leading to a higher rate of exposure to potentially addictive medications, accidental misuse of prescription drugs, and possible worsening of existing mental health issues are all reasons this may happen (NIDA, 2020).

Women

Since the 1970s, much attention has been turned to substance abuse problems in women. Evidence is mounting that alcohol use and abuse affect women much differently from how they affect men. Biological differences in body structure and chemistry cause most women to absorb more alcohol and take longer to metabolize it than men (CDC, 2020a—e). Consequently, after drinking the same amount of alcohol, women tend to have higher blood alcohol levels than men, and the immediate effects of alcohol usually occur more quickly and last longer in women than men. Specific aggregates of women may be more severely affected by substance abuse problems, including those from minority groups, those with low or no income, and those of the working classes. The increased risk stems from economic, social, and cultural factors.

Lesbians are another aggregate of women in whom substance abuse may be associated with marginalization and should be understood within the diversity of lesbians individually and culturally. This issue is especially heightened in periods when homosexuality is demonized through media, churches, and legislation linking homosexuality with pathology and when lesbians and gays are denied the right to marry (e.g., civil unions, partner benefits).

Women who were abused as children are more susceptible to substance abuse problems in adolescence and adulthood than are nonabused women. They also face many more distressing consequences in substance abuse treatment and recovery. There remains work to be done in the research of and care delivery for women who use alcohol or other drugs. For example, though the increasing mortality caused by opioid overdose, including among women, has led to official acknowledgment that opioid abuse represents a public health emergency, resulting in dedicated funding to address the epidemic, resources have been channeled mostly toward law enforcement to reduce drug supply and toward the development of nonopioid treatments for pain (The President's Commission on Combating Drug Addiction and the Opioid Crisis, 2017). However, this agenda lacks expansion of harm reduction services or treatment for women's comorbid medical, psychiatric, and social conditions—including HIV, Hepatitis C, depression, trauma, and homelessness—or acknowledgment of the importance of gender in the context of substance use (Meyer et al., 2019).

Drug-dependent women report frequent physical and medical problems, many related to their reproductive systems (American Addiction Centers, 2019a,b). Women tend to experience cardiac and hepatic pathology sooner than men because they metabolize alcohol at a different rate. They also have higher blood alcohol levels relative to body weight and higher mortality rates from heavy drinking (NIDA, 2020a—r).

Excessive alcohol use, especially binge drinking, during pregnancy continues to have long-term developmental consequences in the newborn (CDC, 2020a—e). Cocaine use during pregnancy is associated with increased risk of miscarriage, low birth weight, spontaneous abortion, premature delivery, and abruptio placentae (American Addiction Centers, 2020). Infants who have been addicted to cocaine in utero are often delivered prematurely, have low birth weights, smaller head circumferences, and are shorter in length than babies born to mothers who do not use cocaine (American Addiction Centers, 2020). Long-term learning disabilities, behavioral problems, limb defects, congenital heart disease, language development problems, and impaired memory are other potential consequences associated with children of cocaine-using mothers (Vertiva Health, 2021).

Getting the pregnant woman into treatment and managing her withdrawal are frequently problematic. The woman's fear of punitive legal actions complicates the process. Additionally, the addiction itself often interferes with obtaining adequate prenatal care. If addiction is linked with risky sexual behavior or sexual assault, there is an increased risk of contracting HIV and hepatitis viruses, which can infect the infant; testing should be recommended.

Ethnocultural Considerations

Community health nurses need to be culturally competent and aware of certain ethnocultural vulnerabilities and differing perspectives when considering treatments for individuals with substance abuse. Data on African Americans, Hispanics, and Native Americans suggest an increased risk for substance abuse in these groups (Hilton et al., 2018; SAMHSA, 2020a–f). However, the usual ethnic/racial categories in research do not consider distinctions within each category. Consequently, there are limited data, especially about middle-class minorities. Creating another stereotype might undermine prevention and treatment strategies. However, it is true that, under the strain of poverty, underemployment, decreased job opportunities, macrolevel and microlevel aggression, and ongoing racism, some members of these aggregates find the relief in using substances, which numb the "social pain" caused by their environments. Racial and ethnic minorities are overrepresented among the economically disenfranchised. Limited financial resources may limit alternatives to public treatment settings, which are often understaffed, underfunded, and filled to capacity and have long waiting lists. The privatization of treatment has further decreased access to treatment.

Theories of stress, social causation, and oppressed status support the belief that discrimination and racism are factors in the generation of mental illness and alcohol and drug problems in members of racial and ethnic minorities. Socioeconomic, political, and historical realities have encouraged some minorities to enter into the illegal drug trade as a means of economic survival. In working with ethnic and racial minorities, health care professionals must recognize the sociopolitical and socioeconomic factors that form the context of substance use, abuse, and dependency. These same factors will have an impact on seeking help, treatment, and outcome. Recovery for minority groups might be contextually and experientially different from that for whites, just as the environment that contributed to the initial abuse was different. Community health nurses will be better positioned to work with diverse individuals, if they are aware of treatment disparities and obstacles for minority groups.

During periods of slavery, alcohol was used as a reward, and it was seen as a way to cope. The value themes for this aggregate are a oneness with nature and spirituality, the importance of extended family, a present orientation, and a spiral concept of time. Barriers to treating African Americans with substance abuse or addiction problems are listed in Box 27.7.

Myths about certain ethnicities must be critically examined. Native Americans, for example, fight the stereotype of the drunken, once-noble warrior. However, alcohol as the predominant drug of choice does pose a threat to this population, particularly among youth and young adults. Lifetime drug use among American Indian youth were higher than among the general NIDA MTF sample at each grade level (8th, 10th, and 12th) for all illicit substances, except for tranquilizers and amphetamines, and 30-day rates of use were higher for nearly all substances (NIDA, 2018a–h). Evidence for a biological predisposition is conflicting, and many stop drinking when

BOX 27.7 Barriers to Treating Substance Abuse and Addiction Problems in African Americans

- Weekend drinking as a reward
- Ongoing sociocultural violence
- Use of substances to escape the emotional pain caused by racism
- Poverty, underemployment, and unemployment
- Prevalence of both drugs and liquor stores within the community
- Cultural and community disintegration, which has altered traditional values and behaviors
- Allure and economic rewards of selling drugs
- Inadequate social support system for recovery
- Internalized racism harming the self-concept, along with anger and frustration
- Greater likelihood of being arrested than treated (three to six times more than whites)
- Limited role models
- Inability to "change people and places" as advocated by 12-step programs

they reach adulthood and their sense of family and social responsibility increases. Interventions for this group must involve long-term outreach that gains respect from the community.

Studies have identified that social support has a positive effect on treatment and outcome. Without this support, the individual completing treatment may return to the original social environment, undermining any gains made within the treatment setting. Environmental cues and conditioned reinforcement for continued drug and alcohol use may be extremely powerful. The individual may return to an environment of nonsupport, characterized by continued use by important members of the individual's social network. The individual needs a well-coordinated aftercare program that addresses these issues. For example, Hispanic youth may have positive recovery outcome with family intervention programs such as "the Familia Adelante Program," a program that looks at and works with HIV prevention, risk, and family intervention (National Network to Eliminate Disparities, 2017).

The treatment of ethnic and racial minority aggregates poses special challenges related to the individuals seeking treatment. Treatment providers must recognize that these vulnerable aggregates will encounter a host of barriers that will make treatment and long-term recovery extremely difficult. For example, providers should understand the effect of rituals, holidays, music, and customs and how they can hinder progress. Providers who work from the public health perspective of "thinking upstream" will examine larger, macrolevel issues that increase the susceptibility of at-risk populations to alcohol and drug problems. Box 27.8 presents helpful information on working with people from diverse cultures.

Other Aggregates

Substance abuse is the most common psychopathological problem in the general population. Within this category is a smaller aggregate of people with one or more psychiatric

BOX 27.8 Intervention Approaches for Working With People From Diverse Cultures

- Show respect for another culture's values and identity
- Improve your ability to connect with your target community
- Increase the relevance of your actions
- Decrease the possibility of unwanted surprises
- Increase the involvement and participation of members of other cultural groups
- Increase support for your program by those cultural group members, even if they don't participate or get directly involved
- Build future trust and cooperation across cultural lines—which should raise the prospects for more successful interventions in the future.

From Work Group for Community Health and Development, University of Kansas: *The community toolbox*, chapter 19, *section 4: adapting community interventions for different cultures and communities*, 2016. Available from: http://ctb.ku.edu/en/tablecontents/sub_section_main_1163.aspx.

diagnoses in addition to substance abuse; this situation is referred to as **dual diagnosis**. Roughly 50% of individuals with severe mental disorders are affected by substance abuse; 37% of alcohol abusers and 53% of drug abusers also have at least one serious mental illness. And, of all people diagnosed as mentally ill, 29% abuse either alcohol or drugs (NAMI, 2017). This may be less readily identified by health care providers, who may fail to recognize that the two problems may coexist. Treatment of the individual with a dual diagnosis is complicated when the individual must take prescribed psychotropic medications. As previously mentioned, it may be perceived as prescription drug abuse or as the substitution of one addiction for another. Special attention and flexibility are needed to meet the needs of the dual-diagnosis aggregate, and such strategies are still in the developmental phase.

In assessing the risks for substance abuse and the extent of its impact on the community, nurses must be aware that are there frequently several bases for the vulnerability in an individual or group. The adolescent, the low-income Hispanic male, the lesbian African American mother receiving public assistance, and the Native American family living on reservation land are all facing multiple sources of vulnerability that contribute to an increased potential for substance abuse.

Special attention must be paid to the impact of sexually transmitted diseases (STDs) (e.g., HIV, herpes, genital warts, and syphilis) and their relationship to substance abuse. Substance abusers are at increased risk of STDs, including HIV, in the following ways:

- Substances may cloud judgment, leading to high-risk sexual practices involving the exchange of body fluids (e.g., sex without the use of appropriate barriers such as condoms).
- Intravenous drug use may involve the sharing of hypodermic needles.
- Chronic substance use (e.g., of alcohol, heroin, amphetamines, nicotine, and cocaine) impairs the immune system and facilitates infection by HIV or by other pathogens that increase the chances of HIV infection.

- Substance abuse may hasten physical and mental deterioration from the condition of seropositivity to an AIDS diagnosis and, eventually, the terminal phase of the disease.
- Chronic substance abusers generally have few supportive relationships available to them in the process of coping with the hardships that accompany severe and chronic illnesses.
- People facing a stigmatizing, terminal, debilitating illness, in themselves or in a significant other, are more prone to experience substance abuse problems in an attempt to cope with distress.

ETHICAL INSIGHTS

Ethical Issues Related to Substance Abuse

Ethical issues regarding substance use and abuse relate to behaviors of the user/abuser that present a risk to the self, coworkers, or the public. A nurse who diverts medication from a patient, thereby depriving the patient of pain relief, is acting both unethically and illegally. Other ethical areas of concern include property theft or damage and the general welfare of others. The American Nurses Association states that up to 10% of the RN workforce could be dependent on drugs or alcohol (Starr, 2015). Access to controlled substances, stress exacerbated by inadequate support and workload, lack of education about substance abuse, pain, and fatigue are risk factors specific to nurses (American Addiction Centers, 2019a,b). Nurses who are living in addiction have more options than ever with assessment and treatment that may not necessarily end their professional careers. Currently 44 states offer some form of substance abuse treatment program to direct nurses to treatment, monitor their reentry into work, and continue their licensure according to the National Council of State Boards of Nursing (National Council of State Boards of Nursing [NCSBN], 2021). Alternative to Discipline programs for Substance Use Disorder enhance a state board of nursing's ability to quickly assure public protection by promoting earlier identification, mandating immediate removal from the workplace, and evidence-based treatment for nurses with substance use disorder. Benefits to the nurse include the opportunity to demonstrate to the board in a nondisciplinary and nonpublic manner that they can become safe and sober and remain so, while retaining their license (NCSBN, 2021).

Finally, substance abuse among health care professionals cannot be ignored. Physicians, nurses, dentists, and pharmacists are vulnerable to substance abuse; alcohol or narcotic use is most common (DrugRehab.com, 2017). Health care professionals are assumed to be "immune" to dependency because they are knowledgeable about medications. However, their increased access to drugs, belief in pharmaceutical solutions, and work-related stress increase their risk for substance abuse. Typically, they gain access to drugs through their work settings by diverting medications for their own use or by abusing drugs obtained by prescription. State regulatory boards discover the abuse by these health care professionals after drug theft or when the effects of the substance abuse impair professional functioning.

Community health nurses should be especially vigilant about this possibility because colleagues are working in isolation and episodes of incompetence may not be easily observed. Most states have rehabilitation programs for health care professionals that consist of treatment and monitoring. They are allowed to retain their professional licenses during treatment. Despite their usually favorable recovery rate, it is difficult to get this population into treatment because they exhibit denial and shame related to their substance abuse. However, the threatened loss of their professional license to practice may be a good motivator to break through denial of the problem and encourage them to seek treatment.

? ACTIVE LEARNING

Visit a treatment program for women, and determine how the particular needs of this population are assessed and addressed.

NURSING PERSPECTIVE ON SUBSTANCE ABUSE

Nurses have encountered substance abuse in clients whose health problems are clearly related to alcohol abuse, such as cirrhosis of the liver, heart disease, neurological syndromes, and nutritional deficits. Unfortunately, alcohol problems were often not addressed in these health encounters in the past because of the stigma of alcoholism and a lack of effective treatments. The nursing literature did not clearly address substance abuse as a nursing problem until the late 1960s and did not address it as a significant problem until the 1970s. Before the 1970s, substance abuse was usually viewed as a moral problem or, if it involved illicit drugs, as a legal problem.

Since the 1970s, nursing has become more involved in the spectrum of compulsive behavior problems, including substance abuse. A specialized organization, the International Nurses Society on Addictions (IntNSA; at http://www.intnsa.org), has been established with the philosophy that alcohol abuse and other drug abuse, eating disorders, sexual and relational addiction, and compulsive gambling, working, and spending are closely related behavior patterns. There is a tendency in society to deal with substance abusers in stigmatizing, devaluing, coercive, and punitive ways. Negative attitudes are ubiquitous in our culture. As part of the larger culture, nurses may reflect these attitudes and have difficulty providing care to these individuals. The moral view of substance abuse implies that individuals choose to become sick, injured, or addicted.

Strong negative feelings that conflict with nursing's humanistic stance may also stem from personal experiences. Being the emotionally or physically abused spouse or child of a substance abuser can have lasting effects on a nurse's attitude toward substance-abusing clients. The nurse who uses alcohol or drugs to relieve stress or to self-medicate a dysphoric state may overidentify with the client and deny the severity of the client's substance abuse.

Frequently, substance abusers are difficult clients in health care settings. When intoxicated, they may be raucous, uncooperative, and antisocial. When not intoxicated, they may exhibit none of these negative behaviors, or they may be manipulative and demanding, using flattery or intimidation to hide drug-seeking behavior. Nurses may initially be warm and understanding, but once aware of manipulative attempts, they may have difficulty maintaining an accepting, nonjudgmental attitude. Realizing that recovery from substance abuse often comes very slowly can help nurses feel less pressured to get patients into treatment and more able simply to raise consciousness by presenting the facts about addictive illness and leaving the decision making to the client.

Nursing Interventions in the Community

The problem of substance abuse is so widespread that it affects every community and its inhabitants to varying degrees. Hence, the community health nurse is often involved with substance abusers or their significant others. Substance abuse nursing interventions with clients and their caregivers are necessary to ensure the success of other health interventions. Ignoring substance abuse problems frequently leads to lack of progress and clients' inability to perform needed health practices. This situation is especially frustrating for the community health nurse and other professionals who have collaborated on a comprehensive plan to allow an individual with a serious health problem to remain at home and avoid placement in an institution.

There are many ways in which community health nurses can assist individuals, families, and groups experiencing substance abuse problems. Community health nurses may be the first to identify or suspect an alcohol or drug problem in the clients and families with whom they are working. Nurses in all care contexts should routinely assess substance use patterns when performing client histories. The client history is a critical assessment and screening tool that can identify those at risk. Using current knowledge and theories about substance abuse etiology and risk factors should help identify those individuals predisposed to alcohol and drug use.

The community health nurse can be alert to environmental cues in the home that indicate substance abuse, such as empty liquor and pill bottles. An indication of prescription medication abuse is the patient's involvement with several physicians from whom narcotic analgesics and tranquilizers are obtained. This type of assessment can help with case finding and treatment referral, although the individual may have denied the existence of a substance abuse problem initially.

Denial of substance abuse or dependence may range from completely blocked awareness of the problem to partial disavowal of the detrimental effects of the substance use and abuse. One of the primary tasks for intervention and treatment with the substance-dependent individual is to increase the individual's awareness of the problem. Family and significant others can assist with this process by being more honest and direct with the individual about the detrimental effects of the substance abuse. Before this occurs, the significant others must overcome their own denial of the problem and its associated shame and guilt. Referrals to community education programs on substance abuse and dependence and mutual help groups such as Al-Anon and Narcotics Anonymous are helpful interventions for families and significant others.

The community health nurse may also involve the social network in getting the client into treatment. Although individuals who are forced to enter treatment may not be willing to admit the severity of the abuse, they can still benefit from exposure to the treatment program and eventually begin recovery. Experiencing serious health consequences related to dependency may constitute "hitting bottom" for the individual. This experience may also break through denial or collusion on the part of the family.

The trust that develops in a caring nursing relationship can support disclosure of substance abuse problems and decrease denial in the client or family members. A realistic and positive attitude toward the person with substance abuse can provide families with hope. Community health nurses must have knowledge of available community resources. One of the primary roles of the community health nurse in helping substance abusers is to facilitate contact with helping agencies such as local treatment programs or mutual help groups. Collaboration with the client's physician is helpful, should medical detoxification be necessary. Community health nurses should assume a validating, nonjudgmental position toward the whole family and should avoid being confrontational so as not to fan the fires of resistance. It is imperative that nurses ascribe a noble intention to their substance-abusing clients and families and avoid negativity and preaching.

Other traditional community health nursing roles and interventions also are appropriate to use with substance abusers. Examples follow:

- Health teaching regarding addictive illness and addictive effects of different substances
- Advocating that evidence-based practice treatment works in special populations through problem-solving courts (drug courts), specialized adolescent treatment, and other community case management programs
- Providing direct care for abuse-related and dependence-related cooccurring medical problems
- Educating clients and families about problems related to substance abuse
- Collaborating with other disciplines to ensure continuity of care

- Coordinating health care services for the client to prevent prescription drug abuse and avoid fragmentation of care
- Providing consultation to nonmedical professionals and lay personnel
- Facilitating care through appropriate referrals and follow-up
- Knowing how to refer to community resources working with substance abuse, mental health, and other issues

Nursing Care Standards Related to the Patients With Substance Abuse Problems

Utilization of the nursing process is critical to quality care of patients with substance abuse problems. Nurses must know how to develop therapeutic alliances with the patient and family to develop trust and rapport. There is no single treatment appropriate for all individuals, and in the development of health teaching for clients, evidence-based models meet the needs for many specific populations may be chosen. Evidence demonstrates that effective treatment must address the multiple holistic needs of the individual. Ongoing assessment is critical for continual assessment in treatment planning and services. Knowledge, skills, and attitudes of the behavioral health workforce must be adequate. More success is noted when patients remain in treatment for adequate periods and when individual and group counseling and other behavioral therapies are utilized. Medications are an important element of treatment for many patients, especially when combined with counseling and other behavioral therapies. Nurses must have the knowledge of treatment in cooccurring mental health disorders and substance use disorders. Addiction recovery usually is a long-term process and frequently requires multiple episodes of treatment.

ACTIVE LEARNING

1. Learn about problem solving courts in your community.
2. Contact mental health services or substance abuse treatment services at the county or city level, and obtain a list of local treatment and education resources.

CASE STUDY Application of the Nursing Process

Kate Gray, 29 years old, was having abdominal pain, nausea, and vomiting. She was admitted to the hospital thorough the emergency department. After 3 days she was discharged and referred to a community clinic and public health department. Kate has been diagnosed with hepatitis C and alcoholism. She weighs 115 pounds. She is taking a multivitamin, cimetidine for symptoms of gastroesophageal reflux disease, gabapentin for chronic pain, and Atarax for pruritus. She had abdominal pain and a low-grade fever on discharge from the hospital. Her appetite is poor and she often is nauseated. She becomes fatigued easily. She agrees to comply with discharge planning from the hospital. She is unemployed and recently started Medicaid benefits.

Kate's drug use history is as follows: Marijuana use starting at age 16, alcohol use starting at age 20, methamphetamine (MA) use at age 26; she has been injecting the drug for 2 years. She was arrested 4 months ago for drug use and mandated to participate in a community felony drug court. She has been abstinent from marijuana and MA since her arrest. However, 2 weeks ago she violated probation by drinking and received 3 days in jail for probation violation.

She has two daughters aged 6 and 8. Her children live with their father in the same city.

Assessment
Individual

The drug court team nurse practitioner sees Kate 2 days after discharge. Kate is still struggling with fatigue and poor appetite. She is afebrile. The nurse practitioner will follow her through drug court. When participating in drug court, Kate will attend **intensive outpatient treatment (IOT)** and Narcotic Anonymous (NA) meetings. She has an NA sponsor.

Family

Kate will meet with her daughters weekly for family therapy through drug court. She meets with her husband, daughters, and pastor weekly for family counseling. Kate's husband attends NA meetings. He has been clean and sober for 1 year. He also is on felony probation and has recently graduated from drug court.

Continued

CASE STUDY   Application of the Nursing Process—cont'd

He works as a mechanic. Their daughters have safe and adequate housing with their father.

Community

Drug court firmly assists with keeping individuals in treatment long enough for it to work while supervising them closely. Participants are held accountable by the drug court judge for meeting their obligations to the court, society, themselves, and their families. Participants are regularly and randomly tested for drug use. Kate is required to appear in court frequently so that the judge may review her progress and reward her for doing well or sanction her when she does not live up to drug court obligations.

Diagnosis
Individual
- Altered gastrointestinal and hepatic status secondary to hepatitis C and alcoholism pain
- Poor nutritional status
- Inadequate coping related to substance abuse history
- Need for patient education regarding hepatitis C, alcoholism, and addiction

Family
- Inadequate knowledge about addictive disease and effects of alcoholism, MA abuse, and polysubstance abuse
- Inadequate knowledge of treatment approaches available for alcohol abuse and the recovery process
- Family dysfunction secondary to poor communication and denial of addiction in client

Community
- Need for understanding of the prevalence of alcohol abuse problems in the older adult community and adverse health effects of alcohol consumption.
- Inadequate knowledge in community agencies that assist alcohol abusers (e.g., local Alcoholics Anonymous [AA] and counselors) regarding the need to make home visits and provide services

Planning
Planning for Kate and her family's care involves collaboration among her family, her case management team through drug court, probation services, her pastor, and other community treatment resources. Case management health promotion teaching, counseling, support, and advocacy are the main approaches used to directly assist the client and her family. Indirect approaches involve networking with community agencies, collaboration, and communications.

Individual
Short-Term Goals
- Kate will follow her posthospitalization IOT attendance, drug court, and case management.
- Kate will be compliant with her medications.

Long-Term Goals
- Kate will continue to be clean and sober.
- Kate's health status will improve and/or stay at optimal health status as indicated by stabilization of weight, and optimal pain control.
- Kate will complete drug court.

Family
Short-Term Goals
- Kate's family will continue family therapy.
- Communication will improve between Kate, her husband, and children.

Long-Term Goals
- Family recovery in abstinence and sobriety

Community
Long-Term Goals
- NA meetings and sponsorship
- Successful completion of and release from probation
- Optimal health status

Intervention
Individual
- Nurse practitioner appointments weekly initially to monitor the client's medication issues or problems as related to maintaining abstinence, gastrointestinal and hepatic functioning, medication compliance, and nutritional status
- Health promotion and patient/family education regarding addiction, hepatitis C, and alcoholism
- Patient teaching about the client's medications, their effects and side effects, and the necessity of following recommended dosing schedules

Family
- Continued support for Kate and her family through early recovery
- Health promotion and education to the family on the course and treatment of addiction, and other medical problems associated with Kate's medical diagnosis
- Nonjudgmental support and advocacy

Community
- List of local and national referral resources for clients with substance abuse problems made available to drug court team and physicians, with a particular focus on resources providing services for drug court participants
- Educating community stakeholders about drug courts, NA and other 12-step programs, and community case management
- Collaboration with community organizations that provide outreach for other individuals and families living with addiction

Evaluation
Individual
Kate was very compliant with drug court, IOT, NA meetings, and following medical treatment.

Family
Kate's family joined her in drug court graduation. Kate continues outpatient drug once weekly, NA meetings, and family therapy.

Community
Drug court case management will follow through with compliance in IOP attendance, NA meeting compliance, family therapy compliance, and other treatment obligations.

Levels of Prevention
Primary
- Health teaching to individuals and groups on the risk factors, early symptoms, and adverse health and social consequences of substance abuse; the addictive disease process; and available treatment services
- Need to gear educational approaches to the more vulnerable aggregates

Secondary
- Screening and earlier treatment approaches aimed at minimizing health and social consequences of substance abuse
- Involvement of physicians, nurses, and other healthcare professionals in various community healthcare settings in this process

Tertiary
- More direct approaches, such as case management, IOT, family therapy, and NA meeting with sponsorship. Goals are to halt the physiologically damaging effects of hepatitis C and alcoholism in Kate's abstinence and sobriety.

CASE STUDY Application of the Nursing Process—cont'd

- Frequent use of medications to treat the symptoms of substance abuse —related disorders or as part of aversion therapy (e.g., disulfiram)
- Services provided by medical practitioners, treatment services, and mutual help organizations generally advocate abstinence from the substance and improving the individual's health status

This case study illustrates the complexity of substance abuse and **cooccurring disorders**. There is hope in treatment through problem-solving courts.

Substance abuse affects patients and their families. Now more than ever, substance abuse may be treated through case management involving multidisciplinary team members. In sobriety, the social situation, living situation, or social acquaintances must change to maintain long-term recovery. However, with patience, persistence, and a caring, nonjudgmental attitude, the nurse can often be effective in helping clients with substance abuse problems attain recovery and improve their health status.

SUMMARY

This chapter provides an overview of the complex, multifaceted phenomenon of substance abuse and its manifestations in the community. The focus is on social, economic, political, and health-related aspects of substance abuse. In addition, the concept of substance abuse is related to the more general concept of addictive behaviors, not just those related to drug or alcohol abuse.

From the review of the various etiological theories, it is clear that there is no one causative factor in the development of substance abuse. Consequently, one treatment approach does not apply to all substance abusers. Multiple factors as well as issues specific to vulnerable aggregates, such as women, adolescents, older adults, and people of color, must be considered in the development of intervention plans and strategies and in the evaluation of outcomes. Resources for prevention and intervention at the individual, family, and community levels are outlined here and should be familiar to nurses practicing in the community.

EVOLVE WEBSITE

http://evolve.elsevier.com/Nies
- NCLEX Review Questions
- Case Studies

BIBLIOGRAPHY

Addiction Policy Forum: *DSM-5 criteria for addiction simplified*, 2020. Retrieved January 15, 2021 from: https://www.addictionpolicy.org/post/dsm-5-facts-and-figures.

AlcoholRehab.Com: *Social support for drinking*, 2022. https://alcoholrehab.com/alcohol-recovery/aftercare/social-support/.

Alcoholism-Statistics.com: *Family alcoholism statistics*, 2013. Retrieved January 16, 2021 from: http://www.alcoholism-statistics.com/family-statistics/.

American Academy of Child & Adolescent Psychiatry: *Alcohol use in families*, 2019. Retrieved January 16, 2021 from: https://www.aacap.org/AACAP/Families_and_Youth/Facts_for_Families/FFF-Guide/Children-Of-Alcoholics-017.aspx.

American Addiction Centers: *Dangers of using cocaine during pregnancy*, 2020. Retrieved January 16, 2021 from: https://americanaddictioncenters.org/cocaine-treatment/dangers-pregnancy.

American Addiction Centers: *Veteran drug & alcohol rehab*, 2021. Retrieved January 19, 2021 from: https://americanaddictioncenters.org/rehab-guide/veterans-resources.

American Addiction Centers: *What role does drug abuse play in the health of the reproductive system?*, 2019. Retrieved January 16, 2021 from: https://americanaddictioncenters.org/health-complications-addiction/reproductive-system.

American Addiction Centers: *Why nurses are at risk for substance abuse*, 2019. Retrieved January 16, 2021 from: https://americanaddictioncenters.org/medical-professionals/nurses-at-a-higher-risk-for-substance-abuse.

American Psychiatric Association: *Diagnostic and statistical manual of mental disorders, DSM-5*, ed 5, Arlington, VA, 2013, APA Publishing.

American Psychiatric Association: *Substance-related and addictive disorders*, 2021. Retrieved January 20, 2021 from: http://dsm.psychiatryonline.org/doi/abs/10.1176/appi.books.9780890425596.dsm16.

American Psychological Association: *Johnson intervention*, 2021. Retrieved January 21, 2021 from: https://www.apa.org/pi/about/publications/caregivers/practice-settings/intervention/johnson-intervention.

Association of Intervention Specialists: *What is an Arise Intervention?*, 2017. Retrieved January 22, 2021 from: http://www.associationofinterventionspecialists.org/arise-gains-more-ground/. Accessed January 22, 2021.

Blume A: Advances in substance abuse prevention and treatment interventions among racial, ethnic, and sexual minority populations, *Alcohol Res Curr Rev* 38(1), 2016. Retrieved January 19, 2021 from: https://www.arcr.niaaa.nih.gov/arcr381/article05.htm. Accessed April 1, 2017.

Buell D, Filewod N, Ailon J, Burns KEA: Practice patterns in the treatment of patients with severe alcohol withdrawal: a multidisciplinary, cross-sectional survey, *J Inten Care Med* 35(11):1250–1256, 2020. https://doi.org/10.1177/0885066619847119.

Center for Behavioral Health Statistics and Quality: *Behavioral health trends in the United States: results from the 2014 National Survey on Drug Use and Health*, HHS Publication No. SMA 15-4927, NSDUH Series H-50, Rockville, MD, 2015, Substance Abuse and Mental Health Services Administration.

Center for Behavioral Health Statistics and Quality: *2015 National Survey on Drug Use and Health: detailed tables*, Rockville, MD, 2016, Substance Abuse and Mental Health Services Administration.

Centers for Disease Control and Prevention: *Age 21 minimum legal drinking age*, 2020. Retrieved December 18, 2020 from: https://www.cdc.gov/alcohol/fact-sheets/minimum-legal-drinking-age.htm.

Centers for Disease Control and Prevention: *Alcohol and public health: alcohol-related disease impact (ARDI)*, Annual average for United States 2011–2015 alcohol-attributable deaths due to excessive alcohol use, all ages, 2019. Retrieved December 14, 2020 from: https://nccd.cdc.gov/DPH_ARDI/Default/Report.aspx?T=AAM&P=1A04A664-0244-42C1-91DE-316F3AF6B447&R=B885BD06-13DF-45CD-8DD8-AA6B178C4ECE&M=32B5FFE7-81D2-43C5-A892-9B9B3C4246C7&F=AAMCauseGenderNew&D=H.

Centers for Disease Control and Prevention: *Alcohol and public health: alcohol-related disease impact (ARDI)*, 2020. Retrieved January 4, 2021 from: https://nccd.cdc.gov/DPH_ARDI/default/default.aspx.

Centers for Disease Control and Prevention: *Alcohol use in pregnancy*, 2020. Retrieved January 16, 2021 from: https://www.cdc.gov/ncbddd/fasd/alcohol-use.html.

Centers for Disease Control and Prevention: *Drug overdose deaths*, 2020. Retrieved December 14, 2020 from: https://www.cdc.gov/drugoverdose/data/statedeaths.html#:~:text=In%202018%2C%2067%2C367%20drug%20overdose,2018%20(20.7%20per%20100%2C000).

Centers for Disease Control and Prevention: *Excessive alcohol use is a risk to women's health*, 2020. Retrieved January 16, 2021 from: https://www.cdc.gov/alcohol/fact-sheets/womens-health.htm.

Centers for Disease Control and Prevention: *Fact sheets—alcohol use and your health*, 2021. Retrieved January 18, 2021 from: http://www.cdc.gov/alcohol/fact-sheets/alcohol-use.htm.

Centers for Disease Control and Prevention: *Youth risk behavior surveillance system (YRBSS)*, 2019. Retrieved January 4, 2021 from: https://www.cdc.gov/healthyyouth/data/yrbs/index.htm.

Center for Motivation and Change: *What is CRAFT*, 2014. Retrieved January 19, 2021 from: http://motivationandchange.com/outpatient-treatment/for-families/craft-overview/.

Center for Substance Abuse Treatment: *Substance abuse treatment: addressing the specific needs of women. treatment improvement protocol (TIP) series 51*, HHS Publication No. (SMA) 09-4426, Rockville, MD, 2015, Substance Abuse and Mental Health Services Administration.

Chen F, Yang H, Bulut, O, Cui X, Xin T: Examining the relation of personality factors to substance use disorder by explanatory item response modeling of DSM-5 symfloridaptoms. *PLoS One* 14(6): e0217630, 2019. https://doi.org/10.1371/journal.pone.0217630.

Close L: *Addiction among different races in the U.S.*, 2020. Retrieved January 13, 2021 from: https://sunrisehouse.com/addiction-demographics/different-races/.

Close L, Thomas S, Kelley R, Stein S, Osbourne N, Ackerman K: *Addiction among Asian Americans*, 2020. Retrieved January 13, 2021 from: https://sunrisehouse.com/addiction-demographics/asian-americans/.

Common Sense for Drug Policy: *Drug war facts*, 2021. Retrieved January 15, 2021 from: https://drugwarfacts.org/chapter/crime_arrests.

De Kock C: Cultural competence and derivatives in substance use treatment for migrants and ethnic minorities: what's the problem represented to be? *Soc Theor Health* 18:358–394, 2020.

Devenyns J: *How the legal drinking age has changed over time*, 2019. Retrieved December 17, 2020 from: https://www.wideopeneats.com/how-the-legal-drinking-age-has-changed-over-time/.

DrugRehab.com: *Doctors and addiction*, 2017. Retrieved January 23, 2021 from: https://www.drugrehab.com/addiction/doctors/.

Drugs.com: *PCP (Phencyclidine)*, 2021. Retrieved January 23, 2021 from: https://www.drugs.com/illicit/pcp.html.

Drugwarfactsorg: *Prisons, jails, and people arrested for drugs*, 2016. Retrieved January 19, 2021 from: http://www.drugwarfacts.org/cms/Prisons_and_Drugs#sthash.OajBAhra.dpbs.

Esser M, Guy G, Zhang K, Brewer R: Binge drinking and prescription opioid misuse in the U.S., 2012–2014 external icon, *Am J Prev Med* 57:197–208, 2019.

Esser M, Sherk A, Liu Y, et al.: Deaths and years of potential life lost from excessive alcohol use—United States, 2011–2015, *Morb Mortal Wkly Rep* 69(39):1428–1433, 2020.

Ewing J: Detecting alcoholism. The CAGE questionnaire, *JAMA* 252(14):1905–1907, 1984. https://doi.org/10.1001/jama.1984.03350140051025. PMID: 6471323.

GenPsych: *Risk factors for substance abuse in adolescents*, 2020. Retrieved January 16, 2021 from: https://www.genpsych.com/post/risk-factors-for-substance-abuse-in-adolescents.

Godinet M, McGlinn L, Nelson D, Vakalahi H: Factors contributing to substance misuse treatment completion among Native Hawaiians, other Pacific Islanders, and Asian Americans, *Subst Use Misuse* 55(1):133–146, 2020. https://doi.org/10.1080/10826084.2019.1657896.

Harm Reduction Coalition: *Principles of harm reduction*, 2020. Retrieved January 23, 2021 from: http://harmreduction.org/about-us/principles-of-harm-reduction/.

Hedegaard H, Miniño A, Warner M: *Drug overdose deaths in the United States, 1999–2018. NCHS data brief, no 356*, Hyattsville, MD, 2020, National Center for Health Statistics. Retrieved December 14, 2020 from: https://www.cdc.gov/nchs/data/databriefs/db356-h.pdf.

Hilton B, Betancourt H, Morrell H, Lee H, Doegy J: Substance abuse among American Indians and Alaska Natives: an integrative cultural framework for advancing research, *Int J Ment Health Addict* 16:507–523, 2018. https://doi.org/10.1007/s11469-017-9869-1.

History.com: *War on drugs*, 2019. Retrieved January 15, 2021 from: https://www.history.com/topics/crime/the-war-on-drugs.

Huhn A, Strain E, Tompkins D, Dunn K: A hidden aspect of the U.S. opioid crisis: Rise in first-time treatment admissions for older adults with opioid use disorder, *Drug Alcohol Depend* 193:142–147, 2018. https://doi.org/10.1016/j.drugalcdep.2018.10.002. Epub 2018 Oct 18. PMID: 30384321; PMCID: PMC6242338.

Jesse S, Bråthen G, Ferrara D, et al.: Alcohol withdrawal syndrome: mechanisms, manifestations, and management, *Acta neurologica Scandinavica* 135(1):1–4, 2017.

Johnston LD, Miech RA, O'Malley PM, Bachman JG, Schulenberg JE, Patrick ME: *Monitoring the future national survey results on drug use, 1975–2017: overview, key findings on adolescent drug use*, 2018, Ann Arbor: Institute for Social Research, The University of Michigan, p 116. Retrieved January 15, 2021 from: http://www.monitoringthefuture.org/pubs/monographs/mtf-overview2017.pdf.

Jones C, Clayton H, Deputy N, et al.: Prescription opioid misuse and use of alcohol and other substances among high school students — Youth Risk Behavior Survey, United States, 2019, *MMWR Suppl* 69(suppl 1):38–46, 2020.

Jones C, Compton W, & Mustaquim D: Patterns and characteristics of methamphetamine use among adults—United States, 2015–2018. *MMWR: Morbidity & Mortality Weekly Report*, 69(12), 317–323. https://doi.org/10.15585/mmwr.mm6912a1.

Kaiser Family Foundation: *Opioid overdose deaths by race/ethnicity*, 2018. Retrieved January 13, 2021 from: https://www.kff.org/other/state-indicator/opioid-overdose-deaths-by-raceethnicity/?currentTimeframe=0&sortModel=%7B%22colId%22:%22Location%22,%22sort%22:%22asc%22%7D.

Kiernan J: *Drug use by state: 2021's problem areas*, 2020. Retrieved January 9, 2021 from: https://wallethub.com/edu/drug-use-by-state/35150.

Kmiec J: *The history and politics of opioid maintenance treatment*, 2017, Training Providers' Clinical Support System. Retrieved December 18, 2020 from: https://pcssnow.org/wp-content/uploads/2017/12/AOAAM-9.20-webinar.pdf.

Matteson M, Lipari R, Hays C, Van Horn S: *A day in the life of older adults: substance use facts*, 2017. Retrieved January 5, 2021 from: https://www.samhsa.gov/data/sites/default/files/report_2792/ShortReport-2792.html#:~:text=Illicit%20drug%20use%20among%20adults,percent%20between%202001%20and%202020.&text=For%20example%2C%20the%20number%20of,to%205.7%20million%20by%202020.

McVay D: *Drug war facts*, 2020. Retrieved December 14, 2020 from: https://www.drugwarfacts.org/chapter/crime_arrests#arrests=&overlay=table/total_arrests.

Meyer J, Isaacs K, El-Shahawy O, Burlew K, Wechsburg W: Research on women with substance use disorders: reviewing progress and developing a research and implementation roadmap, *Drug Alcohol Depend* 197(1):158−163, 2019.

Mohanty S: *U.S. States with legal recreational marijuana use in 2020*, 2020. Retrieved January 4, 2021 from: https://marketrealist.com/p/recreational-marijuana-states-2020/.

National Academies of Sciences, Engineering, and Medicine: *Medications for opioid use disorder save lives*, Washington, DC, 2019, The National Academies Press, https://doi.org/10.17226/25310.

National Alliance on Mental Illness (NAMI): *Dual diagnosis*, 2021. Retrieved January 19, 2021 from: http://www.nami.org/Learn-More/Mental-Health-Conditions/Related-Conditions/Dual-Diagnosis.

National Alliance on Mental Illness: *NAMI*, 2022. Retrieved June 16, 2022 from: https://nami.org/home.

National Conference of State Legislatures: *State medical marijuana laws*, 2021. Retrieved January 4, 2021 from: https://www.ncsl.org/research/health/state-medical-marijuana-laws.aspx.

National Council on State Boards of Nursing: *Alternative to discipline programs for substance use disorder*, 2021. Retrieved January 16, 2021 from: https://www.ncsbn.org/alternative-to-discipline.htm.

National Highway Traffic Safety Administration: *Drug and human performance fact sheets: methamphetamine (and amphetamine)*, 2017. Retrieved March 28, 2017 from: https://one.nhtsa.gov/people/injury/research/job185drugs/methamphetamine.htm.

National Institute on Drug Abuse: *Anabolic steroids drugfacts*, 2018. Retrieved January 15, 2021 from: https://www.drugabuse.gov/publications/drugfacts/anabolic-steroids.

National Institute on Drug Abuse: *Commonly abused drug charts*, 2016. Retrieved January 23, 2021 from: https://www.drugabuse.gov/drugs-abuse/commonly-abused-drugs-charts#LSD.

National Institute on Drug Abuse: *Costs of substance abuse*, 2020. Retrieved December 12, 2020 from: https://www.drugabuse.gov/drug-topics/trends-statistics/costs-substance-abuse.

National Institute on Drug Abuse: *Criminal justice drug facts*, 2020. Retrieved January 18, 2021 from: https://www.drugabuse.gov/publications/drugfacts/criminal-justice.

National Institute on Drug Abuse: *Hallucinogens and dissociative drugs: common hallucinogens and dissociative drugs*, 2015. Retrieved January 23, 2021 from: https://www.drugabuse.gov/publications/research-reports/hallucinogens-dissociative-drugs/what-are-dissociative-drugs.

National Institute on Drug Abuse: *Higher rate of substance use among native American youth on reservations*, 2018. Retrieved January 16, 2021 from: https://www.drugabuse.gov/news-events/news-releases/2018/05/higher-rate-of-substance-use-among-native-american-youth-on-reservations.

National Institute on Drug Abuse: *Inhalants trends and statistics*, 2020. Retrieved January 7, 2021 from: https://www.drugabuse.gov/drug-topics/inhalants/inhalants-trends-statistics.

National Institute on Drug Abuse: *Misuse of prescription drugs research report: what is the scope of prescription drug misuse?*, 2020. Retrieved January 6, 2021 from: https://www.drugabuse.gov/publications/research-reports/misuse-prescription-drugs/what-scope-prescription-drug-misuse.

National Institute on Drug Abuse: *Monitoring the future study: trends in prevalence of various drugs*, 2020. Retrieved January 15, 2021 from: https://www.drugabuse.gov/drug-topics/trends-statistics/monitoring-future/monitoring-future-study-trends-in-prevalence-various-drugs.

National Institute on Drug Abuse: *Nationwide trends*, 2015. Retrieved January 23, 2021 from: https://www.drugabuse.gov/publications/drugfacts/nationwide-trends.

National Institute on Drug Abuse: *Principles of drug addiction treatment: a research-based guide (third edition) preface*, 2020. Retrieved January 15, 2021 from: https://www.drugabuse.gov/publications/principles-drug-addiction-treatment-research-based-guide-third-edition/preface.

National Institute on Drug Abuse (NIDA): *Methamphetamine drug facts*, 2019. Retrieved January 15, 2021 from: https://www.drugabuse.gov/publications/drugfacts/methamphetamine.

National Institute on Drug Abuse (NIDA): *Screening and assessment tools chart*, 2018. Retrieved January 15, 2021 from: https://www.drugabuse.gov/nidamed-medical-health-professionals/screening-tools-resources/chart-screening-tools/.

National Institute on Drug Abuse: *2016−2020 NIDA strategic plan*, 2017. Retrieved January 18, 2021 from: https://www.drugabuse.gov/about-nida/strategic-plan/strategically-supporting-conducting-basic-clinical-research.

National Institute on Drug Abuse (NIDA): *Substance use in older adults drugfacts*, 2020. Retrieved January 16, 2021 from: https://www.drugabuse.gov/publications/substance-use-in-older-adults-drugfacts#ref.

National Institute on Drug Abuse: *Screening, assessment, and drug testing resources*, 2014. Retrieved March 31, 2017 from: https://www.drugabuse.gov/nidamed-medical-health-professionals/tool-resources-your-practice/additional-screening-resources.

National Institute on Drug Abuse: *Substance use in women drugfacts*, 2020. Retrieved January 7, 2021 from: https://www.drugabuse.gov/publications/drugfacts/substance-use-in-women.

National Institute on Drug Abuse: *Substance use in women research report: sex and gender differences in substance use*, 2020. Retrieved January 16, 2021 from: https://www.drugabuse.gov/publications/research-reports/substance-use-in-women/sex-gender-differences-in-substance-use.

National Institute on Drug Abuse: *Trends and statistics*, 2015. Retrieved January 23, 2021 from: https://www.drugabuse.gov/related-topics/trends-statistics.

National Institute on Drug Abuse: *What are anabolic steroids?*, 2016. Retrieved January 23, 2021 from: https://www.drugabuse.gov/publications/drugfacts/anabolic-steroids.

National Institute on Drug Abuse: *What are anabolic steroids?*, 2018. Retrieved January 15, 2021 from: https://www.drugabuse.gov/publications/drugfacts/anabolic-steroids.

National Institutes of Health: *Antabuse-disulfiram tablet*, 2016. Available at: https://dailymed.nlm.nih.gov/dailymed/drugInfo.cfm?setid=f0ca0e1f-9641-48d5-9367-e5d1069e8680. Accessed April 1, 2017.

National Neighborhood Watch: *What your community can do to stop meth*, 2021. Retrieved January 15, 2021 from: https://www.nnw.org/publication/what-your-community-can-do-stop-meth.

National Network to Eliminate Health Disparities: *Familia adelante: multi-risk reduction behavioral health prevention for Latino youth and families*, 2017. Available at: http://nned.net/familia-adelante. Accessed April 1, 2017.

National Wraparound Initiative: *What is wraparound?*, 2017. Available at: http://nwi.pdx.edu/wraparound-basics/#whatisWraparound. Accessed April 1, 2017.

New Beginnings: *The single parent's guide to addiction recovery*, 2021. Retrieved January 19, 2021 from: http://www.newbeginningsdrugrehab.org/drug-addiction/the-single-parents-guide-to-addiction-recovery/.

National Institute on Drug Abuse: *Anabolic steroids drugfacts*, 2018. Retrieved January 15, 2021 from: https://www.drugabuse.gov/publications/drugfacts/anabolic-steroids.

National Institute on Drug Abuse: *Commonly abused drug charts*, 2016. Retrieved January 23, 2021 from: https://www.drugabuse.gov/drugs-abuse/commonly-abused-drugs-charts#LSD.

National Institute on Drug Abuse: *Costs of substance abuse*, 2020. Retrieved December 12, 2020 from: https://www.drugabuse.gov/drug-topics/trends-statistics/costs-substance-abuse.

National Institute on Drug Abuse: *Criminal justice drug facts*, 2020. Retrieved January 18, 2021 from: https://www.drugabuse.gov/publications/drugfacts/criminal-justice.

National Institute on Drug Abuse: *Hallucinogens and dissociative drugs: common hallucinogens and dissociative drugs*, 2015. Retrieved January 23, 2021 from: https://www.drugabuse.gov/publications/research-reports/hallucinogens-dissociative-drugs/what-are-dissociative-drugs.

National Institute on Drug Abuse: *Higher rate of substance use among native American youth on reservations*, 2018. Retrieved January 16, 2021 from: https://www.drugabuse.gov/news-events/news-releases/2018/05/higher-rate-of-substance-use-among-native-american-youth-on-reservations.

National Institute on Drug Abuse: *Inhalants trends and statistics*, 2020. Retrieved January 7, 2021 from: https://www.drugabuse.gov/drug-topics/inhalants/inhalants-trends-statistics.

National Institute on Drug Abuse: *Misuse of prescription drugs research report: what is the scope of prescription drug misuse?*, 2020. Retrieved January 6, 2021 from: https://www.drugabuse.gov/publications/research-reports/misuse-prescription-drugs/what-scope-prescription-drug-misuse.

National Institute on Drug Abuse: *Monitoring the future study: trends in prevalence of various drugs*, 2020. Retrieved January 15, 2021 from: https://www.drugabuse.gov/drug-topics/trends-statistics/monitoring-future/monitoring-future-study-trends-in-prevalence-various-drugs.

National Institute on Drug Abuse; National Institutes of Health; U.S. Department of Health and Human Services: *Monitoring the future 2016 survey results*, 2016. Retrieved March 28, 2017 from: https://www.drugabuse.gov/related-topics/trends-statistics/infographics/monitoring-future-2016-survey-results.

National Institute on Drug Abuse: *Nationwide trends*, 2015. Retrieved January 23, 2021 from: https://www.drugabuse.gov/publications/drugfacts/nationwide-trends.

National Institute on Drug Abuse: *Principles of drug addiction treatment: a research-based guide (third edition) preface*, 2020. Retrieved January 15, 2021 from: https://www.drugabuse.gov/publications/principles-drug-addiction-treatment-research-based-guide-third-edition/preface.

National Institute on Drug Abuse (NIDA): *Methamphetamine drug facts*, 2019. Retrieved January 15, 2021 from: https://www.drugabuse.gov/publications/drugfacts/methamphetamine.

National Institute on Drug Abuse (NIDA): *Screening and assessment tools chart*, 2018. Retrieved January 15, 2021 from: https://www.drugabuse.gov/nidamed-medical-health-professionals/screening-tools-resources/chart-screening-tools/.

National Institute on Drug Abuse: *2016–2020 NIDA strategic plan*, 2017. Retrieved January 18, 2021 from: https://www.drugabuse.gov/about-nida/strategic-plan/strategically-supporting-conducting-basic-clinical-research.

National Institute on Drug Abuse (NIDA): *Substance use in older adults drugfacts*, 2020. Retrieved January 16, 2021 from: https://www.drugabuse.gov/publications/substance-use-in-older-adults-drugfacts#ref.

National Institute on Drug Abuse: *Screening, assessment, and drug testing resources*, 2014. Retrieved March 31, 2017 from: https://www.drugabuse.gov/nidamed-medical-health-professionals/tool-resources-your-practice/additional-screening-resources.

National Institute on Drug Abuse: *Substance use in women drugfacts*, 2020. Retrieved January 7, 2021 from: https://www.drugabuse.gov/publications/drugfacts/substance-use-in-women.

National Institute on Drug Abuse: *Substance use in women research report: sex and gender differences in substance use*, 2020. Retrieved January 16, 2021 from: https://www.drugabuse.gov/publications/research-reports/substance-use-in-women/sex-gender-differences-in-substance-use.

National Institute on Drug Abuse: *Trends and statistics*, 2015. Retrieved January 23, 2021 from: https://www.drugabuse.gov/related-topics/trends-statistics.

National Institute on Drug Abuse: *What are anabolic steroids?*, 2016. Retrieved January 23, 2021 from: https://www.drugabuse.gov/publications/drugfacts/anabolic-steroids.

National Institute on Drug Abuse: *What are hallucinogens?*, 2016. Retrieved January 23, 2021 from: https://www.drugabuse.gov/publications/drugfacts/hallucinogens.

National Institute on Drug Abuse: *What are anabolic steroids?*, 2018. Retrieved January 15, 2021 from: https://www.drugabuse.gov/publications/drugfacts/anabolic-steroids.

National Institute on Drug Abuse: *What are hallucinogens?*, 2016. Retrieved January 23, 2021 from: https://www.drugabuse.gov/publications/drugfacts/hallucinogens.

National Institutes of Health: *Combination treatment for methamphetamine use disorder shows promise in NIH study*, 2021. Retrieved January 15, 2021 from: https://www.nih.gov/news-events/news-releases/combination-treatment-methamphetamine-use-disorder-shows-promise-nih-study.

National Institutes of Health: *Substance use in American Indian youth is worse than we thought*, 2014. Available from: https://www.drugabuse.gov/about-nida/noras-blog/2014/09/substance-use-in-american-indian-youth-worse-than-we-thought. Accessed April 1, 2017.

Office of National Drug Control Policy: *National drug control strategy*, 2020. Retrieved December 19, 2020 from: https://www.whitehouse.gov/wp-content/uploads/2020/02/2020-NDCS.pdf.

Palombi M: *Drugs & alcohol–a symptom of the system*, 2017, The Family Systems Institute. Retrieved January 15, 2021 from: https://www.thefsi.com.au/2017/09/13/drugs-alcohol-symptom-system/.

Patrick M, Schulenberg J, Maggs J, Maslowsky J: Substance use and peers during adolescence and the transition to adulthood: Selection, socialization, and development. In Scher K, editor: *Oxford handbook of substance use and substance use disorders*, vol. 1, https://doi.org/10.1093/oxfordhb/9780199381678.013.004.

PBS: *A social history of America's most popular drugs*, 2014, Frontline. Retrieved January 23, 2021 from: http://www.pbs.org/wgbh/pages/frontline/shows/drugs/buyers/socialhistory.html.

Pew Research Center: *Feds may be rethinking the drug war, but states have been leading the way*, 2014. Retrieved January 15, 2021 from: https://www.pewresearch.org/fact-tank/2014/04/02/feds-may-be-rethinking-the-drug-war-but-states-have-been-leading-the-way/.

Pierce M: *The risk and resistance factors influencing the propensity toward alcoholism among children of alcoholics: an integrative review of the literature*, 2019. Retrieved January 15, 2021 from: https://via.library.depaul.edu/nursing-colloquium/2018/winter/24/.

Ramirez V, Wiers, C, Wang G, Volkow N: Personality traints in substance use disorders and obesity when compared to healthy controls, *Addiction* 115:2130—2130, 2020. https://doi.org/10.1111/add.15062.

Rehab International: *Crystal meth addiction statistics*, 2021. Retrieved January 23, 2021 from: http://rehab-international.org/crystal-meth/addiction-statistics.

Rutman D, Hubberstey C, Poole N, Schmidt R, Van Bibber M: Multiservice prevention programs for pregnant and parenting women with substance use and multiple vulnerabilities: program structure and clients' perspectives on wraparound programming, *BMC Preg Childbirth* 20:441, 2020. https://doi.org/10.1186/s12884-020-03109-1.

Sacks J, Gonzales K, Bouchery E, Tomedi L, Brewer R: 2010 national and state costs of excessive alcohol consumption, *Am J Prev Med* 49(5):e73—e79, 2015.

Sen S, Grgurich P, Tulolo A, et al.: A symptom-triggered benzodiazepine protocol utilizing SAS and CIWA-Ar scoring for the treatment of alcohol withdrawal syndrome in the critically ill, *Ann Pharmacother* 51(2):101—110, 2017.

Shaffer H: *What age group is most likely to use illegal drugs?*, 2020, Sharecare. Retrieved January 15, 2021 from: https://www.sharecare.com/health/illegal-drug-use/what-age-group-illegal-drugs.

Starr K: The sneaky prevalence of substance abuse in nursing, *Nursing* 45(3):16—17, 2015. https://doi.org/10.1097/01.NURSE.0000460727.34118.6a.

Sterling E: *Drug laws and snitching: a primer*, 2021, PBS Frontline. Retrieved January 18, 2021 from: http://www.pbs.org/wgbh/pages/frontline/shows/snitch/primer/.

SAHMSA: *About us*, 2020. Retrieved December 21, 2020 from: https://www.samhsa.gov/about-us.

SAHMSA: *Key substance use and mental health indicators in the United States: results from the 2018 National Survey on Drug Use and Health*, 2018. Retrieved December 22, 2020 from: https://www.samhsa.gov/data/sites/default/files/cbhsq-reports/NSDUHNationalFindingsReport2018/NSDUHNationalFindingsReport2018.pdf.

Substance Abuse and Mental Health Services Administration: *Buprenorphine*, 2020. Retrieved January 22, 2021 from: https://www.samhsa.gov/medication-assisted-treatment/medications-counseling-related-conditions/buprenorphine.

Substance Abuse and Mental Health Services Administration: *Homeless and housing services providers confront opioid overdose*, 2020. Retrieved January 7, 2021 from: https://www.samhsa.gov/homelessness-programs-resources/hpr-resources/homeless-housing-services-providers-confront-opioid.

Substance Abuse and Mental Health Services Administration: *Key substance use and mental health indicators in the United States: results from the 2019 National Survey on Drug Use and Health*, 2020. Retrieved January 15, 2021 from: https://www.samhsa.gov/data/sites/default/files/reports/rpt29393/2019NSDUHFFRPDFWHTML/2019NSDUHFFR1PDFW090120.pdf.

Substance Abuse and Mental Health Services Administration: *National Survey on Drug Use and Health (NSDUH). Table 5.4A—alcohol use disorder in past year among persons aged 12 or older, by age group and demographic characteristics: numbers in thousands, 2018 and 2019*, 2019. Retrieved December 14, 2020 from: https://www.samhsa.gov/data/sites/default/files/cbhsq-reports/NSDUHDetailedTabs2018R2/NSDUHDetTabsSect5pe2018.htm#tab5-4a.

Substance Abuse and Mental Health Services Administration: *Results from the 2018 National Survey on Drug Use and Health: detailed tables*, Rockville, MD, 2019b, Center for Behavioral Health Statistics and Quality, Substance Abuse and Mental Health Services Administration. Retrieved from: https://www.samhsa.gov/data/.

Substance Abuse and Mental Health Services Administration: *Risk and protective factors*, 2021. Retrieved January 18, 2021 from: https://www.samhsa.gov/sites/default/files/20190718-samhsa-risk-protective-factors.pdf.

Substance Abuse and Mental Health Services Administration: *SAMHSA's annual mental health, substance use data provide roadmap for future action*, 2020.

Substance Abuse and Mental Health Services Administration: *The opioid crisis and the Black/African American population: an urgent issue*, 2020. Retrieved January 16, 2021 from: https://store.samhsa.gov/product/The-Opioid-Crisis-and-the-Black-African-American-Population-An-Urgent-Issue/PEP20-05-02-001.

Substance Abuse and Mental Health Services Administration Center for Substance Abuse Treatment: *Substance abuse: clinical issues in intensive outpatient treatment improvement protocol (TIP) series*, Rockville, MD, 2006, Substance Abuse and Mental Health Services Administration. no. 47.

Substance Abuse and Mental Health Services Administration Center for Substance Abuse Treatment: *Behavioral health services for American Indians and Alaska Natives, treatment improvement protocol (TIP) 61*, Rockville, MD, 2019, Substance Abuse and Mental Health Services Administration.

Substance Abuse and Mental Health Services Administration Center for Behavioral Health Statistics and Quality: *Results from the 2018 National Survey on Drug Use and Health: detailed tables*, 2019. Rockville (MD). Retrieved January 6, 2021 from: https://www.samhsa.gov/data/report/2018-nsduh-detailed-tables.

Substance Abuse and Mental Health Services Administration Office of the Surgeon General: Facing addiction in America: the surgeon general's report on alcohol, drugs, and health [Internet]. In *Chapter 4, early intervention, treatment, and management of substance use disorders*, November 2016, Wash Times: US Department of Health and Human Services. Retrieved January 18, 2021 from: https://www.ncbi.nlm.nih.gov/books/NBK424859/.

The president's commission on combating drug addiction and the opioid crisis final report, 2017. Retrieved January 16, 2021 from: https://facesandvoicesofrecovery.org/wp-content/uploads/2019/06/Final-Report-The-Presidents-Commission-on-Combatting-Drug-Addiction-and-The-Opioid-Crisis.pdf.

Trivedi M, Walker R, Ling W, et al.: Bupropion and naltrexone in methamphetamine use disorder, *N Engl J Med* 384:140—153, 2021.

U. S. Department of Health and Human Services (USDHHS) Office of Disease Prevention and Health Promotion: *Healthy people 2030: drug and alcohol use*, 2021. Retrieved January 13, 2021 from: https://health.gov/healthypeople/objectives-and-data/browse-objectives/drug-and-alcohol-use.

U.S. Department of Health and Human Services (USHHS) Office of the Surgeon General: *Facing addiction in America: the surgeon general's report on alcohol, drugs, and healthex*, Washington, DC, 2016, HHS.

United Nations Office on Drugs and Crime: *World drug report 2020*, 2020. Retrieved December 31, 2020 from: https://wdr.unodc.org/wdr2020/index.html.

United States Census Bureau: *Quick Facts United States*, 2019. Retrieved January 12, 2021 from: https://www.census.gov/quickfacts/fact/table/US/PST045219#qf-headnote-b.

Valdez L, Flores M, Ruiz J, Carvajal S, Garcia D: Gender and cultural adaptations for diversity: a systematic review of alcohol and substance abuse interventions for Latino males, *Subst Use Misuse*

53(10):1608–1623, 2018. https://doi.org/10.1080/10826084.2017.1417999.

Vertiva Health: *Cocaine use during pregnancy: effects, risks, and treatment*, 2021. Retrieved January 16, 2021 from: https://vertavahealth.com/cocaine/pregnancy/.

Verywellmind: *What are substance use disorders?*, 2020. Retrieved January 15, 2021 from: https://www.verywellmind.com/dsm-5-criteria-for-substance-use-disorders-21926#citation-1.

Wilkinson S, Yarnell S, Radhakrishnan R, Ball S, Souza D: Marijuana legalization: impact on physicians and public health, *Annu Rev Med* 67:453–466, 2016.

Wilson N, Karlisa M, Seth P, Smith H, Davis N: Drug and opioid-involved overdose deaths — United States, 2017–2018, *Morb Mortal Wkly Rep* 69:290–297, 2020. https://doi.org/10.15585/mmwr.mm6911a4.

Wolf C, Curry A, Nacht J, Simpson SA: Management of alcohol withdrawal in the emergency department: current perspectives, *Open Access Emerg Med: OAEM* 12:53–65, 2020. https://doi.org/10.2147/OAEM.S235288.

Women for Sobriety: *Women for sobriety*, 2021. Retrieved January 23, 2021 from: http://www.womenforsobriety.org/beta2/.

Wong W, Barnett PG: Characteristics of Asian and Pacific Islanders admitted to U.S. drug treatment programs in 2005, *Publ Health Rep* 125(2):250–257, 2010.

Wright L, Leahy M: *Nurses and families: A guide to family assessment and intervention*, ed 7, Philadelphia, 2019, F.A. Davis.

Yockey R, Vidourek R, King K: Trends in LSD use among US adults: 2015–2018, *Drug & Alcohol Depend* 212:108071, 2020. https://doi.org/10.1016/j.drugalcdep.2020.108071. PMID: 32450479.

28

Violence

Kelli M. Galle and C. Paige Owen[a]

OBJECTIVES

Upon completion of this chapter, the reader will be able to do the following:
1. Describe the concepts of interpersonal and community violence.
2. Identify factors that influence violence.
3. Identify populations at risk for violence and the role of public health in dealing with the epidemic of violence.
4. Describe the role of the nurse in primary, secondary, and tertiary prevention of violence.

OUTLINE

KEY TERMS

abusive head trauma
bullying
child maltreatment
date rape drugs
dating violence
elder abuse
emotional abuse
hate crimes
human trafficking
intentional injuries
interpersonal violence
intimate partner violence
neglect
physical abuse
prison violence
sexual abuse
stalking
terrorism
violence
workplace violence
youth-related violence

Violence is a serious national public health problem that affects all ages from the very young to the very old. Violent deaths, however, only tell part of the problem. Although many victims of violence survive, they, their families, and their friends often have permanent emotional and physical scars. Violence exists globally and transpires daily, as evidenced by television and Internet news reports. For example, in the United States:

April 1999: In Columbine High School, Littleton, Colorado, 13 killed by two teenagers who then committed suicide.

September 11, 2001: A total of 2974 people from 90 different countries killed when 19 terrorists hijacked 4 planes and intentionally crashed two of them into the World Trade Center's twin towers, the third into the Pentagon, and the fourth in an empty field in Pennsylvania.

April 2007: 32 killed, 15 wounded at Virginia Tech University in Blacksburg, Virginia, by a student who then committed suicide.

November 2009: 13 killed, 42 injured at a military base in Fort Hood, Texas, by a US Army psychiatrist.

July 2012: 12 killed, 58 injured during a midnight showing of the movie *Batman: The Dark Knight* in Aurora, Colorado.

December 2012: 20 students and 7 adults killed, 2 wounded, at Sandy Hook Elementary School in Newtown, Connecticut.

[a] The authors would like to acknowledge the contributions of Ginette G. Ferszt, Cathi A. Pourciau, and Elaine C. Vallette, who revised this chapter in previous editions.

627

April 2013: 3 killed and an estimated 264 injured when 2 men set 2 pressure-cooker bombs at the finish line of the Boston Marathon.

December 2015: 14 killed and 22 injured at a regional center in San Bernadino, California. The perpetrators—husband and wife—were later killed by police.

June 2016: 49 killed and 58 injured during a mass shooting at a night club in Orlando, Florida, by a man who was killed by the police.

October 2017: 58 killed and 851 injured when a 64-year-old man fired on a crowd of concert-goers in Las Vegas.

February 2018: 17 people killed and 17 more wounded at Marjory Stoneman Douglas High School by a former student in Parkland, Florida.

August 2019: 23 killed and 23 others injured by a 21 year old shooter who appeared to target Latinos at a Walmart Supercenter in El Paso, Texas.

November 2021: 26 people were killed and 62 injured at a Christmas parade in Waukesha Wisconsin when a 39-year-old man intentionally drove his SUV into the crowd.

Finally, in May 2020 the death of George Floyd sparked a wide series of protests and riots nationally, resulting in at least 19 deaths and extensive property damage.

Although the preceding list shows well-publicized acts of extreme violence, violence occurs daily in communities across the country; most instances go unreported or unpublicized. These include situations in which a woman is beaten and killed by her husband, a child kidnapped and murdered by a neighbor, an infant who is shaken to death by his mother, a young woman who is gang raped, children who are sexually abused, and coworkers who are killed by a disgruntled former employee are all examples of the violence that occurs with alarming frequency.

The purpose of this chapter is to explore the influence of violence from a public health perspective as it relates to individuals and communities. It includes discussions of the effects of violence in terms of homicides and suicides, review of the direct influence of violence on individuals and communities, examination of public health interventions to reduce violence, the roles and responsibilities of the community health nurse in dealing with those experiencing violence, and measures to increase awareness of violence in the workplace. An in-depth look at the causes, effects, interventions, and measures to increase awareness of violence is presented.

OVERVIEW OF VIOLENCE

The World Health Organization (WHO) defines **violence** as "the intentional use of physical force or power, threatened or actual against oneself, another person, or against a group or community, which either results in or has a high likelihood of resulting in injury, death, psychological harm, maldevelopment, or deprivation" (WHO, 2021). In the field of public health, injuries from violence are referred to as **intentional injuries**. Violence threatens the health and well-being of people of all ages globally. Worldwide, 1.25 million people lose their

lives annually as a result of violence-related injuries (WHO, 2021). In 2019, 19,141 people were victims of homicide in the United States alone (Centers for Disease Control and Prevention [CDC], 2021a).

The reasons for the high rate of violence in societies are complex. Universally recognized factors that contribute to violence include the following:
1. Poverty, unemployment, economic dependency
2. Substance abuse
3. Mental illness
4. Media influence
5. Access to firearms
6. Political and/or religious ideology
7. Intolerance and ignorance

HISTORY OF VIOLENCE

Violence is a global problem. From prehistoric times humans have dealt violently with other humans. In the Bible, Cain killed his brother Abel out of jealousy and anger. Throughout history, some acts of violence were socially accepted. For instance, sporting events such as the gladiator events in Rome often resulted in death for the audience's pleasure; infanticide, or the killing of unwanted newborn children, has been practiced throughout history. For example, in past eras, a female, a twin, sickly, or deformed child was often left to die of exposure. Children, especially firstborn children, were often sacrificed for religious reasons. Infanticide was not condemned until early in the fifth century; however, this did not protect children in many societies.

Throughout the ages, corporal punishment has been used as a means of controlling the behavior of children. Biblical reference to corporal punishment has often been used as justification for some types of child abuse. To some parents, "spare the rod and spoil the child" (Proverbs 13:24) implies an imperative to abusively discipline an errant child. The idea of "beating some sense into him" was considered necessary to ensure that a lesson was learned. The first anticruelty laws were enacted on behalf of animals rather than children. It wasn't until 1875 that the first organized child protection initiative was established, The New York Society for the Prevention of Cruelty to Children (NYSPCC) was a nongovernmental society that paved the way for the more modern government sponsored child protective services (CPS), which was established in 1962 (Myers, 2008). Even nursery rhymes that adults read to small children seem to condone violence against them. Consider the following Mother Goose nursery rhyme:

> *There was an old woman who lived in a shoe,*
> *She had so many children she didn't know what to do,*
> *She gave them some broth without any bread,*
> *And whipped them all soundly and sent them to bed.*
> ***Mother Goose Nursery Rhymes, 2000, pp. 195—196***

Domestic violence against women was legal in the United States until 1824. Wives were seen as their husbands' property and could be beaten for such offenses as "nagging too much."

In fact, the common phrase "rule of thumb" was derived from English law that allowed a man to beat his wife with a cane no wider than his thumb. Biblical interpretation of "wives be subject to your husband" (Ephesians 5:22) still provides some men with a faulty rationalization for wife beating. Some cultures and religions still allow, and even support, abuse of wives.

The silence that long surrounded domestic violence is derived from the historical perspective of women being considered property of their husbands … Violence against women was not explored in America until the Civil Rights Movement of the 1960s. In fact, marital rape was not considered a criminal offense in the United States for many years. The first state to legislatively change its spousal rape laws was Nebraska in 1976. By 1993, every state had amended its spousal rape law. In the last 3 decades, additional cultural considerations have surfaced regarding domestic abuse which include female circumcision and genital mutilation, abuse between homosexual partners, and the awareness that men are also victims of domestic violence. Even though progress has been made, due to loopholes, differing laws among states, failed repeal efforts, and access to justice, there still exists problematic consent issues, which are at the forefront of the "#MeToo movement," aiming to influence the abolishment of these loopholes (Holmes, 2021).

Elder abuse is also a continuing problem. The problem is of greater magnitude now because people are living longer, resulting in increased numbers of dependent and vulnerable adults. Elder abuse frequently goes undetected because of a lack of awareness on the part of healthcare professionals and society. Elder abuse includes physical, sexual, emotional, neglect, and financial abuse. The exact prevalence of elder abuse is unknown because reporting is not mandatory in all states; however, the CDC estimates from 2002 to 2016, more than 643,000 elders were treated in the emergency department for nonfatal assaults, and over 19,000 homicides occurred as a result of elder abuse (CDC, 2021b).

INTERPERSONAL VIOLENCE

Homicide and Suicide

In the United States, homicide claimed the lives of 19,141 individuals in 2019, with over 14,000 deaths involving the use of firearms (CDC, 2021a). Of note, most homicide offenders and victims are male. When race of the murder victims could be determined, 51% were Black or African American, 44% were Caucasian, and 4% were other races. Approximately 51% of all homicides occurred at a home residence (Federal Bureau of Investigation, 2021). According to the CDC, in 2019, homicide was the third leading cause of death for those in the 10 to 24 age group (at 15.1% of deaths), fourth leading cause for age group 1 to 9 at 7.3%, and the fifth leading cause for age group 25 to 44 at 6.2% (Heron, 2021).

Suicide is also an extremely serious problem in the United States, and its incidence continues to rise at an alarming rate.

Indeed, suicide is the 10th leading cause of death in the United States, accounting for 47,5000 deaths in 2019 (CDC, 2021c). Although females have more suicidal attempts than males, males commit suicide 3.63 times as often when compared to females. In 2019, the most common method of death by suicide was firearms, accounting for 50.39% of suicide deaths. This was followed by suffocation, including hanging at 28.55%, and poisoning, including overdose at 12.89%. Suicide rates vary considerably within different population subgroups. Ethnicity, socioeconomic status, employment status, occupation, veteran status, sexual orientation, and gender identity may disproportionately increase suicide risk. In 2019, for example, the rates of suicide—15.67 per 100,000—were highest among Caucasians accounting. In comparison, suicide rates were 13.64 per 100,000 for American Indians/Alaska Natives, 7.04 per 100,000 for Asians/Pacific Islanders, 7.04 per 100,000 for Black or African Americans, and 7.24 per 100,000 for Hispanics (American Foundation for Suicide Prevention, 2021). Nurses have a key role in identifying individuals who are at risk for suicide. Risk factors for suicide include:

1. History of depression or other psychiatric disorders
2. Alcohol and/or substance abuse
3. Physical illness or disability
4. History of attempted suicide
5. History of violence
6. Age
7. Environmental stressors
8. Veteran status

Refer to Chapter 25 for further discussion on suicide.

Intimate Partner Violence

Intimate partner violence (IPV) is a serious public health problem that affects the lives of millions of people in the United States. IPV is defined as violence that occurs between people in a close relationship, usually spouses, former spouses, and dating partners. According to the CDC, an estimated 1 in 4 women, and 1 in 10 men are victims of sexual violence, physical violence, and/or stalking by an intimate partner each year in the United States (CDC, 2021d).

IPV includes four different types of behavior: physical violence (hitting, kicking, or another type of physical force), sexual violence (forcing a partner to take part in a sex act without his or her consent), psychological aggression (verbal and unwanted attention and contact by a partner with the intent to harm and control another person), and stalking, which will be discussed later in this chapter. IPV is often repetitive, progressive, and escalates in frequency and severity. Because many people are afraid to report IPV to the police, family, or friends, it is hard to capture the exact incidence of this type of violence. IPV has been reported in all types of relationships: women against women in lesbian relationships, men against men in homosexual relationships, and women against men. Box 28.1 presents commonly held myths about IPV.

IPV crosses all ethnic, racial, socioeconomic, and educational lines. The CDC has identified several factors that increase

BOX 28.1   Common Myths Associated With Intimate Partner Violence

- It occurs only in poor, uneducated, minority households.
- It is a private family matter (vs. a societal problem).
- It only occurs in heterosexual relationships.
- Victims deserve the abuse.
- Victims can change the abusers' behavior.
- Abusers will stop the abuse on their own without professional intervention.

the risk of being a victim of IPV: the perpetrator often has a history of being violent or aggressive, witnessing or being a victim of violence as a child themselves, using drugs and/or consuming large amounts of alcohol, and unemployment or other life events that cause stress. Victims of IPV have reported serious negative health outcomes. Physical injuries can include bruising, welts, internal bleeding, disabilities, head trauma, and even death. Victims can also be traumatized and experience depression, chronic pain, sleep difficulties, and a range of other serious mental health problems. IPV can also lead to long-term consequences, including physical injury, poor mental health, and chronic physical health problems. For some people, IPV results in hospitalization, disability, or death. Previous research indicates that victimization as a child or adolescence can increase the likelihood that victimization will continue into adulthood. In order to cope with their suffering, victims may employ maladaptive coping mechanisms such as substance abuse, alcoholism, and/or risky sexual behavior (CDC, 2021d).

Societal awareness of IPV during pregnancy is a relatively recent phenomenon; the mention of abuse during pregnancy began to appear in the literature in the 1980s. The image of a woman being battered during pregnancy shatters the idealized image of pregnancy as a time of nurturing and protection. All pregnant women should be routinely screened for abuse. Common signs of IPV in pregnancy are delay in seeking prenatal care, unexplained bruising or damage to breasts or abdomen, use of harmful substances (cigarettes, alcohol, drugs), recurring psychosomatic illnesses, and lack of participation in prenatal education. Violence during pregnancy can result in hemorrhage, spontaneous abortion, stillbirths, preterm deliveries, low birth weight, and fetal injuries. Indeed, pregnancy may increase stress within the family and provoke the first instances of battering. It is estimated that one in six abused women were first abused during pregnancy. It is estimated more than 320,000 women are abused by their partner during pregnancy annually (March of Dimes, n.d.).

RESEARCH HIGHLIGHTS

Gender-based violence, including IPV, child abuse, elder abuse, sexual assault, stalking and human trafficking, impacts millions of individuals each year. The COVID-19 pandemic has exacerbated risk factors for violence including increased unemployment, financial insecurity, social distancing/quarantining (isolation), depression and anxiety. As a result, the incidence of

IPV and child abuse has increased since the start of the pandemic, though the full extent is unknown. Protective responses to COVID-19, including lockdowns and school closures, designed to protect the community from infectious transmission, have isolated survivors and hinder victim help-seeking. In this survey, over 58% of professionals who serve survivors of violence, reported barriers to helping survivors due to agency closure, maintain staff health, shelter capacity, limited resources (including personal protective equipment), and reduced criminal justice system operations. Most respondents believed IPV (83.7%), child abuse (70.2%), and sexual assault (60.2%) have increased during the pandemic.

Data from Lynch, KR, Logan, TK: *Assessing challenges, needs, and innovations of gender-based violence services during the COVID-19 pandemic: Results summary report.* San Antonio, TX, 2021, University of Texas at San Antonio, College for Health, Community and Policy.

Sexual Assault

Every 68 s an American is sexually assaulted, and every 9 min the victim is a child. Nine out of every 10 sexual assaults occur in females and are often perpetrated by someone they know. The majority occur at or near the victims' homes (Rape, Abuse & Incest National Network [RAINN], 2022). Women may report that they were subjected to forced intercourse when they were ill or had recently given birth. They also report forced anal intercourse and other violent sexual acts. Box 28.2 includes considerations for working with victims of IPV.

BOX 28.2   Considerations for Working With Victims of Violence

1. Working with victims of IPV:
   - Establish rapport and trust.
   - Deal with issues of confidentiality honestly.
   - Provide current information regarding shelters and sources of support.
   - Recognize and accept that clients may "choose" to stay in an abusive relationship.
2. Working with victims of child abuse:
   - Protect the well-being of the child; this is the primary obligation of healthcare providers.
   - Report child abuse; it is a legal and ethical obligation in all states.
   - Establish rapport and trust; this may take time.
   - Remain objective when dealing with suspected family members.
3. Working with victims of elder abuse:
   - Establish rapport and trust; this may take time.
   - Report elder abuse; it is an ethical obligation for healthcare providers and a legal obligation in most states.
   - Remember that competent adults have the right to make decisions about their own care, even if it means staying in an abusive situation.
   - Support efforts to create respite programs and support groups for caregivers.
4. Advocating for the rights of vulnerable populations, which is the responsibility of all healthcare professionals:
   - Support research on effective interventions for violence prevention and reduction.
   - Lobby for a decrease in media violence.
   - Support community efforts to increase resources for victims of violence.
   - Lobby for effective regulation of firearms and cyberstalking.

To address the underreporting and under prosecution of adult sexual assaults, communities throughout the United States have implemented a model using the Sexual Assault Nurse Examiner (SANE). These specially trained nurses provide comprehensive psychological, medical, and forensic services for sexual assault. SANE nurses often work collaboratively with community-based victim advocates assuring continuity of support over time.

The Domestic Abuse Intervention Program (2011) in Duluth, Minnesota, has developed a wheel of violence that depicts how men who batter gain and maintain control over their female partners. The Power and Control Wheel was developed by documenting women's experience of being battered within an intimate relationship. The Power and Control Wheel is therefore not a generic, genderless tool to understand domestic violence. Fig. 28.1 depicts the Power and Control Wheel, "a helpful tool in understanding the overall pattern of abusive and violent behaviors that are used by a batterer to establish and maintain control over his partner. Very often, one or more violent incidents are accompanied by an array of these other types of abuse." The organization has also developed other wheels that focus on domestic abuse that include equality, abuse of children and nurturing children. The Post Separation Wheel is the newest put out by the DAIP and that focuses on the tactics used by men when their partner leaves and they share children.

Dating violence refers to abusive, controlling, or aggressive behavior in an intimate relationship that can take the form of emotional, verbal, physical, or sexual abuse. Dating violence occurs in all types of relationships. Data from CDC's Youth Risk Behavior Survey and the National Intimate Partner and Sexual Violence Survey indicate that 26% of females and 15% of males had ever experienced rape, physical violence, or stalking by an intimate partner; also they first experienced some form of partner violence before the age of 18 (CDC, 2021e).

Teens may not be aware of what constitutes an unhealthy relationship. They may think that teasing and name calling are a "normal" part of a relationship. However, these behaviors can become abusive and develop into more serious forms of violence. Unhealthy, abusive, or violent relationships can have severe consequences with short- and long-term negative effects on developing teens.

Several national initiatives have been developed to address teen dating violence. For example, the CDC's dating violence

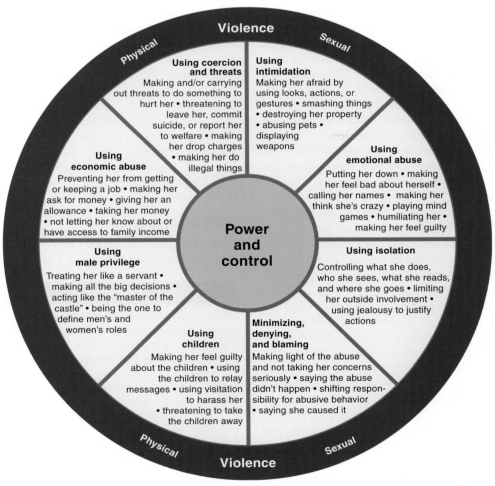

Fig. 28.1 Power and Control Wheel. (Developed by the Domestic Abuse Intervention Project, 206 West Fourth Street, Duluth, MN 55806. Used with permission.)

prevention initiative seeks to reduce dating violence and increase healthy relationships in high-risk urban communities through comprehensive, multisector prevention.

Dating violence can involve the use of **date rape drugs**, also known as *predator drugs*. These include any substances that make rape or sexual assault easier. Nearly 11 million women in the United States have been sexually assaulted while drunk, drugged, or high. Examples of date rape drugs include gamma-hydroxybutyrate (GHB), flunitrazepam (Rohypnol), and ketamine, to reduce inhibitions and promote anesthesia or amnesia in the victim (Office of the Assistant Secretary for Health, 2019). GHB is odorless and colorless and can easily be made at home. Instructions are available in libraries and on the Internet, possibly explaining the drug's rapid rise in popularity. Although illegal in the United States, it has become available in many nightclubs, where it is sold in clear liquid form. GHB has been touted as an aphrodisiac and an anesthetic. It is actually a depressant that slows down the respiratory system and has been responsible for numerous overdoses. When mixed with alcohol, it can be deadly.

Flunitrazepam, which is classified as a benzodiazepine, has been compared with methaqualone (Quaalude), the "love drug" of the 1960 and 1970s. Like GHB, flunitrazepam is not legal in the United States, but many reports have been received of its use at fraternity parties, college gatherings, and in bars. Two other drugs in the benzodiazepine family, alprazolam (Xanax) and clonazepam (Klonopin), are also used as date rape drugs. The ability to provide a quick, cheap high with long-lasting effects may explain their popularity. When they are combined with alcohol, serious side effects, including death, have been reported.

Ketamine (ketamine hydrochloride) is an anesthetic used primarily in veterinary practice and pain management. It causes a lost sense of time and problems with memory. Another drug that is becoming more common as a date rape drug is carisoprodol (Soma), a prescription muscle relaxant and central nervous system depressant.

Studies have also linked alcohol, "a hallmark of college campus social life," with dating violence. Substance abuse is often implicated in sexual assaults on college campuses. Alcohol contributes to sexual assault because it impairs the ability to think clearly, lowers inhibitions, and impairs the ability to evaluate an unsafe situation.

Stalking is a pattern of repeated and unwanted attention, contact, harassment, or any type of conduct directed at a person that instills fear. Like IPV, stalking is a crime of power and control. Types of stalking include unwanted phone calls, waiting at places for the victim, leaving unwanted items such as flowers and gifts, posting information or spreading rumors about the victim, messaging through the Internet or cell phone (cyberstalking), damaging the victim's property, following the victim, obtaining personal information about the victim, and making direct or indirect threats to the victim's family or friends. An estimated 3.8 million persons, aged 16 or older, are victims of stalking in the United States. Nearly 70% of stalking victims knew their offender in some capacity, and approximately one in four victims reported some type of cyberstalking such as email or instant messaging (Office of Justice Programs, Bureau of Justice Statistics, 2021).

Bullying

Bullying is a form of youth violence, and is defined as any "unwanted aggressive behavior(s) by another youth or group of youths who are not siblings or current dating partners that involve an observed or perceived power imbalance" (CDC, 2021f). Bullying is often repeated multiple times or is highly likely to be repeated. Types of bullying include physical threats, hitting, tripping, verbal teasing, spreading rumors, or damage to property of the victim (Box 28.3). The use of technology through email, chat rooms, messaging, cell phones, and even posting videos on social media platforms has contributed to the increase of bullying. Current statistics suggest that 20% of high school students reported being bullied on school property and 17% reported being cyberbullied. Some youth groups experience bullying more than others. For example, an estimated 40% of high school students who identify as LGTBQ experience bullying compared to 22% of heterosexual students. Females are more likely to experience cyberbullying (30%) compared to males (19%). Additionally, 29% of Caucasian students experienced bullying at school compared to 19% of Hispanic and 18% Black or African American students. Bullying can result in physical harm, emotional distress, social isolation, depression, anxiety, poor academic achievement, and self-harm, including suicide (CDC, 2021f).

To address the complex issues of bullying in schools, it has been recommended to develop a school vision and culture that promotes a safe and supportive learning environment. In order to accomplish this, multiple stakeholders must participate in identification and prevention of bullying. These stakeholders should represent the entire school community, including faculty, staff, bus drivers, social workers, students, parents, and their families, so there can be an integrated approach to reduce the incidence of bullying (Karikari & Brown, 2020).

Child Maltreatment

Child maltreatment includes all forms of abuse and neglect of someone under 18 years of age. Children are maltreated more

---

> **BOX 28.3 Bullying**
>
> Bullying includes repeated harmful acts and a real or perceived imbalance of power. Often underreported, bullying creates a climate of fear. Bullying can be physical, verbal, or psychological/relational bullying or cyberbullying.
>
> - Physical bullying involves assault, intimidation, and/or destruction of property.
> - Verbal bullying includes threats and name calling.
> - Psychological/relational bullying can include all of the first two categories and is distinguished by the power imbalance between the victim and the bully.
> - Cyberbullying consists of targeting the victim online.

Modified from Centers of Disease Control and Prevention: *Preventing bullying factsheet* 2021. Available from: https://www.cdc.gov/violenceprevention/pdf/yv/Bullying-factsheet_508_1.pdf.

often by parents, family members, caregivers, clergy, coaches, and teachers. Maltreatment is more commonly seen in families who are under a great deal of stress; are living in poverty or isolation; or when a family member has a history of violence, uses substances, or has a mental illness. Children who increase caregiver burden—for example, children who have a disability (mental impairment, mental illness, and chronic physical illness)—or are under the age of four are at higher risk for being maltreated (CDC, 2021g).

In 2019, one out of seven children in the United States was victim of child abuse and/or neglect, and this is likely an underestimate since many cases go unreported. Aside from physical injuries, consequences of child maltreatment can have a tremendous impact on the victim's lifelong health, increasing their risk for emotional and psychological problems, delayed brain development, lower academic success, substance abuse, future violence victimization, and even death. An estimated 1840 children died of abuse and neglect in 2019 (CDC, 2021g). The fatality rate for boys was slightly higher than that of girls, and children under 3 years of age accounted for 70% of fatalities; almost half (45.4%) of fatalities are younger than 1 year (Children's Bureau, 2019).

The four types of child maltreatment are
- Neglect
- Physical abuse
- Emotional abuse
- Sexual abuse

Although each state is responsible for providing definitions of child abuse and neglect, there is a general consensus of what is included under each category.

Neglect is the failure of the responsible person to provide basic needs such as shelter, food, clothing, education, and access to medical care; permitting the child to use drugs/alcohol; and inattention to the child's emotional needs (Child Welfare Information Gateway, 2019). Failure to provide a nurturing environment for a child to thrive, learn, and develop and to provide for the health needs of a child is also considered neglect. Examples of emotional neglect include failure to cuddle and/or physically stimulate a newborn, failure to give positive feedback, failure to pay attention to the overall emotional needs of a child, and failure to show affection. Poverty and cultural values may contribute to child neglect. Nurses can play a pivotal role in assessing the family's need for information or assistance. In some states abandonment is also considered a form of neglect. This occurs when the parents' identity or whereabouts are unknown, and the child has been left unsupervised and where the child might suffer serious harm.

Physical abuse is intentional physical injury inflicted on a child by another person who has responsibility for the child. Injuries can range from minor bruises to severe fractures or death as a result of beating, kicking, stabbing, choking, burning, biting, throwing, or hitting with a hand, stick, strap, or other object. Spanking or paddling is not considered abuse as long as it does not cause bodily injury to the child. These types of injuries are considered abuse, regardless of whether the caregiver intended to hurt the child (Child Welfare Information Gateway, 2019).

Parents who abuse often have unreasonable expectations of their children and may misinterpret children's behavior as threats to their parental self-esteem and need to control. Patterned injuries may give some clue as to how the child was injured. A child who touches a light cord or light plug might be beaten with it, producing a looped or linear pattern. A child who plays with matches or the stove might have his or her hand placed in the flame. A crying child or a child who talks back might have hot pepper sauce poured into his or her mouth or might be suffocated with a pillow.

Abusive head trauma/inflicted traumatic head injury, also known as *shaken baby syndrome*, is a leading cause of death from abuse in the United States. Most victims are between 2 and 4 months of age. In this form of abuse, violent shaking of the infant causes trauma at the junction of the brainstem and spinal cord that can result in death. Serious and permanent brain damage may occur, with results such as cerebral palsy, seizures, severe retardation, blindness, hearing loss, speech and learning difficulties, problems with memory and attention, and developmental delays. Children with special needs or other medical conditions, including colic or gastroesophageal reflux disease; multiple siblings; and families living in poverty are at greater risk. In most cases of infantile abusive head trauma cases, a male is the perpetrator-biological fathers, stepfathers, and mothers' boyfriends are typically responsible (CDC, Shaken Baby Syndrome).

Emotional abuse, also called *psychological abuse*, is a pattern of behavior that negatively affects a child's self-worth and/or emotional development. This type of abuse may include constant criticism, rejection, and withholding love, affection, and support (Child Welfare Information Gateway, 2019). The child may demonstrate a substantial impairment in behavior, such as being overly compliant or passive, being very aggressive, or being inappropriately adult or infantile. Emotionally abused children frequently do not progress at a normal rate of physical, intellectual, or emotional development. Emotional abuse usually occurs in the home, is not witnessed by others, and is therefore difficult to prove. Impairment in behavior may also occur in children who are not abused; therefore, identification of emotional abuse is difficult.

Sexual abuse involves activities by a parent or caregiver that include fondling a child's genitals, incest, rape, sodomy, exploitation through prostitution, or production of pornographic material (Child Welfare Information Gateway, 2019). The incidence of sexual exploitation of children by Internet pedophiles has increased in recent years. Most research has focused on girls as victims of sexual abuse, but boys are also targets. In such cases, the male victim may refrain from reporting abuse because he is ashamed or because cultural values expect males to be assertive and capable of self-defense.

Child maltreatment can have serious long-term effects. Although physical wounds may heal, the child's ability to cope with life's challenges can be impaired. Childhood trauma may affect the nervous system and development of the immune system, putting the child at a higher risk for health problems as adults. The child may delay reporting the abuse for months or years because it may take that long for him or her to feel safe. Table 28.1 describes physical and behavioral indicators of child abuse and neglect.

All states mandate that healthcare providers and teachers report suspected child abuse. Reporting child abuse may be one of the hardest things a nurse will ever have to do, but may be one of the most rewarding when an abused child is removed from an unsafe and harmful situation.

Elder Abuse

Elder abuse is any form of mistreatment that results in harm or loss to an older person. It occurs in community settings, including private homes, nursing homes, and long-term care facilities. The exact numbers of elders who suffer from abuse and neglect is unknown, however, it is estimated that at least 1 in 10 community dwelling older adults have been victims of abuse (Rosay and Mulford, 2017). Elders may not always report their abuse due to fear of retribution, shame, impaired cognition, or social and physical isolation. Signs of elder abuse may be missed by healthcare professionals due to a lack of awareness and adequate training. Aside from physical injuries, signs of abuse in the elderly may manifest as agitation, withdrawal from activities, lack of self-care, or unusual behaviors often seen in the cognitively impaired adult, including sucking, biting, or rocking (National Center on Elder Abuse [NCEA], 2022). Elders at risk of being abused include those in poor physical or mental health; those dependent on others for physical or financial support; and those who are confused, depressed, or socially isolated. Table 28.2 lists the indicators of possible abuse in older adults.

According to the NCPEA types of abuse and neglect of older adults are categorized as follows:

- Physical abuse (purposeful infliction of physical pain or injury or unnecessary physical or drug-induced restraints).
- Psychological-emotional abuse (verbal assault, threats, provoking fear, or isolation).
- Sexual abuse (unwanted sexual contact or taking pornographic pictures).

TABLE 28.1 Physical and Behavioral Indicators of Child Abuse and Neglect

Physical Indicators	Behavioral Indicators
Physical Abuse	
Unexplained bruises and welts in various stages of healing that may form patterns	Wary of adult contact
Unexplained burns by cigars or cigarettes or immersion burns (e.g., socklike, glovelike, or on buttocks or genitalia)	Apprehensive when other children cry
Burns in the shapes of objects	Constantly on alert
Rope burns	Exhibiting extremes of behavior; aggressive or passive and withdrawn, or overly friendly to strangers
Unexplained lacerations or abrasions	Frightened of parents
Unexplained fractures in various stages of healing; multiple or spiral fractures	Afraid to go home
Unexplained injuries to mouth, lips, gums, eyes, or external genitalia	
Physical and Emotional Neglect	
Hunger	Begging or stealing food
Poor hygiene	Alone at inappropriate times or for prolonged periods
Poor or inappropriate dress	Delinquent behavior
Lack of supervision for prolonged periods	Stealing
Lack of medical or dental care	Arriving early to and departing late from school
Constant fatigue, listlessness, or falling asleep in class	Lack of affection
Sexual Abuse	
Difficulty in walking or sitting	Exhibiting negative self-esteem
Torn, stained, or bloody underwear	Exhibiting inability to trust and function in intimate relationships
Genital pain or itching	Exhibiting cognitive and motor dysfunctions
Bruises in or bleeding from the external genitalia, vaginal, or anal area	Exhibiting deficits in personal and social skills
Sexually transmitted disease	Exhibiting bizarre, sophisticated, or unusual sexual behavior or knowledge
Drug and alcohol abuse	Delinquent or runaway behavior
Developmental delays	Exhibiting suicide ideation
	Reporting sexual assault
	Bed wetting
Emotional Abuse	
Failure to thrive	Exhibiting behavior extremes from passivity to aggression
Lag in physical development	Exhibiting habit and conduct disorders (e.g., antisocial behavior and destructiveness)
Speech disorders	Exhibiting neurotic traits
Developmental delays	Attempting suicide

TABLE 28.2 Indicators of Possible Elder Abuse or Neglect

ABUSE

Physical Indicators	Emotional/Behavioral Indicators
Bruises, black eyes, welts, lacerations, and rope marks	Being emotionally upset or agitated
Bone and skull fractures	Being extremely withdrawn and noncommunicative or nonresponsive
Open wounds, cuts, punctures, untreated injuries in various stages of healing	Unusual behavior usually attributed to dementia (e.g., sucking, biting, rocking)
Sprains, dislocations, and internal injuries/bleeding	Sudden change in behavior
Signs of being subjected to punishment and signs of being restrained	Elder's report of being verbally or emotionally mistreated
Laboratory findings of medication overdose or underutilization of prescribed drugs	
Report of being hit, slapped, kicked, or mistreated	
The caregiver's refusal to allow visitors to see an elder alone	
Unexplained sexually transmitted disease	
Elder's sudden change in behavior	
Elder's report of sexual assault	

Neglect

Physical indicators	Financial indicators (material exploitation)
Dehydration, malnutrition, untreated bedsores, and poor personal hygiene	Sudden changes in bank account or banking practice (e.g., unexplained withdrawal of large sums of money, inclusion of additional names on an elder's bank signature card)
Unattended or untreated health problems	Unauthorized withdrawal of the elder's funds using the elder's automatic teller machine card
Hazardous or unsafe living conditions/arrangements (e.g., improper wiring, no heat, or no running water)	Abrupt changes in a will or other financial documents (e.g., power of attorney)
Unsanitary and unclean living conditions (e.g., dirt, fleas, lice, soiled bedding, fecal/urine smell, inadequate clothing)	Unexplained disappearance of funds or valuables
Elder's report of being mistreated or neglected	Bills unpaid despite the availability of adequate financial resources
Abandonment (desertion of an elder at a hospital, nursing facility, or other similar or public places or institutions)	Elder's signature being forged for financial transactions or for the titles of his or her possessions
	Sudden appearance of previously uninvolved relatives interested in the elder's affairs and possessions
	Unexplained sudden transfer of assets to a family member or someone outside the family
	The provision of services that are not necessary
	Report of financial exploitation

Modified from Administration on Aging/National Center on Elder Abuse: *Types of Abuse*. Available from: https://ncea.acl.gov/Suspect-Abuse/Abuse-Types.aspx.

- Neglect (withholding of personal care, food, or medications; intimidation; humiliation; abandonment). Self-neglect is the failure of the elder who is competent to provide for one's own essential needs.
- Financial exploitation (theft or misuse of money or property).
- Healthcare fraud and abuse (charging for services not delivered or Medicare/Medicaid fraud).

Elder abuse tends to escalate in incidence and severity. When an older adult cannot care for himself or herself because of the physical or mental infirmities of age, what happens to that person may depend on whether relatives can provide care, or whether the person has financial resources to obtain care in his or her own home, a retirement home, or a residential care facility. Caregivers are often adult children or other relatives. The generation of individuals currently in their 40, 50, and 60s is often called the "sandwich generation" because they are caring for their children at the same time they are providing care for their aging parents. As parents age, the role reversal is often painful and demanding for both the elder and the caregiver.

Care of an aging parent requires sacrifice and commitment. As parents age, they may become more physically and cognitively impaired, increasing the likelihood of abuse. Elders who were themselves abusers are more likely to be abused by their caregivers. Older adults may undergo changes in personality that make it difficult for their adult children to care for them. They may need to be lifted, which may be difficult for someone with limited strength. They may need assistance walking, toileting, or eating that requires time the caregiver may not have. There is also an intimacy in caring for a parent that the caregiver may not be comfortable with. All of these factors cause stress, which can be associated with abuse—especially in families in which violence is a response to stress.

The needs of the older adult may exceed the family's ability to meet them. In many ways, helpless older adults are in the same vulnerable position as children because they are dependent on others for care. The population of the United States is aging, and by 2040, the number of adults older than 65 years is expected to climb to 80 million and by 2030, there is an expected 50% increase in the number of elders that will require nursing home care (NCEA, 2022). Recognition of physical and behavioral indicators helps the professional become aware of possible abusive situations. None is conclusive in itself; however, each alerts the professional to the need for careful and complete assessment. Even though nurses are required to report instances of elder abuse, they may be reluctant to do so because assessment is not always conclusive. However, if there is a question of possible abuse, it must be reported to the appropriate authorities for further investigation. In 2008, the state of New York took the lead in passing legislation with its "Granny's Law," which stiffened and increased criminal penalties for assaults on elders.

 ACTIVE LEARNING

Investigate professional responsibilities relative to reporting abuse, neglect, or violence in your state. Share findings with classmates.

COMMUNITY VIOLENCE

The United States is one of the most violent countries in the industrialized world. Every day we hear about some community, region, or state that has been affected by violent crime. Community violence may not affect everyone directly, but it affects all indirectly. In contrast to interpersonal violence, which affects only one or two individuals, community violence usually occurs suddenly and without warning and can potentially destroy entire segments of the population. The health consequences of community violence have become increasingly better understood, demonstrating a concerning and potentially cumulative impact on both physical and mental health conditions. Community violence includes workplace violence, youth violence, gang-related violence, hate crimes, and terrorism as pointed out by the list presented at the beginning of this chapter.

Workplace Violence

Workplace violence is a serious safety and health issue. The Occupational Safety and Health Administration (OSHA) estimates that every year, as many as 2 million Americans report having been victims of workplace violence. Violence in the workplace encompasses acts or threats of violence, including physical assaults such as rape and homicide, muggings, verbal and written threats, and bullying (National Institute for Occupational Safety and Health, 2021). Assaults are currently the fifth leading cause of fatal occupational injuries in the United States, accounting for 20,050 nonfatal work-related injuries in 2020. Unfortunately, this statistic may not accurately reflect the total number of injuries as many are thought to go unreported. In 2020, there were 392 work-related fatalities caused by assaults in the United States, with intentional shooting as the leading cause of work-related homicide (National Safety Council, 2021). Data from 2018 shows that 68% of

women experienced nonfatal workplace violence, but 82% of workplace homicides occurred in men (U.S. Bureau of Labor Statistics, 2018a). Professions prone to experiencing high levels of workplace violence include retail workers, taxi drivers, law enforcement, and nurses.

Examples of risk factors for workplace violence include
- Working in high-crime areas
- Working alone or isolated
- Availability of drugs at the worksite
- Low staffing levels
- Poorly lit parking areas and corridors
- Long waits for service
- Inadequate security
- Increasing numbers of people who use substances
- Access to firearms

Workplace violence has caused specific concern within healthcare and social services. In 2018, healthcare and social service workers were 5 times more likely to experience work-related violence than workers in other sectors, and accounted for 73% of all nonfatal workplace injuries and illnesses resulting in time away from work (U.S. Bureau of Labor Statistics, 2018b). In the healthcare field, frequent areas for the occurrence of violence include emergency departments, psychiatric units, geriatric units, and waiting rooms. Healthcare staff providing patient care is often at risk due to their direct contact with patients and individuals who may exhibit violent behavior.

Beyond injury and death, workplace violence can contribute to low morale, increased job stress and turnover, reduced trust of management and/or coworkers, and hostile work environments. The COVID-19 pandemic has contributed to increased stress levels among the public and is believed to have exacerbated violent incidents in healthcare facilities across the country. In addition to the CDC developing guidance for employers to address workplace violence, protective measures have been introduced through government and accreditation agencies to mitigate and reduce violence in healthcare facilities. In 2021, the US House of Representatives passed the Workplace Violence for Health Care and Social Service Workers Act (HB 1195), supporting OSHA standards that require employers to develop and implement comprehensive workplace violence prevention plans. Additionally, the Joint Commission implemented revised workplace violence prevention requirements to be enacted in all Joint Commission-accredited hospitals in 2022. Nurses must remain aware of the risks they face, and the workplace prevention protocols available to facilitate the safety and well-being of themselves and their patients.

Youth-Related Violence

Violence is taking a toll on American youth. As mentioned, it is the third leading cause of death for young people ages 10 to 24. In 2019, the CDC indicated that 44% of teens experienced violence and that one in seven experienced two or more types of violence (CDC, 2021h). Types of violence most commonly encountered by youth include physical fighting, sexual violence, dating violence, and bullying. Frequent exposure to violence has a cumulative impact on teens' physical and mental health and influence their participation in risky behaviors including tobacco use, binge drinking, sexual activity with multiple partners, and carrying a weapon on school property (CDC, 2021j). Unfortunately, schools are increasingly becoming sites of violent incidents and mass shootings (see Chapter 30 for more information on violence in schools). Directly engaging youth to report and prevent violence is necessary but challenging due to perceived barriers and fears about speaking up.

Youth-related violence occurs across all communities but is more concentrated in minority communities, disproportionately impacting Black or African American youth and young adults. Additionally, sexual minority youth face an increased risk of violence due to stigma and discrimination. The CDC estimates that more than 1000 youth are treated in emergency departments for injuries related to violence, contributing to an estimated annual cost of nearly 21 billion dollars (CDC, 2021h).

Violence among youth is a complicated and multilayered problem influenced by systemic health and social inequities. Adolescents and children exposed to violence are at risk for negative outcomes across the lifespan, thus perpetuating the impact on future generations. Addressing the short- and long-term consequences of youth violence can place significant strain on community resources. Understanding the factors that put youth at risk for experiencing and/or perpetrating violence is key to preventive efforts (Table 28.3). Fostering communities that support healthy family dynamics, quality education, and positive adult relationships with at-risk youth helps promote behavioral changes that can influence protective factors and mitigate violence among youth.

Gangs

Gangs are increasingly responsible for crimes and violence throughout the United States. In the most recent report from 2015, an estimated 1.4 million gang members, representing 33,000 violent street gangs, motorcycle gangs, and prison gangs, are criminally active in the United States and Puerto Rico (FBI, 2017). Gangs are more prevalent in large cities and use violence to control neighborhoods and increase their illegal money-making activities, which include robbery, fraud, drug and gun trafficking, prostitution, and human trafficking. To address this national problem the National Gang Intelligence Center (NGIC) was established in 2005 (FBI, 2017a).

Between 2013 and 2015, the use of social media among gangs increased, providing a platform for increased recruitment and communication (NGIC, 2015). Consequently, young people are at increased risk of exposure to gangs, with the most common age for recruitment being 15 years old. Reasons that young people give for joining gangs include the belief that gangs will provide protection, a sense of belonging, and opportunities to earn money. Unfortunately, youth involved in gangs are less likely to graduate high school, obtain employment, and abstain from drug and alcohol. Additionally, gang-involvement increases the likelihood of committing crimes, being arrested and incarcerated, as well as being a victim of violence (National Gang Center, 2015).

TABLE 28.3 Risk Factors for Youth-Related Violence

Individual risk factors	History of violent victimization
	Attention deficits, hyperactivity, or learning disorders
	History of early aggressive behavior
	Involvement with drugs, alcohol, or tobacco
	Low IQ
	Poor behavioral control
	Deficits in social cognitive or information-processing abilities
	High emotional distress
	History of treatment for emotional problems
	Antisocial beliefs and attitudes
	Exposure to violence and conflict in the family
Family risk factors	Authoritarian childrearing attitudes
	Harsh, lax, or inconsistent disciplinary practices
	Low parental involvement
	Low emotional attachment to parents or caregivers
	Low parental education and income
	Parental substance abuse or criminality
	Poor family functioning
	Poor monitoring and supervision of children
Peer and social risk factors	Association with delinquent peers
	Involvement in gangs
	Social rejection by peers
	Lack of involvement in conventional activities
	Poor academic performance
	Low commitment to school and school failure
Community risk factors	Diminished economic opportunities
	High concentrations of poor residents
	High level of transiency
	High level of family disruption
	Low levels of community participation
	Socially disorganized neighborhoods

Data from Centers for Disease Control and Prevention, National Center for Injury Prevention and Control, Division of Violence Prevention: *youth violence: risk and protective factors*, 2020. www.cdc.gov/ViolencePrevention/youthviolence/riskprotectivefactors.html.

Prison Violence

The United States has one of the world's highest incarceration rates. At the end of 2019, an estimated 634,400 persons were supervised by the US adult correctional systems (U.S. Department of Justice [DOJ], 2021). This number includes persons either incarcerated, on parole, or on probation within federal and state prisons, jails, and community corrections facilities. Compared with 2019, state and federal imprison rates for 2020 decreased by 15%. The COVID-19 pandemic is attributed to the decline, resulting from court closures, delays in trials and sentencing, and expedited releases.

Demographics within the US correctional system are diverse. In 2020, the ethnicity of prisoners under state or federal correctional authority was approximately 30% Caucasian, 33% Black or African American, and 23% Hispanic with the remaining percentages including persons of American Indian, Alaska Native, Asian, or of two or more races. Additionally, women accounted for nearly 7% (79,515 prisoners) of the sentenced federal and state prison population. The prison population is relatively young, as only about 14% were aged 55 or older and 3.5% were aged 65 or older. State prisons had jurisdiction over 352 prisoners aged 17 or younger in 2020 (U.S. DOJ, 2021).

Nearly 60% of prisoners are serving time for violent offenses including murder, manslaughter, rape/sexual assault, robbery, and aggravated assault (U.S. DOJ, 2021). Unfortunately, these same types of violence also occur within prison walls among prisoners or between inmates and prison staff. The public and the judicial system have expressed little sympathy for this population for a variety of reasons, including indifference, disbelief, and denial. Little research exists to reflect the long-term effects on these victims or on society when they are released. See Chapter 32 for more information on forensic and correctional nursing.

Human Trafficking

Human trafficking is a global problem and public health issue both domestically and internationally. It is considered a modern-day form of slavery involving the illegal trade of people for exploitation. Human trafficking is the fastest growing criminal activity in the world. Threats, the use of force, coercion, abduction, fraud, and abuse of power are all methods used by human traffickers to obtain some type of labor or commercial sex act. Adult women represent approximately half of all detected global trafficking victims, while one in every three victims is a child (United Nations Office on Drugs and Crimes [UNODC], 2021). Victims are lured into trafficking through a variety of means including abduction, deceptive job advertisements, false promises of financial or personal gain, or direct threats. While nonviolent deception is the most common method of recruiting victims, traffickers use explicit violence or control to exploit and maintain their victims (UNODC, 2021). Every year, millions of men, women, and children are trafficked in countries around the world, including the United States. It is estimated that human trafficking generates billions of dollars in profit per year, second only to drug trafficking as the most profitable form of transnational crime. Human trafficking is a hidden crime, as victims rarely come forward to seek help because of language barriers, fear of the traffickers, and/or fear of law enforcement. Extreme poverty is a significant risk factor for trafficking because victims are often targeted based on their vulnerability. The economic recession and unemployment stemming from the COVID-19 pandemic is likely to increase the incidence of trafficking. An estimated 46% of victims in low-income countries are children, so there is global concern that traffickers will seek out opportunities to exploit children for forced labor, sexual exploitation, or forced criminality (UNODC, 2021).

Healthcare providers are in a unique position to identify victims of trafficking and provide important physical and psychosocial care. Common health problems among trafficking victims include anxiety, depression, PTSD, substance abuse disorders, headaches, back or stomach pain, dental pain, and sexually transmitted infections including HIV (Ottisova

et al., 2016). There are a number of barriers that can prevent victims from disclosing even to healthcare professionals. Because many victims are undocumented, they may be afraid that they will be deported. If the victim is a minor, the provider has a legal responsibility to phone CPSs. Organized criminal groups are heavily involved in sex trafficking, often for longer durations and using more violence, so victims may not speak up due to fear that harm will be inflicted on themselves or their families (UNODC, 2021). Despite these potential barriers, it is important for nurses to become knowledgeable about this population in order to effectively respond if they do come in contact with a victim who is seeking healthcare.

Hate Crimes

Hate crimes are crimes in which the offender is motivated by factors such as an individual's race, sexual orientation, religious beliefs, ethnic background, or national origin. Hate crimes may include murder, sexual or physical assault, harassment, attacks on homes or on places of worship, or vandalism. Because hate crimes attack an individual's identity, the emotional effects are compounded. It is estimated that only 44% of hate crimes are reported. In 2020, over 8000 hate crimes were reported in the United States, with over 60% of these crimes being motivated by race, ethnicity, or ancestry (U.S. DOJ, 2020).

Terrorism

Terrorism has been present throughout history. The Department of Defense (2021) defines terrorism as "the unlawful use of violence or threat of violence, often motivated by religious, political, or other ideological beliefs, to instill fear and coerce individuals, governments or societies in pursuit of terrorist goals." All terrorist acts include at least three key elements: violence, fear, and intimidation. Nurses need to be prepared for terrorism in whatever form it takes, from an explosion at a local refinery to an act that affects an entire region or country, such as biological, chemical, or nuclear incidents. Mental and physical health issues remain a nursing concern for the victims, responders, and the community long after the act has occurred. See Chapter 29 for a more detailed discussion of terrorism.

FACTORS INFLUENCING VIOLENCE

Controversy surrounds the factors that influence violence in today's society. Three of them are easy access to firearms, the impact of media, and mental illness. These will be discussed briefly.

Firearms

An estimated 393 million privately owned firearms exist in the United States (Karp, 2018). According to the 2021 National Firearms Survey, the overall rate of adult firearm ownership in the United States is 31.9%, suggesting that over 81 million Americans own a gun (English, 2021). The United States ranks number one in privately owned guns worldwide, with statistics indicating firearms as the weapon of choice in homicides. Of the estimated 16,425 murders in the United States in 2019,

73.7% were committed with firearms (Federal Bureau of Investigation [FBI], 2020).

The cost of gun violence is staggering, with direct costs of gun violence related to firearms in the United States estimated at $8.6 billion dollars annually (Follman et al., 2015). Indirect costs, including loss of productivity, mental health treatment, rehabilitation, and legal and judicial costs, add even more.

Despite the majority of gun owners (56.2%) indicating self-defense as the reason for carrying a handgun, laws surrounding gun control are a highly politicized and contentious issue (English, 2021). Research findings are conflicting about whether gun control laws reduce violent crime (Fridel, 2021; McCourt et al., 2020; Kleck et al., 2016). Regardless of the controversial aspects of gun ownership, prevention of firearms-related injury and death is an important public health topic. Therefore, it is important for healthcare professionals to be comfortable speaking with their patients in a nonjudgmental manner about firearms. Nurses are in a prime position to provide patients with factual information about firearms relevant to their health and the health of those around them, fully answer their questions, and advise them on firearms safety.

Media

Media violence is prevalent and is accessible to all age groups. It includes exposure to and participation in violent video games, music and music videos that depict rape or violence, and virtual violence that allows subscribers to harm or kill victims. Television and movies often depict people being tortured or killed in such graphic detail that may make it hard for children and adults to distinguish between reality and fantasy. Media violence has become more pronounced and graphic in nature. The role of social media has raised significant concern in regard to youth violence in particular. Cyberbullying, harassment, dating aggression, and self-harm are recognized as common actions of violence facilitated through social media platforms (Patton et al., 2014). There is concern in the public health community that repeated exposure to media violence leads to emotional desensitization to real-life violence.

Mental Illness

A general consensus exists that severe mental illness (SMI) increases the risk of violence. The media's portrayal of people with mental illness committing violence adds to the belief that a great deal of violence is committed by people with SMI. However, there is little population-level evidence that supports the notion that individuals diagnosed with mental illness are more likely than anyone else to commit gun crimes. The connections between mental illness and gun violence are less causal and more complex than current US public opinion and legislative action allow. It is undeniable that persons who have shown violent tendencies should not have access to weapons that could be used to harm themselves or others. However, notions that mental illness causes increased propensity for violence or that advanced psychiatric attention might prevent these crimes are more complicated than they often seem (Swanson, 2021).

The conundrum of mass-casualty shootings in relation to mental illness have been compared to a "Rubik's cube," illustrating the complexity behind why these tragic events take place (Metzl et al., 2020). In 2021, the United States set a record with 693 mass shootings (incidents killing at least four victims), the most in a single year (Gun Violence Archive, 2022). Catastrophic incidents, particularly school-related shootings at Sandy Hook Elementary (Connecticut in 2012), Santa Fe High School (Texas in 2018), and Oxford High School (Michigan in 2021) have brought to light the need for improved gun safety. Consequently, there has been an increased push for legislation to fund public health strategies that identify and treat mental illness across the country. This is especially important because the budget crisis in the United States has forced many states to eliminate or reduce the availability of mental health services. See Chapter 25 for a more in-depth discussion of mental illness.

ACTIVE LEARNING

1. Call a child abuse center in the community and ask what services they provide.
2. Call a battered women's shelter and determine the procedure for securing shelter placement for a battered victim and her children.
3. Visit a long-term care facility for the elderly and observe the clients and the activities that are provided. Observe behaviors that would contribute to stress in the caregiver.
4. Find out what support groups exist in the community for older adult caregivers.
5. Read your local newspaper for 1 month and clip articles that deal with violence and gun control. Determine how many individuals were killed or injured during that period. How many of the deaths and injuries were gun related?
6. Look up the laws that relate to the reporting of child and elder abuse in your area.

VIOLENCE FROM A PUBLIC HEALTH PERSPECTIVE

Dealing with violence has traditionally been the US criminal justice system's responsibility. However, because violence is also a public health epidemic, efforts are being made to prevent and manage it using public health strategies and community approaches such as church groups, community groups, and local, state, and federal governments. Violence, as discussed previously, has a tremendous influence on morbidity and mortality rates and healthcare resources. The public health system is challenged to go beyond its traditional programs to include prevention and management of violence. As is true with most public health problems, many interrelated factors must be addressed.

Healthy People 2030 and Violence

Violence has been a consistent area of focus since Healthy People 2000, and remains one of the topics addressed by *Healthy People 2030*. Several of the current objectives regarding violence in *Healthy People 2030* can be found in the Healthy People box. These objectives are intended to target causes of violence and abuse, improve national data collection and analysis, provide input for legislative funding, facilitate research efforts, and concentrate public health efforts on models that demonstrate effectiveness.

Many of the *Healthy People 2030* objectives are difficult to achieve because of complex barriers. These include a lack of comparable data sources and standardized definitions, as well as inadequate resources to establish consistent tracking systems and fund prevention programs. Several of the *Healthy People 2030* objectives regarding violence prevention are considered developmental and represent high-priority public health interventions in need of reliable baseline data prior to being determined core objectives. Of the 20 objectives for 2030, half are specifically aimed at reducing violence in children and adolescents.

♥ HEALTHY PEOPLE 2030

Objectives Related to Violence Prevention

Core Objectives

IVP-09: Reduce homicides

IVP-10: Reduce nonfatal physical assault injuries

IVP-11: Reduce physical fighting among adolescents

IVP-12: Reduce gun carrying among adolescents

IVP-13: Reduce firearm-related deaths

IVP-14: Reduce nonfatal firearm-related injuries

IVP-15: Reduce child abuse and neglect deaths

IVP-16: Reduce nonfatal child abuse and neglect

IVP-17: Reduce adolescent sexual violence by anyone

IVP-18: Reduce sexual or physical adolescent dating violence

IVP-19: Reduce emergency department visits for nonfatal intentional self-harm injuries

AH-10: Reduce the rate of minors and young adults committing violent crimes

OSH-05: Reduce work-related assaults

Developmental Objectives

IVP-D01: Increase the number of states where a child fatality team reviews external causes of death in children

IVP-D02: Increase the number of states where a child fatality team reviews sudden and unexpected deaths in infants

IVP-D03: Reduce the number of young adults who report three or more adverse childhood experiences

IVP-D04: Reduce intimate partner violence

IVP-D05: Reduce contact sexual violence

AH-D03: Reduce the proportion of public schools with a serious violent incident

Research Objectives

AH-R11: Reduce the rate of adolescent and young adult victimization from violent crimes

Data from HealthyPeople.gov: *Healthy People 2030: objectives and data: violence prevention.* Available from: https://health.gov/healthypeople/objectives-and-data/browse-objectives/violence-prevention. (Accessed 9 January 2022).

PREVENTION OF VIOLENCE

The nurse who cares for people experiencing violence must be a skilled clinician who is knowledgeable about both the problem and available community resources. Box 28.4 presents tips regarding safety issues for a community health nurse. A considerable body of knowledge has been developed about

BOX 28.4 Safety Issues for the Community Health Nurse

Plan Ahead
- Know the area you are visiting.
- Schedule the visit ahead of time and get the correct address, directions, and information about who will be in the home.
- Tell the office where you will be and check in regularly.
- Carry a cell phone, possibly a pager, and a small amount of money.
- Dress for function and mobility and wear a name tag. Avoid any provocative clothing.
- Ensure that the vehicle you drive is in good repair, has a full gas tank, and has emergency equipment. Always carry two sets of car keys.
- Choose a parking spot that is in the open and near a light if you are there when it is dark.
- Have all personal protective equipment (PPE) available to protect against infectious agents.

Approaching the Home
- Notice the environment, animals, fences, activity, possible indicators of crime, and places you could go for assistance if necessary.
- Walk with confidence and maintain a professional attitude.
- Listen for signs of fighting before knocking. If you hear sounds of fighting, leave!
- Do not enter a home if you suspect an unsafe situation.

In the Home
- Be aware of who is in the home and what is going on. If angry people are in the home, use your professional and social skills. Do not expect the client to protect you.
- Sufficient lighting must be available in order to do your work safely.
- Ensure there is no smoking near anyone using oxygen.
- Note the exits and sit between the client and an exit of the home. Be prepared to leave quickly if the situation changes suddenly.

Handling a Tight Situation
- Do not show fear; control your breathing.
- Speak calmly and in a soothing manner. Be assertive but not aggressive.
- Remind the person that you are there to help, meanwhile planning an escape route.
- If you feel afraid of being harmed, leave the home and call the case manager or local office from a safe place nearby. If you are in immediate danger, call 911.

Leaving the Home
- Take all of your belongings and keep your car keys in your hand.
- Watch for cars following you when you leave. Do not stop. If you feel that you are in danger, go to the nearest police station or well-lighted business and ask for help.
- Trust your instincts. Never forget your own safety.

Modified from Oregon Home Care Commission, Oregon Department of Human Services: *Safety manual for homecare workers and personal support workers,* February 2012.

trends in violence. Table 28.4 provides the components of a comprehensive program to reduce violence in individuals and the community.

Primary Prevention

The goal of primary prevention is to stop violence, abuse, or neglect before it occurs. Education plays a major part in

TABLE 28.4 Examples of Prevention Strategies to Reduce Violence for Individuals and Communities

Individuals	Community
Primary Prevention—Goal: Promotion of Optimal Parenting and Family Wellness	
Life-skills training in schools, churches, and communities	Community education concerning violence
Education of children, adolescents, and adults on methods of conflict resolution	Reduction of media violence
Parenting classes in hospitals, schools, and other community agencies	Development of community support services such as crisis lines, respite care for families with dependent members, shelters for battered women and their children, and development and vigorous enforcement of anti-stalking measures, including cyberstalking
Mental health services for all age groups	
Training for professionals in early detection of violence	Handgun safety education
Secondary Prevention—Goal: Diagnosis of and Service for Families in Stress	
Nursing assessment for evidence of violence in all healthcare settings	Education of all health professionals in assessment of violence and possible protocols for dealing with victims
A safety plan for victims	List of hospital emergency departments and trauma centers with 24-h response
Knowledge of legal options	
Shelter referral for victims	Reporting of different types of abuse
Social services for individuals or families	Coordination with medical authorities
Referral to self-help groups in the community	Coordination with voluntary and social service agencies for provision of services
Referral to appropriate community agencies	Death review teams to review deaths from injury, especially in infants and children
	Public authority involvement by police, district attorneys, and courts
	Epidemiological tracking and evaluation of violence
Tertiary Prevention—Goal: Reeducation and Rehabilitation of Violent Families	
Empowerment strategies for battered women	Foster homes, shelters, and care for dependents
Professional counseling services for individuals	Public authority involvement
Parenting reeducation (i.e., formal training in child rearing)	Follow-up care for known cases of abuse, neglect, or violence
Counseling services for individuals and families	
Self-help groups	

primary prevention and may include life-skills training such as parenting and family wellness, anger management, and/or conflict resolution. Professionals should increase their awareness of violence and identification of cases. The nurse can work in or with the community to educate citizens about the problem of violence, potential causes of violence, and available community services.

Primary prevention must begin at a community level, helping change attitudes about abuse and violence. Primary prevention focuses on stopping the transgenerational aspect of abuse, starting with young children and continuing throughout the life span. Mentoring and peer programs can be designed to promote healthy relationships and decrease conflict. For example, parenting is one of the most difficult jobs that individuals will undertake, yet there is a widespread myth that parenting "comes naturally." Classes for parents should focus on physical care of the infant, including ways to soothe and manage a "fussy" baby, the effect of fatigue on new parents, the need for support, and the fears and questions of new parents. Nurses in the hospital have little time to help new parents learn basic newborn care before discharge. Some hospitals and public health agencies provide follow-up to parents to ensure that they can adequately care for their newborn. This support is especially given to all persons deemed to be high risk for infant abuse, including teenage mothers, mothers without support, or women with a history of spousal abuse.

Secondary Prevention

The goal of secondary prevention is to assess, diagnose, and treat victims and perpetrators of violence. Consideration of the safety of the potential victim is critical.

Secondary prevention begins with assessment. For example, consistent assessment of women during healthcare visits will increase case finding and provide opportunities for early intervention that is particularly crucial during pregnancy. Women should be interviewed in private when asked about abuse. Questions should be asked in a matter-of-fact way, and the healthcare provider should not show shock or dismay at the response.

Victims, once identified, must be offered resources to increase their safety. However, all victims may not be ready or able to leave the situation, and available options must be explored. Victims should have knowledge of legal options and how to access them. The nurse must be ready to intervene when the abuse involves a child or someone who is cognitively impaired. Some states have developed protocols for nurses who deal with victims of violence. Review of these protocols can help the nurse become familiar with the questions to ask and suggestions that should be made to help the victim develop a safety plan.

Another example of secondary prevention involves screening for abuse in the elderly that should occur at every healthcare visit. Elder abuse remains underreported across the United States; therefore, routine screening can facilitate early intervention. Nurses can help raise professional and community consciousness of elder abuse by participating in political activities to create or strengthen mandatory reporting laws and funding of support groups.

The nurse should work with family members or caregivers who provide care for the elderly to promote healthier relationships. Helping the caregiver deal with stress by finding respite care, a home health aide, or counseling may help. Documentation is crucial in meeting medical-legal requirements. The nurse should record observations accurately and refrain from opinions and interpretations because this documentation may be used in court proceedings.

The problem of violence cannot be managed by nurses alone, but rather in combination with other professionals, including physicians, child and adult protective services providers, social workers, clergy, and police. This interdisciplinary approach leads to optimal outcomes. Public health surveillance is important in obtaining accurate numbers of intentional injuries for individuals. Death review teams can analyze records to determine whether an injury was intentional or unintentional.

Tertiary Prevention

Tertiary prevention is aimed at rehabilitation of individuals, families, groups, or communities and includes both victims and perpetrators of violence. Rehabilitation may take months or even years, depending on the situation. For example, the September 11, 2001, attack on the United States disrupted thousands of lives and changed the country's sense of security. This attack affected everyone in the country, not just those in the immediate vicinity. After all these years, the effects continue. The nurse must be able to work in conjunction with a variety of mental health professionals and social service agencies to provide coordinated care. The nurse may have also been a victim and may be experiencing many of the same problems as those he or she is trying to help. Self-care and recognition of the nurse's own limitations or needs are critical.

❓ ACTIVE LEARNING

Using the telephone directory or computer search engine, find three public or private agencies in the community that provide help for victims of violence. Make a list of the telephone numbers and postcopies of it in public areas.

Case Study Application of the Nursing Process

Intimate Partner Violence

Karen, 36 years old, comes to the neighborhood clinic where you are the nurse. She is obviously distraught and is holding her head down when she enters the exam room. As you are getting her vital signs, she lifts her head and you notice multiple bruises on her face, around her left eye, and on her left cheek and the right side of her neck. She sees you looking at her and she begins to cry. You ask her what happened and she tells you that her boyfriend hit her two nights ago. As you question her further, you find out that she is divorced, has custody of her two children, a boy aged 8 and a daughter aged 3, and is unemployed. Her ex-husband lives three states away, about an 8-h drive. She has been with the current boyfriend about 6 months and they have been living together about 3 months. He hit her repeatedly the night before last after he came home upset about a problem at work. The attack ended as abruptly as it started. He apologized repeatedly, hugged her, and left the house. Her children were in bed and did not witness the abuse. She took the children to a friend's house and then went to an after-hours clinic for treatment. While she was at the after-hours clinic, the police were notified, and she pressed charges against her boyfriend. He was arrested later that night and she subsequently filed a restraining order against him.

After further discussion, she tells you that this is not the first time he has hit her; that it has happened twice before, always after something has upset him. She then states that she knows he loves her and that he would not deliberately hurt her—that she must have done something to make him angry. She feels that he does really love her and she regrets having him arrested and filing the restraining order. She felt as if she had no choice once the clinic personnel and the police urged her to do something. He is now in the county jail, and she is considering going to the police station and dropping the charges. She does admit, however, that she is afraid about how angry he is going to be once he gets out.

You tell her about the cycle of domestic violence and how it repeats itself. You give her information about local shelters and explain that abusers usually do not stop their cycle of violence on their own, but only after counseling and support.

You also tell her that she may be in danger of serious harm and even death if she stays with him. You recommend that she leave where she is living, take her children with her, and talk with an attorney before doing anything about the legal situation.

One month later, Karen again appears in your clinic. She tells you that she did leave home and take her two children to her ex-husband's house. She also states that the boyfriend is still in county jail, that she did not drop the restraining order, and that she has moved in with her boyfriend's mother. She visits him every Sunday afternoon and talks to him once a week on the phone. His mother refuses to speak with him.

Assessment
The following are the summary assessment points:
- The boyfriend has a history of IPV—duration unknown.
- Karen is a stay-at-home mom, with two children under the age of 9 years, who currently live with their father in another state.
- Karen does not have close family in the area.
- Karen does not believe that she is in danger.
- Karen believes she lacks employable skills.
- The boyfriend's abuse is aggravated by problems at work.

Diagnoses
- Potential for severe injury or death related to abuse
- High risk for emotional trauma from dysfunctional family dynamics
- High risk for loss of children

Planning
Short-Term Goals
- Boyfriend will be referred for anger management classes once released.
- Strategies will be identified to help Karen regain her children.
- A safe setting will be identified for Karen and the children.

Case Study Application of the Nursing Process—cont'd

Long-Term Goals
- Karen will be free of IPV.
- Karen will enter individual counseling.
- Boyfriend will enter counseling.

Intervention
Individual

Karen was assessed for injuries, and none were found to be life threatening. She was given a referral for counseling at the local counseling center where a community health nurse works. She was also given locations and numbers for local shelters. She did leave the charges against her boyfriend standing and decided not to drop the restraining order.

Karen agreed to enter counseling and continues to live with her boyfriend's mother until other arrangements can be made. She decided to leave her children at her ex-husband's house until she feels more secure about her situation. Karen has spoken with the community health nurse at the local counseling center. The nurse's goals are centered on Karen's ongoing physical and emotional well-being.

During these visits the nurse was able to engage Karen in conversation regarding her future and that of her children. Karen indicated that this most recent episode of violence had frightened her and caused her to question the wisdom of her decision to stay with her boyfriend. Her boyfriend was found guilty of domestic abuse and was released after 2 months with a probation period of 2 years and mandatory anger management classes. She and her ex-husband are discussing child care arrangements and the possibility of her moving closer to him where she should be able to find work.

Community

The community health nurse arranged to speak at the monthly breakfast meeting of community pastors where she presented an informational program on IPV. Within 3 weeks she received speaking invitations from four of the nine churches represented at the meeting. The first of the programs will take place in the next month. In two of the churches, "mother's day out" (a partial day of babysitting) services are available to church members, and after an appeal from the community health nurse, one of the churches has expressed a willingness to open its program to nonchurch members.

Evaluation
Individual and Community

You and the community health nurses jointly focused on safety as a priority of care for Karen. The visit to the after-hours clinic and the medical personnel's call to the police started the chain of events. Karen's injuries created an opportunity for the community health nurse to maintain contact and provide psychosocial support. During visits the nurse was able to speak openly with Karen and offer options to enhance her coping skills. One of the local pastors has encouraged Karen to focus on both her children and her own future.

Karen came back into the clinic where you are working and seems healthier. She states that she is going to move to the same area where her ex-husband is living and will be reconciled with her children. Karen also says that her ex-husband agreed to help her find employment in the area. Her boyfriend continues to fulfill the requirements of his probation, and he acknowledges that this will be an ongoing recovery process.

Levels of Prevention
Primary

Goal: Promote safety and prevent violence.
- Encourage contact with friends in the neighborhood and at church.
- Provide services of the community health nurse.
- Provide community education programs about anger management.
- Provide community education programs about IPV.

Secondary

Goal: Assess for signs of IPV.
- Facilitate healthcare for treatment of injuries.
- Provide both physical and psychosocial support.
- Provide referral for anger management.
- Provide individual and family counseling.
- Provide a 24-h abuse hotline number.

Tertiary

Goal: Promote development of healthy family dynamics.
- Encourage continued use of community resources.
- Encourage community involvement with other young families.
- Provide community education programs on the cycle of violence.

SUMMARY

Violence is a major public health issue in the United States and affects individuals across the life cycle. Morbidity and mortality statistics indicate that violence is epidemic in many communities. Whether it occurs at home, in the neighborhood, or at school, violence affects countless numbers of individuals. The influence of media, easy access to and proliferation of firearms, and mental illness in the United States are considered contributing factors to violence. The cycle of violence will persist if not broken. The abuser is also a victim, and the ultimate victim is society, which must care and pay for the results of violent acts.

There is a wealth of resources that nurses can use to broaden their knowledge of the different types of violence and address best practices for preventing, detecting, and intervening in a timely way. For example, there are free online video training resources for health providers dealing with screening for IPV and effective communication strategies that promote therapeutic conversations with women who experience IPV (Health Cares About IPV, 2018). Several elder abuse screening tools are available from the NCEA (2022) website. Screening tools for human trafficking, including guidelines and victim identification, are available on the Vera Institute of Justice website (2014). The National Domestic Violence Safety Hotline (https://www.thehotline.org/) has excellent resources that nurses can use to help women develop safety plans and legal information that can be discussed with women.

Violence is a public health epidemic, and national objectives for reducing it have been identified. The core public health functions of needs assessment and surveillance, policy development, and assurance are useful methods of combating this epidemic. The literature describes interventions that focus on the three levels of prevention. The need for continued research in violence should be a funding priority at the local, state, and national levels. The reality of violence has been validated. Everyone is affected.

EVOLVE WEBSITE

http://evolve.elsevier.com/Nies/community
- NCLEX Review Questions
- Case Studies

BIBLIOGRAPHY

American Foundation for Suicide Prevention: *Suicide statistics*, 2021. Available from: https://afsp.org/suicide-statistics/.

Centers for Disease Control and Prevention: *Assault or homicide [Fact Sheet]*, 2021a. Available from: https://www.cdc.gov/nchs/fastats/homicide.htm.

Centers for Disease Control and Prevention: *Preventing elder abuse [Fact Sheet]*, 2021b. Available from: https://www.cdc.gov/violenceprevention/elderabuse/fastfact.html.

Centers for Disease Control and Prevention: *Facts about suicide*, 2021c. Available from: https://www.cdc.gov/suicide/facts/index.html.

Centers for Disease Control and Prevention: *Preventing intimate partner violence [Fact Sheet]*, 2021d. Available from: https://www.cdc.gov/violenceprevention/intimatepartnerviolence/fastfact.html.

Centers for Disease Control and Prevention: *Preventing teen dating violence*, 2021e.

Centers for Disease Control and Prevention: *Preventing bullying [Fact Sheet]*, 2021f. Available from: https://www.cdc.gov/violenceprevention/youthviolence/bullyingresearch/fastfact.html.

Centers for Disease Control and Prevention: *Preventing child abuse and neglect*, 2021g. Available from: https://www.cdc.gov/violenceprevention/childabuseandneglect/fastfact.html.

Centers for Disease Control and Prevention: *CDC vitalsigns: violence impacts teens' lives*, 2021h. Available from: https://www.cdc.gov/injury/pdfs/features/teen-violence-impact/VS_Violence_Impacts_Teens_Lives-508.pdf.

Centers for Disease Control and Prevention: *Preventing youth violence*, 2021j. Available from: https://www.cdc.gov/violenceprevention/pdf/yv/YV-factsheet.pdf.

Child Welfare Information Gateway: *What is child abuse and neglect? Recognizing the signs and symptoms*, 2019. Available from: https://www.childwelfare.gov/pubPDFs/whatiscan.pdf.

Children's Bureau: *Administration on Children, Youth and Families, Administration for Children and Families of the U.S. Department of Health and Human Services*, 2019. Child maltreatment 2019, Available from: https://www.acf.hhs.gov/sites/default/files/documents/cb/cm2019.pdf.

Department of Defense: *DOD dictionary of military and associated terms*, 2021. Available from: https://www.jcs.mil/Portals/36/Documents/Doctrine/pubs/dictionary.pdf.

Domestic Abuse Intervention Program: *Wheel gallery*, 2011. Available from: http://www.theduluthmodel.org/index.htm.

English W: *2021 National firearms survey*, 2021, SSRN. Available from: https://ssrn.com/abstract=3887145.

Federal Bureau of Investigation (FBI): What we investigate: Gangs. 2017. Available from: https://www.fbi.gov/investigate/violent-crime/gangs

Federal Bureau of Investigation: *Crime in the United States, 2019: Murder*, 2020. Available from: https://ucr.fbi.gov/crime-in-the-u.s/2019/crime-in-the-u.s.-2019/topic-pages/murder.pdf.

Follman M, Lurie J, Lee J, West J: *The true cost of gun violence in America*, 2015. Available from: https://www.motherjones.com/politics/2015/04/true-cost-of-gun-violence-in-america/.

Fridel E: Comparing the impact of household gun ownership and concealed carry legislation on the frequency of mass shootings and firearms homicide, *Justice Q* 38(5), 2021. Available from: https://doi.org/10.1080/07418825.2020.1789693.

Gun Violence Archive: *Gun violence archive 2021*, 2022. Available from: https://www.gunviolencearchive.org/past-tolls.

Health Cares About IPV: *Intimate partner violence screening and counseling toolkit*, 2018. Available from: http://www.healthcaresaboutipv.org/getting-started/training-resources/.

HealthyPeople.gov: *Healthy people 2030: Violence prevention*. Available from: https://health.gov/healthypeople/objectives-and-data/browse-objectives/violence-prevention. Accessed January 9, 2022.

Heron, M: Deaths: leading causes for 2019, *National vital statistics reports* (70):9, 2021. Available from: https://www.cdc.gov/nchs/data/nvsr/nvsr70/nvsr70-09-508.pdf.

Holmes K: Shining Another Light on Spousal Rape Exemptions: Spousal Sexual Violence Laws in the #MeToo Era. *UC Irvine Law Review*, 11(4), 2021. Available from https://scholarship.law.uci.edu/ucilr/vol11/iss4/11/.

Karikari I, Brown JR, Ashirifi GD, Storms J: Bullying prevention in schools, *Adv Soc Work* 20(1):61—81, 2020. Available from: https://doi.org/10.18060/22928.

Karp A: Estimating global civilian-held firearms numbers, *Small Arms Survey*, 2018. Available from: https://www.smallarmssurvey.org/sites/default/files/resources/SAS-BP-Civilian-Firearms-Numbers.pdf.

Kleck G, Kovandzic T, Bellows J: Does gun control reduce violent crime? *Crim Justice Rev* 41(4):488—513, 2016. Available from: https://doi.org/10.1177/0734016816670457.

March of Dimes: *Abuse during pregnancy, n.d.* Available from: https://www.marchofdimes.org/pregnancy/abuse-during-pregnancy.aspx#.

McCourt AD, Crifasi CK, Stuart EA, Vernick JS, Kagawa RMC, Wintemute GJ, Webster DW: Purchaser licensing, point-of-sale background check laws, and firearm homicide and suicide in 4 US states, 1985—2017, *Am J Publ Health* 110(10):1546—1552, 2020. Available from: https://doi.org/10.2105/AJPH.2020.305822.

Metzl JM, Piemonte J, McKay T: Mental illness, mass shootings, and the future of psychiatric research into American gun violence, *Harv Rev Psychiatr* 29:81—89, 2020. Available from: https://doi.org/10.1097/HRP.0000000000000281.

Mother Goose Nursery Rhymes: Bath, England, 2000, Robert Frederick Publishing.

Myers JEB: A short history of child protection in America, *Fam Law Q* 42(3):449—463, 2008.

National Center on Elder Abuse: *Research, Statistics and Data*, 2022. Available from: https://ncea.acl.gov/What-We-Do/Research/Statistics-and-Data.aspx#signs.

National Gang Center: *Parents' guide to gangs*, 2015. Available from: https://nationalgangcenter.ojp.gov/sites/g/files/xyckuh331/files/media/document/Parents-Guide-to-Gangs.pdf https://nationalgangcenter.ojp.gov/sites/g/files/xyckuh331/files/media/document/Parents-Guide-to-Gangs.pdf.

National Gang Intelligence Center: 2015 National gang report (NGIC, 2015). Available from: https://www.fbi.gov/file-repository/stats-services-publications-national-gang-report-2015.pdf/view.

National Institute for Occupational Safety and Health: *Occupational Violence*, 2021. Available from: https://www.cdc.gov/niosh/topics/violence/.

National Safety Council: *Assault fourth leading cause of workplace deaths*, 2021. Available from: https://www.nsc.org/workplace/safety-topics/workplace-violence.

Office of Justice Programs, Bureau of justice statistics, *Correctional populations in the United States*, 2015. Available from https://www.bjs.gov/index.cfm?ty=pbdetail&iid=5870.

Office of the Assistant Secretary for Health: *Date rape drugs*, 2019. Available from: https://www.womenshealth.gov/a-z-topics/date-rape-drugs.

Office of Justice Programs: Bureau of justice statistics: *Stalking victimization 2016*, 2021. Available from: https://bjs.ojp.gov/content/pub/pdf/sv16_sum.pdf.

Ottisova L, Hemmings S, Howard LM, Zimmerman C, Oram S: Prevalence and risk of violence and the mental, physical and sexual health problems associated with human trafficking: an updated systematic review, *Epidemiol Psychiatr Sci* 25:317–341, 2016. Available from: https://doi.org/10.1017/S2045796016000135.

Patton DU, Hong JS, Ranney M, Patel S, Kelley C, Eschmann R, Washington T: Social media as a vector for youth violence: a review of the literature, *Comput Hum Behav* 35:548–553, 2014. Available from: https://doi.org/10.1016/j.chb.2014.02.043.

Rape, Abuse, & Incest National Network (RAINN): *Victims of sexual violence: statistics*, n.d. Available from: https://www.rainn.org/statistics/victims-sexual-violence 2022.

Rosay AB, Mulford CF: Prevalence estimates and correlates of elder abuse in the United States: the national intimate partner and sexual violence survey, *J Elder Abuse Negl* 29(1):1–14, 2017.

Swanson JW: Introduction: Violence and Mental Illness, *Harv Rev Psychiatry* 29(1):1–5, 2021.

United Nations Office on Drugs and Crimes [UNODC]: *Global Report on Trafficking in Persons 2020*, 2021. Available from: https://www.unodc.org/documents/data-and-analysis/tip/2021/GLOTiP_2020_15jan_web.pdf.

U.S Bureau of Labor Statistics, Fact sheet: Workplace violence in health care, 2018. 2018a Available from: https://www.bls.gov/iif/oshwc/cfoi/workplace-violence-healthcare-2018.htm

U.S Bureau of Labor Statistics, Injuries, Illnesses and Fatalities. 2018b. Available from: https://www.bls.gov/iif/oshwc/osh/case/cd_r4_2019.htm

U.S. Department of Justice: *Bureau of Justice Statistics, Prisoners in*, 2002. Available from: https://bjs.ojp.gov/content/pub/pdf/p20st.pdf.

U.S. Department of Justice: *Hate crime statistics*, 2020. Available from: https://www.justice.gov/hatecrimes/hate-crime-statistics#piechart-description.

Vera Institute of Justice: *Screening for human trafficking, Guidelines for administering the trafficking victim identification tool*, 2014. Available from: https://www.ojp.gov/pdffiles1/nij/grants/246713.pdf.

World Health Organization: *Injuries and violence*, 2021. Available from: https://www.who.int/news-room/fact-sheets/detail/injuries-and-violence.

Natural and Manmade Disasters

Deborah (Debbie) McCrea and Elda Ramirez

OBJECTIVES

Upon completion of this chapter, the reader will be able to do the following:

1. Identify the types of disasters.
2. Discuss the characteristics of disasters.
3. Describe the stages of a disaster.
4. Discuss the stages of disaster management.
5. Describe the roles of federal, state, local, and volunteer agencies involved in disaster management.
6. Identify potential bioterrorist chemical and biological agents.
7. Discuss the impact of disasters on a community.
8. Describe the role and responsibilities of nurses in relation to disasters.

OUTLINE

KEY TERMS

American Red Cross
direct victim
disaster
disaster triage
displaced persons
Federal Emergency Management Agency
first responders
frequency
imminence
indirect victim
mass casualty
mitigation
multiple casualty
natech (natural-technological) disaster
National Incident Management System
National Response Framework
Office of Emergency Management
predictability
preventability
refugees
resource map
risk map
shelter in place
terrorism
U.S. Department of Homeland Security
weapon of mass destruction

Communities throughout the world experience an emergency or disaster incident of one kind or another almost daily. Ritchie and Roser (2021) reported that natural disasters killed an average of 60,000 persons per year and are responsible for 0.1% of global deaths. However, the data indicates that during the last 10 years, there has had a dramatic drop in these fatalities (Ritchie and Roser, 2021).

Emergencies, disasters, and mass casualties can be categorized in several ways. One common way is to describe them based on if they are "natural," "technological," or "manmade." Natural disasters can be subcategorized into biological, geophysical, hydrological, meteorological, and climatological. Technological disasters can be subcategorized into industrial accidents, miscellaneous accidents, and transport accidents (Beerens et al., 2012). Manmade disasters include terrorism (e.g., weapons of mass destruction such as chemical, biological, nuclear, radiological, and explosive devices) and other forms of violence, such as active shooter and mass shooter incidents (Severin and Jacobson, 2020) (Table 29.1). The health of a community can be affected significantly by disasters. For example, natural disasters fairly frequently and in a variety of settings including both urban and rural parts the country, and

TABLE 29.1 Disaster Categories

NATURAL DISASTERS

Biological	Geophysical	Hydrological	Meteorological	Climatological
Epidemics (viral, parasitic, fungal infections)	Earthquakes	Floods	Storms	Extreme temperatures (heat waves/ cold waves)
Insect infestations	Volcanos	Mass movement (wet)	Tropical cyclones and hurricanes	Extreme weather conditions
Animal stampede	Mass movement (dry—e.g., rockslides and landslides)	Avalanche	Extratropical storms	Drought
				Wildfire/forest fires

Technological Disasters

Industrial Accidents	Transport Accidents	Miscellaneous Accidents
Chemical spills	Air	Explosions
Explosions	Sea/boat	Collapse
Radiation leaks	Rail	Fire
Gas leaks	Traffic/road	Other
Fires		

Manmade Disasters

Terrorism	Violence
Weapons of mass destruction (e.g., chemical, biological nuclear, radiation, explosive devices)	Active shooter intendents
	Mass shooter incidents

source: Beerens R, Duyvis M, Heus R: *Aftermath crisis management—Phase I - Acrimas - D3.1 threat/hazard map for EU CM*, 2012; Severin and Jacobson, 2020.

may cover a very wide region. Hurricanes Harvey, Sandy, Katrina, and Rita are recent examples of how communities and their hospitals, clinics, nursing homes, and other healthcare facilities are directly affected by a disaster.

Hurricanes Katrina and Rita which affected the Gulf Coast of the United States 3 weeks apart in 2005 are good examples where access to needed supplies and healthcare was impeded by infrastructure breakdowns due to the storm surge, breach of the New Orleans levy system, winds, tornados, and rainfall all along the Gulf Coast. Disruptions included loss of utilities, road closures due to flooding, inadequate number of first responders and limited number of search and rescue vehicles. Over 1800 persons lost their lives with over $108 billion worth of damages accumulated just from Katrina alone (Medlin et al., 2016).

Patients were evacuated from one hospital to another, sometimes more than once. Healthcare personnel, medicines, and needed supplies were either unavailable, scarce, or even depleted because of the increased demand. Temporary shelters and healthcare services were moved into schools, churches, and a variety of other facilities throughout the area. Panic ensued because of the extensive wind and water damage from Hurricane Katrina. A shortage of food, drinking water and even lifesaving rescue personnel and equipment caused a great deal anxiety from the governmental and healthcare leaders and survivors along the Gulf Coast between New Orleans and Western Florida.

Three weeks after Hurricane Katrina came ashore, Hurricane Rita, became a Category 5 storm in the same region. This caused a large-scale panic and anxiety in the Houston region which ultimately caused the worse freeway gridlock in Houston's history. The traffic jam lasted 18 to 24 h with an estimated 2.5 million people on the roads at the same time. Unfortunately, Hurricane Rita occurred during the very hot and humid September so there were many victims of dehydration and heat exhaustions. This panic exposed huge infrastructure failures including not having contraflow roads set up to help citizens exit the city, inadequate plans for refueling cars who ran of gasoline while fleeing, lack of access to food and water for those stuck in the major traffic jam and the inability for first responders to easily get to the illness/injured persons who were trapped on the highways for sometimes up to a day. More evacuees died because of being on the road and not from the storm. There were 113 deaths in Texas but only 6 from the storm. The rest resulted from the evacuation. This included 24 residents of a nursing home who died while on an evacuation bus that caught fire (Berger, 2015; Levin, 2015).

Hurricane Sandy devastated New York and New Jersey in 2012. It caused damage in 24 states which also struggled with similar infrastructure issues. The lessons learned from these events resulted in changes in disaster plans that have made a significant difference in how subsequent hurricanes were managed. In September 2017, Hurricane Harvey offered more lessons because it became the costliest natural disaster in US history, after more than 60 inches of rainfall fell in Houston and surrounding areas (NOAA, 2017). Because of changes made to disaster response, even though one-third of the city of Houston was under water, only 82 people lost their lives.

Hurricanes, tornadoes, floods, wildfires, and industrial accidents occur yearly throughout the United States. Indeed, fires in California in 2021 burned over 2.5 million acres with damage to 3600 structures and 3 confirmed fatalities (State of California, 2021). Similarly, fires have caused widespread damage in Colorado and Oregon.

Americans are familiar with most of the disasters listed in Table 29.1, but terrorism was largely unknown or unheeded in this country before the bombing of the Alfred P. Murrah Federal Building in Oklahoma City in 1995. The US Code of Federal Regulations defines **terrorism** as violent acts or acts dangerous to human life that appear to be intended to intimidate or coerce the civilian population or to influence the policy or conduct of a government (18 U.S. CFR § 2331, 1992). The FBI is charged with the responsibility for investigating terrorism-related matters in the United States and internationally. According to the Central Intelligence Agency (2022), terrorism "is premeditated, politically motivated violence perpetrated against noncombatant targets by sub-national groups or clandestine agents." International terrorism involves the territory or the citizens of more than one country.

The September 11, 2011 terrorist attacks in several locations including the New York World Trade Center, the Pentagon along with the hijacked plane crash in Pennsylvania resulted in significant fear and ultimately changes in many areas of our lives (e.g., routine screenings prior to commercial flights). Other terrorist attacks include the 2013 Boston Marathon bombings, the 2016 Orlando nightclub shooting, the 2017 Las Vegas music festival shooting, the 2019 El Paso Walmart shooting, and most recently, the SUV that barreled through a parade route in Waukesha Wisconsin, in 2021 which killed six persons and injured many more. These incidents all offered lessons for leaders in both the government and healthcare arenas (Schmidt, 2021).

As suggested by the events described, the potential for mass casualty incidents (MCI) is ever present. Furthermore, they are not confined to the United States.

Other incidents of manmade terrorism included the nerve gas (Sarin) attack in the Tokyo subway in March 1995, which killed 12 and injured more than 6000 people; the bombing of the commuter train in Spain in March 2004, which killed 191 people; the suicide bombings in the London transport system in July 2005, which killed 52 commuters and 4 terrorists; the shooting and bombing attacks in the financial district of Mumbai, India, in November 2008, which killed more than 170; an attack in a Paris theater and nearby neighborhoods in November 2015 that resulted in 137 deaths and injured 368; and a vehicle attack in Nice, France, in July 2016 that killed 86 and injured 434.

Following the September 2001 attacks, concerns have increasingly focused on weapons of mass destruction. **Weapon**

of mass destruction refers to any weapon that is designed or intended to cause death or serious bodily injury through release, dissemination, or impact of toxic or poisonous chemicals, or their precursors; any weapon involving a disease organism; or any weapon that is designed to release radiation or radioactivity at a level dangerous to human life. Biological organisms considered to be potential weapons of mass destruction are shown in Box 29.1. Chemical warfare agents are classified as nerve agents, vesicants, pulmonary agents, and cyanides (formerly "blood agents"). Chemicals that are potential weapons of mass destruction are listed in Table 29.2. These tables also include information about the lethality, treatment, and impact related to each.

BOX 29.1   Bioterrorism Agents/Diseases

Category A

High-priority agents include organisms that pose a risk to national security because they:
- Can be easily disseminated or transmitted from person to person
- Result in high mortality rates and have the potential for major public health impact
- Might cause public panic and social disruption
- Require special action for public health preparedness

Agents/Diseases
- Anthrax (Bacillus anthracis)
- Botulism (Clostridium botulinum toxin)
- Plague (Yersinia pestis)
- Smallpox (Variola major)
- Tularemia (Francisella tularensis)
- Viral hemorrhagic fevers (filoviruses [e.g., Ebola, Marburg]) and arenaviruses [e.g., Lassam, Nacgyoi])

Category B

Second-highest-priority agents include those that:
- Are moderately easy to disseminate
- Result in moderate morbidity rates and low mortality rates
- Require specific enhancements of CDC's diagnostic capacity and enhanced disease surveillance

Agents/Diseases
- Brucellosis (Brucella species)
- Epsilon toxin of Clostridium perfringens
- Food safety threats (e.g., Salmonella species, Escherichia coli 0157:H7, Shigella)

Category C

Third-highest-priority agents include emerging pathogens that could be engineered for mass dissemination in the future because of:
- Availability
- Ease of production and dissemination
- Potential for high morbidity and mortality rates and major health impact

Agents
- Emerging infectious diseases such as Nipah virus and hantavirus

Data from National Center for Environment Health (NCEI): https://www.cdc.gov/nceh/; Agency for Toxic Substances and Disease Registry (ATSDR): http://www.atsdr.cdc.gov/; and National Center for Injury and Violence Prevention and Control (NCIPC): http://www.cdc.gov/injury/.

TABLE 29.2 Chemical Agents of Mass Destruction

Chemical Agent	Lethality	Treatment	Impact
Sarin (nerve agent)	High	Move to fresh air; wash skin; drugs have limited effectiveness	Likely nerve agent; chemicals needed to produce are banned by International Chemical Weapons Convention
VX (nerve agent)	Very high	Move to fresh air; wash skin; drugs have limited effectiveness	Not likely weapon; difficult to manufacture
Tabun (nerve agent)	High	Move to fresh air; wash skin; drugs have limited effectiveness	Easy-to-manufacture nerve agent; likely agent to be used
Chlorine (pulmonary agent)	Low	Move to fresh air; wash skin; no antidote	Readily available; likely agent because of availability; breaks down with water
Hydrogen cyanide (blood agent)	Low to moderate	Move to fresh air; wash skin; some drugs mitigate effects	Industrial product; some chemicals used to produce it are banned; likely agent because of availability

Modified from Cieslak TJ, Eitzen EM: Bioterrorism: agents of concern, *J Public Health Manag Pract* 6(4):19–29, 2000.

Because of the recognition of the need to be prepared, various programs have been created to address the national, state, and local management of disasters. In 2003, President George W. Bush established the US Department of Homeland Security (DHS). The next year the **National Incident Management System** (NIMS) was implemented. The NIMS provides a systematic, proactive way for all levels of governmental and nongovernmental agencies to work seamlessly to prevent, protect against, respond to, recover from, and prevent the effects of disasters (Federal Emergency Management Agency (FEMA), 2022a).

In 2003, "Ready.gov" was launched as a public service campaign to prepare the public to respond to and mitigate disasters through public involvement. Through this effort, Community Emergency Response Teams (CERT) were developed so regular citizens could be trained in fire safety, search and rescue, team organization and disaster medical care (FEMA, 2022b). Other organizations and training programs were also developed through Ready.gov such as "You are the help until help arrives," National Voluntary Organizations Active during Disasters, Volunteer and Receive Training Program, the Teach Preparedness Curriculum for K-12 students' program, and social media sites which encourage emergency preparedness. FEMA also developed an Emergency Management Institute for additional training (FEMA, 2022c; Ready.gov, 2022; https://www.ready.gov/get-involved).

In 2011, President Obama implemented a Presidential Policy Directive which recognized that preparedness is a shared responsibility for security and resilience to respond to terrorism, cyber-attacks, pandemics, and catastrophic natural disasters. This directive tasked the DHS and Counterterrorism to prepare the following missions: (1) Develop a National Preparedness Goal, (2) Set up a National Preparedness System, (3) Build and Sustain Preparedness, (4) Prepare National Preparedness Reports, and (5) Coordinate Roles and Responsibilities (FEMA, 2021; https://www.fema.gov/emergency-managers/national-preparedness).

Efforts to prepare for disasters have also been significantly enhanced at the regional level in most states. In 2003, for example, the Texas Legislature passed a bill requiring nurses to attend a continuing education program related to bioterrorism. In addition, the Emergency System for Advanced Registration of Volunteer Health Professionals (ESAR-VHP) has been implemented by the Texas Department of State Health Services (DSHS) to mobilize volunteers to support communities in times of crisis or disaster (Texas Disaster Volunteer Registry for Medical Public Health and Lay Volunteer Responders, 2022). Similar registries are found in most states.

Nurses have both a personal and a professional role in relation to disasters. Nurses' personal role is to develop a disaster plan for their workplace, home, and family. Disaster kits for survival in each of these settings should be prepared. Professionally, nurses are uniquely positioned to provide valuable information for the development of plans for disaster prevention, preparedness, response, and recovery for the facilities in which they are employed as well as the communities where they live. Nurses, because of their unique breath of knowledge, are excellent choices to collaborate with health and social representatives, government bodies, community groups, and volunteer agencies in disaster planning and preparedness programs (e.g., drills). Using their knowledge of nursing, public health, and cultural-familial structures, as well as their clinical skills and abilities, nurses can actively assist with or participate in all aspects and stages of an emergency or disaster, regardless of the setting in which the event may occur. Disaster nursing requires the application of basic nursing knowledge and skills in difficult environments with scare resources and changing conditions.

DISASTER DEFINITIONS

A **disaster** is any event that causes a level of destruction, death, or injury that affects the abilities of the community to respond to the incident using available resources. Emergencies differ from disasters, in that agencies, communities, families, or individuals can manage emergencies using their own resources. But a disaster event, depending on the characteristics of the disaster, may be beyond the ability of the community to respond and recover from the incident using its own resources. Disasters frequently require assistance from outside the immediate community, known as mutual aid, to help manage resulting infrastructure issues and for recovery.

Some disasters (e.g., a house fire) may affect only a few persons, whereas others (e.g., a hurricane) can affect thousands. An MCI is an event that overwhelms the local healthcare system where the number of casualties exceeds the local resources and capabilities in a short period of time (DeNolf and Kahwaji, 2018).

A casualty can be classified as a direct victim, an indirect victim, a displaced person, or a refugee. A **direct victim** is an individual who is immediately affected by the event; the **indirect victim** may be a family member or friend of the victim or a first responder. Displaced persons and refugees are special categories of direct victims. **Displaced persons** are those who have to evacuate their homes, schools, or businesses as a result of a disaster; **refugees** are a group of people who have fled their homes or even their country as a result of famine, drought, natural disaster, war, or civil unrest.

TYPES OF DISASTERS

The Section Types of Disasters were discussed as seen in Table 29.1. However, it is important to remember there can be combinations of natural, technological, and manmade, disasters. A **natech (natural-technological) disaster** is a natural disaster that creates or results in a widespread technological problem. An example of a natech disaster is an earthquake that causes structural collapse of roadways or bridges, which, in turn, leads to downed electrical wires and subsequent fires. Another example is a chemical spill resulting from a flood.

Injury or death from a disaster may be direct or indirect. For example, injuries from hurricanes occur because people fail to evacuate or take shelter, do not take precautions in securing their property despite adequate warning, and do not follow guidelines on food and water safety or injury prevention during recovery. Drowning, electrocution, lacerations, or punctures from flying debris, and blunt trauma from falling trees or other objects are some of the morbidity concerns. Heart attacks and stress-related disorders also occur. In addition, injuries may occur from activities in the recovery phase, for example, from use of chain saws or other power equipment or from animal, snake, or insect bites.

CHARACTERISTICS OF DISASTERS

Several characteristics have been used to describe disasters (Box 29.2). These characteristics are interdependent and therefore important to consider in plans for managing any disaster event. Each is discussed briefly.

Frequency

Frequency refers to how often a disaster occurs. Some disasters occur relatively often in certain parts of the world. Terrorist activities are occurring on an almost daily basis in some countries. Other examples are hurricanes, which occur with variable frequency between the months of June and November in the

---

> **BOX 29.2** **Characteristics of Disasters**
>
> - Frequency
> - Predictability
> - Preventability
> - Imminence
> - Scope and number of casualties
> - Intensity

Northern Hemisphere and tornados which occur most often in the spring and fall. Earthquakes, occur with varying frequency all around the world. In the United States, earthquakes are generally considered to be a West Coast problem, but 45 states and territories are at moderate to high risk for an earthquake, and they have occurred in every region of the country (DHS, 2019). Other disasters, such as volcanic eruptions, are far less frequent and are geographically limited to certain regions.

Predictability

Predictability relates to the ability to determine when and whether a disaster event will occur. Some disasters, such as floods, may be predicted in the spring through monitoring of the snowmelt and other weather patterns. Weather forecasters can predict when conditions are right for the development of tornadoes; these generally occur between April and June, but they may occur at any time of the year or as secondary results of hurricanes. Weather forecasters can predict hurricanes with increasing accuracy. Other disasters (e.g., fires and industrial explosions) may not be predictable at all.

Preventability/Mitigation

Mitigation refers to actions taken to reduce loss of life and property by lessening the impact of disasters. It means acting now—before the next disaster—to reduce human and financial consequences (FEMA, 2022d). Preventability assumes that all disasters are not inevitable and steps can be taken to prevent them. Some disasters (e.g., hurricanes, tornadoes, and earthquakes) are not preventable, whereas others can be easily controlled, if not prevented entirely. For example, flooding can be controlled or sometimes prevented through construction of dams or levees or deepening bayous.

Primary prevention is aimed at preventing the occurrence of a disaster or limiting consequences when the event itself cannot be prevented (mitigation). Primary prevention occurs in the non-disaster and predisaster stages. The *nondisaster stage* is the period before a disaster occurs, and the *predisaster stage* is the time when a disaster is pending. Preventive actions during the nondisaster stage include assessing communities to determine potential disaster hazards; developing disaster plans at local, state, and federal levels; conducting drills to test the plan; training volunteers and healthcare providers; and providing educational programs of all kinds.

Risk maps and resource maps are developed to aid in planning. A **risk map** is a geographic map of an area that is analyzed

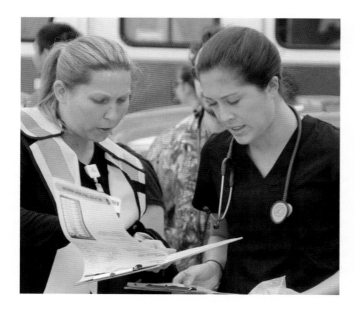

Two emergency nurses in "incident command" for a mass casualty drill in the nondisaster stage.

for the impact of a potential disaster on the population and buildings in the area that would be involved (e.g., an area in a flood plain, an area covered if a nuclear explosion would occur, an area involved in an explosion of an industrial site) (Fig. 29.1). A **resource map** is a geographic map that outlines the resources that would be available in or near the area affected by a potential disaster (e.g., potential shelter sites, potential medical sources, and location of equipment that might be needed) (Fig. 29.2).

The disaster plan is initiated predisaster, or when a disaster is imminent. Primary prevention actions during this stage include notifying the appropriate officials, warning the population, and advising what response to take (e.g., voluntary or mandatory evacuation).

Secondary prevention strategies are implemented once the disaster occurs. They are actions aimed at preventing further injury or destruction. Safety is considered before search and rescue.

Tertiary prevention focuses on recovery of the community—that is, restoring the community to its previous level of functioning and its residents to their maximum functioning. Tertiary prevention is aimed at preventing a recurrence or minimizing the

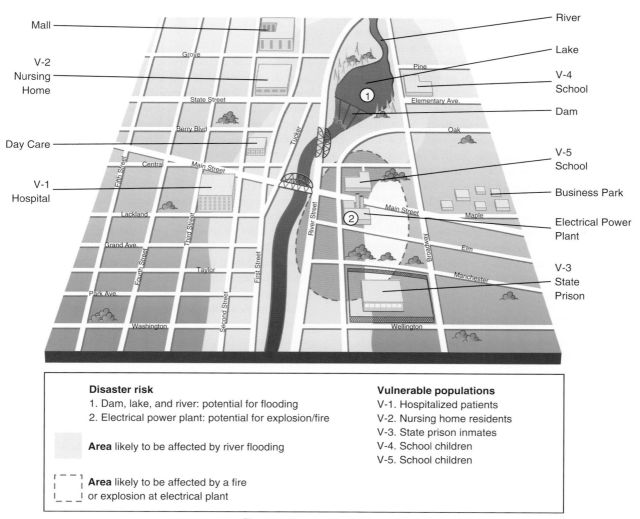

Disaster risk

1. Dam, lake, and river: potential for flooding
2. Electrical power plant: potential for explosion/fire

Area likely to be affected by river flooding

Area likely to be affected by a fire or explosion at electrical plant

Vulnerable populations

V-1. Hospitalized patients
V-2. Nursing home residents
V-3. State prison inmates
V-4. School children
V-5. School children

Fig. 29.1 Community risk map.

effects of future disasters through debriefing meetings to identify problems with the plan and make revisions.

Nurses should be involved in all stages of prevention and related activities. In order to respond effectively, personally, and professionally during different types of disasters, nurses need to know (1) what kind of disasters threaten their communities, (2) what injuries to expect from different disaster scenarios, (3) evacuation routes, (4) locations of shelters, and (5) warning systems. They must be able to educate others about disasters and how to prepare for and respond to them. Finally, nurses need to keep up to date on the latest recommendations and advances in lifesaving measures (e.g., basic first aid, cardiopulmonary resuscitation [CPR], and use of automated external defibrillators).

Imminence

Imminence is the speed of onset of an impending disaster and relates to the extent of forewarning possible and the anticipated duration of the incident. Weather forecasters can tell when a hurricane may be developing days ahead of its expected arrival and can give the time of arrival, the general direction it will take, and an approximate location for its landing and forward movement. Hurricanes, however, are subject to other weather variables and can change direction and intensity several times before making landfall. A warning for a hurricane means it will reach landfall in 24 h or less, whereas a watch means it will reach landfall in 24 to 36 h. A warning for tornadoes means to take shelter immediately, and a watch means to stay alert for possible tornadoes.

Some disastrous incidents (e.g., wildfires, explosions, and terrorist attacks) have no warning time. Bioterrorist attacks are generally silent, and the first awareness may be days or even weeks after exposure. For example, individuals exposed to a pathologic agent (e.g., anthrax, smallpox) may arrive at healthcare facilities at various times and to various providers, making diagnosis and early treatment difficult. Nurses and medical personnel need to know the signs and symptoms of biological, chemical, radiation, and nuclear exposure in order to identify the nature of the threat, report the problem to the Centers for Disease Control and Prevention (CDC), and then treat and control the spread of both biological and chemical agents (see Box 29.1 and Table 29.2).

Scope and Number of Casualties

The *scope* of a disaster indicates the range of its effect. The scope is described in terms of both the geographic area involved and the number of individuals affected, injured, or killed. From a healthcare perspective, the location, type, and timing of a disaster event are predictors of the types of injuries and illnesses that might occur. For example, the October 1989 earthquake in San Francisco occurred while people were on their way to work. Overall, more than 60 people died from a multitude of causes, including a motorcycle officer who was killed after the collapse of a freeway, 16 people who were killed by building collapses, 5 who died as a result of falls, and 9 who died of heart attacks.

In contrast, the earthquake and tsunami occurred in the Indian Ocean in December 2004, killing more than 200,000 people in South Asia, Southeast Asia, and East Africa; most died of drowning (World Vision, 2019).

Another example of the extremely destructive power of earthquakes is the Haitian quake of 2010, which resulted in the death of more than 160,000 people and displacement of more than a million (CDC, 2015).

Hurricanes generally affect a large geographic area. Nevertheless, they may cause few, if any, deaths if sufficient preventive measures are taken. The scope of Hurricane Katrina in September 2005 covered all of New Orleans; most of South Louisiana; and parts of Florida, Alabama, and Mississippi. Hurricane Rita, only a few weeks later, struck New Orleans again as well as South Louisiana and much of Eastern Texas. Remarkably, despite the widespread destruction caused by these storms, the number of dead from Katrina was more than 1300, and the number of dead from Hurricane Rita was 58, including 23 elders who were killed in a bus accident while evacuating. As mentioned previously, Hurricanes Sandy (2012) and Harvey (2017) were much more destructive but resulted in many fewer deaths. Much of the improvement in loss of life can be attributed to better preparation and timely notifications, allowing for evacuations.

Intensity

Intensity is the characteristic describing the level of destruction and devastation of the disaster event. Factors contributing to the amount of damage from a disaster event such as a hurricane are the distance from the zone of maximum winds, how exposed the location is, building standards, vegetation type, and resultant flooding. Parts of New Orleans were under water from the primary effects (storm surge and rain) and secondary effects (levee failure) of Hurricane Katrina. Some buildings and homes were completely destroyed, and others were left in terrible condition by flooding and wind damage.

Various hurricane and tornado scales have been developed on the basis of wind intensity and predicted level of destruction. The Fujita Tornado Intensity Scale, developed in 1971, categorized each tornado by its intensity and the area involved. In 1992, Fujita updated the scale to include an estimate of F-scale damage. The new scale, the Enhanced Fujita Scale (EF Scale), implemented in the United States on February 1, 2007, is still a set of wind estimates (not measurements) based on types of structural damage. The estimates vary with the height of apparent damage above the ground and exposure (National Oceanic and Atmospheric Administration, 2022).

Hurricanes have been categorized since 1975 with use of the Saffir-Simpson Hurricane Scale, which includes sustained wind intensity, storm surge ranges, and flooding references. On an experimental basis for the 2009 tropical cyclone season, the storm surge ranges and flooding references were removed for each of the five categories (Box 29.3) because storm surge information is inaccurate. For example, Hurricane Ike in 2008 was a category 2 hurricane but had a storm surge at Galveston, Texas, equivalent to a category 4 to 5 storm surge. Hurricane

BOX 29.3   The Saffir-Simpson Hurricane Wind Scale

- *Category 1* (74–95 mph): Very dangerous winds will produce some damage.
- *Category 2* (96–110 mph): Extremely dangerous winds will cause extensive damage.
- *Category 3* (111–129 mph): Devastating damage will occur.
- *Category 4* (130–156 mph): Catastrophic damage will occur.
- *Category 5* (157 mph or higher): Catastrophic damage will occur.

Data from National Oceanic and Atmospheric Administration National Weather Service, National Hurricane Center: *Saffir-Simpson hurricane wind scale,* 2022. Available from: http://www.nhc.noaa.gov/aboutsshws.php.–.

Katrina in 2007 was a category 3 hurricane with a storm surge equivalent to a category 5. The scale was revised in 2012 and is now called the *Saffir-Simpson Hurricane Wind Scale.* The new scale does not include storm surge, rainfall-induced floods, and tornadoes (National Oceanic and Atmospheric Administration, 2022a,b).

❓ ACTIVE LEARNING

Assess the community where you live for potential disasters that could result in mass casualties. What disasters are predictable? Are there measures that can be taken to prevent or minimize injuries, death, or destruction?

DISASTER MANAGEMENT

When one is aware of the types and characteristics of disasters, the question then becomes: What can be done to prevent/ mitigate, prepare for, respond to, and recover from disasters? Disaster management requires an interdisciplinary, collaborative team effort and involves a network of agencies and individuals to develop a disaster plan that covers the multiple elements necessary for an effective plan. Communities can respond more quickly, more effectively, and with less confusion if the efforts needed in the event of a disaster have been anticipated and plans for meeting them identified. The result of planning is that more lives are saved and less property is damaged. Planning ensures that resources are available and that roles and responsibilities of all personnel and agencies, both official and unofficial, are delineated.

Nurses need to know their personal, professional, and community responsibilities and obligations. They should realize conflicts may arise between their professional and personal responsibilities. Plans need to be made long in advance of a disaster so the person can resolve the ethical dilemma of volunteering for a disaster especially if they have a family and pets that need care (see the Ethical Insights box).

Nurses may also become direct or indirect victims during the disaster. They may also be displaced as a result of a disaster event. Recognizing that this may be a possibility, nurses need to plan, prepare, practice, and teach their family and significant

others how to respond. Many agencies can help with this from FEMA, CDC, and Ready.gov.

ETHICAL INSIGHTS

Deciding Whether to Care for Family or Care for Patients

During a disaster, a nurse might face an ethical dilemma because of competing responsibilities to their patients, employers, family, self, and even their pets. For example, a nurse who is a single parent with young children and has a limited support system may be forced to decide between her responsibility to care for her children and a mandate to report to work to care for patients. Depending on the choice made, one may end up losing their job or put their children endanger if they do not have adequate caregivers to watch after them. Potential conflicts such as this should be considered and discussed and decisions made in conjunction with the employer before a disaster event.

Local, State, and Federal Governmental Responsibilities

Local Government

The local government is responsible for the safety and welfare of its citizens. Emergencies and disaster incidents are handled at the lowest possible organizational and jurisdictional level. Police, fire, public health, public works, and medical emergency services are the **first responders**, responsible for incident management at the local level. Local officials and agencies are responsible for preparing their citizens for all kinds of emergencies and disasters and for testing disaster plans with mock drills. They manage events during an incident by carrying out evacuation, search and rescue, and maintaining public health and public works responsibilities. Local communities should have contingency operation plans for multiple disaster situations and for various aspects of the plan. For example, landline telephone service and cell phone service may not work because of being restricted for emergency use only or damage to the infrastructure, so other forms of communication need to be available.

In an incident other than a biological, chemical, radiation, or nuclear event, in most cases, it is the 911 communication center or the fire or police department that gets the initial message. The emergency communication center then communicates the incident to the other first responders and the director of the **Office of Emergency Management**, who determines what others may be needed (e.g., ambulances, other officials, and voluntary group representatives). Local hospitals are notified of the incident and the predicted nature of impending casualties. The hospitals may begin to receive victims via private automobiles who have not been triaged at the site of the incident. According to the CDC, a hospital can assess the expected number of victims that it may receive by counting the number that arrive within the first hour and doubling it.

For a biological or chemical terrorist incident, the process is very different. First responders generally are not involved. Rather, nurses and doctors in healthcare facilities may be the first to suspect that a biological or chemical agent has been released into the community. Box 29.4 lists the guidelines for detecting

BOX 29.4 Guidelines for Early Detection of Biochemical Terrorist Incidents

- A rapidly increasing disease incidence (within hours or days) in a normally healthy population.
- An unusual increase in the number of people seeking care, especially with fever, respiratory, or gastrointestinal complaints.
- An endemic disease rapidly emerging at an uncharacteristic time or in an unusual pattern.
- Clusters of patients arriving from a single locale.
- Large numbers of rapidly fatal cases—patients who die within 72 h after admission to the hospital.
- Any patient presenting with a disease that is relatively uncommon and has bioterrorism potential (e.g., pulmonary anthrax, smallpox, or plague).

From Chettle C: Recognizing bioterrorism: nurses on the frontline, *NurseWeek* 6:29–30, 2001.

biochemical incidents. If any of these instances occur in a healthcare provider setting, the suspicion should be immediately reported to the infection control department, the administration of the facility, or both. Each setting should post near the telephone the numbers to be called if a biochemical incident (whether internal or external) is suspected. These numbers should include those of the CDC Bioterrorism Emergency Response, the CDC Hospital Infections program, and the US Army Medical Research Institute of Infectious Diseases.

The Office of Emergency Management involves representatives from all official and unofficial agencies in developing the community disaster plan; developing scenarios to test the plan through drills; and assessing the scope, intensity, and number of casualties once an incident has occurred to initiate the proper response. For those events that are not within the abilities of the local community or in the event of a terrorist-type incident, higher-level agencies and resources must be requested and will become involved.

State Government

When a disaster overwhelms the local community's resources, the state's Department or Office of Emergency Management is called for assistance. Before such an event, state officials provide technical support for prevention, preparedness, response, and recovery. State officials visit local officials to assist and assess local emergency management plans, promote and conduct workshops and training courses, help with training exercises, advise and support local government officials, and are on scene at disaster events to facilitate coordination of state resources and to disseminate information. In some cases, the National Guard may be called in to aid the community. When the scope of the event is so great that local and state resources are not adequate to meet the needs, the state calls on the federal government; at that point, the president may declare the incident a "national disaster." Once the president declares a national disaster, federal aid is made available. The **National Response Framework** is the core operational plan for domestic incident

management for an all-hazards response. It describes best practices for managing incidents "that range from the serious but purely local, to large-scale terrorist attacks or catastrophic natural disasters" (FEMA, 2021).

Federal Government

US Department of Homeland Security. As previously mentioned, the **U.S. DHS** was established in March 2003 to realign the existing federal departments, agencies, groups, and organizations into a single department focused on protecting the American people and their homeland (DHS, 2022a).

There are five homeland security missions: (1) prevent terrorism and enhance security; (2) secure and manage US borders; (3) enforce and administer immigration laws; (4) safeguard and secure cyberspace; and (5) ensure resilience to disasters (DHS, 2022b).

The organizational structure of the DHS has several divisions, and within each of these divisions are multiple offices and centers, listed in Box 29.5.

The DHS established its Homeland Security Advisory System to build a comprehensive and effective communication structure for disseminating threat information to public safety officials and the public at large. The previous color-coded threat level system has been replaced with the National Terrorism Advisory System. "The system provides timely, detailed information to the public, government agencies, first responders, airports and other transportation hubs, and the private sector" (DHS, 2022a–d). The threat alert indicates whether there is an elevated threat (no specific information about timing or location) or imminent threat (impending or very soon). DHS (2022d) has published a public guide with recommended steps that individuals, communities, businesses, and governments can take to help prevent, mitigate, or respond to the threat.

FEMA (2022a–d) has published an in-depth guide for citizen preparedness, *Are You Ready?* The focus of the contents is on how to prepare, practice, and maintain emergency plans

BOX 29.5 Operational and Support Components That Make Up the Department of Homeland Security

United States Citizenship and Immigration Services (USCIS)
United States Customs and Border Protection (CBP)
United States Coast Guard (USCG)
Federal Emergency Management Agency (FEMA)
Federal Law Enforcement Training Center (FLETC)
United States Immigration and Customs Enforcement (ICE)
United States Secret Service (USSS)
Transportation Security Administration (TSA)
Directorate for Management
National Protection and Programs Directorate
Domestic Nuclear Detection Office
Science and Technology Directorate
Office of Health Affairs

From: U.S. Department of Homeland Security: *Operational and support components*, 2020. Available from: https://www.dhs.gov/operational-and-support-components.

that indicate what must be done before, during, and after a disaster. The guide explains how to prepare disaster supplies sufficient in quantity for individuals and families to survive (Box 29.6). Additionally, *Are You Ready?* lists specific natural hazards, technological hazards, and terrorism incidents with detailed information on what to do in each incident (Box 29.7). Nurses could use this guide in developing educational programs and disaster plans related to natural and manmade disasters to which individuals, families, or communities may be exposed.

BOX 29.6 Federal Emergency Management Agency Recommendations for Basic Disaster Supplies Kit

- Three-day supply of nonperishable food
- Three-day supply of water—one gallon of water per person, per day
- Portable, battery-powered radio or television and extrabatteries
- Flashlight and extrabatteries
- First aid kit and manual
- Sanitation and hygiene items (moist towelettes and toilet paper)
- Matches and waterproof container
- Whistle
- Extraclothing
- Kitchen accessories and cooking utensils, including a can opener
- Photocopies of credit and identification cards
- Cash and coins
- Special needs item, such as prescription medications, eye glasses, contact lens solution, and hearing aid batteries
- Items for infants, such as formula, diapers, bottles, and pacifiers
- Other items to meet your unique family needs
- If you live in a cold climate, you must think about warmth. Be sure to include one complete change of clothing and shoes per person, including:
  - Jacket or coat
  - Long pants
  - Long-sleeve shirt
  - Sturdy shoes
  - Hat, mittens, and scarf
  - Sleeping bag or warm blanket (per person)

From: U.S. Department of Homeland Security (2021). https://www.ready.gov/build-a-kit

---

BOX 29.7 What to Do in Different Types of Emergencies

Biological Attack
- Move away quickly.
- Wash with soap and water.
- Contact authorities.
- Listen to the media for official instructions.
- Seek medical attention if you become sick.

Nuclear Blast
- Do not look at the flash or fireball—it can blind you.
- Take cover behind anything that might offer protection.
- Lie flat on the ground and cover your head. If the explosion is some distance away, it could take 30 s or more for the blast to hit.
- Take shelter as soon as you can, even if you are many miles from ground zero—where the attack occurred; radioactive fallout can be carried by the winds for hundreds of miles. Remember the three protective factors: distance, shielding, and time.

Chemical Attack
- If you are instructed to remain in your home or office building, you should:
  - Close doors and windows and turn off all ventilation, including furnaces, air conditioners, vents, and fans.
  - Seek shelter in an internal room and take your disaster supplies kit.
  - Seal the room with duct tape and plastic sheeting.
  - Listen to your radio for instructions from authorities.
- If you are caught in or near a contaminated area, you should:
  - Move away immediately in a direction upwind of the source.
  - Find shelter as quickly as possible.

Radiation Dispersion Device Event
Outdoors
- Seek shelter indoors immediately in the nearest building.
- If appropriate shelter is not available, move as rapidly as is safe upwind and away from the location of the explosive blast. Then seek appropriate shelter as soon as possible.
- Listen for official instructions and follow directions.

Indoors
- If you have time, turn off ventilation and heating systems, and close windows, vents, fireplace dampers, exhaust fans, and clothes dryer vents. Retrieve your disaster supplies kit and a battery-powered radio, and take them to your shelter room.
- Seek shelter immediately, preferably underground or in an interior room of a building, placing as much distance and dense shielding as possible between you and the outdoors where the radioactive material may be.
- Seal windows and external doors that do not fit snugly with duct tape to reduce infiltration of radioactive particles. Plastic sheeting will not provide shielding from radioactivity or from blast effects of a nearby explosion.
- Listen for official instructions, and follow directions.

Explosions
- If there is an explosion, you should:
  - Get under a sturdy table or desk if things are falling around you.
  - When they stop falling, leave quickly, watching for obviously weakened floors and stairways.
  - As you exit from the building, be especially watchful of falling debris.
  - Leave the building as quickly as possible. Do not stop to retrieve personal possessions or make phone calls.
- Do not use elevator. Once you are out:
  - Do not stand in front of windows, glass doors, or other potentially hazardous areas.
  - Move away from sidewalks or streets to be used by emergency officials or others still exiting the building.
- If you are trapped in debris:
  - If possible, use a flashlight to signal your location to rescuers.
  - Avoid unnecessary movement so you don't kick up dust.
  - Cover your nose and mouth with anything you have on hand (Dense-weave cotton material can act as a good filter. Try to breathe through the material).
  - Tap on a pipe or wall so rescuers can hear where you are.
  - If possible, use a whistle to signal rescuers.
  - Shout only as a last resort. Shouting can cause a person to inhale dangerous amounts of dust.

Modified from Federal Emergency Management Agency: *Are you ready? An in-depth guide to citizen preparedness*, 2021. Available from: https://www.fema.gov/related-link/are-you-ready-guide-citizen-preparedness.

The DHS has presented a national preparedness goal. The goal is "a secure and resilient nation with the capabilities required across the whole community to prevent, protect against, mitigate, respond to, and recover from the threats and hazards that pose the greatest risk." The risks cited include natural disaster, pandemic, chemical spills, terrorist attacks, and cyberattacks. The plan identifies and elaborates on the "core capabilities" and target necessary to achieve preparedness across five mission areas: prevention, protection, mitigation, response, and recovery (DHS, 2022c). Thirty-one core capabilities needed to achieve the goal have been identified where they most logically fit. Materials to enhance the capabilities are available from the DHS.

The Federal Emergency Management Agency. The **Federal Emergency Management Agency** became part of DHS in 2003. FEMA's mission is to support citizens and first responders to ensure that as a nation, everyone works together to build, sustain, and improve the capacity to prepare for, protect against, respond to, recover from, and mitigate all hazards. In 2006, President George W. Bush signed into law the Post-Katrina Emergency Reform Act (PL 109–295). The act significantly reorganized FEMA, giving it substantial new authority to remedy gaps that became apparent in the response to Hurricane Katrina in 2005 (FEMA, 2022b).

Centers for Disease Control and Prevention. After the rescue of survivors has been accomplished, the Department of Health and Human Services and sometimes the CDC conducts surveillance to ensure that clean drinking water, food, shelter, and medical care are available for those affected. Whether CDC's involvement is necessary depends on the type of disaster. For example, floods pose risks of contaminated water (e.g., cholera) and food supplies (e.g., *Escherichia coli*); loss of shelter leaves people vulnerable to heat or cold and other environmental hazards (e.g., insects); and earthquakes create traumatic injuries (e.g., broken bones, head injuries) that will need to be addressed.

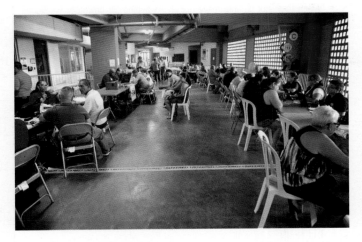

Puerto Rican survivors of Hurricane Maria meet with FEMA and US Small Business Administration officials inside a baseball stadium serving as a disaster recovery center, October 2017. (Photo by Stephen Shepard.)

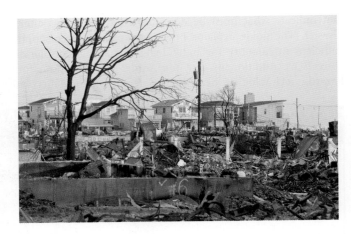

The close-knit community of Breezy Point, New York, lost more than 100 homes to fire during Hurricane Sandy. FEMA is providing ongoing support and resources to the Queens, New York community. (Photo by Andre R. Aragon/FEMA.)

Public Health System

The public health system's mission is the promotion of health, prevention of disease, and protection from threats to health. *Public health system* is a broad term used to describe all of the governmental and nongovernmental organizations and agencies that contribute to the improvement of the health of populations. Public health agencies are the primary agencies for the health and medical responses to disaster incidents and therefore are a part of the initial response activities.

Public health officials provide advice and assistance to other public officials on environmental and health matters. Preparedness includes surveillance and reporting of suspicious illnesses (e.g., signs and symptoms of biological agents, foodborne diseases, and communicable diseases) in the community by physicians and nurses in local healthcare facilities or private offices and clinics. Public health officials then have the responsibility of detecting outbreaks, determining the cause of illness, identifying the risk factors for the population, implementing interventions to control the outbreak, and informing the public of the health risks and preventive measures that need to be taken. These activities relate both directly and indirectly to the 10 essential public health services described in Chapter 1.

📋 NURSING CARE GUIDELINES

Role of Nurses in Disaster

"When disaster strikes, nurses form the backbone of our nations' healthcare response" (RWJF, 2016). Indeed, as Deputy Surgeon General, Rear Admiral, Sylvia Trent-Adams, PhD, RN, noted: "Nurses play an essential role in our nation's ability to prepare for, respond to, and recover from disasters." A report from the Robert Wood Johnson Foundation highlighted how nurses contributed to saving lives during three of the country's recent disasters: the Ebola outbreak, the Joplin, Missouri tornado, and Hurricane Sandy. The report describes how nurses worked within disaster teams to meet both immediate and long-term care needs.

Review the report (the link is provided at the end) to recognize the importance of nurses being prepared to respond during multiple types of disasters and to be encouraged by the leadership of nurses during very challenging circumstances. https://www.rwjf.org/content/dam/farm/reports/issue_briefs/2016/rwjf429036.

American Red Cross

The **American Red Cross** (ARC or Red Cross) is not a governmental agency. It is, however, chartered by Congress to provide disaster relief. The ARC works in partnership with FEMA; DHS; the CDC; and other local, state, and federal agencies to provide and manage needed services (ARC, 2022).

The ARC is primarily a volunteer organization with chapters in all 50 states, Puerto Rico, the Virgin Islands, and the Pacific Rim; its national headquarters is in Washington, DC. Disaster Services is only one of the programs that this agency provides. Others are International Services; Biomedical Services; Armed Forces Emergency Services; and Health, Safety, and Community Services.

The Red Cross places great emphasis on preparedness and participates with communities in developing and testing their disaster plans, maintaining and training personnel for disaster response, and responding during an actual emergency or disaster. The ARC publishes many pamphlets and educational materials to help individuals, families, neighborhoods, schools, and businesses prepare for potential disasters. The key actions the agency recommends are (1) identify potential disaster events, (2) create a disaster plan for sheltering in place or for evacuation, (3) assemble a disaster supplies kit, and (4) practice and maintain the plan. The disaster plan should include an emergency communications plan, a predetermined meeting place for family members or significant others, and plans for care of pets in the event that evacuation is required.

The Red Cross disaster response efforts focus on meeting the immediate disaster-related needs of affected people and providing support services to the emergency rescue and recovery workers (ARC, 2022). The disaster response functions are to provide health services, mental health services, family services, and mass care and to inquire about family well-being. Mass care involves feeding, sheltering, providing basic first aid, bulk distribution, and a Disaster Welfare Information system (ARC, 2022).

🄯 ACTIVE LEARNING

- Find out who is responsible for disaster management in your community. What plans are in place for warning people and for communicating which actions to take in the event of a disaster? Are the people aware of these plans?
- Interview the person or persons in the ARC responsible for disaster services in your area. What is the role of their disaster nurses? What are the requirements to become a disaster nurse for the ARC?
- Speak with police and fire department personnel about their responsibilities during a disaster. Do their roles during a disaster differ from their roles on a day-to-day basis? Do they have special teams and plans for biological, chemical, nuclear, or radiological incidents?

DISASTER MANAGEMENT STAGES

Prevention Stage

The first stage in disaster management occurs before a disaster is imminent and is also known as the *nondisaster stage*. Potential disaster risks should be identified and risk maps created (see Fig. 29.1). The population demographics and vulnerabilities, as well as the community's capabilities, should be analyzed. Primary prevention measures include educating the public regarding what actions to take to prepare for disasters at the individual, family, and community levels. Furthermore, on the basis of the assessment of potential risks, the community must develop a plan for meeting the potential disasters identified.

With regard to bioterrorist attacks, prevention means that healthcare providers need to be knowledgeable about the biological and chemical agents that might be used. In addition, healthcare providers must be able to recognize the signs and symptoms of the various biological and chemical agents that have been recognized as potential threats and must know what to do in the event of exposure for themselves and others. As mentioned, unlike other disasters, biochemical terrorist threats may be identified only when events raise suspicions of healthcare providers rather than by first responders at a particular site.

Early identification of ill or exposed persons, rapid implementation of preventive therapy, special infection control considerations, and collaboration or communication with the public are essential in controlling the spread of cases. Hospitals

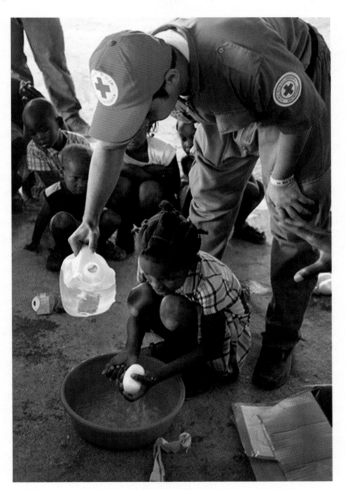

Red Cross volunteers share health and hygiene messages with young earthquake survivors. (Photo by Bonnie Gillespie/American Red Cross.)

need to identify rooms that can be converted into isolation units to meet the demand. Nurses must be instructed in decontamination and reminded of isolation techniques that might be needed, depending on the biological agent. Volunteers and professionals must remain current in first aid, CPR, and advanced lifesaving procedures.

Preparedness and Planning Stage

Individual and family preparedness involves training in first aid, assembling a disaster emergency kit, establishing a predetermined meeting place away from home, and making a family communication plan. Recommendations for what needs to be included in each of these activities are available from many sources (e.g., ARC, DHS, and FEMA). These are guidelines, and each individual and each family must modify the preparations to meet their personal needs. Nurses need to have plans and survival kits for work, family, and evacuation.

Although there will be some variation according to the individual community's needs, all community disaster plans should address the following elements: authority, communication, control, logistical coordination of personnel, supplies and equipment, evacuation, rescue, and care of the dead. The plan should indicate who has the power to declare that there is a disaster and who has the power to initiate the disaster plan.

Authority should be designated by the title of the person; it should not specify a person by name. Backup positions should also be identified in the event the first individual is not available. Every individual should be equally informed about the role and responsibilities that go with this authority. A clear chain of authority for carrying out the plan is critical for its successful implementation. Authority may change, depending on whether the disaster is natural or manmade, and change of authority should be addressed in the plan.

Communication is recognized as a very significant problem during disasters. Misinformation and misinterpretation can occur when communication is ineffective. Reliance on telephone systems or cell phones should not be the sole planned means of communicating because these may not work or the systems might be overwhelmed. The communication section of the disaster plan should address how the authority figure will be notified of the disaster, how the emergency management team members will be notified, how the community residents will be warned about the incident, and what actions to take. This section needs to address how communication between relief workers and authorities will be maintained. Also, it should include information on the role of the media in keeping people informed and in letting people know what assistance and supplies are needed.

The analysis of the population that was completed during the nondisaster stage should identify groups that need special attention as to how they will be notified. These people should be noted in advance and plans developed to meet the varied needs of these vulnerable groups. Such groups include those who speak different languages; are homeless or poor; are without television or other means of communication; and are in institutions such as prisons, nursing homes, day care settings, or schools. Effective communication during a disaster

must be credible, current, and authoritative and must give some indication of future events.

The *logistical* section should specify where supplies and equipment are located or where additional supplies and equipment can be obtained, where they will be stored or found, and how they will be transported to the disaster site (see Fig. 29.2). Essential *human resources* (e.g., emergency and disaster specialists, officials of governmental and voluntary agencies, engineers, weather specialists, and community leaders) should be identified and where they will be located together determined. The plan should include information about transportation for *evacuation and rescue* (particularly taking into account vulnerable groups), documentation and record keeping, and plans for evaluation of the success or failure of the plan.

A disaster plan is a dynamic entity. Planning is a continuous process, and the plan changes with circumstances and when gaps are identified during drills or from actual disaster incidents. The plan should set realistic expectations of effects and needs, should be brief and concise, and should establish priorities and timelines for actions. It should also follow the disaster planning principles listed in Box 29.8.

For a plan to be effective, it must be tested with different disaster scenario drills. The more times realistic scenarios are created to test the plan in actual practice sessions, and not just with tabletop or paper drills, the more problems with the plan will be identified and solutions for those problems found. Without practice drills, a plan may have many unrecognized faults, and as a result, many more individuals may be harmed and communities damaged when an actual disaster occurs.

Response Stage

The response stage begins immediately after the disaster incident occurs. The community preparedness plans that have been developed are initiated. If a disaster occurs, people should remain calm and exert patience, follow the advice of local emergency officials, and listen to the radio or television for news and instructions. If people nearby are injured, one should give first aid, seek help, and check the area for dangerous hazards. Those at home should shut off any damaged utilities, confine or secure pets, call family contact(s), and check on neighbors, especially the elderly or disabled.

The plan may call for people to shelter in place or to evacuate, or for search and rescue to begin. If the only response needed is to shelter in place, people need to know what to do if they are at home, at work, at school, or in their vehicles.

Shelter in Place

The ARC has provided explicit instructions for individuals and families to be followed when told by authorities to "**shelter in place**" in the event of a disaster. Table 29.3 shows these guidelines (CDC, 2018).

If local authorities issue a shelter-in-place communication, instructions that address what actions to take if at home, at work, at school, or in a vehicle should be followed. For example, during a disaster such as hazardous gas emission from

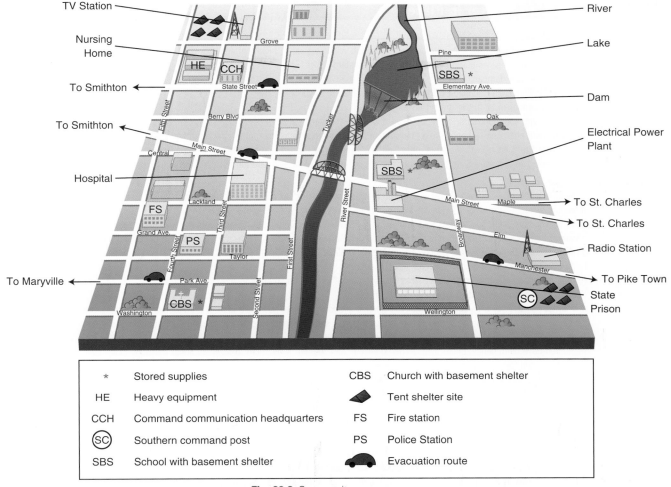

Fig. 29.2 Community resource map.

*	Stored supplies	CBS	Church with basement shelter
HE	Heavy equipment		Tent shelter site
CCH	Command communication headquarters	FS	Fire station
SC	Southern command post	PS	Police Station
SBS	School with basement shelter		Evacuation route

BOX 29.8   Disaster Planning Principles

1. Measures usually taken are not sufficient for major disasters.
2. Plans should be adjusted to people's needs.
3. Planning does not stop with development of a written plan.
4. Lack of information causes inappropriate responses by community members.
5. People should be able to respond with or without direction.
6. Plans should coordinate efforts of the entire community, so large segments of the citizenry should be involved in the planning.
7. Plans should be linked to surrounding areas.
8. Plans should be general enough to cover all potential disaster events.
9. As much as possible, plans should be based on everyday work methods and procedures.
10. Plans should specify a person's responsibility for implementing segments by position or title rather than by name.
11. Plans should develop a record-keeping system before a disaster occurs regarding:
    - Supplies and equipment
    - Records of all present at any given time (to account for everyone and to identify the missing)
    - Identification of victims and deceased, conditions and treatment documented, and to which facility victims are sent
12. Backup plans need to be in place for the following:
    - Disruption of telephone and cell phone lines
    - Disruption of computer data (should be downloaded weekly and stored off-site)
    - Protecting essential public health functions (e.g., vital records and communicable disease data)

an industrial plant, anyone at home, at a business, or in a public building, may be instructed to go inside and follow home or work shelter-in-place recommendations (i.e., close doors, turn off fans and air conditioning, bring children and pets inside, and stay inside until "all clear" has been called).

Evacuation

Each community should have established evacuation routes for the residents to use if evacuation from the area is necessary. In some instances, mandatory evacuation may be implemented. However, there are always some individuals who will not leave

TABLE 29.3   How to Shelter in Place

Location	Instructions
At home	Close and lock all windows and exterior doors close the window shades, blinds, or curtains
	Turn off fans, heating, ventilation, or air conditioning system
	Close the fireplace damper
	Get your family disaster supplies kit and make sure the radio is working
	Go into an interior room above ground level
	Bring pets with you along with additional food and water for them
	Use duct tape and plastic sheeting (e.g., heavy-duty plastic garbage bags) to seal all cracks around the door and any vents into the room;
	A hard-wired telephone in the room is ideal; call your emergency contact and have the phone available
	Keep listening to the radio or television until told all is safe or told to evacuate (do not evacuate unless instructed to do so).
At school	Close the school
	Activate the school's emergency plan and follow reverse evacuation procedures to bring students, faculty, visitors, and staff indoors
	If visitors are in the building, provide for their safety by asking them to stay—not leave.
	Have all children, staff, and visitors take shelter in preselected rooms (preferably interior rooms about the ground floor with the fewest windows or vents. That have phone access, stored disaster supply kits, and, preferably, access to a bathroom; provide a way to communicate among all rooms where people are sheltering in place
	Bring everyone into the room(s); shut and lock the door
	Provide directions to close and lock all windows, exterior doors, and any other openings to the outside
	Seal doors and vents with duct tape and plastic sheeting
	If it is not possible for a person to monitor the telephone and the school has voice mail or an automated attendant, change the recording to indicate that the school is closed and that students and staff are remaining in the building until authorities say it is safe to leave
	Turn off heating, ventilating, and air-conditioning systems
	If children have cell phones, allow them to use them to call a parent or guardian to let them know that they have been asked to remain in school until further notice and that they are safe
	A teacher or staff member in each room should write down the names of everyone in the room and call the designated contact to report who is in that room
	Listen for an official announcement from school officials via the public address system.
	Everyone should stay in the room until school officials announce that all is safe or say everyone must evacuate.
At work	Close the office or business
	If there are customers, clients or visitors in the building, provide for their safety by asking the m to stay (not leave)
	Close and lock all windows, exterior doors, and any other openings to the outside
	A knowledgeable person should use the building's mechanical systems to turn off all heating, ventilating, and air-conditioning systems (systems that automatically provide for exchange of inside air with outside air, in particular, need to be turned off, sealed, or disabled)
	Gather essential disaster supplies (e.g., nonperishable food, bottled water, radios, first aid supplies, flashlights, duct tape, plastic sheeting)
	Select interior room(s) above the ground floor, with the fewest window or vents; when everyone is in, shut and lock the doors
	A hard-wired telephone in the room is ideal
	Turn on call-forwarding or alternative telephone answering systems or services; close any window shades, blinds, or curtains
	Write down names of everyone in the room and call the business's designate emergency contact to report who is in the room
	Monitor radios or TVs for updates until you are told all is safe or you are told to evacuate.
In a vehicle	If very close to home, workplace, or a public building, go there immediately and go inside and follow the shelter in place advice.
	If unable to get indoors quickly and safely, stop the vehicle in the safest place possible (e.g., stop under a bridge or in a shady spot to avoid being overheated)
	Turn off the engine and close windows and vents
	If possible, seal the heating, ventilating, and air-conditioning vents with duct tape or anything else you may have available;
	Listen to the radio periodically for updated advice and instructions
	Stay in place until you are told it is safe to get back on the road, and follow the directions of law enforcement officials.

Modified from American Red Cross: *Shelter-in-place during a chemical or radiation emergency*, 2006. Modified from: shelterinplace.pdf (red-cross.org).

their homes for any number of reasons (e.g., fear of vandalism, denial of the potential extent of the disaster, pride in home and belongings). Education of residents as to the potential damage, deaths, and injuries that will be incurred from the potential disasters that may affect their community needs to be accomplished during the preparedness stage and not when evacuation is ordered. In some extreme cases, it may be necessary for hospitals and other facilities, such as nursing homes, to evacuate patients. This procedure requires significant advance planning, because health practitioners must determine how to move seriously ill, and even critically ill, people and coordinate transportation and placement for their disposition to safe facilities.

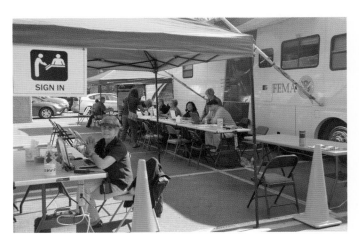

A FEMA mobile disaster recovery unit travels around the state of Georgia to offer assistance in the aftermath of Hurricane Matthew. (Photo by Gary Petty/FEMA.)

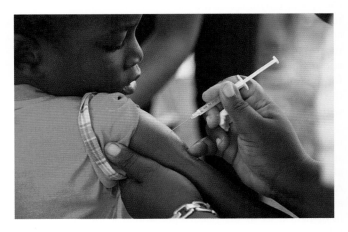

Between February 8 and March 9, 2010, 125,000 earthquake survivors in Port-au-Prince, Haiti, were vaccinated against measles, diphtheria, pertussis, and tetanus. (Photo by Bonnie Gillespie/American Red Cross.)

Search and Rescue

Before search and rescue begin, safety must be considered. In some instances, if a criminal action is suspected as part of the disaster, law officials will be among the first to respond in order to secure the area and possibly gather evidence. While the area is being checked and then cleared of potential threats, a staging area can be set up at or near the site of the incident to direct on-site activities. Search for and rescue of victims can begin once clearance is given, a disaster triage area is established, and an emergency treatment area is set up to provide first aid until transportation for victims to hospitals or healthcare facilities for treatment can be coordinated (Fig. 29.3).

The National Incident Command System (NIMS)

The NIMS is a federal mandate to coordinate, organize the command system and response to a disaster. The incident command structure (ICS) offers an organized approach during a disaster (FEMA, 2022a).

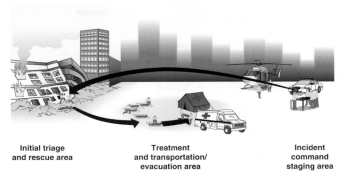

Fig. 29.3 Areas of operation of disaster response.

Initial triage and rescue area · Treatment and transportation/ evacuation area · Incident command staging area

Staging Area

The staging area is the on-site incident command station. The Incident commander is the person in charge and is usually the highest ranked person in the fire service. They are responsible for assigning personnel to each of the sectors.

Disaster responders should report to this area to "check in" so that everyone is accounted for and can be given an assignment. This arrangement allows for the most effective use of the skills and abilities of those responding. No one should go to the disaster site unless directed to do so by the staging area commander. The staging area is also where the authority rests for decisions as to the need for additional resources to manage the disaster incident. Such resources include construction equipment to move building materials; rescue dogs to locate humans who are buried in the debris; and more fire, police, or medical personnel. The Medical Command is normally staffed by an emergency or EMS physician. This person will assign personnel to the Triage, Treatment or Transportation Sector.

Triage Sector

The first sector under the Incident Command System is known as the Disaster Sector. Triage is identifying and separating individuals quickly according to injury severity and treatment needed. Disaster triage focuses on sorting the greatest number of people as fast as possible. Triage performed at the site and again at the treatment area is very different from triage that is routinely conducted in the emergency department. The focus of **disaster triage** is to do the greatest good, for the greatest number, in the shortest time. One triage system that is used by first responders is START system of triage, which stands for "simple triage and rapid treatment." This system describes what to do when first arriving at a multiple casualty or MCI. Disaster triage of an injured person should occur in less than 1 min. This system also describes how to use people with minor injuries to help. As a decision is made regarding the status of an individual, the person is labeled with a colored triage ribbon (Fig. 29.4).

Green on the triage ribbon is for the walking wounded or those with minor injuries (e.g., cuts and abrasions) who can wait several hours before they receive treatment; yellow is for those with systemic but not yet life-threatening complications who can wait 45 to 60 min (e.g., simple fractures); red is considered top

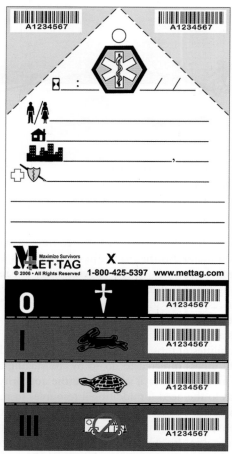

Fig. 29.4 Disaster triage ribbon.

priority or immediate and is for those who have life-threatening conditions but who can be stabilized and have a high probability of survival (e.g., amputations); black is for the deceased or for those whose injuries are is so extensive that nothing can be done to save them (e.g., multiple severe injuries). A new classification of victim, those who are contaminated, will require a hazmat (for "hazardous materials") ribbon.

To assess an individual within the one-minute guideline, the START system uses three characteristics. First, respiration is checked; if the rate is more than 30 per minute, the individual is tagged red or immediate. If the rate is fewer than 30 per minute, the assessor moves to the second step, *perfusion*. The assessor pinches the nail bed and observes the reaction. Color should return to normal within 2 s; if it takes longer, the person is tagged red or immediate. The third step is checking mental status. If the person is able to answer a question, he or she is tagged yellow; the person not able to answer a question is tagged red or immediate. By doing these steps, the individual responsible for triage can very quickly assess an individual and decide which color ribbon fits his or her condition. Furthermore, the steps are easy to remember with the mnemonic "30—2—can do," in which "30" is the number of respirations, "2" is the number of seconds needed to check for perfusion, and "can do" relates to checking mental status.

Treatment Sector

The treatment sector personnel set up a four tarps system (green, yellow, red, and black) while victims are being triaged so they are ready to receive the victims once the process has been completed. After victims are triaged, they are moved to the treatment sector by litter bearers and triage personal. When the victim arrives at the treatment sector that corresponds to their ribbon color, medical personnel reassess the victim and document their findings on a treatment tag. This treatment tag is the official disaster medical documentation tool and will follow the victim all the way to the hospital. Of note, some systems are starting to use electronic treatment tags. Care is rendered as needed and then the transportation sector personnel will move the victim to higher or lower level of care as appropriate.

Transport Sector

The transportation sector leader has many roles including patient transportation unit leader, medical communication, staging area manager, ground ambulance coordinator, and air ambulance coordinator. A variety of transportation methods are used to move patients including ambulances, helicopters, "Ambuses," and regular commercial buses (e.g., commuter buses especially for the walking wounded victims). Victims are usually moved to the higher level of care or to an area where they can be reunited with their families.

In many instances, while search and rescue missions are taking place, other agencies (e.g., public health agencies) are surveilling for threats such as contaminated water, vectors, and air quality. They also disseminate data on findings and then relate health information to officials, the media, and the public as appropriate. Designated agencies gather epidemiological information as to the occurrence and distribution of health-related events associated with the disaster, describe factors contributing to health-related effects, and assess the needs of populations and facilities. They then allocate resources and work to prevent further adverse health problems that might result from the disaster. Resources may be allocated to offer protection to those supporting relief efforts such as gloves and other protective gear as first responders and some of the victims may be exposed potentially harmful substances during evacuation. For example, after Hurricane Katrina, public health officials administered tetanus and hepatitis A immunizations to rescuers and victims.

Although triage of individuals exposed to chemical agents is basically the same as for any multiple or MCI, it poses special challenges. For these events, the triage area is set up in the "hot zone" to assist in determining priorities for resuscitation, decontamination, pharmacological therapy, and site evacuation. Only specially trained emergency personnel who are familiar with chemical agents and the use of personal protection equipment should triage victims of a chemical agent. The same triage categories can be assigned to these victims.

Psychological triage presents the challenge of determining who most needs help and deciding what interventions will help.

Mental health disorders related to disasters include anxiety disorders, exacerbation of existing substance abuse problems, somatic complaints, depression, and later, posttraumatic stress disorder (PTSD). Risks for PTSD include living through dangerous events or traumas; having a history of mental illness; getting hurt; seeing people hurt or killed; feeling horror, helplessness, or extreme fear; having little or no social support after the event; and dealing with extra stress after the event, such as loss of a loved one, pain and injury, or loss of a job or home. Research has identified four key indicators to gauge the mental health impact of such events. Any two of the following factors may result in severe, lasting, and pervasive psychological effects. The key factors include (1) extreme and widespread property damage; (2) serious and ongoing financial problems; (3) high prevalence of trauma in the form of injuries, threat to life, and loss of life; and (4) when human intent caused the disaster. In addition, panic during the disaster, horror, separation from family, and relocation or displacement are factors that may play a part in psychological impairment. Nurses need to continue to evaluate an individual's risk to self or others throughout the disaster.

Box 29.9 is a list of positive coping strategies for survivors in the event of a disaster.

Community Responses to a Disaster
Heroic Phase

The classic four phases of a community's reaction to a disaster include the following: (1) the heroic phase, (2) the honeymoon phase, (3) the disillusionment phase, and (4) the reconstruction phase. During the heroic phase, nearly everyone feels the need to rush to help people survive the disaster. Medical personnel may work hours without sleep, under very dangerous and life-threatening conditions, in order to take care of their patients. Medical personnel may help out in areas with which they are not familiar and have no experience. Disaster Medical Assistance Teams (D-MAT) consist of professional and para-professional medical personnel, who provide emergency relief during a disaster and may travel long distances to help. This was illustrated by the thousands of people who volunteered to help in the immediate aftermaths of September 11 and Hurricanes Katrina and Rita.

Honeymoon Phase

Individuals who have survived the disaster gather together with others who have simultaneously experienced the same event; this is known as the *honeymoon phase.* People begin to tell their stories and review over and over again what has occurred. Bonds are formed among victims and healthcare workers. Gratitude is expressed for being alive.

Disillusionment Phase

When time has elapsed and a delay in receiving help or failure to receive the promised aid has not occurred, feelings of despair arise. Medical personnel and other first responders may begin to experience depression due to exhaustion from many long days of long hours. Depression may set in as a result of knowledge about what has happened to the community, friends, and family. People realize the way things were before the disaster is not the way things are now and may never be again. They recognize that many things are different and much needs to be done to adjust to the current situation.

Reconstruction Phase

Once the community has restored some of the buildings, businesses, homes, and services and some sense of normality is returning, feelings of despair subside. Counseling support for victims and helpers may need to be initiated to help people recover more fully. During this phase, people begin to look to the future.

Common Reactions to a Disaster

The reactions of individuals to a disaster vary greatly. Table 29.4 lists some of the more commonly encountered emotional, cognitive, physical, and interpersonal reactions to a disaster that someone may experience.

Posttraumatic Stress Disorder

The reactions mentioned usually resolve in 1 to 3 months after the disaster event, but, in some cases, may lead to PTSD. PTSD

BOX 29.9   **Positive and Maladaptive Coping Strategies**
Positive Coping Strategies
• Relaxation methods (muscular relaxation, deep breathing, meditation)
• Exercise in moderation
• Talking to another person for support
• Getting adequate rest
• Positive distracting activities
• Trying to maintain a normal schedule (if appropriate)
• Scheduling pleasant activities
• Eating healthy meals
• Taking breaks
• Spending time with others
• Keeping a journal
• Participating in a support group
• Seeking counseling
Maladaptive Coping Strategies
• Use of alcohol or drugs to cope
• Social isolation and withdrawal
• Extreme avoidance of thinking or talking about the event
• "Workaholism"
• Anger or violence

From VA National Center for PTSD: *Psychosocial treatment of disaster-related mental health problems,* 2010.

NATURAL AND MANMADE DISASTERS

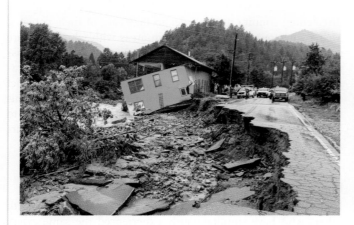

The devastation of the tsunami that occurred in Indonesia in December 2004 (Copyright Associated Press.)

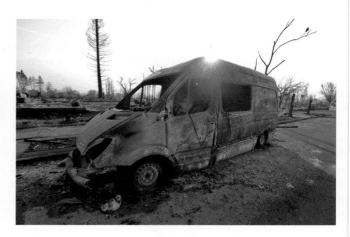

Many homes and vehicles were destroyed in a wildfire in Santa Rosa, California, in October 2017. (Photo by Dominic Del Vecchio/FEMA.)

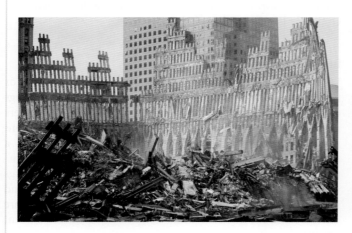

The remaining section of the World Trade Center, New York, City, is surrounded by a mountain of rubble after the September 11, 2001, terrorist attacks. (Photo by Bri Rodriguez/FEMA News Photo.)

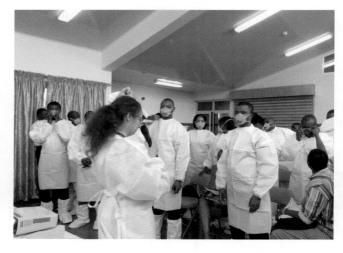

CDC personnel in Sierra Leone teach the proper use of personal protective equipment (PPE) for those working with Ebola patients. (Photo by CDC.)

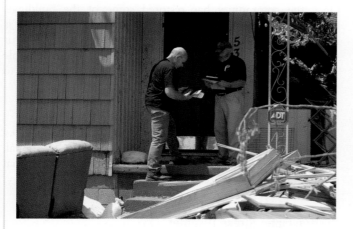

FEMA disaster survivor assistance team members are "boots on the ground," passing out information after tornado devastation in Alabama, 2014.

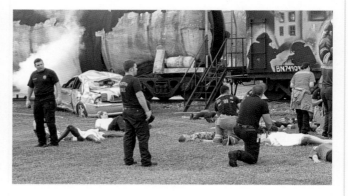

Houston Fire Department cadets and nursing students as victims and providers for a mass casualty drill.

DISASTER RELIEF: HURRICANE HARVEY, AUGUST/SEPTEMBER 2017

When Hurricane Harvey hit the Gulf Coast in late August 2017, more than 30,000 evacuees from the area sought shelter—the vast majority were evacuated to the Houston metropolitan area. Two huge shelters and many smaller shelters were set up to accommodate those displaced, and the needs, as was documented in the media, were massive.

- More than 1 million relief items were distributed.
- More than 3.1 million meals and snacks were served.
- Immediate financial assistance was offered to nearly 320,000 severely affected households.
- More than 98,000 health and mental health contacts were made.
- More than 413,000 people stayed in overnight shelters.

Faculty, staff, and students from the University of Texas Health Science Center at Houston (UT—Houston), personnel from the city and county health departments, and local emergency medical services personnel were joined by thousands of volunteers to care for these disaster victims. Doctors, nurses, and other healthcare providers came to help from across Texas as far away as California, Arizona, Illinois, and New York. To care for the health needs of the evacuees, a clinic was established in the Houston's George R. Brown Convention Center. The clinic was modeled after army field hospitals, with a command center, triage areas, and various clinics. There were sections for trauma and acute care, adult medical care, women's/gynecological care, and pediatric care, as well as an area for people with mental health concerns. A full-service pharmacy was also set up.

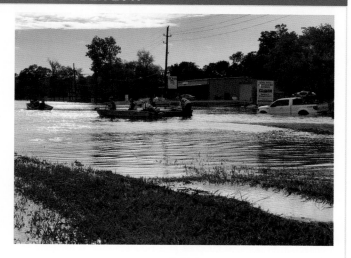

The "Cajun Navy" (civilian boat owners from across the region and even beyond) rescued thousands of stranded people during Hurricane Harvey, September 1, 2017. (Photo courtesy Scott McEwen.)

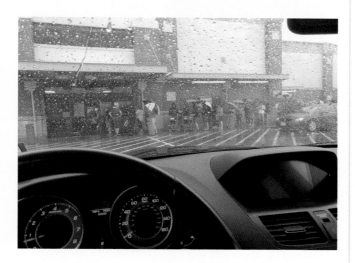

People waiting to get supplies during Hurricane Harvey.

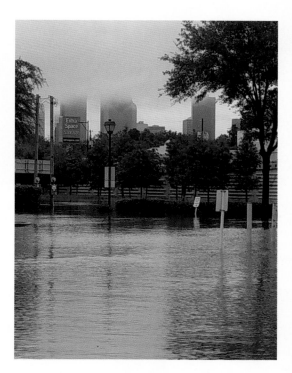

This is the morning after Hurricane Harvey. Most Houston streets were flooded, leading to many water rescues.

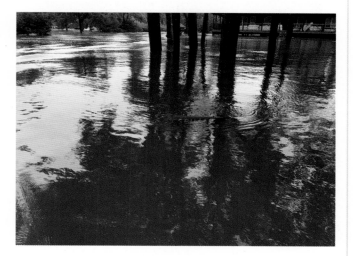

Floodwaters from Hurricane Harvey reached higher than this street sign. (Photo courtesy Scott McEwen.)

Continued

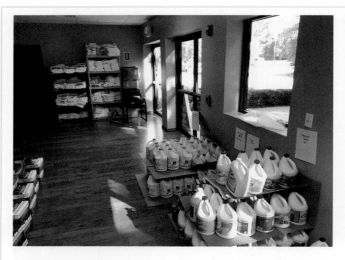

A collection of donated supplies at a Houston church to assist residents with cleanup. (Photo courtesy Scott McEwen.)

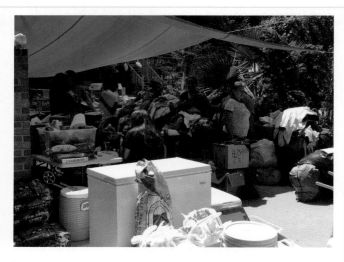

Community-based donation site in one neighborhood hard-hit by Harvey, September 2, 2017. (Photo courtesy Scott McEwen.)

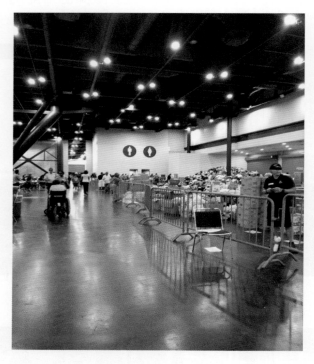

Supplies for evacuees at the George R. Brown Convention Center.

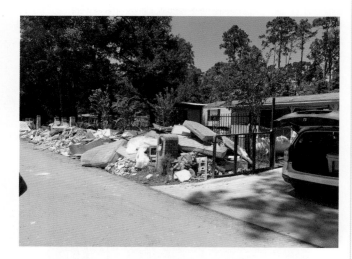

In many neighborhoods, homes were completely destroyed and families were forced to discard all their belongings. Flooded houses had to be taken down to the studs/framing with all appliances, cabinets, sheetrock, and windows removed. Massive piles of debris lined the streets. Houston, Texas, September 2, 2017. (Photo courtesy Scott McEwen.)

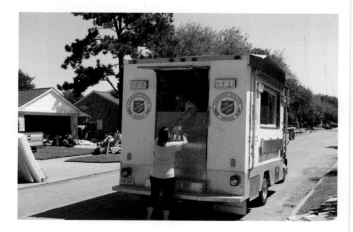

Salvation Army volunteers distribute food to survivors of Hurricane Harvey, September 8, 2017. (Photo by Steve Zumwalt/FEMA.)

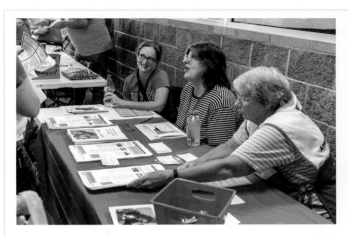

Red Cross volunteers distribute information to survivors of Hurricane Harvey, September 16, 2017. (Photo by Steve Zumwalt/FEMA.)

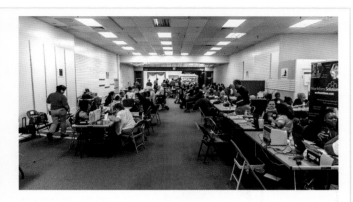

A disaster recovery center in a downtown Houston mall, September 20, 2017. (Photo by Steve Zumwalt/FEMA.)

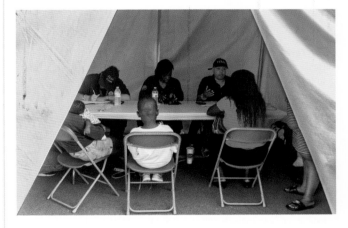

FEMA representatives offer relief to a family of survivors, September 16, 2017. (Photo by Steve Zumwalt/FEMA.)

is a psychiatric disorder that can occur after an individual experiences or witnesses a life-threatening event, such as a disaster. Men and women, adults and children, and all socioeconomic groups can experience PTSD. People who have the disorder often relive the experience through nightmares and flashbacks. The social and psychological symptoms mentioned in Table 29.4 can be severe enough and last long enough to significantly impair a person's daily life. If PTSD occurs in conjunction with related disorders (e.g., depression, substance abuse, and other problems of physical and mental health), the situation becomes more complicated. Individuals experiencing PTSD require medical attention (National Institute of Mental Health, 2022).

❓ ACTIVE LEARNING

1. What social and cultural factors need to be considered in disaster planning in your community? Are there vulnerable populations with special needs (e.g., homeless, imprisoned, mobility impaired)? If evacuation of the community is mandated, have plans for evacuation of these groups been made?
2. Create an emergency plan for yourself, your family, or both. What factors would you consider in deciding whether to stay or leave your home? If evacuation were mandated, what important documents and mementos would you need to take with you?
3. What emergency supplies does your healthcare facility have available in the event of a disaster? What provisions have been made available for vulnerable patients when there is no electricity? How would patients be evacuated from the facility to safe shelters?

CASE STUDY   Application of the Community Assessment Process

Coastal City: Preparedness for Disaster

Assessment

Deer Park, Texas, is a city 20 miles east of Houston, Texas. The population is approximately 32,000 people. The majority of the people are white (80.8%) and Hispanic (15.2%). The median age of the population is 34.7 years, and the median income $61,334. Eighty-nine percent of the population older than 25 years has a high school diploma or higher education degree. The unemployment rate is 5.6%. The city consists of residential homes, apartment complexes, and retail and service businesses. There are nine schools and several churches of all denominations. Many AM and FM radio stations and TV broadcast stations are available to the Deer Park area.

The Federal Communications Commission (FCC) has developed the Emergency Alert System to warn of any emergency (nuclear attack, hurricane, tornado, flood, or chemical release). The FCC has designated KTRH 740 a.m. as the station for the Houston area. The city has a volunteer fire department (5 full-time employees) and a city police department (55 full-time employees). The city government consists of a mayor, city council, and city manager. The city has two emergency committees: the Community Awareness and Emergency Response Committee and the Local Emergency Planning Committee.

There are no hospitals in Deer Park. The closest hospitals are six—seven miles away and take 20 min to reach. The closest level 1 trauma center is 15 miles away, and the nearest adult care burn center is 20 miles away; the pediatric burn center is in Galveston, Texas, which is about 45 miles away.

The city is also the home of the Deer Park Chemical Plant and the Deer Park Refining Company. The company processes 3% of the nation's oil supply into gasoline. The plants are located on 1500 acres in the Houston Ship Channel. The company employs approximately 1100 people and 2200 contract workers. The chemical plant and the refining company have their own fire stations, an internal railroad, docks and transportation networks, small medical facilities (one physician and four nurses, 7 days a week, 24 h a day), first responder teams, two ambulances, and a vehicle that can handle 30 casualties.

Diagnosis

Individual

Because of Deer Park's location on the Gulf Coast and the presence of the Deer Park Refining Company and Deer Park Chemical Plant, the residents are at risk for injury or death due to hurricane disasters and potential industrial incidents from either accidental or terrorist causes.

Family

The families of Deer Park are at risk for losing their homes, separation from family members, and having to evacuate from their homes either temporarily or permanently due to hurricane damages or industrial accidents.

Community

The community of Deer Park is at risk for destruction of buildings and city public works due to hurricane disasters and potential explosions from either accidental or terrorist causes.

Planning

Disaster Management

Deer Park is in the storm surge zone, requiring its residents to evacuate when a category 1 hurricane is predicted to land in or within a 100-mile radius of the Deer Park area. The media sources available to the Deer Park area or the city officials are to give instructions about supplies and equipment to have ready and when to leave. Only one evacuation route is available to the community.

A survey was conducted during the nondisaster stage to identify vulnerable groups that would need help in evacuating.

Individual

Vulnerable individuals who would need to have special consideration for evacuation are the very young (4000 individuals between birth and 10 years), the elderly (2110 individuals aged 65 years and over), and families below the poverty level (1200). It was determined that more than 7000 individuals might need some form of transportation in order to evacuate.

Long-Term Goal

- Residents will have a disaster kit prepared according to ARC and FEMA guidelines.

Short-Term Goals

- Residents will follow officials' instructions for sheltering in place or evacuation.
- Vulnerable individuals will know what to do in the event of an evacuation order or shelter-in-place announcement.

Family

Long-Term Goal

- Family members will continually update their family disaster plans according to family dynamics.

Short-Term Goals

- Families will have a disaster plan in place for communicating.
- Families will have a disaster kit in place to accommodate each family member for a period of at least 3 days.

Community

Long-Term Goals

- Additional evacuation routes will be identified for area residents.
- Central meeting locations will be identified for those needing transportation assistance for evacuation.

Short-Term Goal

- School buses will be used for evacuation of vulnerable individuals and families who need transportation.
- Other sources must be identified that could be called upon to provide transportation.
- School bus drivers should be able to include their family members on the buses with others being evacuated so the drivers will not have to worry about their families.
- If all individuals follow instructions, there should be no injuries to or deaths of Deer Park residents from a hurricane or related storm surge. Homes may be damaged or destroyed, but no lives should be lost. With the help of local, state, and possibly federal agencies, the community should recover.

Long-Term Goal

- City officials will continually update the community disaster plan as gaps are identified and keep the residents informed as the plan changes.

Onsite Management

The following figure summarizes the disaster plan in place for the Deer Park plants for handling any industrial accident that occurs on their property.

CASE STUDY Application of the Community Assessment Process—cont'd

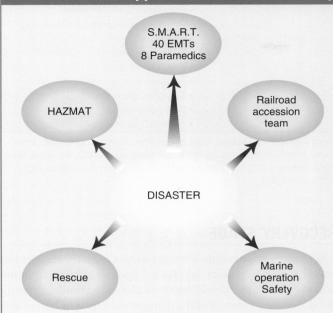

The company has annual drills with the Harris County's Emergency Management and Channel Industries Mutual Aid organization to evaluate emergency response. This group is the company's direct link to support in the event of a disaster. Many buildings on the property can serve as shelters, and no visitor or employee is allowed on the property without having a "safe shelter map" in his or her possession. If an explosion occurs that is confined to the property, and only minor casualties result, the resources available should be sufficient to manage the disaster.

The company has developed a buffer zone between the plants and the city of Deer Park. However, if fumes were to escape as a result of the explosion, a shelter-in-place warning would be issued for Deer Park residents through a specific six-sound message system. Chemical products that are used and that might potentially escape are benzene, toluene, solvent xylene, isoprene butadiene, sulfur, phenol, hydrogen sulfide, and asbestos. Citizens would be advised about actions to take according to the chemical released. Most plants have also installed dedicated fiber-optic telephone lines so that the city and industry can stay in touch even when normal phone circuits are overloaded or out of service.

Community and Local Response Preparedness

Deer Park's police and fire dispatchers have been trained on how to handle calls from industries about a chemical release and how to quickly activate the city's emergency warning systems. The local emergency planning committee has adopted a leveled community awareness and emergency response system to categorize the severity of each chemical release. Level 1 is information only, level 2 is standby alert, and level 3 is full emergency condition, with sheltering in place required. The final level is "all clear." Deer Park has a website featuring Wally Wise Guy, who gives instructions to the citizens about what to do if a shelter-in-place emergency is issued.

The local emergency planning committee hired a consulting group to study the impact of toxic substances on the community to ensure that shelter-in-place procedures are adequate for protecting the residents. The consulting group recommended that each home in the region have a shelter-in-place kit containing 2- to 3-inch—wide masking tape, plastic film or sheets, towels or sheets for sealing under doors, battery-powered radio and extra batteries, flashlight and extra batteries, and bottled water stored inside a designated shelter-in-place room.

The Deer Park Communications Subcommittee works with others to develop detailed procedures on how to notify and warn the public of a chemical release. The city and local industry have invested in six state-of-the-art systems to provide reliable and redundant warning to homes, schools, businesses, and visitors. Siren-type alarms have been mounted on utility poles throughout the city. This system is used only for chemical emergencies, not for tornadoes, hurricanes, or other types of emergencies. In addition, the city has contracted with First Call Interactive Network, an automated telephone notification network that can ring the telephones of homes and businesses in the immediate danger area to give prerecorded instructions about what to do.

Evaluation
Individuals and Families
- Before a hurricane, all residents will be evacuated.
- All vulnerable individuals and families will be evacuated to shelters.
- All residents will know and respond to shelter-in-place warnings as indicated by the siren-type alarm system in place.

Community
- City officials will evaluate and continually update the community disaster plan as gaps are identified.
- Community residents will remain informed and prepared.

The city of Deer Park and the Deer Park plants have detailed plans for prevention, preparedness, and response in the event of an industrial accident. In that event, evaluation of the plan will take place to identify gaps and make appropriate changes. A plan needs to be in place for hurricane preparedness of the plants to avoid industrial accidents, and the plan evaluated for effectiveness. Drills are conducted to test their industrial accident plans; they provide training of personnel; they have identified sites for shelters both on the company property and in the city; and they have elaborate notification and warning systems in place.

Areas that need to be enhanced include readily available city health resources (lack of a nearby trauma hospital or burn center to care for the types of injuries that would occur). Plans for preparing the plants for hurricanes and evacuation need to be developed and made available to the workers.

Prevention
Primary
- Perform periodic education of area residents regarding warning systems in place and appropriate response to take should they be implemented.
- Perform periodic review of plans in response to changing demographics.

Secondary
- Check credentials of first responders for currency.
- Screen first responders for training needs and preparedness to take action during disasters.

Tertiary
- Institute building codes that will reduce the amount of damage to infrastructures.

TABLE 29.4 Common Responses to a Traumatic Event

Cognitive	• Poor concentration • Confusion • Disorientation • Indecisiveness • Shortened attention span • Memory loss • Unwanted memories • Difficulty making decisions
Emotional	• Shock • Numbness • Feeling overwhelmed • Depression • Feeling lost • Fear of harm to self and/or loved ones • Feeling nothing • Feeling abandoned • Uncertainty of feelings • Volatile emotions
Physical	• Nausea • Lightheadedness • Dizziness • Gastrointestinal problems • Rapid heart rate • Tremors • Headaches • Grinding of teeth • Fatigue • Poor sleep • Pain • Hyperarousal • Jumpiness
Behavioral	• Suspicion • Irritability • Arguments with friends and loved ones • Withdrawal • Excessive silence • Inappropriate humor • Increased/decreased eating • Change in sexual desire or functioning • Increased smoking • Increased substance use or abuse

From Centers for Disease Control and Prevention: *Coping with a traumatic event: information for health professionals,* 2005. Available from: https://www.cdc.gov/masstrauma/factsheets/professionals/coping_professional.pdf.

RECOVERY STAGE

The recovery stage begins when the danger from the disaster has passed and all local, state, and federal agencies are present in the area to help victims rebuild their lives and the community restore public services. Cleanup of the damage and repair of homes and businesses begin. Evaluation and revision of the disaster plans based on lessons learned from the experience are made. Understanding the financial impact on the community and agencies involved is essential in developing future public health policy.

Research is needed on all aspects of prevention, preparedness, response, and recovery stages of disasters. Research is also needed on the education and training needs of first responders, healthcare providers, and community populations. Nurse researchers, in partnership with researchers from other disciplines, can play a significant role in conducting research on disaster management.

SUMMARY

Communities must be aware of potential disasters that may affect their residents. Comprehensive disaster plans need to be developed at all levels of government and by all communities, families, and individuals. Having disaster plans in place increases the likelihood of an effective response, resulting in saved lives and minimized destruction to the community.

Nurses have a role in, and contribution to make, at every stage of disaster management. Nurses need to have personal and professional plans in place for any disaster. All medical personnel must keep their credentials current and must learn the signs and symptoms of exposure to weapons of mass destruction so that they will recognize people who may have been exposed. They should learn what injuries may be sustained from various disasters and know which types of disasters are most likely to affect their communities so that disaster triage and treatment can save lives. Finally, they must take drills in their respective healthcare facilities seriously. The more prepared the population and healthcare providers are for all kinds of disasters, the fewer lives will be lost.

EVOLVE WEBSITE

http://evolve.elsevier.com/Nies/community

- NCLEX Review Questions
- Case Studies

BIBLIOGRAPHY

18 U.S. code 18 U.S. code § 2331: *Definitions*. 1992.

Adini B, Goldberg A, Cohen R, Laor D, Bar-Dayan Y: Evidence-based support for the all-hazards approach to emergency preparedness, *Isr J Health Pol Res* 1(1):40, 2012. https://doi.org/10.1186/2045-4015-1-40.

American Red Cross (ARC): *Our federal charter*, 2022. Available from: https://www.redcross.org/about-us/who-we-are/history/federal-charter.html-.

American Red Cross (ARC): *Disaster service program review, fiscal year 2020*, 2021. Available from: https://www.redcross.org/local/florida/central-florida/about-us/news-and-events/press-releases/2020-year-in-review.html–.

Beerens R, Duyvis M, Heus R: *Aftermath crisis management—phase I - Acrimas - D3.1 threat/hazard map for EU CM*, 2012.

Berger E: *Ten years ago, Houston was a living hell*, 2015. Available from: https://blog.chron.com/weather/2015/09/ten-years-ago-houston-was-a-living-hell/.

Centers for Disease Control and Prevention: *Looking back: a local emergency response to the 2010 Haiti earthquake*, 2015. https://blogs.cdc.gov/publichealthmatters/2015/10/looking-back-a-local-emergency-response-to-the-2010-haiti-earthquake/.

Centers for disease Control and Prevention: *Facts about sheltering in place*, 2018. https://emergency.cdc.gov/planning/Shelteringfacts.asp.

Centers for Disease Control and Prevention: *Emergency preparedness and response*, 2022. Available from: https://www.cdc.gov/disasters/index.html–.

Central Intelligence Agency: *Terrorism FAQs*, 2022. Available from: https://www.cia.gov/the-world-factbook/references/terrorist-organizations/.

Chettle C: Recognizing bioterrorism: nurses on the frontline, *Nurse-Week* 6:29—30, 2001.

DeNolf RL, Kahwaji CI: *EMS mass casualty management*, Treasure Island (FL), 2018, StatPearls Publishing.

Federal Bureau of Investigation: *What we investigate: terrorism*, 2022. Available from: https://www.fbi.gov/investigate/terrorism.

Federal Emergence Management Agency: *Emergency Management - Presidential Policy Directive*, 2021. Available from: National Preparedness, FEMA.gov.

Federal Emergency Management Agency: *National incident management system*, 2022. Available from: https://training.fema.gov/nims/.

Federal Emergency Management Agency: *Post-Katrina Emergency Management Reform Act*, 2022. Available from: https://www.congress.gov/bill/109th-congress/senate-bill/3721.

Federal Emergency Management Agency: *Are you ready?* 2022. Available from: https://www.ready.gov/sites/default/files/2021-11/are-you-ready-guide.pdf.

Federal Emergency Management Agency: *What is mitigation?* 2022. Available from: https://www.fema.gov/emergency-managers/risk-management/hazard-mitigation-planning.

Landesman LY, Burke RV: *Landesman's public health management of disasters: the practice guide*, ed 4, Washington, DC, 2017, American Public Health Association.

Levin M: *How Hurricane Rita anxiety led to the worst gridlock in Houston history*, 2015. Available from: https://www.chron.com/news/houston-texas/houston/article/Hurricane-Rita-anxiety-leads-to-hellish-fatal-6521994.php.

Medlin J, Ball R, Beeler G: *Extremely powerful hurricane Katrina leaves a historic mark on the Northern Gulf Coast*, 2016. Available from: https://www.weather.gov/mob/katrina.

Morris M: *Katrina evacuees fled to Houston*, 2016. Available from: https://www.chron.com/local/history/major-stories-events/article/Katrina-evacuees-fled-to-Houston-9974175.php.

National Institute of Mental Health: *Post-traumatic stress disorder (PTSD)*, 2022. Available from: https://www.nimh.nih.gov/health/topics/post-traumatic-stress-disorder-ptsd-.

National Oceanic and Atmospheric Administration, National Weather Service, National Hurricane Center: *Saffir-Simpson hurricane wind scale*, 2022. Available from: https://www.nhc.noaa.gov/aboutsshws.php.

National Oceanic and Atmospheric Administration: *National Hurricane Center tropical cyclone report Hurricane Harvey*, 2017. Available from: https://www.nhc.noaa.gov/data/tcr/AL092017_Harvey.pdf.

Robert Wood Johnson Foundation (RWJF): *When disaster strikes*, 2016. Available from: When Disaster Strikes: Nurse Leadership, Nursing Care, and Teamwork Save Lives - RWJF.

Ready.gov: *Citizen corps*, 2022. Available at: https://www.ready.gov/citizen-corps.

Ritchie H, Roser M: *Natural disasters*, 2021. Available from: https://ourworldindata.org/natural-disasters#natural-disasters-kill-on-average-60-000-people-per-year-and-are-responsible-for-0-1-of-global-deaths.

Schmidt R: *Parade became a nightmare: 5 dead, 48 injured after SUV barrels through Waukesha Christmas Parade*, 2021. Available from: https://cbs58.com/news/police-confirm-5-dead-and-more-than-40-injured-after-car-barrels-through-waukesha-holiday-parade.

Severin PN, Jacobson PA: Types of disasters. In Goodhue CJ, Blake N, editors: *Nursing Management of Pediatric Disaster*, 2020, Springer International Publishing, pp 85—197.

State of California: *Cal fire—active incidents*, 2021. Available from: https://www.fire.ca.gov/incidents/2021/.

Texas Disaster Volunteer Registry for Medical, Public Health and Lay Volunteer Responders, 2022. Available from: TDVR, texasdisastervolunteerregistry.org.

U.S. Department of Homeland Security: *National response framework*, ed 3, 2022. Available from: https://www.fema.gov/emergency-managers/national-preparedness/frameworks/response.

U.S. Department of Homeland Security: *National Response Framework*, ed 4, 2019. Available from National Response Framework (fema.gov).

U.S. Department of Homeland Security: *Our mission*, 2022. Available from: https://www.dhs.gov/our-mission.

U.S. Department of Homeland Security: *National preparedness goal*, 2022. Available from: https://www.dhs.gov/national-preparedness-goal.

U.S. Department of Homeland Security: *National terrorism advisory system*, 2022. Available from: https://www.dhs.gov/topic/ntas.

World Vision: *2004 Indian Ocean earthquake and tsunami: facts, FAQs, and how to help*, 2019.

30

School Health

Anitra Frederick and Christina N. DesOrmeaux

OBJECTIVES

Upon completion of this chapter, the reader will be able to do the following:

1. Discuss how *Healthy People 2030* can be used to shape the care given in a school health setting.
2. Identify and discuss the eight components of a comprehensive school health program.
3. Recognize the major stressors that can negatively affect an adolescent's mental and physical health.
4. Identify common health concerns of school-age children and associated health interventions.
5. Explore the various roles of the nurse in the school setting.
6. Be familiar with the standards according to which school nurses practice.
7. Cite several resources available to the school nurse.

OUTLINE

KEY TERMS

Early and Periodic Screening, Diagnosis, and Treatment
emergency care plan
Family Educational Rights and Privacy Act
Health Insurance Portability and Accountability Act of 1996

individualized healthcare plan
Individuals With Disabilities Education Act of 1990
Public Law 99-142
school emergency plan
school health

school nurse
school-based health centers
Shattuck Report
Youth Risk Behavior Surveillance System

According to the Centers for Disease Control and Prevention (CDC, 2019b), the healthy development of children and adolescents is influenced by many societal institutions, and after the family, the school is the primary institution responsible for the development of young people in the United States. The school environment is also a key setting in which students' behaviors and ideas are shaped. Just as schools are critical to preparing students academically and socially, they are also vital partners in helping young people take responsibility for their

health and adopting health-enhancing attitudes and behaviors that can last a lifetime (CDC, 2019b).

Academic success and healthy children and youth are closely intertwined. It is impossible to achieve success in school without maximizing the health of the students. School-age children and adolescents face increasingly difficult challenges related to health. Many of today's health challenges are different from those of the past and include behaviors and risks linked to the leading causes of death such as heart disease, injuries, and cancer. Examples of behaviors that often begin during youth and increase the risk for serious health problems are the use of tobacco, vaping, alcohol, and drugs; poor nutritional habits; inadequate physical activity; irresponsible sexual behavior; violence; suicide; and reckless/texting driving (Box 30.1).

In the United States, approximately 56.4 million children attend school every day (National Center for Educational Statistics, 2020). Their presence creates a unique opportunity for **school nurses** to have a positive impact on the nation's youth. The primary providers of health services in schools are school nurses, and there are approximately 95,776 registered nurses working in schools in the United States (National Association of School Nurses [NASN], 2020b).

School nursing is a specialized practice of professional nursing that advances the well-being, academic success, and lifelong achievement and health of students. To that end, school nurses facilitate positive student responses to normal development; promote health and safety, including a healthy environment; intervene with actual and potential health problems; provide case management services; and actively collaborate with others to build student and family capacity for adaptation, self-management, self-advocacy, and learning (NASN, 2017). Appropriate staffing (NASN, 2020b) of school nurses is imperative to ensuring the healthy and well-being of children in the United States. When determining nurse staffing, schools review: students' health needs and medical acuity; social determinants of health in the student population; nurses educational experience and practice; and culture and context of the school's systems.

More than 10% of the nation's children live in poverty (National Center for Children in Poverty, 2021). Poverty is defined as an annual income below $26,500 for a family of four (U.S. Census Bureau, 2021). Decreased or inferior healthcare has been linked to serious health problems, resulting in an increase in absenteeism that may be correlated with failure in school. The school nurse can effectively manage many complaints and illnesses, allowing these children to return to or remain in class.

Indeed, on a daily basis, school nurses see students with a variety of complaints. Increasing numbers of children are being seen in the school setting because they lack a source of regular preventative and medical care. According to the Children's Defense Fund (2021), nearly 4.4 million children under the age

of 19 in the United States do not have health insurance. Nearly one in seven live in poverty in the the United States.

This is a decrease from the nearly 12 million in previous years. Poor academic performance is strongly correlated with the uninsured status of youth, and conversely, acquisition of health insurance leads to an improvement in school performance. Through education, counseling, advocacy, and direct care across all levels of prevention, the nurse can improve the immediate and long-term health of this population.

There is a need for mental and physical health services for students of all ages to improve both their academic performance and their sense of well-being. This chapter provides an overview of **school health** and the role of the nurse in the provision of health services and health education. It also offers an in-depth look at the components of a successful school health program and the major health problems of today's youth.

HISTORY OF SCHOOL HEALTH

Before 1840, education of children in the United States was uncoordinated and sparse. In 1840, Rhode Island passed legislation that made education mandatory, and other states soon followed. In 1850, a teacher and school committee member, Lemuel Shattuck, spearheaded the legendary report that has become a public health classic. This report, known as the **Shattuck Report**, has had a profound impact on school health because it proposed that health education was a vital component in the prevention of disease.

Public health officials and others soon realized that schools played an important part in the prevention of communicable disease. When smallpox broke out in New York City in the 1860s, health officials were faced with trying to implement a widespread prevention program. They chose to target the schools and began vaccinating children. This experience led to the 1870 requirement that all children be vaccinated against smallpox before entering school (Allensworth et al., 1997).

At that time, schools were frequently poorly ventilated and lacked fresh air, effectively spreading diseases among the children. Late in the nineteenth century, a practice of inspecting schools began to identify children who were ill and exclude them until it was deemed they were no longer infectious. Soon thereafter, compulsory vision examinations became a requirement to identify children who might have difficulty in school. In 1902, New York City hired the first nurses to help inspect children, educate families, and ensure follow-up treatment. Within a few years the renowned nurse Lillian Wald was able to show that the presence of school nurses could reduce absenteeism by 50%. By 1911, more than 100 cities were using school nurses, and by 1913, New York City employed 176 school nurses (Allensworth et al., 1997).

As they became more comfortable in their positions, early school nurses began to take on more active roles in the assessment of children, treatment of minor conditions, and referral for more serious problems. In addition to identification, treatment, and exclusion for communicable diseases and

---

BOX 30.1 Youth at Risk

- High school students reporting they had ever had sex 38.4% in 2019 (46.0% in 2009).
- High school students currently use alcohol 29.8% in 2017 (47.1% in 2001)
- High school students ever used marijuana 35.6% in 2017 (42.4% in 2001)
- High school students ever misused opioids 14.3% in 2019
- High school students had been electronically bullied 15.7% in 2019
- Each day in the United States about 1600 youth smoke their first cigarette

From Youth Risk Behavior Survey Data Summary & Trends Report 2009–2019. Accessed from: https://www.cdc.gov/healthyyouth/data/yrbs/pdf/YRBSDataSummaryTrendsReport2019-508.pdf, 2021.

screening for problems that might affect learning, other issues quickly became part of school nurses' practice. In the early part of the twentieth century, the temperance movement led schools to teach children about the effects of alcohol and tobacco. Also, early in the twentieth century, "gymnastics" was introduced in schools in an effort to promote physical activity. World War I was a pivotal point for school health services, and the call for a national effort to improve the health of schoolchildren emerged. In 1918 the National Education Association joined forces with the American Medical Association (AMA) to form the Joint Committee on Health Problems and publish the report *Minimum Health Requirements for Rural Schools*. This group also called for the coordination of health education programs, medical supervision, and physical education. By 1921 nearly every state had laws that required physical and health education in schools. Additionally, fire drills became part of safety education programs introduced during and after World War I (Allensworth et al., 1997).

Even though emphasis was placed on health services in schools, barriers still existed. Many schools and cities were unwilling to take on the task of providing primary health care for all children. The idea that schools should simply identify and refer problems to physicians was a common practice backed by the AMA. By the 1920s, medical services and preventive health services were clearly separated in the public health arena and in the schools, thereby largely supported by each state, which focused more attention on "health education." The federal government did not get involved with school health until the passage of the National School Lunch Program in 1946. The School Breakfast Program was implemented 30 years later (Allensworth et al., 1997).

There was no impetus to change the direction of school health programs until the 1960 and 1970s. During these decades there was increasing publicity about children living in poverty and the move to mainstream children with disabilities. These two issues, along with an increase in the number of children of immigrants, contributed to changes in school health programs.

During the 1960s the first nurse practitioner training programs opened and made the inclusion of primary care services in schools possible. In 1976 the first National School Conference, supported by the Robert Wood Johnson Foundation, was held in Galveston, Texas. After this conference a variety of school health service models began to emerge with new partnerships and ideas created to provide the most comprehensive healthcare services for school-age children. In addition, the Education for the Handicapped Act in 1975 mandated that all children, regardless of disabilities, have access to educational services.

The 1980 and 1990s saw several measures aimed at improving the health of schoolchildren. The Drug-Free Schools and Community Act was implemented in 1986 to fight substance abuse through education and was expanded in 1994 to include violence prevention measures. During this period, the Centers for Disease Control and Prevention (CDC), Division of Adolescent and School Health, began funding state education agencies to develop and implement programs aimed at alcohol and tobacco use, physical education, and the reduction of sexually transmitted diseases (STDs) and HIV infection among the nation's youth. Also, the federal government encouraged states to use part of their maternal and child block grant monies to fund school-based health centers.

The No Child Left Behind Act (NCLB) was signed into law by President Bush in 2002. As part of the NCLB, the Safe and Drug Free Schools and Communities Act (SDFSC) became effective that same year. SDFSC supports programs that focus on prevention of school violence and illegal use of alcohol, tobacco, and drugs. This legislation promotes the involvement of parents and communities in efforts and resources to create a safe and drug-free environment in order to enhance student academic achievement.

The Patient Protection and Affordable Care Act was signed into law March 23, 2010, by President Obama. Under this act, an initial 95 million dollars was awarded to 278 school-based health centers (SBHCs) as part of a capital program to create new sites and expand existing services in 2011. See later discussion of SBHCs.

School health services vary widely among states and school districts. There continues to be a lack of coordination among providers, with no single agency responsible for tracking services. Recognizing that there are differences among schools in the United States and that important health information must be delivered to children and adolescents, the United States Health and Human Services (USDHHS) addressed many related issues in the *Healthy People 2030* program. Objectives targeting children and adolescents are written for diverse areas, including physical activity, sex education and HIV prevention, nutrition, smoking/vaping, prevention, injury prevention, and school absences related to asthma. The *Healthy People 2030* box lists a few of these objectives related to school health.

SCHOOL HEALTH SERVICES

The School Health Policies and Programs Study describes school health services as a "coordinated system that ensures a continuum of care from school to home to community health care provider and back" (Allensworth et al., 1997, p. 153). School health services goals and objectives vary from state to state, community to community, and school to school. These differences reflect wide variations in student needs, community resources, funding sources, and school leadership preferences. Many organizations, such as the American School Health Association and NASN, are involved in the care and welfare of school-age children and have compiled and adopted definitions, standards, and statistics related to school health.

According to the School-Based Health Alliance (2017), there are 2584 SBHCs located in 49 out of 50 states, including the District of Columbia. Most SBHCs are staffed with a nurse, a nurse practitioner, or physician assistant. The following services provided in these centers typically include first aid, medication administration, and preventive screenings (vision, hearing, scoliosis, blood pressure, weight, and acanthosis nigricans).

Nearly all schools maintain health records on students and, at a minimum, monitor immunization status per federal and state laws. Most authorities agree that comprehensive school health programs should have the following eight components (Fig. 30.1): health education; physical education; health services; nutrition services; counseling, psychological, and social services; healthy school environment; health promotion for staff; and family and community involvement.

♥ HEALTHY PEOPLE 2030

Selected General Objectives for Schools

ECBP-D09: Increase core clinical prevention and population health education in medical schools

ECBP-D10: Increase core clinical prevention and population health education in nursing schools

ECBP-D11: Increase core clinical prevention and population health education in physician assistant training programs

ECBP-D12: Increase core clinical prevention and population health education in pharmacy schools

ECBP-D13: Increase core clinical prevention and population health education in dental schools

AH-R07: Increase the proportion of secondary schools with a start time of 8:30 a.m. or later

AH-R09: Increase the proportion of public schools with a counselor, social worker, and psychologist

From HealthyPeople.gov: *Healthy People 2030: Topics & objectives.* Available from: https://health.gov/healthypeople/objectives-and-data/browse-objectives/schools. Accessed May 28, 2021.

Health Education

An objective of *Healthy People 2030* sets a goal that middle, junior, and senior high schools provide health education courses in priority areas. The CDC (2020a,b,c,d,e) identified the following six high-risk behaviors, utilizing the Youth Risk

Behavior Surveillance System (YRBSS), as needing to be targeted in health education courses:

1. Alcohol and drug use
2. Unintentional injuries and violence
3. Tobacco use
4. Poor nutrition
5. Lack of physical activity
6. Sexual behavior that results in STIs or unwanted pregnancies

These problems and behaviors are preventable and often coexist. They also lead to both social and educational problems that contribute to our nation's dropout rates, unemployment rates, and crime statistics.

The National Health Education Standards were established to promote positive health behaviors for students in all grades (CDC, 2019a,b). These standards give educators, administrators, and policy makers a framework for developing and designing health education programs in schools. The standards are written to promote personal, family, and community health in students, targeting grades 2, 5, 8, and 12. The standards provide a guide for curricula development in health education and specify that the students will (1) comprehend concepts related to health promotion and disease prevention to enhance health; (2) analyze the influence of family, peers, culture, media, technology, and other factors on health behaviors; (3) demonstrate the ability to access valid information, products, and services to enhance health; (4) demonstrate the ability to use interpersonal communication skills to enhance health and avoid or reduce health risks; (5) demonstrate the ability to use decision-making skills to enhance health; (6) demonstrate the ability to use goal-setting skills to enhance health; (7) demonstrate the ability to practice health-enhancing behaviors and avoid or reduce health risks; and (8) demonstrate the ability to advocate for personal, family, and community health.

In 1990, to learn more about high-risk behaviors among youth, the (CDC , 2020e) instituted the **Youth Risk Behavior Surveillance System** The YRBSS survey is conducted every 2 years among selected high school students throughout the United States in both private and public schools. Box 30.2 lists the purposes of the YRBSS. Reports from the survey provide

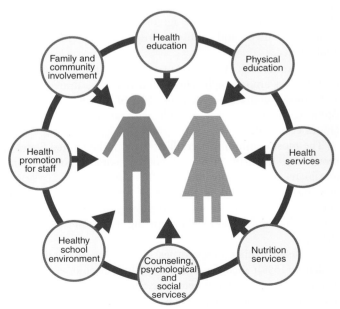

Fig. 30.1 The eight components of school health programs.

BOX 30.2 Purposes of the Youth Risk Behavior Survey System

- Determine the prevalence of health risk behaviors.
- Assess whether health risk behaviors increase, decrease, or remain the same over time.
- Examine the cooccurrence of health risk behaviors.
- Provide comparable data among subpopulations of youth.
- Provide comparable national, state, territorial, tribal, and local data.
- Monitor progress toward achieving the *Healthy People 2020* objectives and other program indicators.

From Kann L, McManus T, Harris WA, et al.: Youth risk behavior surveillance—United States, 2015, *MMWR Surveill Summ* 65(No. SS-6):1–174, 2016.

valuable information that can help improve health education programs in schools.

Injury Prevention

Injury prevention should be taught early in schools, and the information should be age appropriate. For example, bicycle safety, including the importance of wearing a helmet and the proper use of backpacks, must be stressed beginning in elementary schools. Safety on the schoolyard and playground is also important for this age group, because from 2009 to 2014, 1.5 million children were injured on playgrounds in the United States (U.S. Consumer Product Safety Commission, 2016). Motor vehicle safety should be included in programs for adolescents who are beginning to drive. These motor vehicle safety programs should include the hazards of distracted driving (e.g., cell phones, texting), which are issues affecting all drivers.

Sports safety is particularly important among adolescents as participation in sports continues to grow, especially among girls. More than 1.35 million children are seen for treatment in emergency rooms each year related to sports-related injuries (Safe Kids USA, 2013). Injuries occur most commonly on playgrounds, on athletic fields, and in gymnasiums. Orthopedic injuries (e.g., strains, sprains, fractures, and dislocations), dental injuries, neurological problems (e.g., traumatic brain injury [TBI] and concussion), ophthalmic injuries, cuts, abrasions, and bruises are frequently seen. TBI's account for more than 20,000 of these injuries and continues to be a significant concern for health care providers and school nurses (Cheng et al., 2016).

Use of proper equipment should be mandatory for children and adolescents participating in sports activities. Fitted mouth guards, shin guards, pads, helmets, and other protective gear should be required to prevent injury. Regular hydration and frequent rest periods should be required to prevent heat-related illnesses, especially during hot weather. Effective warm-up and cool-down exercises should be encouraged to prevent muscle strain. Schools that participate in aquatic sports should include pool safety. The school nurse has a unique opportunity to work with the athletic staff to promote these kinds of policies.

The sports physical is a good time for the school nurse to counsel the student about the risk of health problems related to physical activity. This is also an appropriate setting for the nurse to question girls about menstrual irregularities and to ask all students about their eating behaviors, feelings about their weight, depression/anxiety, and history of musculoskeletal injuries. The nurse can use this setting to teach the importance of stretching exercises to help prevent injuries.

Many school districts have school safety committees that make recommendations for sports-related safety. These committees collect data on injuries, develop safety inspection policies, and plan staff training and student education related to school environmental factors. Nurses are vital members of school health teams and committees from instituting injury prevention programs to injury response on the athletic field.

Tobacco/Vaping Use

For the past several decades, major concerns have been raised about long-term health problems associated with adolescents' use of tobacco, vaping, alcohol, and illegal substances. There is an increased likelihood that these youthful abusers will ultimately engage in other high-risk behaviors. Adolescent smoking/vaping has been closely correlated with alcohol use and other drugs. Smoking/vaping by young people can cause serious health problems, such as heart disease; chronic lung disease; and cancers of the lung, pharynx, esophagus, and bladder. Factors that have been associated with youth tobacco/vaping use include low economic status, peer pressure, smoking by parents, a perception that tobacco use is the norm, low levels of academic achievement, exposure of advertising, and history of aggressive behavior such as membership in gangs (CDC, 2020b).

Although there has been improvement over the last decades, smoking remains a major problem in this country and is the single leading preventable cause of death in the United States. Cigarette smoking has declined significantly, but the usage of other forms of tobacco has emerged; this includes electronic cigarettes (vaping), hookah, pipes, bidis, flavored tobacco, and smokeless tobacco (CDC, 2020d). Prevention should be a priority in youth because 9 out of 10 cigarette smokers first tried smoking/vaping by 18 years of age (CDC, 2020d). While tobacco use has declined significantly, e-cigarette use has increased dramatically. Indeed, in 2020, 85% of high school students/74% of middle school students who used tobacco products in the past 30 days reported using a flavored tobacco product during that time (Wang et al., 2020).

Substance Abuse

The use of alcohol and other drugs is associated with problems in school, injuries, violence, and motor vehicle deaths. All 50 states and the District of Columbia have outlawed the sale of alcohol to anyone under the age of 21, yet it is still the most commonly used and abused drug among children and adolescents.

The Youth Risk Behavior Survey (2020) found that in the past 30 days among high school students: 29% drank alcohol, 14% binge drank (+5 drinks), 5% of drivers drove after drinking alcohol, and 17% rode with an intoxicated driver (Jones et al., 2020).

The most commonly used illicit drug in the United States is marijuana. In 2019, 36.8% of young people reported using marijuana one or more times in their lives (CDC, 2019a). A new disturbing trend is the use of synthetic marijuana as known as *K2*, *Spice*, *fake weed*, *King Kong*, or *Moon Rocks*, with 7.3% of high school students reporting its use in 2019 (CDC, 2019a).

The use of other illegal drugs is common in high school students (15%): includes cocaine, hallucinogenic, ecstasy, inhalants, heroin, methamphetamine, steroids, and prescription drugs (opioids, depressants, or stimulants) (CDC, 2019a). Of significant concern is the growing abuse of prescription drugs.

Opioids (e.g., Vicodin or OxyContin), depressants or anti-anxiety medications (e.g., Valium or Xanax), and stimulants (e.g., Ritalin or Adderall) are the most commonly abused. Many times, students obtain these drugs from other family members who have been prescribed the medication or from the illegal sale on the streets or through the Internet.

The use of anabolic steroids has decreased somewhat among high school students, declining from 3.6% in 2011 to 3.0% in 2015, but the issue should remain a concern to school health nurses because of the number of athletes who abuse the drugs (CDC, 2017a). Many athletes believe that anabolic steroids will produce an increase in strength and muscle mass and enhance their performance. There are more than 100 different types of anabolic steroids, and all require a prescription. Abuse or improper use of anabolic steroids can result in severe problems, including renal impairment or failure; liver cancer; cardiovascular problems such as high blood pressure and elevated cholesterol levels; and sexual changes such as testicular shrinkage, clitoral enlargement, and accelerated puberty (National Institute on Drug Abuse, 2018).

Sex Education

A number of objectives of *Healthy People 2030* address issues of human sexuality and prevention of pregnancy, STIs, and HIV. These issues are important for the nurse working with older children and adolescents.

Many teens become sexually active at an early age, and despite recent declines, pregnancy rates continue to be high (Box 30.3). Data obtained from the YRBSS reveals a decrease from 47.4% in 2011 to 41.2% in 2015 of adolescents in grades 9 through 12 who have had sexual intercourse (CDC and YRBSS, 2016c).

Sex education in the school setting is a controversial topic. Opponents of sex education believe that parents have the responsibility for teaching this content to their children. Laws in certain states prohibit or dramatically limit sex education in public schools. However, 30 states and the District of Columbia mandate that public schools teach sex education (National Conference of State Legislatures, 2020). Proponents argue that for many children sex education will not be addressed in the

BOX 30.3 Teen Pregnancy

- The US teen birth rate is one of the highest among developed countries.
- 194,377 babies were born to teenagers aged 15–19 in 2017.
- American Indian/Alaska Native, Black, and Hispanic youth have a disproportionately high rate of teen pregnancy.
- Teen mothers are less likely to complete high school.
- Teen mothers are more likely to be single parents and to live in poverty.
- Children of teenage mothers are more likely to have lower school achievement, to drop out of school, to be incarcerated during adolescence, and to face unemployment as an adult
- Birth rates among teenagers vary substantially from state to state.

Data from Centers for Disease Control and Prevention: *About teen pregnancy*, 2019. https://www.cdc.gov/teenpregnancy/about/.

home. If this information is not taught in schools, children may receive inadequate or incorrect information from peers, media, or other sources. Contrary to some concerns, there is no research that concludes that sex education in the schools increases sexual activity. According to the Future of Sex Education Initiative (2012) the following seven topics are considered fundamental to a comprehensive sex education curriculum: anatomy and physiology, puberty and adolescent development, identity (sexual orientation), pregnancy and reproduction, STIs and HIV, healthy relationships, and personal safety. School nurses have been caught in the center of this controversy but historically have advocated for education on normal human sexuality that encourages discussion in an objective, nonjudgmental manner and in which students are free to ask questions and receive correct answers.

Tattoos and Body Piercings

Tattoos and body piercings are a form of self-expression. Their popularity has risen dramatically in the last decade. The procedures are often done at home, on the streets, or in parlors where sterile technique and safety precautions are not practiced. Both hepatitis C and methicillin-resistant *Staphylococcus aureus* have been linked to tattoos and body piercings. This fact presents an opportunity for the school nurse to teach students the importance of making healthy decisions on whether to have such procedures done and, if so, under what conditions they will be performed.

Dental Health

One of the most common complaints of school-age children is dental caries. There are numerous contributing factors, including poor oral hygiene, lack of fluoridated water, and lack of funds or insurance for dental care. More than half of children have dental caries by the time they are 8 years of age. This disease is more common in lower-income children, and approximately 66% of those between the ages of 12 and 19 have had tooth decay. Untreated cavities can greatly affect a child's quality of life and cause pain, absence from school, and decreased self-worth (CDC, 2015). Proper brushing of teeth should be taught along with good nutritional habits and the importance of regular dental checkups. Children should also be taught the relationship between high-sugar foods and dental caries.

Physical Education

One of the major objectives of *Healthy People 2030* is improvement of health and fitness through regular physical activity. Children today are less active than children in the past. Daily enrollment in physical education classes among high school students dropped considerably over the last few decades. Children are becoming more sedentary as a result of increased use of computers and television and decreasing requirements for physical education. Screen time and use of electronic devices has increased dramatically over the past few years. Today children between 8 and 18 years average 7.5 h of screen time per day (CDC, 2018a,b,c).

A sedentary lifestyle is associated with obesity, hypertension, heart disease, and diabetes. Studies show that people who are active have a better quality of life and outlive those who are inactive. Habits in childhood are likely to continue into adulthood, making it imperative that children are taught the importance of being physically active at a young age. Studies also show that children and adolescents who are physically active have increased self-confidence and self-esteem and decreased anxiety, stress, and depression. Regular physical activity helps build and maintain healthy bones and muscles.

Physical education should focus on activities that children can continue into their adult years, such as walking, swimming, biking, and jogging. The educational content should change as the child ages. For example, what may appeal to a young child, such as playing on the playground with friends, is different from what motivates an adolescent, such as competitive sports and aerobic exercise. The CDC has made 10 recommendations for the promotion of lifelong physical activity (Box 30.4).

Health Services

Health care provided in schools includes preventive services such as immunizations and health screenings. This component of a comprehensive school health program may also involve

---

BOX 30.4   Guidelines for School Programs: Promoting Healthy Eating and Physical Activity

- Use a coordinated approach to develop, implement, and evaluate healthy eating and physical activity policies and practices.
- Establish school environments that support healthy eating and physical activity.
- Provide a quality school meal program and ensure that students are offered only appealing, healthy food and beverage choices outside the school meal program.
- Implement a comprehensive physical activity program with quality physical education as the cornerstone.
- Implement health education that provides students with the knowledge, attitudes, skills, and experiences needed for healthy eating and physical activity.
- Provide students with health, mental health, and social services to address healthy eating, physical activity, and related chronic disease prevention.
- Partner with families and community members in the development and implementation of healthy eating and physical activity policies, practices, and programs.
- Provide a school employee wellness program that includes healthy eating and physical activity services for all school staff members.
- Employ qualified persons and provide professional development opportunities for physical education; health education; nutrition services; and health, mental health, and social services staff members, as well staff members who supervise recess, cafeteria time, and out-of-school-time programs.

From Centers for Disease Control and Prevention: School health guidelines to promote healthy eating and physical activity, *MMWR Recomm Rep* 60(RR-5):1–76, 2011. www.cdc.gov/mmwr/pdf/rr/rr6005.pdf.

---

emergency care, management of acute and chronic health conditions, appropriate referrals, health counseling, education about healthy lifestyles, and medication administration.

Immunizations

Immunizations are a vital component of routine health care, providing long-lasting protection against many diseases. Vaccine-preventable deaths are at record-low levels. Many communicable diseases have been reduced by more than 99% as a result of immunizations. Under vaccination of children, especially those in large urban areas, is a concern because of the potential for disease outbreaks.

All states now require proof of immunization status or evidence of immunity before a child can enter school. Certain exceptions based on religious and philosophical beliefs or medical contraindications may apply. The school nurse plays an important role in verifying compliance with immunization requirements and in educating children and parents about the benefits of immunization. See the CDC website (https://www.cdc.gov/vaccines/schedules/hcp/index.html) for current immunization schedules.

Health Screenings

Many children in the United States are not appropriately screened for certain treatable conditions. Impaired vision and hearing can result in poor academic performance, slowed emotional development, and stress-related disorders. Early identification and treatment of these problems is highly effective and less costly. Vision and hearing screenings are provided at most schools according to a schedule set by the state or school district. These screenings usually occur upon a child's initial entry to school and at least once during elementary, middle, and high school. Children and adolescents may need to be screened more often on the basis of family history, developmental delays, speech, recurrent ear infections, or exposure to loud noise.

Vision screening is required in most states, with referrals as needed. The standard Snellen vision chart is the usual screening tool. Screening for strabismus is a nursing responsibility, and this condition must be identified and treated early to prevent amblyopia. If left untreated, amblyopia may result in loss of vision. Referral to an eye specialist is a critical component of all abnormal eye examination results.

Scoliosis or postural screening should be done to identify spinal deviations in an effort to prevent secondary problems. Spinal problems may lead to cosmetic, functional, or emotional problems. Scoliosis screening in the school consists primarily of a visual inspection of the back. The American Academy of Pediatrics and the American Academy of Orthopedic Surgeons recommend screening of all girls at 10 and 12 years and boys once at either 13 or 14 years (United States Preventative Services [USPS], 2018).

The assessment of high blood pressure during childhood is important in identifying children who have hypertension and who will benefit from early intervention and follow-up. Vascular and end-organ damage from hypertension can begin in early childhood. Periodic blood pressure measurements are inexpensive and should be performed routinely for all children. Other periodic screenings may be mandated by various state or district regulations. These include body mass index (BMI) (height and weight) and dental screenings.

The Children's Health Insurance Program is a national program designed for children of families who earn too much money to qualify for Medicaid but cannot afford the high cost of health insurance. Medicaid-eligible children are guaranteed access to comprehensive health care services and routine dental examinations. Medicaid created the **Early and Periodic Screening, Diagnosis, and Treatment** (EPSDT) service because of the large number of uninsured children. EPSDT, a comprehensive child health program for the uninsured under the age of 21, includes health education and periodic screening. Services provided under the EPSDT program are often performed through the public health offices in each state, but may occur in community health clinics and schools. Screening services must include a comprehensive health and developmental history, an unclothed physical examination, immunizations and laboratory testing that are age appropriate, and lead toxicity screenings (Centers for Medicare and Medicaid Services, 2021).

Emergency Care

Schools are a common site of injuries ranging from minor scrapes, bruises, and fractures, to more severe life-threatening events such as seizures, head injuries, diabetic ketoacidosis, severe asthma attacks, and mass casualty incidents. Injuries may occur in school buildings or classrooms or during physical education classes or athletic events. Emergencies can include natural events, such as hurricanes, tornadoes, and earthquakes, or manmade disasters, such as hazardous material spills, fires, and acts of terror. Basic first aid equipment should be available in all schools. The school nurse must be knowledgeable about standard first aid and certified in cardiopulmonary resuscitation and use of an automated external defibrillator. The school nurse must also be responsible for the development of a **school emergency plan** that provides school staff with a guide to facilitate quick response in case of a student or school emergency.

Care of the Ill Child

The school nurse is responsible for monitoring the health of all students. For students with acute or chronic illnesses, administration of medications or treatments may be necessary. The nurse is often required to assess an ill child to determine the type of illness or health problem and develop a management plan. Two commonly encountered chronic illnesses are asthma and diabetes.

Asthma is one of the leading causes of chronic illness among school-aged children; approximately 1 in 12 children having the

diagnosis. Thus, asthma is a leading cause of school absenteeism (CDC, 2018b). Because asthma is so prevalent, school-based support for affected children is recommended. Actions undertaken by some schools across the country include immediate access to asthma medications, development and implementation of asthma action plans, and student and staff education on asthma. An assessment tool has been developed to determine how well schools assist children with asthma (Box 30.5). Answers to all the questions in the assessment tool should be "yes." "No" answers indicate that students may not be in an environment conducive to asthma control.

According to the American Association of Diabetes Educators (AADE, 2016), diabetes is prevalent in school-age children, affecting around 190,000 people younger than 20 years. Most cases of diabetes in this cohort is type 1, but type 2 diabetes is being diagnosed with increasing frequency in children. Further, cases of both are disproportionately larger in minority populations (CDC, 2020a). Childhood obesity and the decline in physical activity are considered major factors in this development. In general, teachers are inadequately prepared to care for children with diabetes and must rely on the school nurse. Children should be able to participate in their care to the extent that they are able. With the growing number of children who have diabetes, it is imperative that the nurse recognize the signs and symptoms of hypoglycemia and hyperglycemia in order to assist children in the monitoring of glucose levels and the administration of insulin or glucagon. The American Diabetes Association (ADA) has specific recommendations based on age, as shown in Box 30.6.

Medication Administration

Administration of medications is a service provided almost universally by school districts across the country. The use of medications by school-age children has increased over the last several years, allowing many children to attend school despite serious health problems.

Medication administration in the schools is a serious undertaking. Issues facing the school nurse include safety, monitoring of both therapeutic and side effects, proper documentation, confidentiality, and ongoing communication with the student and family. Only those medications considered necessary are administered at school.

The following guidelines from NASN (2017) should be included in school medication policies:
- Delegation (including training and supervision of unlicensed assistive personnel)
- Medication orders
- Prescription and over-the-counter medications
- Proper labeling, storage, disposal, and transportation of medication
- Documentation of medication administration
- Rescue and emergency medications
- Off-label medications and investigational drugs
- Complementary and alternative medications
- Psychotropic medications and controlled substances

BOX 30.5 How Asthma-Friendly Is Your School? Checklist

Children with asthma need proper support at school to keep their asthma under control and be fully active. Use the following questions to find out how well your school assists children with asthma.

☐ Yes ☐ No   Is your school free of tobacco smoke at all times, including during school-sponsored events and on school buses?

☐ Yes ☐ No   Does the school maintain good indoor air quality? Does it reduce or eliminate allergens and irritants that can make asthma worse?
      Check if any of the following are present:
        ☐ Cockroaches
        ☐ Dust mites (commonly found in humid climates in pillows, carpets, upholstery, and stuffed toys)
        ☐ Mold
        ☐ Pets with fur or feathers
        ☐ Strong odors or fumes from art and craft supplies, pesticides, paint, perfumes, air fresheners, and cleaning chemicals

☐ Yes ☐ No   Is there a school nurse in your school all day, every day? If not, is a nurse regularly available to help the school write plans and give the school guidance on medicines, physical education, and field trips for students with asthma?

☐ Yes ☐ No   Can children take medicines at school as recommended by their doctor and parents? May children carry their own asthma medicines?

☐ Yes ☐ No   Does your school have a written, individualized emergency plan for teachers and staff in case of a severe asthma episode (attack)? Does the plan make clear what action to take under different emergency situations such as fire, weather, or lock-down? Whom to call? When to call?

☐ Yes ☐ No   Does someone teach school staff about asthma, asthma action plans, and asthma medicines? Does someone teach all students about asthma and how to help a classmate who has it?

☐ Yes ☐ No   Can students actively participate in physical education class and recess? (For example, do students have access to their medicine before exercise? Can they choose modified or alternative activities when medically necessary?)

If the answer to any question is "no," students in your school may be facing obstacles to asthma control. Uncontrolled asthma can hinder a student's attendance, participation, and progress in school. School staff, health professionals, and parents can work together to remove obstacles and promote students' health and education.

From National Heart, Lung, and Blood Institute, National Asthma Education and Prevention Program, NAEPP School Asthma Education Subcommittee: *How asthma friendly is your school?* 2008. www.nhlbi.nih.gov/health/public/lung/asthma/friendly.pdf.

BOX 30.6 Expectations of the Child With Diabetes

Toddler and Preschool Age
- The child should be able to determine which finger to prick.
- The child can usually choose an injection site.
- The child is generally cooperative.

Elementary School Age
- The child should be able to assist in all diabetes tasks at school.
- The child is usually able to perform his or her own fingerstick glucose monitoring.
- The child can administer his or her own insulin with supervision.
- The child is usually able to let an adult know when he or she is experiencing a hypoglycemic episode.

Middle School and High School Age
- The child should be able to perform self-monitoring of blood glucose.
- Most children should be able to administer their own insulin with supervision; adolescents should be able to administer insulin without supervision.
- All children may need assistance with blood glucose testing when the glucose level is low.

Data from American Diabetes Association: Diabetes care in the school and day care setting, *Diabetes Care* 35:S76–S80, 2012.

- Medication doses that exceed manufacturer's guidelines
- Student confidentiality

Medications commonly given in schools include analgesics and antipyretics (e.g., acetaminophen [Tylenol] or ibuprofen [Advil]), antacids, antitussives, anticonvulsants, antiemetics and antidiarrheals, antifungals, antihistamines, and antibiotics. Medications used to treat attention-deficit hyperactivity disorder (ADHD) are among the most commonly administered. It has been estimated that more than 10% of children in the United States between 4 and 17 years have been diagnosed with ADHD, and this number has been steadily increasing (Xu et al., 2018).

Alternative and complementary medicine includes practices and products outside the realm of conventional medicine. Medication administration policies should exist that reflect local and state laws that address these products. The request for the administration of any of these medications provides the nurse with an excellent health teaching opportunity.

School nurses must be aware of medications that are being self-administered on school grounds and must provide education as needed to both children and parents. Rescue medications such as albuterol for asthma or an EpiPen for a child with a severe allergic reaction must be administered quickly to affect asthma symptoms, and the nurse must be familiar with its expected effects to properly assist the child who needs it. It is now legal in all 50 states for students to carry and self-administer asthma medications (NASN, 2017).

Children With Special Health Needs

In 1976, **Public Law 99-142** was enacted, giving all students, including those who are severely handicapped, the right to public education in the least restrictive environment possible, regardless of mental or physical disabilities. The Education for All Handicapped Children Act of 1973 and the subsequent **Individuals with Disabilities Education Act (IDEA) of 1990** enhanced the opportunities for children previously served in acute care and long-term care settings to have access to public education. Children affected by these laws include those who are hearing impaired, mentally challenged, multi-handicapped, orthopedically impaired, "other" health impaired (e.g., chronic or acute health problems such as a heart condition or epilepsy), seriously emotionally disturbed, speech impaired, visually handicapped, or who have a specific learning disability.

The development of healthcare services and technology has enabled students whose conditions may have prevented them in the past from leaving an institution or controlled environment to attend public school. Many of these children need nursing services of varied types (e.g., tube feedings, suctioning, catheterization) to continue their progression in school. Public Law 94–142 requires school nurses to screen or identify children in need of special education and related services and to participate in the development of an interdisciplinary individualized education program that includes educational goals and specific services to be provided. The nurse is also responsible for the development of an **individualized healthcare plan** (IHP) for all students requiring continuous nursing management while at school.

Student Records

Health records are maintained for all students according to individual school district policy. At a minimum, student health records should include immunization status, pertinent history, results of screenings and examinations, and IHPs. The **Family Educational Rights and Privacy Act**, a strong privacy protection act, protects student education and health records. Student health records should be afforded the same level of confidentiality as that given to clients and patients in other settings (i.e., sharing confidential information with others without approval is considered unethical and improper except in emergency situations).

The **Health Insurance Portability and Accountability Act of 1996** (HIPAA) was instituted in 2003. A major component of HIPAA is ensuring confidentiality of personal health information. Public schools that provide health care services fall under HIPAA regulations. Private schools that do not receive federal funding but engage in HIPAA-related activities are also governed by this act.

Delegation of Tasks

Not every school has a full-time nurse available on site. A nurse may be assigned to three or four schools, resulting in delegation of certain tasks to unlicensed personnel. Each state's Nurse Practice Act stipulates which procedures may be delegated. The responsibility for assessment, diagnosis, goal setting, and evaluation may never be delegated. When tasks are delegated, the nurse must provide appropriate education,

written procedures, and ongoing supervision and evaluation of the caregivers.

Nutrition

School-age children are undergoing periods of rapid growth and development and have complex nutritional needs. They must eat a variety of foods to meet their daily requirements. Diets should include a proper balance of carbohydrates, protein, and fat, with sufficient intake of vitamins and minerals. Children and adolescents share a well-known preference for junk food (Box 30.7), and their diet is often high in fat and sugar and frequently consists of fast-food items, such as hamburgers and French fries, instead of fruits and vegetables. Skipping meals, especially breakfast, and eating unhealthy snacks contribute to poor childhood nutrition. Identifying nutritional problems, counseling, and making appropriate referrals are important in the school setting. The school nurse should consider cultural influences on diet when teaching students and assessing their nutritional status.

Poor nutritional status is closely associated with poverty. Federally funded programs such as the School Breakfast Program and National School Lunch Program were initiated to ensure that all children have access to these meals during the school day.

Eating Disorders

It is imperative that the school nurse recognize the association between feelings of inadequacy and unhealthy eating practices in adolescents and young people. These self-perceptions begin early in life; therefore, education and counseling must begin in elementary school. Prevention should concentrate on eliminating misconceptions surrounding nutrition, dieting, and body composition and should stress optimal health and personal performance. Outside influences such as social media, celebrity admiration, commercials, and advertisements make this a serious problem.

School nurses must also be aware of eating disorders and related risk factors. Anorexia, bulimia, and binge eating are the three most common eating disorders in adolescents (NIMH, 2021). *Binge eating* is defined as recurrent, out-of-control eating of large amounts of food whether a person is hungry or not. *Anorexia* is a severely restricted intake of food based on an extreme fear of weight gain. Literature has shown that anorexia

---

BOX 30.7   Vending Machine Food Choices

In 2004, the National Association of School Nurses addressed the issue of unhealthy foods found in school vending machines and sold in school fundraising projects. The organization specifically resolved that schools should provide healthy food choices in school vending machines and for sale in fundraising projects.

Data from National Association of School Nurses: *Resolution: vending machines and healthy food choices in schools,* 2004. Available from: www.nasn.org.

is multifactorial, seen primarily in females, and often correlated with family dysfunction or a history of sexual abuse. *Bulimia* is a form of anorexia characterized by a chaotic eating pattern with recurrent episodes of binge eating followed by purging. Health consequences of eating disorders may include reduction of bone density, severe dehydration, tooth decay, and potentially fatal electrolyte imbalances.

Female Athlete Triad. The "female athlete triad" is a syndrome consisting of eating disorders, amenorrhea, and osteoporosis. Pressure to attain a particular body shape or weight considered desirable in a selected sport may put the female athlete at risk for development of this disorder. The triad is a complex problem with psychological and physiological factors. It can result in menstrual irregularities, premature osteoporosis, and decreased bone mineral density; if taken to the extreme, it can become life threatening.

Obesity

Obesity is the fastest-rising public health concern in the nation and will likely overtake tobacco use as the single leading preventable cause of death. The obesity rate has more than doubled in children and tripled in adolescents over the past three decades. Alarmingly, currently, about 20% of 6- to 11-year-olds and 21% of 12- to 19-year-olds are considered obese (CDC, 2021). Statistics show that obese children and adolescents are more likely to become obese adults. Thus, obesity and its prevention or management must be of concern to the school nurse.

Although many of the underlying causes of obesity are not well understood, several contributing factors have been identified; they include reduced access to and affordability of nutritious foods, decreased physical activity, and cultural and genetic influences. Obesity is associated with development of diabetes, dyslipidemia, hypertension, and other disorders, such as osteoarthritis, sleep apnea, different cancers, and cholelithiasis. In addition, obesity may result in social and quality-of-life impairment, and obese children often have low self-esteem and may be labeled by their peers and ridiculed. The school nurse should determine the BMI for all adolescents. A BMI greater than the 85th percentile for age and gender suggests the need for further assessment and perhaps referral. To be successful, the treatment of obesity must begin early and must be multifaceted. Some of the solutions include improved health education related to nutrition and dietary behavior, increased physical activity and physical education programs, healthier school environments, and better nutrition services.

Nutritional Education Programs

Nutritional education is essential and must include parents, teachers, and the child. Children need to know the basics of good nutrition, how to make healthy snack choices, and the importance of balancing physical activity with food intake. Obesity, dental caries, anemia, and heart disease can be reduced or prevented with proper education and lifestyle changes. In addition, all adolescents and school-age children should receive counseling regarding intake of saturated fat.

The United States Department of Agriculture (USDA) Food and Nutrition Service (FNS) provide nutritional education for food service educators, professionals, parents, and child care providers, The USDA and FNS have a number of resources, including *MyPlate*, Team Nutrition, Let's Move, and SNAP-Ed Connection. These programs focus on healthy nutritional choices and health promotion and disease prevention topics in school and child care settings. Comprehensive school-based nutrition programs and services should be provided to all students. The ultimate goal of these efforts is that children will make healthy nutritional choices both inside and outside the school setting.

Counseling, Psychological, and Social Services

The mental health of a child or adolescent is affected by physical, economic, social, psychological, and environmental factors. Children, like adults, often hide problems from others. They may see problems as a sign of weakness or as a lack of control. Children may also be trying to protect themselves or someone they love and so do not seek help, with tragic results. Promotion of mental health and reduction or removal of threats to mental health is important to children and adolescents. This can be an enormous challenge for school nurses as mental health is difficult, yet essential, to assess.

Children and teens often struggle with depression, substance abuse, conduct disorders, self-esteem issues, suicidal ideation, eating disorders, and underachievement or overachievement. They may also have to cope with physical or mental abuse, chronic health conditions, or pregnancy. Common warning signs of stress in children are presented in Box 30.8. Drugs and alcohol can enter a child's life as early as elementary school. Many children live in single-parent households with little social or economic support. They may not have enough to eat or a safe, warm place to sleep, yet are expected to come to school each day ready to learn. Services aimed at helping children cope with these problems are often lacking or too costly for many families.

BOX 30.8   Warning Signs of Stress

- Problems eating or sleeping
- Use of alcohol or other substances (e.g., sedatives, sleep enhancers)
- Problems making decisions
- Persistent anger or hostile feelings
- Inability to concentrate
- Increased boredom
- Frequent headaches and ailments
- Inconsistent school attendance

ETHICAL INSIGHTS

An Ethical Dilemma: What Would You Do?

You are working as the school nurse in a rural high school when Grace, a 15-year-old female student, enters the clinic. Grace appears very worried, and, after several hesitant starts, she begins to cry and tells you that she is sexually active with a 17-year-old senior. She goes on to tell you that she has missed her last period and that her home pregnancy test result was positive. She states that she is afraid to tell her parents because she feels that they will be very disappointed in her and because she is afraid of what her father will do. She asks you where she can go to get an abortion. You speak with Grace for quite a while and encourage her to speak with her parents. She leaves the clinic a little more composed and promises you that she will think about what you have said. The next day Jenny, Grace's mother, comes into the clinic and asks to speak with you. She confides that she is worried about Grace and asks whether you know what is going on with her child. What would you do in this situation?

Although maintaining confidentiality and a professional relationship respectful of the student's wishes is vital, state laws and school district policies determine what a school nurse may do, and in some cases is required to do, when providing care to minor children. In order to deal with personal and sensitive information such as described here, the school nurse should be well versed in relevant laws and policies and should follow them. When in doubt, contact a supervisor.

BOX 30.9 Truths About Adolescent Suicides

- Most adolescents who attempt suicide are ambivalent and torn between wanting to die and wanting to live.
- Any threat of suicide should be taken seriously.
- Warning signs usually precede a suicide attempt; they may include depression, substance abuse, decreased activity, isolation, and appetite and sleep changes.
- Suicide is more common in adolescents who are dealing with bisexuality or homosexuality without support or in a hostile school environment.
- Education concerning suicide does not lead to an increased number of attempts.
- Females are more likely to consider or attempt suicide, and males are more likely to complete a suicide attempt.
- One suicide attempt is more likely to result in a subsequent attempt.
- 60% of completed suicides in children and adolescents are committed with guns.
- Most adolescents who have attempted or completed suicide have not been diagnosed as having a mental disorder.
- Suicide affects all socioeconomic groups.

The nurse or teacher may be the only stable adult in a child's life who will listen without being judgmental. Therefore, one of the most important roles of the school nurse is to act as counselor. Children may come to the school nurse with various vague complaints, such as recurrent stomachaches, headaches, and history of sexually promiscuous behavior, and the nurse must look beyond the initial complaint to identify underlying problems.

Major depressive disorders often have their onset in adolescence and are associated with an increased risk of suicide. In 2018 suicide was the first leading cause in both the 10- to 14-year and 15- to 19-year age groups (CDC, 2018a). Suicide attempts are more common than completed suicides. A recent survey of students in grades 9 through 12 showed that 7.4% attempted suicide in the preceding year and 17.2% seriously considered suicide (CDC, 2017a). The nurse and other school personnel must be on the alert for suicide clusters that are often known to follow a successful suicide. Adolescents may approach school nurses and other school professionals for help before a suicide attempt. The call for help may be subtle and not recognized as such. Therefore, it is important for the school nurse to be cognizant of the warning signs associated with suicide and to recognize and refer at-risk adolescents to appropriate mental health professionals (Box 30.9).

Unfortunately, a large number of children are victims of abuse. Physical and psychological abuse and neglect are usually a result of many interacting factors, such as poverty, social isolation, and drug and alcohol abuse. School nurses and other school personnel are mandated to report suspected cases of child maltreatment and neglect. The nurse must be alert to subtle changes in behavior or physical appearance that may

point to abuse. Box 30.10 outlines some of the signs and symptoms of child maltreatment.

In cases of child abuse or neglect, the school nurse may help the child learn problem solving, coping mechanisms, and steps to build self-esteem. The role of the nurse may extend outside the school campus. The nurse may need to work closely with families and social services to develop an appropriate health plan for a particular child.

Healthy School Environment

A healthy school environment is one in which distractions are minimized and that is free of physical hazards and psychological health risks. The NASN believes that all students and staff have an inherent right to learn and work in a healthy school environment. The school environment is a social of health in the school community. The school nurse is to assess for "environmental health hazards, implements and coordinates individual health and social interventions and addresses social determinants of health, to positively influence children's environmental health" (NASN, 2021).

Violence

Violence is a major public health problem because it threatens the health and well-being, both physical and psychological, of many children and adolescents. Nearly one in five high school students have reported being bullied on school property in the last year. Students also reported one in seven were electronically bullied via computer or cell phone involving posts on Instagram, Facebook, or other social media (CDC, 2020c).

Of great concern, homicide is the third leading cause of death for young people ages 10 to 24. It is estimated that about 13 young people are victims of homicide each day and over

BOX 30.10 Possible Signs of Abuse and Neglect

Physical Abuse
- Has unexplained injuries such as burns, bites, bruises, black eyes, or broken bones
- Has fading bruises or other noticeable marks after an absence from school
- Seems scared, anxious, depressed, withdrawn, or aggressive
- Seems frightened of parents and protests or cries when it is time to go home
- Shrinks at the approach of adults
- Shows changes in eating and sleeping habits
- Reports injury by a parent or another adult caregiver
- Abuses animals or pets

Neglect
- Is frequently absent from school
- Begs or steals food or money
- Lacks needed medical care, dental care, or glasses
- Is consistently dirty or has severe body odor
- Lacks sufficient clothing for the weather
- Abuses alcohol or other drugs
- States that there is no one at home to provide care

Sexual Abuse
- Has difficulty walking or sitting
- Experiences bleeding, bruising, or swelling in their private parts

- Suddenly refuses to go to school
- Reports nightmares or bedwetting
- Experiences a sudden change in appetite
- Demonstrates bizarre, sophisticated or unusual sexual knowledge or behavior
- Becomes pregnant or has a sexually transmitted disease, particularly if under age 14
- Runs away
- Reports sexual abuse by a parent or another adult caregiver
- Attaches very quickly to strangers or new adults in their environment

Emotional Abuse
- Shows extremes in behavior, such as being overly compliant or demanding, extremely passive or aggressive
- Is either inappropriately adult (e.g., parenting other children) or inappropriately infantile (e.g., frequently rocking or head-banging)
- Is delayed in physical or emotional development
- Shows signs of depression or suicidal thoughts
- Reports an inability to develop emotional bonds with others

Data from Child Information Gateway: *What is child abuse and neglect? Recognizing the signs and symptoms,* 2019. https://www.childwelfare.gov/pubPDFs/whatiscan.pdf.

1100 are seen in emergency departments for nonfatal assault-related injuries (CDC, 2020c).

In recent years, there have been a number of shootings and other acts of serious violence in schools. The CDC (2016a,b,c,d) reported that 4.1% of children admitted to having carried a weapon at least 1 day out of the last 30 and that 6.0% had been threatened or injured with a weapon on school property within the last year. The school shooting at Columbine High School in Littleton, Colorado, in 1999 was probably the first time that people in this country realized how unsafe schools could be. More recently, the mass shooting, in Newtown, Connecticut, killed 20 children and six adults, making it the nation's worst K–12 school shooting.

School nurses and other school personnel should be aware of risk factors and signs that could indicate a tendency to violence. Factors common in those who commit violent acts in school include being male and having a history of being ostracized or bullied in school. Media influences such as movies and video games that desensitize the impact of violence are being studied more closely as a possible cause of increased violence among children and adolescents. Children involved in school shootings often have a need for instant gratification, have easy access to guns, and may have a history of discipline problems.

Although the number of students who commit violent acts is small, these random acts are frightening, and school officials struggle with ways to prevent their occurrence and to recognize the signs of troubled youth. Violence prevention programs should begin in elementary schools. Children who exhibit aggressive behavior in elementary school are more likely to

exhibit antisocial and violent behavior as adolescents and adults. Programs should target stress management, conflict and anger resolution, and personal and self-esteem development. Nurses should use data collected through the YRBSS and other local data as a means of assessment when developing violence policies and prevention programs in the school and community. Additionally, nurses should initiate and participate in research that examines the complex developmental, social, and psychological factors surrounding violence.

Terrorism

Schools may not be the primary target in an act of terrorism, but they will be affected. Events following the September 11, 2001, terrorist attack illustrate potential problems facing schools, which may include fear and panic among students, teachers, and parents and anxiety among those directly affected.

Every school is expected to have an emergency management plan. In fact, many states mandate that schools develop plans to address the potential threat of a terrorist attack or natural or manmade disaster. School nurses must be prepared to act after any form of terrorism has occurred. The school nurse has an important role as a potential first responder in any emergency situation and should be an active participant in planning and policy development.

Health Promotion for School Staff

Although specific numbers vary, it is estimated that schools in the United States employ more than 5.5 million teachers and other employees. Health promotion programs at the work site have beneficial results, including positive effects on blood pressure control, daily physical activity, smoking cessation, stress and mental health management, and weight control. Staff who participate in health promotion programs increase their knowledge and positively change their attitudes and behaviors relative to smoking practices, nutrition, physical activity, stress, and emotional health. Health promotion programs improve morale, reduce job stress and absenteeism, and heighten interest in teaching health-related topics to students. School nurses play an important role in all levels of prevention through assessment, planning, intervention, and evaluation. The school nurse can assist the faculty and staff by giving workshops on exercise and nutrition, screening for increased blood pressure, and establishing weight management programs.

Family and Community Involvement

School nurses are often asked to provide health education to family, parents, and the community on a variety of topics, such as sexuality, STIs, health promotion, communicable diseases, and substance abuse. Health education in the community consists of programs that are designed to positively influence parents, staff, and others in matters related to health. School nurses are a resource in the community and can take a leadership role in developing programs that positively affect the community. School nurses may also serve as consultants and advocates for other community health programs.

Programs that engage the parents in school activities should be based on community needs and resources. Studies show that students who have parental support are more successful, experience less emotional distress, eat healthier, and are more actively engaged in learning. School nurses can promote parental involvement through the establishment of clear communication, involving parents as volunteers and including them in the planning of health-related events at schools. The nurse must also recognize that an increasing number of children are being raised in nontraditional families—single parents, grandparents, gay or lesbian couples, and interracial couples. When addressing issues with families, the nurse cannot let personal feelings alter the plan of care and must be aware that what worked with one family situation will not necessarily work for another.

School nurses need to understand the needs of families and how these needs may affect children in the school setting. The Annie E. Casey Foundation (AECF) looks at some of these key needs using the KIDS COUNT Index. The index looks at four domains that kids need in order to thrive: (1) economic well-being, (2) education, (3) health, and (4) family and community (AECF, 2020). Using these, the AECF measures the status of child well-being at both state and national levels. In 2020, Massachusetts ranked first among all states in overall child well-being, with New Mexico coming in last (AECF, 2020). During the past 6 years, there has been progress in some of the domains of child well-being (health and education) but setbacks in others (economic well-being, family, and community).

Nurses should become adept at working in the public sphere by increasing their visibility and becoming skilled in working with the media and legislators. The media can be useful in assisting school nurses with health education advocacy.

? ACTIVE LEARNING

1. Explain how the *Healthy People 2030* objectives can be used to shape school-based health care.
2. Log on to one of the websites for school nurses such as http://www.schoolnurse.com/ or https://www.nasn.org/ and review the many resources available.
3. Interview a member of the local school board about controversial subjects in health education (e.g., sex education).
4. Review the most common diseases and reported injuries in school-age children in your area. Develop a plan for how the school and the community can work together to decrease their incidence.
5. Interview the parents of several school-age children. Ask what health services they would like to see provided in the school setting.
6. Arrange with the principal of a local school to have a discussion session with children in a particular grade level. Ascertain what their eating habits are and then develop a class that can enhance healthy eating.

SCHOOL NURSING PRACTICE

School nursing is a specialty practice. School nurses need education in specific areas, such as growth and development, public health, mental health nursing, case management, program management, family theory, leadership, and cultural sensitivity, to effectively perform their roles. They must be prepared to work with children of all ages and cultures and under variable circumstances. The nurse must also keep abreast of issues affecting children and must participate in research that explores and expands the role. The school nurse's practice is relatively independent and autonomous, even though the school nurse functions as a member of an interdisciplinary team. For entry into school nursing, it is recommended that nurses hold a minimum of a bachelor's degree. The school nurse must be able to identify and access professional development opportunities in order to maintain competency in the care of children and adolescents.

School nurses' function in many roles. Among these are care provider, student advocate, educator, community liaison, and case manager. Additional skills needed by school nurses include the ability to supervise others, to practice relatively independently, and to delegate care. The National Association of School Nurses and the American Nurses Association have collaborated to develop standards of practice and competencies relevant to school nurses (2017) (see https://www.nasn.org/nasn/nasn-resources/professional-topics/scope-standards).

The school setting is a perfect place to conduct research on how children adapt to life transitions such as divorce, illness or death of a loved one, illness of either themselves or a peer, and domestic violence. The health-related behaviors of the young are a rich source of research opportunities. The school nurse must be aware of and interested in participating in different research studies.

RESEARCH HIGHLIGHTS

Research Priorities for School Nursing

The National Association of School Nursing (NASN) has identified critical areas for needed research in which there is no evidence supporting or identifying best practices and the cost-effectiveness of nursing practice in school (NASN, 2020). These critical areas are:

- The impact of infrastructure, financing (including Medicaid), policy, and systems on school healthcare processes and outcomes.
- Cost benefit analyses related to school nursing services.
- Testing the impact of NASN guidelines on student health and well-being.
- Analysis of effective implementation strategies to improve the number of school nurses using evidence-based practices.
- Studies (including analysis of existing data) that examine the structural measures of school health services or school nursing interventions (process measures) on individual and population-based student outcomes (i.e., chronic absenteeism, chronic condition management, seat time, early dismissal, errors). Examples of structural measures may include (but are not limited to) education level of school nurse, certification, supervision, using an electronic health record, and time management.

Additionally, Gordon and Barry (2006) surveyed 263 school nurses to identify what the nurses believed to be the top research priorities for the specialty. Ten areas were identified as being priority research topics. These priority areas, and examples for each, are presented here:

- Obesity/Nutrition: Nutrition and weight-loss counseling programs, eating disorders, obesity in children and teens, important of exercise
- Legal/Ethical Issues: Legal liability when delegating to nonmedical personnel, ethical issues related to children with Do Not Resuscitate orders, confidentiality, HIPAA mandates
- Emergencies: Emergency preparedness, administering epinephrine auto-injectors (EpiPen's) in school, standing orders for emergencies
- Health Education: Effective curricula for health promotion on hot topics (drugs, sexual activity, nutrition, exercise)
- Absenteeism/Attendance: The school nurse's impact on student attendance, impact of absenteeism on educational success, strategies to decrease absenteeism
- Injuries: Playground safety, sports injuries
- Health Services: Funding of school health services by using matching reimbursement (Medicaid), access to health services for students and their families, benefits and cost-effectiveness of school health services

Data from Gordon SC, Barry CD: Development of a school nursing research agenda in Florida: a Delphi study. *J Sch Nurs* 22(2):114–119, 2006.

? ACTIVE LEARNING

Attend a meeting of the school nurse association in your area. Identify the major pros and cons of being a school nurse. Look at factors such as working conditions, number of children assigned to each nurse, job functions, and job satisfaction.

SCHOOL-BASED HEALTH CENTERS

School-based health centers are one of the best ways to offer comprehensive health care services to school-age children and adolescents. It is important to note that the center or clinic works in collaboration with, but does not take the place of, the school nurse. The collaboration between the school nurse and the SBHC staff prevents fragmented care and duplication of services. SBHCs provide an interdisciplinary team approach with personnel such as nurse practitioners, social workers, psychologists, and physicians. Services provided in these centers include nutrition education, injury treatment, general and sports physicals, prescriptions, pregnancy testing, laboratory services, immunizations, gynecological examinations, medication dispensing, social work services, and management of chronic illnesses. Close collaboration must exist within and among the community, the educational board, and the families for such a center to develop and flourish.

? ACTIVE LEARNING

1. Visit a comprehensive school-based clinic in your area. Discuss how the care given in this type of clinic differs from the care that a school nurse can provide. Review the protocols of both settings and see how they differ.
2. What is the cultural makeup of your local area? How should this knowledge influence the school nurses' practice?

FUTURE ISSUES AFFECTING THE SCHOOL NURSE

Our nation's youth are our greatest asset and our hope for the future. The school nurse's role must constantly evolve to meet the demands of this future hope. Issues that will face the school nurse of tomorrow include ethical dilemmas, use of telehealth, continued threat of school violence, threat of bioterrorism, new and emerging infectious diseases, and increase in antibiotic-resistant diseases. The school nurse will need to understand and appreciate the multicultural community in which he or she will practice.

■ SUMMARY

Components of a comprehensive school health program have been clearly identified and discussed. Many of the *Healthy People 2030* objectives specifically relate to issues that can be addressed in the school setting. The role of the school nurse has changed dramatically since its inception and continues to evolve to meet the demands of school-age children, their parents, and the communities in which they live. School nurses continue to reduce the number of days and the frequency with which students miss school related to illness. They have become child advocates, counselors, health promoters and collaborators, educators, researchers, and resources in both the school and the community.

Case Study Application of the Nursing Process

Student With Lice

The nursing process is a systematic, organized approach to problem solving that nurses use when working with clients. It is neither fixed nor stagnant. It is a flexible process that allows for ongoing changes. This case study illustrates the use of the nursing process in a school setting.

Sandra Baker is a nurse at an elementary school in a small town. A second-grade teacher brought Carrie Broussard to the clinic and told Sandra that Carrie had been scratching her head all day and she was worried that Carrie might have an infection.

Assessment

Carrie was 7 years old. Her shoulder-length blond hair appeared neat and clean. When questioned by Sandra, Carrie replied that her head had been itching for 2 or 3 days, but she denied any pain or trauma. Sandra noted that Carrie did not have a fever or swollen lymph nodes, but examination of her scalp revealed multiple excoriated areas. Carrie's hair was examined with a Wood's light, and Sandra saw adult lice at the base of the hair follicles on the back of her head, near the nape of the neck. She also saw multiple nits. Sandra learned that Carrie had two brothers in the school and one sister who was a toddler at home.

On Carrie's initial visit to the clinic, Sandra assessed the following:
- Temperature
- Lymph nodes
- Scalp for any abnormal findings

Diagnosis
Individual
- Head lice

Family and Community (School)
- Potential for spread of infestation in both family and school
- Educational opportunity to prevent the spread of lice by teachers and family members

Planning

Sandra was familiar with the school district's policy that covers head lice in schoolchildren. According to the policy, the nurse must do the following:

Individual
Long-Term Goal
- Carrie's return to school after successful treatment

Short-Term Goals
- Contact Carrie's parents to tell them about the lice.
- Inform Carrie's parents that she must be picked up from school.
- Recommend treatment based on school protocol.
- Provide guidelines for returning to school.

Family and Community
Long-Term Goal
- Ensure that the teachers, staff, and family members have the necessary education relative to prevention and treatment of head lice.

Short-Term Goals
- Examine the hair of all other children in Carrie's class for lice, and treat each according to the school protocol.

- Check the hair of all siblings who attend the school for lice.
- Check the hair of all students in the siblings' classes if lice are identified.

Intervention
Family

Carrie's brothers, David and Paul, were brought to the clinic for examination. Both brothers had lice. Sandra contacted Mrs. Broussard, explained the situation to her, and requested that she come to the school to pick up her children. When Mrs. Broussard arrived at the school, Sandra gave her written information on treatment and prevention of lice and showed her what nits and lice look like. Mrs. Broussard was also instructed to check other members of the family not attending this school, especially those who share hairbrushes, pillowcases, and towels, because all family members with lice must be treated or the lice would continue to be passed from member to member. Sandra also explained procedures for cleaning combs, brushes, bedding, and potentially contaminated clothing and toys. Finally, Mrs. Broussard was informed that the children could return to school the day after treatment.

It was obvious to Sandra that Mrs. Broussard was embarrassed. To ease her mind, Sandra carefully explained that head lice are highly contagious, are easily passed from child to child, and are not an indication of poor hygiene. Mrs. Broussard repeated the instructions and left with her three children.

Community

Sandra examined all of the students from each of the Broussard children's classes for head lice. From the three classes, she identified five more children with head lice and notified their parents. Those children had siblings in three additional classrooms and she repeated the procedure for each of them. At the end of the day, she had identified a total of 15 children with head lice and contacted all parents.

Sandra investigated whether the teachers and staff desired an information session on the transmission and spread of head lice because so many students had lice. She discovered that it had been 2 years since this was done, and so she arranged a class for the coming week for the teachers and teachers' aides to learn how to identify and treat head lice.

Evaluation
Individual and Family

Mrs. Broussard brought Carrie, David, and Paul to school the following day, and on examination Sandra found their hair to be free of lice and nits. Mrs. Broussard expressed her appreciation for the nurse's help and nonjudgmental approach to the problem.

Community

Over the next 2 days, Sandra reexamined all of the children in the affected classrooms and found that the infected children had been successfully treated and that there were no new cases. New cases were not identified during the remainder of the semester. The teachers and staff gave her positive feedback about the head lice education class and asked for it to be repeated at the beginning of each school year.

Levels of Prevention and School Health

School nursing encompasses all three levels of prevention (i.e., primary, secondary, and tertiary), and all three may be practiced individually or concurrently. Table 30.1 lists examples of school nursing interventions for each of the three levels of prevention.

TABLE 30.1   Examples of Prevention and the Role of the Nurse in the School Setting

Example	Nurse's Role
Primary Prevention	
Nutrition education	Provide education to children and parent(s); consult with dietary staff
Immunizations	Provide for or refer to source(s) for immunizations; offer consultation for immunization in special circumstances
Safety	Provide safety education; inspect playgrounds and buildings for safety hazards
Health education	Teach healthy lifestyle education; develop health education curriculum for appropriate grade levels; provide health education to parents, faculty, and staff; develop suicide prevention and sex education programs
Secondary Prevention	
Screenings	Schedule routine screenings for scoliosis, vision and hearing problems, eating disorders, obesity, depression, anger, dental problems, and abuse
Case finding	Identify at-risk students
Treatment	Administer medications; develop individualized health plan; implement procedures and tasks necessary for students with special health needs; administer first aid
Home visits	Assist with family counseling and assess special and at-risk students
Tertiary Prevention	
Referral of student for substance abuse or behavior problems	Serve as an advocate; assist with resource referrals; assist parents, faculty, and staff; consult with neighborhood and law enforcement officials; initiate outreach programs
Prevention of complications and adverse effects	Follow-up and referral for students with eating disorders and obesity; participate with faculty and staff to reduce recurrence and risk factors; serve as a case manager
Faculty and staff monitoring	Follow-up for faculty and staff experiencing chronic or serious illness; follow-up of work-related injuries and accidents

EVOLVE WEBSITE

http://evolve.elsevier.com/Nies/community

- NCLEX Review Questions
- Case Studies

BIBLIOGRAPHY

Allensworth D, Lawson E, Nicholson L, Wyche J, editors: *Schools and health: our nation's investment*, Washington, DC, 1997, National Academies Press.

American Diabetes Association: Diabetes care in the school and day care setting, *Diabetes Care* 35:S76–S80, 2012.

American Association of Diabetes Educators: *Management of children with diabetes in the school setting: AADE Position Statement*, 2016. Available from: www.diabeteseducator.org/docs/default-source/practice/practice-resources/position-statements/diabetes-in-the-school-setting-position-statement_final.pdf.

Centers for Disease Control and Prevention: *10 Leading cause of injury deaths by age group, United States—2018*, 2018a. Available at: https://www.cdc.gov/injury/images/lc-charts/leading_causes_of_death_by_age_group_unintentional_2018_1100w850h.jpg.

Centers for Disease Control and Prevention: *Alcohol and other drug use, questions*, 2019a. Available from: https://nccd.cdc.gov/youthonline/App/QuestionsOrLocations.aspx?CategoryId=C03.

Centers for Disease Control and Prevention: *Childhood obesity facts*, 2021. Available at: https://www.cdc.gov/obesity/data/childhood.html.

Centers for Disease Control and Prevention: Trends in incidence of Type 1 and Type 2 diabetes among youths—Selected counties and Indian reservations, United States, 2002–2015. *MMWR*, 69-6. 2020a. Accessed from: https://www.cdc.gov/mmwr/volumes/69/wr/pdfs/mm6906a3-H.pdf.

Centers for Disease Control and Prevention: *Controlling asthma in schools*, 2018b. Available from: https://www.cdc.gov/asthma/controlling_asthma_factsheet.html.

Centers for Disease Control and Prevention: *Division of nutrition, physical activity, and obesity*, 2018c. Available from: https://www.cdc.gov/nccdphp/dnpao/multimedia/infographics/getmoving.html.

Centers for Disease Control and Prevention: *HIV/STD prevention at a glance*, 2017a. Available from: www.cdc.gov/healthyyouth/about/hivstd_prevention.htm.

Centers for Disease Control and Prevention: *National health education standards*, 2019. Available from: https://www.cdc.gov/healthyschools/sher/standards/index.htm.

Centers for Disease Control and Prevention: *Dental caries and sealant prevalence in children and adolescents in the United States, 2011–2012*, 2015. Available from: https://www.cdc.gov/nchs/products/databriefs/db191.htm.

Centers for Disease Control and Prevention: *High risk substance use among youth*, 2020. Available from: https://www.cdc.gov/healthyyouth/substance-use/index.htm.

Centers for Disease Control and Prevention: *Preventing school violence*, 2020c. Available from: https://www.cdc.gov/violenceprevention/youthviolence/schoolviolence/fastfact.html.

Centers for Disease Control and Prevention: *School health guidelines*, 2017. Available at: www.cdc.gov/healthyschools/npao/strategies.htm.

Centers for Disease Control and Prevention: *Suicide: facts at a glance*, 2015. Available from: www.cdc.gov/violenceprevention/pdf/suicide-datasheet-a.pdf.

Centers for Disease Control and Prevention: *Teen pregnancy in the United States*, 2016a. Available from: www.cdc.gov/teenpregnancy/about/.

Centers for Disease Control and Prevention: *The case for coordinated school health*, 2015. Available from: www.cdc.gov/healthyyouth/cshp/case.htm.

Centers for Disease Control and Prevention: Tobacco use among middle and high school students—United States, 2011–2015, *Morb Mortal Wkly Rep* 65(14):361–367, 2016b. Available from: https://www.cdc.gov/mmwr/volumes/65/wr/mm6514a1.htm?s_cid=mm6514a1_w.

Centers for Disease Control and Prevention: *Trends in the prevalence of sexual behaviors and HIV testing national YRBS: 1991–2015*, 2016. Available from: https://www.cdc.gov/healthyyouth/data/yrbs/pdf/trends/2015_us_sexual_trend_yrbs.pdf.

Centers for Disease Control and Prevention: *Understanding school violence: fact sheet*, 2016c. Available from: www.cdc.gov/violenceprevention/pdf/school_violence_fact_sheet-a.pdf.

Centers for Disease Control and Prevention: *Youth and tobacco use*, 2020. Available from: https://www.cdc.gov/tobacco/data_statistics/fact_sheets/youth_data/tobacco_use/index.htm.

Centers for Disease Control and Prevention: Youth Risk Behavior Surveillance—United States, 2017, *MMWR (Morb Mortal Wkly Rep)* 67(8), 2018.

Centers for Disease Control and Prevention: *Youth risk behavior surveillance system (YRBSS) overview*, 2020. Available from: https://www.cdc.gov/healthyyouth/data/yrbs/overview.htm.

Centers for Medicare & Medicaid Services: *Early and periodic screening, diagnostic, and treatment*, 2021. Available from: https://www.medicaid.gov/medicaid/benefits/early-and-periodic-screening-diagnostic-and-treatment/index.html.

Cheng TA, Bell JM, Haileyesus T, et al.: *Nonfatal playground-related traumatic brain injuries among children, 2001–2013*, Pediatrics publish0ed online, May 2, 2016, https://doi.org/10.1542/peds.2015-2721.R3.

Children's Defense Fund: *The state of America's Children 2021*, 2021. Available from: https://www.childrensdefense.org/wp-content/uploads/2021/04/The-State-of-Americas-Children-2021.pdf.

Future of Sex Education Initiative: *National sexuality education standards: core content and skills, K–12*, 2012. Available from: http://www.futureofsexed.org/documents/josh-fose-standards-web.pdf.

Gordon SC, Barry CD: Development of a school nursing research agenda in Florida: a Delphi study, *J Sch Nurs* 22(2):114–119, 2006.

Jones CM, Clayton HB, Deputy NP, Roehler DR, et al.: Prescription opioid misuse and use of alcohol and other substances among high school students—Youth risk behavior survey—2019, *MMWR (Morb Mortal Wkly Rep)* 69(S1):38–46, 2020.

National Association of School Nurses: *Medication administration in schools*, 2017a. Available from: https://schoolnursenet.nasn.org/blogs/nasn-profile/2017/03/13/medication-administration-in-schools.

National Association of School Nurses: *Role of the school nurse*, 2017b. Available from: https://schoolnursenet.nasn.org/blogs/nasn-profile/2017/03/13/the-role-of-the-21st-century-school-nurse.

National Association of School Nurses: *Environmental health*, 2021. Available from: www.nasn.org/nasn/advocacy/professional-practice-documents/position-statements/ps-environmental-health.

National Association of School Nurses: *Research priorities*, 2020a. Available from: https://www.nasn.org/research/research-priorities.

National Association of School Nurses: *School nurse workload: staffing for safe care*, 2020b. Available from: https://www.nasn.org/nasn/advocacy/professional-practice-documents/position-statements/ps-workload.

National Center for Children in Poverty: *Basic facts about low-income children*, 2021. Available from: https://www.nccp.org/wp-content/uploads/2021/03/NCCP_FactSheets_All-Kids_FINAL-2.pdf.

National Center for Education Statistics: *Fast facts: back to school statistics*, 2020. Available from: https://nces.ed.gov/fastfacts/display.asp?id=372#PK12_enrollment.

National Conference of State Legislatures: *State policies on sex education in schools*, 2020. Available from: https://www.ncsl.org/research/health/state-policies-on-sex-education-in-schools.aspx.

National Institute on Drug Abuse: *Drugfacts: anabolic steroids*, 2018. Available from: www.drugabuse.gov/publications/drugfacts/anabolic-steroids.

National Institute of Mental Health: *Eating disorders*, 2021. Available: https://www.nimh.nih.gov/health/topics/eating-disorders.

Safe Kids USA: *Game Changers: Stats, stories, and what communities are doing to protect young athletes*, 2013. Available from: https://www.safekids.org/sites/default/files/documents/ResearchReports/game_changers_-_stats_stories_and_what_communites_are_doing_to_protect_young_athletes.pdf.

School-based Health Alliance: *National survey of SBCSs*, 2017. Available from: http://www.sbh4all.org/school-health-care/national-census-of-school-based-health-centers/.

The Annie E: Casey Foundation (AECF): *KIDS COUNT Data book: state trends in child well-being*, 2020. Available from: http://www.aecf.org/m/resourcedoc/aecf-the2016kidscountdatabook-2016.pdf.

U.S. Census Bureau: *Poverty threshold*, 2021. Available from: www.census.gov/topics/income-poverty/poverty.html.

U.S. Consumer Product Safety Commission: *Injuries and investigated deaths associated with playground equipment, 2009–2014*, 2016. Available from: https://www.cpsc.gov/s3fs-public/Injuries%20and%20Investigated%20Deaths%20Associated%20with%20Playground%20Equipment%202009%20to%202014_1.pdf?29GwYlhQ6fUwXskAQxLoGaHaE8aHZSsY.

United States Preventive Services (USPS), Task Force: *Adolescent idiopathic scoliosis: screening*, 2018. Available from: https://www.uspreventiveservicestaskforce.org/uspstf/recommendation/adolescent-idiopathic-scoliosis-screening#fullrecommendationstart.

Wang TW, Neff LJ, Park-Lee E, Ren C, Cullen KA, King BA: E-cigarette use among middle and high school students—United States, *MMWR (Morb Mortal Wkly Rep)* 69(37):1310–1312, 2020. Available from: https://www.cdc.gov/mmwr/volumes/69/wr/mm6937e1.htm.

Xu G, Lane S, Buyun L, et al.: Twenty-year trends in diagnosed attention-deficit/hyperactivity disorder among US children and adolescents, 1997–2016, *JAMA Open Network* 1(4):e181471, 2018.

31

Occupational Health

*Melanie McEwen**

*The author would like to acknowledge Dr. Bonnie Rogers, whose authorship of this chapter is unparalleled.

OBJECTIVES

Upon completion of this chapter, the reader will be able to do the following:

1. Describe the historical perspective of occupational health nursing.
2. Discuss emerging demographic trends that will influence occupational health nursing practice.
3. Identify the skills and competencies relevant to occupational health nursing.
4. Apply the nursing process and public health principles to worker and workplace health issues.
5. Discuss federal and state regulations that affect occupational health.
6. Describe a multidisciplinary approach for resolution of occupational health issues.

OUTLINE

KEY TERMS

Ada Mayo Stewart
Americans With Disabilities Act
ergonomics
industrial hygiene

National Institute for Occupational Safety and Health
occupational health nursing
Occupational Safety and Health Administration

safety
toxicology
Workers' Compensation Acts

Occupational health nursing, a subspecialty of public health nursing. The American Association of Occupational Health Nurses (AAOHN) employs the following definition:

> *Occupational and environmental health nursing practice focuses on health promotion and restoration, client protection, and disease and injury prevention within the workplace.*

> *AAOHN (2019)*

As depicted in Fig. 31.1, occupational health nursing derives its theoretical, conceptual, and factual framework from a multidisciplinary base. Elements of this multidisciplinary base include the following (Rogers, 2017):

Nursing science, which provides the context for healthcare delivery and recognizes the needs of individuals, groups, and populations within the framework of prevention, health promotion, and illness and injury care management, including risk assessment, risk management, and risk communication

Medical science specific to treatment and management of occupational health illness and injury, integrated with nursing health surveillance activities

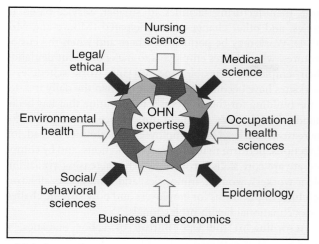

Fig. 31.1 Occupational health nursing knowledge domains. (From Rogers B: Occupational health nursing expertise, *AAOHN J* 46:477–483, 1998. Copyright Bonnie Rogers, 1998.)

Occupational health sciences, including toxicology, to recognize routes of exposure, examine relationships between chemical exposures in the workplace and acute and latent health effects such as burns or cancer and understand dose–response relationships; industrial hygiene, to identify and evaluate workplace hazards so control mechanisms can be implemented for exposure reduction; safety, to identify and control workplace injuries through active safeguards and worker training and education programs about job safety; and ergonomics, to match the job to the worker, emphasizing capabilities and minimizing limitations

Epidemiology, to study health and illness trends and characteristics of the worker population, investigate work-related illness and injury episodes, and apply epidemiological methods to analyze and interpret risk data to determine causal relationships and to participate in epidemiological research

Business and economic theories, concepts, and principles for strategic and operational planning, for valuing quality and cost-effective services and for management of occupational health and safety programs

Social and behavioral sciences, to explore influences of various environments (e.g., work and home), relationships, and lifestyle factors on worker health and determine the interactions affecting worker health

Environmental health, to systematically examine interrelationships between the worker and the extended environment as a basis for the development of prevention and control strategies

Legal and ethical issues, to ensure compliance with regulatory mandates and contend with ethical concerns that may arise in competitive environments

EVOLUTION OF OCCUPATIONAL HEALTH NURSING

The evolution of occupational health nursing in the United States has mirrored the societal changes in moving from an agrarian-based to an industrial-based economy and then as we entered the 21st century, to a service-based economy. Occupational health nursing dates to the late 1800s with the employment of Betty Moulder and Ada Mayo Stewart (Parker-Conrad, 2002; Rogers, 2017).

A group of coal-mining companies hired Betty Moulder in 1888 to care for coal miners and their families (American Association of Industrial Nurses [AAIN], 1976). Seven years later, the Vermont Marble Company hired Ada Mayo Stewart to care for workers and their families. Stewart is often referred to as the first "industrial nurse," and her activities are well documented (Parker-Conrad, 1988). In 1897, Anna B. Duncan was employed by the John Wanamaker Company to visit sick employees at home; then, in 1899, a nursing service was established for employees of the Frederick Loeser department store in Brooklyn, New York (AAIN, 1976).

At the turn of the 20th century, the industrial revolution was well under way, and the concept of health care for employees spread rapidly. Companies hiring industrial nurses in the early 1900s included the Emporium in San Francisco; Plymouth Cordage Company in Massachusetts; Anaconda Mining Company in Montana; Broadway Store in Los Angeles; Chase Metal Works in Connecticut; Hale Brothers in San Francisco; Filene's in Boston; Carson, Pirie, Scott in Chicago; Fulton Cotton Mills in Georgia; and Bullock's in Los Angeles (McGrath, 1946; Parker-Conrad, 1988). The cost-effectiveness of providing health care to employees achieved greater recognition, and by 1912, following implementation of workers' compensation legislation, 38 nurses were employed by business firms (McGrath, 1946; Parker-Conrad, 1988). The following year, a registry of industrial nurses was initiated, and in 1915, the Boston Industrial Nurses Club was formed; this group evolved into the Massachusetts Industrial Nurses Organization.

In 1916, the Factory Nurses Conference was organized. This group was open only to graduate, state-registered nurses affiliated with the American Nurses Association (ANA), and their efforts identified the industrial nurses' need to explore the uniqueness of this evolving specialty area (AAIN, 1976). More importantly, industrial nurses were practicing in single-nurse settings and recognized the benefit of uniting as a group for the purpose of sharing ideas with peers practicing in the same nursing arena. In 1917, the first educational course for industrial nurses was offered at Boston University's College of Business Administration.

During and after the Great Depression, many nurses lost jobs because employers and business managers viewed industrial nursing as a nonessential aspect of business (Felton, 1985,

1986). The focus of health care for employees again changed as a result of many factors, including the impact of the two world wars. During World War I, the government demanded health services for workers at factories and shipyards holding defense contracts. Demographics in the workplace were also dramatically different during World War II, because higher numbers of women entered the workforce. In 1942, the U.S. Surgeon General told an audience of nurses that the health conservation of the "industrial army" was the most urgent civilian need during the war (Felton, 1985).

From 1938 to 1943, the number of occupational health nurses increased by more than 10,000. In 1942, some 300 nurses from 16 states voted to create a national association for the specialty. Catherine R. Dempsey, a nurse at Simplex Wire and Cable Company in Cambridge, Massachusetts, was elected president of the national association. By 1943, approximately 11,000 nurses were employed in industry (AAIN, 1976).

Nine years later, members of AAIN voted to remain an independent, autonomous association rather than merge with the National League for Nursing or the ANA. In 1953, another important step was taken toward formalizing this specialty area of nursing practice when the *Industrial Nurses Journal* (now the *AAOHN Journal*) began publishing. In 1977, the organization changed its name to the AAOHN, reflecting a broader, more diverse scope of practice.

In the 1980s and 1990s, occupational health nursing rapidly increased its role in health promotion, policy development, management, and research while maintaining traditional occupational health nursing practice. In 1989, AAOHN developed its first research agenda, and in 1993, the **Occupational Safety and Health Administration** (OSHA) established the Office of Occupational Health Nursing, reenergizing the concept of occupational health into practice. In 1999, the AAOHN Foundation was established, and competencies in the specialty were delineated. In the 21st century, the AAOHN continues to expand specialty borders, emphasizing the importance of occupational health concepts and population-based practice. National Institute for Occupational Safety and Health (NIOSH) Centers for Excellence to Promote a Healthier Workforce were established in 2006. In 2007, the first occupational and environmental health nurse (OHN) Academic Certificate was established at the University of North Carolina School of Public Health. This led the way for the establishment of NIOSH-funded multidisciplinary academic certificate programs throughout the United States (Wachs, 2017).

DEMOGRAPHIC TRENDS AND ACCESS ISSUES RELATED TO OCCUPATIONAL HEALTH CARE

Sweeping transformations in industry have influenced the direction of occupational health nursing. These transformations include changing workforce demographics, rising healthcare costs, diversity of healthcare systems with the integration of managed care, influence of the world economy, shift in production from goods to services, and proliferation of advanced technologies. The focus of US industry is moving away from large manufacturing facilities to smaller, service-based businesses, and other changes are anticipated (Moore and Moore, 2014). Work may be performed where and when the customer requires, which forces employers to make different demands on their employees. Flexible and varying work schedules and worksites have become more common than the daily trek to the same building for the 40-hour, 9 to 5 routine that has been the standard for decades. Of major importance is the demand for an increase in skill level of all employees. The abilities to read, follow directions, perform mathematical calculations, and be computer literate are core skills for workers. The increasing availability of older workers, women, minorities, and immigrants all have far-reaching implications for employers and pose specific challenges for occupational health professionals.

According to the U.S. Bureau of Labor Statistics, total employment is expected to increase by almost 12 million jobs from 2020 to 2030. Industries and occupations related to leisure and hospitality is expected to increase the fastest driven by post-COVID-19 recovery growth. Increases in health care, personal care and social assistance, and construction are expected to grow rapidly. Service-producing industries are anticipated to continue to produce the greatest majority of the new jobs, with employment in health care—related occupations expected to grow fastest, followed by personal care and service, largely because an aging population will require more medical care. Furthermore, patients increasingly are seeking home care as an alternative to costly hospital or residential care stays (U.S. Bureau of Labor Statistics, 2021). These trends are important to understand because they have a direct impact on the national rate of economic growth, especially in the area of population-sensitive products such as food; automobiles; housing units; household goods; and services such as health care, education, and transportation. With expansion of each of these sectors, there are concomitant hazards.

Within the context of these evolving organizational trends, key characteristics include a focus on a shared vision, strategy, and long-term objectives in an environment composed of individuals working in teams. Occupational health nurses have enhanced opportunities to work on cross-functional teams to shape decisions in areas such as benefits, research, safety, and legal matters. Specifically, occupational health nurses have opportunities to positively affect the transformation of the healthcare delivery system, establish policies within the managed care environment and within corporations, and assume leadership positions on legislative staffs and in governmental agencies.

It is important that the occupational health nurse remain informed about the various healthcare options available to the workforce such as telehealth and on-site health care as rapid changes occur regarding corporate benefits and structures. This issue is of particular importance when the nurse is considering the referral of an employee to a health resource. Participation in one of the managed care plans requires that treatment takes place according to the organization's guidelines and within its health service delivery system. Managed care plans have replaced traditional indemnity plans. Access to care is closely managed and often limited. As this trend continues, the role of the occupational health nurse will take on added importance. The nurse may be called upon to accept increasing responsibilities as a primary care provider as well as a tertiary care coordinator/case manager.

As businesses seek ways to maximize the value of the dollars they spend on healthcare services, occupational health nurses and other health professionals must validate the services they provide in order to demonstrate contributions to the health of the workforce and the company (Randolph et al., 2014). This includes a focus on cost-effectiveness and value to companies to demonstrate a return on the investment for quality health care.

OCCUPATIONAL HEALTH NURSING PRACTICE AND PROFESSIONALISM

As workplaces have continued to change over the past few decades, the role of the occupational health nurse has become even more diversified and complex (Rogers, 2012). Occupational health nurses work in a variety of settings including manufacturing such as meat packing, food production, battery manufacturing, and textiles; hospital employee health institutions; and service industries such as banking and government and academic centers. Often working as the only on-site healthcare professional, the occupational health nurse collaborates with workers, employers, and other professionals to identify health problems or needs, prioritize interventions, develop and implement programs, and evaluate services delivered. The occupational health nurse is in a unique and critical position to coordinate a holistic approach to the delivery of quality, comprehensive occupational health services. The Standards of Occupational and Environmental Health Nursing, the Code of Ethics, and AAOHN practice competencies guide the nurse.

AAOHN's Standards of Occupational and Environmental Health Nursing Practice form the basis of the profession's responsibilities and accountabilities (AAOHN, 2019). The 11 standard statements are listed in Table 31.1. For each standard, identifiable criteria are detailed that can be used to evaluate practice relative to the standard. Refer to the complete standards document from the AAOHN for this information.

Guided by an ethical framework made explicit in the AAOHN Code of Ethics, occupational health nurses encourage and enable individuals to make informed decisions about healthcare concerns (AAOHN, 2016) (Box 31.1). The occupational health nurse is a worker advocate and has the responsibility to uphold professional standards and codes. The occupational health nurse is also responsible to management, is usually compensated by management, and must practice within a framework of company policies and guidelines (Rogers, 2017). Ethical dilemmas arise because the nurse is loyal to both workers and management. Issues such as screening, drug testing, informing employees about hazardous exposures, and confidentiality of health information, which is integral and central to the practice base, often create ethical debates. As advocates for workers, occupational health nurses foster equitable and quality healthcare services and safe and healthy work environments.

TABLE 31.1 Standards of Occupational and Environmental Health Nursing

Standard I: Assessment	The occupational health nurse systematically assesses the health status of the client(s).
Standard II: Diagnosis	The occupational health nurse analyzes assessment data to establish relevant diagnoses.
Standard III: Outcome identification	The occupational health nurse identifies outcomes specific to the client(s) outcome identification.
Standard IV: Planning	The occupational health nurse develops a comprehensive and goal-directed plan and formulates interventions to attain expected outcomes.
Standard V: Implementation	The occupational health nurse implements evidence-based interventions to attain desired outcomes identified in the plan.
Standard VI: Evaluation	The occupational health nurse systematically and continuously evaluates responses to interventions and progress toward achievement of desired outcomes.
Standard VII: Resource management	The occupational health nurse secures and manages the resources to support occupational health and safety programs and services.
Standard VIII: Professional development	The occupational health nurse is accountable for professional development to enhance growth and maintain competency.
Standard IX: Collaboration	The occupational health nurse collaborates clients for health promotion, restoration and disease and injury prevention within the conduct of a safe and healthy work environment.
Standard X: Research	The occupational health nurse uses evidence-based research findings in practice, and contributes to the scientific base in occupational and environmental health nursing to improve practice and advance the profession.
Standard XI: Ethics	The occupational health nurse uses an ethical framework as a basis for practice.

Data from American Association of Occupational Health Nurses: *Standards of occupational and environmental health nursing*, 2019. Copyright American Association of Occupational Health Nurses. http://www.aaohn.org.

Occupational health nurses make up the largest professional group providing healthcare services to employees in highly complex work environments. The roles of occupational health nurses are changing as a result of many factors, including rising health care costs, increased recognition of health effects associated with various exposures, emphasis on health promotion and wellness, health surveillance, women's issues, ergonomics, reproductive issues, company downsizing, trends in managed care, and multicultural workforces. Box 31.2 reflects this growth in scope of practice and outlines the occupational health nursing services currently mandated by state and federal regulations and those generally mandated by company policies.

ETHICAL INSIGHTS

Confidentiality of Employee Health Information

The occupational health nurse sometimes experiences ethical dilemmas because of dual responsibility to both the employer and the employees. In dealing with health information, the employee has the right to privacy; however, exceptions to legal protection of health information may require the nurse to provide health-related records without the worker's knowledge or consent. These exceptions are cases in which public benefit from disclosure outweighs loss of individual privacy. Specific circumstances include life-threatening emergencies; workers' compensation situations in which state regulations limiting information to carriers and/or employers are followed; examination for drug and alcohol testing in some circumstances; compliance with government regulations; OSHA-mandated surveillance and/or occupational injury or illness evaluations; and other situations as required by law (e.g., public health purposes, law enforcement, judicial proceedings, or court order).

From American Association of Occupational Health Nurses: *Position statement: confidentiality of medical records and worker health information in the occupational health setting*, 2018. http://aaohn.org/page/position-statements. Accessed December 2021.

BOX 31.1 American Association of Occupational Health Nurses Code of Ethics

I. The American Association of Occupational health Nurses (AAOHN) articulates occupational and environmental health nursing values, maintains the integrity of our specialty practice area and the nursing profession, and integrates principles of social justice into nursing and health policy.

II. The occupational and environmental health nurse (OHN) practices with compassion and respect for the inherent dignity, worth and unique attributes of every person. The OHN's commitment is to the client, whether an individual, group, community or population.

III. The OHN promotes, advocates for, and protects the rights, health, and safety of the client.

IV. The OHN has authority, accountability, and responsibility for nursing practice; makes decisions; and takes action consistent with the obligation to prevent illness and injury, promote health, and provide optimal care.

V. The OHN owes the same duties to self and others, including the responsibility to promote health and safety, preserve wholeness of character and integrity, maintain competence, and continue personal and professional growth.

VI. The OHN, through individual and collective effort, establishes, maintains, and improves the ethical environment of the work setting and conditions of employment that are conducive to safe, quality health care.

VII. OHN help advance the nursing profession and our specialty practice through research and scholarly inquiry, professional standards development, and the generation of nursing and health policy.

VIII. The OHN collaborates with other health professionals and the public to protect human rights, promote health, and reduce health disparities.

From American Association of Occupational Health Nurses: *AAOHN Code of Ethics and interpretive statements*, 2016. Available from: http://aaohn.org/p/cm/ld/fid=1350.

According to the most recent National Nursing Workforce Survey, slightly less than 1% of the total nursing population practices in the occupational health field in the United States (Smiley et al., 2021). Approximately 70% of these occupational health nurses work alone, making decisions about health and safety issues, influencing policy in health and safety, and planning and implementing myriad health programs. More than 70% of nurses practicing in occupational health are prepared at the baccalaureate level or higher, and a majority have been practicing in the field of occupational health for at least 6 years (AAOHN, 2018).

The occupational health nurse's strengths are embedded in assessing, planning, implementing, and evaluating health programs for populations, creating plans for individuals, and health education activities for worker aggregates. Often, lack of understanding or misconceptions about the occupational health nurse's role have fostered the invisibility of the nurse, both within the nursing profession itself and within the business environment, thereby exacerbating the difficulties the nurses face in being the lone provider of health care for workers in many companies. Empowered, well-trained, educated OHNs can help bring about crucial changes in the areas of primary, secondary, and tertiary prevention in occupational health.

In response to societal changes and historical events, the practice of occupational health nursing has changed dramatically, demanding a sophisticated knowledge base and problem-solving skills that are empirically grounded and multidisciplinary in nature (Rogers, 2017). For example, demographic changes with an aging, multiethnic, or largely female workforce requires enhanced knowledge and skills about managing health issues and potential problems specific to each aggregate. The roles and responsibilities of the occupational health nurse must be clearly articulated to lay people, managers, workers, union representatives, and colleagues in occupational health, nursing, and medicine to ensure that occupational health nursing can continue to positively affect workers' health, contribute to reducing healthcare costs, and foster reduction in health risks. Occupational health nurses must seize opportunities in areas such as program planning, research, and policy making during this era fraught with a health care system in crisis. Issues to be addressed and managed include nursing shortages in many areas of the country, ongoing influence of the COVID-19 pandemic including dramatic changes in the business environment, employees' awareness of workplace hazards, and the need to demonstrate the cost-effectiveness of occupational health nursing care and services.

Research is an integral component of occupational and environmental health nursing practice because it provides the basis for scientific discovery that improves practice. That National Occupational Research Agenda (**National Institute for Occupational Safety and Health [NIOSH]**) first set the priorities for research in the occupational health field in 1996. They have been updated periodically to serve as the scientific basis to continue to build the body of knowledge in

BOX 31.2 Occupational Health Nursing Services

Services Mandated by Federal and State Regulations
- Safe and healthful workplace
- Emergency medical response
- First aid responder selection and training
- First aid space, supplies, protocols, and records
- Designated medical resources for incident response
- Workers' compensation
- Confidentiality of medical records
- Compliance with medical record retention requirements
- Occupational Safety and Health Administration (OSHA) compliance
- Medical personnel requirement (29 *CFR* 1910.15)
- Injury and illness reporting and recording
- Accident and injury investigation
- Cumulative trauma disorder prevention
- Employee access to medical and exposure records
- Medical surveillance and hazardous work qualification
- Personal protective equipment evaluation and training
- Infection control
- Employee Right-to-Know Act notification and training
- Community Right-to-Know Act compliance
- Americans With Disabilities Act (ADA) compliance
- Rehabilitation Act: handicap, preplacement, fitness for duty evaluations, accommodations
- Department of Defense, Department of Transportation, Nuclear Regulatory Commission, and Drug-Free Workplace Act compliance
- Policy development
- Drug awareness education
- Drug testing and technical support
- Employee Assistance Program services
- Threat of violence and duty to warn

- Video display terminal (VDT) local regulations
- State and local public health regulations
- Nursing practice acts
- Board of Pharmacy and Drug Enforcement Agency regulations
- Continuing professional education required for licensure

Services Often Mandated by Company Policy
- Clinical supervision of on-site health services
- Health strategy development
- Health services standards
- Space, staffing, and operational standards
- Occupational illness and injury assessment, diagnosis, treatment, and referral
- Nonoccupational illness and injury assessment, diagnosis, treatment, and referral
- Disability and return-to-work evaluations and accommodations
- Impaired employee fitness-for-duty evaluation
- Preplacement evaluation and medical accommodation
- Handicap evaluation, placement, and accommodation
- Employee Assistance Program standards
- International health: travel, medical advisory, and immunizations
- Data collection and analysis
- Medical consultation
- Pregnancy placement in hazardous environments
- Professional education and development
- Audit and quality assurance

Optional Services
- Health education and health promotion
- Medical screening for early detection and disease prevention
- Physical fitness programs
- Allergy injection programs

occupational and environmental health nursing for practice improvement and expansion (Box 31.3).

OCCUPATIONAL HEALTH AND PREVENTION STRATEGIES

Like the practice of all community health professionals, the occupational health nurse's practice is based on the concept of prevention. Promotion, protection, maintenance, and restoration of worker health are priority goals set forth in the definition of occupational health nursing. Prevention of exposure to occupational and environmental safety hazards and specific strategies for each level of prevention are described along with objectives from the *Healthy People 2030* initiative.

Healthy People 2030 and Occupational Health

One topic area of *Healthy People 2030* concentrates on is termed "Workforce" (U.S. Department of Health and Human Services [USDHHS], 2021). A focus on the health and well-being is seen as vital to the economy. Objectives from this priority area cover work-related injuries and deaths, repetitive-motion injuries, work-related assaults, lead exposure, skin disorders, indoor smoking and hearing loss. In addition, objectives from other topic areas address issues related to occupational health and

BOX 31.3 Research Priorities in Occupational Health Nursing

- Effectiveness of primary healthcare delivery at the worksite
- Effectiveness of health promotion nursing intervention strategies
- Nature and effects of stress and workplace stressors on worker health
- Strategies that minimize work-related adverse health outcomes (e.g., respiratory disease)
- Health effects resulting from chemical exposures in the workplace
- Occupational hazards of healthcare workers (e.g., latex allergy and bloodborne pathogens)
- Factors that influence workers' rehabilitation and return to work
- Effectiveness of ergonomic strategies to reduce worker injury and illness
- Health effects resulting from the interaction between aging and workplace hazards
- Evaluation of critical pathways to effectively improve worker health and safety and enhance maximum recovery and safe return to work
- Evaluation of intervention strategies to improve worker health and safety
- Strategies for increasing compliance with or motivating workers to use personal protective equipment
- Emergency/pandemic preparedness in the workplace
- Impact of occupational health nursing interventions on workers' compensation claims

From American Association of Occupational Health Nurses: *Research priorities in occupational and environmental health nursing,* 2012. Available from: http://aaohn.org/page/aaohn-research-priorities.

safety. The *Healthy People 2030* box lists a few of the objectives that are specific to occupational health.

From Healthy People.gov: *Healthy People 2030: workforce objectives.* Accessed December 29, 2021.

HEALTHY PEOPLE 2030

Occupational Health Objectives

ECBP-D03—Increase the proportion of worksites that offer an employee health promotion program

ECBP-D05—Increase the proportion of worksites that offer an employee nutrition program.

OSH-01—Reduce deaths from work-related injuries

OSH-06—Reduce new cases of work-related hearing loss

OSH-05—Reduce work-related assaults

OSH-03—Reduce work-related skin diseases

ECBP-D04—Increase the proportion of worksites that offer and employee physical activity program

TU-17—Increase the number of states, territories, and DC that prohibit smoking in worksites, restaurants, and bars

Prevention of Exposure to Potential Hazards

To prevent occupational and environmental safety hazards in the work environment, it is important to identify work-related agents and exposures that are potentially hazardous. These can be categorized as follows:

Biological-infectious hazards: Agents such as bacteria, viruses, fungi, and parasites that may be transmitted via contact with infected clients or contaminated objects or substances

Chemical hazards: Various forms of chemical agents, including medications, solutions, and gases, that interact with body tissues and cells and are potentially toxic or irritating to body systems

Enviromechanical hazards: Factors encountered in work environments that cause accidents, injuries, strain, or discomfort (e.g., poor equipment or lifting devices and slippery floors)

Physical hazards: Agents within work environments, such as radiation, electricity, extreme temperatures, and noise that can cause tissue trauma through transfer of energy from these sources

Psychosocial hazards: Factors and situations encountered or associated with the job or work environment that create stress, emotional strain, or interpersonal problems

Table 31.2 provides examples of work-related exposures in each of these areas. Having a good understanding of the nature of these hazards allows for the development of health promotion and prevention strategies to mitigate exposure risk.

Levels of Prevention and Occupational Health Nursing

Because occupational health nurses typically practice autonomously in their role as healthcare providers, their activities in primary, secondary, and tertiary prevention strategies are expected to assume an even more important role in the

TABLE 31.2 Types of Occupational Hazards and Associated Health Effects

Category	Exposures	Health effects
Biological	Blood or body fluids	Bacterial, fungal, and viral infections (e.g., hepatitis B)
Chemical	Solvents	Headache and central nervous system dysfunction
	Lead	Central nervous system disturbances
	Asbestos	Asbestosis
	Acids	Burns
	Glycol ethers	Reproductive problems
	Mercury	Ataxia
	Arsenic	Peripheral neuropathy
Enviromechanical	Static or non-neutral postures	Musculoskeletal disorders
	Repetitive or forceful exertions	Back injuries
	Lighting	Headache and eye strain
	Shift work	Sleep disorders
	Electrical	Electrocution
	Slips and falls	Musculoskeletal conditions
	Struck by or against object	Injury
Physical	Noise	Hearing loss
	Radiation	Reproductive effects and cancer
	Vibration	Raynaud disease
	Heat	Heat exhaustion and heat stroke
Psychosocial	Stress	Anxiety reactions and a variety of physical symptoms
	Work–home balance	

prevention and treatment of illness, injury, and chronic disease in the future. NIOSH has embarked on an initiative, Total Worker Health. Total Worker Health is defined as "policies, programs, and practices that integrate protection from work-related safety and health hazards with promotion of injury and illness prevention efforts to advance worker well-being" (NIOSH, 2020). This initiative is designed to integrate health protection and health promotion and is important for occupational health nurses to engage. Additional information can be found at https://www.cdc.gov/niosh/twh/default.html.

Primary Prevention

In the area of primary prevention, the occupational health nurse is involved in both health promotion and disease

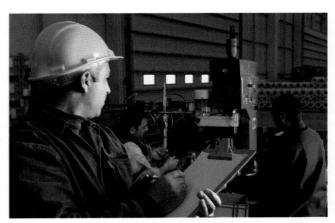

Fig. 31.2 Occupational health nurses often perform "walk-throughs" in the workplace to look for potential hazards and maintain communication with workers to prevent illness and injury.

prevention. O'Donnell (2009) describes health promotion as follows:

> *The art and science of helping people discover the synergies between their core passions and optimal health, enhancing their motivation to strive for optimal health, and supporting them in changing lifestyle to move toward a state of optimal health. Optimal health is a dynamic balance of physical, emotional, social, spiritual and intellectual health. Lifestyle change can be facilitated through a combination of learning experiences that enhance awareness, increase motivation, and build skills and most importantly, through creating opportunities that open access to environments that make positive health practices the easiest choice (p. iv).*

Primary prevention, then, begins with recognition of a health risk, a disease, or an environmental hazard. This recognition is followed by measures to protect as many people as possible from harmful consequences of that risk.

The occupational health nurse uses a variety of primary prevention methods, with one-on-one interaction as an important strategy for evaluating risk reduction behavior for individuals. The occupational health nurse has daily contact with numerous employees for many reasons (e.g., assessment and treatment of episodic illness or injury, health surveillance); therefore, this contact is an important method of promoting health. The phrase "seize the moment" aptly describes the opportunity that exists with every employee encounter.

The occupational health nurse plans and implements programs covering topics such as: weight and cholesterol reduction, promoting AIDS awareness, training in ergonomics, and smoking cessation. Performing "walk-throughs" in the workplace on a regular basis, recognizing potential and existing hazards, and maintaining communications with safety and industrial hygiene resources to prevent illness and injury from occurring will continue to be critical work for the occupational health nurse (Levy et al., 2018) (Fig. 31.2).

For overall *health promotion*, the nurse may plan, implement, and evaluate a health fair, a multifaceted health promotion strategy that usually includes a number of community health resources to provide expertise on a wide range of health issues and community services. As part of an overall health and wellness strategy, the occupational health nurse may negotiate with the employer for an on-site fitness center or area with fitness equipment; if cost or space is prohibitive, the employer may choose to partially subsidize membership at a local fitness center (Rogers et al., 2018).

⚡ SAFETY ALERT

Violence has emerged as an important safety and health issue in the workplace. According to NIOSH, *workplace violence* is defined as a violent act, including physical assault, a threat of assault, harassment, intimidation, other threatening disruptive behavior, or homicide directed toward persons at work or on duty. The violent incident may threaten the safety of an employee, customer, or vendor; have an impact on an employee's physical or psychological well-being; or cause damage to company property. Violence can also involve an assault; an aggressive act of hitting, kicking, pushing, scratching; a sexual act or attempt, with or without a weapon; or any physical or verbal attacks or threats or bullying directed to a worker by a coworker, client, relative, customer, patient, or work-associated individual that arises during or as a result of the performance of duties and that results in death, physical injury, or mental harm.

Risk factors for workplace violence include working alone or in small numbers, exchanging money with the public, working late at night or during early-morning hours, having a mobile workplace such as taxi cab, working in high-crime areas, guarding valuable property or possessions, and dealing with violent people or volatile situations. Health care professionals, public service workers, law enforcement personnel, delivery drivers, and customer service agents are also at higher risk.

The occupational health nurse works collaboratively with others to develop and implement an effective violence prevention program. Responsibilities might include participating as a member of the threat assessment team, including representatives from senior management, operations, employees, security, finance, legal, human resources, and health and safety; identifying prevention and control strategies; assisting or providing guidance in dealing with difficult or disgruntled employees or customers; and coordination of care. The nurse also provides direct care and emotional support to the victimized worker and/or worker who witnessed the violent incident, including referral to employee assistance programs or other community agencies. In addition, the nurse assists the employee with return to work. Accurate and complete documentation of violence incidents is critical for preventing future incidents and for legal purposes.

Types of *nonoccupational programs* included in the area of primary prevention are cardiovascular health, cancer awareness, personal safety, immunization, prenatal and postpartum health, accident prevention, retirement health, stress management, and relaxation techniques. Occupational health programs could include topics such as emergency response, first aid and cardiopulmonary resuscitation training, right-to-know training, immunization programs for international business travelers, prevention of back injury through knowledge of proper lifting techniques, ergonomics, and other programs targeted to the specific hazards identified in the workplace (Burgel and Childre, 2012; Rogers et al., 2018).

Women's health and safety issues such as maternal-child health, reproductive health, breast cancer education and early detection, stress management, and work—home balance issues

TABLE 31.3   Work-Related Diseases and Injuries

Work-Related Disease(s) or Injury	Example(s)
Occupational lung disease	Cancer and asthma
Musculoskeletal injuries	Back, upper extremity, and musculoskeletal disorders
Occupational cancers	Leukemia, bladder, and skin
Trauma	Death, amputation, and fracture
Cardiovascular diseases	Hypertension and heart disease
Reproductive disorders	Infertility and miscarriage
Neurotoxic disorders	Neuropathy and toxic psychosis
Noise-induced hearing loss	Loss of hearing
Dermatological conditions	Chemical burns and allergies
Psychological disorders	Neurosis; alcohol or substance abuse

are very significant as more women have entered the workforce. Thirty percent of women currently in the workforce are between ages 16 and 44 years, and each year approximately one million infants are born to these women. Interest in workplace safety and the relationship to reproductive outcomes continues to grow as women of childbearing age enter the workplace in greater proportions than ever before.

The occupational health nurse can play a key role in the development and delivery of prenatal, postpartum, and childhood programs in the workplace. Of primary importance is the ability to serve as a change agent to initiate needed programs in the work environment. Employers must be educated regarding strategies not only to reduce healthcare costs for women and infants but also to improve the work environment for mothers. Women who believe their employers are interested in the well-being of themselves and their families are more apt to be productive and satisfied employees. The occupational health nurse can play a critical role in the shaping of supportive policies and practices to accommodate the needs of families, including flexible working hours, parental leave, and on-site child care (Rogers et al., 2018).

Members of *racial and ethnic minority* groups make up a large share of the labor force, and as the number of minority and ethnic workers in the workforce increases, so will the illnesses traditionally associated with these groups of workers (e.g., heart disease and stroke, hypertension, cancer, cirrhosis, and diabetes) (Rogers et al., 2018). In addition to basic health concerns for this population, available statistics indicate that minority workers have been disproportionately concentrated in some of the most dangerous work, and they are at greater risk for experiencing many of the leading occupation-related diseases and injuries. Table 31.3 illustrates examples of common occupational diseases and injuries.

The occupational health nurse may face challenges in developing programs that are culturally and linguistically appropriate. The occupational health nurse may be in an advocacy role to negotiate with the employer for changes in the work environment that will reduce or eliminate existing or potential occupational exposure to risk factors and assist with literacy efforts that can be offered at the worksite.

Finally, veterans of our uniformed services are being employed at noteworthy numbers as they return to civilian life. Occupational health nurses should be aware of health problems—both physical and mental—that are sometimes encountered among this aggregate. Nurses should ensure that information for education for potential and anticipated problems is readily available. Furthermore, they can collect and maintain resources for referral to help assist with the most serious issues.

Secondary Prevention

Secondary prevention strategies are aimed at early diagnosis, early treatment interventions, and attempts to limit disability. The focus at this level of prevention is on identification of health needs, health problems, and employees at risk.

As with primary prevention, the occupational health nurse uses a number of different secondary prevention strategies (Rogers, 2017). By providing direct care for episodic illness and injury, the occupational health nurse is afforded the opportunity to conduct assessments and provide treatment and referrals for a variety of physical and psychological conditions. The occupational health nurse can offer health screenings, which are designed for early detection of disease, at the worksite with relative ease and at minimal cost. During the COVID-19 pandemic, wide-spread onsite testing for the virus has become commonplace and necessary for early identification of the disease as well as return to work. In addition, commonly used screenings conducted in occupational health settings may focus on vision, cancer, cholesterol, hypertension, diabetes, tuberculosis, and pulmonary function. Other types of screening, such as mammography, may be contracted with a vendor who uses mobile equipment.

Secondary prevention efforts provided by the occupational health nurse include *preplacement, periodic,* and *job transfer evaluations* to ensure that a worker is being placed or is continuing to work in a job that is safe for him or her (Rogers, 2017). The preplacement evaluation is performed before the worker begins employment in a new company or is placed in a different job (Fig. 31.3). The evaluation is a baseline examination that consists of a health history, an occupational health history, and a physical assessment that should target the type of work that the employee will be performing. For example, if the employee is going to be lifting materials in a warehouse, special attention should be paid to any history of musculoskeletal problems. Strength testing and range of motion should be performed for all muscle groups.

The preplacement examination may also include tests to determine specific organ functions that may be affected by exposure to existing agents in the employee's workplace. For example, if the employee is working with a chemical that is a known liver toxin, baseline liver function tests may be

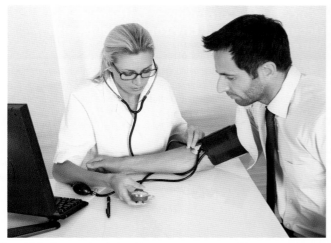

Fig. 31.3 Occupational health nurses may provide preemployment physical examinations or monitor health problems.

appropriate to determine the current health status of the liver and its ability to handle this specific chemical exposure. However, the preplacement examination must be carefully evaluated to ensure compliance with the Americans With Disabilities Act (ADA), which is discussed later in the chapter.

Periodic assessments usually occur at regular intervals (e.g., annual and biannual) and are based on specific protocols for those exposed to substances or irritants such as lead, asbestos, noise, and various chemicals. Examinations of individuals transferring to other jobs are critical to document any changes in health that may have occurred while the employee was working in a specific area or with a specific process. Such examinations are usually done to comply with OSHA regulations or NIOSH recommendations. (See **Resource Tool 30C** for an example of an OSHA screening and surveillance guide.) For full details of compliance requirements, OSHA standards must be consulted.

Activities must continue to focus on prevention and early detection by increasing awareness of the incidence of commonly occurring health conditions such as breast cancer and providing accessible and affordable screening programs. For example, it is estimated that in 2021, invasive breast cancer will be diagnosed in more than 281,000 women and that about 43,600 women will die of the disease each year, making breast cancer one of the most commonly diagnosed malignancies among women in the United States and the second leading cause of cancer death, after lung cancer (American Cancer Society, 2021). By detecting early malignancies, breast cancer screening reduces the mortality rate in women between ages 50 and 69 years. Mammography is the most effective method for detecting these early malignancies. The occupational health nurse is in an excellent position to play a key role in reducing morbidity and mortality associated with breast cancer. Increasingly, the occupational health nurse will be expected to document the return on investment for these and other related activities in the workplace.

Tertiary Prevention

On a tertiary level, the occupational health nurse plays a key role in the rehabilitation and restoration of the worker to an optimal level of functioning. Case management is complex, and the goal is to return the employee to gainful employment as soon as possible, but taking care to not reinjure the employee (AAOHN, 2015a). Strategies include negotiation of workplace accommodations, and counseling and support for workers who will continue to be affected by chronic disease and disability (Rogers, 2017).

Knowledge of the workplace, the ability to negotiate with the employer for appropriate accommodations, early intervention, and comprehensive case management skills have been and will continue to be essential to the disabled employee's successful return to work. The process of returning an individual to work begins with the onset of injury or illness (Rogers, 2017). Regardless of whether an occupational or a nonoccupational condition is involved, the occupational health nurse is the center of case management (Levy et al., 2018). The nurse works closely with the primary care provider to monitor the progress of the ill or injured worker and to identify and eliminate potential barriers in the return-to-work process. The nurse has a comprehensive understanding of the workplace and of the physical requirements necessary for the employee to work. The physical demands analysis (Randolph and Dalton, 1989) is a useful tool for objectively assessing the physical demands of any job. (See **Resource Tool 30D**, Physical Demands Analysis.) Once the assessment is completed, the occupational health nurse can relay this information to community health professionals caring for the employee.

For workers needing special accommodations, the occupational health nurse can negotiate and facilitate those appropriate to the employee's health limitations (AAOHN, 2015a). The nurse is often the driving force behind the employer's creation of a transitional duty pool. The goal of this type of program is to provide temporary work that is less physically demanding in nature than the employee's regular work. It facilitates the employee's return to the workplace earlier than if he or she was required to wait until after regaining full strength.

The occupational health nurse can monitor and support the health of employees returning to work who continue to experience adverse health effects of chronic disease. For example, the employee who is returning to work after sustaining a myocardial infarction may undergo blood pressure monitoring on a routine basis. Counseling regarding adjustment to normal work life and support for behavior modification (e.g., smoking cessation) also may be provided.

In addition, because the workforce is aging and because older workers are more prone to chronic disease, the occupational health nurse can implement and monitor treatment protocols and help workers live and work at their optimum comfort level while managing their diseases. Responsibilities for the care of elderly parents or significant others will influence the balance of work and home for older workers. The occupational health nurse's role as counselor, referral resource for workers, and consultant to management can influence future beneficial changes.

❓ ACTIVE LEARNING

1. A weight loss program was conducted during August. Ten people participated in the 6-week program. The total weight loss for the group was 185 pounds. The following chart indicates the weight loss for the individuals:

Weight before program (lb)	Weight after program (lb)
215	190
175	160
139	129
275	245
145	120
198	183
120	115
243	233
185	145
210	200

Is there a more effective way to show the results of the program? Assume a peer distributed this report for critique. Be creative, filling in any data, facts, figures, or other information that may be missing. Redesign a report to send to management.

2. Take an occupational history on five currently employed workers. Identify the occupation, associated job tasks, and potential health hazards. Describe control strategies that could minimize or eliminate the risk of adverse health effects.

3. Conduct a literature review to identify critical concepts in occupational health nursing, epidemiology, ergonomics, safety, industrial hygiene, and medicine, and describe how these disciplines work together to achieve optimal ends.

SKILLS AND COMPETENCIES OF THE OCCUPATIONAL HEALTH NURSE

Although clinical and emergency care remains an important tenet of occupational health nursing, the current and future practice must focus on a proactive approach with the goal of preventing illness and injury and promoting health. Therefore, the occupational health nurse must possess competencies necessary to recognize and evaluate potential and existing health hazards in the workplace. Management and budgeting skills and knowledge of legal and regulatory requirements, toxicology, ergonomics, epidemiology, environmental health, safety, counseling, and health promotion and education are essential to meet the present and future demands of occupational health nursing practice.

Competencies in occupational and environmental health nursing have been outlined by AAOHN (2015b) (Box 31.4). Each competency delineates comprehensive performance criteria at the competent, proficient, and expert levels. Each level is described here, followed by a description of occupational health nursing practice at that level.

BOX 31.4   Competency Categories in Occupational and Environmental Health Nursing

1. Manages total worker health independently and with other team members
2. Adheres to principles of professional practice
3. Demonstrates understanding of the business climate and its impact on the health of the community
4. Practices culturally appropriate, evidence-based nursing care within licensed scope of practice

From American Association of Occupational Health Nurses: *Competencies in occupational and environmental health nursing,* 2015. Can be purchased at: http://aaohn.org/p/cm/ld/fid=1350.

Competent

At the "competent" level of practice, the nurse has gained confidence and his or her perception of the role is one of mastery and an ability to cope with specific situations. There is less of a need to rely on the judgments of peers and other professionals. Work habits tend to stress consistency rather than routine tailoring of care to encompass individual differences (Benner, 1984).

The competent OHN has sufficient experience to recognize a range of practice issues and to function comfortably in such roles as clinician, occupational health services coordinator, and case manager. This nurse follows company procedures and relies on assessment checklists and clinical protocols to provide treatment.

Proficient

The "proficient" nurse has an increased ability to perceive client situations as a whole on the basis of past experiences, focusing on the relevant aspects of the situation. The nurse is able to predict the events to expect in a particular situation and can recognize that protocols sometimes must be altered to meet the needs of the client (Benner, 1984).

Occupational and environmental health nursing example: A proficient OHN is able to quickly obtain the information needed for accurate assessment and move rapidly to the critical aspects of the problem. Structured goals are replaced by priority setting in response to the situation. The proficient nurse usually possesses sophisticated clinical or managerial skills in the occupational health setting.

Expert

The "expert" nurse has extensive experience and a broad knowledge base and is able to grasp a situation quickly and initiate appropriate action. The nurse has a sense of salience grounded in practice guiding actions and priorities (Benner, 1984).

Occupational and environmental health nursing example: OHNs at the expert level include those providing leadership in developing occupational and environmental health policy within an organization, those functioning in upper executive or management roles, those serving as consultants to business and government, and those designing and conducting significant research in the field.

Examples of Skills and Competencies for Occupational Health Nursing

As described, numerous skills and competencies are necessary for occupational health nursing practice. Examples of some of these are outlined here, according to four of the defined areas of competence.

- Manages total worker health independently and with other team members
  - Identifies hazards and exposures and recommends control strategies for their mitigation
  - Plans, implements, and evaluates occupational health and safety programs and services for the target populations
- Adheres to principles of professional nursing practice
  - Practices nursing ethically, competently, and within the legal scope of practice
  - Stays current with evidence-based occupational health nursing practice and interventions
- Demonstrates understanding of the business climate and its impact on the health of the community
  - Works with interdisciplinary teams to provide services to workforces and with those who provide disaster services in times of emergencies
  - Manages budgets
- Practices culturally appropriate, evidence-based nursing care within a licensed scope of practice
  - Gathers information related to occupational health history, conducts assessments, and informs decision making regarding fitness for duty and return to work (see Fig. 31.3)
  - Provides education and counsels on strategies for risk identification and elimination

IMPACT OF FEDERAL LEGISLATION ON OCCUPATIONAL HEALTH

Legislation and associated activities have influenced the practice of occupational health in the United States. Table 31.4 presents a historical perspective of some of the major pieces of legislation that have had, and will continue to have, a direct impact on the general practice of occupational and environmental health nursing. The Occupational Safety and Health Act, Workers' Compensation Acts, and the ADA are highlighted here.

Occupational Safety and Health Act

The Occupational Safety and Health Act of 1970 was enacted 2 years after a major coal-mining disaster in West Virginia. The passage of this legislation came about because of concerns about workers' health, a burgeoning environmental awareness, union activities, and a greater knowledge about workplace

TABLE 31.4 Historical Perspective of Legislation Affecting Occupational Health in the United States

Year	Legislation
1836	First restrictive child labor law enacted (Massachusetts)
1877	State legislation passed requiring factory safeguards (Massachusetts)
1879	State legislation passed requiring factory inspections (Massachusetts)
1886	State legislation passed requiring reporting of industrial accidents (Massachusetts)
1910	State legislation passed requiring formation of an Occupational Disease Commission (Illinois)
1911	Workmen's Compensation Act passed (New Jersey)
1935	Social Security Act Passed (state and federal unemployment insurance program)
1936	Walsh-Healey Act (federal legislation setting occupational safety and health standards for certain government contract workers)
1938	Fair Labor Standards Act (setting minimum age for child labor)
1948	All states now have Workers' Compensation Acts
1964	Civil Rights Act
1965	McNamara-O'Hara Act (extends protection of the Walsh-Healey Act to include suppliers of government services)
1966	Mine Safety Act (mandatory inspections and health and safety standards in mining industry)
1969	Coal Mine Health and Safety Act (mandatory health and safety standards for underground mines)
1970	Occupational Safety and Health Act
1970	Environmental Protection Agency established
1970	Consumer Protection Agency established
1972	Equal Employment Opportunity Act
1972	Noise Control Act
1972	Clean Water Act
1973	HMO Act
1973	Rehabilitation Act
1976	Toxic Substances Control Act
1976	Resources Conservation and Recovery Act
1977	Federal Mine Safety and Health Act
1990	Americans With Disabilities Act
1991	Bloodborne Pathogens Standard
1993	Family Medical Leave Act
1996	National Occupational Research Agenda (NIOSH) established
1996	Health Insurance Portability and Accountability Act (HIPPA)
2000	Needlestick Safety and Prevention Act
2002	Recordkeeping rule amended
2008	Genetic Information Nondiscrimination Act
2010	Patient Protection and Affordable Care Act
2012	Whistleblower Protection Enhancement Act
2020	Pandemic and All-Hazards Preparedness and Advancing Innovation Act
2020	CARES Act (Coronavirus Aid Relief and Economic Security Act)

hazards. The general duty clause of the act (section 5) states that employers must "furnish a place of employment free from recognized hazards that are causing or likely to cause death or serious physical harm to employees" (OSHA, 1970). The act also identifies the roles of the various governmental agencies; provides for the establishment of federal occupational safety and health standards; and identifies a structure of penalties, fines, and sentences for violations of regulations. Under the act, any state has the right to implement its own occupational safety and health administration. The only requirement is that the state standards meet or exceed federal standards. Currently, 25 states and the Virgin Islands operate state occupational safety and health administrations. The following organizations were formed under the provisions of the act:

- Under the jurisdiction of the Department of Labor, the OSHA is responsible for promulgating and enforcing occupational safety and health standards.
- Under the jurisdiction of the USDHHS, NIOSH is responsible for funding and conducting research, making recommendations for occupational safety and health standards to OSHA, and for funding Occupational Safety and Health Education and Research Centers for the training of occupational health professionals.
- The Occupational Safety and Health Review Commission, which is appointed by the president, is responsible for advising OSHA and NIOSH regarding the legal implications of decisions or actions in the course of performing their duties.
- The National Advisory Committee on Occupational Safety and Health, which is also appointed by the president, is a group of consumers and professionals who are responsible for making recommendations to OSHA and NIOSH regarding occupational health and safety.
- The National Commission on State Workers' Compensation Laws, appointed by the president as well, was tasked with studying the adequacy of state workers' compensation laws and making recommendations to the president on its findings. This commission's work ended as of October 30, 1972.

Since it was instituted, OSHA has promulgated occupational health and safety standards. These are published in the *Code of Federal Regulations* (CFR) and updated on a regular basis. Having access to the most recent publication of these standards is a responsibility of the occupational health nurse.

The occupational health nurse must be knowledgeable of Title 29 of the *Code,* part 1910 (29 CFR 1910) (OSHA, 2021a), and other sections that apply to specific hazards in the workplace. For example, 29 CFR 1904 (OSHA, 2021b) pertains to OSHA's record-keeping requirements and mandates the employer's responsibility to keep records of work-related injuries, illnesses, and deaths. These records must be posted in the workplace for 1 month per year and made available for review by OSHA at any time. In many cases, the occupational health nurse has full responsibility for compliance with this standard.

OSHA has 10 regional offices throughout the United States. Inspectors are assigned to each region to enforce the standards and to provide consultation to industries. An OSHA inspection can be initiated in one of several ways. Each office plans a schedule of routine visits to the industries in their respective regions. In the past, funding has been an issue, and inspections have not taken place in the number or frequency originally intended. An inspection will occur if a major health or safety problem, such as a death, occurs at the worksite, or if three or more workers are sent to the hospital as a result of the same incident. Inspection also may occur by employer request. A request is not usually made unless the employer has an exemplary occupational health and safety program and wishes to participate in OSHA's voluntary inspection program. Inspection also may be initiated by an employee request if there is concern about a suspected hazardous condition. In this case, OSHA is mandated to respond, and it must keep the employee's name confidential at the employee's request. In the past, penalties for violations have been inconsequential, and sentences have rarely been served. However, events now indicate that fines have increased, and OSHA has made public its intention to criminally prosecute company executives for serious and willful violations.

In many organizations, the occupational health nurse is the interface with the OSHA inspector. This position requires the nurse to be knowledgeable about the potential hazards in the workplace and about the appropriate control measures designed to eliminate or minimize exposure. The nurse should know that employees or their union representatives have the right to accompany the OSHA investigators.

Workers' Compensation Acts

Workers' Compensation Acts are state mandated and state funded. Workers' compensation programs provide income replacement and pay for health care services for workers who sustain a work-related injury, temporary or permanent disability, or death. Workers' Compensation Acts also protect the employer if the compensation received by the employee precludes legal suits against the employer. Each state regulates its own workers' compensation program that is unique to that state. The employer can self-insure, contract with commercial insurance carriers, or purchase a policy with the state-operated insurance fund. Workers receive an average of 66% of their take-home pay before taxes as compensation. Some disabled workers and their families are eligible for other benefit programs, including old age, survivors, disability, and health insurance; supplemental security income; and any other disability arrangement that they may have purchased through the company or on an individual basis.

In an era of high healthcare costs and a propensity for injured workers to engage the services of lawyers to represent them in negotiating financial settlements, many employers are claiming that workers' compensation costs are harming their ability to compete in an international marketplace. The occupational health nurse has a unique opportunity to support both the employee and employer in this arena. For the employee, the nurse may be the initial person to whom the work-related injury or illness is reported. Accurate assessment of the injury or illness and appropriate treatment are essential. Community resources must be identified to ensure that the injured worker is provided with high-quality health care and appropriate medical follow-up.

The occupational health nurse educates the employee regarding benefits under the Workers' Compensation Act and is often the one who files the claim. If the employee is unable to work for a period, the nurse provides case management support and remains in contact with the employee until they return to work. If the employer uses an insurance carrier, the nurse works closely with the claims adjuster to manage the case. The need for light duty or other workplace accommodations is determined before the employee's return. In most cases, the nurse facilitates this process with the employer.

For the employer, the occupational health nurse provides the expertise in early intervention and case management. The goal is to limit the worker's disability and provide an opportunity for early return to work through appropriate workplace accommodations. The desired outcome is a productive employee with optimum health and productivity, with reduced health care and workers' compensation costs.

Americans With Disabilities Act

The Americans With Disabilities Act, enacted by Congress in July 1990, is a comprehensive act that prohibits discrimination on the basis of disability. The core of this law requires employers to adjust facilities and practices for the purpose of making "reasonable accommodations" to enhance opportunities for individuals with disabilities.

The ADA defines disability as "physical or mental impairment that substantially limits one or more major life activities, having record of such an impairment, or being regarded as having such an impairment" (Kaminshine, 1991, p. 249). Physical or mental impairment guidelines are the same as those described by the Federal Rehabilitation Act and include "any physiologic disorder or condition, cosmetic disfigurement, anatomical loss affecting any of the major body systems, or any mental or psychological disorder" (Kaminshine, 1991, p. 249). Major life activities include caring for self, walking, seeing, hearing, and speaking. The ADA excludes conditions relating to sexual preference and gender identity, compulsive gambling, kleptomania, and pyromania. The ADA also denies protection for individuals who are currently involved in illegal drug use.

With regard to the ADA, the occupational health nurse has particular responsibility in two areas. The first involves the duty to provide or facilitate reasonable accommodations. This duty is facilitated by the nurse's familiarity with the physical requirements of the jobs at the particular workplace. The second involves preplacement inquiries and health examinations. Preplacement health examinations will be permitted only if phrased in terms of the applicant's general ability to perform job-related functions rather than in terms of a disability and after a job offer has been made. The examination must be job related and consistently conducted for all applicants performing similar work.

As illustrated in this discussion of specific laws pertinent to occupational health, the legal context for occupational health

nursing practice is broad and involves many arenas. The occupational health nurse must be knowledgeable about all laws and regulations that govern any industry in which the nurse provides health care to employees (e.g., laboratories, transportation, and utilities).

LEGAL ISSUES IN OCCUPATIONAL HEALTH

In recognition of the dynamic nature of occupational health nursing practice, coupled with the influences and impact of larger policy issues, the occupational health nurse must know the legal parameters of practice and must respond to legislative mandates that govern worker health and safety. Professionally, the occupational health nurse is primarily accountable to workers and worker populations and to the employer, the profession, and self (AAOHN, 2019). In particular, the occupational health nurse must be aware of liability and legal issues related to the following:

- The employee—nurse relationship
- The employment capacity of the occupational health nurse
- Any acts of negligence

The employee—nurse relationship can be confusing when the employer hires the nurse to provide services to the employee. The concern is whether a professional relationship exists under the law or the relationship is based on a coworker status.

MULTIDISCIPLINARY TEAMWORK

As workplaces have become more complex, a diverse array of expertise has emerged in many functional and technical areas. To be successful, the occupational health nurse must recognize the need to work as part of an interdisciplinary team. The nurse may interact with occupational medicine professionals, industrial hygienists, safety and ergonomic professionals, employee assistance counselors, personnel professionals, and union representatives (Fig. 31.4). Community health professionals, insurance carriers, and other support agencies in the community are also critical links.

? ACTIVE LEARNING

A large automobile manufacturer needs a program designed to control respiratory disease among foundry workers. Workers in different areas of ferrous foundries are exposed to different respiratory hazards. The main problems are exposures to silica and formaldehyde. The corporation would like to develop a pilot program for one of its foundries that will then be applied to its other foundries. Health and industrial hygiene data will be collected. Both the corporation and the workers support the project, and both see the project as having the following three purposes:

- Detecting health effects in individuals who may benefit from intervention
- Determining the relationship of health effects with environmental exposures
- Identifying control strategies as appropriate

Outline a pilot program. Discuss the implications of discovering adverse health effects among current workers. Describe the roles of the occupational health nurse, physician, industrial hygienist, safety professional, manager, and employee.

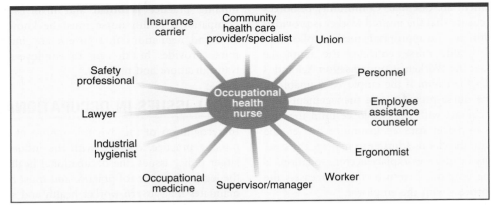

Fig. 31.4 The occupational health nurse's professional links in the workplace and community.

CASE STUDY   Application of the Nursing Process

Employee With Exposure to Chemicals

Leslie Johnston is a 23-year-old woman who was transferred by her employer into a job that required her to work with chemicals used in photolithography. Leslie became concerned when she noticed that the label on one of the pieces of equipment warned of possible adverse effects on reproduction. Because of her concern and related issues, she went to the on-site health clinic to talk with Peter Mitchell, the occupational health nurse.

Peter invited Leslie into his office to ask her questions and do a brief health history. Leslie reported that her health had been "excellent" until recently but that she had not felt well since transferring to her new position. She explained that she was newly married and thought she may be pregnant, but this was unconfirmed. She questioned whether her vague physical complaints (fatigue, headaches, and occasional queasiness) might be related to working with chemicals, a pregnancy, or another reason.

Peter reassured Leslie that he had been employed at the company for 8 years, and he was aware that there were no restrictions in Leslie's work area for pregnant women. He pulled up her health file from his computerized database and gave her a set of health history forms to complete. He also had her read and sign several forms related to confidentiality and assured her that none of her health information would be shared with their employer without her consent.

Assessment

To obtain needed information, Peter:
- Completed general health and occupational health histories.
- Performed a modified physical assessment and discussed the symptoms Leslie was experiencing.
- Referred Leslie to her personal healthcare provider for further evaluation and to obtain a pregnancy test. (NOTE: In some cases, on-site clinics will be equipped for basic procedures such as this. If this is not a service provided by the occupational health nurse, referral must be made to the employee's health care provider. If the employee does not have one, referral must be made to an appropriate community health resource.) Peter encouraged Leslie to inform her supervisor and himself if the pregnancy test result was positive so they could adapt her assignments to her condition.
- Assessed Leslie's work area with an industrial hygienist to determine whether there might be problems, such as leaking equipment or problems with ventilation.
- Reviewed the most current industrial hygiene data appropriate to the area.

Diagnosis

Individual
- At risk for chemical exposure
- Vague physical complaints of unknown etiology

- Possible pregnancy
- At risk for possible adverse pregnancy outcomes
- Stress related to concern regarding possible exposure to harmful chemicals

Community
- Potential for exposure of employees to unsafe chemicals and/or working conditions

Planning
- Peter developed a plan of care based on Leslie's health history and concerns. Together they set the following goals:

Individual

Short-Term Goals
- Determine pregnancy status.
- Determine potential exposure levels and review side effects of chemicals.
- Determine reason for her vague physical complaints.
- Reduce stress experiences.

Long-Term Goals
- Ensure that the work environment is safe for future pregnancies (if Leslie is not pregnant at present).
- Collaborate with Leslie and her supervisor on possible work restrictions.

Community (Workplace)

Short-Term Goals
- Company personnel (e.g., the occupational health nurse, the industrial hygienist, and all others who are directly affected) will be knowledgeable in safe handling of all hazardous chemicals.
- All company policies regarding safety and exposure will be followed.

Long-Term Goals
- Policies on handling of chemicals and related information will be reviewed periodically as required by law.
- All employees who work with and around potentially hazardous chemicals will undergo periodic instruction and instruction in and confirmation of knowledge about proper procedures.
- Work areas will be monitored per policy for compliance with safe practices.
- There will be no incidents involving worker exposure to chemicals.

Intervention

Individual

Peter conducted a brief physical examination and did not identify any obvious physical abnormalities. Because Leslie's chief complaints were fatigue, occasional

CASE STUDY   Application of the Nursing Process—cont'd

headaches, and queasiness, he encouraged her to make an appointment with her primary care provider or gynecologist for a more extensive workup and to assess for pregnancy.

With her permission, he called the industrial hygienist to counsel Leslie regarding the policies of the company, to explain what chemicals might potentially be hazardous, and to review procedures and restrictions. The hygienist also stated that he would send a team to Leslie's work area to take air samples, check lighting, and perform other tests to ensure there were no problems.

Community (Workplace)

The assigned industrial hygiene team sampled the environment for chemical exposure per established procedure. They also set up a plan to have the area more frequently observed pending the results of the tests. The hygienist assured Peter and Leslie that he would communicate any work restrictions or changes to the personnel department and Leslie's supervisor if needed.

Evaluation
Individual

After the meeting with Peter and the industrial hygienist, Leslie stated that she felt reassured. She agreed to make an appointment as soon as possible with her

doctor for an evaluation and pregnancy test. She also agreed to inform Peter and her direct supervisor if she learned that she was pregnant.

Community (Workplace)

The industrial hygienist and his assistants performed several tests in close proximity to Leslie's work station; they found no abnormal readings, and all equipment was in good working order. Per agency policy and following OSHA regulations, they charted all findings and submitted reports.

Levels of Prevention
Primary
- Teach about chemicals, exposures, etc.
- Instruct about chemical avoidance.
- Remove employee from environment through work restrictions.

Secondary
- Assess employee for signs and symptoms.
- Assess work environment for exposure.
- Refer for evaluation of possible health problems as needed.

Tertiary
- Provide reproductive counseling.

■ SUMMARY

This chapter describes the evolution of occupational health nursing. It also highlighted current and future demographics as well as business and industry trends as they relate to this nursing specialty area. Aging workers, escalating health care costs, increasing numbers of women and minorities in the workforce, and the competitive international marketplace are key factors shaping occupational health nursing practice.

The occupational health nursing role is challenging and can have a tremendous impact on the quality and delivery of health

care to workers and their families. Nurses working in occupational settings should have an excellent understanding of all levels of prevention and possess the skills and competencies outlined here.

For the public health nurse who works in other settings, such as home health, clinics, and schools, knowledge of occupational health nursing practice is also important. Many companies do not have on-site occupational health nurses and therefore must rely on community health nurses to support their occupational health and safety needs.

EVOLVE WEBSITE

http://evolve.elsevier.com/Nies/community
- NCLEX Review Questions
- Case Studies

BIBLIOGRAPHY

American Association of Industrial Nurses: *The nurse in industry*, 1976. New York.

American Association of Occupational Health Nurses: *Case management: the occupational and environmental health nurse role*, 2015a. Chicago, Case Management The Occupational and Environmental Health Nurse Role Position Statement (1).pdf.

American Association of Occupational Health Nurses: *2018 Compensation & benefits survey*, 2018. Atlanta, GA, 2018 Salary Survey Executive Summary.pdf.

American Association of Occupational Health Nurses: Competencies in occupational and environmental health nursing, *AAOHN J* 55:442–447, 2015b. Available from: http://www.aaohn.org.

American Association of Occupational Health Nurses: *AAOHN Code of Ethics and interpretive statements*, 2016. Available from: www.aaohn. org.

American Association of Occupational Health Nurses: *Standards of occupational and environmental health nursing*, 2019.

American Cancer Society: *How common is breast cancer?*, 2021. Available from: https://www.cancer.org/cancer/breast-cancer/about/how-common-is-breast-cancer.html.

Benner P: *From novice to expert: excellence and power in clinical nursing practice*, Menlo Park, CA, 1984, Addison-Wesley.

Burgel B, Childre F: The occupational health nurse as the trusted physician in the 21st century, *AAOHN J* 60:143–150, 2012.

Felton JS: The genesis of occupational health nursing: Part I, *Occup Health Nurs* 30:45–49, 1985.

Felton JS: The genesis of occupational health nursing: Part II, *AAOHN J* 34:210–215, 1986.

Kaminshine S: New rights for the disabled: the Americans with Disabilities Act of 1990, *AAOHN J* 39:249–251, 1991.

Levy BS, Wegman DH, Baron SL, Sokas R. In *Occupational and environmental health*, ed 7, New York, 2018, Oxford University Press.

McGrath BJ: *Nursing in commerce and industry*, New York, 1946, The Commonwealth Fund.

Moore P, Moore R. In *Core curriculum for occupational and environmental health nursing*, ed 4, Chicago, 2014, AAOHN.

National Institute for Occupational Safety and Health (NIOSH): *NIOSH total woker health program*, 2020. Available from: Total Worker Health | NIOSH | CDC.

Occupational Health and Safety Administration (OSHA): *Occupational Safety Act*, 1970 (P.L. 91—596).

Occupational Health and Safety Administration (OSHA): *Reglations (Standards—29): 1910*, 2021a. Available from: 1910 | Occupational Safety and Health Administration (osha.gov), https://www.osha.gov/pls/oshaweb/owasrch.search_form?p_doc_type=STANDARDS&p_toc_level=1&p_keyvalue=1910.

Occupational Health and Safety Administration (OSHA): *Regulations (Standards—29): 1904*, 2021b. Available from: Record-keeping - Detailed Guidance for OSHA's Injury and Illness Recordkeeping Rule | Occupational Safety and Health Administration, https://www.osha.gov/pls/oshaweb/owasrch.search_form?p_doc_type=STANDARDS&p_toc_level=1&p_keyvalue=1904.

O'Donnell M: Editor's notes: definition of health promotion 2.0: embracing passion, enhancing motivation, recognizing dynamic balance, and creating opportunities, *Am J Health Promot* 24(Iv), 2009.

Parker-Conrad JE: A century of practice: occupational health nursing, *AAOHN J* 36:156—161, 1988.

Parker-Conrad JE: Celebrating our past, *AAOHN J* 50:537—541, 2002.

Randolph SA, Dalton PC: Limited duty work: an innovative approach to early return to work, *AAOHN J* 37:446—452, 1989.

Randolph S, Scully A, Bertsche P: Economic, political, and business factors. In Moore P, Moore R, editors: *Core curriculum for occupational and environmental health nursing*, ed 3, Chicago, 2014, AAOHN, pp 67—143.

Rogers B: Occupational health nursing expertise, *AAOHN J* 46:477—483, 1998.

Rogers B. In *Occupational health nursing: concepts and practice*, ed 3, Beverly, MA, 2017, OEM Press.

Rogers B: Occupational and environmental health nursing: ethics and professionalism, *AAOHN J* 60:177—182, 2012.

Rogers B, Randolph S, Mastrianno K. In *Occupational health nursing guidelines for primary clinical conditions*, ed 5, Beverly, MA, 2018, OEM Press.

Smiley RA, Ruttinger C, Oliveira CM, et al.: The 2020 national nursing workforce survey, *J Nur Regul* 12(1S):S2—S96, 2021.

Thompson M: Professional autonomy of occupational health nurses un the United States, *AAOHN J* 60:159—166, 2012.

U.S. Bureau of Labor Statistics: Employment Projections: 2020—2030 Summary, Employment Projections 2020—2030 (bls.gov), https://www.bls.gov/news.release/ecopro.nr0.htm.

U.S. Department of Health and Human Services: *Healthy people 2030*, 2021. www.healthypeople.gov.

Wachs JE: The American Association of Occupational Health Nurses: seventy-five years of education, practice and research, *Workplace Health & Saf* 65:148—153, 2017.

32

Forensic and Correctional Nursing

Stacy A. Drake

OBJECTIVES

Upon completion of this chapter, the reader will be able to do the following:

1. Define forensic nursing.
2. Describe specialties of forensic nurses.
3. Explain issues important to each of the subspecialty areas of forensic nursing.
4. Describe interventions and services forensic nurses perform.
5. Discuss factors affecting health and wellness in a correctional setting.

OUTLINE

KEY TERMS

child abuse
clinical forensic nurse
coroner
correctional nursing
elder abuse
forensic

forensic nurse death investigator
forensic nurse examiner
forensic nursing
forensic psychiatric nurse
legal nurse consultant
living forensics

medical examiner
medicolegal death investigator
nurse attorney
nurse coroner
sexual assault nurse examiner

In the United States, in 2019, the FBI's Uniform Crime Reporting Program reported over one million violent crimes occurred; this was a slight decrease from the number of violent crimes in 2018; but higher than the 5 year trend (https://ucr.fbi.gov/crime-in-the-u.s/2019/crime-in-the-u.s.-2019/topic-pages/violent-crime). The crimes ranged from robbery, and rape, to aggravated assault and murder. The estimated medical and economic burdens of violence (homicide, child and elder maltreatment, youth violence, intimate partner violence, and other assaults) and self-directed violence (suicide, substance abuse) on society are staggering.

Because of the intersection between healthcare and violence, healthcare professionals are recommended to identify and assess victims of violence and provide proper care and referrals as needed. Indeed, screening for violence is now considered to be a minimum standard of care for all patients, as is vigilance in looking for indications of abuse among children, and older, or vulnerable adults. Additionally, given the growing burden of

violence and injury on the healthcare system a growing body of science is shifting toward injury prevention programs (USPSTF, 2018).

The term **forensic** means "pertaining to the law, legal" (Lynch and Duval, 2011, p. 5). It refers to instances, activities, or information used in or suitable to courts of law. Healthcare providers, especially nurses, frequently care for both victims and perpetrators of crime, and they should be prepared to assess for indications of violence, neglect, and abuse and to intervene as needed.

Forensic nursing is defined as "application of the nursing process to public or legal proceedings, and the application of forensic healthcare in the scientific investigation of trauma and/or death related to abuse, violence, criminal activity, liability, and accidents" (Lynch and Duval, 2011, p. 5). Forensic nursing combines the disciplines of nursing science, forensic science, medical science, sociology, and psychology with law enforcement and the criminal justice system. The specialty of forensic nursing was officially recognized by the American Nurses Association (ANA) in 1995, and the *Scope and Standards of Forensic Nursing Practice* was published in 1997 (ANA, 2015; Amar and Sekula, 2017) and revised in 2009 (ANA, 2009). More recently, the International Association of Forensic Nurses (Price and Maguire, 2016), recognizing the need to provide accurate and reliable knowledge, skills, and scope of practice education to the new forensic nurse, endorsed the Core Curriculum for Forensic Nurses.

Forensic nursing has evolved in nursing practice with the development of a Middle Range Theory—The Constructed Theory of Forensic Nursing Care. This theory affirms the practice of forensic nursing that fills a gap between the healthcare system and the criminal justice system (Lynch and Duval, 2011; Valentine et al., 2020).

Forensic nurses practice in multiple areas and settings in both the healthcare and public health systems. Their responsibilities may include screening, assessment and documentation of injuries, and collection of evidence, and may also include expert witness testimony for victims and perpetrators across a variety of settings such as hospitals, community clinics, and death scenes. In addition to working with victims and perpetrators, forensic nurses may be involved in paternity disputes and cases involving workplace injuries, medical malpractice, vehicle collisions, food or drug tampering, and medical equipment defects (Fig. 32.1) (Lynch and Duval, 2011). The advanced or certified forensic nurse may take the lead in developing and implementing protocols and policies and procedures to assist victims or perpetrators of violent occurrences, aid in research and policy changes, develop and supervise systems of care for complex health issues, and provide essential education to others. The *Healthy People 2030* box lists some objectives related to this highly specialized practice area.

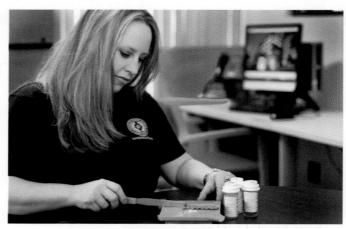

Fig. 32.1 A forensic nurse counting medications.

♥HEALTHY PEOPLE 2030

Goals Related to Forensic Nursing that includes a wide range of the *Healthy People 2030* topics, settings, and populations:
  Injury Prevention Goals: Prevent injuries; 30 objectives all applicable to forensic nursing Violence Prevention Goals: Prevent violence and related injuries and death; 20 objectives all applicable to forensic nursing.

From HealthyPeople.gov: *Healthy People 2030: topics & objectives*, 2020. https://health.gov/healthypeople/objectives-and-data/browse-objectives. Accessed June 22, 2021.

SUBSPECIALTIES OF FORENSIC NURSING

The International Association of Forensic Nurses (IAFN) and Academy of Forensic Nursing (AFN) recognize core specialties within forensic nursing (Box 32.1). Each of the subspecialties will be briefly discussed.

SEXUAL ASSAULT NURSE EXAMINER

The **sexual assault nurse examiner** (SANE) is the most widely recognized subspecialty in forensic nursing. In the 1970s,

emergency department (ED) registered nurses identified a special client population—sexual assault victims—who were not receiving the appropriate, compassionate care after a terrifying traumatic event (Ledray and Arndt, 1994). They observed that in many cases the staff did not know how to compassionately but objectively approach the sexual assault victim entering the ED; to properly assess, document, and collect evidence; or to provide testimony in a court of law. Therefore, the SANE role was developed.

A SANE is a specially trained registered nurse who applies the nursing process during forensic examinations to victims or perpetrators of sexual assault. Recognizing cultural and developmental differences, as well as the impact of trauma of victims, the SANE assesses and documents detailed physical examination findings, collects forensic evidence related to a reported crime, and frequently testifies as an expert witness at subsequent trials (Office for Victims of Crime, 2017). SANEs are usually employed in EDs and community clinics dedicated to victims of interpersonal violence. SANEs may also be employed to complete forensic examinations on deceased individuals for whom sexual assault is presumed.

If the client is medically stable, the SANE is responsible for conducting a thorough examination, including obtaining a history, performing the physical assessment, and collecting forensic evidence (Box 32.2). If the client is medically unstable, he or she will be assessed and stabilized by a provider before the forensic examination. Other responsibilities of the SANE are crisis intervention referral, pregnancy risk assessment and

---

BOX 32.1   Specialties of Forensic Nurses

- Sexual assault nurse examiner
- Nurse coroner and death investigator
- Legal nurse consultant and nurse attorney
- Forensic nurse educator and consultant
- Forensic psychiatric nurse
- Forensic nurse examiner
- Correctional nurse

BOX 32.2 Examples of Evidence Collected From a Victim of Sexual Assault

- Documentation of history of the event
- Documentation of injuries (photographic, diagram, and written)
- All clothing worn at the time of incident
- Trace evidence (fiber, glass, soil, particulate matter)
- Biological evidence for DNA comparison (patient's oral swab)
- Swabs and smears from various anatomical locations dependent upon patient history
- Pubic hair combings

Data from *A national protocol for sexual assault medical forensic examinations—adults/adolescents*, ed 2, at page 72; Shaw J., et al.: Bringing Research into practice: an evaluation of Michigan's Sexual Assault Kit, *J Interpers Violence*, 31(8):1476–1500, 2016.

interception as needed, and client referral for additional support (Ledray, 2011). The role of SANE are expanding to encompass the growing field of clinical forensic nursing to include strangulation examinations, child and elder maltreatment, human trafficking, firearm injuries, and interpersonal violence.

A registered nurse caring for sexual assault victims may receive SANE certification offered through the IAFN and the AFN. Both adult and pediatric certifications are available. The requirements for a registered nurse or advanced practice nurse to be eligible for the SANE adult and/or pediatric certification examinations are that the nurse must (1) be in practice for a minimum of 2 years, (2) have successfully completed 40 h of didactic instruction or academic course equivalent, and (3) demonstrate competency in sexual assault examinations within a clinical setting (IAFN, 2015).

Medicolegal Death Investigation

According to Hanzlick (2007), there are four different types of death investigation: medicolegal, institution-based, private, and public health. Medicolegal death investigations are usually conducted to clarify the sudden unexpected, and often nonnatural circumstances in which death occurred. Institution-based death investigations are usually those that occur in the hospital or nursing home setting. Private death investigations are family initiated and are focused on answering questions the family may have surrounding the death. Public health investigations are frequently conducted in cooperation with the medicolegal and/or are retrospective studies. An example of public health death investigation would be sudden unexpected infant deaths. The medicolegal death investigation system falls within the purview of the public health system as defined by the Centers for Disease Control and Prevention. One of the outputs of death investigation is death certificates. In the United States, medicolegal death investigation systems are characterized as medical examiner, coroner/justices of the peace, or mixed (Hanzlick, 2007; Lynch and Duval, 2011; Drake et al., 2020).

Typically, **medical examiners** are licensed physicians who are board certified in anatomic and forensic pathology (Hanzlick, 2007). Usually a medical examiner is appointed for an unspecified term and serves a county, district, region, or state as determined by law. The **coroners**/justices of the peace are usually elected laypersons; that is, persons who have little or no training in medicine or science who conduct medicolegal investigations and certify cause and manner of death. However, specific eligibility requirements vary greatly across the nation (CDC, 2015). A mixed medicolegal system is a combination of medical examiner and coroners/justices of the peace systems, depending on state law (Hanzlick, 2007).

Most medicolegal death investigation agencies are responsible for issuing death certificates that state the cause and manner of death. These data are collected at city, county, state, and national levels and are used to determine the health of the nation and how best to allocate financial resources. The *cause of death* is the event that initiated the progression of events that ended in death (Hanzlick, 2007). The *manner of death* is categorization that relates to the circumstances in which the cause of death occurred (Hanzlick, 2007). The National Association of Medical Examiners identifies five acceptable options for recording manner of death: natural, accident, suicide, homicide, and "undetermined" (Hanzlick et al., 2002).

Role of a Forensic Nurse Death Investigator

Typically the forensic nurse is employed in the medicolegal death investigation or public health setting. Forensic nurses enter the death investigation arena possessing knowledge of anatomy, physiology, pharmacology, growth and development; and skilled in conducting the physical examination, and health history interviewing techniques and obtaining specimens while recognizing chain of custody, all of which are needed to conduct a comprehensive death investigation (Lynch and Koehler, 2011; Mitchell and Drake, 2017; Drake et al., 2020). In most cases related to a death investigation, the role of the death investigator varies to include police officers or homicide detectives or forensic scientists—members of professions without foundational medical knowledge. The **forensic nurse death investigator** (FNDI) or medicolegal death investigator evaluates the death scene from a holistic nursing perspective and might interpret the scene differently (Clinical Example 32.1 and Fig. 32.2). The requirements for being an FNDI vary; however, most employers ask for a minimum of 2 years of experience, preferably in the setting of critical care or emergency or requisite medicolegal death investigation training from a reputable entity (ABMDI, 2021).

Clinical Example 32.1

A police officer entering a house observes several pools of blood located throughout the residence and discovers a deceased male, nude, and lying in bed; the police officer suspects foul play or homicide. The FNDI entering the same death scene notices the same findings as the initial police officer, but also notes bloody emesis in the toilet, blood-soaked towels in the washing machine, and empty alcohol bottles in the trash and throughout the residence. A preliminary examination of the decedent by the FNDI reveals

Continued

Clinical Example 32.1—cont'd

ascites, jaundice, and multiple contusions on the body. Through communication with family members, the FNDI discovers the decedent was an alcoholic with many health problems; the FNDI suspects that he had ruptured esophageal varices. This suspicion was confirmed by an autopsy, and the manner of death was determined to be from natural causes rather than homicide, as initially believed.

Role of Nurse Coroner

In coroner systems in which the chief medicolegal death investigator is elected and often state laws do not have specific requirements of the office, nurses may decide to run for the position of coroner or **nurse coroner**. The coroner is responsible for ensuring that appropriate measures are taken to perform death investigations and to certify death certificates. A nurse coroner's educational background, knowledge, and skills enable him or her to identify disease processes that the lay coroner may not recognize or may misinterpret as foul play, as in the preceding clinical example. Additionally, the nurse coroner is well versed in the healthcare system and competent in reviewing medical records, that often assist in a medicolegal death investigation.

FNDIs and nurse coroners exhibit communication skills when dealing with grieving families. Nurses are provided education in therapeutic communication and trauma informed care and are able to practice those skills in any setting. They are acutely aware of the importance of using open-ended questions, listening attentively, and being fully present with family and friends. The use of these techniques allows family and friends to openly share the feelings and thoughts experienced with the death of a loved one (Potter and Perry, 2019; SAMHSA, 2014). Additionally, nurses are guided by their nursing code of ethics (ANA, 2015). These codes cross all settings for the nurse and are the foundation for providing ethical values and obligations across the life span.

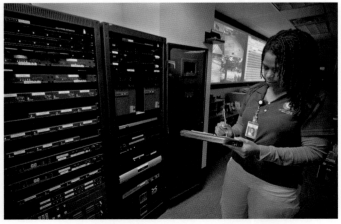

Fig. 32.2 A forensic nurse plans her day.

Nurse coroners and FNDIs may apply to become board certified in death investigation through the American Board of Medicolegal Death Investigators (ABMDI). ABMDI requires applicants to (1) acknowledge the code of ethics, (2) be currently employed at an agency with the job responsibility to conduct scene investigations, and have a minimum of 640 h of experience in the last 6 years, (3) provide a professional reference letter, and (4) demonstrate skills via completion of the Performance Training Guidebook Checklist (ABMDI, 2021). Once an investigator satisfies these requirements, he or she may take a standardized examination and to become qualified with a registered certification from the ABMDI. Advanced board certification is also available.

Legal Nurse Consultant and Nurse Attorney

Legal nurse consultants (LNCs) and nurse attorneys are nurses who provide assistance within the legal system using specialized nursing knowledge and expertise when interaction between law and healthcare quality and safety issues arise (Geissler-Murr and Moorhouse, 2011; Pagliaro and Cewe, 2013). Among many activities, LNCs evaluate, analyze, and render informed opinions on the delivery of healthcare and its outcomes, based on their area of expertise (American Association of Legal Nurse Consultants [AALNC], 2021). Many law firms hire LNCs to review and interpret medical records and charts, provide objective opinions based on standards of care, and possibly to testify in court as expert witnesses. A forensic nurse practicing as an LNC may apply for certification through the American Legal Nurse Consultant Certification Board (ALNCCB). The candidate must have (1) a current nursing license full and unrestricted, (2) a minimum of 5 years' experience as a registered nurse, and (3) evidence of 2000 h of legal nurse consulting experience within the last 5 years (ALNCCB, 2020). Once the candidate meets these requirements, he or she may sit for a standardized examination, and once having passed the examination, he or she earns the Legal Nurse Consultant Certified credential.

Nurse attorneys are academically educated in both law and nursing. They may practice in a variety of law settings to include healthcare, public health, or criminal or civil law, which would include malpractice cases. Malpractice cases may require participation of a nurse attorney on either the plaintiff's or the defendant's side and may involve licensure disciplinary action or agency oversight (Collins and Halpern, 2005). Some practitioners have differing opinions regarding LNCs and nurse attorneys. They may be perceived as either defending the profession or prosecuting peers by testifying against professional colleagues. By providing services as experts and by testifying, nurses serving as legal consultants help hold accountable practitioners who are unsafe to the public. In contrast, meticulous practitioners who are wrongfully accused of negligence are defended by these nurses' actions.

According to the AALNC (2021), an LNC performs many different services and activities, as follows:

- Participate in client interviews
- Identify, organize, and analyze pertinent medical records

- Prepare a chronology, timeline, or other summaries of documentation in medical records
- Conduct medical literature searches and assist in other research
- Identify applicable standards of care in medical malpractice cases
- Identify, screen, and facilitate review by expert witnesses
- Evaluate case strengths and weaknesses
- Draft or analyze medical portions of legal documents
- Evaluate causation and damage issues
- Educate attorneys and clients regarding relevant medical issues
- Identify plaintiff's future medical needs and associated costs
- Participate in case management and case strategy discussions
- Attend independent medical exams
- Serve as a nurse expert witness
- Perform cost of care estimates for long-term care treatment and catastrophic case management scenarios
- Locate or prepare demonstrative evidence for trial
- Assist with preparation for and support during deposition, trial, or ADR

LNCs read reports and records and determine whether the standards of care were met or breached. In general, if working for a plaintiff in a malpractice case, the LNC will look for breaches in the standards of care; if working for the defense, the LNC will look for nursing care that is given within the standards of care related to the complaint. It is essential that the attorneys be kept informed of all findings—even those that might negatively affect their case (Robson, 2009).

When providing services, the LNC may submit an affidavit, a written statement explaining the expert's credentials, background, and licensing or certification(s). It also provides a list of the materials read and considered in the case, and the findings of the review are summarized into a case analysis. After the submission of an affidavit, the LNC may be asked to provide a deposition. The *deposition* is a pretrial discovery process that allows the attorneys on both sides to learn more about what the courtroom testimony will be. It is given to a court reporter, and the respondent is under oath.

During the deposition, the LNC presents the facts of the case and is questioned by attorneys from both sides. This process may be quite lengthy and stressful. It is essential that the LNC be prepared, having reviewed everything thoroughly. After this process, the LNC is given a written transcript of the deposition, which needs to be carefully reviewed for accuracy. If the case goes to trial, the LNC will then testify in court (Robson, 2009; Ruiz-Contreras, 2005).

In some cases, the forensic nurse is called on to testify in court, not as an expert witness as described previously, but as a factual witness—one who has firsthand knowledge of the case in question. In these cases, the forensic nurse provides factual statements about the evidence collected and what was observed (Pagliaro and Cewe, 2013). Box 32.3 lists tips that will be helpful for nurses to review before testifying in court.

Clinical Forensic Nurse Examiner
Emergency and Critical Care
Registered nurses may be employed in a variety of healthcare settings; however, are often within EDs and critical care units as **forensic nurse examiners**. In this role they deliver care to living patients who present with health conditions often intersecting with the legal system, and their services may include several subspecialties such as SANE services. The term **living forensics** refers to individuals who are subject to forensic investigations, including but not limited to survivors of physical and mental trauma, toxicology emergencies, interpersonal violence, transportation crashes, and police detention (Lynch and Duval, 2011).

As illustrated in Clinical Example 32.2, the ED is frequently the initial location of the forensic nursing examination (Doughtery, 2011). It is imperative that registered nurses identify forensic patients; initiate the proper collection, preservation, and chain of custody of evidence; and then provide accurate documentation for this unique population. The recognition, collection, and documentation of evidence collected within the ED may have an important role in the investigation of crimes and can have a major impact on legal decisions. Box 32.4 lists types of evidence.

BOX 32.3 Tips for Testifying at a Deposition or in Court

Do's
- Dress professionally and conservatively.
- Tell the truth at all times.
- Listen to the complete question before responding.
- Speak slowly, clearly, and concisely when answering.
- Take a few seconds to formulate an answer before responding.
- Minimize "ums" or "uhs" by pausing at the end of sentences.
- If there is an objection, stop talking and wait for the judge to make a ruling.
- When answering questions, make eye contact with the jury members.
- Remain calm.
- Respond confidently.
- Practice difficult words.
- Avoid nervous gestures; keep your hands in your lap.
- Discuss with the attorney ways to translate medical testimony that is translatable to the general person.

Don'ts
- Avoid saying "I think" and "I believe."
- Avoid absolutes, thus saying "in all cases" or "everytime."
- Avoid interrupting.
- Avoid answering a question that you do not understand; instead ask the attorney to repeat question(s) as needed.
- Avoid being defensive or angry.
- Avoid facial or other gestures/actions that may be distracting.

Data from Ruiz-Contreras A: The nurse as an expert witness, *Top Emerg Med* 27(1):27–35, 2005; https://www.expertinstitute.com/resources/insights/preparing-expert-witness-trial-testimony/.

BOX 32.4   Types of Evidence

Tangible (touchable) evidence—recognized on sight:
- Weapons/tools
- Bullets, casing, wadding, gunshot residue
- Matches, lighters, or other ignition sources
- Blood, semen, saliva, tissue
- Soil, paint
- Clothing or personal effects
- Notes or messages
- Photographs

Transient evidence—temporary and may be lost, destroyed, or damaged:
- Physical findings such as bruises, swelling, bleeding, tenderness
- Odors (e.g., marijuana, alcohol, gasoline)

Trace evidence—may not be visible; identified by microscope or alternative light sources:
- Fibers
- Biological specimens: blood, semen stains
- DNA

Data from Hammer RM, Moynihan B, Pagliaro EM: *Forensic nursing: a handbook for practice*, ed 2, Burlington, MA, 2013, Jones & Bartlett Learning; Lynch VA, Duval JB: *Forensic nursing science*, ed 2, St. Louis, 2011, Elsevier/Mosby; and Saferstein R: *Criminalistics: an introduction to forensic science*, ed 10, Upper Saddle River, NJ, 2010, Pearson.

Clinical Example 32.2

A 72-year-old male arrived at the ED via emergency medical services from an unlicensed group home after the patient was found unresponsive on the floor. The patient was admitted to the critical care unit with urosepsis and bilateral pneumonia. Upon physical examination the body was odorous, malnourished; based on low BMI, low albumin, and abnormal chemistry; multiple unstageable decuibitus ulcers were identified on the sacral, bilateral heels, and back. The wounds were seeping thick pussy fluid and had neurosis. Based upon these findings the nurse contacted Adult Protective Services and the on-call forensic nurse examiner. Case management made arrangements for the patient to be discharged to a nursing home.

Organ and Tissue Donation and Transplantation

Forensic nurses also have a role in providing a detailed physical examination of patients who may be organ and tissue donors. This area of care is complex and requires detailed understanding of related legal and ethical issues. When a patient is declared brain dead or donation after cardiac death (DCD), federal law states that the legal next of kin shall be approached for organ and tissue donation. A forensic nurse is able to conduct and provide a detailed physical examination and to collect any evidence that may be required. A thorough death investigation at the hospital may be required for sudden unexpected, and nonnatural deaths. This involves reviewing medical records and documenting injuries, which is essential for the medicolegal investigation agency to identify acceptable candidates and potential organs and tissues for harvest. The nurse involved in this process must be knowledgeable about legal specifications related to organ donation and be familiar with agency policies and procedures for determining brain death and DCD. The nurse must also have excellent communication skills as well as the ability to relate empathetically to grieving families. In this capacity, the forensic nurse working harmoniously with organ and tissue procurement agencies can obtain release authorization for lifesaving organs (Shafer, 2011).

Care of Vulnerable Populations

The youngest, oldest, and disabled populations are the most vulnerable to maltreatment. Nurses dedicating their practice to these vulnerable populations often are required to collaborate with other agencies to ensure adequate resources are available. Often advocacy groups are referred to for assistance.

Child Abuse and Neglect. **Child abuse** and neglect (child maltreatment) are major concerns for society; therefore, the role of a forensic nurse examiner is especially imperative. The Federal Child Abuse Prevention and Treatment Act defines child abuse and neglect as minimum of:

> *Any recent act or failure to act on the part of a parent or caretaker which results in death, serious physical or emotional harm, sexual abuse or exploitation; or an act or failure to act which presents an imminent risk of serious harm.*
>
> *(42 U.S.C.A. §5106g, as amended and reauthorized by the CAPTA Reauthorization Act of 2010 & 2015).*

In 2019, approximately 656,000 children were victims of child abuse and neglect, a number slightly decreased from previous years. . However, the reported cases of child abuse or neglect resulting in death in were estimated to be 1840 children, which were somewhat higher than 2018 estimates (U.S. Department of Health and Human Services [USDHHS], Administration for Children and Families [ACF], 2019).

States have varying definitions of what constitutes or determines child abuse and neglect. If a forensic nurse suspects that a child is being abused or neglected, the nurse should refer to the state's legislation surrounding the reporting of these suspicions. The following definitions are provided by the Child Abuse Prevention and Treatment Act (CAPTA) (P.L. 100–294), as amended by the CAPTA Reauthorization Act of 2010 (P.L. 111–320) of which human trafficking is now included:

"Any recent act or failure to act on the part of a parent or caretaker which results in death, serious physical or emotional harm, sexual abuse or exploitation [ ]; or an act or failure to act, which presents an imminent risk of serious harm" (USDHHS, ACF, 2019).

In broad terms, although the definition and/or arrangement varies by state, Neglect, Sexual Abuse, Physical Abuse, and Emotional Abuse are defined as here:

Neglect: Failure of a parent, guardian, or caregiver to provide basic needs. Neglect may be physical (deprivation of adequate food, clothing, shelter, or supervision); medical (failure to provide necessary medical treatment);

educational (failure to educate a child or attend to special education needs); or emotional (failure to attend to emotional needs or provide psychological care or allowing the usage of alcohol or other drugs).

Sexual abuse: Range of activities from noncontact indecent exposure to production of pornographic materials, to incest, rape, fondling, and genital contact to actual adult–child sexual intercourse.

Physical abuse: Intentional physical injury, including striking, kicking, burning, and biting.

Emotional abuse (or psychological abuse): A pattern of behavior that impairs the child's emotional development or sense of self-worth, including constant criticism, threats, and rejection.

For the well-being and safety of the child, a nurse ensures that abuse and neglect are swiftly identified and reported to the proper authorities, including the consultation of a forensic nurse examiner (Finn, 2011; Lewis-O'Connor and Latimore, 2017). The nurse obtains a thorough history and assessment, focusing on several facets of abuse and neglect. These include child–parent interaction, the child's appearance and behavior, child–child interaction, and the environment.

A forensic nurse may be employed in a variety of clinical settings that assess, diagnose, and treat children. These settings may include pediatric or general EDs, hospitals, physician offices, schools, home health, hospice, and child advocacy centers.

Elder Maltreatment. Forensic nurse examiners caring for the geriatric population play an important role similar to that of those providing services for the pediatric population. Elder maltreatment is thought to be one of the most underdiagnosed and underreported crimes in the United States (Pickens and Dyer, 2016). Unfortunately, there is no exact accounting of elder mistreatment cases, for several reasons: an absence of standardized reporting systems, no consistency in state definition of elder mistreatment, and lack of national data collection (NCEA, 2021). Regardless, elder maltreatment is an act of violence or the nonconsented withdrawal of necessary care to sustain life (Pickens and Dyer, 2016)

There are several forms of **elder abuse**: physical, psychological or emotional, financial, neglect, and sexual abuse (Pickens and Dyer, 2016). Physical abuse is the intentional harm or injury of another person resulting in injury, pain, or impairment (Pickens and Dyer, 2016). Rosen and Colleagues (2020) compared physical examination findings of adjudicated elder physical abuse cases within unintentional fall and identified that those being physically abused were more likely to have injuries of the maxifacial, dental, and neck area than nonabused patients (67% vs. 28%). Of note, those dwelling with others in a community setting accounted for 65% of the injuries. Additionally, only one-third had received care in an ED; the majority refused care at the scene. This was a small study, and the actual prevalence of elder abuse is unknown (Yon et al., 2017).

Psychological or emotional abuse occurs when there is mental or emotional anguish (e.g., verbal or nonverbal inflic-

tion of anguish, pain, or distress) (Pickens and Dyer, 2016). Estimates of elders residing in the community versus institution experienced of range of emotional abuse, identified by self-report (11.6%), other older adult (33.4%) and by staff (32.5%). The growing concern of financial exploitation of elders is becoming apparent with billions of dollars lost annually (NAPSA, 2016; Burnes et al., 2017). Financial exploitation refers to situations in which the elder person's financial assets, property, or funds are utilized for another person's benefit without the elder's consent. The majority of known cases occurred among strangers (51%), followed by family/caregiver/neighbor (34%) and 16% occurring among business or Medicaid/Medicare fraud. The prevalence in various settings of community and institutional ranges from 6.8% to 13.8%; however, it is noted that all seniors, regardless of income level, are at risk (WHO; NAPSA, 2016).

Sexual abuse is recognized as a form or elder maltreatment; however, is less common than other forms. Sexual abuse is the nonconsensual contact of any kind with an elderly person (Pickens and Dyer, 2016). The elder population is at risk for sexual abuse because of inability to resist pursuit or inability to recognize the abuse due to mental illness or other advanced disease processes. Less than 1% of elderly living in the community report sexual abuse and 1.7% of elders residing in an institution report sexual abuse (WHO).

Finally, neglect is the most common form of elder abuse. . Neglect may be carried out by a perpetrator in form of medical neglect or neglect of other activities of daily living; this can include delay in seeking care of medical emergency (Murphy et al., 2013). Caregiver neglect occurs when the obligated caregiver fails to provide appropriate clothing, food, or health services either via refusal to fulfill these requirements or abandonment of the elder client (Pickens and Dyer, 2016).

Elder abuse is a public health issue. With estimated reports occurring within one in 24 adults. The elderly client, if cognitively capable, is often hesitant to report abuse, ask for assistance, or acknowledge the maltreatment because the abuser might be a spouse and/or partner, child, or close relative, or because the disclosure would possibly result in litigation and institutionalization (WHO). Providing nursing services within the elderly population affords nurses the opportunity to identify and report concerns of elder maltreatment. Forensic nurses may be consulted to offer services for injury documentation or evidence collection (Clinical Example 32.3).

Clinical Example 32.3

A home healthcare nurse has received a referral from the hospital for an 80-year-old female residing at her home with her son. The patient had been discharged from the hospital with the diagnosis of urinary tract infection and pneumonia. Her son reports she was confused and coughing for 2 months before he took her to the hospital. Her past medical history includes dementia, impaired mobility, and dysphasia from a prior stroke. Upon arrival at the residence, the nurse greets the patient, who is lying in bed. The home is cluttered and dirty, with visible roaches, and the refrigerator/freezer is filled

Continued

Clinical Example 32.3—cont'd

with meat, cheese, milk, and beer. The nurse's assessment findings include the following: clothing is loose fitting and adult brief is soiled, strong body and urine odor present, body is emaciated with upper and lower extremity contractures, contusions of various coloring are located on the left eye, cervical area of neck, upper thighs and posterior torso, stage II decubitus ulcers are present on the right hip and sacral areas (both are covered with soiled dressing), and dentition is poor. The son explains that the patient obtained the contusions because at times she becomes confused and strikes out, hitting things. This happens during times that he attempts to bathe and turn the patient. Furthermore, he indicated the decedent has not been taking her medications and the son has not had time to have them refilled for past 2 months.

Upon leaving the residence, the nurse contacts her supervisor to discuss the findings and her concerns about physical, financial, sexual abuse and medical neglect. The supervisor agrees, and the patient is returned to the ED for a forensic nurse examination, at which time the forensic nurse places a call to Adult Protective Services for further evaluation and investigation. The hospital is also contacted to discuss why the patient was discharged back into the unsafe environment.

Disabled Population. It is well documented that persons with disabilities are more likely to be mistreated. Disabilities occur across the lifespan to include hearing, visual impairments to mobility impairments and several cognitive/behavior disorders and birth defects. The community or forensic nurse should be aware of the mandatory laws addressing the identification of and reporting of abuse or neglect of a disabled person varies within states. Throughout their life span, the risk for one or more forms of mistreatment of individuals with disabilities is three times higher than that for individuals without disabilities (Harrell, 2017).

Forensic Psychiatric Nurse

As mentioned, the **forensic psychiatric nurse** often bridges the gap between the criminal justice, legal, and mental health systems. Forensic psychiatric nurses apply the nursing process to clients who await a criminal hearing or trial while maintaining a neutral, objective, and detached position (Mason, 2011). Forensic psychiatric nurses collect evidence by determining intent or diminished capacity in the client's thinking at the time of the incident. To do so, they often spend several hours interviewing and observing the client, carefully documenting conversations and observations.

The forensic psychiatric nurse may be called to court to testify as an expert witness in a variety mental health issues. Roles filled by or activities performed by psychiatric forensic nurses include the following (Mason, 2011):

- Sanity or competency evaluation (for legal purposes)
- Assessment of violence potential
- Assessment of capacity to formulate intent
- Parole and probation considerations

- Assessment of racial or cultural factors in crime
- Assistance in jury selection
- Sexual predator screening
- Provision of expert witness testimony

?ACTIVE LEARNING

Spend a few hours observing or interview a forensic nurse in a clinical setting. Observe the nurse's interventions and processes related to forensic interviewing, trauma informed care, physical examination, evidence collection and preservation, documentation, and collaboration with, for example, police officers or adult protective services. Take note of the techniques used for interviewing, discharge planning, referrals, and counseling.

CORRECTIONAL NURSING

Correctional nursing is a specialized subset of forensic nursing. It requires a significant amount of knowledge as well as an understanding and awareness of the unique needs and perspective of the clients served. The Bureau of Justice Statistics provides an exceptional overview of the justice system that offers details visualizations of the process and the communities and publics role in such (BJS, 2021). Several issues specific to correctional nursing and related issues are described in this section.

Unlike in any other care setting, clients are inmates, and care is negotiated and provided with recognition of safety and security issues for the nurse and the constitutional right of prisoners to receive adequate and timely healthcare. The primary goal in correctional facilities is to maintain a safe, secure, and humane environment for inmates. Healthcare, including nursing care, is a necessary and essential part of that environment.

Maintenance of a Safe Environment

Correctional facilities are violent environments, and nurses practicing in correctional settings must continually negotiate personal safety and nursing care (Clinical Example 32.4). Nurses in this setting must be aware that medical supplies issued to inmates can be a safety threat to the environment. For example, a simple elastic bandage can be used to improve the grip on a homemade weapon. Virtually any prescribed medication can have value on the prison "black market." Furthermore, nurses are subject to manipulation by inmates, who may seek nursing care for reasons other than health (Kaminski, 2003). As the following clinical example illustrates, the nurse must maintain an escape route to use if a situation of personal violence is imminent. In addition, no nursing care in a correctional environment requires a nurse to be locked in an enclosed environment with an inmate. Although it might appear that providing humane, therapeutic nursing care in an environment of potential violence is contradictory, it is ultimately a prerequisite for nursing practice in correctional settings.

Clinical Example 32.4
Safety in Correctional Facilities
In a state penitentiary in 2021, a nurse and correctional officer were killed by an inmate who was in the medical infirmary ostensibly seeking care. This incidence illustrates the risk within the environment and the need to be alert (https://www.nbcnews.com/video/nurse-and-correctional-officer-killed-by-iowa-prison-inmate-during-attack-109034053556). In a similar instance, a nurse was attacked while administering medications in an open section of the medical infirmary in Cuyahoga County Jail in 2019 (https://youtu.be/ecftyTTAEOc).

RESEARCH HIGHLIGHTS

Public Health Role in Death Investigation
Drake et al. (2015) assessed the practice differences of the public health role of two death investigation systems in Texas. The authors utilized a previously validated instrument adapted from the Public Health Essential Services and sent it to 723 justice of the peace offices and 12 medical examiner offices in the 254 counties of Texas. Ten medical examiners and 112 justices of the peace responded. The study found that medical examiners are more likely than justices of the peace to fulfill the essential medicolegal death investigation services. Specifically, the researchers indicated that medical examiners have formal processes and follow set guidelines for carrying out their role versus the justice of the peace. In terms of formally evaluating or trending quality and effectiveness of their work product, no statistical differences were found between the two systems. Drake and colleagues proposed improving the Texas medicolegal death investigation system by restructuring it into a regionalization system. This could ensure optimal standards, accreditation, training, education, and quality and economy of scale service were being provided to the public.

HEALTH ISSUES IN PRISON POPULATIONS

Today's prison inmate often enters prison with healthcare issues. Nurses employed in the correctional setting are likely to see healthcare problems that are similar to those in an acute care setting or a community outpatient clinic. The daily operation of a correctional clinic includes management of acute and chronic illness. Most healthcare clinics in correctional environments screen each inmate upon entry into the facility. The healthcare triage process generally includes a physical and a mental health history. Many significant healthcare issues are recognized during the screening process, often for the first time.

Chronic and Communicable Diseases

The most critical heathcare issues among the incarcerated population are chronic and communicable diseases. Of continuous concern are HIV, hepatitis, and tuberculosis. According to the Bureau of Justice Statistics, the rate of HIV infection decreased slightly from 146 cases per 10,000 inmates in 2010 to 143 per 10,000 at year end in 2012 (Maruschak et al., 2015), but remains very high. Likewise, hepatitis is a serious healthcare issue in correctional facilities. According to the Bureau of Justice Statistics, 6.5% of inmates reported hepatitis

as a health problem in 2012 (Maruschak et al., 2015). The rate of these and other communicable diseases among the incarcerated population is associated with high-risk behaviors, including current and previous drug use, unprotected sexual intercourse, and tattooing.

Of recent concern were documented outbreaks of COVID-19 among various prison systems (CIDRAP, 2021). Some of the sources of disease transmission occurred among incoming new inmates and outside healthcare providers. Zawitz, et al. (2020) concluded that effective mitigation of transmitting COVID 19 was decreased via discontinuing programs, visiting, and converting cells into single units. Additionally, widespread testing of both staff and inmates and screening of staff for fever was implemented.

Of continuous concern is the rates of chronic conditions such as hypertension and diabetes (Maruschak et al., 2015). Both prisoners and inmates are more likely to report chronic conditions than the general public. For example, in 2012 about one-quarter of inmates were of normal weight, with the majority being overweight (46%) to morbidly obese (2%). As it is for the general population, managing inmates/prisoners with multiple chronic conditions, including infectious and noninfectious, will continue to be a major threat to the health of those incarcerated.

Women in Prison

As of 2019, more than one million women were under supervision of the criminal justice system, with about 20% of them being currently incarcerated (The Sentencing Project, 2020). In 2019, 26% of women in state prisons were held for drug offenses compared with 13% for males (Carson, 2020). Of note, the rate of imprisonment for white women rose by 41% between 2000 and 2019 during the same timeframe a decline of 60% for black women (Carson, 2020).

Children of those incarcerated offer additional opportunities for the forensic and community nurses. An estimated 684,500 state and federal prisoners were parents of at least one minor child in 2016. This represents nearly half of state prisoners (47%) and more than half of federal prisoners (58%) (Maruschak et al., 2021).

The National Commission on Correctional Healthcare (NCCHC, 2020) provides several white papers or position statements that address a wider variety of concerns within the correctional setting. Of which, the following offers a guide for the provision of healthcare among women:

- Correctional institutions' healthcare intake procedures should include comprehensive, age appropriate, and trauma informed gynecological history gathering and examination procedures in accordance with NCCHC standard.
- Comprehensive healthcare services should be available to incarcerated women that give special consideration to the age-appropriate reproductive health needs of women, menopausal needs, screening for sexual and physical abuse, counseling related to sexual transmitted infection risk factors, parenting issues, and accessibility to drug or alcohol treatment.

Inmates' Refusal of Medications

An inmate's right to refuse treatment is a legal and ethical issue that nurses working in a correctional environment sometimes experience. The right to refuse treatment and the state's power to enforce treatment are both highly charged legal and political issues and have gained attention in state and local courts (Treatment Advocacy Center, 2014). The issue of forced medication and competence to stand trial is of particular concern. The legal and ethical principles that guide forced treatment against the will of an inmate have historically been potential safety issues toward self or others in the environment. The Supreme Court decision in *Harper v. Turner* in 1987 permits the violation of the rights of the incarcerated so long as the prison policy is reasonably related to repressing violence within the prison system (Black, 2008).

Unlike in nursing practice with the general population, prison inmates who refuse healthcare do not leave the facility and return home. Nurses practicing in correctional facilities continue to provide care and address the consequences of an inmate's refusal of treatment. For example, an inmate who refuses to adhere to treatment protocols for schizophrenia may affect the safety of the environment and in fact create a "ripple effect," thus undermining prisoner administration (LGIT, 2009). Nurses are obliged to treat any resultant health issues. However, individuals who are incarcerated by the state have a constitutional right to refuse and receive healthcare. Nurses practicing in correctional settings must recognize that involuntary medical treatment is undertaken after internal review and judicial proceedings; however, a hearing is not necessary (Treatment Advocacy Center, 2014).

MENTAL HEALTH ISSUES IN CORRECTIONAL SETTINGS

It is widely recognized that the correctional setting houses a fair number of individuals with mental health needs. Approximately 37% of prisoners, and 44% of jail inmates had been informed by a mental health professional that they had a mental health disorder (Bronson and Berzofsky, 2017). According to recent data, more females and whites met the criteria for serious phycological distress (Bronson and Berzofsky, 2017). Being in prison with a mental illness such as schizophrenia, bipolar affective disorder, major depressive disorder, or personality disorder makes adjustment to incarceration extremely difficult. The high number of diagnosed inmates and lack of resources to address mental illness in today's prisons makes it difficult to meet the needs of this population.

In the late 1950s and early 1960s, deinstitutionalization moved people with mental illness out of state hospitals into communities that were often ill prepared to care for them. As a result, many people with a mental illness reside in nursing homes, residential homes, prisons, or jails. People with mental illness, in a variety of setting to include middle and high school, are more likely to encounter law enforcement than a healthcare

Adolescents in Prison

Increasing numbers of adolescents are committing violent crimes (Bureau of Justice Statistics, 2016), and many states have lowered the age limit at which adolescents may be tried and sentenced as adults. Thus, adolescents who have been convicted of violent crimes are often incarcerated in adult facilities. Incarcerating adolescents presents barriers to meeting the distinct developmental needs of adolescents. These developmental needs include rapid physical and emotional growth and nutritional needs, heavily influenced by environment, genetics, and family experiences. Adult correctional facilities are not generally equipped to deal with the challenges of adolescent development. Adolescents in an adult correctional facility are the highest at risk than any other incarcerated group to commit suicide (Radeloff et al., 2019).

To ensure the safety of adolescents in any facility, adult or juvenile, the nurse must be aware of their individual vulnerability. A mechanism for adolescents to access medical and mental healthcare is essential. Services and interventions should be provided that consider the developmental stage and the experience of adolescence.

?ACTIVE LEARNING

Spend a day in a jail or correctional facility working with a correctional nurse. Pay particular attention to differences in care delivery related to legal and ethical issues unique to this subspecialty versus the delivery of care within a general clinic within a community setting. Develop impressions into a reflection paper regarding your personnel perceptions (tactile and nontactile) of the experience.

TABLE 32.1   Example of Basic Curricula for Forensic Nursing Programs

Subject	Topic(s)
Fundamentals for forensic nursing	Evidence collection
	Documentation
	Forensic photography, written descriptions, diagrams, sketches
	Forensic interviewing skills
	Trauma informed care
	Basic criminal, procedural, and constitutional law
	Scope of practice
	Interdisciplinary collaboration
	Testifying in court as an expert witness
	Wound identification
	Wound healing
	Injury investigation
Forensic law	Legal concepts (culpability, burden of proof, rationale for punishment, mitigating circumstance)
	Defense issues (justification, insanity, entrapment, duress)
Forensic science	Interpretation of DNA and laboratory reports
	Forensic chemistry, biology,
	Forensic toxicology/pharmacology
	Forensic pathology

Data from Burgess AW, Berger AD, Boersma RR: Forensic nursing: investigating the career potential in this emerging graduate specialty, *Am J Nurs* 104(3):58–64, 2004; Texas A&M University Core Curriculum (https://catalog.tamu.edu/graduate/colleges-schools-interdisciplinary/nursing/msn-forensic-nursing/).

BOX 32.5 Schools Offering Programs in Forensic Nursing (Graduate and Certificate Programs)

Alabama
University of Alabama Birmingham, Birmingham, Alabama

California
University of California at Riverside, Riverside, California

Colorado
Aspen University, Denver, Colorado

Florida
St. Petersburg College, St. Petersburg, Floridaa

Iowa
Mount Mercy University, Cedar Rapids, Iowa

Massachusetts
Fitchburg State College, Fitchburg, Massachusetts

New Jersey
Fairleigh Dickinson University, Teaneck, New Jersey
Monmouth University, West Long Branch, New Jersey

New York
Binghamton University, Binghamton, New York

Ohio
Cleveland State University, Cleveland, Ohio
Xavier University, Cincinnati, Ohio

Pennsylvania
Duquesne University, Pittsburgh, Pennsylvania
Desales University, Center Valley, Pennsylvania
Penn State World Campus, University Park, Pennsylvania

Texas
Texas A&M University, College Station, Texas

Aspen University	Denver	CO	MSN	Online
Binghamton University (SUNY)	Binghamton	NY	Graduate Certificate in Forensic Health	Campus
Cleveland State University	Cleveland	OH	MSN	Campus
DeSales University	Center Valley	PA	MSN	Online
Duquesne University	Pittsburgh	PA	MSN	Online
Fairleigh Dickinson University	Teaneck	NJ	MSN	Campus
Fitchburg State	Fitchburg	MA	MSN	Online
Monmouth University	West Long Branch	NJ	MSN	Online
Mount Mercy University	Cedar Rapids	IA	MSN	Online
Oakland University	Rochester	MI	MSN/Graduate Certificate	Campus
Penn State World Campus	University Park	PA	Undergraduate Certificate	Online
St. Petersburg College	St. Petersburg	FL	MSN	Online
Texas A&M University	College Station	TX	MSN	Online
			Certificate in Forensic Health	
University of Alabama at Birmingham	Birmingham	AL	MSN	Campus
University of California, Riverside	Riverside	CA	Certificate	Online
Xavier University	Cincinnatti	OH	MSN	Online

Note several Nursing Schools offer various forensic electives; however, not an official degree or certificate within the area of forensic nursing. From IAFN website: https://www.forensicnurses.org/page/ForensicNursingSchools.

provider when in the midst of acute mental distress. This results in more than two million people a year going to jails, with the vast majority not the result of criminal activity (National Alliance for the Mentally Ill [NAMI], 2021).

According to NAMI, most jail inmates with symptoms of mental illness are charged with minor crimes. A far smaller number of inmates with severe mental illness commit more serious crimes, again frequently a consequence of either prior or existing inadequate or no treatment within the community in which they came. NAMI (2021) takes the position that many dangerous or violent acts by people with severe mental illness are a result of inappropriate or inadequate treatment. The following strategies have been proposed to address the criminal justice and forensic issues facing mental illness:

- Effectiveness—using trauma informed, culturally competent, evidenced based, and patient-centered care
- Equity—communities can create avenues to decrease these barriers
- Accessibility—community services made available

Two additional core needs have been identitied that of ensuring peer support along the mental health continuum and intersection with legal system and case management strategies that ensure open communication and collaboration.

Nurses employed in correctional settings must always be aware of the vulnerabilities of people with mental illness who are incarcerated. Depression, schizophrenia, bipolar disorder, and other neurobiological disorders can be readily treated with newer-generation psychiatric medications that reduce or ameliorate symptoms, but the unique vulnerabilities of incarceration often remain. Nurses must ensure that early planning and frequent screening for those incarcerated with mental illness occurs.

EDUCATION AND FORENSIC NURSING

According to Kent-Wilkinson (2011), because of the amount and depth of knowledge and skills needed by forensic nurses, whatever their subspecialty area, simply completing a continuing education course is not adequate for practice. As a result, several colleges and universities offer a variety of programs to educate practitioners, future educators, and researchers of forensic nursing. The core curriculum for forensic nursing was published recently (Price and Maguire, 2016) to provide guidance across settings. This is the direct result of the identified need and growing knowledge base for practice of this specialty area. Table 32.1 gives an overview of basic curricula for forensic nursing programs. In addition, during the formal programs of study, the student usually completes a minimum specified number of supervised clinical hours; a clinical internship or fellowship also may be required.

For those interested in seeking additional education in the growing specialty of forensic nursing, Box 32.5 lists nursing colleges and universities that have programs in forensic nursing. It should be noted that some of these programs offer a certificate in forensic nursing, whereas others provide a minor or concentration, and still others grant a graduate degree (typically a master of science in nursing degree) or postgraduate certificate.

SUMMARY

Forensic nursing is a rapidly expanding subspecialty that intersects nursing science into the care of patients, families, community, and the public presenting in a variety of settings with the forensic or legal system. Most often, the forensic nurse is employed in a hospital, clinic, correctional facility, or death investigation setting. Specialized knowledge, competencies, and skills are essential to the practice and require advanced or additional education and training.

As mentioned previously, screening for evidence of violence and intervening by reporting concerns to the appropriate agency are fundamental requirements of care that all nurses must perform. Therefore, every nurse has the potential to interact with a client, patient, or population with forensic needs, regardless of the client population or setting of care.

Case Study Application of the Nursing Process

Correctional Nursing

Mr. Smith is a 65-year-old white female serving a sentence for aggravated assault and intent to distribute. Ms. Smith has a medical history of diabetes mellitus, hypertension, coronary artery disease, and peripheral vascular disease. Less than a month before, her right foot was amputated because of gangrene. Ms. Smith had been admitted to the infirmary six times following the procedure, presenting, with vague concerns of "Not feeling well."

The incision site at all visits was reported as healing well, and her blood sugar levels were within normal ranges with adequate medication. Ms. Smith takes her medications as prescribed, and her provider indicated she is doing well.

Ms. Smith's son visits her only once every 6 months because he lives out of state. Her daughter is also in prison but at another location. Ms. Smith's grandson recently died of injuries related to a motor vehicle crash, and she was unable to attend the funeral.

Assessment

Ms. Smith has a flat affect and does not make eye contact. She constantly looks at the ground and does not speak clearly when asked questions. Many times the nurse must ask her to repeat herself. According to medical records, she has lost approximately 18 pounds since surgery and she says, "I'm not hungry." When asked about her sleeping habits, Ms. Smith states she sleeps all day except when the guards make her get up. She says she has not played board games with her buddies in more than a week. She also reports that she has been buying Soma "from them" and has not taken a bath in 3 days.

Diagnosis
Individual
- Despair, gloom, hopelessness
- Inability to overcome mental and emotional difficulties
- Powerlessness

Family
- Situational crises

Community
- Lack of mental health services
- Lack of grief (death and dying) services

Planning
Ms. Smith will set goals with the healthcare provider and will ask for assistance with communication with her son and attend grief service sessions, if available.

Individual
Long-Term Goal
- Client will reestablish positive relationships with fellow inmates within 2 weeks.

Short-Term Goal
- Client will verbalize and recognize her feelings.
- Client will participate in activities of her choice (e.g., playing cards).

Family
Long-Term Goal
- Family will demonstrate coping skills appropriate to the situation.

Short-Term Goal
- Family will verbalize and recognize feelings.

Community
Long-Term Goal
- Program will be available for all individuals.

Short-Term Goal
- Begin mental health peer support programs.

Intervention
Individual
- Ms. Smith will be encouraged to express her feelings in an open and nonjudgmental environment, allowing for the development of a therapeutic relationship.
- The nurse will schedule several visits to the clinic and encourage Ms. Smith to participate in activities, such as board games, with her friends.

Family
- Ms. Smith's son will be included in the plan of care and encouraged to express his thoughts and feelings relating to his mother's imprisonment.

Community
- The nurse will coordinate with other agencies/professionals to enable several activities for inmates suffering from grief, depression, and other mental illness including group activities and group talk.

Evaluation
Individual
Ms. Smith slowly engaged the nurse individually and in group therapy. She gained 5 pounds over 2 weeks and was able to make eye contact. Ms. Smith expressed her grief for the death of her grandson. She gradually stopped buying Soma and spent more time with her friends.

Family
Ms. Smith's son continued to visit only once every 6 months, but was able to start to express his thoughts and feelings about his mother's incarceration. The time the son spent with his mother was more meaningful.

Community
A nurse was on constant duty to assist inmates with acute or chronic mental health illnesses.

Levels of Prevention
Primary
- Encourage interaction with colleagues and family.
- Promote participation in prison activities.

Secondary
- Screen for depression.
- Screen for grief.
- Provide outreach services to inmates with mental illness.

Tertiary
- Encourage therapy to reduce symptoms of mental illness.

Case Study Application of the Nursing Process

Forensic Nursing

Transcript of a 911 telephone call:

- *Emergency operator.* "This is 911, what is your emergency?"
- *Caller.* "My daughter isn't breathing, she's not moving, I need help!"
- *Emergency operator.* Provides information regarding placement of body on firm surface and initiation of bystander CPR. Stating, "We will send an ambulance to assist you."
- *Caller.* Screams, "Please hurry!"

Emergency medical personnel arrived at the house to discover JO, a 14-year-old white female, lying face up next to her bed. The female was unresponsive and not breathing. Emergency medical personnel immediately began lifesaving interventions, but despite all efforts, they were unsuccessful. JO was pronounced dead at her home.

Police officers arrived at the residence during the rescue attempt and secured the scene. They then notified homicide detectives and the medical examiner's office. Teresa Fernandez, an FNDI, was dispatched to the residence to work in collaboration with law enforcement, to investigate the death.

The police determined that there was no indication of foul play and homicide detectives declined to attend the scene. The house was in order, there was no evidence of a robbery, and all the doors and windows were locked. A PlayStation was attached to the television, various clothes were strewn about the room, and schoolbooks were on the desk.

The decedent's mother, informed the FNDI that JO was in fine health. She explained that she had undergone a physical examination last week for athletics and that the findings were unremarkable. JO had an older brother and younger sister, both in excellent health. JO's father had hypertension and a history of heart disease, and diabetes and cancer had been present in maternal grandparents.

Teresa turned to the decedent's father who was also present who reported that other parents and teachers had been concerned about rumors of the increasing use of "bars" in area schools. Teresa questioned him further about what he meant; he confirmed that the school kids were reportedly buying and using the antianxiety medication Xanax. Neither parent reported prior suicide attempts or ideation.

Assessment

Teresa performed an assessment of the decedent. Her examination findings consisted of: "Livor mortis is consistent with body position and blanchable; rigor mortis is breakable in the jaw, arms, and legs. Frothy white foam cone was present at mouth and within bilateral nares. There are no visible signs of trauma."

In addition to providing details on the next steps, information regarding grief services and various community resources were offered. The body of JO was removed from the residence by the medical examiner's office, and an autopsy was performed the next day. The pathologist reported that the physical findings from the autopsy were unremarkable. During the autopsy, toxicology samples were collected from the heart, liver, and stomach.

Toxicology results were returned and were positive for an extremely large amount of alprazolam (Xanax). The final official cause of death for JO was alprazolam toxicity; the manner of death was accidental.

JO's parents were informed of the cause and manner of death. Both were devastated by the news. Grief resources were again made available.

Diagnosis
Family

- Mental and emotional distress
- Grief
- Excessive stress

Community

- Readiness for healing

Planning
Family

- The family will initiate counseling to assist with acceptance of and coping with death.

Long-Term Goal

- Family will identify need for outside support and seek such support.

Short-Term Goals

- Family will verbalize and recognize feelings surrounding the death.
- Family will express feelings honestly.

Community
Long-Term Goal

- Members of the community will establish a plan to deal with problems and stressors, including sudden unexpected deaths.

Short-Term Goal

- Members of the community, including school personnel and students, will identify positive and negative factors affecting management of current and future problems and stressors.

Intervention
Family

- Listen to the family's comments, remarks, and expression of concerns, noting nonverbal behaviors and responses
- Encourage family members to verbalize feelings openly and clearly
- Refer family to appropriate resources for assistance as indicated.

Community

- Reviewed the community plan for dealing with substance abuse problems among schoolchildren and assessed the related stressors
- Determined the community's strengths and weaknesses
- Identified available resources
- Established a mechanism for selfmonitoring of community needs and evaluation of efforts

Evaluation
Family

- The family began family counseling and slowly accepted death.
- JO's siblings began educating fellow classmates about the ill effects of abusing prescription medications.

Community

- The community implemented quarterly meetings for grieving families that included licensed counselors.
- The community members initiated peer review support groups

Levels of Prevention
Primary

- Initiate drug teaching in middle and high schools, focusing on resilience training, social skills, and personal management.
- Support programs that encourage students to role-play and apply life skills to deal with peer pressure.
- Provide life-skills training (e.g., skills to cope with peer pressure, improve self-esteem/confidence).

Case Study Application of the Nursing Process—cont'd

Secondary
- Organize group sessions in school to discuss illegal prescription medication abuse.
- Provide information to school personnel and parents on how to identify or screen for evidence of use of drugs and alcohol among school-aged children.
- Provide information on area groups that provide support for students who want to avoid using drugs or want to stop using drugs.

- Reduce or stop harm that is done to individuals or groups while they are using drugs.

Tertiary
- Reduce risk that additional students will abuse prescription medication.
- Provide support to those who are abusing such substances.
- Refer to support systems (e.g., Narcotic Anonymous).

EVOLVE WEBSITE

http://evolve.elsevier.com/Nies/community
- NCLEX Review Questions
- Case Studies

BIBLIOGRAPHY

42 U.S.C.A: *42 U.S.C.A. §5106g, as amended and reauthorized by the CAPTA Reauthorization Act of 2010*, 2015. https://www.law.cornell.edu/uscode/text/42/5106g.

Amar AF, Sekula LK: *A practical guide to forensic nursing incorporating forensic principles into nursing practice Sigma Theta Tau International*, 2017.

American Association of Legal Nurse Consultants (AALNC): *What is an LNC?*, 2021. Available from: http://www.aalnc.org/page/what-is-an-lnc.

American Board of Medicolegal Death Investigators (ABMDI): *Board certification (advanced)*, 2021. Available from: http://www.abmdi.org/board_certification.

American Legal Nurse Consultant Certification Board (ALNCC): *Eligibility criteria*, 2020. Available from: http://www.aalnc.org/page/become-an-lnc.

American Nurses Association: *Scope and standards of forensic nursing practice*, Washington, DC, 2009, American Nurses Publishing.

American Nurses Association (ANA): *Code of ethics with interpretive statement*, Washington, DC, 2015, American Nurses Publishing.

Black L: Forced medication of prison inmates, *Virtual Mentor AMA J Ethics* 10(2):106—109, 2008.

Bronson J, Berzofsky M: *Indicators of mental health problems reported by prisoners and jail inmates, 2011—12*, 2017. Accessed from: https://bjs.ojp.gov/content/pub/pdf/imhprpji1112.pdf.

Bureau of Justice Statistics (BJS): *The justice system*, 2021. Accessed from: https://bjs.ojp.gov/justice-system.

Bureau of Justice Statistics (BJS): *Co-offending among adolescents in violent victimizations, 2004—13*, 2016. Accessed from: https://bjs.ojp.gov/library/publications/co-offending-among-adolescents-violent-victimizations-2004-13.

Burgess AW, Berger AD, Boersma RR: Forensic nursing: investigating the career potential in this emerging graduate specialty, *Am J Nurs* 104(3):58—64, 2004.

Burnes D, Henderson CR, Sheppard C, Zhao R, Pillemer K, Lachs MS: Prevalence of financial fraud and scams among older adults in the united states: a systematic review and Meta-Analysis, *Am J Publ Health* 107(8):e13—e21, 2017. https://doi.org/10.2105/AJPH.2017.303821.

Carson EA: *Prisoners in 2019*, Washington, DC, 2020, Bureau of Justice Statistics. Accessed from: https://bjs.ojp.gov/library/publications/prisoners-2019.

Centers for Disease Control and Prevention (CDC): *Death Investigation System*, 2015. Retrieved at: https://www.cdc.gov/phlp/publications/coroner/death.htmlhttps://www.cdc.gov/phlp/publications/coroner/death.html.

Center for Infectious Disease Research and Policy (CIDRAP): *Studies detail large COVID outbreaks at US prisons, jails*, 2021. Retrieved at: https://www.cidrap.umn.edu/news-perspective/2021/04/studies-detail-large-covid-outbreaks-us-prisons-jails.

Collins SE, Halpern KJ: Forensic nursing: a collaborative practice paradigm, *J Nurs Law* 10(1):11—19, 2005.

Doughtery CM: Evidence collection in the emergency department. In Lynch V, Duval JB, editors: *Forensic nursing science*, St. Louis, 2011, Mosby.

Drake SA, Tabor P, Hamilton H, Cannon A: Nurses and Medicolegal Death Investigation, *J Forensic Nurs* 16(4):207—214, 2020. https://doi.org/10.1097/JFN.0000000000000310.

Drake SA, Cron S, Giardino A, Nolte KB: Comparative analysis of the public health role of two types of death investigation in Texas: application of the essential services, *J Forensic Sci* 60(4):914—919, 2015. https://doi.org/10.1111/1556-4029.12748.

Finn O: Child maltreatment: forensic biomarkers. In Lynch V, Duval JB, editors: *Forensic nursing science*, St. Louis, 2011, Mosby.

Geissler-Murr A, Moorhouse MF: Legal nurse consulting. In Lynch V, editor: *Forensic nursing*, St. Louis, 2011, Mosby.

Hanzlick R: *Death investigation systems and procedures*, Boca Raton, FL, 2007, CRC Press.

Hanzlick R, Hunsaker III JC, Davis GJ: *National association of medical examiners: a guide for manner of death classification*, 2002. Available from: https://netforum.avectra.com/Public/DocumentGenerate.aspx?wbn_key=38c0f1d2-11ec-45c7-80ca-ff872d0b22bc&SITE=NAME.

Harrell E: *Crime against persons with disabilities, 2009—2015 — Statistical tables (Bureau of Justice Statistics Rep No NCJ250632)*, 2017. Available from: https://bjs.ojp.gov/content/pub/pdf/capd0915st.pdf.

International Association of Forensic Nurses: *Sexual assault nurse examiner (SANE) educational guidelines handbook*, 2015. Available from: http://c.ymcdn.com/sites/www.forensicnurses.org/resource/resmgr/2015_SANE_ED_GUIDELINES.pdf.

Kaminski M: Games prisoners play, *Ration Soc* 15:188—217, 2003. https://doi.org/10.1177/1043463103015002002.

Kent-Wilkinson A: Forensic nursing educational development: an integrated review of the literature, *J Psychiatr Ment Health Nurs* 18(3):236—246, 2011.

Ledray LE: Sexual violence. In Lynch V, Duval JB, editors: *Forensic nursing science*, ed 2, St. Louis, 2011, Mosby.

Ledray LE, Arndt S: Examining the sexual assault victim: a new model for nursing care, *J Psychosoc Nurs* 32(2):7—12, 1994.

Local Government Insurance Trust (LGIT): *Right of inmates to refuse medical treatment*, 2009. Retrieved at: http://www.lgit.org/DocumentCenter/Home/View/356.

Lewis-O'Connor A, Latimore A, Amar AF, Sekula LK, editors: *A practical guide to forensic nursing incorporating forensic principles into nursing practice Sigma Theta Tau International*, 2017.

Lynch V: Evolution of forensic nursing science. In Lynch V, Duval JB, editors: *Forensic nursing science*, St. Louis, 2011, Mosby.

Lynch V, Koehler SA: Forensic investigation of death. In Lynch V, Duval JB, editors: *Forensic nursing science*, ed 2, St. Louis, 2011, Mosby.

Maruschak LM, Bronson J, Alper M: *Parents in prison and their minor children: Survey of prison inmates, 2016*, 2021. Accessed from: https://bjs.ojp.gov/library/publications/parents-prison-and-their-minor-children-survey-prison-inmates-2016.

Maruschak LA, Berzofsky M, Unangst J: *Medical problems of state and federal prisoners and jail inmates, 2011–12 (Bureau of Justice Statistics Rep No NCJ 248491)*, February 2015. Available from: https://www.bjs.gov/content/pub/pdf/mpsfpji1112.pdf.

Mason T: Psychiatric forensic nursing. In Lynch V, Duval JB, editors: *Forensic nursing*, ed 2, St. Louis, 2011, Mosby.

Mitchell S, Drake SA: Death investigation. In Amar AF, Sekula LK, editors: *A practical guide to forensic nursing incorporating forensic principles into nursing practice Sigma Theta Tau International*, 2017.

Murphy K, Waa S, Jaffer H, Sauter A, Chan A: A literature review of findings in physical elder abuse, *Can Assoc Radiol J = Journal l'Association canadienne des radiologistes* 64(1):10–14, 2013. https://doi.org/10.1016/j.carj.2012.12.001.

National Center on Elder Abuse (NCEA): *Research, statistics and data*, 2021. Access from: https://ncea.acl.gov/What-We-Do/Research/Statistics-and-Data.aspx#prevalence.

National Commission on Correctional Health Care (NCCHC): *Women's health care in correctional settings*, 2020. Available from: https://www.ncchc.org/filebin/Positions/Womens-Health-Care-in-Correctional-Settings-2020.pdf.

National Alliance for the Mentally Ill [NAMI]: *Mental illness and the Criminal Justice System*, 2021. Available from: https://nami.org/NAMI/media/NAMI-Media/Infographics/NAMI_CriminalJustice System-v5.pdf.

National Adult Protective Services (NAPSA): *Just the facts senior financial fraud and abuse*, 2016. Accessed from: http://www.napsa-now.org/wp-content/uploads/2016/11/senior-scams-financial-fraud-and-abuse-2016.pdf.

Office for victims of crime, 2017. Available from: https://www.ovcttac.gov/saneguide/introduction/what-is-a-sane/.

Pagliaro EM: Cewe BRB: The forensic nurse witness in the American Justice System. In Hammer RM, Moynihan B, Pagliaro EM, editors: *Forensic nursing: a handbook for practice*, ed 2, Burlington, MA, 2013, Jones and Bartlett.

Potter PA, Perry AG: *Fundamentals of nursing*, ed 10, St. Louis, 2019, Mosby.

Price B, Maguire K: *Core curriculum for forensic nursing*, 2016, Lippincott Williams & Wilkins.

Pickens S, Dyer CB: Elder abuse in America, *Open Med J* 3:188–193, 2016. https://doi.org/10.2174/1874220301603010188.

Radeloff D, Stoeber F, Lempp T, Kettner M, Bennefeld-Kersten K: Murderers or thieves at risk? Offence-related suicide rates in adolescent and adult prison populations, *PLoS One* 14(4):e0214936, 2019. Accessed from: https://doi.org/10.1371/journal.pone.0214936.

Robson B: From emergency nurse to legal nurse consultant and independent practitioner: legal nurse consulting? What is that? *NENA Outlook* 32(2):24–26, 2009.

Rosen T, LoFaso VM, Bloemen EM, Clark S, McCarthy TJ, Reisig C, et al.: Identifying injury patterns associated with physical elder abuse: analysis of legally adjudicated cases, *Ann Emerg Med* 76(3):266–276, 2020.

Ruiz-Contreras A: The nurse as an expert witness, *Top Emerg Med* 27(1):27–35, 2005.

Shafer TJ: Organ donation. In Lynch V, Duval JB, editors: *Forensic nursing science*, ed 2, St. Louis, 2011, Mosby.

Substance Abuse and Mental Health Services Administration (SAMHSA): *SAMHSA's concept of trauma and guidance for a trauma-informed approach*, 2014. Available from: https://ncsacw.samhsa.gov/userfiles/files/SAMHSA_Trauma.pdf.

The sentencing project: *Fact Sheet: Trends in U.S. Corrections*, 2020. https://www.sentencingproject.org/wp-content/uploads/2021/07/Trends-in-US-Corrections.pdf.

Treatment Advocacy Center: *The treatment of persons with mental illness in prisons and jails: A state survey*, 2014. Accessed from: https://www.treatmentadvocacycenter.org/storage/documents/treatment-behind-bars/treatment-behind-bars.pdf.

U.S. Department of Health and Human Services: *Administration for Children and Families; Administration on Children; Youth and Families Children's Bureau (USDHHS): Child maltreatment, 2019*, Washington, DC, 2019, Author. https://www.acf.hhs.gov/sites/default/files/documents/cb/cm2019.pdf#page=11.

U.S. Preventive Services Task Force (USPSTF): *Intimate Partner Violence, elder abuse and abuse of vulnerable adults: screening*, 2018. Recommendation: Intimate Partner Violence, Elder Abuse, and Abuse of Vulnerable Adults: Screening | United States Preventive Services Taskforce (uspreventiveservicestaskforce.org). Available from: https://uspreventiveservicestaskforce.org/uspstf/recommendation/intimate-partner-violence-and-abuse-of-elderly-and-vulnerable-adults-screening.

Valentine JL, Sekula LK, Lynch V: Evolution of forensic nursing theory- Introduction of the constructed theory of forensic nursing care: a middle-range theory, *J Forensic Nurs* 16(4):188–198, 2020.

Yon Y, Mikton CR, Gassoumis ZD, Wilber KH: Elder abuse prevalence in community settings: a systematic review and meta-analysis, *Lancet Global Health* 5(2):e147–e156, 2017. https://doi.org/10.1016/S2214-109X(17)30006-2.

Zawitz C, Welbel S, Ghinai I, et al.: Outbreak of COVID-19 and interventions in a large jail — cook county, IL, United States, *Am J Infect Control* 49(9):1129–1135, 2020.

33

Faith Community Nursing

Allison Findlay*

OBJECTIVES

Upon completion of this chapter, the reader will be able to do the following:

1. Understand the potential role of faith communities in improving the health of Americans.
2. Describe the philosophy and historical basis of faith community nursing.
3. Define the roles, functions, and education of the faith community nurse.
4. Discuss faith communities as clients of the community health nurse.

5. Describe the role of the faith community nurse in the spiritual health and wellness of faith communities.
6. Discuss contemporary issues in faith community nursing, such as working with vulnerable populations and facing ethical and legal issues.
7. Apply the nursing process to a case study related to a faith community practice.

OUTLINE

KEY TERMS

advocate

Faith Community Nurse

health educator

volunteer coordinator

spirituality

FAITH COMMUNITY NURSING

The purpose of this chapter is to present an overview of Faith Community Nursing (FCN) and the implications for this growing specialty as perspectives shift from the physiologic management of care to a more holistic mind-body-spirit approach. Foundational to nursing is evidenced-based care and holistic care of individuals, populations, and groups. Nurses working in faith-based church congregations and communities are in a unique position to support and educate diverse populations and bridge the gap to the healthcare system to improve health outcomes. Clinical examples 1 and 2 illustrate models of FCN in the United States and the role of the FCN.

Clinical Example 33.1

Sandra Mills began her faith community nurse (FCN) practice as a volunteer when her parish priest recruited her to help establish a cancer support group and coordinate classes for caregivers. Within 6 months, her church's social concerns committee established a paid position on their ministry team and employed her as a full-time, paid staff member. After completing an FCN program through a local university, she began to develop a health ministry in her church. She describes her days as full and rewarding. Each day, she visits ill or homebound parish members and provides support through prayer, education, and listening. She is challenged to locate and refer community resources, provide health education to church groups (e.g., mother's day out and the over-55 group), and coordinate the efforts of other volunteers in the church. She is

Continued

* The author would like to acknowledge the contribution of Beverly Cook Siegrist, who revised this chapter for the previous edition.

Clinical Example 33.1—cont'd

practicing holistic nursing for the first time in her 15 years of practice. She found that the church, as a healing community, allows her to focus on the body-mind-spirit connection she believes is necessary to improve the health of congregation members.

Clinical Example 33.2

Marilyn Michaels is a former home care and hospice nurse who works as an FCN coordinator for St. Luke's Hospital, which is a 400-bed medical center serving a Midwestern rural population. Her position was created to assist community churches in developing and maintaining parish nurse (PN) programs. She coordinates educational programs, including a 30-h preparation program for beginning FCNs, an advanced program for FCN coordinators in individual churches, and monthly educational programs offered through an FCN support group. Marilyn developed the support group and facilitates communication among the 200 nurses and 100 church communities that St. Luke's Hospital serves. She also assists the many faith community programs by connecting them with other services that the hospital and community agencies provide (e.g., screening, support groups, and speakers). The program at St. Luke's Hospital is self-supporting from grants and educational programs.

These examples illustrate the role of the Faith Community Nurse. According to the Westberg Institute (WI) (2022, p. 1), **Faith Community Nurses** (FCNs) are "... licensed, registered nurses who practice wholistic health for self, individuals and the community using nursing knowledge combined with spiritual care. They function in paid and unpaid positions as members of the pastoral team in a variety of religious faiths, cultures, and countries. The focus of their work is on the intentional care of the spirit, assisting the members of the faith community and other faith-based organizations to maintain and/or regain wholeness in body, mind, and spirit." Although similar to other community-based nursing specialties, FCN is distinct in its intentional emphasis on the spiritual as part of health promotion and prevention and minimizing illness (American Nurses Association & Health Ministries Association [ANA & HMA], 2017; Westberg Institute, 2019). In addition to facilitating physical and psychological functioning and lifestyle change, FCN emphasizes care of the family, coping assistance, referrals to the healthcare system, and educational programs to improve the health of the congregation and community (Solari-Twadell & Ziebarth, 2019). Religion and spirituality are considered important social determinants of health and FCNs have an important role to play in public health practice (Ransome, 2020).

Faith Communities: Role in Health and Wellness

Faith-based communities are made up of people of diverse cultures, values, and beliefs. The majority of the US population (70.6%), identify themselves as Christian, followed by Jewish (1.9%), Muslims (0.9%), Buddhists (0.7%), and Hindus (0.7%)

according to the *2014 Religious Landscape Study* (Pew Research Center, 2014). Globally, approximately one-third of the population, 1.6 billion (31.5%) identify themselves as Christian, followed by Muslim (1.6 billion, 23%), Hindus (1 billion, 15%), Buddhists (500 million, 7%), and Jews (14 million, 0.2%) (Hackett & Grim 2012). This diversity in norms, beliefs and practices, even within subcultures of the populations, related to health, healing, and spirituality, present opportunities and challenges. Faith-based organizations (FBOs) have a long history of community outreach, providing basic needs such as food, clothing, and shelter, spiritual counseling, social services, health education, and locations for interventions. Health ministry is traditionally part of the holistic mission of FBOs, who tailor programs to the needs of their communities in culturally appropriate ways. Organized religions are using multi-faceted approaches to connect with congregational members of all ages, such as online services, support and connect groups, youth and children's programs, and music and drama incorporated into worship. Established relationships between FBOs and their community members provide a unique setting for FCNs to implement health promotion and prevention programs. Poor underserved faith-based communities with less resources and access to health services can partner with FBOs that provide economic and functional support for FCNs to design programs that will address health inequalities.

Over the last decade, FBOs have reached out to research universities to form partnerships to address health disparities. Academic organizations collaborate with ministry teams and FCNs to assess needs and programming priorities, investigate funding sources, and design interventions that are tailored to the needs and wants of the faith community. FCNs and ministry teams implement programs that are evaluated by researchers, who measure health outcomes. Advanced practice FCNs have community nursing experience and educational training that can ensure health information and programming is accurate and accessible. One example of a successful academic-community partnership was described by De Marco et al. (2014). A rural Black church in North Carolina collaborated with a research university to design and implement a church-based pilot garden project to improve food access and reduce chronic illness with healthy food. The project, called "Harvest of Hope," was composed of 44 youth and adults. Both organizations worked together on study design, project aims, budget, recruitment, programming, and reporting of results. The project increased community ownership and was culturally appropriate. The researchers cited challenges such as adequate communication and managing expectations of diverse parties. The success of the project led to a larger "Faith, Farming, and the Future" project, funded by the NIH to include four churches and 60 youth (De Marco et al., 2014).

Religion and Health

There is growing evidence that religiosity and spirituality are associated with better healthcare practices and outcomes. The terms religion and spirituality may be used interchangeably in the literature, but they have separate and distinct meanings. Religion is commonly defined as "a social institution with an organized system of beliefs, practices, rituals, and symbols that enables a person's closeness or submission to a higher power or God." (Lalani & Chen, 2021, p. 207).

Spirituality can be defined as a personal search for meaning or purpose in life and may represent a relationship to God or another higher power that could include healing by means of prayer, meditation or other practices (Thoresen, 1999). In Western traditions it is a connection to God, Allah, HaShem, or a Higher Power, and in Eastern traditions may be called Brahman, manifestations of Brahman, Buddha, Dao, or ultimate truth/reality (Koenig, 2012). In the Old Testament, *Shalom* denotes a state of completeness or well-being, God's desire for health and wholeness. The New Testament discusses Jesus' healing people in relation to the whole spirit, soul, and body. The Talmud describes the importance of health prevention practices and the responsibility of the person and the Rabbi to maintain physical health as God's will in their lives. Followers of Buddhism believe in maintaining physical and mental health and following a healthy lifestyle as a spiritual path to Enlightenment. The majority of religions view health holistically, and discuss the importance of maintaining physical, mental, and spiritual wholeness. Religions prescribe spiritual methods of healing such as prayer, chanting, meditation, good deeds and other rituals and ceremonies that include the leaders of the faith community. The majority of religions also recognize community health is an important part of individual health. Spirituality and religion are an integral part of health (Ketchell & Canda, n.d.).

Garssen et al. (2021) conducted a meta-analysis of 48 longitudinal studies related to religion and spirituality and the effect on mental health. Among the studies, the frequency of church visits and other religious activities, and the importance of religion in one's life were predictive of mental health. Overall, studies demonstrated religion and spirituality were associated with distress and life satisfaction.

Coping with chronic illness can be particularly challenging for health status and quality of life (QoL). Alvarez et al. (2016) cited an association between spirituality, religiosity, and personal beliefs and better adherence to health management, in a cohort of 130 outpatients with heart failure. In addition, the authors found a positive correlation between religiosity and QoL. Parks et al. (2016) reported experiencing spiritual peace and adherence to a healthy lifestyle were better predictors of mortality risk than physical health measures such as functional status and comorbidity in individuals with heart failure. High levels of self-rated religiosity and spirituality were associated with higher self-rated health among South Asians living in the United States (Stroope et al., 2020). Research findings support the belief that spiritual resources can have a beneficial effect on QoL. Counted et al. (2018) conducted an Integrative Review of 20 studies from 2007 to 2017 examining Relational Spirituality and QoL. Twelve studies reported positive associations between RS and QoL, three studies showed a negative association, and two of five studies that did not show an association supported indirect associations between RS and QoL. In these studies, RS is associated with better outcomes of QoL in the areas of physical health, psychological well-being, social relationship quality, and spiritual functioning, and serve as an important coping strategy for managing stress of illness.

The relationship between religion and spirituality and health highlight that individuals have spiritual needs related to biopsychosocial conditions that, if not met, can lead to adverse health outcomes and increasing mortality. Spirituality and faith are found to be major resources of resilience and coping dealing with feelings of loneliness, isolation, anxiety, and depression and physical illness. FCNs need to assess spiritual and religious beliefs and be aware of factors that influence healthcare decisions and health. Faith communities are a source of social support that can promote health behaviors and adherence to medical treatments for members of the faith community (Counted et al., 2018; Koenig, 2012).

? ACTIVE LEARNING

Speak with FCN in the community about congregational health needs. Discuss how the roles of the FCN are implemented through FCN programs and ministry. Observe the nurse in their daily activities and identify how spirituality is a basis for congregational nursing care.

RESEARCH HIGHLIGHTS

Faith-Placed Cardiovascular Health Promotion: A Framework for Contextual and Organizational Factors Underlying Program Success

Best practices in planning and implementing programs related to cardiovascular health are a frequent topic among FCNs. Many comprehensive programs are being implemented to improve positive health behaviors among congregational members across all ethnic groups and ages. The purpose of this study was to review all current faith-placed cardiovascular health promotion programs and to construct a framework of factors to increase the effectiveness of existing programs. The sample included current, published reports of programs in the literature from 1984 to 2004. Variables were identified and characterized by identifying clusters from the literature that describe factors contributing to the success of any program. The significant variables for the model are defined as faith support, community support, community partnerships, faith organization capabilities, secular organization capabilities (other healthcare system support), and caring interventions. For example, the faith support variable required activation of family, peer, pastor, volunteer, and nurse support. Secular support includes increasing awareness through education, such as helping the community understand the connection among spiritual health, cardiovascular health, and success in a health promotion program. The construct of caring interventions is significant to FCNs implementing a cardiovascular health promotion program. The authors found that caring included "visible involvement" on many levels such as engaging staff and members in health conversations, providing group and individual support, and being highly visible to church members. The results of this study provide a useful model for successful implementation of health promotion programs for the nurse and health ministry team.

From Sternberg Z, Munchauer FE, Carrow SS et al.: Faith-placed cardiovascular health promotion: a framework for contextual and organizational factors underlying program success, *Health Educ Res* 22(5):619–629, 2007.

Foundations of Faith Community Nursing

In 1984 Reverend Dr. Granger Westberg, a Lutheran pastor, founded the parish nurse (PN) movement, an approach based on the concept of holistic care by doctors, clergy, chaplains, and nurses, to address the physical, emotional, and spiritual health needs within the faith community. A year later the Parish Nurse Resource Center began in the Chicago area, sponsored by a Lutheran General Hospital, now Advocate Health. Six FCNs were hired, with salaries provided by the hospital and churches. The establishment of the PN was influenced by Dr. Westberg's partnership with the Kellogg foundation and Department of Medicine at the University of Chicago College of Medicine in 1976, to create "wholistic health centers" partnering family physicians with churches and teams of nurses and Clergy. The success of the centers was due in part to the nurses, who were trained in spiritual and community nursing practice, and acted as a bridge between the faith team and primary physicians (Holistic Health Centers, 1976). In 1988, the American Nurses Association (ANA) in collaboration with the Health Ministries Association, Parish Nurse Division, published the first Scope and Standards of Parish Nurse Practice, establishing PN as a nurse specialty. The standards were revised in 2012 to include clearer definition of practice and advanced nursing practice. As the PN role grew and expanded outside of the United States, it evolved to the International Parish Nurse Resource Center (IPNRC) and was moved to the St. Louis Missouri Deaconess Foundation in 2002. In 2004, the field of palliative care cited spiritual, religious, and existential issues as a required component of care (Puchalski et al., 2009). The organization moved to the Church Health Center in Memphis Tennessee in 2011, and the name was changed to the WI for FCN. Recognizing the diverse nature of parish nursing across denominations and faith communities, the name was changed to FCN. Other names for FCN are congregational nurses or church nurses, depending on their individual faith communities.

The Church Health Center was founded in 1987 by Dr. Scott Morris, a physician and ordained minister, to provide quality and affordable healthcare for working uninsured people and their families. His mission was to reestablish the Church's role in caring for people physically and spiritually, which had been overshadowed by technological advances in Medicine and emphasis on physical care. The Center assembled a volunteer interprofessional team of nurse practitioners, dentists, and others, to provide care for people for a small fee based on a sliding scale. Thirty years and 70,000 patients later, Dr. Morris' vision still serves as a model of wellness today. Fig. 33.1 is an illustration of the Wellness Model and the vision, mission, and programs of the Model.

The WI moved to New York in 2020 and is continuing to support the professional practice of FCNs through education, resources, and knowledge sharing. Its partner organization, the Spiritual Care Association Nursing Division, was developed to "support best-practice spiritual nursing care and self-care through education, mentoring, and resources, for healthcare

The Church Health Center Model for Healthy Living

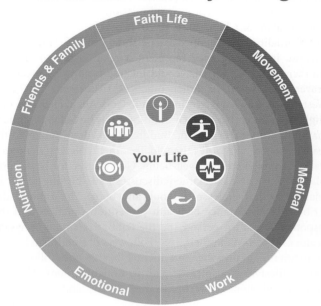

 Faith Life
Building a relationship with God, your neighbors, and yourself.

 Movement
Discovering ways to enjoy physical activity.

 Medical
Partnering with your healthcare provider to manage your medical care.

 Work
Appreciating your skills, talents, and gifts.

 Emotional
Managing stress and understanding your feelings to better care for yourself.

 Nutrition
Making smart food choices and developing healthy eating habits.

 Family & Friends
Giving and receiving support through relationships.

Fig. 33.1 The church health center model for healthy living. (From Church Health Center: *Model for Healthy Living*, n.d. Aailable from: https://chreader.org/model-healthy-living2/. Accessed 2021.)

professionals and nursing-related organizations." (Westberg Institute, 2022). The Association focuses on the spiritual dimension of professional nursing practice for registered nurses and advanced and specialty practice nurses, in hospital and non-hospital settings. The professional Faith Community Nurses International (FCNI) organization was established to promote FCN research, education and policy and realize their mission of connecting, supporting and promoting a global community of FCNs to positively affect the health of faith communities and the community as a whole (ANA, 2017). The organization has an open-access online journal for publications, titled the *International Journal of Faith Community Nursing* (FCNI, 2017). As of 2017, FCNs now practice in 29 countries, including Australia, Canada, England, New Zealand, Bahamas, Ghana, Kenya, South Korea, Madagascar, Malawi, Malaysia, Nigeria, South Africa, Switzerland, Singapore, etc., serving Muslim, Jewish, and Christian faith communities.

The Philosophy of the FCN is rooted in Abrahamic Faith traditions and professional nursing practice and is based on five key elements:

1. The spiritual dimension is essential to practice.
2. The role balances nursing science and technology with service and spiritual care.
3. The nurse's clients are members of the faith-based community defined by the church and its public service philosophy.
4. Parish nursing services are built upon principles of self-care and capacity building, with a focus on understanding the connections between health and the individual's relationship with God, faith traditions, nursing, and the broader society.
5. The PN understands that holistic health is a dynamic process that requires connections among the person's spiritual. Psychological, physical, and social dimensions.

The Westberg Institute's (2022) philosophy of FCN recognizes it as a specialty practice combining nursing and health ministry within the faith community for health and healing. Central to the philosophy are four concepts: spiritual formation; professionalism; shalom as health and wholeness; and community, incorporating culture and diversity.

The unique nature of this nursing specialty is embodied in the philosophy of care towards wholeness of body and spirit, the underpinning of FCN practice (Solari-Twadell & McDermott, 1999; Westberg Institute, 2022). The unique nature of this nursing specialty is embodied in the philosophy of care underpinning FCN practice.

Roles or Functions of the Faith Community Nurse

The purpose of the FCN is to provide health education, connect people with resources, facilitate referrals for services, help people navigate the healthcare system, intentionally care for the spirit and integrate spiritual care into health promotion, organize support groups and systems, and assist in creating conversations around end-of-life care and other critical healthcare decision-making. The FCN functions as a health educator, personal health advisor, referral agent, health advocate, coordinator of volunteers, developer of support groups, and integrator of health and healing (Westberg Institute, 2022).

As a **health educator**, the FCN assesses the educational needs of the faith community members and identifies resources and teaching strategies tailored to the health literacy, age, and developmental stage of the members. The selection of educational topics is based on needs assessments, priorities of the organization and members, and public health agency priorities as outlined in *Healthy People 2020/2030*. Participants can be recruited through events, church bulletin articles, or activities, for topics targeting healthy lifestyles such as nutrition and exercise, CPR classes for new mothers, management of chronic illnesses such as diabetes, values topics such as disability awareness, and many others (Langdon & Hinton, 2019). The FCN can function as a personal health advisor as part of an educational program or informally while interacting at events, or on a one-to-one basis. Active listening, presence, anticipatory guidance, emotional and spiritual support, decision-making support, coping enhancement, grief work facilitation, and consultation are part of the advisor role. The FCN may be asked about health problems and disease management, or visit homes, hospitals, or nursing homes (Langdon & Hinton, 2019).

The FCN utilizes referral skills and knowledge of community resources to guide individuals in accessing resources that may be available online, in the faith community, governmental and public health service agencies, or healthcare providers. FCNs can develop working relationships with community coalitions, hospital-based community initiatives, and other community-based groups to build connections. FCNs may make referrals to clinics, specialists, a counseling center, support group, food pantry, or hospice, for example. The FCN serves as an **advocate** for individuals, families and groups and speaks on their behalf. Navigating the healthcare system can be challenging. Assistance to obtain health services and appropriate care or management plans or coaching and educating about questions to ask empowers members of the community to speak for themselves and make the best choices when utilizing health services. In a broader context, FCN advocacy at the community and organizational level promotes community awareness of significant health problems, lobbies for beneficial public policies, and represents the holistic perspectives of faith-based healthcare providers on topics such as birth control, stem cell technology and sex education for teens and youth (Langdon & Hinton, 2019).

The role of a **volunteer coordinator** involves recruiting, training, and directing volunteers to work with the FCN program or health ministry. Training volunteers develops workers for the ministry who can be delegated to manage existing programs. Volunteerism provides a sense of giving back to the community, an important part of spiritual health and missions involvement. Facilitating outside resources for the community such as health screenings, flu shots, and immunizations through the health department for example, connects volunteers with broader communities and provides opportunities for involvement with other FBOs. Development of support groups requires skills in community assessment and program evaluation skills. Support groups for people experiencing similar problems or experiences such as bereavement groups, new mother groups, self-help, and addiction groups (e.g., AA) can provide additional resources for the ministry team and create social support networks among group members with similar values and beliefs. The FCN may develop the group or make a referral to outside sources (Langdon & Hinton, 2019).

Education of the Faith Community Nurse

FCNs are registered nurses that must have an active license in the state of practice. FCNs should have a baccalaureate degree with experience in community nursing and educational courses that provide specialized knowledge in the spiritual beliefs and practices of the faith community they serve (Westberg Institute, 2022.). FCNs practice "wholistic" health, a whole-person approach that includes intentional care for the spirit and recognizes the inter-relationship between faith and health; they practice in faith communities or FBOs and help their patients maintain or regain wholeness in mind, body, and spirit (ANA & HMA 2017; Solari-Twadell & Ziebarth, 2019; Westberg Institute, 2021).

Foundations for Faith Community Nursing (2019) is a comprehensive, evidence-based curriculum that prepares licensed registered nurses for the specialized practice of FCN. This curriculum focuses on the intentional care of the spirit and promotion of whole-person health and the prevention or minimization of illness within the community. Wholistic health and prevention or minimization of illness within the context of faith communities is foundational. Fifteen modules contain essential content that is aligned with the FCN and the ANA and the Health Ministries Association Scope and Standards for Practice (2017). Practicing FCNs with advanced degrees share their knowledge and experience, and develop FCN skills with critical thinking questions, group learning activities, case studies, and practical resources (Church Health Organization, 2022).

FCN curriculums are based on four concepts: Wholistic health, Spiritual Dimension, Community, and Professionalism. Wholistic Health is embodied in the meaning of "shalom," representing wholism, health and healing within education, prevention and teaching and learning principles. Wholistic health is multi-faceted, addressing diverse issues such as suffering, grief and loss, and family violence. The Spiritual Dimension is described as "the need for meaning, purpose and fulfillment in life, the hope or will to live, and belief and faith." (Jacob & Solari-Twadell, 2019, p. 81). The spiritual dimension is essential for attaining an overall sense of health, well-being, and QoL. The community includes the faith community, professional nursing community, geographic community, global community, demographic community, or other communities. Professionalism defines the scope and standards of practice outlined in state nursing boards, and by the ANA (2015) Scope and Standards of Practice and Code of Ethics for Nurses with Interpretive Statements (2008), and the FCN: Scope and Standards of Practice (ANA & HMA, 2012; 2017; Jacob & Solari-Twadell, 2019). The International Council of Nursing and the Joint Commission on Accreditation of Healthcare Organizations require healthcare organizations to incorporate spirituality as an essential component of care for patients and families (Lalani et al., 2021).

The Faith Community Nurse and Spirituality

The Westburg Institute (n.d) describes an FCN as one who has personal spiritual maturity and specialized knowledge of the spiritual beliefs and practices of the faith community and the ability to apply spiritual aspects to the health of the community served. Often there is a confusion in the literature between religion and spirituality; however, most authors agree that religion and spirituality are separate constructs and spirituality is a broader concept than religion. Religion is commonly defined as an organized system of beliefs, practices, rituals, and symbols that enables a person's closeness or submission to a higher power or God, whereas spirituality is defined as a personal search for meaning or purpose in life (Lalani & Chen, 2021). A common definition found in the nursing literature by Puchalski et al. (2009) states that **spirituality** is an aspect of humanity that refers to the way individuals seek and express meaning and purpose, the way they experience their connectedness to the moment, to self, to others, to nature, and to the significant or sacred. FCNs must have an in-depth knowledge and understanding of the spiritual context of nursing in order to meet the needs and concerns of the community they serve. Models have been developed, such as the HOPE Model and the Jarel Spiritual Well-Being Scale (McEwan, 2005).

Clinical Example 33.3

Sue James is a member of an FCN group from five inner-city churches in south-central Indiana. This group of nurses came together from five different church denominations to meet their congregation members' health needs. The nurses are unpaid within their own congregations. They came together to share their resources because their churches are small in membership and they identified similar and unmet health needs in each of the churches. Primarily, the group serves an aging population that represents the few remaining individuals and families living in the inner-city area. Sue agreed to serve as the group coordinator, a position that has been shared among their group. In this position, she plans biweekly meetings for the nurses at alternating churches and serves as a community liaison for participating churches. The group's PN effort began 2 years earlier, supported by a local hospital grant and matched with small donations from the participating churches. Each nurse volunteers at least 10 h each week. On the basis of the health and wellness assessment completed in each church, they arranged a health fair that included health screening and referral information at one church and began educational classes on topics related to depression and healthy aging. They focus on health promotion, and their individual churches recognize them as the FCN, the congregational nurse, and the health minister.

ISSUES IN FAITH COMMUNITY NURSE PRACTICE

The strong connection between health messages and the spiritual mission of the FBO, in addition to its reach into underserved communities, further justify the church as an effective health promotion setting.

Providing Care to Vulnerable Populations

Faith communities historically care for vulnerable populations such as refugees, migrant workers, homeless individuals and families, offer assistance to low-income families, and provide resources during times of disaster such as fire or flood. FCNs can be instrumental in helping people access services, often in partnership with established health agencies and programs. FCNs can build a community of caring for vulnerable groups by educating faith communities about the people or population and their spiritual, emotional and physical needs, and providing opportunities to volunteer with programs to meet them. His model of leadership has been referred to as the *Nehemiah approach*, meaning that people collectively share their talents and desires to do the work. (Leadership Lessons from Nehemiah, 2019)

Riza et al. (2020) identified 15 effective healthcare best practices and tools in community-based healthcare for migrants and refugees. The study found good communication, overcoming linguistic barriers and understanding cultural differences are necessary ingredients for interventions to be effective. Close collaboration of organizational and community stakeholders, the local communities, the migrant/refugee communities, and the partnerships is a key element in the successful implementation of primary healthcare provision. FCNs are particularly suited to the best practice interventions in the literature review, such as community outreach, cultural sensitivity training for staff and community, health promotion education among migrants, and advocacy. FCNs are able to provide care in these diverse populations using skills in assessment, planning, and interventions.

End-of-Life Issues: Grief and Loss

Faith communities are often the first to offer assistance and support when a person or family is experiencing loss, grief and end-of-life. An increasingly aging population and increased prevalence of chronic illnesses such as cardiovascular disease and cancer has led to a greater awareness of end-of-life care. Health education for this population may include living wills, advanced directives, healthcare proxies, and understanding of hospice and palliative care. FCNs can partner with hospice and palliative care programs and home care nurses to assist faith community members in managing end-of-life care. Older adults from cultural and ethnic minorities are less likely to have advanced care planning in addition to palliative and end-of-life care management. Health literacy, religiosity, and spirituality are significant contributors to this problem, and lead to substandard care (de Vries et al., 2019). FCNs can bridge the gap in these vulnerable populations through health education interventions incorporating faith and spirituality with end-of-life decisions. FCNs roles also conduct home visits to dying congregational members, provide emotional support to family and survivors, and develop grief support groups. FCN plays an essential role in meeting the needs of gerontological and chronical illness populations in their faith community.

Family Violence Prevention

Nurses must be knowledgeable about identifying and treating abuse against women, family, children, and elders in their faith community. Education and prevention of family violence is part of *Healthy People 2030* objectives, who recommend that healthcare providers screen all women of reproductive age for intimate partner violence (IPV) and provide access to support services for women who screen positive for IPV (also known as domestic abuse, spouse abuse, courtship violence, battery, marital rape, or date rape). Proper training and continuing education for FCNs will enable early recognition and effective interventions and support. In the United States there are no standard reporting laws. However, it is essential that FCNs have an intervention plan that includes providing support, establishing a trusting relationship, discussing safety issues, making appropriate referrals to counseling and shelters, and documenting the abuse according to the faith organizations policy (Saletti-Cuesta et al., 2018).

Child abuse and neglect are reportable in all 50 states (DHHS, 2022). Nurses are required to do the following:
1. Report to the proper authority.
2. Provide resources and referrals.
3. Establish a trusting relationship with child or adolescent.
4. Provide presence.
5. Listen.
6. Document according to policy, law, or both.

The National Center on Elder Abuse (n.d.) reported that at least one in 10 community-dwelling older adults in the United States experienced some form of abuse in the prior year. Globally it is estimated that one in six elders (15.7%) in the community experienced past year abuse. psychological (11.6%), physical (2.6%), financial (6.8%), neglect (4.2%), and sexual (0.9%) abuse. All states have laws against elder abuse, and FCNs should be knowledgeable about laws governing elder abuse in their state and making the appropriate reports and referrals. FCNs may be the first to notice signs of abuse. Assessment and screening tools are available to aid in identifying at risk and victims of abuse that can be shared with faith community clergy and volunteers. Establishing a trusting relationship with the elder and being present (as needed) and providing spiritual and emotional support are valuable nursing interventions.

Confidentiality

The Code of Ethics for Nurses (ANA, 2015) and the Scope and Standards of Faith Community Nursing Practice (HMA and ANA, 2012) provide ethical guidance for nurses. FCNs are accountable to their state board of nursing and faith community employers and the community they serve. FNCs share many of the ethical and legal issues encountered in general nursing practice; however, due to the nature of the nurse-organization-community relationship, confidentiality can be potentially problematic in a church community. The nurse should protect the client's rights to confidentiality concerning health and health related conditions. Although the nurse must share information with the church minister at times, church leadership and prayer groups should not be given private client information unless given permission by the client. Exceptions are found in circumstances where a religious practice gives permission or requires public confession of behaviors or conditions and other private information. FCNs should follow general guidelines for medical record management including procedures for storing records and requesting medical information and making or receiving referrals. FCN programs with the faith community are not required to follow the Health Insurance Portability and Accountability Act (HIPPA) related to medical and records and confidentiality, because churches are not recognized as healthcare providers. However, if the nurse is working under a licensed healthcare provider such as a hospital, HIPPA regulations would apply. It is important for the FCN to have a thorough understanding of policies and procedures governing confidentiality in the faith community setting and faith organizations.

Accountability

FCNs must be in compliance with professional standards and state board of nursing requirements, as well as the American Nurses Association-Health Ministries Association (ANA-HMA) standards of practice for FCN. FCNs should carry personal liability insurance and be covered under the faith community's liability policy. To decrease FCN liability, the WI (n.d.) recommends maintaining a strong line of communication between the FCN and church, staff and stakeholders, have a well-defined job description, comply with Faith Community Scopes of Practice, and maintain a documentation system that supports actions. Volunteers are held to church laws to the same degree of accountability as paid employees, subject to discrimination laws. Ministers, both ordained and nonordained may be required to disclose confidential information in court. The nurse should be familiar with all policies and procedures that may affect the scope of their professional practice. The FCN should be knowledgeable of the faith organizations position and beliefs on topics that may conflict with secular nursing health promotion and programs and create policies that establish a program's position on a particular issue.

It is important to have policies and procedures in place that clearly outline the FCNs responsibilities, organizational structures, professional and administrative expectations, reporting guidelines, protection of client's rights and information, such as referrals and documentation records, and personnel management, work and environment safety. The FCN can use expectations and responsibilities in annual performance reviews, to be accountable to the faith community and organization. Nurses are accountable to the nursing standards and civil laws designed to protect individuals from abuse, neglect and discrimination. In addition to administrative concerns, FCNs should ensure policies and procedures are in place for issues that may arise in nursing programs such as blood pressure screenings, medical emergencies, transportation, home visitations, and cases of abuse and neglect.

FCNs as nonordained ministers do not have client-professional privileges and should follow appropriate standards in documenting provided services. Documentation should be thorough and consistent format and thoroughly. Look for universal formatting examples as a template. Follow guidelines for record keeping and storage. Many churches do not have file storage systems that lock and can keep information in a secure location. Keep simple records of individuals information gathered for blood pressure screenings or other health education programs. For example, the screening could include the number of attendees or blood pressure results categorized by the American Heart Association standards as hypertensive, borderline, or normal. Also in documentation, keep a record the number of individuals referred to services. The handbooks, brochures, or programs that church-related institutions offer are contracts. The FCN should ensure that health information is current and based on accepted practices and standards. Following the boundaries and guidelines set out for professional practice and administrative and nursing programs and planning ahead can decrease professional liability and ensure accountability in practice.

? ACTIVE LEARNING

1. Speak with a minister, priest, rabbi, or church leader in the community from a faith belief system different from your own. Explore the philosophical basis for the church's role in health and healing
2. Visit websites devoted to FCN and identify the models of FCN programs or read the descriptions of their practice. Share these with the clinical group.

CASE STUDY   Application of the Nursing Process

Needs Assessment of a Faith Community

Nancy Elliot, an FCN at Living Hope Baptist Church, just completed a needs assessment of her faith community of 200 families. Nancy is new to the FCN role, having recently been hired. Living Hope, considered a moderate-sized church, is located in a rural community of 40,000. Nancy decided to perform the needs assessment of the congregation and community before planning programs and services for the community.

Assessment

The community has one hospital and a variety of voluntary and official community agencies. Many private practitioners are available, either in the town or within a 1-h drive in a larger city. Recently the town was awarded a grant to develop community parks and recreational facilities. Nancy is surprised by the demographic picture she finds after completing an assessment. Young families with toddlers to young school-age children comprise more than 70% of the congregation. She notes that these families are in the childbearing developmental stage of family growth and development. The remaining 30% of the members reported having no health insurance.

A discussion with the minister provides additional information. Two new industries have recently located to the area. The parent home of both of those industries was formerly located in distant states. Many new members have relocated to the area. Nancy understands that these young families may have decreased family and social support and little knowledge of existing community resources. The minister also informs her that the current church ministry focus on the elderly members and that new services are needed. Nancy schedules a meeting with the young parents after a church social

CASE STUDY Application of the Nursing Process—cont'd

gathering. Fifty mothers and fathers attend the session to discuss the health-related needs of the families. They identify that a "mothers' day out" program is a priority and also request information on community resources, parenting classes, and health and wellness programs for the children and parents. On the basis of the needs assessment and sessions with the parents, the FCN determines the following goals, nursing diagnoses and population-focused interventions.

Diagnoses
Individual
- Readiness for health promotion, as evidenced by requests for health information related to parenting, health, and wellness.
- Potential for community building, as evidenced by individual concerns related to limited social support and lack of social networks

Family
- Potential needs for family support, related to recent relocation to new community and lack of social network

Community (Faith Community)
- At risk for community (congregation) disorganization, related to recent change in membership demographics, lack of developed resources, and new or developing FCN role

Planning
- A plan of care is developed to address the needs of the individuals, families and the Living Hope faith community. Goals suggested by the FCN are mutually agreed upon by the ministerial team and congregational members.

Individual
Long-Term Goals
- Monthly educational programs will be offered addressing current issues in parenting and health and wellness of young families
- Congregations will establish a social network for young parents
- Ministerial leaders will dedicate funds to increase resources for children and young adults.

Short-Term Goals
- Establish parent steering committee for educational program ideas, identification of parent talents, (assist with education programs)
- Explore development of mothers' day out program

Family
Long-Term Goals
- Parent members will report increased social networks
- Parent members will identify adequate resources to support growing family

Short-Term Goal
- Identify community and congregation support for new and growing families

Community (Faith Community)
Long-Term Goal
- Program will be established to support growing families

Short-Term Goal
- Implement one new program (educational, social) or resource for families each quarter of the church year

Interventions
Nancy utilized diverse interventions to meet the goals established for families of Living Hope

Individual
Nancy asked the parents to complete a talent survey to identify the resources available within the families of Living Hope. From this survey, Nancy identified two RNs willing to help provide educational programs and three previously certifies early childhood teachers. The teachers were willing to develop a committee to explore the development of a mothers' day out program, a play-group, and a new parent support group. Additional members were willing to begin a ministry to provide meals to new parents. Community resources were identified at the local health department to help teach parenting classes and provide immunizations. A plan was established to begin the mothers' day out program part-time within 2 months. The playgroup and educational programs were implemented immediately.

Family
The ministerial team and a parent advisory group were formed to identify family needs. Family social events were planned, including a church picnic. Planning was made for age-appropriate activities, such as the development of a soccer team for the youth, a soft ball team for the young adults, and a literary club for those interested. The advisory committee developed a budget to submit to the ministerial team, requesting financial support to develop a playground for the children attending the mothers' day out programs and the hiring of a part-time employee to supervise the related activities. The families reported greater feelings of support from the faith community, increased social support and networks, and a feeling of belonging to the greater community.

Community (Faith Community)
The faith community developed a budget to support individual and family requests. Monthly health education programs became the standard, with topics noted on the monthly calendar. Members reported increased feelings of "community" not only among the young families but also across generational lines, as new members increasingly participated in leadership roles within the congregation. The minister documented an increase in weekly attendance, which had a positive impact on the long-range goals identified by the congregational members.

Evaluation
Individual and the Family
Attendance at the health and wellness and parenting sessions increased with each educational session offered. Initial attendance was five—seven people for each session, and after 6 months attendance was 15—20 people for each session. The request from attendees changed from offering additional education sessions to planning intervention programs such as a yoga class and a weight reduction program. The playground was completed in less than the planned time because of the increased budget. The mothers' day out program, which began as a part-time, 3-day-per-week program, grew to a Monday-Friday program within 12 months. The program became self-sufficient by the end of the year because of established fees, parent volunteers, and donations. Men and women verbalized an increased satisfaction with their spiritual growth and support from the faith community. Nancy developed a health ministry committee of volunteers from within the church and was able to increase the number and variety of related FCN nurse activities.

Community (Faith Community)
The health and wellness activities attracted the attention of sister churches, and a grant was offered to increase the number of family support services and wellness programs offered within the church. Health and wellness programs were expanded to include additional methods for reaching congregational members such as through a website. The greater attendance and participation of congregational members positively affected all members, who benefited from the leadership and positive environment. The educational offerings and intervention programs were developed on the basis of *Healthy People 2020* goals, in particular, increasing activity and exercise, healthy eating, and obesity prevention (DHHS, 2022).

Continued

CASE STUDY   Application of the Nursing Process—cont'd

Levels of Prevention

The roles of the FCN direct the interventions and programs planned for faith communities. The following are examples of all three levels of prevention applied to this case study.

Primary

- Assessment and teaching about parenting, health, and wellness
- Development of programs and social support systems to prevent social isolation and increase resources for successful parenting and healthy behaviors

Secondary

- FCN assessment and screening to identify individuals and families at risk
- Congregational resources and educational programs developed to meet individual and family needs

Tertiary

- FCN either provides or refers to resources for rehabilitation for families coping with children with disabilities or chronic health problems (parents and children).

SUMMARY

This chapter provides an overview of the FCNs' role in providing nursing care for faith communities. FCN is now a growing specialty, differentiated from other community nursing by the philosophical underpinning that spirituality is integral to nursing and health. FCNs are licensed nurses trained in community health practices, with specialized knowledge of integrating spirituality into care. FCN is a "wholistic" approach that is practiced in FBOs such as churches, to help individuals and groups maintain or regain wholeness in mind, body, and spirit. Research supports the interrelationship between faith and health, to improve physical, psychological, spiritual and emotional health, coping, QoL, and health outcomes. The integration of intentional spirituality to nursing practice gives meaningful and person-centered care to faith community members in programs and practice.

FCNs are in a unique position as frontline community nurses to plan and implement nursing programs and groups that are tailored to the distinct needs of their faith community and suited to their age, developmental stage and preferences. FCNs are advisors, educators, advocates, referral agents, volunteer coordinators and much more, with multi-faceted interventions for diverse groups of people. Many nursing education programs, continuing education classes and training workshops are available for nurses to increase skills and knowledge in this specialty. FCN is relatively new to nursing specialties. Faith community nurses have the opportunity to minister and educate the mind, body, and spirit of faith community members, and build community connections among FBOs and clergy, public health agencies, healthcare providers, and other stakeholders, to promote health and healing.

BIBLIOGRAPHY

Alvarez JS, Goldraich LA, Nunes AH, et al.: Association between spirituality and adherence to management in outpatients with heart failure, *Arq Bras Cardiol*, 2016. https://doi.org/10.5935/abc.20160076.

American Nurses Association & Health Ministries Association: *Faith community nursing: scope and standards of practice*, ed 3, Silver Springs, MD, 2017, Nursebooks.org.

Church Health Organization, 2022. https://churchhealth.org/about/history/.

Counted V, Possamai A, Meade T: Relational spirituality and quality of life 2007 to 2017: an integrative research review, *Health Qual Life Outcome* 16(1):75, 2018. https://doi.org/10.1186/s12955-018-0895-x.

Thoresen CE: Spirituality and health: is there a relationship, *J Health Psychol* 4(3):291–300, 1999. https://doi.org/10.1177/135910539900400314.

de Vries K, Banister E, Dening KH, Ochieng B: Advance care planning for older people: the influence of ethnicity, religiosity, spirituality and health literacy, *Nurs Ethics* 26(7–8):1946–1954, 2019. https://doi.org/10.1177/0969733019833130.

De Marco M, Kearney W, Smith T, Jones C, Kearney-Powell A, Ammerman A: Growing partners: building a community-academic partnership to address health disparities in rural North Carolina, *Progress Community Health Partnerships: Res Education Action* 8(2):181–186, 2014. https://doi.org/10.1353/cpr.2014.0021.

Faith Community Nurses International (FCNI), (n.d.). Available from: https://www.fcninternational.org/.

Garssen B, Visser A, Pool G: Does spirituality or religion positively affect mental health? Meta-analysis of longitudinal studies, *Int J Psychol Relig* 31(1):4–20, 2021. https://doi.org/10.1080/10508619.2020.1729570.

Hackett C, Grim BJ: *The Global Religious Landscape. Pew Research Center's Religion & Public Life Project*, 2012, Pew Research Center. https://www.pewresearch.org/religion/2012/12/18/global-religious-landscape-exec/.

Holistic Health Centers: *Survey research report*, Hinsdale IL, 1976, Society for Holistic Medicine.

Jacob S, Solari-Twadell AP: Standardization of educational preparation of faith community nurses. In Solari-Twadell PA, Ziebarth DJ, editors: *Faith Community Nursing: an international specialty practice changing the understanding of health*, 2019, Springer International Publishing. https://doi.org/10.1007/978-3-030-16126-2.

Ketchell L, Canda E: *World religious views of health and healing*, n.d. Available from: https://spiritualdiversity.ku.edu/sites/spiritualitydiversity.drupal.ku.edu/files/docs/Health/World%20Religious%20Views%20of%20Health%20and%20Healing.pdf.

Koenig HG: Religion, spirituality, and health: the research and clinical implications, *ISRN Psychiatry* 2012:1–33, 2012. https://doi.org/10.5402/2012/278730.

Lalani N, Chen A: Spirituality in nursing and health: a historical context, challenges, and way forward, *Holist Nurs Pract* 35(4):206–210, 2021. https://doi.org/10.1097/HNP.0000000000000454.

Langdon AT, Hinton ST: Faith community nursing: as health ministry. In Solari-Twadell PA, Ziebarth DJ, editors: *Faith community nursing: an international specialty practice changing the understanding of health*, 2019, Springer International Publishing. https://doi.org/10.1007/978-3-030-16126-2.

Leadership Lessons from Nehemiah. (2019, April 17). Lewis Center for Church Leadership. https://www.churchleadership.com/leading-ideas/ten-leadership-lessons-from-nehemiah/.

Hackett C, Grim BJ: *The Global Religious Landscape. Pew Research Center's Religion & Public Life Project*, 2012, Pew Research Center. https://www.pewresearch.org/religion/2012/12/18/global-religious-landscape-exec/.

McEwen M. Spiritual nursing care: State of the art. *Holist Nurs Pract.* 19(4):161-168. https://doi.org/10.1097/00004650-200507000-00007. PMID: 16006830.

National Center on Elder Abuse, n.d. Available from: https://ncea.acl.gov/What-We-Do/Research/Statistics-and-Data.aspx.

Park CL, Aldwin CM, Choun S, George L, Suresh DP, Bliss D: Spiritual peace predicts 5-year mortality in congestive heart failure patients, *Health Psychol: Official J Division Health Psychol Am Psychol Assoc* 35(3):203—210, 2016. https://doi.org/10.1037/hea0000271.

Pew Research Center: *Religion in America: U.S. Religious Data, Demographics and Statistics, Pew Research Center's Religion & Public Life Project*, 2014. Available from: https://www.pewforum.org/religious-landscape-study/.

Puchalski C, Ferrell B, Virani R, et al.: Improving the quality of spiritual care as a dimension of palliative care: the report of the consensus conference, *J Palliat Med* 12(10):885—904, 2009. https://doi.org/10.1089/jpm.2009.0142.

Ransome Y: Religion, spirituality, and health: new considerations for epidemiology, *Am J Epidemiol* 189(8):755—758, 2020. https://doi.org/10.1093/aje/kwaa022.

Riza E, Kalkman S, Coritsidis A, et al.: Community-based healthcare for migrants and refugees: a scoping literature review of best practices, *Healthcare* 8(2):115, 2020.

Saletti-Cuesta L, Aizenberg L, Ricci-Cabello I: Opinions and experiences of primary healthcare providers regarding violence against women: a systematic review of qualitative studies, *J Fam Violence* 33(6):405—420, 2018. https://doi.org/10.1007/s10896-018-9971-6.

Solari-Twadell PA, McDermott A, Parish N: *Promoting whole person health within faith communities*, Thousand Oaks CA, 1999, Sage.

Solari-Twadell PA, Ziebarth DJ, editors: *Faith Community Nursing: an international specialty practice changing the understanding of health,* 2019, Springer International Publishing. https://doi.org/10.1007/978-3-030-16126-2.

Stroope S, Kent BV, Zhang Y, Kandula NR, Kanaya AM, Shields AE: Self-rated religiosity/spirituality and four health outcomes among US South Asians, *J Nerv Ment Dis* 208(2):165—168, 2020. https://doi.org/10.1097/NMD.0000000000001128.

Westberg Institute: *Position statement, faith community nursing compared to other nursing specialties*, 2019. Available from: https://www.fcninternational.org/resources/Documents/POSITION%20STATEMENT%20Comparing%20Other%20Nursing%20Specialties%20Dec2019.pdf.

Westberg Institute: *Faith community nursing*, 2022. Available from: https://westberginstitute.org/.

FURTHER READINGS

Church Health: Care for one another (2022) https://churchhealth.org/.

Healthy People 2030: *Intimate partner violence*, n.d. Accessed from: https://health.gov/healthypeople/tools-action/browse-evidence-based-resources/intimate-partner-violence-elder-abuse-and-abuse-vulnerable-adults-screening.

Hixson LB, Loeb SJ: Promoting successful aging through faith community nursing, *J Christ Nurs* 35(4):242—249, 2018. https://doi.org/10.1097/CNJ.0000000000000528.

Interfaith Health Program: *Strong partners interfaith health program*, Atlanta GA, 2005, Emory University.

Kruse-Diehr AJ, Lee MJ, Shackelford J, Saidou Hangadoumbo F: The state of research on faith community nursing in public health interventions: results from a systematic review, *J Relig Health* 60(2):1339—1374, 2021. https://doi.org/10.1007/s10943-020-01168-4.

National Consensus Conference for Palliative Care: *Clinical practice guidelines for quality palliative care*, ed 2, 2009.

Solari-Twadell PA, Hackbarth DP: Evidence for a new paradigm of the ministry of parish nursing practice using the nursing intervention classification system, *Nurs Outlook* 58(2):69—75, 2010.

U.S Department of Health and Human Services. Children's Bureau: *Child Abuse & Neglect*, 2022. https://www.acf.hhs.gov/cb/focus-areas/child-abuse-neglect.

34

Home Health and Hospice

Tanna Woods and Mary A. Nies

OBJECTIVES

Upon completion of this chapter, the reader will be able to do the following:

1. Define home health care.
2. Discuss the purpose of home health services.
3. Differentiate between the purpose of a public health nursing visit, a home health nursing visit, and a hospice nursing visit.
4. Use the nursing process in outlining the steps involved in conducting a home visit.
5. Identify the types of home health agencies.
6. Apply the nursing process to a home health client situation.

OUTLINE

KEY TERMS

advance directive
durable power of attorney

home health care
living will

Home visits have been an integral part of nursing for more than a century, originating with Florence Nightingale's "health nurses" in England. Following Nightingale's vision, Lillian Wald founded the Henry Street Settlement in 1893. In addition, Wald, the "mother of public health nursing," launched the Visiting Nurse Service of New York, which has become one of the nation's largest nonprofit home- and community-based healthcare organizations (Visiting Nurse Service of New York, 2021).

Home health care includes a wide range of healthcare services provided to people in their homes to help them through an illness or injury (Medicare.gov, 2021). Home health care is typically more affordable than and just as effective as care that people receive in a hospital or skilled nursing facility. In addition, home health care is more convenient for people and their families, as the care they need is brought to them. Examples of home healthcare services include wound care, education, IV therapy, nutrition therapy, follow-up with a patient after discharge from the hospital, and monitoring of an unstable or chronic illness. Home health care allows people to stay in their homes while receiving treatment for illnesses and injuries and regaining as much independence as possible (Medicare.gov, 2021).

Hospice care focuses on caring for people facing a terminal illness when the goal is no longer curing the disease (National Hospice and Palliative Care Organization [NHPCO], 2021). Most hospice care occurs in the home with support given to clients and their families. The goal of hospice care is that each person will die pain free and with dignity. Ongoing support is provided to the family after the patient dies (NHPCO, 2021).

PURPOSE OF HOME HEALTH SERVICES

The primary purpose of home health services is to provide nursing care to individuals and their families in their homes. The specific objectives and services nurses offer vary according to the type of agency providing services and the population served. Nurses who work for public health departments, visiting nurse associations, home health agencies, hospice agencies, or school districts usually provide home visits. Nurses who make home visits receive referrals from a variety of sources, including the patient's physician, nurse practitioner (NP) or nurse midwife, hospital discharge planner or case manager, schoolteacher, and clinic health care provider. The patient or the patient's family can also originate requests for nursing visits to assess and assist in the client's health care.

Nurses from clinics or health departments often conduct home visits as part of patient follow-up. These public health nurses (PHN) make visits to follow patients with communicable diseases and to provide health education and community referrals to patients with identified health problems. Home health nurses who work for home health agencies that are affiliated with hospitals or nursing registries often make home visits to assist patients in their transition from the hospital to home. In addition, health care providers in private practice may order these visits when patients experience exacerbation of chronic conditions.

The focus of all home visits is on the individual for whom the referral is received. In addition, the nurse assesses the individual–family interaction and provides education and interventions for the family and the client. The nurse evaluates how the individual and family interact as part of an aggregate group in the community. The nurse identifies the need for referrals to community services and performs the referrals as necessary.

 HEALTHY PEOPLE 2030

2030 Objectives for Home Health and Hospice Care

> *MICH-HP2030-20:* Increase the proportion of children and adolescents with special health care needs who have a system of care.
> *MICH HP2030-D01:* Increase the proportion of women who get screened for postpartum depression.

From HealthyPeople.gov: *Healthy People 2030: objectives and data*, 2021. Available from: https://health.gov/healthypeople/objectives-and-data.

Home health care has changed dramatically in the last 20 years in relation to changes in Medicare home health reimbursement. "The Balanced Budget Act of 1997 (BBA) (Public Law 105-33), which was enacted on August 5, 1997, significantly changed the way Medicare pays for home health services" (Department of Health and Human Services [DHHS], 2017, p. 3). Prior to the BBA, home healthcare agencies (HHAs) were reimbursed using a retrospective payment system for services rendered. HHAs are now reimbursed using the home health prospective payment system (PPS). Under the PPS, HHAs receive a fixed amount of money based on reasonable cost given the client's diagnosis and plan of care. Since the PPS

was implemented in 2000, the Centers for Medicare & Medicaid Services (CMS) made revisions in 2008, 2012, and 2018. The changes included providing coverage for more diagnosis groups and certain secondary diagnoses, different resource costs depending on the timing of the home health episodes as well as certain wound and skin conditions, and changes to the therapy schedule from a single 10-visit threshold to multiple thresholds to allow for more visits if needed (DHHS, 2017). The most recent changes in 2018 were part of the Bipartisan Budget Act of 2018, which was effective January 1, 2020 (CMS, 2021a). This act removed the payment incentive to overprovide therapy and refocused on clinical characteristics and patient information to align services with client needs and allow outlier provisions of payment for more complex patients (CMS, 2021a).

Home healthcare services have changed to address the needs of the population. Home health nurses visit clients of all ages and races. They visit clients who are acutely, chronically, or terminally ill; were recently discharged from the hospital or a rehabilitation facility; need wound care or intravenous therapy; have a feeding tube or tracheostomy; or high-risk pregnant women. Home health care continues to focus on the care of sick patients and is expanding to include health promotion and disease prevention interventions, including client and family education. Currently, most reimbursement for nursing services is based on the patient's need for skilled nursing. On each patient visit, the nurse must document that the care provided is of a skilled nature that requires the knowledge and assessment skills of a nurse and must verify that the patient or a family member could not provide the same level of care.

Services coordinated in the home include not only skilled nursing care provided by registered nurses (RNs), but also the services of physical, occupational, and speech therapists; social workers; and home health aides. The broader home care industry definition of *home health care* includes supportive social services, respite care, community nursing centers, group boarding homes, homeless shelters, adult day care, intermediate-skilled extended care facilities, and assisted living facilities (American Nurses Association [ANA], 2014).

In addition, telephone support services are becoming an increasingly important aspect of home health care (Dewsbury, 2019). Telephone triage is used to help improve outcomes by identifying signs of issues early and providing timely treatment. Telephone support programs allow nurses to contact clients through regularly scheduled telephone calls to assess how the client is doing, how well they are following the plan of care, and if they need additional support services or a home visit. Telephone support programs are beneficial in improving client outcomes and enabling better communication (Dewsbury, 2019).

TYPES OF HOME HEALTH AGENCIES

Home health agencies differ in financial structure, organizational structure, governing board, and population served. The most common types of home health agencies are official (i.e., public), nonprofit, proprietary, chains, and hospital-based agencies. The number of Medicare home health agencies in the United States has increased from 1890 in 1967 to 11,317 in 2018 (Elflein, 2018). The freestanding proprietary agencies have grown faster than that of any other type of Medicare-certified home health agency. Freestanding proprietary agencies now account for 85% of all home health agencies (Medicare Payment Advisory Commission [MEDPAC], 2018).

There continues to be an increase in the number of managed care agencies, which may have any type of financial structure. Managed care agencies contract with payers, such as insurance companies, to provide specified services to the enrolled clients at predetermined prices. Managed care agencies receive payment before offering services and are responsible for taking the financial risk of providing care to patients within the budgeted allotment. This arrangement works well with large numbers of enrolled clients, because the financial risk is spread across a larger number of people, many of whom are healthy and will not require skilled services.

Official Agencies

Local or state governments organize, operate, and fund official (i.e., public) home health agencies. These agencies may be part of a county public health nursing service or a home health agency that operates separately from the public health nursing service but is located within the county public health system. Taxpayers fund official home health agencies, but the agencies also receive reimbursement from third-party payers such as Medicare, Medicaid, and private insurance companies.

Nonprofit Agencies

Nonprofit home health agencies include all home health agencies that are not required to pay federal taxes because of their exempt tax status. Nonprofit groups reinvest any profits into the agencies. Nonprofit home health agencies include independent home health agencies and hospital-based home health agencies. Not all hospital-based home health agencies are nonprofit, even if the hospital is nonprofit. The home health agency can be established as a profit-generating service and serve as a source of revenue for the hospital or medical center. In this situation, the home health agency is categorized organizationally as for-profit and it pays federal taxes on the profits.

Proprietary Agencies

Proprietary home health agencies are classified as for-profit and pay federal taxes on the profits generated. Proprietary agencies can be individually owned agencies, profit partnerships, or profit corporations. Provided that the agencies make profits, investors in corporate proprietary partnerships receive financial returns on their investments in the agencies. A percentage of the profits generated are also reinvested into the agencies. Agencies within chains have a financial advantage over single agencies. The chains have lower administrative costs, because a larger single corporate structure provides many services. For example, a multiagency corporation has greater purchasing power for supplies and equipment because it purchases a larger volume. A single corporate office can provide administrative services such as payroll and employee benefits for all chain employees, thereby avoiding duplication of these services at each location. Criticism of proprietary and chain agencies includes concerns over the quality of services provided by agencies that are profit driven.

Hospital-Based Agencies

With the implementation of the home health PPS, the number of hospital-based home health agencies significantly increased (NAHC, 2010). This trend is not surprising in light of the fixed reimbursement under PPS and the hospitals' incentive to decrease patients' length of stay. By establishing home health agencies, hospitals are able to discharge patients who have skilled health care needs, provide the necessary services to the patients, and receive reimbursement through third-party payers such as Medicare, Medicaid, and private insurance companies. The rising number of home health agencies affiliated with hospitals indicates that these agencies are profitable endeavors that provide hospitals with an additional revenue source.

CERTIFIED AND NONCERTIFIED AGENCIES

Certified home health agencies meet federal standards; therefore, they are able to receive Medicare payments for services provided to eligible individuals. Not all home health agencies are certified. The noncertified home care agencies, home care aide organizations, and hospices remain outside the Medicare system. Some operate outside the system because they provide non—Medicare-covered services. For example, they do not provide skilled nursing care and are not eligible to receive Medicare reimbursement.

> **❓ ACTIVE LEARNING**
>
> Contact a local home health agency and interview the agency director. Ask what type of agency it is, the profit status, and whether it is Medicare certified. Report findings to classmates.

SPECIAL HOME HEALTH PROGRAMS

Many home health agencies offer special, high-technology home care services. Offering high-tech services at home is both beneficial to the patient's health and financially advantageous. Through the implementation of these special programs, patients who require continuous skilled care in an acute or skilled nursing institution are able to return to receive care in their homes. From the financial perspective, skilled services provided at home are less costly than hospitalization.

Examples of special services are home intravenous therapy programs for patients who require daily infusions of total parenteral nutrition or antibiotic therapy, pediatric services for children with chronic health problems, follow-up for premature infants who are at risk for complications, ventilator therapy, and home dialysis programs. The key to the success of all these programs is the patient's, family's, or caregiver's ability to learn the care necessary for a successful home program and the motivation of these individuals to provide the care. If family or caregiver support is not available in the home, the patient cannot be a candidate for any of these programs, and other arrangements for care must be found.

Home dialysis programs are a growing trend. Through such programs, patients learn how to do dialysis at home with a helper who is often a family member or friend. Patients and their helpers receive 3 to 8 weeks of training from the dialysis clinic to learn how to use the equipment, monitor their vital signs, and keep good records of their treatment. The clinic provides the machine and all of the supplies and furnishes 24-h telephone support. The patient follows up at the clinic monthly to ensure that treatments are working and to discuss any issues or concerns (National Institute of Diabetes and Digestive and Kidney Diseases, 2018).

REIMBURSEMENT FOR HOME CARE

Any individual older than 65 years who is homebound, under the care of a physician, and requires medically necessary skilled nursing care or therapy services may be eligible for home care through a Medicare-certified home health agency. These services must be intermittent or part-time and require physician authorization and periodic review of the plan of care. The only exception is hospice care. Any individual older than 65 years who is certified by a physician or an NP to be terminally ill with a life expectancy of 6 months or less is eligible to receive the Medicare Hospice Benefit (Medicare Learning Network [MLN], 2019). There is no requirement for the individual to be homebound or in need of skilled care or for the services to be intermittent or part-time. The hospice physician or hospice NP must recertify the patient after the first 90 days and then every 60 days to determine whether he or she is still eligible for hospice care (MLN, 2019).

The rapid growth of the home health market is reflective of the following:

- Increasing proportion of people aged 65 years and older
- Lower average cost of home health care compared with institutional costs
- Active insurer support for home care
- Medicare promotion of home health care as an alternative to institutionalization

Patient or family payments comprise 46% of the private financing (12% of total spending) for home health services. Private health insurance and nonpatient revenue pay the remaining private financing. Private health insurance includes managed care plans that often involve preapproval of services and referrals from primary care providers. Private insurance companies require precertification to verify patient eligibility for services. The home care RN speaks to the RN at the insurance company, who determines the number of visits that the insurance company covers. In contrast, for Medicare patients, the home care RN determines the schedule and number of visits without calling Medicare to get preapproval. Medicare pays the home care agency a predetermined amount based on the health

condition and needs of the patient; there is also a special outlier provision to provide appropriate payment amounts for beneficiaries with expensive care needs. Medicare pays for home care services based on 30-day episodes. If a patient is still eligible for home care services after the first episode, a second episode can begin. There are no limits to the number of episodes for each patient. However, if the patient receives four visits or fewer per episode, the HHA is paid a standardized per-visit amount instead of an episode payment. These payment adjustments are called *low utilization payment adjustments* (CMS, 2021a).

Between 1967 and 1985, the number of home health agencies certified to provide care to Medicare recipients tripled, from 1753 to 5983 (NAHC, 2010). In the mid-1980s, this number leveled off at 5900 as a result of an increase in the volume of paperwork required and unreliable payment policies. This led to a lawsuit against the Health Care Financing Administration (HCFA) charged by Representatives Harley Staggers and Claude Pepper and a coalition of members of the US Congress, consumer groups, and the NAHC. The successful conclusion of the lawsuit gave NAHC the opportunity to participate in rewriting the Medicare home care payment policies. New payment policies brought an increase in the home health benefit and increased the number of Medicare-certified home health agencies to more than 10,000. The number is now declining as a direct result of the changes in Medicare home health reimbursement enacted as part of the Balanced Budget Act of 1997. However, because of this decline, the CMS enacted a new payment system whereby home care agencies are reimbursed on a PPS based on the patient's diagnosis. The amount provided to home health agencies is determined on the basis of the average national cost of treating a home health client for 60 days. This was changed when the Bipartisan Budget Act of 2018 (BBA of 2018) became effective on January 1, 2020. Changes included removing therapy thresholds for case-mix adjustment and moving from a 60-day unit of payment to a 30-day period payment rate (CMS, 2021b).

The goal of the PPS is to encourage efficient use of home health services without sacrificing quality (MLN, 2019). Further improvements were made with the CARES Act that amended regulations and allowed for NPs, clinical nurse specialists, and physician assistants (PAs) to certify and order home health care (CMS, 2021b). Additionally, the CARES Act allowed for telecommunications technology to be used as part of home health care plans, so long as the technology does not replace ordered in-person visits in the plan of care (CMS, 2021b).

OASIS

The Outcome and Assessment Information Set (OASIS) is a data set that determines Medicare pay rate and measures outcomes for adult home care patients to monitor outcome-based quality improvement (CMS, 2021a,b). The data set includes sociodemographic, environmental, support system, health status, and functional status attributes of adult patients as well as information about service utilization. These items are used to monitor outcomes, plan patient care, provide reports on patient characteristics for each agency, and evaluate and improve clinical performance. Nurses must use OASIS for all patients receiving skilled care that is reimbursed by Medicare and Medicaid (CMS, 2021b).

NURSING STANDARDS AND EDUCATIONAL PREPARATION OF HOME HEALTH NURSES

According to the ANA (2014), the generalist home care nurse should be educated at the baccalaureate level because of the autonomy and critical thinking skills that are necessary in home care. The generalist home health nurse must have community health assessment skills to assess client and caregiver needs, provide client and caregiver education, perform nursing actions following the client's plan of care, manage resources to facilitate the best possible outcomes, provide and monitor care, collaborate with other disciplines and providers to coordinate client care, and supervise ancillary staff and caregivers. In home care, the nurse has a primary function of managing an interdisciplinary team that includes physical therapists, occupational therapists, social workers, nurse assistants, chaplains, and so on. In addition, the responsibilities of the generalist home health nurse include, but are not limited to, performing holistic, periodic assessments of client, and family/caregiver resources; participating in performance improvement activities; collecting and using research findings to evaluate the plan of care; educating clients and families on health promotion and self-care activities; being a client advocate; promoting continuity of care; using the *Scope and Standards of Home Health Nursing Practice* to guide clinical practice; and identifying ethical issues and exploring options with the necessary individuals and staff members to achieve resolution (ANA, 2014).

In addition to the ANA standards, home health nurses should use the competencies developed by the QSEN (Quality and Safety Education for Nurses) Institute as a guide for best practices in home care (QSEN Institute, 2020). The QSEN competencies were developed by a national advisory board that included distinguished faculty to establish effective teaching approaches to ensure that nurses graduate with essential competencies in (1) patient-centered care, (2) teamwork and collaboration, (3) evidence-based practice, (4) quality improvement, (5) safety, and (6) informatics. These six competencies in QSEN are being used by several health care institutions to monitor and ensure that their nurses are providing safe, high-quality patient care (QSEN Institute, 2020).

The advanced practice home health nurse has a master's or doctoral degree in nursing and can perform all of the duties of the generalist home health nurse (ANA, 2014). In addition, the advanced practice nurse contributes significant clinical expertise to home health patients and their families; demonstrates proficiency in care management and consultation; and is an expert in implementing and evaluating health programs, resources, services, and research for clients with complex conditions. The duties of the advanced practice home health nurse

include, but are not limited to, prescribing pharmacological and nonpharmacological treatment to manage chronic illnesses, providing consultation and serving as a resource to the generalist home health nurse, participating at all levels of quality improvement and research, educating all members of the health care team about emerging trends in home health care, performing direct care of the client and family, managing and evaluating the care the client is receiving from caregivers, monitoring trends in reimbursement for home health services, consulting with staff about any ethical issues that may arise, managing an interdisciplinary team, and disseminating practice and research findings to colleagues (ANA, 2014).

Albrecht's conceptual model (1990) for home care clearly identifies educational content areas for students in undergraduate and graduate nursing programs that have specialties in home health care. An underlying premise of the model is that professional satisfaction and effective patient outcomes depend on the education and experience of the home health nurse. Implications that are apparent in the model include the following (Albrecht, 1990, p. 125):

- Nursing programs at the undergraduate and graduate levels must prepare competent providers of home health care.
- Curricula must include concepts related to the suprasystem, health service delivery system, and home subsystem, which includes structural, process, and outcome elements.
- Students at the undergraduate level need at least one clinical observation or experience in a home care agency.
- Graduate-level students need specific courses that cover concepts present in the model, including knowledge of education; preventive, supportive, therapeutic, and high-tech nursing interventions for home health care; a multidisciplinary approach to home health care; health law and ethics; systems theory; economics covering supply, demand, and productivity; and case management and coordination.

The home health nurse serves as a case manager for patients who receive care either from the staff of the home health agency or through contract services. The success of the case management plan is contingent upon the nurse's ability to use the nursing process to develop a plan of treatment that best fits the individual needs of the patient and the patient's family or caregiver. Patient and family assessment is the first step in developing the treatment plan and nursing care plan.

The Albrecht nursing model for home health care provides a framework for nurses, patients, and their families to interact and identify mutual goals of interventions and promote the patient's self-care capability at home (Fig. 34.1) (Albrecht, 1990). Three major elements for measuring the quality of home health care patient outcomes are structural, process, and outcome elements.

Structural elements include the client, family, provider agency, health team, and professional nurse. The process elements include the type of care, coordination of care, and intervention. Outcome elements consist of patient and family satisfaction with care, quality of care, cost-effectiveness of care, health status, and self-care capability.

In the Albrecht model for home care, the relationship between the structural elements and the process elements directs

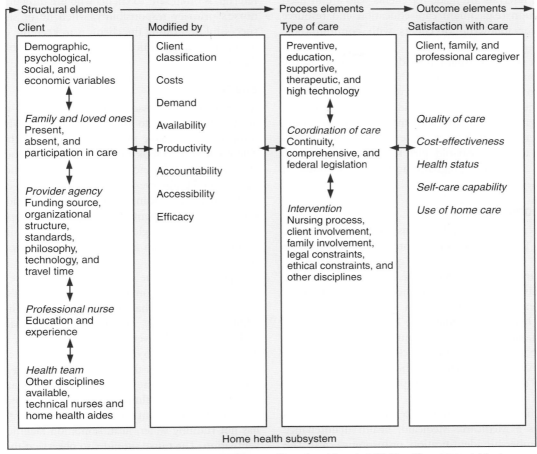

Fig. 34.1 Albrecht nursing model for home health care. (Based on Albrecht MN: The Albrecht model for home health care: implications for research, practice, and education. *Public Health Nurs* 7:118–126, 1990. Reprinted by permission of Blackwell Scientific Publications, Inc.)

the interventions. The nurse executes the nursing process, including assessment, nursing diagnosis, planning, intervention, and evaluation, and then the nurse coordinates patient care (Albrecht, 1990).

CONDUCTING A HOME VISIT

Visit Preparation

It is important that the nurse prepare for the home visit by reviewing the referral form, which should furnish the purpose of the visit, the geographic residence of the family, and any other pertinent information. The first home visit gives the nurse the opportunity to establish a trust relationship with the client and family to establish credibility as a resource for health information and community referrals in a nonthreatening environment.

The Referral

The referral is a formal request for a home visit. Referrals come from a variety of sources, including hospitals, clinics, health care providers, individuals, and families. The type of agency

that receives the referral varies, depending on the necessary client services. Home health referrals are requested to provide clients with short-term, intermittent, skilled services and rehabilitation. Visits can last from 30 to 90 minutes and are scheduled on an intermittent basis according to the specific needs of the client. For example, a client who had a stroke requires skilled nursing assessments, physical therapy visits for gait training, speech therapy for speech deficit improvement, and occupational therapy for retraining in activities of daily living (ADLs) such as bathing and cooking.

By reviewing the referral form before the first visit, the community health nurse (CHN) obtains basic information about the client, such as name, age, diagnosis or health status, address, telephone number, insurance coverage, and reason for the referral. The form also specifies the source of the referral—clinician, health care provider, communicable disease service, hospital, client, or client's family. Additional information provided in the home health referral includes current client medications, prescribed diet, physician's orders, care plan goals, and other disciplines involved in the client's care. This information is important because it helps the nurse become familiar with the client's condition.

Public health referrals are made for clients who are in need of health education (e.g., infant care education and resource allocation) or for follow-up of clients with communicable diseases.

Public health referrals usually provide information on the client's condition that necessitates PHN visits. For example, for a client who is positive for tuberculosis (TB), the PHN is notified of the client's place of residence, type and location of employment, and any known contacts, including family and friends. Another example of a public health referral is one to a 16-year-old girl for antepartum visits because she is 7 months' pregnant and has just initiated prenatal care.

Initial Telephone Contact

The nurse contacts the client and informs him or her about the service referral. The first telephone contact with the client or family consists of an exchange of essential information, including an introduction by the nurse, identification of the agency that received the referral, and the purpose of the visit. After the initial exchange of information, the nurse informs the client of his or her desire to make the home visit, the client gives permission, and the group sets a mutually acceptable time for the visit. The nurse is a guest in the client's home; therefore it is important that the client agrees to the visit. The nurse then verifies the client's address and asks for specific directions to the client's home.

During a home health visit, the nurse requests proof of insurance, such as a Medicare, Medicaid, health maintenance organization membership identification, or insurance card. The nurse should forewarn the client so the client or family can locate the information before the visit. If the client is unable to provide this verification, the nurse assists with locating the information during the visit. Clients who receive a public health home visit do not require evidence of insurance coverage because these services are not billed directly. County public health budgets or state or federally funded programs generally cover these visits.

Not all clients have telephones. For a client without one, the nurse should check the referral for a telephone number where messages can be left. It is also worthwhile to contact the health care provider who made the referral to see whether the telephone number was omitted unintentionally. If the client does not have a telephone, the nurse may choose to make a drop-in visit. This type of visit consists of an unannounced visit to the client's home, during which the nurse explains the purpose of the referral, receives the client's permission for the visit, and appoints a time for a future visit with the client. The client may agree to have the first visit while the nurse is there.

If the client is not at home for the drop-in visit, the nurse should leave an official agency card and a brief message asking the client to contact the agency to schedule a nursing visit. The nurse informs the referring agency that the visit was attempted but that the client was not available for contact. A formal agency letter, identifying the agency and the reason for the referral, is often sent to clients who are difficult to contact. The nurse's primary responsibility, when he or she has been unsuccessful in locating the client, is to keep the clinic, physician, or referring agency informed of efforts to establish contact with the client.

Environment

An environmental assessment begins as the nurse leaves the agency and travels to the client's home. While driving, the nurse should observe the area surrounding the client's home. The nurse should look for the location of grocery stores, drug stores, gas stations, etc., in relation to the client's home. The nurse should observe the condition of the client's home as well as the surrounding neighborhood. In addition, the nurse should note the client's dwelling; for example, whether the client lives in a single-family home, in a single room in a home or hotel, in an apartment, or in a shared apartment or house.

Upon arrival to the client's home, the nurse should note the accessibility of the home relative to the client's condition such as stairs, railings, handicapped facilities, lighting, etc. In addition, the nurse should note potential trip hazards, including uneven pavement, cracked cement, small rocks, etc. The nurse should also observe potential safety concerns, such as the client lives alone, the neighborhood has a high crime rate, the building or home is not secure, trip hazards inside the home (such as rugs, clutter on the floor), unclean environment, etc. It is also important for the nurse to note if the client's home has hot running water, heat, sanitation facilities, and adequate ventilation. The nurse should also observe if the client has food in the home and should make note of the client's primary caregiver and support system.

Improving Communication

When the nurse meets with the client, whether in the home or at another mutually agreeable location, the initial conversation revolves around social topics. The nurse assumes a friendly manner and asks general questions about the client, the client's family, and health care services that will benefit the client. These questions help the nurse assess the client's needs and create a comfortable atmosphere for communication.

Building Trust

Many clients in need of nursing visits do not trust the health care system and are uncomfortable with the representative from an agency visiting their home. For example, a client who is pregnant and does not have legal status in the United States will be hesitant to allow a nurse to visit; the client will be afraid of being reported to immigration authorities. The nurse's role in visiting this client is to focus on the health and safety of the client and her fetus. The nurse must build a trust relationship early in the visit or the client will not allow additional visits. If a trust relationship is not established and the client believes that the nurse will report her to immigration authorities, it is highly probable that the client will move to another location to avoid future contact.

DOCUMENTATION OF HOME CARE

Many home health nurses would probably identify documentation issues as the most frustrating part of providing home health care. The nurse documents assessment data and interventions for all home visits. The patient record also contains a copy of the nursing care plan. "A patient MUST meet these Conditions of Participation to qualify for home health care: (1) confined to home, (2) under the care of a physician, (3) receiving services under a plan of care established and reviewed by a physician, and (4) need of skilled nursing care on an intermittent basis" (MLN, 2019). It is critical that the nurse document that the patient meets all of these criteria at each visit.

Medicare holds a prominent position as a home health care payer; therefore the HCFA's regulations determine the home health industry's documentation. Correct and accurate completion of required Medicare forms is the key to reimbursement. For more information, the reader should visit http://www.cms.gov/Medicare/CMS-Forms/CMS-Forms/CMS-Forms-List.html. Payment or denial of payment for visits is based on the information presented on the forms. If the nurse does not clearly document the provided skilled care in the electronic nursing notes, the fiscal intermediaries will argue that the care was either unnecessary or not performed and will deny reimbursement. The home health nurse must have an excellent clinical foundation and the ability to identify and document actual and potential patient problems that require skilled nursing interventions (Acello and Brown, 2015).

Documenting the care provided to record the patient's quality of care is just as important as documenting for reimbursement purposes. The documentation of home visits records the nurse's observations, assessments of the patient's condition, provided interventions, and the patient's and family's ability to manage the care at home. In addition, documentation of patient visits serves as a formal communication system among other home health professionals who also interact with the patient and family.

APPLICATION OF THE NURSING PROCESS

Assessment

During the first home visit, the type of client assessment will vary depending on the purpose of the home visit. The home health nurse assesses the client's knowledge of his or her health status. The nurse identifies knowledge deficits and uses this information to develop a care plan.

Subjective information is obtained from the client and the client's family and includes the client's perception of the situation and what the client identifies as problems. The nurse assesses whether the client is isolated from others physically or socially and whether the client is a member of a close-knit, nurturing, supportive family or kinship network. The amount of support the client perceives as available may or may not be accurate; therefore the nurse asks several questions about the client's family, friends, and daily routine to assess the client's level of social support.

During the first home visit, the home health nurse assesses the client's health knowledge; his or her physical, functional, and psychosocial status; physical environment; and social support. The nurse collects information through observations and questions the patient and family or caregivers in the home environment. It is not unusual to find inconsistencies between information the patient provides during hospitalization about the amount of physical and emotional support available to the patient in the home and the amount of help actually available to the patient in the home. The nurse validates or modifies the referral information to reflect the actual home situation. Home health nurses often use contracts that the nurse, patient, and family jointly develop to delineate the responsibilities of the patient in the home.

The client's physical assessment is generally performed in the home health visit and includes a review of all systems, with an emphasis on the systems affected by the client's present condition. The nurse obtains objective data through the use of essential physical assessment skills such as observation, palpation, auscultation, and percussion. The physical assessment also includes information regarding the client's functional status. Assessment of the functional status is important for Medicare reimbursement and for the development of an individualized plan of care. This assessment includes information regarding the client's ability to ambulate, to perform ADLs independently, and to use an assistive device such as a cane or wheelchair. Specific functional limitations, such as shortness of breath and muscle weakness, are assessed at this time.

Information obtained during the assessment phase is used to identify nursing diagnoses and develop a plan of care. Data collection continues while the patient receives home health services. Changes in the patient's condition, environment, or social structure necessitate modifications in the treatment plan and the nursing care plan.

There are differences between the treatment plan and the nursing care plan. The plan of treatment includes the type of home health services received, the projected frequency of visits by each discipline, and the necessary interventions (Medicare.gov, 2021). The nursing care plan addresses specific nursing interventions designed to treat the patient's actual or potential problems and includes identified goals with measurable outcomes.

Diagnosis and Planning
Develop a Plan for the Client and Family

After the assessment phase of the home visit, the nurse identifies the nursing diagnoses that address the patient's problems and identifies actual or potential problems. The identification of nursing diagnoses serves as the basis for the nursing care plan. This plan is developed in consultation with the client and the family. The plan identifies short-term and long-term goals and measurable outcomes for the patient. Goals are identified that the client is willing to work toward with the nurse's assistance. The plan identifies nursing interventions that are necessary and additional home health services that are appropriate to help the patient achieve the identified goals. To maximize the plan's success, it is important that the patient and family are involved in the planning process and that they access community resources. Planning is a dynamic process that continues while the patient receives nursing services. The plan is modified as needed, depending on the patient's condition, until the identified goals are met.

Outline the Client and Family Roles

The goal of home visits for both public health and home health nursing is to involve the client and family in taking an active role in health promotion. The nurse is careful not to allow the client to become dependent on the nurse's interventions, because the nurse's involvement is short term. The nurse leaves a written copy of the plan of care with the client as a reminder for the client and family of their role as well as the nurse's role in the plan of care.

Intervention

Implementation of the plan of care begins during the first home visit. The nurse begins to provide the client and family with health information concerning the client's health status and informs them about the availability of and access to community resources. In the case of the home health visit, the nurse provides skilled nursing care. At the end of the initial home visit, the nurse discusses the need for another home visit. The nurse and client discuss the goal of the next visit; specifically, they discuss what the client should do before the visit. The nurse informs the client and family about any information or skills he or she will provide during the next visit, and the nurse and client agree on a day for the next visit.

Referral for Community Services

During the first visit, the nurse provides the client and family with information regarding community resources, including the purpose of the resources, their eligibility for the services provided, any involved expense, and agency telephone numbers. Referrals depend on the availability of community resources, the client's eligibility for the services, the client's and the family's willingness to use the services, and the resources' suitability for the client and family. Examples of such services are immunization clinics for children in the family; adult day care or senior centers for elderly clients who could benefit from socialization; adult education classes or continuation of high school for pregnant teen clients who have dropped out of high school; meals on wheels (MOW) services for clients who are not able to prepare meals; homeless shelters for men, women, and families; soup kitchens; resources for clothing and housing; mental health clinics; resources for battered spouses; and primary care clinics for low-income clients with and without insurance.

If necessary, the client or client's family may request the nurse's assistance in contacting the community resources. The client and family are encouraged to make the contacts, but if the client and family are unable to make the calls or do not speak English, the nurse needs to intervene on behalf of the

client. By providing referral information during the first home visit, the nurse can follow up on the client's or the family's success in contacting and using community services.

Terminating the Visit

The nurse terminates the first visit when the assessment is completed and a care plan has been established with the client. The average visit should not exceed 1 h. The client receives a great deal of information during that hour, and the nurse collects a great deal of information. Most clients are tired at the end of a 1-h visit and often cannot retain additional information. It is preferable to set a date for another home visit to reinforce the information provided and to work progressively toward achieving goals.

Evaluation
Evaluation of Progress Toward Goals

The evaluation phase occurs when the nurse can determine whether the mutually established goals are realistic and achievable for the patient and the patient's family. The evaluation process is continuous and allows the nurse to determine the success or progress toward the patient's identified goals. The nurse can identify the need for revisions in the nursing care plan and treatment plan through the collection of additional data during the evaluation phase. The nurse can intervene to make necessary changes. An example is an elderly wife who, during the initial home visit, stated that she preferred to provide the physical care for her frail, nonambulatory husband. On a subsequent visit, the nurse assessed that the patient was not receiving the care required for the patient's personal care, specifically bathing. The nurse discussed the problem with the wife and presented her with available options. These included the services of a home health aide to provide personal care and bathing three times a week. A new plan was developed, and it included the home health aide. The plan was implemented and evaluated during future visits. Input from the client is critical to determine whether the goals established are realistic and achievable for the client.

Modification of the Plan as Needed

The evaluation process also allows the nurse and client or family to discuss what is working well and where modifications are necessary in the plan. Evaluation occurs through open communication between the nurse and client, and the nurse asks questions about specific parts of the care plan. If a trust relationship exists, the client feels comfortable telling the nurse about problems in the care plan.

When Goals Are Achieved

The overall purpose of home visits is to assist the client with necessary information and nursing care to enable the client to function successfully without nursing interventions. When the plan-of-care goals are achieved, the client does not need the nurse any longer. The client knows what community resources are available and how to access health care services for primary, secondary, and tertiary interventions.

Formal and Informal Caregivers

Formal caregivers include professionals and paraprofessionals who provide in–home health care and personal services. They are compensated for the services they provide. The largest number of employees consists of home care aides and RNs. Informal caregivers are family members who are caring for the client. The presence or absence of an involved family member can make the difference between the successful completion of the plan of treatment, with the patient remaining in the home, and the need to transfer the patient to an extended-care facility or board-and-care facility. When a capable family member or caregiver is available to assist the patient, the home health nurse spends much of the visit assessing the skills of the caregiver. The home health nurse instructs the caregiver in the correct procedures for providing care and in recognizing the signs and symptoms of problems that must be reported to the health care provider. The goal of the home health nurse's instruction is to provide the caregiver with the skills necessary to care for the patient successfully in the home without intervention of the nurse or other members of the home health team.

The home health nurse faces a special challenge with patients who lack a family member or caregiver capable of learning and providing necessary care. When the patient lives alone and does not have caregivers, the nurse explores other resources available to supplement the patient's self-care activities in the home. For example, if the patient has extensive physical care needs and sufficient financial resources, the nurse may suggest hiring an attendant. Medicare and private insurance companies do not pay for attendant care. If the patient's income is low enough, in–home county support services may be an option. The nurse may consider other services for the patient, such as MOW for nutritious meals delivered to the patient's home. Friendly Visitors, a volunteer service, sends a volunteer to the patient's home once a week or more to provide socialization for the patient. Other options that are available in some communities are adult day health centers and senior service centers. Both of these options require arranged patient transportation to and from the centers. A variety of transportation methods are available in different communities; volunteers may transport patients to the centers, or public transportation systems may be available, such as minivans, that provide door-to-door service. Selected services and referrals are based on the patient's individual needs and on the patient's level of functional ability.

ETHICAL INSIGHTS

Home Health and Hospice Care
- Most legal and ethical issues in home health care involve the care of terminally ill patients.
- Early education about these issues is essential to the prevention of problems.

- Early education also gives patients the opportunity to make decisions for themselves and to communicate those decisions to family members and health care providers.
- All competent adults have the right to make decisions that will direct health care providers in the type of care they administer.
- This communication can occur through the completion of advance directives, durable power of attorney for health care, and living wills.

Advance Directive
An **advance directive** is a written document in which a competent person gives instructions about future health care in the event that the individual is unable to make decisions. These directives are completed on a voluntary basis. Medicare-certified health care agencies must ask patients about advance directives and must provide the patient with the advance directive form if the patient is interested in completing it.

Durable Power of Attorney for Health Care
A **durable power of attorney** for health care is one type of advance directive. Also called a *health care proxy*, the durable power of attorney for health care gives another person the power to make medical decisions related to care of the patient. This person, as identified by the patient, acts as the patient's agent in all decisions regarding health care, personal care, and custody in the event that the patient becomes incompetent or disabled and is unable to make decisions.

Living Will
A **living will** is a written document in which a patient voluntarily informs doctors and family members about the type of medical care desired should the patient become terminally ill or permanently unconscious and unable to communicate. In the living will, the patient can describe the type of care desired, depending on the clinical situation. For example, if the patient is terminally ill and unconscious, the patient can direct the health care team to perform only those measures that will provide comfort and nothing further. The patient can specifically indicate his or her opposition to lifesaving measures; for example, the patient may request the denial of cardiopulmonary life support in the event of a cardiac arrest. Other examples are indicating the exclusion of chemotherapy, blood transfusions, and respirator use in an attempt to prolong life.

HOSPICE HOME CARE

Hospice and palliative nursing care is becoming increasingly important, as there is a tremendous need to improve end-of-life care for the terminally ill. Nurses who work with the terminally ill seek to enhance the patient's quality of life by focusing on relieving suffering throughout the illness, supporting the patient and family through the dying process, and providing grief support to the family after the patient has died (ANA, 2007). Hospice and palliative care nurses have a holistic approach to their patients and are responsible for taking a comprehensive health history and physical examination, including an evaluation of mental status; evaluating functional abilities; performing appropriate laboratory and diagnostic studies; determining effective pharmacological and nonpharmacological therapies to manage symptoms; identifying patient and/or family/caregiver goals; providing culturally competent care that is consistent with the patient's health beliefs, values, and practices;

evaluating the patient's emotional state and the response to his or her illness and impending death; identifying coping strategies and support systems; evaluating financial resources; and conducting a spiritual assessment (ANA, 2007).

The advanced practice hospice and palliative nurse is an important role for nurses with a master's degree or higher in nursing (ANA, 2007). The advanced practice hospice and palliative nurse functions as an expert clinician who performs the duties of the generalist hospice nurse in addition to assuming the responsibilities of advanced-level care, which may include prescribing pharmacological treatment to manage symptoms. It is recommended that all advanced practice hospice and palliative nurses obtain certification in advanced practice hospice and palliative nursing (ANA, 2007).

Patients are admitted into hospice care when they have a life expectancy of 6 months or less, and the focus of care shifts from curative to comfort care. However, many patients with terminal illnesses want to continue curative treatments and are not ready to be admitted into a hospice program. Those patients who do not have a life expectancy of 6 months or less and/or want to continue curative treatment can receive the benefits of palliative care. Palliative care focuses on symptom management while the patient is still receiving other treatments, such as chemotherapy. It is important to note that Medicare fully covers all hospice-related expenses, including medications, related to the terminal diagnosis. However, Medicare does not cover any expenses, including medications, related to other diagnoses.

Hospice and palliative nursing care is provided in a variety of settings, including hospitals, nursing homes, residential homes, and palliative care clinics. For the patient receiving hospice services in the home, the goal is to keep the client as comfortable at home as long as possible and to provide support and instruction to caregivers. Some patients stay home until they die, and for others their caregivers decide whether they should remain at home or be admitted to an extended-care facility or a hospital. Each family unit has different needs, and each must be supported in its decisions. Home death should not be the standard that determines excellence in any case, nor should home death be the ultimate measure of "successful" home care. It is vital to realize that caring for a terminally ill person also includes caring for the family or caregivers. Not all caregivers want their loved one to die at home, and not all caregivers are capable of allowing that to happen. The goal of having a home death must be the goal of the patient and family, regardless of the nurse's personal preference.

When caring for a terminally ill person at home, the hospice nurse must be skilled in physical and psychosocial care for both the patient and the caregiver. The patient is viewed as a whole person, not as an isolated disease. Caring for a terminally ill person at home demands that the nurse view the family system as a unit. In addition, it is important to note that hospice care is a team approach. Each patient has a physician, a nurse, a social worker, a nurse assistant, and a spiritual counselor to provide a multidisciplinary, holistic approach to caring for that patient and his or her family. The team coordinates care with each other and additional resources, such as pain management, as necessary. Furthermore, many hospice agencies have weekly interdisciplinary meetings in which the various members of the hospice team meet to discuss the patients and work together to resolve issues and make sure the patients are receiving the best possible care.

Caring for the Caregiver

Although the dying patient is the focus of all skilled nursing care, the experienced home care nurse knows that a careful assessment of the caregiver's mental and physical health is important. The spouse, lover, children, friends, and neighbors who have made the commitment to stay until the end need the nurse's time and attention as much as, if not more than, the patient. Although the patient's wishes are important, all decisions regarding care are made considering the health of the caregivers. Unsar et al. (2021) found that caregivers are at increased risk for developing mental health problems, including anxiety and depression. Caregiver burden is a significant concern; therefore nursing interventions must be directed toward preventing a decline in the caregiver's health.

Caregivers need reassurance that their judgment is sound, and they need reminders that they cannot do anything "wrong" if it is done for the patient's comfort. The caregivers must understand that they will not mistakenly overdose the patient, and they must be reminded repeatedly that the patient will not die from something they did or did not do. Caring for the terminally ill requires that the home care nurse is willing to nurse the entire family. In addition, the nurse must involve all members of the hospice team to ensure that the caregivers receive the care they need.

Pain Control and Symptom Management

Pain control is an important goal for home health/hospice nurses and their patients. Hospice nurses perform regular pain assessments that involve asking patients the following questions about their pain: (1) history; (2) character (such as sharp, dull, aching); (3) severity or intensity, which is most commonly rated on a pain intensity scale from 0 to 10, with 0 being no pain and 10 being the worst pain imaginable; (4) location; (5) effects on quality of life; (6) precipitating factors; and (7) relieving factors (The Joint Commission, 2018). It is vital that the nurses not only performs regular pain assessments but also remembers that pain is highly subjective and every person experiences pain differently and uniquely; therefore the patient's pain is whatever he or she says it is, regardless of the nurse's objective evaluation of the situation.

Pain medication is administered in doses sufficient to keep the patient free of pain and is administered on a regular schedule to prevent pain from recurring before the next dose Norlander (2008). Hospice methods of pain control are particularly well suited to home care. The vast majority of patients can be pain free until their deaths. The key to successful pain control for the terminally ill is to persuade patients to take their medications on a regular basis, not just when they "can't stand it any longer." Generally, these medications are long acting and are administered every 8 to 12 h. In addition, patients have fast-acting pain medications to take for "breakthrough pain," which happens when the patient experiences an increase in pain before it is time for the next dose of scheduled pain medication. The fast-acting medications are generally administered every 1 to 2 h as needed.

Many patients, especially the elderly, are afraid of becoming addicted and want to delay using pain medication until they "get really bad." Many people believe that using these medications signals "the end of the line," and they are amazed to learn that patients do well while receiving such agents for months, even years, before death occurs. Almost every family must learn that addiction is not the same as tolerance and that their physicians will not "cut off the supply" if they "take too much."

In addition to pain control, hospice nurses help in managing other symptoms such as nausea and vomiting, constipation, diarrhea, fatigue, and decreased appetite. Nurses assist patients in management of these symptoms through medications and/or strategies to help cope with the symptoms. Strategies include such things as increasing fluids to prevent constipation, frequent rest periods to minimize fatigue, and eating small amounts as desired to cope with the decrease in appetite. In addition, the nurse educates the patient and family that some of these symptoms, such as fatigue and decreased appetite, are related to the dying process and are signs that the patient is declining.

Furthermore, the nurse, along with other members of the hospice team, provides emotional support to patients and families as they adjust to the patient's impending death. The nurse educates the patient and family about what physical symptoms the patient will most likely experience as he or she approaches death. In addition, the nurse, along with the social worker and spiritual counselor, provides emotional support and helps the patient and family work through any anxiety or fears they have about dying. Finally, the nurse is there to support the family immediately after the patient dies, and hospice provides bereavement support to families up to a year after the patient's death.

Cultural Differences Related to Death and Dying

When caring for patients and their families in hospice, the nurse must remember that beliefs, attitudes, and values about death, dying, grief, and loss are influenced by society and culture (Cancer.net, 2018). However, these societal and cultural influences are often difficult to recognize. Furthermore, many individual differences within a cultural group, such as spirituality, age, and gender, affect a person's interpretation about the meaning of death. Although there are these individual differences, some general characteristics regarding death and dying are common to people of a certain cultural group. It is important to understand some of these differences to provide culturally sensitive care and ensure a peaceful and dignified death.

African Americans generally care for dying elders at home until death is imminent and then they bring their loved one to the hospital, because some believe that death in the house brings bad luck. Among Mexican Americans, the extended family takes care of the sick and dying person, and there are often several family members present at the same time. In general, Mexican Americans prefer to die at home because the hospital environment may be too restrictive in meeting the needs of the extended family and because some believe that their spirit may get "lost" if they die at the hospital. In comparison, among American Indians, some tribes prefer to remain close to the dying person, but other tribes avoid contact with the dying. Similarly, those tribes that prefer to avoid contact may prefer that their loved one dies in the hospital, whereas those tribes that prefer to remain close may prefer to have the person die at home.

These are just some examples of cultural characteristics that influence death and dying beliefs and practices. It is important to understand and respect the differing values and beliefs of patients and their families. Furthermore, it is essential to ask patients and/or families about their beliefs and practices to avoid overgeneralizations and to ensure that nursing care is patient centered and culturally sensitive.

? ACTIVE LEARNING

1. Make arrangements to accompany a PHN, a home health nurse, and/or a hospice nurse on home visits.
2. Interview a PHN about the types of client referrals received, and ask what interventions are usually performed. Repeat this activity with a home health nurse and a hospice nurse. Ask the nurses what they like best about their jobs.
3. Attend a team meeting in a home health agency or a hospice program to see how the roles of the various team members blend together to provide family-centered care.
4. Interview a PHN and a home health nurse, and ask how the community affects the care they provide.

CASE STUDY Public Health Visit

Communicable Disease Follow-Up

The PHN received a referral from the county hospital to see Ray, a 57-year-old white man with newly diagnosed TB. The first purpose of the referral was for the PHN to meet with the client to ensure that he received the appropriate information about TB and received follow-up medical care on a regular basis. The second purpose of the referral was for the PHN to meet with Ray and identify the people with whom he had been in close contact. The nurse then established contact with these people, notified them that they had been exposed to TB, and encouraged them to have follow-up tests for TB.

The nurse contacted Ray and established a time for the home visit. The nurse noted that he resided in a residential hotel in a lower-middle-class neighborhood of a large urban area. During the initial visit, the nurse discovered that the client was an unemployed construction worker. He did not know where he might have contracted TB. Ray assured the nurse that he was taking his medication as directed. He gave the nurse the names of the friends he played poker with every week at a hotel and told the nurse that he advised his friends to be tested for TB. The nurse made a note of the names and later talked with them individually by telephone. During these subsequent conversations, the nurse was very

Continued

CASE STUDY Public Health Visit—cont'd

careful to maintain the client's confidentiality. The nurse informed these individuals that they could have been exposed to TB and that they should seek testing through their health care providers or through their local health department.

Ray indicated that he did not have family and he had minimal contact with other people besides his friends at the hotel. The nurse recorded this information on the communicable disease form and returned the information to the public health department's communicable disease division.

Assessment

The PHN's assessment of the client with a communicable disease involved the individual, family, and community. The PHN assessed whether the client received appropriate information and regular medical care for TB and whether the client followed the prescribed treatment regimen.

Although Ray stated that he did not have family, his friends in the hotel constituted a working support network. The PHN knows that the client's support network is whomever the client identifies. Nursing assessment of Ray's support network involved determining whether the members were tested for TB. In addition, the PHN assessed the client's network for the following:

- Network composition
- Network's knowledge of TB
- Functional capacity
- Network stressors
- Network strengths and weaknesses
- Network's ability to provide support for Ray
- Health beliefs and practices
- Use of health services

The PHN was aware that the number of new cases of TB in the community had increased over the past 12 months. The PHN further noted that there was an increase in the number of area residents immigrating from various developing countries and that this population might be at increased risk for development of TB.

Diagnosis
Individual

Lack of awareness regarding the disease process and transmission of TB.

Family

Lack of awareness regarding the disease process and transmission of TB, location of communicable disease clinics, and the importance of screening those exposed to TB.

Community

Potential for development of TB among community residents, indicated by an increased incidence of new cases of TB over the past 12 months.

Planning

A plan of care is established with mutually agreed-upon goals based on the nurse's assessment of the individual, family, and community.

Individual
Long-Term Goal

- Client will perform self-care activities related to treatment of TB and follow up as necessary with appropriate health care professionals.

Short-Term Goal

- Client will verbalize knowledge of transmission of TB; signs and symptoms of complications of TB; purpose, administration schedule, and side effects of medications.

Family
Long-Term Goal

Support network members with positive test results will receive appropriate treatment.

Short-Term Goal

Support network members will demonstrate basic knowledge of cause and transmission of TB and will agree to be tested for TB.

Community
Long-Term Goal

Incidence of TB in the community will decrease over the next 3 years.

Short-Term Goal

Community members will demonstrate knowledge of increased incidence of TB in their community and of available community resources for treatment and prevention of TB.

Intervention

Implementation of the plan of care for the client with TB occurs at the individual, family, and community levels.

Individual

The PHN referred Ray to the communicable disease clinic at the local health department. TB is a reportable communicable disease; therefore the PHN obtained information from the client regarding people with whom he had been in close contact.

Family

The PHN contacted members of Ray's support network and referred them to the communicable disease clinic as appropriate. The nurse provided these people with information concerning TB transmission and the importance of early treatment and follow-up.

Community

The PHN met with professionals from the communicable disease clinic and the health department and with members of the community to establish a program to raise public awareness about the increased incidence of TB in the community. The public was informed about the importance of preventive measures, the availability of community screening services for TB, and the existing health care resources in the community.

Evaluation
Individual

The client's knowledge of the disease process, transmission, treatment, and signs and symptoms of TB is an indicator in evaluating the care plan. Confirmation of the client's follow-up with the communicable disease clinic can also be used for evaluation.

Family

The support network's knowledge of the disease process, transmission, treatment, and signs and symptoms of TB is an indicator in evaluating the care plan. Confirmation of the support network's follow-up with the communicable disease clinic can also be used for evaluation.

Community

The incidence rate of TB in the community and the rate at which TB clinics and related resources are used are measures that can be used to evaluate the effectiveness of interventions at the aggregate level.

CASE STUDY Public Health Visit—cont'd

Levels of Prevention

The PHN is actively involved in all three levels of prevention through education programs, early detection programs, and appropriate referrals for patients with TB. Examples of each of these levels of prevention are as follows:

Primary

Goal: Prevention of specific disease occurrence such as TB.
- Development of programs that increase public awareness of the disease process and of the transmission, diagnosis, and treatment of TB.

Secondary

Goal: Early detection of existing conditions.
- Tuberculin skin testing and subsequent follow-up of positive test results.

Tertiary

Goal: To reduce the effects and spread of TB.
- Referral for early, effective treatment and education of clients for self-care.

CASE STUDY

Public Health Home Visit: Antepartum Client

The PHN received a referral to see a 17-year-old African American woman named Ali, who was referred by the county prenatal clinic. Ali was 5 months pregnant with her third pregnancy within the past year. Ali miscarried the previous two pregnancies during the first trimester.

When the nurse made the home visit, she noted that Ali was 5 feet 9 inches tall and weighed 120 lb. She resided in a two-room apartment with her boyfriend, who was the father of the baby. The nurse began the first visit with social talk, asking Ali general questions about her employment, education, and the duration of her residence in the area. Ali appeared to be pleased that the nurse was interested in her. Once a trusting relationship was initiated, the nurse asked Ali how she felt about the pregnancy. Ali revealed that she was happy about the pregnancy but was worried that there would be problems because she had had two previous miscarriages. She had not planned any of the pregnancies, but she did not use contraceptives to prevent the pregnancies either. Ali's boyfriend worked and was able to pay the rent and buy food for her. Ali dropped out of high school during her junior year, but she wanted to complete her high school education. She had Medicaid coverage for her health care.

During the initial home visit, the nurse assessed that Ali was underweight and had several knowledge deficits in the areas of prenatal nutrition, infant care, breastfeeding, and contraception. The nurse also identified the need for a referral to the public school for the continuation of Ali's high school education. The nurse briefly discussed her assessment with Ali in a nonthreatening, nonjudgmental manner. The nurse informed Ali that, if she was interested, she could schedule future home visits to provide Ali with more information and answer her questions. Ali agreed to receive future visits to discuss the topics the nurse identified during the assessment phase. They mutually agreed upon the plan for future visits. As the visits progressed, the nurse and Ali modified the plan on the basis of progress evaluation.

The nurse terminated home visits with Ali when the mutually established goals were achieved. The nurse scheduled a postpartum visit with Ali after the baby was born to assess infant care and answer any questions Ali had concerning infant care.

Assessment

Although it was important to perform an individual assessment of Ali, the PHN assessed Ali as a member of a family and as a member of the community. *Community* in this case referred to the aggregate of publicly insured adolescent pregnant women. Assessment of Ali revealed an underweight 17-year-old pregnant woman who was unable to demonstrate knowledge of nutrition in pregnancy, infant care, breastfeeding, contraception, or educational options for pregnant teenagers.

An individual assessment of Ali mandated the need for an assessment of the composition and function of Ali's family. The PHN assessed the following factors with regard to Ali's family:

- Family composition and support network
- Family's and support network's attitude toward mental and physical health and use of health care services
- Family's and support network's attitude toward Ali's physical, mental, social, spiritual, and economic support
- Family's and support network's beliefs and attitudes regarding infant care, breastfeeding/bottle feeding, immunizations, and nutrition
- Attitude of infant's father regarding involvement with Ali and their baby, his health beliefs, and his ability to assume the role of parent

The PHN was aware of the need to see the larger, aggregate picture. Identifying the aggregate as the pregnant adolescent community, the PHN used the following techniques in an ongoing assessment (Lewenson and Truglio-Londrigan, 2010):
- Observations
- Resource analysis
- Key informant interviews
- Environmental indexes

Using these techniques, the PHN gathered information regarding the following:
- Educational and employment options for pregnant teens and teens with infants
- Availability of health services targeting low-birth-weight infants
- Availability of support groups for this aggregate
- Availability of teen parenting classes

Diagnosis

The PHN formulated nursing diagnoses based on thorough individual, family, and community assessments.

Individual
- Lack of awareness regarding nutrition in pregnancy, infant care and feeding, contraception, availability of community resources, and educational options for pregnant teenagers
- Inadequate nutritional support related to low-income status and inadequate knowledge of nutritional requirement for pregnancy

Family
- Lack of family support related to Ali's living away from home
- Altered family communication patterns related to role confusion among family members

Community
- Minimal availability of health care services, parenting classes, contraception counseling, and educational opportunities for pregnant teenagers
- Lack of coordination of existing services

Continued

CASE STUDY—cont'd

Planning

Planning health services and interventions for pregnant teenagers involves formulation of mutually agreed-upon short-term and long-term goals for the individual, family, and community.

Individual
Long-Term Goal
- Ali will carry her infant to term without evidence of maternal or fetal complications.

Short-Term Goals
- Ali will gain at least 3 lb per month.
- Ali will demonstrate knowledge of community resources for pregnant adolescents by the next nursing visit.

Family
Long-Term Goal
- Ali, her partner, and other family members will be able to perform mutually determined role responsibilities.

Short-Term Goal
- Ali and her partner will attend teen parenting classes.

Community
Long-Term Goals
- Establishment of effective, comprehensive prenatal health, contraception, and education services for pregnant teenagers
- Decline in rate of teen pregnancies and birth of compromised neonates over the next 24 months

Short-Term Goals
- Increased community awareness of resources for pregnant teenagers
- Increased awareness of contraception counseling services for adolescents

Intervention
Individual
Implementation of Ali's individual care plan involved visits by the PHN with a referral to existing prenatal services for pregnant teenagers.

Family
Family intervention was composed of Ali's and the father's referral to a support group for pregnant teenagers and partners.

Community
Implementation of the care plan for the aggregate of adolescent pregnant women included the following:
- Meeting with community leaders
- Meeting with local school administrators and faculty to disseminate information for pregnant teenagers
- Formation of community organizing groups

Evaluation
Individual
Evaluation included measures of the client's nutritional status and her use of support groups and educational and nutritional services.

Family
Evaluation included measures of the family's use of support groups and educational and services.

Community
Evaluation of the effectiveness of interventions at the aggregate level focused on measurement of available options for pregnant teenagers, measures of teen awareness and use of services, and determination of changes in incidence rates of teen pregnancy and compromised neonates.

Levels of Prevention
The PHN not only works with the patient and the patient's support network, but also provides care to the entire community through education and intervention programs. The PHN is actively involved in working with individual teenagers, their friends and families, and the community in reducing the incidence of teenage pregnancy and assisting pregnant teenagers with prenatal care and available resources. Examples of providing care at the three levels of prevention are listed here.

Primary
- Activities that prevent teen pregnancy from occurring, such as individual and family counseling and school and community education programs

Secondary
- Interventions for early detection of teen pregnancy and early intervention, such as counseling for prenatal care

Tertiary
Goal: To reduce the effects of adolescent pregnancy
- Provision of prenatal education in areas such as nutrition, parenting, and infant care

CASE STUDY

Hospice Home Visit
Anne McMillan is 80 years old and is terminally ill with metastatic breast cancer. She has been a widow for 5 years and has three daughters and two sons. All of her children are married with kids of their own, except one son who is handicapped and lives with Anne. Anne is too weak to care for herself and is moving in with her youngest daughter. Her daughter's house is a colonial with all bedrooms upstairs. There is a first-floor bathroom. During her first visit, the hospice nurse talks with Anne and her daughter and explains what hospice is all about. The nurse then admits Anne into the hospice program and begins her initial assessment. Anne's primary physical complaints are back pain and constipation. She is still eating and drinking regularly. The nurse immediately recognizes that Anne will need a hospital bed. Anne already has a walker, but the nurse informed Anne and her daughter that they could have a bedside commode if needed in the future as Anne becomes weaker. Anne's biggest concern is her handicapped son, saying, "He can't be by himself for long, and I don't know where he can go now that I can't take care of him." Except for the handicapped son, all of her children and many of her grandchildren are active in her care.

Assessment
On her initial visit, the hospice nurse collects the following data about Anne, her family, and her community. In this case, the community consists of Anne's social support outside of her family, such as her neighborhood and church.
- Pain assessment, including history, character, severity, location, effects on quality of life, precipitating factors, and relieving factors
- Other physical symptoms, such as fatigue, nausea, vomiting, constipation, diarrhea, decreased appetite, and decreased mobility

- Client and family fears, anxiety about dying and the dying process
- Support network and family dynamics
- Client's anxiety about situation concerning handicapped son
- Additional support network outside of family
- Effect of diagnosis and prognosis on Anne's social support, including her neighbors and her church community

Diagnosis
Individual
- Pain related to disease process
- Potential for constipation and discomfort related to decreased mobility
- Apprehension related to concerns about safety and well-being of handicapped son

Family
- Strong support system indicated by active family participation in Anne's care

Community
- Anticipatory grieving related to social isolation after leaving neighborhood and moving in with daughter

Planning
Individual
Long-Term Goals
- Pain will remain controlled until client expires.
- Client will have regular bowel movements for the next 2 months.
- Client will verbalize satisfaction about resolution of situation concerning handicapped son.

Short-Term Goals
- Pain will be well controlled within 24—48 h.
- Client will have a bowel movement within 24—48 h.
- Client will have decreased anxiety about handicapped son within 24—48 h because the social worker will have found a place for the son to live.

Family
Long-Term Goals
- Family will remain active in Anne's care until she is buried.
- Family will provide a support network for each other and use hospice services for continued support through Anne's death and burial and for months afterward.

Short-Term Goal
- Family will actively participate in Anne's care.

Community
Long-Term Goal
- Client will continue to receive support from friends.

Short-Term Goal
- Client will verbalize feelings about moving in with daughter and leaving friends behind.

Intervention
Individual
After talking with the doctor, the hospice nurse starts Anne on methadone 20 mg daily and Roxanol 5 mg as needed for breakthrough pain. The nurse

explains to Anne and her daughter that she is constipated because of her decrease in mobility. The nurse obtains an order for a stool softener and instructs Anne to take it twice daily. The nurse also explains to Anne and her daughter that, as Anne declines, her appetite will decrease and she will eat less and less and may not have bowel movements very frequently. Anne should let the nurse know if she ever feels uncomfortable because she has not had a bowel movement in a few days. The nurse talks to the social worker, who finds a group home for Anne's handicapped son.

Family
The nurse and social worker talk with the family and help them develop a system so that Anne always has someone with her and to help ensure that all of the responsibility for Anne's care does not fall on one person. They also inform the family about resources to support them.

Community
Anne has a nurse, social worker, spiritual counselor, and nurse assistant assigned to her care. Each of these hospice workers helps Anne discuss her feelings about her situation and works with her to continue to receive support from her friends and neighbors.

Evaluation
Individual
All of Anne's goals are met, because she has good pain control until she dies, she no longer experiences discomfort and problems with constipation, and she expresses less anxiety and worry about her handicapped son. Although she still has some concerns, she feels much better about the situation.

Family
The family's goals are met, because they remain active in Anne's care until she dies. In addition, they use hospice resources appropriately and as necessary, and they support one another through the entire process.

Community
The goals are met, because Anne expresses her feelings about her situation, and her closest friends remain supportive to Anne through visits and phone calls.

Levels of Prevention
In this case, the three levels of prevention focus on helping the client and family through all phases of hospice care from admission until death. Some examples are as follows.

Primary
- Anticipating needs and intervening early on to prevent problems such as skin breakdown and lack of pain control
- Educating the client and family about hospice and the dying process

Secondary
- Responding quickly to needs as they arise
- Continued education about the hospice and dying experience

Tertiary
- Assisting the client and family through the active phase of dying
- Providing follow-up bereavement support to the family

SUMMARY

This chapter presents information on performing public health, home health, and hospice nursing visits to clients in their homes. A general overview of the nursing process for clients in the home setting is presented and expanded to include the individual, family, and community. Case studies involving communicable disease, teen pregnancy, and terminal cancer are described. The home visit is the foundation of community health nursing and provides a forum for important interventions with individuals, families, and communities. The CHN is responsible for bringing the concerns of individuals and families into the community.

EVOLVE WEBSITE

http://evolve.elsevier.com/Nies/community
- NCLEX Review Questions
- Case Studies

BIBLIOGRAPHY

Acello B, Brown LR: *Home health assessment criteria: 75 checklists for skilled nursing documentation*, 2015. Available from: https://hcmarketplace.com/aitdownloadablefiles/download/aitfile_id/1678.pdf.

Albrecht MN: The Albrecht nursing model for home health care: implications for research, practice, and education, *Publ Health Nurs* 7:118–126, 1990.

American Nurses Association: *Scope and standards of hospice and palliative nursing practice*, Washington, DC, 2007, American Nurses Association.

American Nurses Association: *Scope and standards of home health nursing practice*, ed 2, Washington, DC, 2014, American Nurses Association.

Cancer.net: *Understanding grief within a cultural context*, 2018. Available from: https://www.cancer.net/coping-with-cancer/managing-emotions/grief-and-loss/understanding-grief-within-cultural-contextt.

Centers for Medicare and Medicaid Services: *Home health quality reporting program*, 2021a. Available from: https://www.cms.gov/Medicare/Quality-Initiatives-Patient-Assessment-Instruments/HomeHealthQualityInits.

Centers for Medicare and Medicaid Services: *Home health PPS*, 2021b. Available from: http://www.cms.gov/Medicare/Medicare-Fee-for-Service-Payment/HomeHealthPPS/index.html?redirect=/home-healthpps/.

Department of Health and Human Services: *Centers for Medicare and Medicaid Services: home health prospective payment system*, 2017. Available from: https://www.cms.gov/Outreach-and-Education/Medicare-Learning-Network-MLN/MLNProducts/Downloads/Home-Health-PPS-Fact-Sheet-ICN006816.pdf.

Dewsbury G: Use of information and communication technology in nursing services, *Br J Community Nurs* 24(12):604–607, 2019. https://doi.org/10.12968/bjcn.2019.24.12.604.

Elflein, J: *Medicare: number of home health agencies in the U.S. 1967-2018*. Available from: https://www.statista.com/statistics/195318/number-of-medicare-home-health-agencies-in-the-us/.

Lewenson SB, Truglio-Londrigan M: *Public health nursing assessment tool*, 2010. Available from: http://samples.jbpub.com/9780763766542/41764_trugliolondrigan_appendix.pdf.

Medicare.gov: *What's a home health care plan?*, 2021b. Available from: https://www.medicare.gov/whats-a-home-health-care-plan.

Medicare Learning Network: *Hospice payment system*, 2019. Available from: https://www.cms.gov/Outreach-and-Education/Medicare-Learning-Network-MLN/MLNProducts/downloads/hospice_pay_sys_fs.pdf.

Medicare Payment Advisory Commission: *A data book: health care spending and the Medicare Program*, 2018. Available from: http://medpac.gov/docs/default-source/data-book/july2020_databook_entirereport_sec.pdf?sfvrsn=0.

National Association for Home Care and Hospice: *Homecare online: basic statistics about home care*, 2010. Available from: http://www.nahc.org/assets/1/7/10HC_Stats.pdf.

National Hospice and Palliative Care Organization: *About hospice care*, 2021. Available from: https://www.nhpco.org/patients-and-caregivers/about-hospice-care/.

National Institute of Diabetes and Digestive and Kidney Diseases: *Hemodialysis*, 2018. Available from: www.niddk.nih.gov/health-information/kidney-disease/kidney-failure/hemodialysis.

Norlander L: *To comfort always: a nurse's guide to end of life care*, Indianapolis, IN, 2008, Sigma Theta Tau International.

QSEN Institute: *QSEN competencies*, 2020. Available from: http://qsen.org/competencies/.

The Joint Commission: *R3 reports: requirement, rationale, reference*, 2018. Available from: https://www.jointcommission.org/-/media/tjc/documents/standards/r3-reports/r3_22_pain_standards_hc_12_21_18_final.pdf.

Unsar S, Erol O, Ozdemir O: Caregiving burden, depression, and anxiety in family caregivers with cancer, *Eur J Oncol Nurs* 50, 2021. Available from: https://www.sciencedirect.com/science/article/abs/pii/S1462388920301629.

Visiting Nurse Service of New York: *Lillian Wald*. Available from: https://www.vnsny.org/who-we-are/about-us/history/lillian-wald/.

FURTHER READING

Department of Health and Human Services: *Centers for Medicare and Medicaid services: Hospice payment system*, 2016. Available from: https://www.cms.gov/Outreach-and-Education/Medicare-Learning-Network-MLN/MLNProducts/downloads/hospice_pay_wgsys_fs.pdf.

HealthyPeople.gov: *Healthy People 2030: how has healthy people changed?* Available from: https://health.gov/healthypeople/about/how-has-healthy-people-changed; http://www.healthypeople.gov/2020/topicsobjectives2020/default.aspx.

INDEX

HEALTHY PEOPLE 2020

ETHICAL INSIGHTS

RESEARCH HIGHLIGHTS